Comprehensive Respiratory Medicine

Richard K Albert
Professor of Medicine, University of Colorado
Chief, Medical Service
Denver Health Medical Center
Denver, Colorado
USA

Stephen G Spiro
Professor of Respiratory Medicine
Consultant Physician General and Thoracic
Medicine
University College London Hospitals NHS Trust
The Middlesex Hospital
London
UK

James R Jett
Professor of Medicine, Mayo Medical School
Consultant in Pulmonary Medicine and Medical
Oncology
Mayo Clinic
Rochester, Minnesota
USA

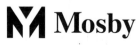 Mosby

London   Philadelphia   St Louis   Sydney   Tokyo

MOSBY
An imprint of Harcourt Brace and Company Limited

©Harcourt Brace and Company Limited 1999

ISBN: 0 7234 3118 3

Reproduction by Prospect Litho, Basildon, UK.
Printed and bound by Grafos SA Arte sobre papel, Barcelona, Spain

Cataloging-in-Publication Data:
Catalogue records for this book are available from the US Library of Congress and the British Library

Drug Notice
The contributors, the editors, and the publishers have made every effort to ensure the accuracy and appropriateness of the drug dosages presented in this textbook. The medications described do not necessarily have specific approval by drug regulatory authorities in all countries for use in the diseases and dosages for which they are recommended. The package insert for each drug should be consulted for use and dosage as approved by the relevant drug regulatory authority. Because standards for usage change, it is advisable to keep abreast of revised recommendations, particularly those concerning new drugs.

Copyright
Every effort has been made to contact holders of copyright to obtain permission to reproduce copyright material. However, if any have been inadvertently overlooked, the publisher will be pleased to make the necessary arrangements at the first opportunity.

Medical Editor	Maria Khan
	Gina Almond
Development Editor	Filipa Maia
Project Manager	Kim Benson
Illustration Manager	Danny Pyne
Senior Designer	Ian Spick
Layout and Illustration	The EDI Partnership:
	Mark Willey and Lee Smith
Cover design	Ian Spick and Danny Pyne
Copyeditor	John Ormiston
Proofreader	Andrew Baker
Production	Andrea Ford
Index	Janine Ross

Preface

The amount of time required to publish a new comprehensive textbook in any discipline is extraordinary. To justify such an undertaking mandates that the rationale for doing so be equally extraordinary. The recent expansion of the community of science and medicine to include practitioners throughout the world provides us with just such a rationale. We believe it is parochial to consider respiratory medicine from an American, Canadian, British, Asian, or European perspective. Many 'national' respiratory meetings are now international in scope. This world-wide perspective should be similarly presented in our textbooks, and this was our primary objective. Comprehensive Respiratory Medicine is written by 120 authors from 10 different countries. We consider it a first attempt at bringing the world community of respiratory medicine together in a single publication. Appreciation of this world perspective can only serve to improve the understanding and practice of our discipline.

Advances in computer graphics and publishing processes provides a secondary rationale for this textbook: the ability to emphasize visual presentation. With the assistance of the artists at Mosby, as much material as possible is presented in graphic rather than textural formats. We believe that the visual appearance of the book will facilitate its use.

Comprehensive Respiratory Medicine has a broad strategy and the book is clearly divided into separate sections. The initial section covers structure and function in considerable detail because respiratory medicine is strongly founded in physiology and is also perhaps more dependent on imaging techniques than most disciplines. The book, therefore, begins with comprehensive chapters on these topics. The subsequent section details with the practical approach to techniques such as bronchoscopy, pleural biopsy, intercostal drainage, and their indications. Part three involves the principles of the major aspects of respiratory care, including invasive ventilation, non-invasive mechanical ventilation, and intensive care unit management. This is followed by a section on the main respiratory symptoms, and then the rest of the book details a systematic approach to each of the respiratory diseases, allowing the entire field of respiratory medicine to be covered in a concise, yet informative, fashion.

The book is intended to be used by students and house officers, trainees in respiratory medicine, physicians practicing general or family medicine, and for respiratory clinicians. Although newer cell and molecular biologic concepts are briefly discussed when appropriate, the book is not designed to provide comprehensive reviews of basic science in the various diseases or conditions considered. Similarly, the topics included in the section pertaining to critical care are limited to those in which respiratory specialists should have special knowledge, above that of a general intensivist.

RKA, SGS, and JRJ

Dedication

To our teachers

Contents

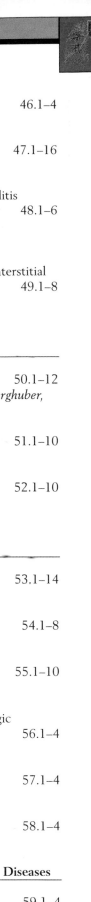

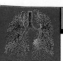

Contents

Contributors

Loutfi S Aboussouan
Assistant Professor of Medicine, Wayne State University, Detroit, Michigan, USA

Carlo Agostini
Senior Investigator also Deputy, Clinical Immunology Branch, Department of Clinical and Experimental Medicine, Padua University School of Medicine, Padova, Italy

Richard K Albert
Professor of Medicine, University of Colorado, Chief, Medical Service, Denver Health Medical Center, Denver, Colorado, USA

Thomas K Aldrich
Director, Unified Pulmonary Medicine Division, Albert Einstein College of Medicine and Montefiore Medical Center, Montefiore Medical Center, New York, New York, USA

Selim M Arcasoy
Pulmonary and Critical Care Division, Hospital of the University of Pennsylvania, Philadelphia, Pennsylvania, USA

Charles W Atwood Jr
Assistant Professor of Medicine, University of Pittsburgh and Veterans Affairs Medical Centers, Pittsburgh, Pennsylvania, USA

Alexander A Bankier
Associate Professor of Radiology, Department of Dignostic Radiology I, University of Vienna - AKH, Vienna, Austria

Daniel Banks
N. LeRoy Lapp Professor and Chief, Section of Pulmonary & Critical Care Medicine, West Virginia University School of Medicine, Morgantown, West Virginia, USA

Neil C Barnes
Consultant in Respiratory Medicine, The London Chest Hospital, London, UK

Peter J Barnes
Professor of Thoracic Medicine, National Heart & Lung Institute, Imperial College, London, UK

John B Bass Jr
University of South Alabama, Mobile, Alabama, USA

Joshua O Benditt
Associate Professor, Pulmonary & Critical Care Medicine, University of Washington Medical Center, Seattle, Washington, USA

Luca Brazzi
Assistant Professor in Anesthesia and Intensive Care, University of Milan, Clinical Assistant, Istituto di Anestesia e Rianimazione, Ospedale Policlinico, Milano, Italy

John R Britton
Professor of Respiratory Medicine, University of Nottingham, City Hospital, Nottingham, UK

William A Broughton
Associate Professor of Medicine, University of South Alabama College of Medicine, USA/KPH Sleep Disorders Center, Mobile, Alabama, USA

Roy G Brower
Associate Professor of Medicine, Johns Hopkins University, Baltimore, Maryland, USA

Otto C Burghuber
Professor of Medicine, Chief, Department of Medicine, Krankenhaus Korneuburg, Korneuburg, Austria

Philippe Camus
Professor of Pulmonary Medicine, Department of Pulmonary Medicine, University Hospital, Dijon, France

Bartolome R Celli
Chief, Pulmonary & Critical Care, St Elizabeths Medical Center, Boston, MA, USA

Moira Chan-Yeung
Department of Medicine, Vancouver General Hospital, Vancouver, Canada

William W L Chang
Professor of Pathology, West Virginia University School of Medicine, Morgantown, West Virginia, USA

G Mac Cochrane
Consultant Chest Physician, Guy's and St Thomas' Hospital Trust, Guy's Hospital, London, UK

Thomas V Colby
Department of Pathology, Mayo Clinic, Scottsdale, Arizona, USA

Chris J Corrigan
Clinical Senior Lecturer/Honorary Consultant Physician, Department of Respiratory Medicine, Imperial College School of Medicine, Charing Cross Hospital, London, UK

Paul A Corris
Reader in Thoracic Medicine and Consultant Physician, Freeman Hospital, Newcastle-upon-Tyne, UK

Stephen W Crawford
Associate Clinical Professor of Medicine, Pulmunary and Critical Care Medicine, UCSD Medical Center, San Diego, California, USA

Bruce H Culver
Associate Professor of Medicine Division of Pulmonary & Critical Care Medicine, University of Washington School of Medicine, Seattle, Washington USA

James Dauber
Medical Director of Pulmonary Transplantation, Professor of Medicine, Division of Pulmonary, Allergy & Critical Care Medicine, University of Pittsburgh, Pittsburgh, Pennsylvania, USA

Roland M du Bois
Consultant Physician, Interstitial Lung Disease Unit, Royal Brompton Hospital, London, UK

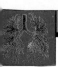

Contributors

Jim Egan
Consultant Respiratory Physician and
Honorary Clinical Lecturer,
Wythenshawe Hospital, Manchester, UK

Mustafa El-Ebiary
Servei de Pneumologia, Hospital Clinic,
Barcelona, Spain

Andrew Evans
Consultant Radiologist, City Hospital,
Nottingham, UK

Timothy W Evans
Professor of Intensive Care Medicine,
Unit of Critical Care, Imperial College
School of Medicine & NHLI, Royal
Brompton Hospital, London, UK

Stanley Fiel
Professor & Chief, Division of
Pulmonary & Critical Care, MCP-
Hahnemann School of Medicine,
Philadelphia, Pennsylvania, USA

Jean-William Fitting
Associate Professor, Division de
Pneumologie, Centre Hospitalier
Universitaire Vaudois, Lausanne,
Switzerland

Luciano Gattinoni
Chief Professor in Anesthesia and
Intensive Care, University of Milan,
Istituto di Anestesia e Rianimazione,
Ospedale Maggiore Policlinico, Milano,
Italy

Paul Goddard
Consultant Radiologist, Bristol Royal
Infirmary, Bristol, UK

E Brigitte Gottschall
Fellow, Pulmonary and Occupational
Medicine, University of Colorado Health
Sciences Center, Division of
Environmental and Occupational Health
Sciences, National Jewish Medical and
Research Center, Denver, Colorado,
USA

Michael M Graham
University of Washington Medical
Center, Seattle, Washington, USA

Margaret Hall-Craggs
Consultant Radiologist, MR Unit,
Department of Imaging, The Middlesex
Hospital, UCLHT, London, UK

David M Hansell
Professor of Thoracic Imaging, Royal
Brompton Hospital, London, UK

Christian J Herold
Professor of Radiology, Director,
Department of Diagnostic Radiology I,
University of Vienna - AKH, Vienna,
Austria

Nicholas S Hill
Professor of Medicine, Director of
Critical Care Medicine, Pulmonary
Division, Rhode Island Hospital,
Providence, Rhode Island, USA

Gérard J Huchon
Professor of Medicine, Université de
Paris, René Descartes, Chef de Service,
Service de Pneumologie, Hopital
Ambroise Paré, Boulougne, France

Richard S Irwin
Professor of Medicine and Director,
Division of Pulmonary Allergy and
Clinical Care Medicine, University of
Massachusetts Medical School,
Worcester, Massachusetts, USA

James R Jett
Professor of Medicine, Mayo Medical
School, Consultant in Pulmonary
Medicine and Medical Oncology, Mayo
Clinic, Rochester, Minnesota, USA

Andrew T Jones
Smith and Nephew Research Fellow in
Intensive Care Medicine
Unit of Critical Care, Imperial College
School of Medicine & NHLI, Royal
Brompton Hospital, London, UK

Sanjay Kalra
Division of Pulmonary and Critical Care
Medicine, Mayo Clinic, Rochester,
Minnesota, USA

Huib A M Kerstjens
Department of Pulmonology, University
Hospital Groningen, Groningen, The
Netherlands

John W Kreit
Assistant Professor of Medicine, Division
of Pulmonary and Critical Care
Medicine, University of Pittsburgh
School of Medicine, Pittsburgh,
Pennsylvania, USA

Stephen E Lapinsky
Assistant Professor of Medicine, Mount
Sinai Hospital, Toronto, Ontario, Canada

Marc C I Lipman
Consultant Physician, Royal Free
Hospital, London, UK

Robert Loddenkemper
Chefarzt der Pneumologischen Abteilung
II, Lungenklinik Heckeshorn, Berlin,
Germany

J Mark Madison
Associate Professor of Medicine and
Physiology, Pulmonary, Allergy and
Critical Care Medicine, University of
Massachusetts Medical School,
Worcester, Massachusetts, USA

Helgo Magnussen
Direktor, Zentrum fur Pneumologie &
Thoraxchirurgie, Krankenhaus
Grosshansdorf, Grosshandorf, Germany

Lisa A Maier
Staff Physician, Division of
Environmental & Occupational Health
Sciences, Department of Medicine,
NJMRC, Instructor, Division of
Pulmonary & Critical Care Medicine,
Dept of Medicine, University of
Colorado Health Science Center,
National Jewish Medical and Research
Center, Denver, Colorado, USA

Jean-Luc Malo
Vancouver General Hospital, Vancouver,
Canada

David E Midthun
Assistant Professor of Medicine, Mayo
Medical School, Consultant in
Pulmonary and Critical Care Medicine,
Mayo Clinic, Mayo Clinic, Rochester,
Minnesota, USA

Rob F Miller
Reader in Clinical Infection, Royal Free
and University College Medical School,
London, UK

Peter R Mills
Pulmonary Fellow, St. Bartholomew's
and Royal London School of Medicine &
Dentistry, London Chest Hospital,
London, UK

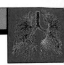

Erich Minar
Associate Professor of Medicine,
Department of Medicine II, Division of
Angiology, University of Vienna - AKH,
Vienna, Austria

David M Mitchell
Consultant Physician and Hon Senior
Lecturer in Medicine, Chest & Allergy
Clinic, St Mary's Hospital and Imperial
College School of Medicine, London,
UK

David R Moller
Associate Professor of Medicine,
Division of Pulmonary & Critical Care
Medicine, The Johns Hopkins University
School of Medicine, Baltimore,
Maryland, USA

Ernest E Moore
Professor & Vice Chairman, Department
of Surgery, University of Colorado
Health Sciences Center Chief of Surgery
Denver Health Medical Center, Denver,
Colorado, USA

Jeffrey L Myers
Mayo Clinic, Rochester, Minnesota,
USA

Lee S Newman
Associate Professor of Medicine and of
Preventive Medicine and Biometrics,
University of Colorado School of
Medicine, Head, Division of
Environmental and Occupational Health
Sciences, NJMRC, National Jewish
Medical and Research Center, Denver,
Colorado, USA

Anthony J Newman-Taylor
Professor of Occupational and
Environmental Medicine, Royal
Brompton Hospital, London, UK

Paul M O'Byrne
EJ Moran Campbell Professor of
Medicine, Faculty of Health Sciences,
McMaster University, Hamilton,
Ontario, Canada

Patrick J Offner
Associate Professor, Department of
Surgery, University of Colorado Health
Sciences Center, Chief of Surgical
Critical Care, Denver Health Medical
Center, Denver, Colorado, USA

Eric J Olson
Assistant Professor of Medicine, Senior
Associate Consultant, Department of
Internal Medicine, Division of
Pulmonary and Critical Care Medicine,
Mayo Clinic, Rochester, Minnesota,
USA

Simon Padley
Consultant Radiologist, Chelsea &
Westminster Hospital, London, UK

Martyn R Partridge
Consultant Chest Physician
Chest Clinic, Whipps Cross Hospital,
London, UK

Paolo Pelosi
Assistant Professor in Anesthesia and
Intensive Care, University of Milan,
Clinical Assistant, Istituto di Anestesia e
Rianimazione, Ospedale Policlinico,
Milano, Italy

Anthony C Pickering
Professor of Occupational Medicine,
Department of Thoracic Medicine,
North West Lung Centre, Wythenshawe
Hospital, Manchester, UK

David J Pierson
Medical Director of Respiratory Care,
Harborview Medical Center, Professor
of Medicine, Division of Pulmonary adn
Critical Care Medicine, University of
Washington, Harborview Medical
Center, Seattle, Washington, USA

Venerino Poletti
Department of Pulmonary Medicine,
Ospedale Maggiore, Bologna, Italy

Dirkje S Postma
Professor of Pulmonology, University
Hospital Groningen, Groningen, The
Netherlands

Udaya B S Prakash
Scripps Professor of Medicine, Mayo
Medical School, Consultant in
Pulmonary, Critical Care and Internal
Medicine, Director of Bronchoscopy,
Mayo Medical Center, Mayo Clinic,
Rochester, Minnesota, USA

Nicolas Roche
Assistant Professor of Medicine,
Université de Paris, Rene Descartes,
Service de Pneumologie, Hopital
Ambroise Paré, Hopital Ambroise Paré,
Boulogne, France

Roberto Rodríguez-Roisin
Professor of Medicine, Universitat de
Barcelona, Head, Servei de Pneumologia
i Allergia Respiratoria, Department de
Medicina, Institut d'Investigacions
Biomèdiques August Pi i Sunyer
(IDIBAPS), Hospital Clinic, Barcelona,
Spain

Melissa L Rosado De Christenson
Department of Radiologic Pathology,
Armed Forces Institute of Pathology,
Washington, DC, USA

Robin M Rudd
Consultant Physician, Department of
Respiratory Medicine, London Chest
Hospital, London, UK

Jay H Ryu
Mayo Clinic, Rochester, Minnesota,
USA

Daniel V Schidlow
Professor and Acting Chair, Department
of Pediatrics, MCP Hahnemann
University School of Medicine,
Executive Vice President for Medical
and Academic Affairs, Director, Cystic
Fibrosis Center, St. Christopher's
Hospital for Children, Philadelphia,
Pennsylvania, USA

Marvin I Schwarz
The James C. Campbell Professor of
Pulmonary Medicine, Head, Division of
Pulmonary Sciences & Critical Care
Medicine, University of Colorado Health
Sciences Center, University of Colorado
Health Sciences Center, Denver,
Colorado, USA

Gianpietro Semenzato
Chief, Clinical Immunology Branch,
Department of Clinical and
Experimental Medicine, Padua
University School of Medicine, Padova,
Italy

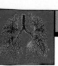

Jonathan Sevransky
Fellow, Pulmonary and Critical Care
Medicine, Johns Hopkins University,
Johns Hopkins Hospital, Baltimore,
Maryland, USA

Thomas E Shaughnessy
Assistant Professor of Anesthesia, UCSF
Medical Center, San Francisco,
California, USA

Penny Shaw
Consultant Radiologist
The University College London
Hospital, London, UK

Anita K Simonds
Consultant in Respiratory Medicine,
Royal Brompton and Harefield NHS
Trust, Royal Brompton Hospital,
London, UK

Arthur S Slutsky
Department of Medicine, Mount Sinai
Hospital, University of Toronto, Toronto,
Ontario, Canada

Stephen G Spiro
Professor of Respiratory Medicine,
Consultant Physician in General and
Thoracic Medicine, University College
London Hospitals NHS Trust, The
Middlesex Hospital, London, UK

Robert G Stirling
Thoracic Medicine, National Heart and
Lung Institute, London, UK

James K Stoller
Professor of Medicine, Vice-Chairman,
Division of Medicine, Head, Section of
Respiratory Therapy, Department of
Pulmonary and Critical Care Medicine,
Cleveland Clinic Foundation, Cleveland,
Ohio, USA

Diane C Strollo
Department of Radiology, University of
Pittsburgh, Pittsburgh, Pennsylvania,
USA

Patrick J Strollo Jr
Associate Professor of Medicine,
Division of Pulmonary, Allergy and
Critical Care Medicine, Medical
Director, Pulmonary Sleep Disorders
Laboratory, University of Pittsburgh
Medical Center, Pittsburgh,
Pennsylvania, USA

Nick HT Ten Hacken
Department of Pulmonology, University
Hospital Groningen, Groningen, The
Netherlands

Galen B Toews
Chief, Division of Pulmonary and
Critical Care Medicine
Professor of Internal Medicine,
University of Michigan Health System,
Ann Arbor, Michigan, USA

Antoni Torres
Director Respiratory Intensive Care
Unit, Servei de Pneumologia,
Coordinator, Instituto de Molalties
Respiratorias, Hospital Clinic, Barcelona,
Spain

Franco Valenza
Clinical Assistant, Istituto di Anestesia e
Rianimazione, Ospedale Policlinico,
Milano, Italy

Roland Vanderschueren
Head of the Department of Pulmonary
Diseases, St Antonius Ziekenhuis,
Nieuwegein, The Netherlands

William S Walker
Consultant Cardiothoracic Surgeon, The
Royal Infirmary of Edinburgh,
Edinburgh, Scotland, UK

Herbert H Watzke
Associate Professor of Medicine,
Department of Medicine I, Division of
Hematology and Hemostaseology,
University of Vienna - AKH, Vienna,
Austria

Jadwiga A Wedzicha
Reader in Respiratory Medicine, St.
Bartholomew's and Royal London School
of Medicine & Dentistry, London Chest
Hospital, London, UK

Dorothy A White
Cardiology and Pulmonary Medicine,
Memorial Sloan-Kettering Cancer
Center, New York, New York, USA

Jeanine P Wiener-Kronish
Vice-Chairman, Department of
Anesthesia, Critical Care, and
Perioperative Care, University of
California, San Francisco, California,
USA

Ashley A Woodcock
Professor of Respiratory Medicine,
North West Lung Centre, Department
of Respiratory Physiology, Wythenshawe
Hospital, Manchester, UK

Mark A Woodhead
Consultant in General & Respiratory
Medicine, Manchester Royal Infirmary,
Manchester, UK

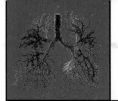

Section 1 Structure and Function

Chapter 1

Imaging

David Hansell and Simon Padley

IMAGING TECHNIQUES

Today, clinicians have two main imaging techniques at their disposal for the investigation of patients with chest disease – the chest radiograph, which produces a projectional image, and computed tomography (CT), which provides a cross-sectional view. Other techniques, such as magnetic resonance imaging (MRI), radionuclide scanning, and ultrasonography, can provide valuable additional information (see Chapters 1.2, 1.3, and 2.8), but are rarely performed without prior chest radiography or CT. Since imaging is an integral part of the practice of respiratory medicine, an understanding of the strengths and weaknesses of these various techniques is vital. The advent of high-resolution and spiral CT has lent further precision to the investigation of patients with suspected chest disease, but the use of such sophisticated tests should not be indiscriminate; accurate interpretation of the chest radiograph remains the mainstay of thoracic imaging.

Plain chest radiography
Technical considerations
The views of the chest most frequently performed are the erect posteroanterior (PA) and lateral projections, taken with the patient breath held at total lung capacity. On a frontal PA chest radiograph just under half of the lung is free from overlying structures, such as the ribs or diaphragm. Many technical factors, notably the kilovoltage and film–screen combination used, determine how well the lungs are shown. The characteristics of radiographic film make it impossible to obtain perfect exposure of the least and most dense parts of the chest in a single radiograph. Methods to overcome this handicap of radiographic film include the use of high-kilovoltage techniques, asymmetric film–screen combinations, and sophisticated devices that control regional X-ray exposure.

Since the coefficients of X-ray absorption of bone and soft tissue approach one another at high kilovoltage, the skeletal structures do not obscure the lungs on a higher kilovoltage radiograph to the same degree as on low-kilovoltage radiographs (Fig. 1.1). The high-kilovoltage radiograph thus demonstrates much more of the lung. Improved penetration of the mediastinum also allows some of the central airways to be seen. Although high-kilovoltage radiographs are preferable for routine examinations of the lungs and mediastinum, low-kilovoltage radiographs provide good detail of unobscured lung because of the improved contrast between lung vessels and surrounding lung. Furthermore, dense lesions, for example calcified pleural plaques, are particularly well demonstrated on low-kilovoltage films.

One of the most important major advances in plain-film radiography in recent times was the introduction of more sensitive phosphorescent screens. Screens luminesce when an X-ray beam falls on them, and are in contact with the radiographic film, which records the image. The improved light emission from the latest rare-earth phosphors compared with older calcium screens results in shorter exposure times and thus sharper images. A significant advance in film–screen combinations for chest imaging was the development of an asymmetric combination of a thin front screen and high-contrast film emulsion and, on the reverse side of the film base, a thicker back screen and a low-contrast film emulsion. In this way the wide spectrum of transmission of X-rays through the thorax can be accommodated. Such a film–screen combination shows significantly more detail in the mediastinum and lung obscured by the diaphragm and heart.

To overcome the considerable density differences between the mediastinum and lungs, attempts have been made to produce a more uniformly exposed chest radiograph (see Fig. 1.2). Newer devices modulate the exposure for each part of the

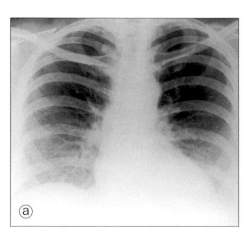

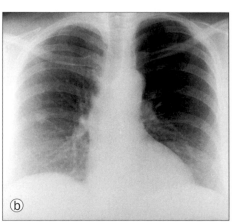

Figure 1.1 The effect of low and high kilovoltage on the chest radiograph. (a) Low-kilovoltage chest radiograph showing good detail of the bones, such that a small nodule in the right mid zone is obscured by an overlying rib. (b) A high-kilovoltage radiograph of the same patient shows better penetration of the mediastinum and allows clear demonstration of a small carcinoid tumor in the right mid zone.

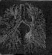
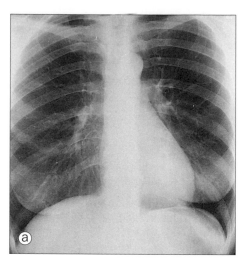

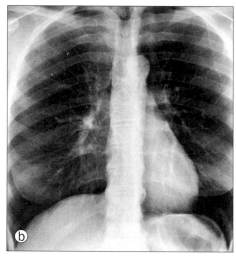

Figure 1.2
Comparison of conventional and advanced multiple beam equalization radiographs.
(a) Conventional high-kilovoltage chest radiograph.
(b) Advanced multiple beam equalization radiograph (scanning equalization radiograph) of the same patient revealing increased lung detail behind the heart and right hemidiaphragm.

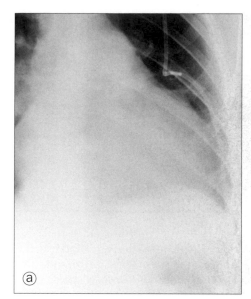

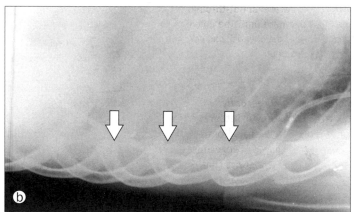

Figure 1.3
Demonstration of small effusions. (a) Posteroanterior chest radiograph of a patient who has a ventriculoperitoneal shunt. More soft tissue than usual occurs between the gastric air bubble and the base of the lung, because of a subpulmonic effusion.
(b) Decubitus film shows redistribution of fluid to the dependent part of the chest (arrows).

chest through an electronic feedback system. One of the mostly widely used is the advanced multiple beam equalization radiography (AMBER) system. The AMBER unit uses a horizontal scanning slit-beam which is divided into segments, each being modulated by an electronic feedback loop from corresponding detectors on the far side of the patient. Such a system is particularly good at demonstrating lung pathology obscured by the heart and diaphragm.

The frontal and lateral projections are sufficient for most purposes in chest radiography. Other radiographic views are less frequently required, but they should not be overlooked since they may solve a particular problem quickly and cheaply. The lateral decubitus view is not, as its name implies, a lateral view. It is a frontal view taken with a horizontal beam and the patient lying on his or her side. Its main purpose is to demonstrate the movement of fluid in the pleural space (Fig. 1.3). An adaptation of this is the 'lateral shoot-through' sometimes used in bed bound patients – a lateral radiograph of the supine patient is taken to show an anterior pneumothorax behind the sternum (not always visible on a frontal chest radiograph; Fig. 1.4). If a pleural effusion is not loculated it gravitates, to some extent, to the dependent part of the pleural cavity. If the patient lies on his or her side, the fluid layers between the chest wall and the lung edge. This view may also be useful for demonstrating a small pneumothorax, because the visceral pleural edge of the lung falls away from the chest walls in the nondependent hemithorax.

The lordotic view, now rarely performed, is taken by angling the X-ray beam 15° cranially, either by positioning the patient upright and angling the beam up or by leaving the beam horizontal and leaning the patient backward. In this way, the lung apices are demonstrated free from the superimposed clavicle and first rib. It may be useful to differentiate pulmonary shadows from incidental calcification of the costochondral junctions (Fig. 1.5).

Portable chest radiography

Portable or mobile chest radiography has the obvious advantage that the examination can be carried out without moving the patient from the ward. However, the portable radiograph has many disadvantages. The shorter-focus film distance results in undesirable magnification, and high-kilovoltage techniques cannot be used because portable machines are unable to deliver high kilovoltage. Furthermore, the maximum current is limited so that long exposure times are needed, which potentially increases blurring of the image. Portable lateral radiographs are even less likely to be successful because of the extremely long exposure times required.

It is difficult to position patients for portable radiography and the resultant radiographs are often suboptimal. Even in the so-called erect position, in which the patient sits up, the chest is rarely as vertical as it is in a standing patient. Since many patients are unable to move to the radiography department for a formal radiograph, any method of improving the quality of a portable chest radiograph, such as digital radiography, represents a significant advance.

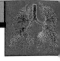

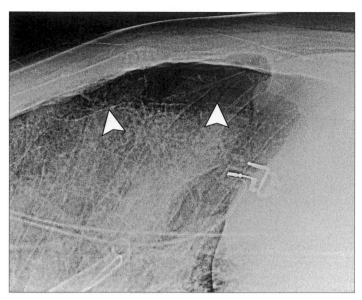

Figure 1.4 Lateral shoot-through digital radiograph of a patient in the intensive care unit. The anterior pneumothorax (note the visceral pleural edge – arrowheads) was not obvious on the anteroposterior portable radiograph.

Digital chest radiography

Digital technology is integral to techniques such as CT and MRI. Conventional film radiography as a means of image capture, storage, and display represents something of a compromise, and it has become apparent that digital image acquisition, transmission, display, and storage can, with advantage, be applied to chest radiography[1].

There are three methods of producing a digital chest radiograph. The first is to digitize conventional film radiographs using optical drum scanners or laser scanners. Although there are few reasons for adopting this approach, much useful information has been derived from observer performance studies of digitized conventional film to establish the parameters for clinically acceptable digital radiographs. The second technique is to use a dedicated digital chest unit which allows digital acquisition of the image (rather than digitization of a conventional radiograph). The prototype device was described more than 10 years ago and used a scanning slit beam and 1024 solid-state detectors. The number of detectors limited the spatial resolution of this system and it has not been further developed.

The third type of system uses conventional radiographic equipment but employs a reusable photostimulable plate (selenium or phosphor derivatives) instead of conventional film. Phosphor-plate computed, or digital, radiography has been installed in many hospitals, often as a substitute for portable film radiography. The phosphor plate is housed in a 'filmless' cassette, and stores some of the energy of the incident X-ray as a latent image. On scanning the plate with a laser beam, the stored energy is emitted as light that is detected by a photo-multiplier and converted into a digital signal. The digital information is then manipulated, displayed, and stored in whatever format is desired. The phosphor plate can be reused once the latent image has been erased by exposure to light. Most currently available computed radiography systems produce a digital radiograph with a picture element (pixel) size of 0.2mm. The fundamental requirement to segment the image into a finite number of pixels has resulted in much work to determine the relationship between pixel size, which affects spatial resolution, and the detectability of focal abnormalities. Although it might seem desirable to aim for an image composed of pixels of the smallest possible size, an inverse relationship occurs between pixel size and the cost and speed of data handling. Thus, pixel size is ultimately a compromise between image quality and ease of data processing and storage.

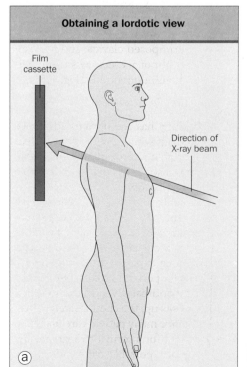

Obtaining a lordotic view

Film cassette

Direction of X-ray beam

(a)

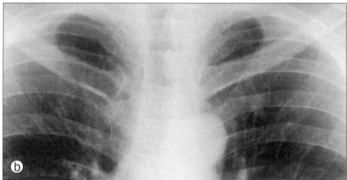

(b)

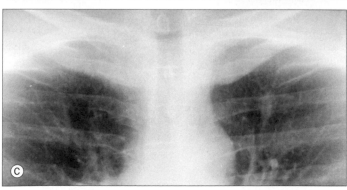

(c)

Figure 1.5 The value of lordotic views. (a) Method of obtaining a lordotic view of the lung apices: the X-ray beam is angled upward. (b) Selective view of the upper zones of a patient who presented with hemoptysis, with a suggestion of a small opacity projected over the anterior end of the left first rib. (c) A lordotic view confirms that the small opacity is intrapulmonary (rather than calcified costochondral cartilage).

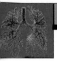

An unequivocal advantage of digital computed radiography over conventional film radiography is the linear photoluminescence-dose response, which is much greater than that of conventional film. This extremely wide latitude coupled with the facility for image processing produces diagnostic images over a wide range of exposures.

Observer performance studies have shown that computed radiography can equal conventional film radiography in virtually any task. However, postprocessing of the digital image has to be used to match the digital radiograph to the specific task. Enhancement of the image for one purpose often degrades it for another. Reports conflict as to whether digital chest radiographs can be satisfactorily interpreted on television monitors, as opposed to laser-printed film, but it is increasingly apparent that high-resolution monitors are adequate for making primary diagnoses from digital chest radiographs.

Computed tomography

The same basic principles as for film radiography apply to CT, namely the absorption of X-rays by tissues that contain constituents of different atomic number. Using multiple projections and computed calculations of radiographic density, slight differences in X-ray absorption are displayed as a cross-sectional image. The components of a CT scanner are an X-ray tube, which rotates around the patient, and an array of X-ray detectors opposite the tube. The speed with which a mechanical CT scanner acquires an image depends upon the time it takes to rotate the anode around the patient. Modern CT machines have scan times of below 2 seconds and some scanners are capable of millisecond scan times. The signal from the X-ray detectors is reconstructed by a computer and displayed on the computer console, and may be laser printed onto film.

Spiral (also known as volume or helical) scanning entails continuous scanning and table movement into the CT gantry. In this way a continuous data set or 'spiral' of information may be acquired in a single breath hold (Fig. 1.6)[2]. The information is reconstructed into axial sections, perpendicular to the long axis of the patient, identical to conventional CT sections. The main advantage of spiral CT is that truly contiguous scanning is possible, so that small pulmonary nodules are not missed for example. Since a continuous data set is acquired with spiral scanning, a three-dimensional reconstruction of complex anatomic areas can be produced (Fig. 1.7).

An alternative technology that dispenses with the mechanical rotating anode is electron beam, ultrafast CT scanning, in which the patient is surrounded by a tungsten target ring and a focused electron beam sweeps around the tungsten ring at high speed to produce an X-ray beam. Such machines can acquire an image in 100ms or less and thus real-time studies are possible, with images acquired at 17 frames per second at a given level. Rapid-acquisition studies allow the evaluation of normal and abnormal dynamic structural changes, for example lung density during the respiratory cycle or the excursion of the tracheal wall during forced respiratory maneuvers.

Technical considerations

The CT image is composed of a matrix of picture elements (pixels). A fixed number of pixels makes up the matrix, so the size of each pixel varies according to the diameter of the circle to be scanned. The smaller the circle size, the smaller the area represented by a pixel and the higher the spatial resolution of the image. In practical terms, the field of view size is adjusted to the size of area of interest, usually the chest diameter.

Often a marked difference occurs in the 'look' of the CT images obtained on different CT scanners. This is largely the result of differences in the software reconstruction algorithms used to smooth the image, to a greater or lesser extent, by averaging the density of neighboring pixels. The lung is a high-contrast environment so less smoothing is needed than in other parts of the body. High spatial-resolution algorithms (which make image noise – a granular appearance – more conspicuous) are generally more desirable for lung work.

Section thickness

Although a CT section is viewed as a two-dimensional image, it has a third dimension of depth. The depth, or section thickness, is determined by the width of the slit through which the X-ray beam passes (beam collimation). Since a section has a predetermined thickness, each pixel has a volume and this three-

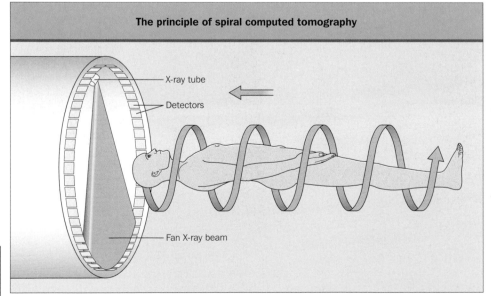

The principle of spiral computed tomography

X-ray tube

Detectors

Fan X-ray beam

Figure 1.6. The principle of spiral computed tomography. The patient moves into the scanner with the X-ray tube continuously rotating and the detectors acquiring information. The rapidity of data acquisition allows a complete examination of the thorax to be performed in a single breath hold.

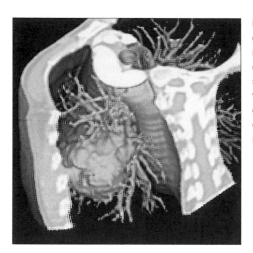

Figure 1.7 Three-dimensional reconstruction of data from a routine spiral computed tomography of the chest. A large tumor occupies much of the right lower lobe.

dimensional element is referred to as a voxel. The computer calculates the average radiographic density of tissue within each voxel and the final CT image consists of a representation of the numerous voxels (not individually visible without magnification) in the section. The single attenuation value of a voxel represents the average of the attenuation values of all the various structures within the voxel. The thicker the section, the greater the chance that different structures will be included within the voxel and so the greater the averaging that occurs. This is known as the partial volume effect; the easiest way to reduce this effect is to use thinner sections (Fig. 1.8).

When the whole chest is examined, contiguous sections 7–10mm thick are usually employed. Thinner sections are occasionally required to study complex areas of anatomy, such as the aortopulmonary window and subcarinal regions. Another specific example for which narrow sections may be useful to display differential densities (which would otherwise be lost because of the partial volume effect) is the small foci of fat or calcium that are sometimes seen within a hamartoma. There is a striking difference in the radiation dose to the patient between contiguous standard section and interspaced fine section scanning. The effective dose to the patient with interspaced fine sections (e.g. 1 or 2mm) is considerably less than that imposed by spiral CT of the entire chest volume.

Window settings

The average density of each voxel is measured in Hounsfield units (HU); the units have been arbitrarily chosen so that zero is water density and –1000 is air density. The span of Hounsfield units in the thorax is wider than in any other part of the body, ranging from aerated lung (approximately –800HU) to ribs (+700HU). Two variables are employed, which allow the operator to select the range of densities to be viewed – window width and window center (or level).

The window width determines the number of Hounsfield units to be displayed. Any densities greater than the upper limit of the window width are displayed as white, and any below the limit of the window are displayed as black. Between these two limits, the densities are displayed in shades of gray. The median density of the window chosen is the center or level, and this center can be moved higher or lower at will, thus moving the window up or down through the range. The narrower the window width the greater the contrast discrimination within the window. No single window setting can depict the wide range of densities encountered in the chest on a single image. For this reason, at least two sets of images are required to demonstrate the lung parenchyma and soft tissues of the mediastinum, respectively (see Fig. 1.9). Standard window widths and centers for thoracic CT vary between departments, but generally for the soft tissues of the mediastinum a window width of 400–600HU and a center of +30HU is appropriate. For the lungs, a wide window of 1000HU or more at a center of approximately –600HU is usually satisfactory. For bones, the widest possible window setting at a center of 30HU is best.

Window settings have a profound influence on the size and conspicuity of normal and abnormal structures. Nonetheless, it is impossible to prescribe precise window settings, since there is an element of observer preference and there are differences between machines. The most accurate representation of an object is achieved if the value of the window level is half way between the density of the structure to be measured and the density of the surrounding tissue. For example the diameter of a pulmonary nodule, measured on soft-tissue settings appropriate for the mediastinum, will be grossly underestimated. When inappropriate window settings are used, smaller structures (e.g. peripheral pulmonary vessels) are affected proportionately much more than larger structures.

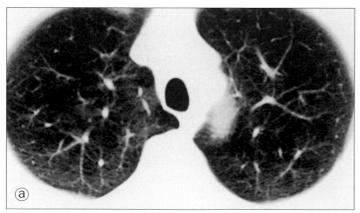

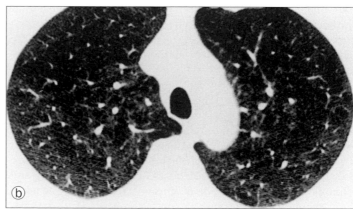

Figure 1.8 The partial volume effect on computed tomography. (a) This 10mm computed tomography section shows a poorly defined opacity, adjacent to the left superior mediastinum, apparently within the lung. (b) The 1.5mm section through the same region reveals that the appearance in (a) results from a partial volume effect, that is, the aortic arch is partially included in the 10mm-thick section.

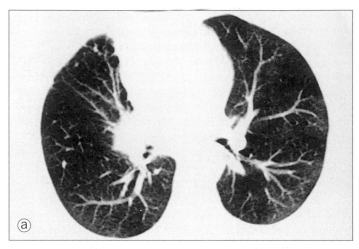

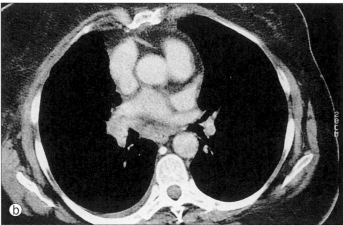

Figure 1.9 The effect of window settings on computed tomography scans. A 6mm thick computed tomography section displayed on different window settings. (a) On lung windows (center 600HU, width 1000HU) nodules in the right lung and pulmonary vessels are clearly visible. Note the lack of mediastinal detail. (b) On soft-tissue windows (center 35HU, width 400HU), the contrast-enhanced chambers of the heart and a small right pleural effusion are visible.

Intravenous contrast enhancement

Intravenous contrast enhancement only needs to be given in specific instances, because of the high contrast on CT between vessels and surrounding air in the lung, and between vessels and surrounding fat within the mediastinum. One such instance is to aid the distinction between hilar vessels and a soft-tissue mass. The exact timing of the injection of contrast media depends most on the time the CT scanner takes to scan the thorax. With fast spiral CT scanners, the circulation time of the patient becomes an important factor.

Contrast medium rapidly diffuses out of the vascular space into the extravascular space, so that opacification of the vasculature following a bolus injection quickly declines and structures such as lymph nodes steadily increase in density over time. Such dynamics result in a point at which a solid structure may have exactly the same density as an adjacent vessel. The timing and duration of the contrast medium infusion must therefore be taken into account when interpreting a contrast-enhanced CT examination. Rapid scanning protocols with automated injectors tend to improve contrast enhancement of vascular structures at the expense of enhancement of solid lesions because of the rapidity of

scanning. With spiral CT it is possible to achieve good opacification of all the thoracic vascular structures using small volumes of contrast media. Optimal contrast enhancement of the pulmonary arteries is a prerequisite for the diagnosis of pulmonary embolism (PE). When examining inflammatory lesions, such as the reaction around an empyema, it may be necessary to delay scanning by 30 seconds to allow contrast to diffuse into the extravascular space.

High-resolution computed tomography
Technical considerations

In the past 10 years the development of high-resolution computed tomography (HRCT) has had a great impact on the approach to the imaging of diffuse interstitial lung disease and bronchiectasis. Images of the lung produced by HRCT correlate closely with the macroscopic appearances of pathologic specimens, so in the context of diffuse lung disease, HRCT represents a substantial improvement over chest radiography. Three factors significantly improve the spatial resolution of CT and so confer the description 'high resolution' CT – narrow beam collimation, a high spatial reconstruction algorithm, and a small field of view[3].

Narrow collimation of the X-ray beam reduces volume averaging within the section and so increases spatial resolution compared with standard 10mm collimation. For routine HRCT scanning, 1.5mm beam collimation is generally regarded as optimal. Narrow collimation has a marked effect on the appearance of the lungs, notably the vessels and bronchi – the branching vascular pattern seen particularly in the mid zones on standard 10mm sections has a more nodular appearance with narrow sections, because shorter segments of the obliquely running vessels are included in the section (Fig. 1.10).

In HRCT lung work, a high spatial-frequency algorithm is used to take advantage of the inherently high-contrast environment of the lung. The high spatial-frequency algorithm (also known as the edge-enhancing, sharp, or formerly 'bone' algorithm) reduces image smoothing and makes structures visibly sharper, but at the same time makes image noise more obvious.

Several artifacts are consistently identified on HRCT images, but they do not usually degrade the diagnostic content of the images. Nevertheless, it is useful to be able to recognize the more common ones. Probably the most frequently encountered is a streaking appearance that arises from patient motion. Cardiac motion sometimes causes movement of the adjacent lung and hence degradation of image quality. The size of the patient has a direct effect on the quality of the lung image – the larger the patient the more conspicuous the noise, which is seen as granular streaks, because of increased X-ray absorption by the patient. This artifact is particularly evident in the posterior lung adjacent to the vertebral column. The phenomenon of aliasing results in a fine, streak-like pattern radiating from sharp, high-contrast interfaces. The severity of the aliasing artifact is related to the geometry of the CT scanner and, unlike quantum mottle, aliasing is independent of the radiation dose. These artifacts are exaggerated by the non-smoothing, high spatial-resolution reconstruction algorithm, but do not mimic normal anatomic structures and are rarely severe enough to obscure important detail in the lung parenchyma (Fig. 1.11).

The degree to which HRCT samples the lung depends primarily on the spacing between the thin sections. An HRCT examination also may vary in terms of the number of sections, the position of the patient, the phase in which respiration is suspended, the window settings at which the images are displayed,

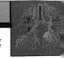

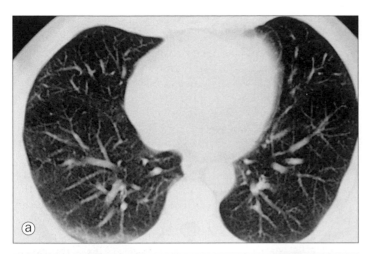

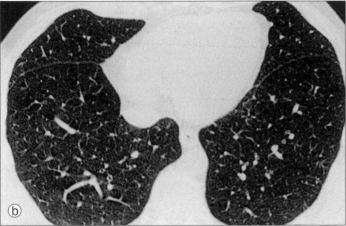

Figure 1.10 The effect of computed tomography section thickness on resolution. (a) This 10mm computed tomography section through the lower lobes shows normal lung parenchyma and vessels. (b) In the 1.5mm high-resolution computed tomography at the same level as (a), the vessels are sharper and appear as more nodular opacities (less of their length is included in the plane of section). Note the increased clarity of the oblique fissures and bronchi. The opacification in the dependent parts of the lungs, more obvious in the right lung, is a normal phenomenon.

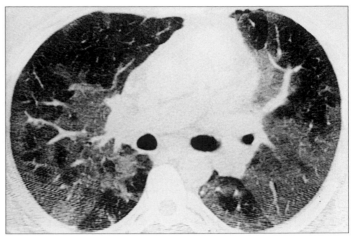

Figure 1.11 High-resolution computed tomography image demonstrating artifact caused by aliasing and quantum mottle. Detail is obscured in the posterior parts of the lungs. The patchy parenchymal opacification was due to desquamative interstitial pneumonitis.

and the manipulation of the image by postprocessing. No single protocol can be recommended to cover every eventuality. However, the simplest protocol entails 1.5mm collimation sections at 20mm intervals from apex to lung bases. Any given scanning protocol may need to be modified – a patient referred with unexplained hemoptysis ideally is scanned with contiguous standard sections through the major airways (to show a small endobronchial abnormality) and interspaced narrow sections through the remainder of the lungs (to identify bronchiectasis).

When early interstitial disease is suspected, for example in asbestos-exposed individuals who have an apparently normal chest radiograph, HRCT scans are often performed in the prone position to prevent any confusion with the increased opacification seen in the dependent posterior–basal segments of many normal individuals scanned in the usual supine position (Fig. 1.10). The increased density seen in the posterior dependent lung in the supine position disappears in normal individuals when the scan is repeated at the same level with the patient in the prone position. No advantage is gained by scanning a patient in the prone position if no obvious diffuse lung disease is found on a contemporary chest radiograph.

A limited number of scans taken at end expiration can reveal evidence of air trapping caused by small airways disease, which may not be detectable on routine inspiratory scans. Areas of air trapping range from a single secondary pulmonary lobule to a cluster of lobules that give a patchwork appearance of low attenuation areas adjacent to higher attenuation, normal lung parenchyma (see Fig. 1.12).

Alterations of the window settings of HRCT images sometimes makes detection of parenchymal abnormalities impossible when there is a subtle increase or decrease in attenuation of the lung parenchyma. Uniformity of window settings from patient to patient aids consistent interpretation of the lung images. In general, a window level of −500 to −800HU and a width of between 900 and 1500HU are usually satisfactory. Modification of the window settings for particular tasks is often desirable; for example, in looking for pleuroparenchymal abnormalities in asbestos-exposed individuals, a wider window of up to 2000HU may be useful. Conversely, a narrower window of approximately 600HU may emphasize the subtle density differences that characterize emphysema and small airways disease.

The relatively high radiation dose to the patient inherent in all CT scanning needs to be appreciated. The radiation burden to the patient is considerably less with HRCT than with conventional CT scanning. It has been estimated that the mean radiation dose delivered to the skin with HRCT using 1.5mm sections at 20mm intervals is 6% that of conventional 10mm contiguous-scanning protocols. A further method of reducing the radiation burden to the patient is to decrease the milliamperage; it is possible to reduce the milliamperage by up to 10-fold and still obtain comparably diagnostic images[4]. Although future refinements in CT technology may reduce the radiation burden to patients, CT still represent a relatively high radiation dose to patients, and as such must not be performed indiscriminately.

Clinical applications of high-resolution computed tomography
Increasingly, HRCT is used to confirm or refute the impression of an abnormality seen on a chest radiograph. It may also be used to achieve a histospecific diagnosis in some patients who have obvious but nonspecific radiographic abnormalities[5,6].

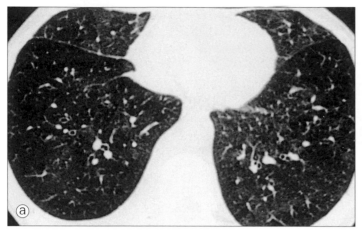

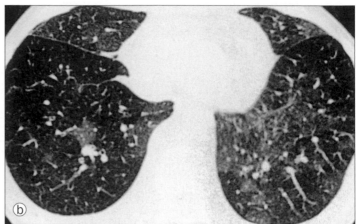

Figure 1.12 High-resolution computed tomography through the lower lobes of a patient who has severe dyspnea and rheumatoid arthritis. (a) Minor inhomogeneity of the density of the lung parenchyma and some dilatation of the bronchi. (b) A high-resolution computed tomography taken at end expiration emphasizes the density differences. Appearances are consistent with obliterative bronchiolitis.

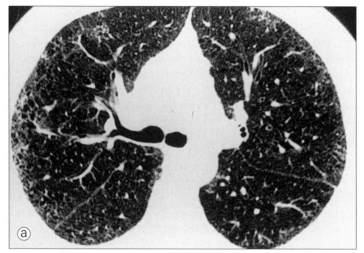

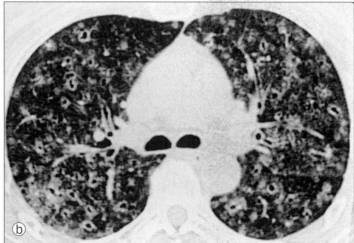

Figure 1.13 High-resolution computed tomography patterns. (a) Subpleural reticular pattern typical of established fibrosing alveolitis. (b) Numerous cavitating nodules, several of which have odd shapes; sections through the lung bases were normal. This high-resolution computed tomography pattern and distribution is virtually pathognomonic of Langerhans' cell histiocytosis.

It is probably impossible to determine the frequency with which HRCT will show significant parenchymal abnormalities when the chest radiograph appears normal. Studies of individual diseases show that HRCT demonstrates abnormalities despite normal chest radiographs in 29% of patients who have systemic sclerosis, and in up to 30% of asbestosis patients. For subacute hypersensitivity pneumonitis, the proportion may be even higher. Taking the average sensitivity results of several studies, HRCT appears to have a sensitivity of approximately 94% compared with 80% for chest radiography; this increased sensitivity does not seem to be achieved at the expense of decreased specificity.

In patients with clinical, radiographic, and lung function evidence of diffuse lung disease, much evidence now indicates that HRCT correctly predicts more often, and with a greater degree of confidence than chest radiography allows, the correct histologic diagnosis. In the original study that compared the diagnostic accuracy of chest radiography and CT in the prediction of specific histologic diagnoses in patients with diffuse lung disease, Mathieson et al. showed that three observers could make a confident diagnosis in 23% of cases on the basis of chest radiographs and in 49% of cases using CT; the correct diagnoses were made in 77 and 93% of these readings, respectively (Fig. 1.13)[7].

In a later study, Grenier et al. showed that, for each of three observers, the high-confidence diagnoses that were correct from chest radiography findings alone were 29, 34, and 19%, respectively, whereas in HRCT the results were 57, 55, and 47%, respectively[8]. Moreover, the intraobserver agreement for the proposed diagnosis was improved with HRCT compared with chest radiography. These studies show that HRCT is clearly useful in the assessment of patients suspected of having diffuse lung disease but for whom the clinical features and chest radiograph do not allow a confident diagnosis to be made. Even without clinical information, a number of diffuse lung diseases can, in the hands of experienced chest radiologists, have a 'diagnostic' appearance on HRCT; these include fibrosing alveolitis, sarcoidosis, Langerhans' cell histiocytosis, lymphangioleiomyomatosis, pneumoconiosis, and hypersensitivity pneumonitis (Fig. 1.14). Intriguingly, the ability of HRCT to allow observers to provide correct histospecific diagnoses appears to be maintained in advanced 'end-stage' disease[9].

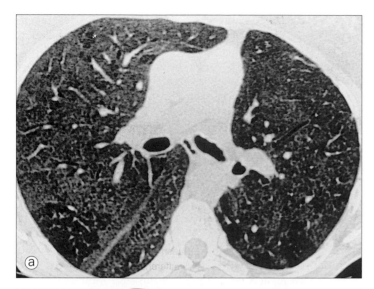

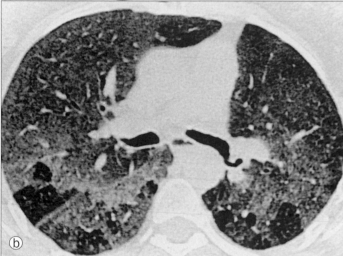

Figure 1.14 High-resolution computed tomography of a patient with subacute hypersensitivity pneumonitis. (a) Widespread nodular and ground-glass patterns. (b) Note the areas of decreased attenuation posteriorly, made more obvious on this scan obtained in expiration.

However, HRCT is sometimes used indiscriminately for patients in whom the high certainty of diagnosis from clinical and radiographic findings do not justify the extra cost and radiation burden. No evidence shows that an HRCT examination adds anything of diagnostic value for a patient who has progressive shortness of breath, finger clubbing, crackles at the lung bases, and the typical radiographic pattern and lung-function profile of fibrosing alveolitis. Nevertheless, the ability of HRCT to characterize disease, and often to deliver a definite and correct diagnosis in patients with nonspecific radiographic shadowing, is frequently helpful.

Much interest has been shown in defining the role of HRCT in staging disease activity, particularly for fibrosing alveolitis, in which cellular histology indicates disease activity and is used to predict both responses to treatment and prognosis. There is now evidence that a predominance of ground-glass opacification in fibrosing alveolitis predicts a good response to treatment and increased actuarial survival compared with patients with a more reticular pattern, which denotes established fibrosis. Similar observations about the potential reversibility of disease can be made

using HRCT on patients who have sarcoidosis, in whom a ground-glass or a nodular pattern predominates. In other conditions, the identification of ground-glass opacification on HRCT, although nonspecific, almost invariably indicates a potentially reversible disease, for example extrinsic allergic alveolitis, diffuse pulmonary hemorrhage, and *Pneumocystis carinii* pneumonia (Fig. 1.15). An important exception is bronchioloalveolar cell carcinoma, in which there may be areas of ground-glass opacification that merge into areas of frank consolidation or a more nodular pattern. Another caveat is the situation in which fine, intralobular fibrosis is seen on HRCT as widespread ground-glass opacification; in this rare occurrence evidence of traction bronchiectasis is usually present within the areas of ground-glass opacification.

The ability of CT to discriminate between various patterns of disease has clarified the reasons for the sometimes complex mixed obstructive and restrictive functional deficits found in some diffuse lung diseases. A good example is hypersensitivity pneumonitis, in which both interstitial and small airways disease coexist – patterns caused by these different pathologic processes can readily be appreciated on HRCT (Fig. 1.14). The extent of the various HRCT patterns correlates with the expected functional indices of restriction and obstruction. Other conditions in which CT is able to tease out the morphologic abnormalities responsible for complex functional deficits include fibrosing alveolitis, when there is coexisting emphysema, and sarcoidosis, when there may be a combination of interstitial fibrosis and small airways obstruction by peribronchiolar granulomata.

In patients for whom lung biopsy is deemed necessary, HRCT may be invaluable for indicating which type of biopsy procedure is likely to be successful in obtaining diagnostic material. The broad distinction between peripheral disease versus central and bronchocentric disease is easily made on HRCT. Thus, disease with a subpleural distribution, such as fibrosing alveolitis, is most unlikely to be sampled by transbronchial biopsy, whereas diseases with a bronchocentric distribution on HRCT, such as sarcoidosis and lymphangitis carcinomatosa, are consistently accessible to transbronchial biopsy. In patients for whom an open or thoracoscopic lung biopsy is contemplated, HRCT assists in determining the optimal biopsy site. Pathologic examination of a lung biopsy can still justifiably be regarded as the final arbiter for the presence or absence of subtle interstitial lung disease. Since HRCT images provide an 'in-vivo big picture', many lung pathologists now combine the imaging and pathologic information before assigning a

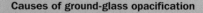

Causes of ground-glass opacification
Pneumocystis carinii or cytomegalovirus pneumonia
Acute respiratory distress syndrome/acute interstitial pneumonia
Hypersensitivity pneumonitis – subacute
Desquamative interstitial pneumonitis
Pulmonary edema
Idiopathic pulmonary hemorrhage
Bronchioloalveolar cell carcinoma
Alveolar proteinosis
Lymphocytic interstitial pneumonia
Respiratory bronchiolitis – interstitial lung disease

Figure 1.15 Causes of ground-glass opacification.

final diagnosis, and in many centers the benefits of a team approach to the diagnosis of diffuse lung disease are recognized[10,11]. The indications for HRCT that have been developed over the past 10 years are summarized in Figure 1.16[12,13].

Pulmonary angiography

Pulmonary angiography is used to investigate the pulmonary circulation when other, less invasive methods have failed to provide the requisite information. The most frequent indication is for suspected PE, usually following a nondiagnostic ventilation–perfusion scan ($\dot{V}/\dot{Q}$). Ideally, the angiogram is undertaken within 24 hours of an acute presentation of suspected embolism. However, a delay of 48–72 hours should not preclude the use of pulmonary angiography, although the diagnostic yield progressively declines because of fragmentation of thrombi over time, especially if anticoagulation has been instituted.

Pulmonary angiography is a technique that tends to be under used for a variety of reasons. Apart from the relatively expensive and invasive nature of angiography, it is perceived to have a high complication rate (although this is not supported by the published evidence). The imbalance between the rates of $\dot{V}/\dot{Q}$ scan and angiography is striking and it has been estimated that only one angiogram is requested for every 100 $\dot{V}/\dot{Q}$ scans. This is a ratio that flatters the diagnostic abilities of $\dot{V}/\dot{Q}$ scanning, which in most series yields an equivocal result in 30–60% of patients[14]. The frequently quoted complications of angiography, namely respiratory compromise, arrhythmia, renal failure, and transient hypersensitivity reactions, are based on historical data that suggested a mortality rate of up to 0.5%, a major nonfatal complication rate of 1%, and a minor complication rate of 5%[3]. More recent evaluation suggests pulmonary angiography is much safer[4]. This improvement is attributed predominantly to the change from ionic contrast media to low, osmolar nonionic agents. Secondly, more flexible, small-gauge pigtail catheters have reduced the incidence of myocardial injury[15].

The technique of pulmonary angiography involves fluoroscopically directed insertion of a guide wire, followed by a modified pigtail catheter into the right and left main pulmonary arteries in turn, with injection of a nonionic contrast at an appropriate flow rate. At least two views per side are required, with additional oblique or magnification views as necessary. Catheter access is usually via the femoral vein, with the internal jugular and subclavian veins as possible alternatives. Despite the desirable high resolution of conventional film–screen angiography, most departments now undertake angiography with digital subtraction vascular equipment (Fig. 1.17). Problems with misregistration artifact, inherent in digital subtraction systems, and caused by respiratory or cardiac cycle-phase differences between the mask image and the contrast image, can usually be overcome by acquiring a series of mask views prior to contrast injection. Crossing the tricuspid valve may induce an arrhythmia that is usually transient. Therefore, electrocardiogram (ECG) monitoring is mandatory and the use of prophylactic, antiarrhythmic agents or temporary pacing-wire insertion is common practice in some centers.

When a pulmonary embolus is present, it is most frequently situated in the posterior segments of the lower lobe. Thrombi beyond the segmental vessel level are detected less reliably than more central thrombi. However, the significance of thrombi confined to subsegmental vessels is unclear. The typical angiographic findings of PE are vascular cut-off or, when vascular occlusion is not complete, an intraluminal filling defect with contrast passing around and beyond the clot. Indirect signs of embolism include areas of relatively delayed or reduced perfusion, late filling of the venous circulation, and vessel tortuosity. When the angiogram is undertaken to investigate suspected chronic thromboembolic disease, the vascular changes include local stenosis or thin webs, luminal ectasia, and irregularities of the normal tapering pattern.

The high threshold for proceeding to pulmonary angiography when the diagnosis of PE remains in doubt has advanced the developing role of contrast-enhanced spiral CT scanning for the diagnosis of PE.

Bronchial artery embolization

Bronchial artery embolization is usually performed to stop massive hemoptysis[16]. The most common causes of bronchial artery hypertrophy and consequent hemorrhage are suppurative lung diseases (particularly bronchiectasis) and fibrocavitary disease

Indications for high-resolution computed tomography of the lungs
Narrow the differential diagnosis or make a histospecific diagnosis in patients with obvious but nonspecific radiographic abnormalities
Detect diffuse lung disease in patients with normal or equivocal radiographic abnormalities
Elucidate unexpected pulmonary function test results
Investigate patients presenting with hemoptysis
Evaluate disease reversibility, particularly in patients who have fibrosing alveolitis
Guide the type and site of lung biopsy

Figure 1.16 Indications for high-resolution computed tomography of the lungs.

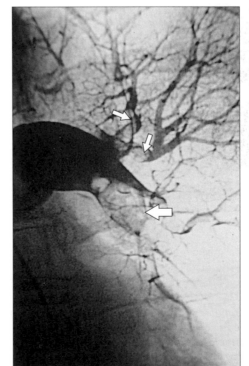

Figure 1.17 Digital subtraction pulmonary angiogram. A large thrombus causes a filling defect within the contrast in the artery of the left lower lobe (large arrow). Smaller thrombi are present within the proximal branches to the upper lobe (small arrows).

containing mycetomas. Less common causes of hemorrhage from the bronchial circulation include bronchial carcinoma, chronic pulmonary abscess, and congenital cyanotic heart disease. No absolute contraindications to bronchial artery embolization are known, although the patient should be hemodynamically stable and able to cooperate.

The most common anatomic arrangement on bronchial arteriography is one main right bronchial artery arising from a common intercostobronchial trunk, which comes off the thoracic aorta at approximately the level of T5, and two left bronchial arteries arising more inferiorly. However, bronchial arteries may arise from the thyrocervical trunk, internal mammary artery, costocervical trunk, subclavian artery, a lower intercostal artery, inferior phrenic artery, or even the abdominal aorta. The right intercostal bronchial trunk takes off from the aorta at an acute upward angle, whereas the left bronchial arteries leave the aorta more or less at right angles, and special catheters have been designed to facilitate selective catheterization. Superselective catheterization of the bronchial circulation allows precise delivery of embolic material and so prevents spillover into the aorta or inadvertent embolization of the spinal artery.

Fiberoptic bronchoscopy is often advocated prior to bronchial artery embolization to establish the site of hemorrhage. However, a large hemoptysis almost invariably results in vigorous coughing and so blood is spread throughout the bronchial tree, which makes localization impossible. Few criteria exist to determine which angiographically demonstrated bronchial arteries should be embolized. Guidelines are particularly relevant when several bronchial arteries have been identified and the site of hemorrhage is not obvious from prior thoracic imaging. Embolization is directed at the vessels considered most likely to be the source of hemorrhage (Fig. 1.18). Bronchial arteries of diameter >3mm may be considered pathologically enlarged. In patients with diffuse, suppurative lung disease, most commonly cystic fibrosis,

attempts are made to embolize all significantly enlarged bronchial arteries bilaterally. If no abnormal bronchial arteries are identified, a systematic search is made for aberrant bronchial arteries. When a patient continues to have hemoptysis after embolization of all suspicious systemic arteries, it may be necessary to investigate the pulmonary circulation for a source of hemorrhage.

A variety of embolic materials have been used for the embolization of bronchial arteries, ranging from particles of polyvinyl foam to small pieces of gelfoam. Although coils lodged proximally in the bronchial artery have been used, they prevent subsequent catheterization.

Following bronchial artery embolization, many patients experience transient fever and chest pain; after 2 days some patients cough up a small amount of blood, which possibly arises from limited infarction of the bronchial mucosa. Serious complications after bronchial artery embolization are rare, the most serious being transverse myelitis, probably caused by contrast toxicity rather than inadvertent embolization. Inadvertent spillover of embolization material into the thoracic aorta may cause distant ischemia in the legs or abdominal organs.

The aim of bronchial artery embolization is the immediate control of life-threatening hemoptysis, which is achieved in over 75% of patients. Failures usually result from nonidentification of significant bronchial arteries and an inability to maintain the catheter position and proceed to embolization. Up to 20% of patients re-bleed within 6 months of an initially successful bronchial artery embolization. The reasons cited for recurrent hemorrhage are recanalization of previously embolized vessels, incomplete initial embolization, and hypertrophy of small bronchial arteries not initially embolized. However, bronchial artery embolization usually can be satisfactorily repeated in patients who re-bleed.

Superior vena cava stents

Superior vena cava (SVC) obstruction (SVCO) is characterized by facial and upper limb swelling, headache, and shortness of breath, and is usually caused by advanced mediastinal malignancy. Conventional palliative treatment relies on radiotherapy, chemotherapy, and sometimes surgery. Radiotherapy usually produces an initial improvement, although subsequent recurrence of symptoms is frequent. Balloon angioplasty of both benign and malignant causes of SVCO has been reported, but not surprisingly symptoms are liable to recur soon after angioplasty alone.

The percutaneous placement of metallic stents for the treatment of SVCO has several attractions. With increasing experience, reliable and successful palliation of SVCO has been reported using various stent designs[17]. A superior venacavogram is necessary to identify the length of the stenosis, and its site in relation to the confluence of the brachiocephalic veins and the right atrium. Identification of intraluminal thrombus or tumor is an absolute contraindication to the procedure. Following balloon dilatation of the SVC stricture, the stent is positioned across the stricture and a postplacement venocavogram is performed to confirm free flow of blood into the right atrium (see Fig. 1.19). After angioplasty and stent placement, relief of SVCO symptoms is usually rapid and dramatic. Recurrence of symptoms may be caused by venous thrombosis or tumor progression distal to the stent. Although rupture of the SVC at the time of angioplasty is a risk, this complication seems to be extremely rare, possibly because of the tamponade provided by surrounding tumor or postirradiation fibrosis.

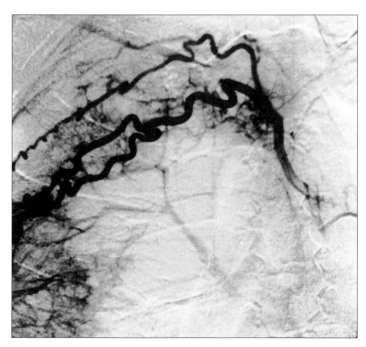

Figure 1.18 Bronchial arteriogram in a patient with hemoptysis.
There is marked hypertrophy of the intercostal and bronchial arteries. These changes were caused by chronic thromboembolic disease.

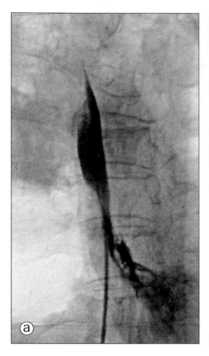
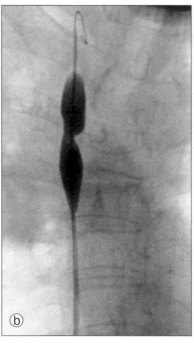
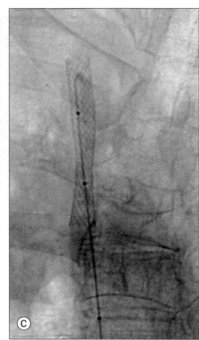

(a) (b) (c)

Figure 1.19 Stenting of superior vena cava obstruction. The patient had a superior vena cava obstruction caused by mediastinal malignancy. (a) Superior venacavogram showing a tight stricture in the mid superior vena cava. (b) Balloon dilatation of the stricture. (c) Placement of a meshed-wire stent in the patent superior vena cava.

The role of intravascular stents in nonmalignant SVCO has not yet been defined. Patients who have SVCO caused by benign fibrosing mediastinitis have been treated successfully, although occlusion of the stent by the progression of the mediastinal fibrosis or by endothelial proliferation may occur.

NORMAL RADIOGRAPHIC ANATOMY

The mediastinum and hilar structures

The mediastinum is delineated by the lungs on either side, the thoracic inlet above, the diaphragm below, and the vertebral column posteriorly. Since the various structures that make up the mediastinum are superimposed on each other, they cannot be separately identified on a two-dimensional chest radiograph; for this reason the normal anatomy of the individual components of the mediastinum is considered in more detail in the section on CT of the mediastinum. Nevertheless, because a chest radiograph is usually the first imaging investigation, it is necessary to appreciate the normal appearances of the mediastinum and the considerable possible variations, which are influenced by the patient's body habitus and age.

The mediastinum is conventionally divided into superior, anterior, middle, and posterior compartments (Fig. 1.20). The practical use of these arbitrary divisions is that specific mediastinal pathologies show a definite predilection for individual compartments (e.g. a superior mediastinal mass is most frequently caused by intrathoracic extension of the thyroid gland; a middle mediastinal mass usually results from enlarged lymph nodes). However, localization of a mass within one of these compartments does not normally allow a specific diagnosis to be made, and neither do the arbitrary boundaries preclude disease from involving more than one compartment.

Only the outline of the mediastinum and the air-containing trachea and bronchi (and sometimes esophagus) are clearly seen on a normal PA chest radiograph. On a chest radiograph, the right brachiocephalic vein and SVC form the right superior mediastinal border. This border is usually vertical and straight (in contrast to the situation in which there is right paratracheal lymphadenopathy, when the right superior mediastinal border tends to be undulate), and it becomes less distinct as it reaches the thoracic inlet. The right side of the superior mediastinum can appear to be considerably widened in patients who have an abundance of mediastinal fat (Fig. 1.21); these individuals often have prominent cardiophrenic fat pads. The mediastinal border to the left of the trachea above the aortic arch is the result of summation of the left carotid and left subclavian arteries, together with the left brachiocephalic and jugular veins. The left cardiac border comprises the left atrial appendage that merges inferiorly with the left ventricle. The silhouette of the heart should always be sharply outlined. Any blurring of the border results from loss of immediately adjacent aerated lung, usually by collapse or consolidation.

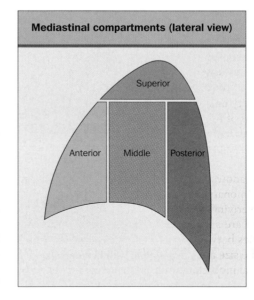

Mediastinal compartments (lateral view)

Superior

Anterior Middle Posterior

Figure 1.20 The mediastinal compartments. Note that the separation between the compartments is arbitrary – there are no definite anatomic boundaries.

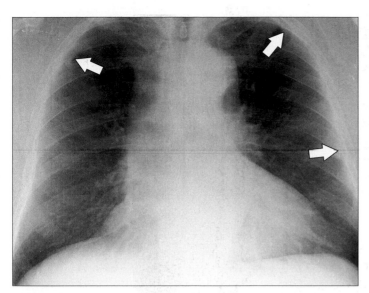

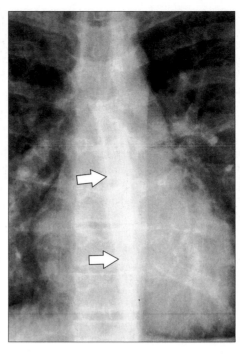

Figure 1.22 Amber chest radiograph. The normal azygoesophageal line is demonstrated (arrows).

Figure 1.21 Widening of the superior mediastinum caused by abundance of mediastinal fat. In addition, bilateral cardiophrenic fat pads are present. The apparent pleural thickening (arrows) results from extrapleural fat.

The density of the heart shadow to the left and right of the vertebral column should be identical – any difference indicates pathology (e.g. an area of consolidation or a mass in a lower lobe). On a well-penetrated film, a density with a convex lateral border is frequently seen through the right heart border – this apparent mass is caused by the confluence of the right pulmonary veins as they enter the left atrium and is of no clinical significance.

The trachea and main bronchi should be visible through the upper and middle mediastinum. The trachea is rarely straight and is often to the right of the midline at its midpoint. In older individuals, the trachea may be markedly displaced by a dilated aortic arch below. In approximately 60% of normal subjects the right wall of the trachea (the right paratracheal stripe) can be identified as a line of uniform thickness (<4mm in width); when visible, it excludes the presence of any adjacent space-occupying lesion, most usually lymphadenopathy. The angle between the main bronchus, which forms the carina, is usually somewhat less than 80°. Splaying of the carina is a relatively crude sign of subcarinal disease, either in the form of a massive subcarinal lymphadenopathy or a markedly enlarged left atrium. A more sensitive sign of subcarinal disease is obscuration of the upper part of the azygoesophageal line, which is usually visible in its entirety on a well-penetrated chest radiograph (Fig. 1.22). The origins of the lobar bronchi, when they are projected over the mediastinal shadow, can usually be identified, but segmental bronchi within the lungs generally are not seen on plain radiography.

The normal hilar shadows on a chest radiograph represent the summation of the pulmonary arteries and veins, with little contribution from the overlying bronchial walls or lymph nodes of normal size. The hilae are approximately the same size and the left hilum normally lies between 0.5 and 1.5cm above the level of the right hilum. The size and shape of the hilae show remarkable variation in normal individuals, making subtle abnormalities difficult to identify.

Pulmonary fissures, vessels, and bronchi

The two lungs are separated by the four layers of pleura behind and in front of the mediastinum. The resultant posterior and anterior junction lines are often visible on frontal chest radiographs as nearly vertical stripes, the posterior junction line lying higher than the anterior (Fig. 1.23). Since these junction lines are not invariably seen (their visibility is largely dependent on whether the pleural reflections are tangential to the X-ray beam), their presence or absence is not usually of significance.

The lobes of lung are surrounded by visceral pleura – the major (or oblique) fissure separates the upper and lower lobes of the left lung. The major (or oblique) fissure and the minor (hor-

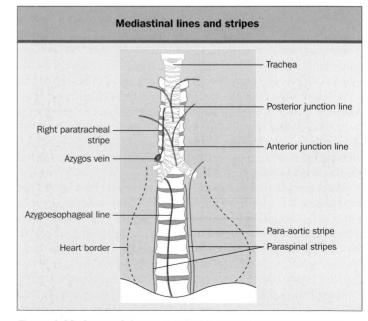

Mediastinal lines and stripes

Trachea
Posterior junction line
Right paratracheal stripe
Anterior junction line
Azygos vein
Azygoesophageal line
Para-aortic stripe
Heart border
Paraspinal stripes

Figure 1.23 Some of the mediastinal lines and stripes frequently seen on a frontal chest radiograph.

izontal or transverse) fissure separate the upper, middle, and lower lobes of the right lung. The minor fissure is visible in over half of normal PA chest radiographs. In normal individuals, the minor fissure is slightly bowed upward and runs horizontally; any deviation from this configuration is usually caused by loss of volume of a lobe. The major fissures are not visible on a frontal radiograph and are inconsistently identifiable on lateral radiographs. Inability to detect a fissure usually means that the fissure is not exactly in the line of the X-ray beam. However, in a few individuals, fissures are incompletely developed, a point familiar to thoracic surgeons who sometimes encounter difficulty in performing a lobectomy because of incomplete cleavage between lobes. Accessory fissures are occasionally seen, for example in the left lung a minor fissure can be present, which separates the lingula from the remainder of the upper lobe.

All of the branching structures seen within normal lungs on a chest radiograph represent pulmonary arteries or veins. The pulmonary veins may sometimes be differentiated from the pulmonary arteries – the superior pulmonary veins have a distinctly vertical course. However, it is usually impossible to differentiate arteries from veins in the lung periphery. On a chest radiograph taken in the erect position, a gradual increase in the diameter of the vessels is seen, at equidistant points from the hilum, traveling from lung apex to base; this gravity-dependent effect disappears if the patient is supine or in cardiac failure.

The lobes of the lung are divided into segments, each of which are supplied by their own segmental pulmonary artery and accompanying bronchus. The walls of the segmental bronchi are rarely seen on the chest radiograph, except when lying parallel with the X-ray beam, in which case they are seen end-on as ring shadows that measure up to 8mm in diameter. The most frequently identified segmental airways are the anterior segmental bronchi of the upper lobes.

The diaphragm and thoracic cage

The interface between aerated lung and the hemidiaphragms is sharp, and the highest point of each dome is normally medial to the midclavicular line. The right dome of the diaphragm is higher than the left by up to 2cm in the erect position, unless the left dome is elevated by air in the stomach. Laterally, the hemidiaphragm forms an acute angle with the chest wall. Filling in or blunting of these costophrenic angles usually represents pleural disease, either pleural thickening or an effusion. In the elderly, localized humps on the dome of the diaphragm, particularly posteriorly (thus most obvious on a lateral radiograph) are common and represent minor weaknesses or defects of the diaphragm. Interposition of the colon in front of the right lobe of the liver is a frequently seen normal variant (so-called Chilaiditi syndrome).

Apparent pleural thickening along the lateral chest wall in the mid zones is a frequent observation in obese individuals; it is caused by subpleural fat bulging inward (see Fig. 1.21). Deformities of the thoracic cage may cause distortion of the normal mediastinum and so simulate disease. One of the most common deformities is pectus excavatum which, by compressing the heart between the depressed sternum and vertebral column, causes displacement of the apparently enlarged heart to the left and blurring of the right heart border (Fig. 1.24). A similar appearance may arise from an unusually straight thoracic spine, referred to as straight back syndrome (Fig. 1.25).

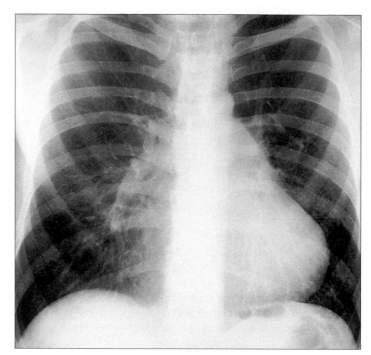

Figure 1.24 Frontal chest radiograph of a patient who has marked pectus excavatum. The blurring of the right heart border and apparent increase in heart size are a direct consequence of a depressed sternum. Note the '7' configuration of the ribs.

Anatomy on the lateral chest radiograph

Viewing lateral chest radiographs consistently in the same orientation, whether a right or left lateral projection, improves the ability to detect deviations from normal. In the lateral view, the trachea is angled slightly posteriorly as it runs toward the carina, and its posterior wall is always visible as a fine stripe (Fig. 1.26). The posterior walls of the right main bronchus and the right intermediate bronchus are outlined by air, and are also seen as a continuous stripe on the lateral radiograph. The overlying scapulae are invariably seen running almost vertically in the upper part of the lateral radiograph (and may be misinterpreted as intrathoracic structures). Further confusing shadows are formed by the soft tissues of the outstretched arms, which project over the upper mediastinum. The carina is not visible as such on the lateral radiograph, and the two transradiancies projected over the lower trachea represent the right main bronchus (superiorly) and the left main bronchus (inferiorly).

Overlying structures on a lateral radiograph obscure most of the lung. In normal individuals, the unobscured lung in the retrosternal and retrocardiac regions should be of the same transradiancy. Furthermore, as the eye travels down the spine, a gradual increase in transradiancy should be apparent. The loss of this phenomenon suggests the presence of disease in the posterior–basal segments of the lower lobes, for example fibrosing alveolitis (Fig. 1.27).

The two major fissures are seen as diagonal lines, of a hair's breadth, that run from the upper dorsal spine to the anterior surface of the diaphragm. Care must be taken not to confuse the obliquely running rib edges with fissures. The minor fissure extends horizontally from the mid right major fissure. It is often not possible to differentiate the right from the left major fissures with confidence. Similarly, although the two hemi-diaphragms

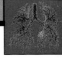

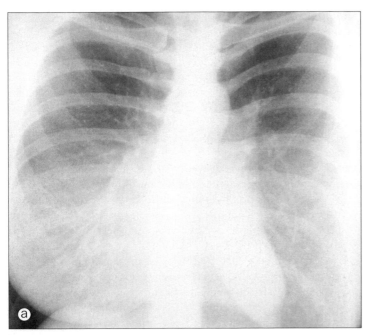

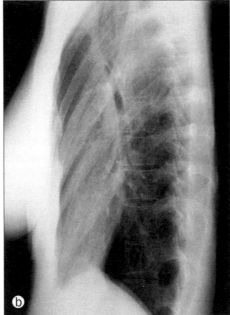

Figure 1.25 The effect of a straight spine. (a) Loss of the right heart border occurs. (b) The loss is caused by complete lack of the normal spinal kyphosis, which results in a reduction of the anteroposterior diameter of the chest.

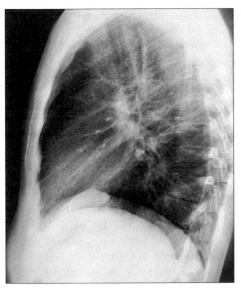

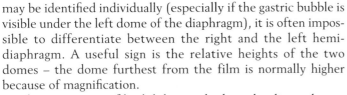

Figure 1.26 The lateral radiograph in a normal subject.

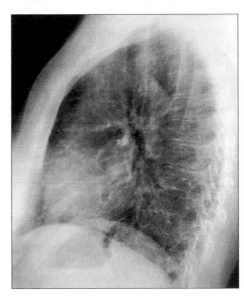

Figure 1.27 Loss of the normal increase in transradiancy toward the lower part of the dorsal spine in a patient with fibrosing alveolitis.

may be identified individually (especially if the gastric bubble is visible under the left dome of the diaphragm), it is often impossible to differentiate between the right and the left hemidiaphragm. A useful sign is the relative heights of the two domes – the dome furthest from the film is normally higher because of magnification.

The summation of both hilae on the lateral radiograph generates a complex shadow. However, one general point is useful in the interpretation of this difficult area – the right pulmonary artery lies anterior to the trachea and right main bronchus, whereas the left pulmonary artery arches over the left main bronchus so that a large part of it lies posterior to the major bronchi (Fig. 1.28).

A band-like opacity is often seen along the lower third of the anterior chest wall behind the sternum. It represents a normal density and occurs because less aerated lung is in contact with the chest wall, since the space is occupied by the heart; it should not be confused with pleural disease.

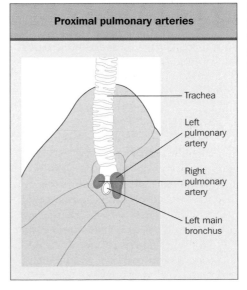

Proximal pulmonary arteries

Trachea

Left pulmonary artery

Right pulmonary artery

Left main bronchus

Figure 1.28 The position of the proximal pulmonary arteries seen on a lateral chest radiograph.

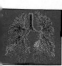

POINTS IN THE INTERPRETATION OF A CHEST RADIOGRAPH

Even when an obvious radiographic abnormality is present, it is necessary to review a chest radiograph using a systematic method. With increasing experience, appreciation of deviation from normal appearances becomes rapid, which leads quickly to a directed search for related abnormalities. Before interpreting a chest radiograph, it is vital to establish whether any previous radiographs are available for comparison – the sequence and pattern of change is often as important as the identification of a radiographic abnormality. Information gained from preceding radiographs, particularly the lack of serial change, often prevents needless further investigation.

A check that the radiograph is of satisfactory quality includes an estimation of the adequacy of radiographic exposure, depth of inspiration, and position of the patient. The intervertebral disc spaces of the entire dorsal spine should be visible on a correctly exposed chest radiograph, and the midpoint of the right hemidiaphragm lies at the level of the anterior end of the sixth rib if the (normal) subject has taken a satisfactory breath in. The medial ends of the clavicles should be equidistant from the spinous processes of the cervical vertebral bodies.

The order in which the various parts of a chest radiograph are examined is unimportant. A suggested sequence is to start with a check of the position of the trachea, mediastinal contour (which should be sharply outlined in its entirety), and then the position, outline, and density of the hilar shadows. The certain identification of a hilar abnormality often requires comparison with a previous radiograph; any suspicion of a hilar abnormality necessitates the retrieval of any previous chest radiographs. At least as important as an abnormal contour in detecting a mass at the hilum is a discrepancy in density between the two sides – both hilar shadows, at equivalent points, should be of equal density, and a mass at the hilum (or an intrapulmonary mass projected over the hilum) is evident as an increased density of the affected hilum. For a questionably abnormal hilum, the lateral radiograph is sometimes helpful in clarifying the situation, providing the normal anatomy is remembered (i.e. most of the right pulmonary artery lies anterior to the trachea and the bulk of the left pulmonary artery lies behind the trachea) (Fig. 1.28). Thus, a suspected right hilar mass on a frontal radiograph that appears to be behind the trachea on a lateral view is unlikely to represent a prominent right pulmonary artery, and is therefore most likely to be an abnormal mass (the converse rule applies to a suspicious left hilum).

The lungs may then be examined in terms of their size, the relative transradiancy of each zone, and the position of the horizontal fissure. Pulmonary vessels are seen as far out as the outer third of the lung and the number of vessels should be roughly symmetric on the two sides. Next, the position and clarity of the hemidiaphragms should be noted, followed by an assessment of the ribs and soft tissues of the chest wall. Before regarding a chest radiograph as normal, it is useful to review areas that are poorly demonstrated or sometimes misinterpreted; these include the central mediastinum (where even a large mass may be invisible on the PA view), the lungs behind the diaphragm and heart, the lung apices (often obscured by the overlying clavicles and ribs), and the lung and pleura just inside the chest wall.

Radiographic signs
Consolidation

Consolidation, or synonymously air-space shadowing, is caused by opacification of the air-containing spaces of the lung. The causes of consolidation are numerous (Fig. 1.29), and include almost any pathologic process that results in the filling of the normal alveolar spaces and small airways. The responsible material is almost invariably of fluid density, and usually the volume of the displacing fluid equals the volume of air displaced. This normally results in no net change in size of the lobar anatomy. Typically it is not possible to tell from the radiologic appearances what has caused the air-space filling, especially in the absence of a clinical history. The possible exception to this generalization is air-space shadowing because of cardiogenic alveolar edema, when associated signs of congestive cardiac failure are found. When analyzing an area of pulmonary opacification, the presence of a number of radiologic characteristics allows the confident characterization of air-space shadowing.

Typically, the shadowing is ill-defined, except where it directly abuts a pleural surface (including the interlobar fissures), in which case it is sharply demarcated (Fig. 1.30). Although consolidation respects lobar boundaries, there are no such barriers to spread into adjacent lung segments, which are frequently contiguously involved. Thus, an area of consolidation within a single lobe often enlarges in an irregular manner, and a discrete, well-defined opacity (so-called round pneumonia) is the exception and not the rule (Fig. 1.31).

The vascular markings within an area of consolidation usually become obscured, as the contrast between the air-containing lung and the soft-tissue density vascular markings is lost. By contrast, the bronchi, which are usually too thin walled to be differentiated from the surrounding lung parenchyma, become apparent in negative contrast to the air-space opacification, to produce the true hallmark of consolidation, the air bronchogram (Fig. 1.32). A relatively uncommon, but very suggestive, radiologic sign of consolidation is the acinar shadow, where an individual or cluster of acini become opacified but remain surrounded by normally aerated lung. The resultant soft-tissue density nodule is usually on the periphery of a more confluent area of consolidation, and normally measures 0.5–1 cm in diameter. These acinar opacities are most commonly seen in association with mycobacterial and varicella-zoster pneumonias, but can occur in any other cause of consolidation (Fig. 1.33). Occasionally, an acinus is left normally aerated but surrounded by opacified air spaces. When

Causes of consolidation	
Common	**Rare**
Infection	Allergic lung diseases
Infarction	Connective tissue diseases
Cardiogenic pulmonary edema	Drug reactions
Noncardiogenic pulmonary edema	Hemorrhage
Adult respiratory distress syndrome	Lymphoma
Neurogenic edema	Radiation
Drug-induced edema	Amyloid
Miscellaneous	Eosinophilic lung disease
	Sarcoid
	Alveolar proteinosis

Figure 1.29 Causes of pulmonary consolidation.

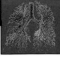

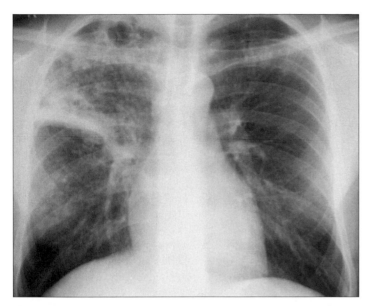

Figure 1.30 Patchy consolidation caused by tuberculosis. Where this abuts the horizontal fissure, the inferior surface of the consolidation is sharply defined.

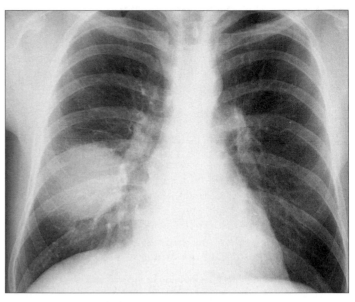

Figure 1.31 Well-defined, rounded opacity in the right mid zone, which fades out peripherally. Round pneumonia caused by pneumococcal infection.

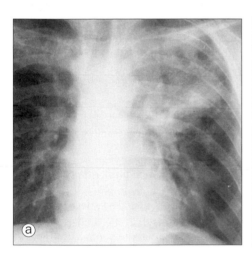

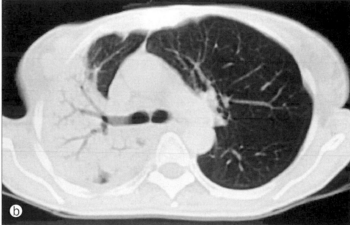

Figure 1.32 Air bronchogram in consolidation. (a) Left, upper zone tuberculosis demonstrating an air bronchogram. (b) Computed tomography scan through the carina demonstrates an extensive air bronchogram in a different patient who has lobar pneumonia.

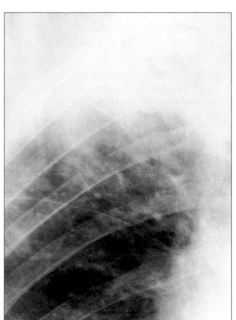

Figure 1.33 Acinar opacities seen at the periphery of confluent right upper lobe consolidation in a patient who has tuberculosis. Note the elevation of the horizontal fissure.

consolidation is not fully developed and has caused only partial filling of the air spaces, the resultant radiographic appearance is ground-glass opacification (see Fig. 1.34). Again, there is a wide range of possible causes, and in addition to causes of consolidation this pattern may result from interstitial lung infiltration.

When an area of consolidation undergoes necrosis, because of either infection or infarction, liquefaction may result, and if either a gas-forming organism or communication with the bronchial tree is present, an air–fluid level may develop in addition to cavity formation (see Fig. 1.35). Consolidation frequently produces a silhouette sign, as described by Felson and Felson[18]. Although this radiographic sign may be seen in association with a wide number of intrapulmonary pathologic processes, it is the relatively transitory nature of many forms of consolidation that best demonstrate the features of this finding. The original description stated that when an intrathoracic lesion touched a border of the heart, aorta, or diaphragm, it obliterated that border on the radiograph. Furthermore, a small area of consolidation may obliterate a normal air–soft tissue interface as effectively as a large area. This is demonstrated well by the obliteration of the right

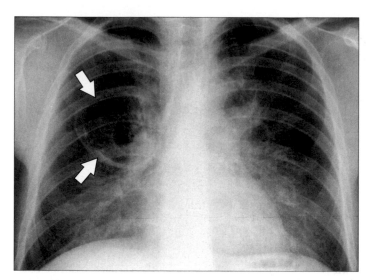

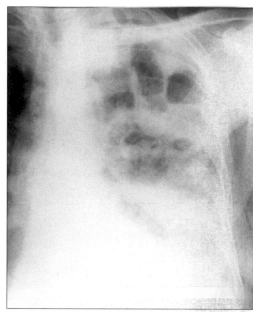

Figure 1.35 **Multiple cavities, some containing air–fluid levels within the left lung.** The patient has necrotizing pneumonia.

Figure 1.34 Ground-glass opacification in the mid and lower zones in a patient who has *Pneumocystis carinii* pneumonia. Note the development of cysts within the lungs, for example in the right mid zone (arrows).

heart border by subtle middle-lobe consolidation that might otherwise be overlooked.

Understanding the significance of the silhouette sign allows the observer to localize an area of consolidation or other pulmonary opacity. Only if an area of consolidation lies in direct contact with a normal structure is the silhouette of that structure lost. If an area of consolidation and a normal structure–lung interface merely lie along the same X-ray path, then they are superimposed on the radiograph but do not demonstrate the silhouette sign. Thus, lingular or right middle lower lobe consolidation is likely to obscure the heart border, but lower lobe consolidation usually does not (Figs 1.36 & 1.37). There are several potential causes for a falsely positive silhouette sign. Some relatively common anatomic variants that result in a reduced anteroposterior (AP) diameter of the thorax, such as pectus excavatum or straight back syndrome, cause loss of the right heart border as the depressed sternum distorts the normal anatomy (see Fig. 1.24). Occasionally a scoliosis, usually concave to the left, and which may be relatively trivial, causes the right heart border to be projected over the spine. It is only when the heart border is projected over the right lung that the silhouette sign can be elicited. Underexposed radiographs may appear to demonstrate the silhouette sign, so it is imperative that the technical quality of the radiograph is taken into account.

Collapse
When there is partial or complete volume loss in a lung or lobe, this is referred to as collapse or atelectasis. The terms are essentially interchangeable, and they imply a diminished volume of air in the lung with associated reduction of lung volume. Several different mechanisms result in lung or lobar collapse.

Relaxation or passive collapse
The lung retracts toward its hilum when air or an abnormal amount of fluid accumulates in the pleural space.

Cicatrization collapse
The normal expansion of the lung, to contact the parietal pleura, depends upon a balance between outward forces in the chest

wall and opposite elastic forces in the lung. If the lung is abnormally stiff, this balance is disturbed, lung compliance is decreased, and the volume of the affected lung is reduced. The best example of this phenomenon is volume loss associated with pulmonary fibrosis.

Adhesive collapse
In the normal lung, the forces that govern surface tension become more pronounced as the surface area of the air space is reduced. Hence, the collapse of smaller airways and alveoli tends to occur at lower lung volumes, a tendency that is offset by surfactant, which reduces the surface tension of the fluid that lines the alveoli. This reduction is usually sufficient to overcome the tendency to collapse in the normal lung. However, if the mechanism is disturbed, as in respiratory distress syndrome, collapse of the alveoli occurs, and typically the larger airways remain patent.

Reabsorption collapse
In acute bronchial obstruction, gases in the alveoli are steadily taken up by the blood in the pulmonary capillaries and are not replenished, which causes alveolar collapse. The degree of collapse may be counteracted by collateral air drift if the obstruction is distal to the main bronchus, and also by infection and accumulation of secretions. If the obstruction becomes chronic, subsequent reabsorption of intra-alveolar secretions and exudate may result in complete collapse, the usual mechanism of collapse seen in carcinoma of the bronchus. When the cause of collapse is a proximal obstructing mass, the S sign of Golden may be apparent[19] (see Fig. 1.40). This sign refers to the 'S'- shape made by the relevant fissure as the distal part of a lobe collapses, but the proximal part of a lobe maintains its bulk due the presence of a tumor.

Radiographic signs of lobar collapse
The radiographic appearance in pulmonary collapse depends upon a number of factors, which include the mechanism of collapse, the extent of collapse, the presence or absence of consolidation in the affected lung, and the pre-existing state of the pleura. This last factor includes the presence of underlying pleural

Chapter 1

Imaging

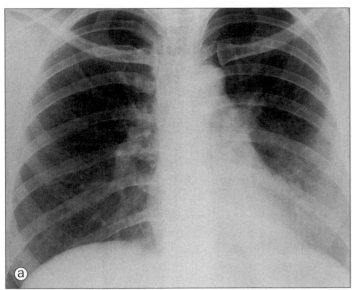

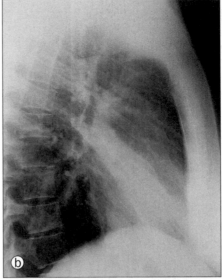

Figure 1.36 Lower lobe and lingular collapse.
(a) Loss of the left heart border with a diffuse pulmonary infiltrate in the left mid and lower zone. The outer aspect of the left diaphragm is preserved. (b) Lateral view of the same patient as in (a), showing consolidation within the lingula and delineated posteriorly by the major fissure. (c) In comparison, mid and lower zone consolidation in the left lower lobe in a different patient. There is preservation of the left heart border, but loss of the left hemidiaphragm. (d) Lateral view of the same patient as in (c), showing the consolidation in the lower lobe delineated anteriorly by the major fissure.

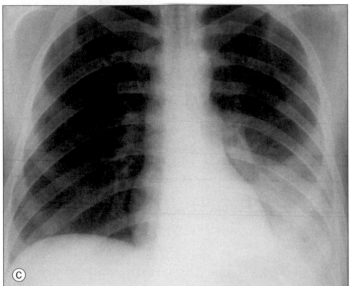

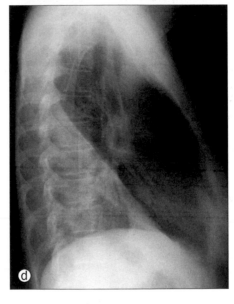

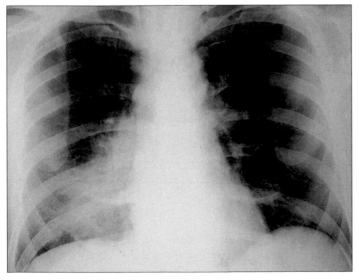

Figure 1.37 Right lower lobe consolidation. The right heart border is clearly defined. Since the consolidation is not complete the hemidiaphragm has not been effaced.

tethering or thickening and the presence of pleural fluid. Pre-existing lung disease, such as fibrosis and pleural adhesions, may alter the expected displacement of anatomic landmarks in lung collapse. An air bronchogram is rare in reabsorption collapse, but is usual in passive and adhesive collapse, and may be seen in cicatrization collapse if fibrosis is particularly dense.

Signs of collapse may be direct or indirect. Indirect signs are the result of compensatory changes that occur as a consequence of the volume loss.

The direct signs of collapse include:
- displacement of interlobar fissures;
- loss of aeration;
- vascular and bronchial crowding.

Indirect signs include:
- elevation of the hemi-diaphragm;
- mediastinal displacement;
- hilar displacement;
- compensatory hyperinflation;
- crowding of the ribs.

There tends to be a reciprocal relationship between the individual compensatory signs of collapse, so that if there is mediastinal shift to the side of collapse, there is unlikely to be significant diaphragmatic elevation. For example in lower lobe collapse, if hemidiaphragmatic elevation is marked, hilar depression is less marked.

Displacement of interlobar fissures
Displacement of interlobar fissures is the most reliable sign, and the degree of displacement depends on the extent of collapse.

Loss of aeration
The increased density of a collapsed area of lung may not become apparent until collapse is almost complete. However, if the collapsed lung is adjacent to the mediastinum or diaphragm, the presence of the silhouette sign may indicate loss of aeration.

Vascular and bronchial crowding
If a lobe is partially collapsed, crowding of its vessels may be visible; also, if an air bronchogram is visible, the bronchi may appear crowded together.

Elevation of the hemidiaphragm
Elevation of the hemidiaphragm may be seen in lower lobe collapse, but is uncommon in collapse of the other lobes.

Mediastinal displacement
In upper lobe collapse, the trachea is often displaced toward the affected side; in lower lobe collapse, the heart may be displaced to the same side.

Hilar displacement
The hilum may be elevated in upper lobe collapse, and depressed in lower lobe collapse.

Compensatory hyperinflation
The remaining normal lung may become hyperinflated, and thus may appear more transradiant, with the vessels more widely spaced than in the corresponding area of the contralateral lung. With considerable collapse of a lung, compensatory hyperinflation of the contralateral lung may occur, with herniation of lung across the midline.

Crowding of the ribs
On the side of the collapse there is often narrowing of the intercostal spaces with crowding together of the ribs, which reflects the diminished overall volume of the affected hemithorax.

Complete lung collapse
When there is complete collapse of an entire lung (in the absence of an accompanying pneumothorax, large pleural effusion, or extensive consolidation), complete opacification of that hemithorax is seen, with displacement of the mediastinum to the affected side and elevation of the hemidiaphragm. Compensatory hyperinflation of the contralateral lung occurs, often with herniation across the midline. Herniation is most often in the retrosternal space, anterior to the ascending aorta, but may occur posterior to the heart (Fig. 1.38).

Individual or combined lobar collapse
The descriptions below apply to collapse of individual lobes, uncomplicated by pre-existing pulmonary or pleural disease. The alterations to the positions of the fissures, mediastinal structures, and diaphragms are shown in Figure 1.39.

Right upper lobe collapse
As the right upper lobe collapses (see Fig. 1.40), the horizontal fissure rotates around the hilum and the lateral end moves upward and medially toward the superior mediastinum. The anterior end moves upward, toward the apex. The upper half of the oblique fissure moves anteriorly. The two fissures become concave superiorly. In severe collapse, the lobe may be flattened against the superior mediastinum, and may obscure the upper pole of the hilum. The hilum is elevated, and its lower pole may be prominent. Deviation of the trachea to the right is usual, and compensatory hyperinflation of the right middle and lower lobes may be apparent.

Middle lobe collapse
In right middle lobe collapse (see Fig. 1.41), the horizontal fissure and lower half of the oblique fissure move toward each other, a feature best seen on the lateral projection. Since the horizontal fissure tends to be more mobile, it usually shows the greater displacement. On the frontal radiograph, middle lobe collapse may be subtle since the horizontal fissure may not be visible, and increased opacity does not become apparent until collapse is almost complete. Critical analysis of the radiograph sometimes reveals obscuration of the right heart border as the only clue. The lordotic AP projection is rarely required, but may be used to bring the displaced fissure into the line of the X-ray beam, and occasionally may elegantly demonstrate middle lobe collapse. Since the volume of this lobe is relatively small, indirect signs of volume loss are rarely obvious.

Left lower lobe collapse
In left lower lobe collapse (see Fig. 1.42), the normal oblique fissures extend from the level of the fourth thoracic vertebra posteriorly to the diaphragm, close to the sternum anteriorly. The position of these fissures on the lateral projection is the best index of lower lobe volumes. When a lower lobe collapses, the oblique fissure moves posteriorly but maintains its normal slope. In addition to posterior movement, the collapsing lower lobe causes medial displacement of the oblique fissure, which may become visible in places on the frontal projection. In left lower lobe collapse the heart may obscure the wedge-like opacity, and a penetrated view may be required to demonstrate it.

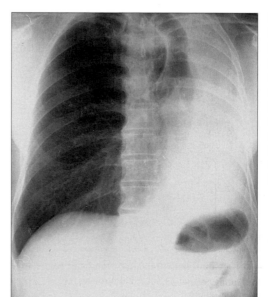

**Figure 1.38
Collapse of the left lung.** There is a proximal obstructing tumor within the left main bronchus, with complete collapse of the left lung and a mediastinal shift to the left.

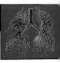

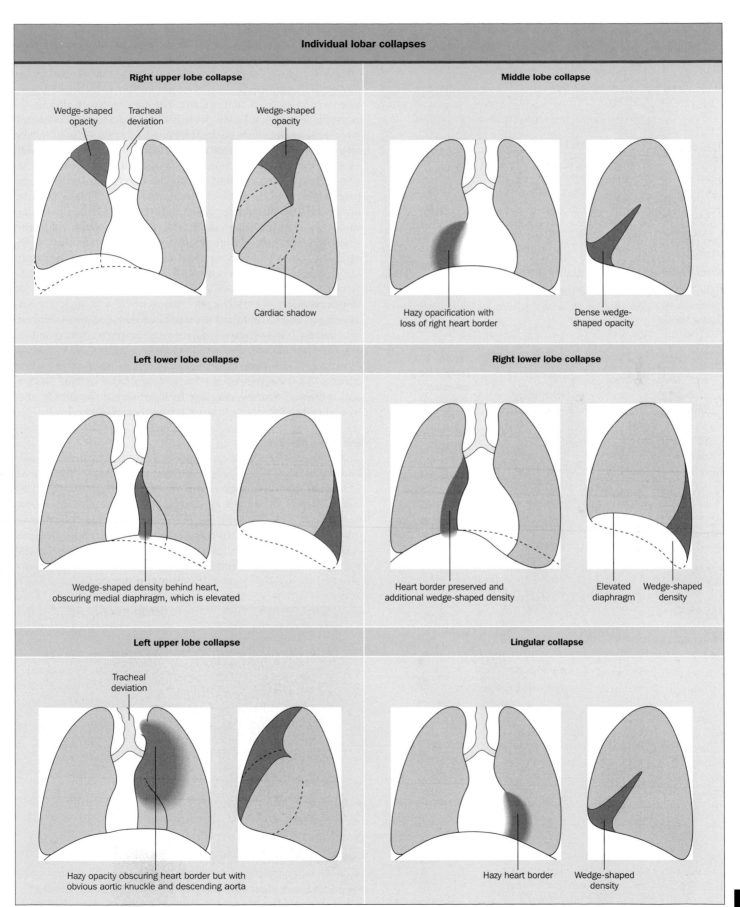

Figure 1.39 Individual lobar collapses. Compare these representations with the radiographic examples (see Figs 1.40–1.44).

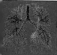
Right lower lobe collapse

Right lower lobe collapse (Fig. 1.43) causes partial depression of the horizontal fissure, which may be apparent on the frontal projection. Increased opacity of a collapsed lower lobe is usually visible on the frontal projection also. A completely collapsed lower lobe may be so small that it flattens and merges with the mediastinum, to produce a thin, wedge-shaped shadow. Mediastinal structures and parts of the diaphragm adjacent to the nonaerated lobe are obscured. When significant lower lobe collapse occurs, especially when the collapsed lobe is so small as to be invisible as a separate opacity, confirmatory evidence is usually apparent from close inspection of the relevant hilum. This is usually depressed and rotated medially, with loss of the normal hilar vascular structures, which is made all the more obvious if a previous film is available for comparison. In addition, indirect signs of collapse, such as upper lobe hyperinflation, are present. Diaphragmatic elevation is unusual.

Lingula collapse

The lingula is often involved in collapse of the left upper lobe, but occasionally it may collapse individually, in which case the radiographic features are similar to those of middle lobe collapse. However, the absence of a horizontal fissure on the left makes anterior displacement of the lower half of the oblique fissure and increased opacity anterior to it important signs. On the frontal projection, the left heart border becomes obscured.

Left upper lobe collapse

The pattern of upper lobe collapse is different in the two lungs. Left upper lobe collapse (Fig. 1.44) is apparent on the lateral projection as anterior displacement of the entire oblique fissure, which becomes oriented almost parallel to the anterior chest wall. With increasing collapse the upper lobe retracts posteriorly and loses contact with the anterior chest wall. With complete collapse, the left upper lobe may lose contact with the chest wall and diaphragm and retract medially against the mediastinum.

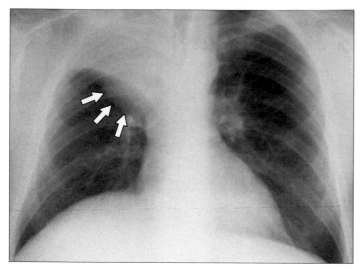

Figure 1.40 Right upper lobe collapse caused by a right hilar tumor. The horizontal fissure takes on an 'S' configuration, known as the S sign of Golden (arrows).

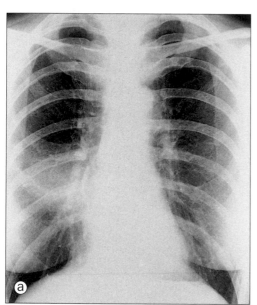

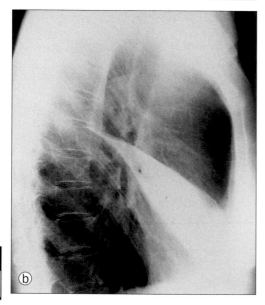

Figure 1.41 Middle lobe collapse. (a) Loss of the right heart border is seen on the frontal radiograph. (b) A well-defined wedge-shaped opacity on the lateral radiograph is delineated by the horizontal and oblique fissures.

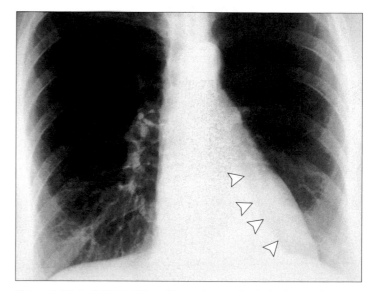

Figure 1.42 Left lower lobe collapse in a patient who has asthma and mucus plugging. The left hemithorax is of reduced volume, and there is loss of the normal silhouette of the left lower lobe pulmonary artery. The left lower lobe has contracted behind the cardiac silhouette (arrowheads).

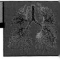

On a lateral film, therefore, left upper lobe collapse appears as an elongated opacity that extends from the apex and reaches, or almost reaches, the diaphragm; it is anterior to the hilum and is bounded by the displaced oblique fissure posteriorly, and by hyperinflated lower lobe.

A collapsed left upper lobe does not produce a sharp outline on the frontal view. An ill-defined, hazy opacity is present in the upper, mid, and sometimes lower zones, the opacity being densest near the hilum. Pulmonary vessels in the hyperinflated lower lobe are usually visible through the haze. The aortic knuckle is usually obscured, unless the upper lobe has collapsed anterior to it, in which case hyperexpansion of the lower lobe apical segment may occur and separate the collapsed upper lobe from the mediastinal silhouette and aortic knuckle. This produces an unusual but characteristic medial crescent of lucency (termed the Luftsichel sign). If the lingula is involved, the left heart border is obscured. The hilum is often elevated, and the trachea deviated to the left.

Combined lobar collapses
Right lower and middle lobe collapse
Since the right lower and middle lobes take their origin from the bronchus intermedius, an extensive lesion at that site may cause combined collapse. The appearances are similar to right lower lobe collapse (Fig. 1.45), except that the horizontal fissure is not apparent, the opacification reaches the lateral chest wall on the frontal radiograph, and similarly extends to the anterior chest wall on the lateral view.

Right upper and middle lobe collapse
Combined collapse of the right upper and middle lobes is unusual because of the distance between the origins of their bronchi; combined collapse can generally be taken to imply the presence of more than one lesion. This combination produces appearances (Fig. 1.46) almost identical to those of left upper lobe collapse. On occasion, isolated right upper lobe collapse also produces appearances that are identical to those of left upper lobe collapse.

Rounded atelectasis
Rounded atelectasis is an unusual form of pulmonary collapse which may be misdiagnosed as a pulmonary tumor. On the plain film there is an opacity that may be of several centimeters in diameter, frequently with ill-defined edges. Rounded atelectasis is always pleurally based and associated with pleural thickening. Vessels may radiate from part of the opacity, and are said to resemble a comet's

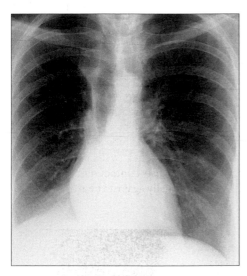

Figure 1.43 Right lower lobe collapse in the same patient as shown in Figure 1.42, admitted on a different occasion. There is preservation of the right heart border, but reduction in volume of the right hemithorax, obstruction of the right hemidiaphragm, and shift of the trachea to the right side.

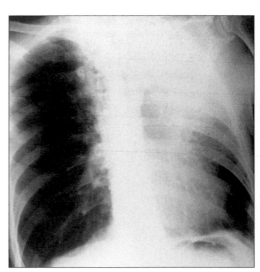

Figure 1.44 Left upper lobe collapse with shift of the mediastinum to the left and loss of definition of the mediastinal structures. The opacification fades out more inferiorly.

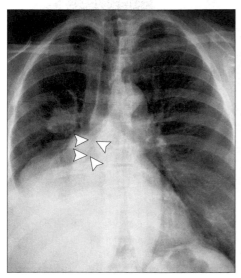

Figure 1.45 Right middle and lower lobe collapse caused by an obstructing lesion in the bronchus intermedius. A bronchial cutoff sign is visible (arrowheads). A separate pulmonary mass is present in the right upper lobe.

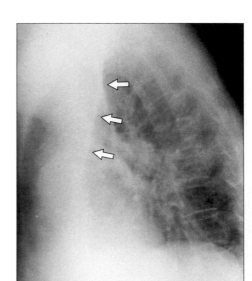

Figure 1.46 Right middle and upper lobe collapse. Lateral radiographic changes are similar to those seen on the opposite side with a left upper lobe collapse. The major fissure shifts anteriorly (arrows) and extends from the lung apex to the anterior costophrenic recess.

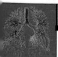
tail (Fig. 1.47). The appearance is caused by peripheral lung tissue folding in on itself. Rounded atelectasis is usually related to previous asbestos exposure, but may also occur secondary to any exudative pleural effusion. It is not of any other pathologic significance, although when present often raises the question of a malignancy. The CT appearance is usually sufficiently diagnostic to allow differentiation from other pulmonary masses (Fig. 1.48).

Unilateral increased transradiancy

The most common causes of increased unilateral transradiancy are technical factors, such as patient rotation, poor beam centering, or an offset grid. Usually, hypertransradiancy caused by technical factors can be identified by comparison of the soft tissues around the shoulder girdle, and particularly over the axillae. Nevertheless, there are a number of pathologic causes of unilateral increased transradiancy.

Chest wall

A hemithorax may appear to be of increased transradiancy (blacker) if the X-rays are less attenuated because of a reduction in the amount of overlying soft tissue. The most common cause for this is a mastectomy. Rarely, the same phenomenon

may be seen in patients who have congenital unilateral absence of pectoral muscles, known as Poland's syndrome (Fig. 1.49). This may be accompanied by associated skeletal abnormalities in the ipsilateral ribs, but may be recognized by loss of the normal axillary skin fold.

Reduced vascularity

Interruption or significant reduction in the blood supply to one lung, either congenital or acquired, results in increased transradiancy in that lung (Fig. 1.50).

Lung hyperexpansion

If a lung is over expanded, because of either air trapping secondary to the presence of a foreign body or asymmetric emphysema, then that hemithorax may appear to be of increased transradiancy. When the whole lung is affected, the hemithorax is usually relatively larger than the opposite side. However, the same phenomenon may occur with compensatory emphysema, because of collapse or removal of an ipsilateral lobe. In this case, the transradiant hemithorax may be of normal volume, and the presence of the increased transradiancy should prompt a search for other evidence of collapse or prior surgery.

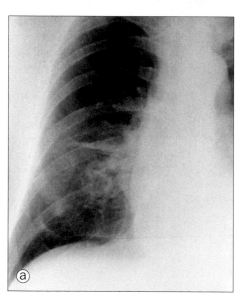

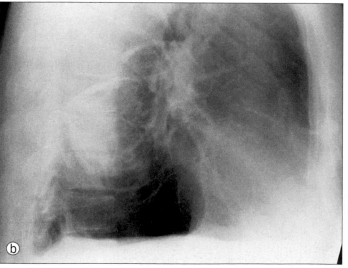

Figure 1.47 Rounded atelectasis. (a) A poorly defined opacity is visible on the frontal radiograph. (b) On the lateral film, this is seen to be caused by a radiating parenchymal band that extends from the posterior chest wall.

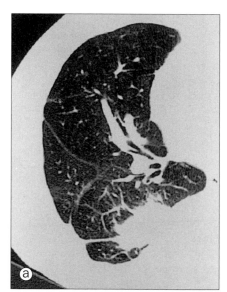

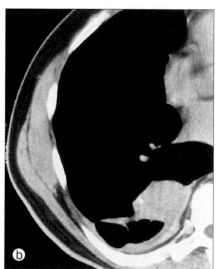

Figure 1.48 Rounded atelectasis. (a) Computed tomography scan reveals the characteristic pleurally based mass with radiating bronchovascular strands. (b) Mediastinal window settings demonstrate a fleck of calcification, in keeping with previous asbestos exposure.

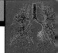

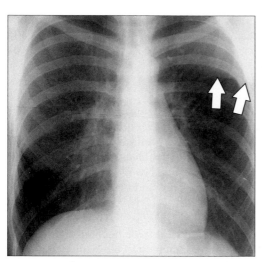

**Figure 1.49
Poland's
syndrome.**
Incidental finding
on a chest
radiograph of
congenital
absence of the left
pectoralis major
muscle. Note the
alteration in the
left axillary skin
fold compared
with the right
(arrows).

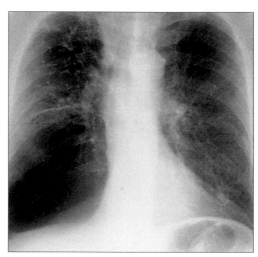

**Figure 1.50
Increased
transradiancy in
the right lower
zone.** A large
emphysematous
bulla occupies the
lower half of the
right lung and the
apical changes are
in keeping with
previous
tuberculosis.

A relatively increased transradiancy of one hemithorax with no obvious cause suggests the possibility of a generalized increase in radio-opacity of the opposite side; for example, the posterior layering of a pleural effusion in a supine patient (Fig. 1.51).

The pulmonary mass

The finding of a solitary pulmonary nodule on the chest radiograph requires careful analysis, since the diagnostic possibilities are numerous. Once a pulmonary mass has been identified, the observer must first decide if the lesion is genuine and second whether the lesion is truly intrapulmonary. The possibility of a cutaneous lesion should not be forgotten, especially if only a part of the nodule is well defined. If doubt remains repeat radiographs are obtained, with a lateral view and, if relevant, nipple markers. What appears at first glance to represent a solitary pulmonary mass may, on closer inspection, actually represent the most obvious of a number of pulmonary nodules. The radiology of multiple pulmonary nodules is discussed later.

When a pulmonary mass is clearly defined around its entire circumference, and is projected over the lung on frontal and lateral projections, the mass is truly intrapulmonary (see Fig. 1.52). However, if a surface is in contact with another soft-tissue structure, the possibility of an extrapulmonary mass projecting into the lung must be considered. Analysis of the

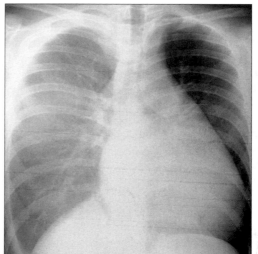

**Figure 1.51
Supine
radiograph of a
patient who has
a large right
pleural effusion.**
The generalized
increase in radio-
opacity of the
right side is
caused by
posterior layering
of a pleural
effusion.

breadth of the base of the lesion, the angle made with the adjacent structure, and the presence of bone destruction often allows the observer to differentiate between an extrapulmonary mass that extends into the adjacent lung from an intrapulmonary mass that has grown to contact the mediastinum, diaphragm, or chest wall.

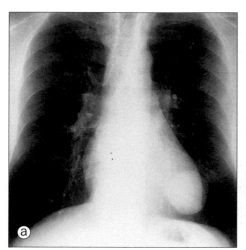
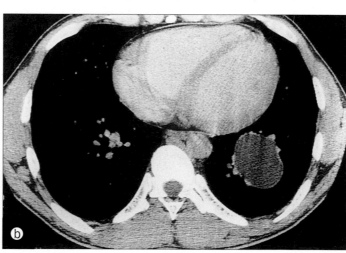

**Figure 1.52 A rounded
pulmonary mass.**
(a) Posteroanterior
radiograph of a patient
who has a well-defined
pulmonary mass. The
entire circumference is
visualized on the film,
which indicates no
surface of contact with
the mediastinal
structures. (b) Computed
tomography of this mass
demonstrates it is of fluid
density (hydatid cyst).

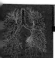

The analysis of a solitary pulmonary mass relies on a number of radiologic and clinical factors. The latter include patient age, geographic and ethnic origins, smoking history, and past medical history. The likelihood that a pulmonary nodule represents a malignancy in a young nonsmoker who comes from an area where histoplasmosis is endemic is clearly different to that for an elderly patient with a lifetime history of smoking.

Radiographic features of a pulmonary nodule that should be analyzed include size, density, margins, vascular markings, and growth rate.

Size

Generally, the likelihood of malignancy is greater with increasing size, although the opposite argument is not reliable.

Density

Most pulmonary masses are of soft-tissue density. However, careful inspection must be made for the presence of calcification, since certain patterns of calcification are typical of benign lesions that may be safely observed rather than resected. A completely or centrally calcified nodule is diagnostic of a tuberculoma or histoplasmoma. Often, CT is required to confirm this pattern of calcification. Likewise, concentric rings of calcification are typical of healed histoplasmosis infection. Popcorn calcification, within the matrix of a pulmonary nodule, is highly suggestive of a hamartoma (Fig. 1.53). Other forms of calcification do not reliably indicate whether a nodule is benign or malignant, and dystrophic calcification within a pulmonary malignancy is relatively common.

Margins

Perfectly smooth, round lesions are likely to be benign (see Fig. 1.52). However, this is not a completely reliable rule since some primary lung malignancies and secondary deposits, particularly from soft-tissue sarcomas, may be perfectly spherical. By contrast, lobulated or spiculated masses are much more likely to represent malignancy.

Vascular markings

A rare, benign, but important cause of a pulmonary nodule is an arteriovenous malformation. The diagnosis may be suggested on the plain radiograph if a prominent feeding artery or draining vein is identified.

Growth rate

Review of the previous radiographs, when available, may establish whether a lesion is static or increasing in size. It is usual practice to express the growth of a pulmonary tumor in terms of the time taken for it to double in volume, which equates to an increase in diameter of 25%, assuming that the tumor is roughly spherical, as is usually the case. Tumors with a doubling time of <30 days or >2 years are very unlikely to be caused by malignancy[20]. However, often no previous films are available, and thus the use of growth rate as a diagnostic aid is limited.

When a solitary lung mass is evident on the chest radiograph, and no features suggest whether it is of benign etiology or a malignant lesion, it should be assumed to be a primary lung carcinoma until proved otherwise. In the assessment of a potential lung primary tumor, certain guidelines may be helpful.

Approximately half of primary lung carcinomas arise centrally in a proximal or segmental bronchus and as a result present as a hilar mass.

Since carcinoma of the bronchus arises in the bronchial mucosa, the tumor is likely to grow into the bronchial lumen and around the bronchus. As the bronchial lumen narrows, the distal lung may become consolidated and lose volume. Depending on the site of the tumor, a malignant solitary lung mass may be associated with lobar or segmental collapse (Fig. 1.54) or even collapse of an entire lung (see Fig. 1.38).

Peripheral tumors usually appear as solitary nodules or masses, but no features on plain films reliably differentiate a benign from a malignant pulmonary nodule. As described above, malignant tumors are often larger, poorly defined, spiculated, or lobulated. Satellite opacities around a mass are more commonly seen with benign lesions, notably granulomatous diseases (see Fig. 1.33). At least 5% of bronchial carcinomas cavitate because of central necrosis or abscess formation; the resultant cavity is typically thick-walled with an irregular inner margin (Fig. 1.55). Peripheral tumors may invade the ribs or spine directly. Bone destruction must be specifically looked for and, when present, almost invariably indicates malignancy (Fig. 1.56).

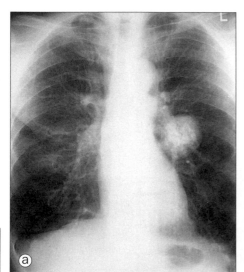

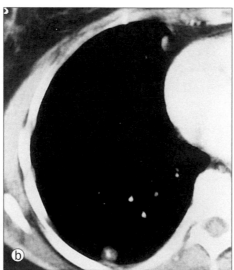

Figure 1.53 Examples of pulmonary calcification. (a) Posteroanterior chest radiograph of a mass that projects over the left hilum. This is smoothly marginated and contains central popcorn calcification; it is unusually large but otherwise a typical pulmonary hamartoma. (b) Computed tomography scan through a small, peripherally based lung nodule. A well-defined fleck of central calcification is visible. These are the typical appearances of subacute histoplasmosis.

(a)

(b)

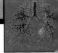

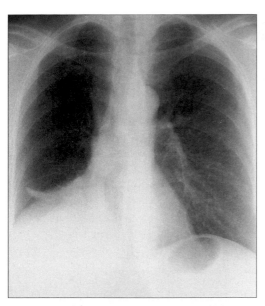

Figure 1.54 Right lower and partial middle lobe collapse secondary to a proximal bronchogenic carcinoma.

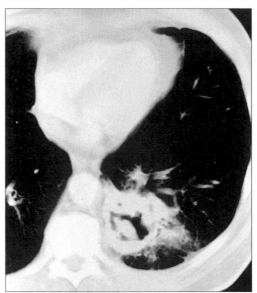

Figure 1.55 Computed tomography scan of a left lower lobe bronchogenic carcinoma with central necrosis and cavitation. The cavity wall is thick and irregular.

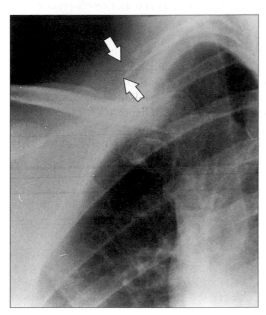

Figure 1.56 Oblique view of the right apex demonstrating bone destruction within the first rib (arrows). The patient has peripheral bronchogenic carcinoma.

Causes of acquired pulmonary nodules	
Acquired	
Neoplastic	**Inflammatory**
Benign	Infectious
Hamartomas	Granulomatous infections
Papillomatosis	Multiple embolic abscesses
Bronchogenic cysts	Round pneumonias
Malignant	Viral infections – chickenpox and measles
Metastases	Parasites – hydatid and paragonimiasis
Lymphoma	Noninfectious
Multifocal tumor	Caplan's syndrome and rheumatoid nodules
Kaposi's sarcoma	Wegener's granulomatosis
Bronchoalveolar cell carcinoma	Sarcoid
	Others
	Progressive massive fibrosis
	Amyloid
	Infarcts
	Bronchial impaction

Figure 1.57 Multiple pulmonary nodules.

Multiple pulmonary nodules

The differential diagnosis of multiple pulmonary nodules is wide (Fig. 1.57), but analysis of the chest radiograph and a review of the clinical status of the patient rapidly narrows the number of possibilities. Many of the radiographic features used in the analysis of the solitary pulmonary nodule can be employed usefully in the assessment of multiple lesions.

Multiple nodules are described in terms of size, number, distribution, density, definition, cavitation, speed of growth (if serial films are available), and accompanying pleural, mediastinal, or skeletal abnormalities. Further important clinical clues may come from the clinical status of the patient. Specifically, evidence of infection, systemic illness, and prior malignancy is sought (Fig. 1.58 and see Figs 1.59 & 1.60).

Diffuse shadowing

Many diseases cause diffuse lung shadowing on chest radiography. Careful analysis is required to determine correctly the nature of the abnormality and narrow the differential diagnosis.

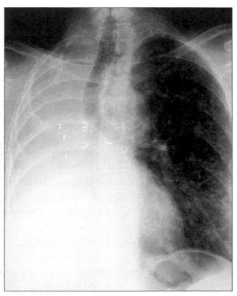

Figure 1.58 Chest radiograph of a patient who had a previous right pneumonectomy for adenocarcinoma. Multiple pulmonary nodules are now within the lung because of secondary deposits.

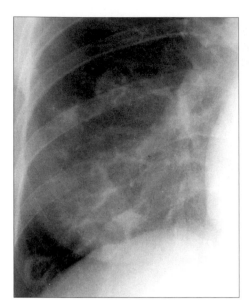

Figure 1.59
Magnified view of the right lower zone.
The multiple pulmonary nodules are cavitating in this case of multiple staphylococcal abscesses in an intravenous drug abuser.

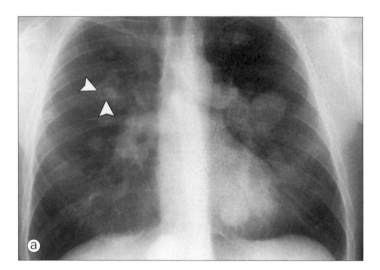

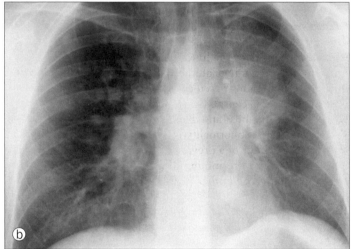

Figure 1.60 Multiple pulmonary nodules. (a) The multiple pulmonary nodules are smoothly defined and vary in size; some are cavitating (arrowheads). (b) Subsequent chest radiograph obtained shortly afterward. The left perihilar nodules are no longer visible because they lie within the now collapsed left upper lobe. The patient has multiple metastases from soft-tissue sarcoma.

Appearances on the chest radiograph can be misleading, and the pattern of disease demonstrated at pathologic or HRCT examination may differ considerably from the pattern of abnormality suggested by the chest radiograph[21]. The summation of multiple, small, linear opacities on the chest radiograph may produce the appearance of multiple small nodules. Likewise, the superimposition of multiple small nodules may produce a granular or ground-glass pattern. A variety of descriptive terms are used in the analysis of a chest radiograph in this context and frequently appearances are classified as being either interstitial or air space. However, a number of processes are capable of producing both patterns, so that the differential diagnosis may be erroneously narrowed at an early stage of analysis. Thus, it is preferable to analyze the pattern in purely descriptive terms, such as reticular or nodular shadowing, to avoid this pitfall.

Reticular shadowing

Reticular or linear shadowing (Fig. 1.61) is made up of multiple, short, irregular linear densities, usually randomly oriented, and often overlapping to produce a net-like pattern. When profuse they may summate to form ring shadows or sometimes a nodular pattern. Occasionally, the linear shadows may be oriented at right angles to the pleural surface, so-called Kerley's B lines (Fig. 1.62), which indicates thickening of the interlobular septa. When the linear opacities are extremely profuse or coarse, the impression of a ring or honeycomb pattern is given.

Nodular opacities

Nodules may be well or poorly defined and of varying density, ranging from soft tissue to calcific (Fig. 1.63). They may be discrete or coalescent, with areas of confluence producing consolidation. When the nodules are greater than a few millimeters in diameter the differential diagnosis changes. Larger discrete nodules are discussed above.

Reticulonodular shadowing

Often it is impossible to assign confidently a pattern of diffuse shadowing to one of the two categories above because they overlap. The reticulonodular pattern is probably the most common form of diffuse lung shadowing.

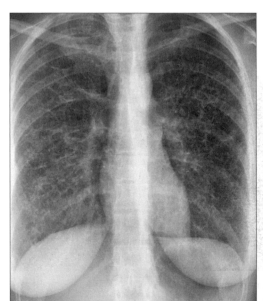

Figure 1.61
Extensive reticular infiltrate in a patient who has normal-volume lungs. The patient has Langerhans' cell histiocytosis.

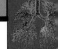

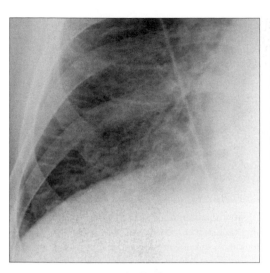

Figure 1.62 Kerley's B lines in a patient who has heart failure. Note how the reticular opacities are oriented at right angles to the pleural surface.

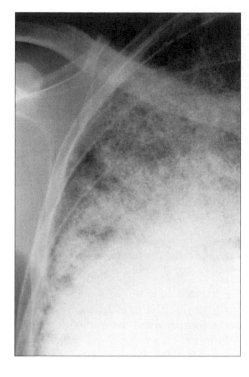

Figure 1.63 Very profuse dense nodular shadowing, coalescent in the mid and lower zone. The individual nodules are of high density. The patient has alveolar microlithiasis.

Ground-glass shadowing

Ground-glass shadowing (see Fig. 1.34) refers to a generalized increase in density of the lung, which may be diffuse or patchy, but is most commonly bilateral and mid and lower zonal or perihilar. The underlying vascular branching pattern is not totally obscured, as it is in consolidation, but the vessels become less distinct; likewise the hilar and diaphragms may appear slightly less sharp. This subtle abnormality is considerably easier to appreciate with the benefit of a previous normal film for comparison.

In addition to determining the radiographic pattern of diffuse abnormality, a number of other features must be sought, including whether the distribution of disease is central or peripheral, in the upper, mid, or lower zone, and if distortion of the lung architecture is associated. Additional important features include signs of cardiac failure or fluid overload, such as increased heart size, equalization of upper and lower lobe vein size, and pleural effusions. Hilar or mediastinal enlargement caused by lymph nodes or vascular enlargement should also be specifically sought. The bones and soft tissues of the chest wall may also provide important clues, such as evidence of previous breast surgery or an erosive arthritis. The accuracy of radiographic analysis is reduced in the absence of appropriate clinical information. For example, ascertaining whether the patient is well, acutely or chronically unwell, of normal immune status, or immunocompromised can dramatically narrow a wide radiologic differential diagnosis.

Airway disease

Plain tomography has been replaced by CT as the investigation of choice for the examination of airway abnormalities.

Tracheal narrowing

Tracheal narrowing may be caused by an extrinsic mass, mediastinal fibrosis, or an intrinsic abnormality of the tracheal wall[22]. Chronic inflammatory causes include fibrosing mediastinitis, sarcoidosis, chronic relapsing polychondritis (Fig. 1.64), and Wegener's granulomatosis. Primary tumors of the trachea are rare. Benign tumors present as small, well-defined, intraluminal nodules that are difficult or impossible to visualize on the chest radiograph. Malignant tumors of the trachea tend to occur close to the carina (Fig. 1.65), although they may be quite extensive and cause a long stricture (see Fig. 1.66). Tracheal wall thickening and tracheal

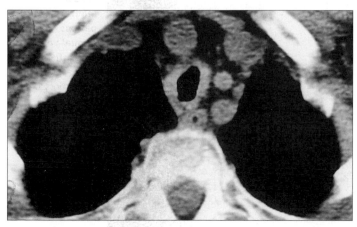

Figure 1.64 Circumferential tracheal wall thickening with tracheal narrowing. This is a case of relapsing polychondritis.

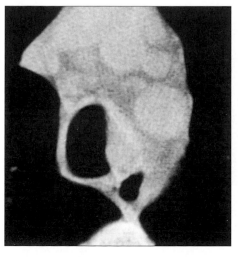

Figure 1.65 Focal carcinoma within the tracheal wall.

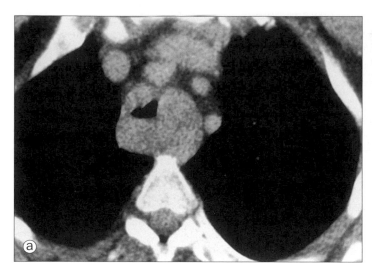

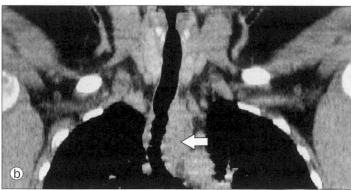

Figure 1.66 Adenoid cystic carcinoma. Extensive tracheal tumor. (a) Circumferential soft-tissue tumor of the trachea at the level of the great vessels. (b) Coronal reformation showing extensive tracheal wall thickening measuring, on the left, almost 2cm (arrow).

luminal narrowing can be detected on the plain chest radiograph, especially when specifically sought. The right lateral wall of the trachea (the right paratracheal stripe) above the level of the azygos vein is typically a 2mm-thick, soft-tissue stripe, and tracheal wall thickening is easily appreciated if this portion of the airway is involved [Fig. 1.67; see also Mediastinal lymphadenopathy (Fig. 1.71)].

Tracheal widening

The normal dimensions of the trachea have been assessed using a variety of techniques, most recently CT. The trachea becomes slightly larger with increasing age. On CT scanning, the maximal coronal diameter of the trachea is 23mm in a man and 20mm in a woman. Dilatation of the trachea is rare, and may result from a generalized defect of connective tissue (Fig. 1.68). On the plain radiograph, shift of the right paratracheal stripe to the right is often the only sign of tracheal widening, and since the trachea is frequently not central, it is only if the left wall of the trachea is also identified that tracheal widening can be recognized.

Bronchiectasis

The chest radiograph is relatively insensitive for the detection of bronchiectasis, and in most series a significant portion of plain

radiographs of patients who have bronchiectasis are judged to be normal (Fig. 1.69). The use of HRCT is discussed below, and is now the investigation of choice for bronchiectasis. Abnormalities present on the chest radiograph are as follows.

Bronchial wall thickening is evident as parallel, linear opacities radiating from the hilum, with lack of the normal convergence more peripherally. Ring shadows occur when the dilated airway is seen end on, and may be thick or thin walled and may contain

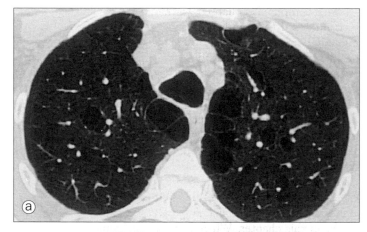

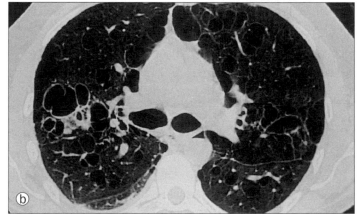

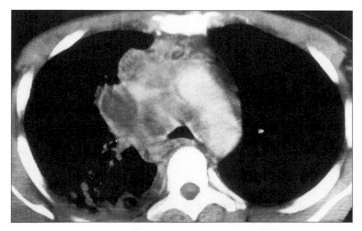

Figure 1.67 Computed tomography scan demonstrating an extensive necrotic mediastinal lymph-node mass that is causing tracheal narrowing.

Figure 1.68 Tracheobronchomegaly. Computed tomography scans showing diffuse moderate dilatation of the trachea and main bronchi in association with cystic bronchiectasis. (a) At the level of the trachea. (b) At the level of the carina.

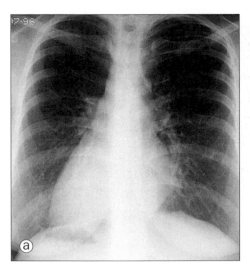

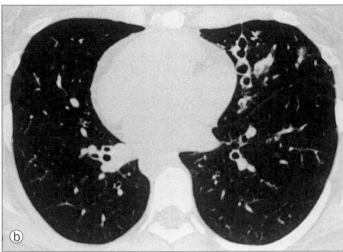

Figure 1.69
Bronchiectasis. (a) The chest radiograph of a patient who has primary ciliary dyskinesia. There is dextrocardia, and some questionable bronchial wall thickening adjacent to the left heart border, which is obscured. (b) The changes of bronchiectasis are much more convincingly demonstrated on high-resolution computed tomography.

secretions that produce an air–fluid level. Bronchiectatic airways that become plugged with secretions may produce tubular, soft-tissue density opacities radiating from the hilum, more commonly in the lower lobes.

Distortion of the lobar anatomy with volume loss and crowding together of bronchovascular structures may be associated. However, patients who have cystic fibrosis, also characterized by bronchiectasis, may have significant air trapping, which results in overexpansion. Even severe bronchiectasis may be invisible within a completely collapsed lobe.

Cylindrical (or tubular) bronchiectasis produces a dilated bronchus with parallel walls, in varicose bronchiectasis the walls are irregular, and in saccular (or cystic) bronchiectasis the airways terminate as round cysts. In an individual patient it is usual to see more than one pattern. Bronchiectasis usually involves the peripheral bronchi more severely than the central bronchi. Although it has long been held that this pattern may be reversed in allergic bronchopulmonary aspergillosis, overall the distribution and morphology demonstrated by CT are not usually helpful in predicting the underlying etiology.

Mediastinal abnormalities

The normal radiographic anatomy of the mediastinum is discussed earlier in this chapter. When a mediastinal abnormality is present on the PA radiograph, a lateral view should be obtained to aid anatomic localization. The imaging of mediastinal masses nowadays depends heavily on CT scanning, which is discussed in Chapter 74. However, familiarity with normal anatomy is required to detect mediastinal masses that at first appear as a subtle distortion of the normal mediastinal contours. A considerable volume of mediastinal tumor or lymph-node enlargement may be present in the face of an apparently normal chest radiograph.

The most common cause of mediastinal enlargement visible on the chest radiograph in children is the normal thymus, which may enlarge and contract in certain disease states, but normally remains relatively prominent, especially on CT scans, until puberty (Fig. 1.70). Lymphadenopathy, tumor, hiatus hernia, and vascular abnormalities account for most mediastinal masses seen in adults.

Mediastinal lymphadenopathy

Lymph nodes are present in all compartments of the mediastinum, but are visible on the chest radiograph only when they are calcified

or enlarged. Causes of mediastinal nodal enlargement are discussed in the Computed tomography section. The chest radiograph is a relatively insensitive indicator of lymphadenopathy. Enlargement of right paratracheal nodes is identified more easily than that of left paratracheal, aorto–pulmonary, or subcarinal lymph nodes (see Fig. 1.71). Barium swallow is a simple method of identifying some cases of subcarinal lymphadenopathy, but CT is the most comprehensive and accurate method of assessing mediastinal nodes.

Abnormalities of the thoracic aorta

The thoracic aorta arises in the middle mediastinum and then arches through the anterior, middle, and posterior mediastinal compartments. The great vessels arise from the aortic arch in the superior mediastinum (see Fig. 1.72). Dilatation or tortuosity of the aortic arch or its branches may cause widening of the mediastinal shadow. So-called 'unfolding of the aorta' is a common finding in the chest radiograph of elderly or hypertensive patients. Aneurysm of the aorta most often results from atherosclerosis

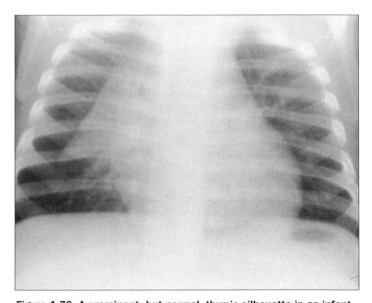

Figure 1.70 A prominent, but normal, thymic silhouette in an infant. Note the characteristic sail shape of the thymus as it projects over the right lung, and the typically slightly lobulated contour as it conforms to the overlying ribs.

(Fig. 1.73). Cystic medial necrosis (Marfan's syndrome), infection (mycotic aneurysm), syphilitic aortitis, and previous trauma are less common causes. Most aortic aneurysms are asymptomatic and present as a mediastinal opacity on the radiograph, sometimes with curvilinear calcification visible in the wall. Aneurysms of the ascending aorta are best appreciated on the lateral radiograph as a filling in of the retrosternal window. Aneurysms of the arch and descending aorta are frequently evident on the frontal radiograph, but a lateral view is often required for more accurate localization, and cross-sectional imaging is often required to confirm that the mediastinal abnormality in question is of vascular origin.

In the acutely injured patient, traumatic aortic rupture may be suspected from chest radiographic findings, and confirmation of injury usually requires angiography (Fig. 1.74). However, when the chest radiograph is equivocal and the degree of trauma less than that usually associated with aortic injury, a spiral CT scan may be performed in the stable patient to exclude a mediastinal hematoma. If any doubt remains, the patient should proceed to angiography. If the aortic injury remains undetected and the patient survives, an aneurysm secondary to the trauma may develop subsequently. This is almost always confined to the junction of arch and descending aorta. Aortic abnormalities may produce pressure changes in adjacent skeletal structures.

Aneurysm of the ascending aorta may erode the posterior surface of the sternum, and descending aortic aneurysms may cause scalloping of the spine. Tortuosity of the inominate artery is a common cause of widening of the superior mediastinum in the elderly. Right-sided aortic arch (Fig. 1.75) and pseudocoarctation of the aorta are two anomalies that may alter the appearance of the mediastinum and suggest a mass.

Dilatation of central veins

The superior vena cava and azygos veins may dilate because of increased pressure, increased flow, obstruction, or congenital abnormality. Increased flow in the superior vena cava is seen in

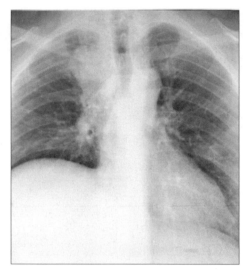

Figure 1.71 Right paratracheal lymph-node enlargement caused by bronchogenic carcinoma. A right phrenic nerve palsy results in elevation of the right hemidiaphragm.

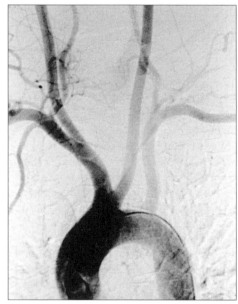

Figure 1.72 Digital subtraction arch aortogram. This patient has two vessels arising from the arch, a common variant of the normal three vessels. The image was obtained with the patient in a 30° left anterior oblique position.

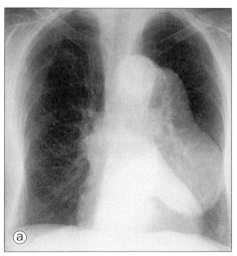
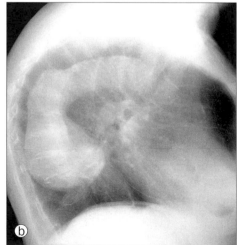
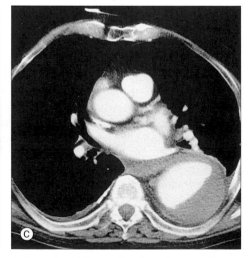

Figure 1.73 Thoracic aortic aneurysm. (a) Marked dilatation and tortuosity of the descending thoracic aorta is present. Note how the left heart border is still evident, indicating the abnormality is likely to lie in the posterior thorax. (b) Lateral view in the same patient demonstrates that the aneurysm involves the posterior arch and descending thoracic aorta. Note calcification within the ascending aorta. (c) Computed tomography demonstrating extensive mural thrombus.

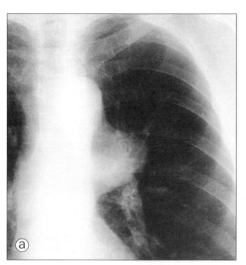
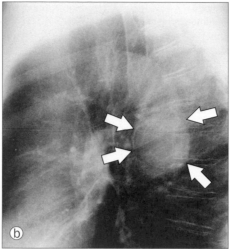
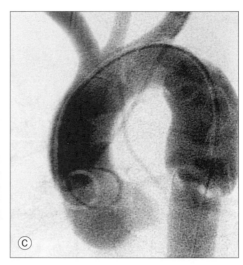

Figure 1.74 Traumatic aortic aneurysm. (a) On the posteroanterior radiograph, a soft-tissue density mass projects over the left hilum. Note how the left lower lobe artery is still visible through this mass, which indicates that it is separate from the hilum. The medial surface blends smoothly with the mediastinal structures indicating it is likely to be extrapulmonary. (b) The lateral view confirms an aneurysm secondary to previous trauma at the typical site, the junction of the posterior arch and descending thoracic aorta (arrows). (c) Acute aortic injury in a different patient. The arch aortogram confirms the diagnosis of an acute aortic injury at the typical site.

supracardiac, total, anomalous pulmonary venous drainage (Fig. 1.76), and in the azygos vein in congenital absence of the inferior vena cava. Rarely, aneurysmal dilatation of the superior mediastinal veins produces an abnormal mediastinal silhouette. Likewise, obstruction of the superior vena cava may cause dilatation of the great veins in the superior mediastinum, which results in widening of the mediastinal contour. However, the clinical features are likely to be obvious by the time radiographic abnormalities become significant.

Other mediastinal abnormalities

Pneumomediastinum or mediastinal emphysema is the presence of air between the tissue planes of the mediastinum. This may occur secondary to interstitial pulmonary emphysema (most often caused by mechanical ventilation), to perforation of the esophagus, trachea, or a bronchus, or to a penetrating chest injury. Chest radiography may show vertical, translucent streaks in the mediastinum, which represent air separating the soft-tissue planes (see Fig. 1.77). The air may extend up into the neck and over the chest wall (causing subcutaneous emphysema), and also over the diaphragm. The mediastinal pleura may be displaced laterally and then be visible as a thin stripe alongside the mediastinum.

Acute mediastinitis is usually caused by perforation of the esophagus, pharynx, or trachea, and a chest radiograph usually shows widening of the mediastinum. A pneumomediastinum is often apparent, and fluid levels may be visible in the mediastinum. Chronic or fibrosing mediastinitis usually presents as SVCO. Mediastinal hemorrhage may occur from venous or arterial bleeding. The mediastinum appears widened, and blood may be seen to track over the lung apices. It is obviously imperative to identify a life-threatening cause such as aortic rupture.

Hilar abnormalities

Having identified a hilar abnormality, the observer must differentiate between a vascular and a nonvascular cause. Vascular prominence is often bilateral and accompanied by enlargement

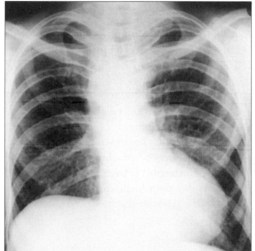

Figure 1.75 Tetralogy of Fallot. There is a right-sided aortic arch in addition to elevation of the ventricular apex because of right ventricular hypertrophy.

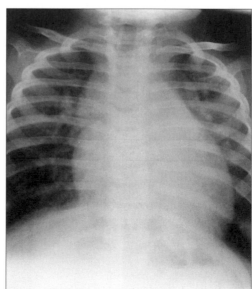

Figure 1.76 Total anomalous pulmonary venous drainage. Widening of the superior mediastinum caused by dilatation of the superior vena cava.

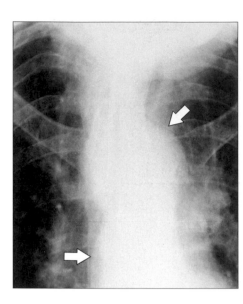

Figure 1.77
Pneumomediastinum.
Air separates the tissue
planes within the
mediastinum, visible
over the aortic arch and
right heart border
(arrows), for example.

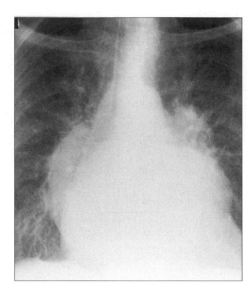

Figure 1.78
**Atrioseptal defect
results in marked
dilatation of the
proximal pulmonary
arteries.** The cardiac
silhouette is enlarged.

of the main pulmonary artery (Fig. 1.78). Although the hilae are large, they are of relatively normal density, and it is usually possible to trace the pulmonary artery branches in continuity from the adjacent lung to their point of convergence with the interlobar arteries, known as the 'hilar convergence' sign. By comparison, enlargement caused by lymph nodes or hilar tumor usually produces a lobulated hilar contour, with discernible lateral or inferior borders. Frequently, the normal hilar point is obliterated and, on the left, the aortopulmonary angle is filled in (Fig. 1.79).

Occasionally, a pulmonary lesion is superimposed directly on the hilum on the frontal radiograph, which produces a spuriously large or dense hilum. The true position of the abnormality is revealed on the lateral radiograph (see Fig. 1.74). A further pitfall is encountered when the vessels to the lingula or, more commonly, the right middle lobe are superimposed on the lower part of the hilar shadow, particularly when the film is taken anteroposteriorly, in a lordotic projection, or with a poor inspiratory effort. A lateral radiograph usually confirms the vascular nature of the shadowing.

Pleural disease
Pleural fluid
The most dependent recess of the pleural space is the posterior costophrenic angle, which is where a small effusion tends to col-

lect. As little as 100–200ml of fluid accumulated in this recess can be seen above the dome of the diaphragm on the frontal view. Even smaller effusions may be seen on a lateral radiograph, and it is possible to identify effusions of only a few milliliters using decubitus views with a horizontal beam, ultrasound, or CT. Eventually, the costophrenic angle on the frontal view fills in, and with increasing fluid a homogeneous opacity spreads upward, obscuring the lung base (Fig. 1.80). The fluid usually demonstrates a concave upper edge, higher laterally than medially, and obscures the diaphragm. Fluid may track into the fissures. A massive effusion may cause complete opacification of a hemithorax with passive atelectasis. The space-occupying effect of the effusion may push the mediastinum toward the opposite side, especially when the lung does not collapse significantly (Fig. 1.81).

Lamellar effusions are shallow collections between the lung surface and the visceral pleura, sometimes sparing the costophrenic angle. Subpulmonary effusions accumulate between the diaphragm and under surface of a lung, mimicking elevation of the hemidiaphragm (see Fig. 1.3). Usually, the contour to the top of such an effusion differs from the normal diaphragmatic contour, the apparent apex being more lateral than usual. Also, some blunting of the costophrenic angle or tracking of fluid into fissures may be visible. On the left side, increased distance between

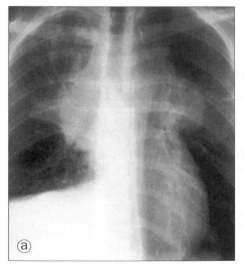

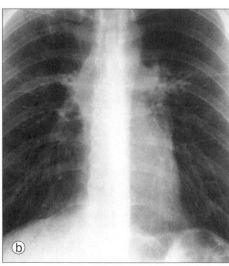

Figure 1.79 Non-Hodgkin's lymphoma.
(a) Bilateral hilar lymph-node enlargement, with obliteration of the normal aortopulmonary angle and subcarinal nodes. A right-sided pleural effusion is present. (b) The same patient showing residual abnormality after chemotherapy.

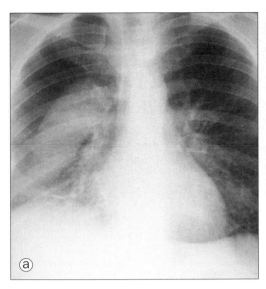

(a)

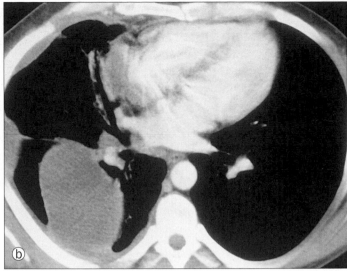

(b)

Figure 1.80 Small, right pleural effusion. (a) The lentiform opacity in the right mid zone is caused by a loculated interlobar effusion. (b) Computed tomography scan on mediastinal settings demonstrating the position of the loculated fluid within the oblique fissure.

the gastric air-bubble and lung base may be apparent. A subpulmonary effusion may be confirmed by ultrasound. However, since the fluid is free to shift within the pleural cavity with changes in patient position, a decubitus film may be needed for confirmation.

Encapsulated or encysted fluid may be difficult to differentiate from an extrapleural opacity, parenchymal lung disease, or mediastinal mass. However, an encysted effusion is often associated with free pleural fluid or other pleural shadowing, and may extend into a fissure (see Fig. 1.80). Loculated effusions tend to have comparatively little depth, but considerable width, rather like a biconvex lens. Their appearance, therefore, depends on whether they are viewed face on, in profile, or obliquely. Extrapleural opacities tend to have a much sharper outline, with tapered, sometimes concave edges where they meet the chest wall. Peripheral, pleurally based lung lesions may show an air bronchogram that differentiates them from true pleural disease. The differentiation between pleural thickening or mass and loculated pleural fluid may be difficult on plain films; CT and ultrasound are particularly useful in this context.

Fluid may become loculated in the interlobar fissures and is most frequently seen in heart failure. Fluid that collects in the horizontal fissure produces a lenticular, oval, or round shadow, with well-demarcated edges. Loculated fluid in an oblique fissure may be poorly defined on a frontal radiograph, but a lateral film

is usually diagnostic since the fissure is seen tangentially, and the typical lenticular configuration of the effusion is demonstrated. Loculated interlobar effusions can appear rounded on two views and may disappear rapidly. Hence they are sometimes known as pulmonary pseudotumors (Fig. 1.82). With subsequent episodes of heart failure they may return at the same site.

Diagnosis of an empyema usually requires thoracentesis. Nevertheless, radiographically the diagnosis may be suspected on a plain film by the spontaneous appearance of an air–fluid level in a pleural effusion, since this usually equates with loculation and communication with the tracheobronchial tree. Loculation is best demonstrated with ultrasound.

Pneumothorax

A small pneumothorax is easily overlooked and, in an erect patient, usually collects at the apex. The lung retracts toward the hilum and on a frontal chest film the sharp white line of the visceral pleura are visible, separated from the chest wall by the radiolucent pleural space, which is devoid of lung markings. This should not be confused with a skin fold (see Fig. 1.83). The lung usually remains aerated, although perfusion is reduced in proportion to ventilation and therefore the radiodensity of the partially collapsed lung remains relatively normal. A closed

Figure 1.81 Large, left pleural effusion. There has been a previous mastectomy on the right and the pleural effusion is malignant. The mediastinal shift to the right results from the space-occupying effects of the fluid.

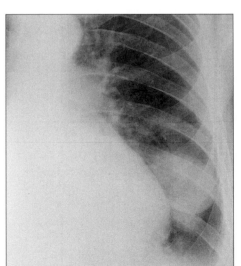

Figure 1.82 Small, left basal pleural effusion. The opacity in the left mid zone is caused by fluid loculated in the oblique fissure.

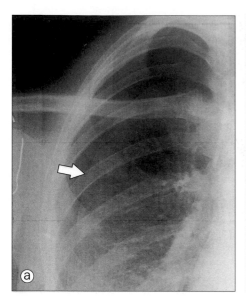

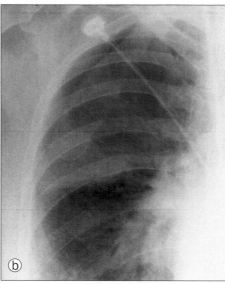

Figure 1.83 Shallow right pneumothorax. (a) A discrete pleural white line is seen (arrow). Peripheral to this, there are no lung markings. (b) In this film, although a change in density parallels the chest wall, no discrete pleural line is present, and lung markings are seen to extend beyond the apparent lung edge. This appearance is caused by a fold of skin produced by the X-ray cassette.

pneumothorax is easier to see on an expiratory film, although expiratory radiographs are not routinely required to detect clinically significant pneumothoraces. A lateral decubitus film with the affected side uppermost is occasionally helpful, as the pleural air can be seen along the lateral chest wall. This view is particularly useful in infants, since small pneumothoraces are difficult to see on supine AP films, as the air tends to collect anteriorly and medially.

A large pneumothorax may lead to complete relaxation and retraction of the lung, with some mediastinal shift toward the normal side (Fig. 1.84). As it is a medical emergency, tension pneumothorax is often treated before a chest radiograph is obtained. However if a radiograph is taken in this situation it shows marked displacement of the mediastinum (Fig. 1.85). Radiographically, the lung may be squashed against the mediastinum, or herniate across the midline, and the ipsilateral hemidiaphragm is depressed.

Complications of pneumothorax

Pleural adhesions may limit the distribution of a pneumothorax and result in a loculated or encysted pneumothorax. The usual appearance is an ovoid air collection adjacent to the chest wall, which may

be radiographically indistinguishable from a thin-walled, subpleural pulmonary cyst or bulla. Pleural adhesions are occasionally seen as line shadows that stretch between the two pleural layers; they prevent relaxation of the underlying lung. Rupture of an adhesion may produce a hemopneumothorax. Collapse or consolidation of a lobe or lung in association with a pneumothorax is important because it may delay re-expansion of the lung.

Since the normal pleural space contains a small volume of fluid, blunting of the costophrenic angle by a short fluid level is commonly seen in a pneumothorax (see Fig. 1.84). In a small pneumothorax, this fluid level may be the most obvious radiologic sign. A larger fluid level usually signifies a complication and represents exudate, pus, or blood, depending on the etiology of the pneumothorax (Fig. 1.86).

The usual radiographic appearance of a hydropneumothorax is that of a pneumothorax containing a horizontal fluid level which separates opaque fluid below from lucent air above. A hydro- or pyopneumothorax may arise as a result of a bronchopleural fistula (an abnormal communication between the bronchial tree and the pleural space). This may be a complication of surgery, but may also occur as a result of a subpleural lung tumor (Fig. 1.87).

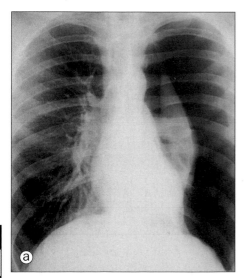

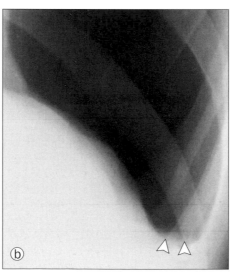

Figure 1.84 Left-sided pneumothorax.
(a) Complete collapse of the left lung, which is retracted to the left hilum. (b) Magnified view of the left lower zone demonstrates the short air–fluid level commonly seen in a costophrenic angle when a pneumothorax is present (arrowheads).

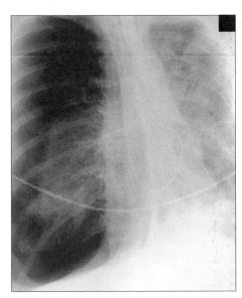

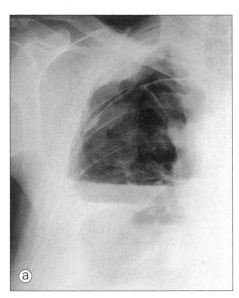

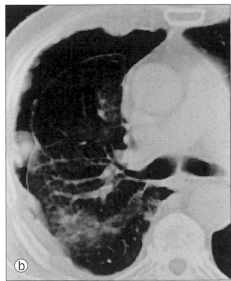

Figure 1.85 Tension pneumothorax following insertion of a Swan–Ganz catheter. Note the shift of the mediastinum toward the left and reversal of the normal contour of the right hemidiaphragm.

Figure 1.86 Hydropneumothorax in a patient with a mesothelioma. (a) Note the normal thickness of the visceral pleura, but the lobulated soft-tissue shadowing caused by tumor within the parietal pleura. (b) Computed tomography scan in the same patient that demonstrates the lobulated pleural tumor.

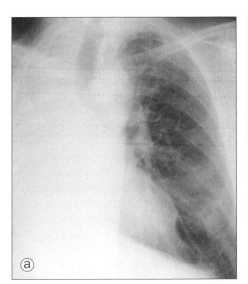

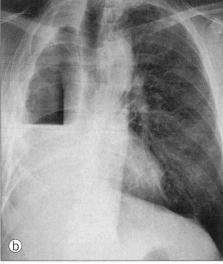

Figure 1.87 Pneumonectomy – appearances and complications. (a) Chest radiograph showing the normal appearances following a right pneumonectomy. (b) Spontaneous development of an air–fluid level caused by a bronchopleural fistula from local recurrence.

Pleural thickening

Blunting of a costophrenic angle is a common observation, and is usually caused by localized pleural thickening secondary to previous pleuritis. In the asymptomatic patient and in the absence of other radiologic abnormalities, it is of no significance other than that it may simulate a pleural effusion. When relevant, the possibility of pleural fluid may have to be excluded by other techniques. Localized pleural thickening that extends into the inferior end of an oblique fissure may produce so-called tenting of the diaphragm, and is of similar significance, although a similar appearance may result from scarring caused by previous pulmonary infection or infarction.

Bilateral apical pleural thickening is common, usually symmetric, more frequent in elderly patients, and does not necessarily indicate previous tuberculosis. The etiology is uncertain, but in some individuals the caps represent extrapleural fat that has descended because of scarring and consequent retraction of the upper lobes. In contrast, asymmetric or unilateral apical pleural thickening may be highly significant, especially if associated with pain. Asymmetric apical pleural shadowing may represent a Pancoast's tumor and bone destruction should be specifically sought (see Fig. 1.88).

More extensive unilateral pleural thickening is usually the result of a previous thoracotomy, or an exudative pleural effusion. A simple transudate usually resolves completely, but empyema and hemothorax are likely to resolve with pleural fibrosis. The thickened pleura may calcify (see Fig. 1.89), and the entire lung may become surrounded by fibrotic pleura, which may be as much as a few centimeters thick (see Fig. 1.90). Bilateral (parietal) pleural plaques are a common manifestation of asbestos exposure, and occasionally more diffuse, visceral pleural thickening is seen.

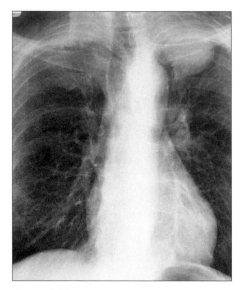

Figure 1.88 Apical abnormalities. Benign apical pleural thickening on the right. On the left there is a Pancoast's tumor.

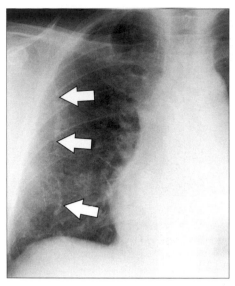

Figure 1.89 Previous thoracotomy (note sternotomy sutures) for mitral valve replacement. Pleural calcification is seen on the right side (arrows).

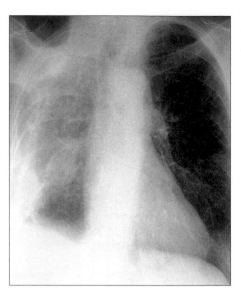

Figure 1.90 Previous tuberculosis. Extensive right-sided pleural thickening and calcification, with reduction in volume of the right hemithorax.

Pleural calcification

In general, pleural calcification has the same causes as pleural thickening. Unilateral pleural calcification is, therefore, likely to be the result of previous empyema or hemothorax, and bilateral calcification occurs after asbestos exposure (Fig. 1.91). Pleural calcification may be discovered in a patient who is not aware of previous chest disease.

The calcification associated with previous pleurisy, empyema, or hemothorax occurs in the visceral pleura (Fig. 1.92); associated pleural thickening is almost always present, and separates the calcium from the ribs. The calcium may be in a continuous sheet or in discrete plaques, which usually produce dense, coarse, irregular shadows, often sharply demarcated laterally. When a plaque is viewed face on, it may be less well defined and mimic a pulmonary infiltrate.

Pleural masses

Primary tumors of the pleura are rare. Benign tumors of the pleura include pleural fibroma and lipoma (Fig. 1.93). The most common malignant disease of the pleura is metastatic, usually adenocarcinoma from the bronchus or breast. Malignant mesothelioma is usually associated with prior asbestos exposure (Fig. 1.94).

COMPUTED TOMOGRAPHY

Anatomy of the mediastinum

The soft-tissue contrast provided by CT, as well as its cross-sectional nature, makes the diagnostic information available from CT far superior to that provided by two-dimensional radiography. Modern CT scanners can acquire a volume of information that

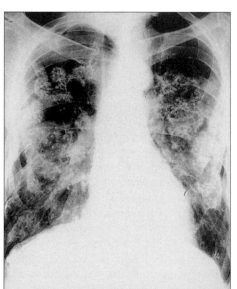

Figure 1.91 Extensive bilateral pleural thickening secondary to asbestos exposure.

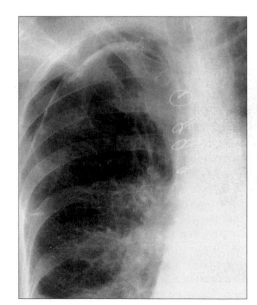

Figure 1.92 Previous sternotomy-associated hemothorax resulting in pleural thickening and calcification. A small pneumothorax is visible. Note the visceral pleural thickening.

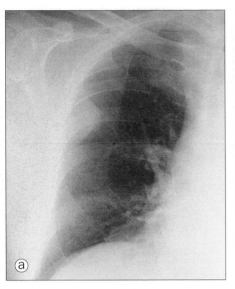

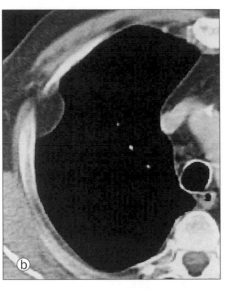

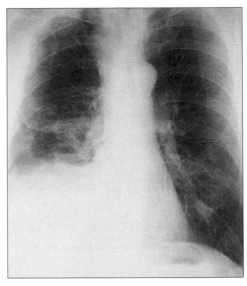

Figure 1.93 The appearances of a pleural lipoma. (a) Localized view of the right lung from a posteroanterior chest radiograph. There is a pleurally based opacity in the right mid zone, well-defined medially but fading out laterally. (b) Computed tomography scan of the same. The opacity is caused by a pleural lipoma. Note the identical computed tomography attenuation of this mass compared with the subcutaneous fat.

Figure 1.94 Malignant mesothelioma. A lobulated pleural thickening extends from the right apex down to the right diaphragm, which appears elevated. The overall volume of the right hemithorax is reduced.

includes the whole of the mediastinum within the time of a single breath hold. This three-dimensional data set can then be displayed as continuous or overlapping axial slices, free from breathing movement artifact. Usually, a collimation and slice width of between 5 and 10mm is used, and it is usual, but not always essential, to give intravenous contrast. The normal mediastinal anatomy is demonstrated in Figs 1.95–1.99.

Great vessels

The great vessels form the most familiar anatomic landmarks within the mediastinum. Knowledge of the relationships of these vessels to other mediastinal components allows accurate description of the location of pathology, and has important implications for planning the approach to either open operation or mediastinoscopy. The most common branching pattern of the aortic arch is for three arteries to arise from the upper arch – the right inominate, left common carotid, and left subclavian (Fig. 1.95). However, many variations to this basic anatomy exist (see Fig. 1.72). The transverse portion of the aortic arch is the most readily recognizable vascular structure within the mediastinum (see Fig. 1.96). The great veins lie anterior to the arterial structures. The left brachiocephalic vein is situated above and anterior to the aortic arch and aortic branches, although its position is variable. The right brachiocephalic vein descends more directly in the anterior right mediastinum to merge with its counterpart to form the superior vena cava. As CT contrast is given from one arm, one brachiocephalic vein is heavily opacified while the other remains of soft-tissue density.

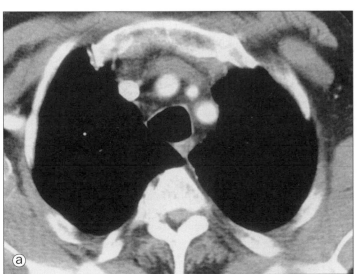

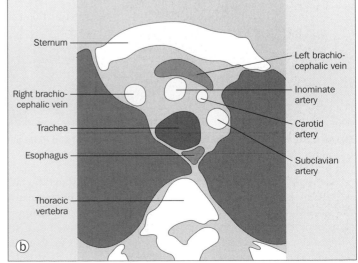

Sternum
Left brachio-cephalic vein
Right brachio-cephalic vein
Inominate artery
Trachea
Carotid artery
Esophagus
Subclavian artery
Thoracic vertebra

Figure 1.95 Mediastinal anatomy at the level of the great vessels.

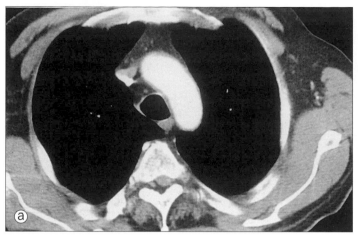

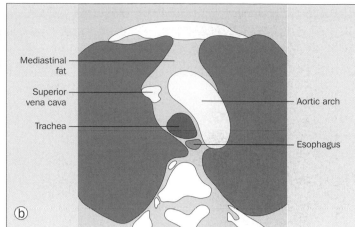

Figure 1.96 Mediastinal anatomy at the level of the aortic arch.

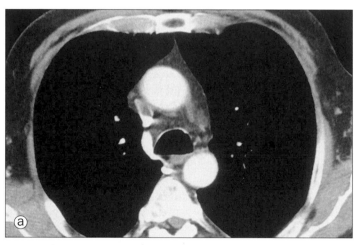

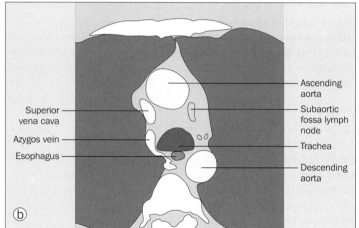

Figure 1.97 Mediastinal anatomy at the level of the subaortic fossa.

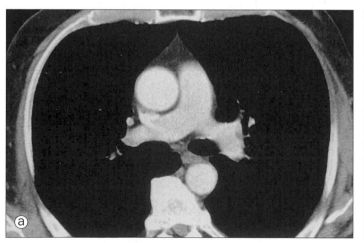

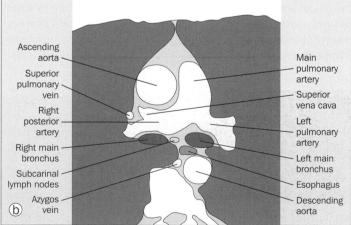

Figure 1.98 Mediastinal anatomy through the division of the main pulmonary artery.

The pulmonary outflow tract ascends, usually outlined by fat within the pericardium, to divide adjacent and just posterior to the ascending aorta. Usually the main pulmonary artery diameter is equal to or less than the ascending aorta as measured on CT. When the pulmonary artery diameter exceeds the aortic diameter, underlying pulmonary hypertension is likely. The right pulmonary artery swings dorsally and to the right, behind the ascending aorta and SVC and anterior to the right main bronchus (Fig. 1.98). After giving a branch to the upper lobe, it descends posterolaterally to the bronchus intermedius. The left pulmonary artery follows a shorter course and arches up and over the left main bronchus.

Hilar anatomy is well demonstrated on contrast-enhanced CT, especially when vascular structures are traced sequentially

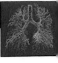

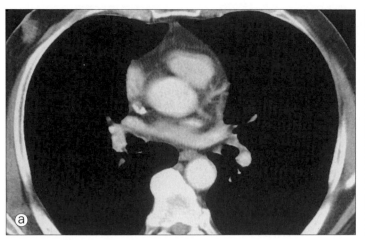

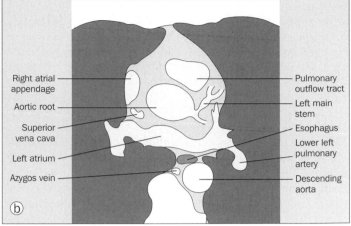

Figure 1.99 Mediastinal anatomy through the aortic root.

over contiguous images. Knowledge of normal anatomy enables differentiation of vascular structures from normal or enlarged mediastinal lymph nodes, even on unenhanced scans; however, if there is any cause for doubt, intravenous contrast clarifies the situation (Fig. 1.100).

Airways

The trachea descends through the thoracic inlet, where reduction in caliber may occur, and usually appears rounded on scans obtained in full inspiration. If scans are obtained during expiration, the membranous posterior wall of the trachea is seen to bow forward into the tracheal lumen. The wall of the trachea is only 2mm thick, and any intramural thickening is well demonstrated on CT. Modern scanners also allow reformatting of the data in sagittal or coronal planes, thus providing more elegant demonstration of tracheal abnormalities. The anatomy of the bronchial tree can be traced from the tracheal carina out into the lungs, at least to segmental level, with excellent correlation between CT and bronchoscopic findings. Furthermore, the three-dimensional data set acquired on modern spiral scanners can be manipulated to provide a computer simulation of the bronchoscopic appearances (Fig. 1.101).

Thymus

The thymus, in the normal state, is not visible on the chest radiograph of the adult patient, but the thymic remnant is frequently evident on CT. The thymus reduces in size after puberty. It lies in the anterior mediastinum, just in front of the root of the aorta; it is bilobed, with the left lobe usually being the larger. Generally, the thymus is assessed by examining the contours of the gland, which should be concave, and the thickness of the individual lobes. In childhood, the thymus is of soft-tissue density on CT scanning, but after puberty as it starts to involute, and the gland undergoes atrophy and fatty replacement. Traces of thymic tissue within the anterior mediastinal fat are frequently identifiable on CT in young adults.

Thyroid

Usually the thyroid is confined to the neck, but frequently mediastinal extension occurs with thyroid enlargement (see below). Typically, the thyroid lies on either side of the extrathoracic trachea, and is bounded laterally by the carotid artery and internal jugular vein. On contrast enhancement, normal thyroid tissue enhances avidly, and is usually of relatively high attenuation on unenhanced scans because of its relatively high iodine content.

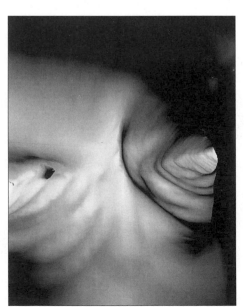

Figure 1.101 Computer-generated view of the carina derived from a three-dimensional spiral computed tomography data set. Surface shading allows appreciation of contour irregularity. (Courtesy of Dr Roger Chinn, Royal Brompton Hospital.)

Figure 1.100 Contrast-enhanced computed tomography scan. Left hilar lymph-node enlargement with extension of abnormal tissue anterior to the descending aorta.

Esophagus

Often the esophagus is completely collapsed on CT scanning and is thus inconspicuous, but is easily identified if it contains air or contrast. Initially, the esophagus lies directly posterior to the trachea, and below the bifurcation it usually deviates slightly to the left and lies adjacent to the aorta. The esophageal wall is usually only 2–3mm in thickness.

Lymph nodes

Numerous lymph nodes occur within the mediastinum, usually <1cm in long axis and discrete; they may not be visible on CT scanning. Previous granulomatous disease may result in extensive mediastinal lymph-node calcification, which reveals the true extent of normal mediastinal lymph-node distribution (Fig. 1.102). An extensive chain of lymph nodes also accompanies the internal mammary vessels bilaterally. Further nodes are present in the intercostal chain adjacent to the heads of the ribs in a posterior, paraspinal position, and alongside the esophagus and descending thoracic aorta. These merge with the retrocrural lymph-node chain, and the para-aortic nodes on the abdomen.

Pericardium

The pericardial membrane is composed of visceral and parietal layers and surrounds the heart. The visceral layer is separated from the myocardium by a variable amount of epicardial fat. The parietal layer is variably fused with the mediastinal pleura. Where they are separate, mediastinal fat may accumulate (such as in the epiphrenic fat pad). Fluid within the pericardial sac may be evident on the chest radiograph, CT, or ultrasound.

Evaluation of mediastinal masses

Most patients who have a mediastinal mass present with symptoms from the local compressive or invasive effects of the mediastinal mass, but in a surprising number the mass is discovered on a chest radiograph taken for an unrelated cause. Generally, the PA and lateral chest radiographs enable localization of the mass to one of the compartments of the mediastinum, which refines the differential diagnosis. However, current practice is for patients who present with a mediastinal mass to undergo a contrast-enhanced CT scan, or sometimes MRI.

The differential diagnosis of a mediastinal mass is wide[23]. Masses can arise from any of the normal structures in the mediastinum, as well as from metastatic disease from a distant primary. In addition, mediastinal abscesses may also present as a mass. The diagnosis is considerably narrowed by CT, which enables the organ of origin of the mass to be assessed, defines the attenuation and enhancement characteristics, and detects evidence of invasion of adjacent structures. It is usual to classify mediastinal masses according to the anatomic portion of the mediastinum from which they appear to arise (Fig. 1.103).

Superior mediastinal masses

Thyroid

An enlarged thyroid may extend inferiorly into the superior mediastinum, and may be large enough to reach into the middle mediastinum. However, this rarely presents a diagnostic problem since the mass is obviously continuous with the cervical thyroid tissue, and enhances avidly following intravenous contrast. Frequently, the enlarged gland contains low-density cysts and areas of calcification,

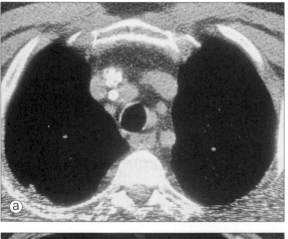
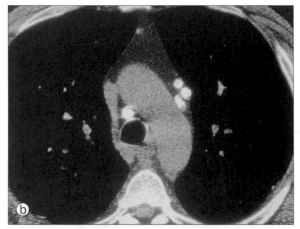
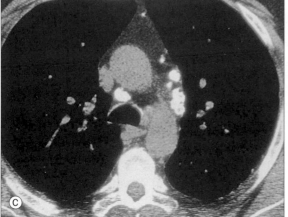
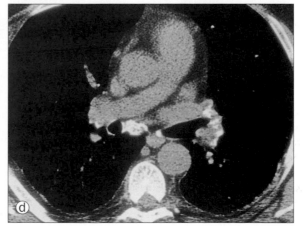

Figure 1.102 Calcified mediastinal lymph nodes secondary to previous granulomatous disease. Unenhanced computed tomography scan through the thorax. Compare (a)–(d) with Figs 1.95–1.98 respectively.

Mediastinal masses

Solid masses

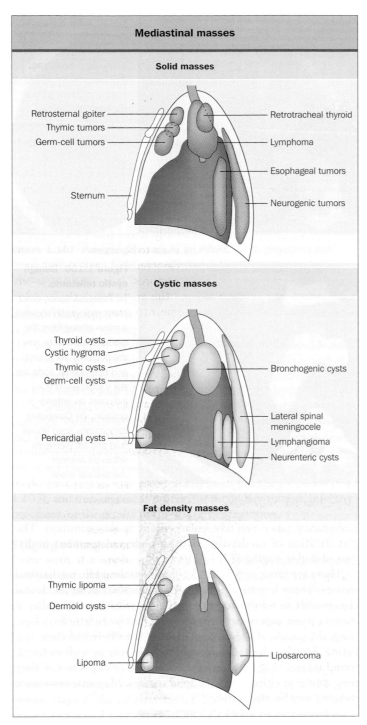

Retrosternal goiter

Thymic tumors

Germ-cell tumors

Sternum

Retrotracheal thyroid

Lymphoma

Esophageal tumors

Neurogenic tumors

Cystic masses

Thyroid cysts

Cystic hygroma

Thymic cysts

Germ-cell cysts

Pericardial cysts

Bronchogenic cysts

Lateral spinal meningocele

Lymphangioma

Neurenteric cysts

Fat density masses

Thymic lipoma

Dermoid cysts

Lipoma

Liposarcoma

Figure 1.103 Distribution and classification of mediastinal masses depending on density derived from computed tomography.

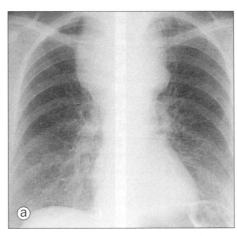

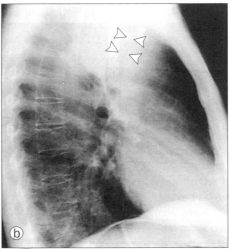

Figure 1.104 Retrosternal thyroid mass.
(a) Posteroanterior chest radiograph with a large superior mediastinal mass mainly to the right of the trachea. (b) The lateral view demonstrates an extension behind the trachea, which is narrowed in its anteroposterior dimension (arrow heads). The thyroid frequently extends into a retrotracheal position in the upper mediastinum.

particularly within cyst walls. Large thyroid masses may cause tracheal deviation or narrowing, and may enlarge acutely if there is hemorrhage into the gland (Fig. 1.104). Although the thyroid originates anterior to the trachea, there may be extension to the right and even posterior to the trachea within the upper mediastinum.

Lymphatic malformations
Lymphatic malformations are rare and may present in the superior mediastinum. The most common of these is the cystic

hygroma, which usually presents in infants as a cervical mass with an extensive intrathoracic component. Although considered benign, these lesions are difficult to resect completely because of a tendency to spread around normal structures.

Anterior mediastinal masses
The majority of anterior mediastinal masses arise from the thymus, thyroid (see above), germ-cell tumors, and enlarged lymph nodes.

Thymus
The normal thymus involutes after puberty, but may show reactive enlargement in certain disease states or following chemotherapy. However, intrinsic neoplasia of the thymus is a relatively common cause of an anterior mediastinal mass in adult life. Causes of thymic neoplasia include thymoma, thymic carcinoma, thymic cysts (see Fig. 1.105), thymic lipoma, thymic carcinoid, and thymic lymphoma. With CT, fat or fluid elements may be identified within a thymic mass, and invasion of adjacent structures can be shown. With the exception of thymolipoma and thymic cysts, histology is usually required for definitive diagnosis.

Teratomas and germ-cell tumors
Teratomas and germ-cell tumors originate from primitive stem cell rests. It is useful to separate these neoplasms into benign and malignant forms – the former is the benign cystic teratoma (synonymous with dermoid cysts). Benign cystic teratomas (see Fig. 1.106) may contain differentiated elements and so on CT

tree for the duration of the scan, so revealing any thrombus within the central pulmonary vessels (Fig. 1.108). Subsequently, a series of studies have evaluated helical and electron beam CT in the diagnosis of acute pulmonary embolus, with excellent reported sensitivity and specificity for the detection of emboli down to the segmental level. Most of these studies also identified an important additional advantage of CT: the ability to provide an alternative diagnosis that explains the symptoms of chest pain or dyspnea in those patients who do not have PE[26].

When CT detection of subsegmental embolus is assessed against pulmonary angiography, the sensitivity and specificity of CT is not as good. Isolated, subsegmental thrombus may be relatively common. Indeed, in one series 30% of the patients had emboli confined to the subsegmental vessels and many would have been missed on CT. By comparison, the PIOPED study suggested a prevalence of only 6% for isolated subsegmental emboli (see Chapter 50). The clinical significance of isolated subsegmental emboli remains uncertain.

The case for a major role for CT within the diagnostic algorithm for PE has been proposed recently[27]. While some authorities have suggested that $\dot{V}/\dot{Q}$ scanning may be omitted as part of the diagnostic workup, others have highlighted a continuing role for $\dot{V}/\dot{Q}$ scanning in patients who have a normal chest radiograph. The rationale is that the $\dot{V}/\dot{Q}$ scan, with its lower cost and radiation dose, is likely to be conclusive in patients who have otherwise normal lungs.

Cost is always an issue in the acceptability of any new test. A cost–effectiveness analysis of 15 combinations of five commonly utilized tests in PE, which included angiography, CT, and $\dot{V}/\dot{Q}$ scanning, revealed all the best outcomes included helical CT, when both effectiveness (mortality) and marginal cost–effectiveness (cost per life saved) were assessed. Even when the assumed sensitivity fell below 85%, CT maintained its economic advantage[28].

Despite the rapid developments in this area (including a potential role for MRI), it seems likely that spiral CT scanning will have an important role in the diagnosis of PE for some time to come, especially in view of the generally high threshold for performing pulmonary angiography.

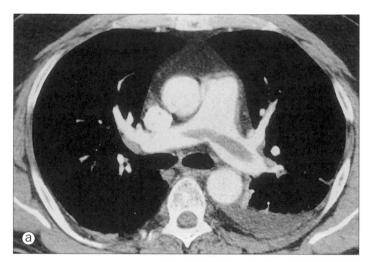

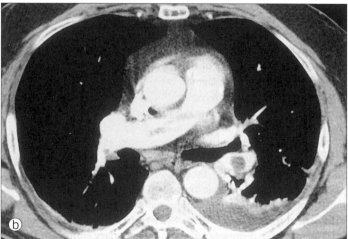

Figure 1.108 Spiral computed tomography for pulmonary embolism. (a) Contrast-enhanced computed tomography scan through the division of the main pulmonary artery showing a saddle thrombus. (b) Sections slightly more inferiorly showing further thrombus extending down into the left main pulmonary artery.

INTERPRETATION OF HIGH-RESOLUTION COMPUTED TOMOGRAPHY OF THE LUNGS

Appearance of normal lung anatomy

Accurate interpretation of HRCT of the lung requires an understanding of the normal appearances of the bronchi, blood vessels, and the secondary pulmonary lobule. The close correspondence between the appearances of gross pathologic specimens and HRCT features enables the use of anatomic terms to describe the patterns of lung disease depicted by HRCT.

Throughout the lung, the bronchi and pulmonary arteries run together and taper slightly as they travel radially; this is easiest to appreciate in the bronchovascular bundles that run within and parallel to the plane of HRCT section. At any given point, the diameter of the bronchus is the same as its accompanying pulmonary artery. The bronchovascular bundle is surrounded by connective tissue from the hilum to the bronchioles in the lung periphery. The concept of connected components making up the lung interstitium is useful for the understanding of HRCT findings in interstitial lung disease – the peripheral interstitium around the surface of the lung beneath the visceral pleura extends into the lung to surround the secondary pulmonary lobules. Within the lobules, a finer network of septal, connective-tissue fibers support the alveoli. The 'axial' fibers form a sheath around the bronchovascular bundles. Thus, the connective tissue stroma of these three separate components is in continuity and so form a fibrous skeleton for the lungs.

In normal individuals, HRCT shows a clear and definite interface between the bronchovascular bundle and surrounding lung. Any thickening of the connective tissue interstitium results in apparent bronchial wall thickening and blurring of this interface. The size of the smallest subsegmental bronchi visible on HRCT is determined by the thickness of the bronchial wall, rather than by the bronchial diameter. In general, bronchi with a diameter <3mm and walls less than 300μm thick are not consistently identifiable on HRCT. Airways reach this critical size at about 2–3cm from the pleural surface. The secondary pulmonary lobule is the smallest anatomic unit of the lung that is surrounded by a connective tissue septum (Fig. 1.109). Within the septa lie lymphatic vessels and venules. The lobule contains between five and 12 acini, each of which measures approximately 6–10mm in diameter. Each lobule is approximately 2cm in diameter and

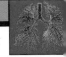

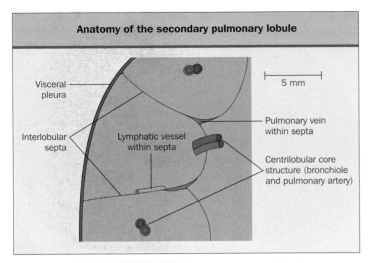

Anatomy of the secondary pulmonary lobule

Visceral pleura

Interlobular septa

Lymphatic vessel within septa

5 mm

Pulmonary vein within septa

Centrilobular core structure (bronchiole and pulmonary artery)

Figure 1.109 Anatomy of the secondary pulmonary lobule.

polyhedral in shape, and often resemble a truncated cone. In the lung periphery, the bases of the cone-shaped lobules lie on a visceral pleural surface. In the central parts of the lung, the interlobular septa, and thus the lobules, are less well developed. The centrilobular bronchiole and accompanying pulmonary artery enter through the apex of the lobule.

The interlobular septa measure approximately 100μm in thickness. The lower limit of resolution of HRCT is approximately 200μm, so normal septa are infrequently identified on HRCT. The few interlobular septa that are visible in normal individuals are seen as straight lines 1–2cm in length that terminate at a visceral pleural surface. Sometimes several septa that join end to end are seen as a nonbranching, linear structure, which can measure up to 4cm in length; these are most frequent at the lung bases, just above the diaphragmatic surface.

The secondary pulmonary lobule is supplied by a centrilobular artery and bronchiole that are approximately 1mm in diameter as they enter the lobule. In the normal state, the core structures, effectively the 500μm diameter centrilobular artery, are visible as dots 1cm deep to the pleural surface. On standard window settings, the lung parenchyma is of almost homogeneous low density, marginally greater than that of air.

Patterns of parenchymal disease

Vague terms traditionally used in the lexicon of plain chest radiography can be replaced by precise descriptions derived from an understanding of HRCT anatomy. Abnormal patterns on HRCT that represent pulmonary disease can usually be categorized into one of four patterns – reticular and linear opacities, nodular opacities, increased lung density, and cystic air spaces with areas of decreased lung density.

While these HRCT patterns generally have a corresponding pattern on chest radiography, they are seen with much greater clarity on the cross-sectional images of HRCT and the precise distribution of disease can be more readily appreciated[29]. There is increasing conformity in the terminology used to describe the HRCT abnormalities of diffuse, infiltrative lung diseases[30].

Reticular pattern

A reticular pattern on HRCT always indicates significant pathology. A reticular pattern caused by thickening of interlobular

septa is a cardinal sign of many interstitial lung diseases. Numerous interlobular septa that join up to form an obvious network indicate an extensive interstitial abnormality caused by infiltration with fibrosis, abnormal cells, or fluid (e.g. fibrosing alveolitis, lymphangitis carcinomatosa, and pulmonary edema, respectively). Interlobular septal thickening that results from fibrosing alveolitis is often associated with intralobular, interstitial thickening (beyond the resolution of HRCT) and a coarse reticular pattern that contains cystic air spaces and produces the 'honeycomb' of destroyed lung. Thickening of the interlobular septa may be smooth or irregular, but this distinction is not always obvious. Irregular septal thickening is a feature of lymphangitic spread of tumor, whereas pulmonary edema and alveolar proteinosis cause smooth thickening. Sarcoidosis is typified by some nodular septal thickening, although widespread septal thickening is not characteristic of this condition.

Since the various parts of the lung interstitium are in continuity, widespread interstitial disease that causes interlobular septal thickening also results in bronchovascular interstitial thickening (e.g. by lymphangitis carcinomatosa). The bronchovascular thickening seen on HRCT is equivalent to the peribronchial 'cuffing' seen around end-on bronchi on chest radiography. The HRCT finding of peribronchovascular thickening in isolation must be interpreted with caution, since it may be seen in reversible pure airways disease, for example asthma. Thickening of the subsegmental and segmental bronchovascular bundles, for example caused by lymphangitis carcinomatosa, sometimes gives the interface between the thickened bronchial wall and surrounding lung a 'feathery' appearance (Fig. 1.110).

The coarseness of the network that makes up the reticular pattern on HRCT is determined by the level at which the interstitial thickening is most severe. Thickening of the intralobular septa results in a very fine reticular pattern on HRCT, only visible on an optimal HRCT scan. Some of the very delicate linear structures that make up such a fine reticular pattern are so small as to be below the resolution limits of HRCT, even with the narrowest collimation. The result is an amorphous increase in lung density ('ground-glass' opacification, see later) caused by volume averaging within the section.

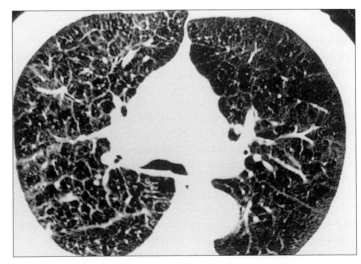

Figure 1.110 High-resolution computed tomography showing generalized, irregular thickening of the interlobular septa in both lungs. The patient has lymphangitis carcinomatosa.

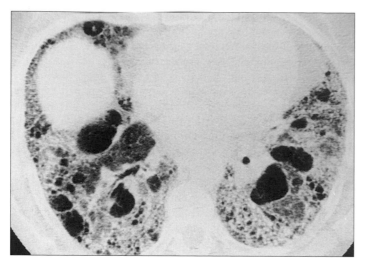

Figure 1.111 High-resolution computed tomography of end-stage pulmonary fibrosis. Large cystic air spaces are visible within the destroyed lung.

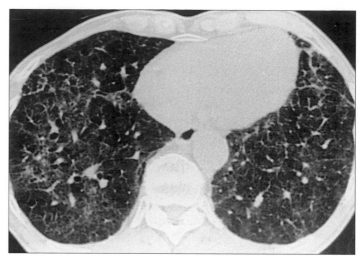

Figure 1.112 Widespread reticular pattern with architectural distortion. The patient has pulmonary fibrosis caused by chronic hypersensitivity pneumonitis. In the right lower lobe the airways are dilated ('traction bronchiectasis').

Extensive pulmonary fibrosis causes complete destruction of the architecture of the secondary pulmonary lobules, which results in a coarse reticular pattern made up of irregular, linear opacities. The reticular pattern of end-stage fibrotic or honeycomb lung mirrors the appearances on chest radiography and is characterized by cystic spaces that measure a few millimeters to several centimeters across and are surrounded by discernible walls (Fig. 1.111). Paradoxically, thickened interlobular septa are not an obvious feature of advanced fibrosing alveolitis, probably because of the severe disturbance of the normal lung architecture. The distortion that accompanies interstitial fibrosis may result in irregular dilatation of the segmental and subsegmental bronchi, a phenomenon termed traction bronchiectasis (Fig. 1.112).

Nodular pattern

A nodular pattern on HRCT comprises innumerable, small, discrete opacities that range in diameter from 1mm to 10mm, and is a feature of both interstitial and air-space diseases. The location of nodules in relation to the lobules and bronchovascular bundles, as well as their density, clarity of outline, and uniformity of size may indicate whether the nodules lie predominantly within the interstitium or air spaces. Since most diffuse lung pathologies have both interstitial and air-space components, this distinction does not always aid in the diagnosis. Whether pulmonary nodules can be detected on CT depends upon their size, profusion, density, and the scanning technique. Narrow collimation HRCT is clearly superior to conventional CT for the detection of micronodular disease, because there is less partial-volume effect, which can average out the attenuation of tiny nodules. A further refinement is the use of maximum-intensity projection images obtained with spiral CT to detect extremely subtle micronodular disease. Nodules within the lung interstitium are seen in the interlobular septa, subpleural regions (particularly in relation to the fissures), and in a peribronchovascular distribution. Nodular thickening of the bronchovascular interstitium results in an irregular interface between the margins of the bronchovascular bundles and the surrounding lung parenchyma. These features are most pro-

nounced in cases of sarcoidosis, in which coalescent, perilymphatic granulomas cause a beaded appearance of the thickened bronchovascular bundles. The bronchovascular distribution of nodules, in conjunction with a perihilar concentration of disease, is virtually pathognomonic of sarcoidosis (Fig. 1.113).

The nodular pattern seen in coal-worker's pneumoconiosis and silicosis is generally more uniform in distribution; the distribution of centrilobular nodules may be more in the upper zone and subpleurally, but overall they tend to be more evenly spread throughout the lung parenchyma than those seen in sarcoidosis.

When the air spaces are filled, or partially filled, with exudate, individual acini may become visible as poorly defined nodules approximately 8mm in diameter. Acinar nodules may merge with

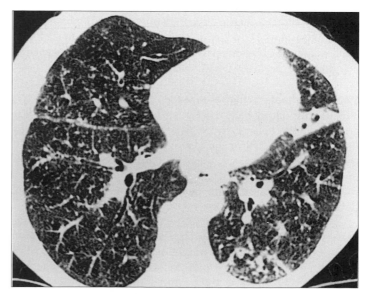

Figure 1.113 High-resolution computed tomography of sarcoidosis. Thickening and beading of the bronchovascular bundles is typical of sarcoidosis. Subpleural nodularity is evident along the right oblique fissure. On a mediastinal window setting, extensive mediastinal and hilar lymphadenopathy was found.

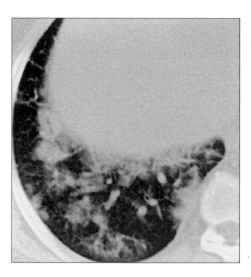

Figure 1.114 Poorly defined acinar nodules and patchy consolidation. The patient has cardiogenic pulmonary edema.

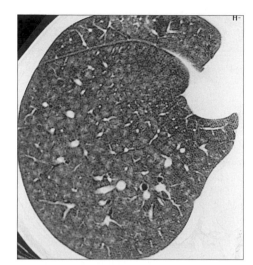

Figure 1.115 High-resolution computed tomography showing poorly defined nodular opacities merging with ground-glass opacification. The patient has subacute hypersensitivity pneumonitis.

areas of ground-glass opacification and are sometimes seen around the periphery of areas of dense parenchymal consolidation (Fig. 1.114). Such nodules are usually centrilobular, although this may be difficult to appreciate if the nodules are very profuse. Conditions in which this nonspecific pattern is seen include organizing pneumonia, hypersensitivity pneumonitis (Fig. 1.115), endobronchial spread of tuberculosis, idiopathic pulmonary hemorrhage, and some cases of bronchoalveolar cell carcinoma.

Increased lung density

An amorphous increase in lung density on HRCT is often described as a ground-glass opacification appearance (Fig. 1.116). Unlike the equivalent abnormality on chest radiography, in which the pulmonary vessels are often indistinct, a ground-glass pattern on HRCT does not obscure the pulmonary vasculature. In cases in which the presence of a ground-glass pattern is equivocal, HRCT is often useful to compare the density of the lung parenchyma with air in the bronchi – in the normal state, the difference in density is marginal. Although this HRCT abnormality is usually easily recognizable, particularly when it is interspersed with areas of normal lung parenchyma, subtle degrees of increased parenchymal opacification may not be obvious. It is important to recognize that a normal increase in parenchymal density, indistinguishable from a generalized opacification caused by infiltrative lung disease, a ground-glass pattern is seen in patients who breath hold at end expiration.

On a pathologic level, the changes responsible for ground-glass opacification are complex and include partial filling of the air spaces and thickening of the interstitium, or a combination of the two(see Fig. 1.117). Conditions that are characterized by these pathologic changes and result in the nonspecific pattern of ground-glass opacification include fibrosing alveolitis in the active cellular phase, *Pneumocystis carinii* pneumonia, subacute hypersensitivity pneumonitis, sarcoidosis, drug-induced lung damage, diffuse pulmonary hemorrhage, and acute lung injury. The amorphous ground-glass density seen on HRCT in these conditions usually represents a potentially reversible process. However, mild thickening of the intralobular interstitium by irreversible fibrosis may rarely produce a ground-glass appearance in fibrosing alveolitis. Furthermore, ground-glass opacification may be seen in areas of bronchoalveolar cell carcinoma, usually in conjunction with patches of denser, consolidated lung (see Fig. 1.118).

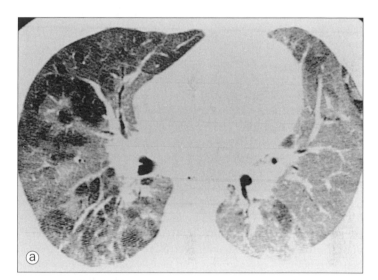

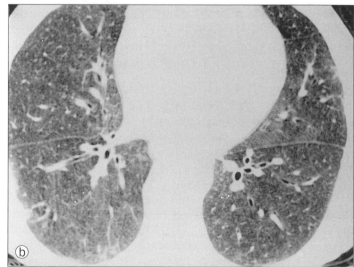

Figure 1.116 Ground glass-appearance on high-resolution computed tomography. (a) Extensive ground-glass opacification in a patient who has desquamative interstitial pneumonitis. Note that the vessels are visible within the areas of ground-glass opacification. (b) Generalized ground-glass opacification in a patient who has lymphocytic pneumonitis (note the marked contrast between the density of air within the bronchi and the density of the lung parenchyma).

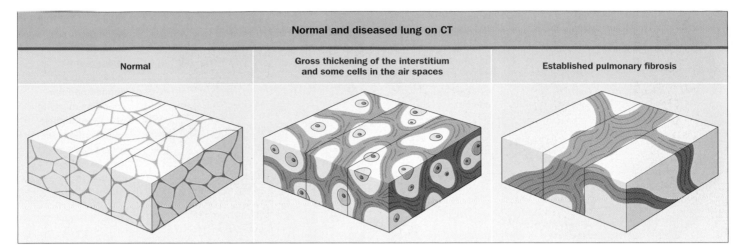

Normal and diseased lung on CT

Normal	Gross thickening of the interstitium and some cells in the air spaces	Established pulmonary fibrosis

Figure 1.117 Normal and diseased lung on computed tomography (CT). In the normal state, most of the volume of these voxels is made up of air (left). Gross thickening of the interstitium and some cells within the air spaces causes displacement of air and thus an increase in density within the voxels (middle) – this produces ground-glass opacification on a high-resolution CT image. In established pulmonary fibrosis, the strands of fibrotic lung occupy much of the volume of individual voxels (see middle voxel), which is reflected in their density (right); pulmonary fibrosis thus has a reticular pattern on high-resolution CT.

A pitfall in identifying a ground-glass pattern on HRCT occurs when regional differences in pulmonary perfusion are present – regional alterations in pulmonary blood flow, caused by thromboembolism, for example, may result in striking differences in lung density (Fig. 1.119). The density difference between the underperfused lung and normal lung may give the appearance of a ground-glass density in normal (but relatively overperfused) lung parenchyma. These areas of different density have been given the term 'mosaic pattern'. A similar appearance is seen in patients who have patchy air-trapping caused by small airways disease, for example an obliterative bronchiolitis; the relatively transradiant areas of underventilated and thus underperfused lung make the normal lung parenchyma appear more than usually dense and thus simulate a ground-glass infiltrate. This potential pitfall can often be recognized for what it is by the relative paucity of vessels in the underventilated parts of the lungs caused by hypoxic vasoconstriction. The vessels in the relatively normal lung of higher density are engorged because of shunting of blood to these regions (Fig. 1.119).

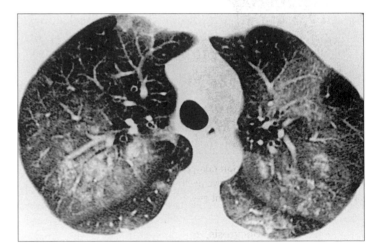

Figure 1.118 Patchy areas of ground-glass opacification in a patient who had biopsy-proved bronchoalveolar cell carcinoma.

Cystic air spaces

The term cystic air space describes a clearly defined, air-containing space that has a definable wall 1–3mm thick. Many conditions are characterized by a profusion of cystic air spaces, which may not be recognizable as such on chest radiography (Fig. 1.120), whereas the size and distribution of these cysts on HRCT may suggest the diagnosis.

The destruction of alveolar walls that characterizes emphysema produces areas of low attenuation on HRCT, which often merge imperceptibly with normal lung (Fig. 1.121). In patients who have predominantly centrilobular emphysema, circular areas of lung destruction may resemble cysts; however, the centrilobular core is usually visible as a dot-like structure in the center of the apparent cyst[31]. Although bullae of varying sizes are clearly seen on HRCT in patients who suffer emphysema, usually a background permeative, destructive parenchyma prevents confusion with other conditions in which cystic air spaces are a prominent feature.

Cystic air spaces as the dominant abnormality are seen in only a few conditions, which include lymphangioleiomyomatosis,

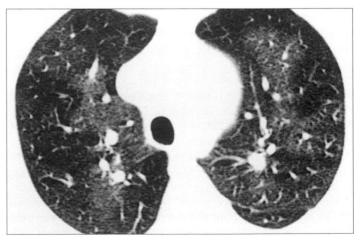

Figure 1.119 Uneven density of the lung parenchyma (mosaic pattern) caused by perfusion inhomogeneity. The patient has chronic thromboembolism (note the dilatation of the segmental pulmonary arteries). The denser (relatively overperfused) lung has a ground-glass appearance.

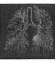

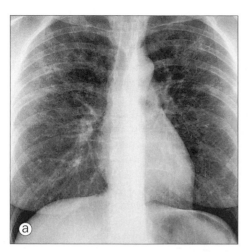

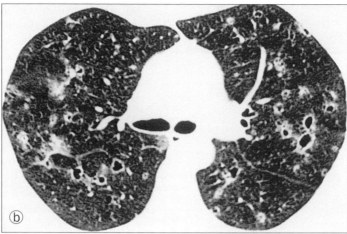

Figure 1.120 Cystic air spaces.
(a) Nonspecific shadowing on a chest radiograph, with the suggestion of a cavitating nodule in the right upper zone.
(b) High-resolution computed tomography through the upper lobes reveals multiple, curious-shaped, cavitating lesions, typical of Langerhans' cell histiocytosis.

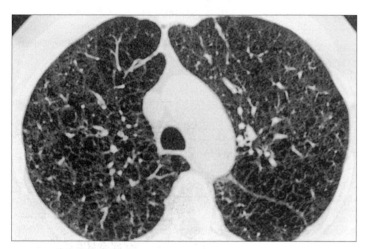

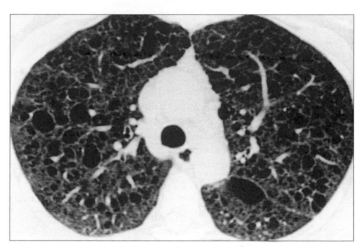

Figure 1.121 High-resolution computed tomography of centrilobular emphysema. Note the permeative destruction of the lung parenchyma with scattered centrilobular lucent areas.

Figure 1.122 High-resolution computed tomography of advanced lymphangioleiomyomatosis. Note the coalescence of cystic air spaces, which resembles severe centrilobular emphysema.

Langerhans' cell histiocytosis, end-stage fibrosing alveolitis, and postinfective pneumatoceles. In lymphangioleiomyomatosis, the cysts are usually uniformly scattered throughout the lungs, with normal lung parenchyma intervening; the individual cysts are rarely larger than 4cm in diameter (Fig. 1.122). As the disease progresses, the larger cystic air spaces coalesce, the circumferential, well-defined walls of the cysts become disrupted, and the HRCT pattern of advanced lymphangioleiomyomatosis, and indeed of Langerhans' cell histiocytosis, may be practically indistinguishable from severe centrilobular emphysema. Distinction of the delicate, 'lace-like' reticular pattern of lymphangioleiomyomatosis on HRCT from that of end-stage fibrosing alveolitis is usually possible because the cystic air spaces in a fibrotic honeycomb lung are smaller and have thicker walls. Furthermore, the tendency for fibrosing alveolitis to have a peripheral distribution, even in its end stage, is usually still obvious in the upper zones.

Similar, confluent cystic air spaces that give a delicate pattern on HRCT are seen in patients who have advanced Langerhans' cell histiocytosis. However, earlier in the disease, a nodular component is present and some of the nodules cavitate. The combination of cavitating nodules, some of which have curious shapes (e.g. cloverleaf shape), and cystic air spaces with a predominantly upper zone distribution is virtually pathognomonic for the diagnosis (see Fig. 1.120). Serial HRCT scans show the natural history of nod-

ules, which cavitate, become cystic air spaces, and, in the end stages, coalesce. In a few cases, the cavitating nodules and cystic air spaces may resolve, with the lung parenchyma reverting to a normal appearance. Some of the cavitating nodules in Langerhans' cell histiocytosis superficially resemble bronchiectatic airways, but there is a lack of continuity between these lesions on adjacent sections, and the segmental bronchi, where they can be identified, do not have any of the HRCT features of bronchiectasis.

Diseases of the airways
The imaging test of choice for the detection of bronchiectasis is now HRCT. The diagnosis of bronchiectasis on chest radiography can rarely be made with certainty unless the disease is severe. The opportunity for prospective studies to compare the accuracy of HRCT with what used to be the gold standard, bronchography, has passed. Most of the evidence that suggests HRCT is at least as good as bronchography is based on small, retrospective studies with different bronchographic and CT techniques. However, now that bronchography is rarely performed, no other imaging technique begins to compare with the sensitivity and specificity of an optimal HRCT examination[32].

Bronchiectasis is defined as damage to the bronchial wall that results in irreversible dilatation of the bronchi, whatever the cause. Thus, the main feature of bronchiectasis on HRCT is

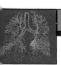
High-resolution computed tomography features of bronchiectosis

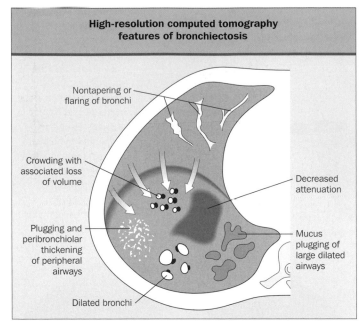

Nontapering or flaring of bronchi

Crowding with associated loss of volume

Plugging and peribronchiolar thickening of peripheral airways

Dilated bronchi

Decreased attenuation

Mucus plugging of large dilated airways

Figure 1.123 High-resolution computed tomography features of bronchiectasis. Nontapering or flaring of bronchi lying within the plane of section. 'Signet ring' sign of dilated bronchi running perpendicular to the plane of computed tomography section. Mucus plugging of large, dilated airways. Plugging and peribronchiolar thickening of small peripheral airways. Crowding with associated loss of volume (see position of oblique fissure). Areas of decreased attenuation, which reflect associated small airways disease.

dilatation of the bronchi with or without bronchial wall thickening. Criteria for the HRCT identification of abnormally dilated bronchi depend on the orientation of the bronchi in relation to the plane of the HRCT section (Fig. 1.123).

Vertically oriented bronchi are seen in the transverse section, so reference can be made to the accompanying pulmonary artery that in normal individuals is of approximately the same caliber; any dilatation of the bronchus results in the so-called signet ring sign (Fig. 1.124). Although this is generally a reliable sign of abnormal

bronchial dilatation, care must be taken when comparing the diameter of the bronchi and adjacent pulmonary arteries just below the division of the lower lobe bronchus. At this level, pairs of segmental and sometimes subsegmental bronchi converge and the resulting fusion of the two bronchi may give the spurious impression of an abnormally dilated bronchus. Bronchi that have a more horizontal course on CT, particularly the anterior segmental bronchi of the upper lobes and the segmental bronchi of the lingula and right middle lobe, are demonstrated along their length and abnormal dilatation is seen as nontapering parallel walls or even flaring of the bronchi as they course distally (Fig. 1.125). In more severe cases of bronchiectasis, the bronchi are obviously dilated and have a varicose or cystic appearance (Fig. 1.126).

Bronchial wall thickening is a frequent, but not invariable, feature of bronchiectasis. The definition of what constitutes abnormal bronchial-wall thickening remains contentious, particularly since mild degrees of wall thickening are seen in normal subjects, asymptomatic smokers, asthmatic individuals, and patients affected by an acute, lower respiratory tract, viral infection. In brief, no robust and reproducible criterion for the identification of abnormal bronchial wall thickening exists, so bronchial wall thickening remains a subjective sign with an attendant high variation in observer interpretation. However, it is the presence of peribronchial thickening that renders the smaller peripheral airways visible on HRCT. Although there is no exact level beyond which visualization of the bronchi can be regarded as abnormal on HRCT, normal bronchi should not be visible within 2–3cm of the pleural surface. The appearance of large elliptical and circular opacities, which represent secretion-filled, dilated bronchi, is a sign of gross bronchiectasis and is almost invariably seen in the presence of other obviously dilated bronchi, some of which may contain air–fluid levels (Fig. 1.127). When mucus plugging of the smaller airways occurs, minute branching structures or dots in the lung periphery may be identifiable. In some cases, plugging of the numerous centrilobular bronchioles gives a curious nodular appearance to the lungs (Fig. 1.128).

Supplementary HRCT signs of bronchiectasis are crowding of the affected bronchi, with obvious volume loss of the lobe as

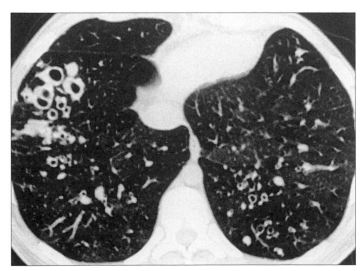

Figure 1.124 Severe bronchiectasis in the right lower lobe with plugging of the dilated bronchi. Mild, cylindrical bronchiectasis in the left lower lobe showing the signet ring sign.

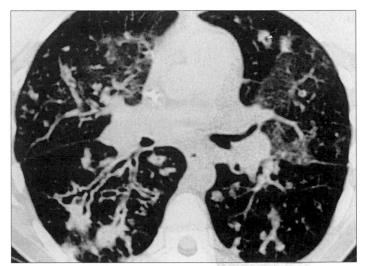

Figure 1.125 High-resolution computed tomography of a patient who had cystic fibrosis. Nontapering and flaring of the bronchiectatic airways is visible in the apical segment of the right lower lobe. In addition, mosaic perfusion is present, reflecting associated small airways disease.

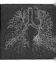

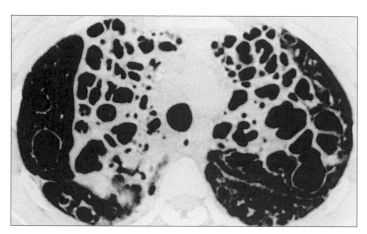

Figure 1.126 Severe cystic bronchiectasis in the upper lobes. The patient has idiopathic (probably post-tuberculous) bronchiectasis.

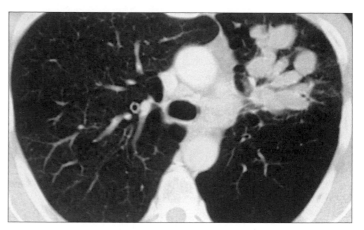

Figure 1.127 Severe bronchiectasis in the left upper lobe. The bronchi are completely filled with fluid, which results in multiple round and elliptical opacities. The patient has allergic bronchopulmonary aspergillosis.

shown by the position of the major fissures. In many lobes affected by bronchiectasis, areas of decreased attenuation of the lung parenchyma adjacent to the abnormal airways can be identified; this pattern of mosaic attenuation is thought to reflect accompanying small airways disease, and the extent of the pattern correlates well with functional evidence of airflow obstruction, particularly indices of small airways dysfunction.

A positive diagnosis of bronchiectasis on HRCT is straightforward in patients who have moderate and severe disease. However, in some situations subtle signs of bronchiectasis may be obscured by technical artifacts. Conversely, the HRCT appearances of bronchiectasis may be mimicked by other lung pathologies. Some of the causes of false negative and false positive diagnoses of bronchiectasis are listed in Fig. 1.129.

Interest in the ability of HRCT to detect small airways disease is increasing[33]. In the exudative form of bronchiolar disease (typified by Japanese panbronchiolitis), HRCT directly shows the plugged small airways as small irregular branching opacities. The HRCT signs of constrictive obliterative bronchiolitis (e.g.

in patients who have rheumatoid arthritis or postviral obliterative bronchiolitis) are indirect – areas of decreased attenuation occur within which the vessels are of reduced caliber (but not distorted, in contrast to emphysema). The areas of decreased attenuation may merge with those of more normal lung or may have sharply demarcated, 'geographic' boundaries (mosaic attenuation pattern). The density differences that characterize constrictive obliterative bronchiolitis may be extremely subtle, but because they represent areas of reduced ventilation, and thus air trapping, they may be dramatically emphasized on scans performed at end expiration. The majority of patients affected by small airways disease have some bronchiectatic changes on HRCT, which tend to be more severe in those who have immunologically mediated obliterative bronchiolitis (e.g. following lung transplantation).

High-resolution computed tomography in the immunocompromised host
Pulmonary infections in immunocompromised patients
Pulmonary opportunistic infections are a common complication in immunocompromised patients[34]. The radiographic appearances are often nonspecific, and high morbidity and mortality are associated with chest infection in these patients. To maximize the diagnostic yield of radiography and HRCT, the

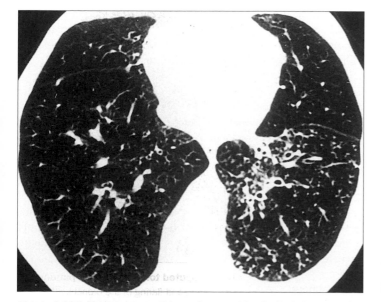

Figure 1.128 Numerous small irregular opacities in the left lower lobe representing plugged bronchioles. This is a case of panbronchiolitis.

Causes of false-positive and false-negative diagnoses of bronchiectasis on high-resolution computed tomography	
False negatives	**False positives**
Inappropriately thick computed tomography section	Cardiac pulsation causing 'double vessels'
Movement artifact obscures lung detail	Confluence of subsegmental bronchi may give spurious impression of bronchiectasis, at a single level (particularly in the lower lobes)
Focal, inconspicuous, thin-walled bronchiectasis	Cavitating nodules mimicking bronchiectasis (e.g. Langerhans' cell histiocytosis)
Bronchiectatic airways masked by surrounding fibrosis	Reversible dilatation of bronchi with acute pneumonic consolidation

Figure 1.129 Causes of false positive and false negative diagnosis of bronchiectasis on high-resolution computed tomography.

underlying cause of immunodeficiency, type of immunosuppressive therapy, white blood cell count, and overall medical status of the patient must be known. The introduction of HRCT now makes it possible to offer earlier and more specific diagnostic information. Furthermore, HRCT allows prediction of the relative chances of obtaining a positive diagnosis from transbronchial versus percutaneous biopsy, particularly when other techniques have proved nondiagnostic.

Bacterial pneumonias are the most frequent pulmonary infection in the immunocompromised patient. Usually, HRCT is reserved for those patients in whom the chest radiograph is equivocal for the presence of abnormality or in whom infective complications require further assessment. Invasive aspergillosis may occur in patients following solid organ or bone marrow transplantation. Diagnosis may be difficult, and an early CT scan has been suggested in the investigation of the immunocompromised patient who has clinical evidence of chest infection but a normal chest radiograph.

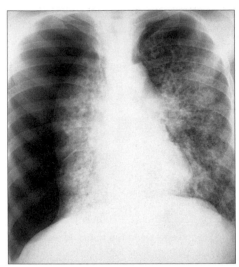

Figure 1.130 A case of *Pneumocystis carinii* pneumonia. The bilateral pneumothoraces are smaller on the left than on the right. Extensive cystic changes are present throughout both lungs.

Acquired immune deficiency syndrome

Although a wide variety of infectious and noninfectious pulmonary diseases occur in acquired immune deficiency syndrome (AIDS), the most common remains opportunistic infection[35]. The role of HRCT in AIDS varies from institution to institution. Although a wide variety of different pathologies have been characterized on HRCT, the diagnosis is more usually made from a combination of clinical and laboratory features, coupled with typical radiology. If necessary, more invasive tests, such as induced sputum analysis or bronchoscopy with biopsy or washings, can establish the diagnosis. Although HRCT is able to characterize an abnormality or confirm that an abnormality is present when the chest radiograph is equivocal, it does not in general allow a specific diagnosis, even though its diagnostic performance is superior to that of plain chest radiography.

Pneumocystis carinii pneumonia

Pneumocystis carinii pneumonia (PCP) is a protozoal infection that occurs in all groups of immunocompromised patients who have reduced cell-mediated immunity, but is particularly common in AIDS. On HRCT scanning the characteristic appearances are ground-glass infiltrates that extend from the hilar regions into the surrounding lung, and occasionally demonstrate a geographic pattern. Cavities, usually thin walled, but occasionally with a wall up to several millimeters thick, may develop (see Fig. 1.34). Appearances may return entirely to normal, although some residual scarring and cyst formation is common. Pneumothoraces often occur late in the course of the disease, tube drainage may be ineffective, and pleurodesis may be required (Fig. 1.130). Many less common manifestations of PCP are described on HRCT, which include miliary disease, discrete pulmonary nodules, pleural effusions, and mediastinal lymphadenopathy. While the radiographic changes may be highly suggestive of PCP (Fig. 1.131), the diagnosis is usually made on examination of induced sputum, which has a reported yield of approximately 80–90%.

Bacterial pneumonia

Patients who suffer AIDS are prone to community-acquired pneumonias such as those caused by *Streptococcus pneumoniae*, *Staphylococcus aureus*, and *Pseudomonas aeruginosa*. While disease progression may be unusually rapid and severe in this patient

group, with cavitation and pleural effusions being more frequent than in nonimmunocompromised patients (Fig. 1.132), most commonly the pattern of disease is the same as in the normal population. There may be a role for HRCT in the detection of additional complications, such as abscess formation, bronchopleural fistula, and empyema.

Tuberculosis

Radiologic manifestations of tuberculosis caused by *Mycobacterium tuberculosis* depend on the degree of immunosuppression. In the early stages of human immunodeficiency virus (HIV) infection, appearances are similar to those of reactivation tuberculosis in the normal population (Fig. 1.133). When the CD4+-lymphocyte count falls in the later stages of HIV disease, radiographic appearances become more in keeping with primary tuberculosis. Cavitation becomes less common and, on CT scanning, mediastinal nodal enlargement typically shows marked, central, low density change with a rim of enhancing tissue. Changes on HRCT include nonspecific areas of pulmonary consolidation and the presence of pulmonary nodules, which are frequently centrilobular and branching.

Within the chest, appearances of *Mycobacterium avium-intracellulare* infection are similar to those of *M. tuberculosis* infection, although pleural effusions are more common with the former and miliary disease is particularly uncommon.

Cytomegalovirus

Although cytomegalovirus (CMV) inclusion bodies are a frequent finding in lung material from AIDS patients, CMV rarely causes clinical infection; when identified in patients affected by acute pulmonary disease, it is often in association with other pathogenic organisms.

Toxoplasmosis

A high prevalence of previous exposure to toxoplasmosis exists in the HIV-positive adult population. However, significant pulmonary involvement is distinctly unusual, despite the frequent occurrence of central nervous system toxoplasmosis.

Histoplasmosis

Histoplasma capsulatum infection occurs in patients who have visited or reside in areas where the organism is endemic, such as

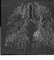

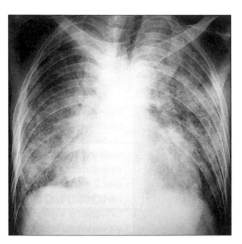

Figure 1.131 Diffuse and severe ground-glass and air-space infiltrate from *Pneumocystis carinii* pneumonia.

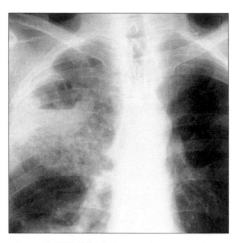

Figure 1.132 Staphylococcal pneumonia. An air–fluid level within a cavity is surrounded by more confluent consolidation.

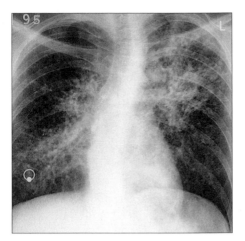

Figure 1.133 Reactivation tuberculosis in an HIV-positive patient. Bilateral bronchopneumonia shows multiple nodules up to 5mm in diameter.

the central United States and Central and South America. The diagnosis is usually made from bone marrow aspirate and culture.

Coccidioidomycosis

Coccidioides immitis is also widespread in the central United States and occasionally causes disease in exposed AIDS patients. The radiographic features are nonspecific. Occasionally, solitary pulmonary nodules occur with this infection.

Cryptococcosis

When *Cryptococcus neoformans* causes clinical disease in the HIV population, usually the brain or meninges is infected, and when pulmonary disease occurs it is usually in association with central nervous system disease. Radiographic changes are nonspecific and include single or multiple nodules, consolidation with or without cavitation, interstitial infiltrates, and mediastinal lymph nodes.

Aspergillosis

Aspergillus fumigatus is an infrequent fungal infection in the HIV population, and occasionally causes pneumonic disease or discrete pulmonary nodules.

Noninfectious pulmonary disease in acquired immune deficiency syndrome
Kaposi's sarcoma
Kaposi's sarcoma occurs in approximately 10% of patients who have AIDS. Usually, cutaneous or visceral disease is evident when the lung is involved (Fig. 1.134) and HRCT is reserved for difficult diagnostic cases that do not show typical radiographic or bronchoscopic appearances. On the chest radiograph, Kaposi's sarcoma usually appears as ill-defined nodules, sometimes associated with pleural effusions and lymphadenopathy.

Miscellaneous lymphoproliferative disorders
A variety of lymphoproliferative disorders are associated with AIDS, including lymphocytic interstitial pneumonitis (seen most frequently in the non-AIDS population in association with Sjögren's syndrome and systemic lupus erythematosus). In the AIDS population, this occurs most frequently in children, although adult cases are regularly encountered. The radiologic appearances are most commonly a mid and lower zone reticular or reticulonodular infiltrate. Although radiographically indistinguishable from opportunistic infection, slow progression of radiologic

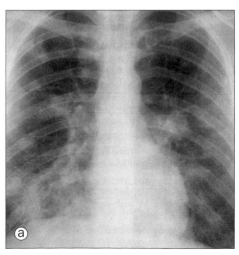

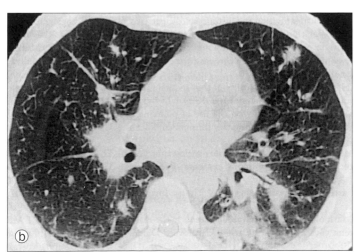

Figure 1.134 Kaposi's sarcoma in an HIV-positive patient. (a) Multiple, poorly defined pulmonary nodules are becoming confluent in the right lower zone. A small lamellar effusion is present bilaterally. (b) Computed tomography scan of the same patient as in (a) demonstrates the irregular outline to the pulmonary nodules, which are often related to bronchovascular bundles.

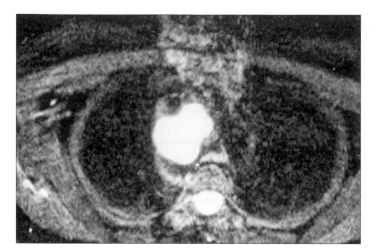

Figure 2.1 Mediastinal cyst. Transverse, T2-weighted image at the level of the aortic arch. A right-sided mediastinal mass lies anterior to the trachea and posterior to the superior vena cava. The mass shows homogeneous, very high signal similar to that of cerebrospinal fluid in the spine. These features confirm that it is a cyst.

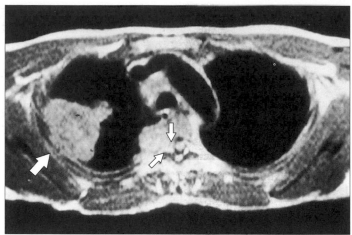

Figure 2.2 Squamous cell carcinoma of the lung with chest wall, spinal, and mediastinal invasion. Transverse, T1-weighted image at the level of the aortic arch shows a peripheral tumor invading the chest wall (arrow). Further mediastinal disease is invading the vertebral body and the right intervertebral foramen (small arrows). Enlarged mediastinal nodes are visible anterior to the trachea.

tumors, the reliability of MRI to show invasion of the chest wall (Figs 2.2–2.4) and mediastinum (as compared with opposition of the tumor and these structures) is at least as good as that of CT, and sometimes better. In a comprehensive review of the literature on staging malignant disease of the chest, Grover concluded that MRI performed better than CT for staging superior sulcus tumors, those that involved the aortopulmonary window, chest wall and diaphragm, and hilar nodes, as well as in patients with equivocal CT examinations[4]. However, the clinical benefit of using MRI rather than CT is questionable and commensurate improvements in outcome to compensate for the more lengthy and expensive procedure have not been shown. Some preliminary data suggest that MRI may be able to predict poor outcome of lung cancer better than can CT or surgical staging.

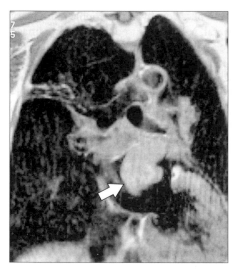

Figure 2.3 Adenocarcinoma with invasion of the mediastinum and left atrium. Coronal, T1-weighted images show extensive left intrapulmonary and mediastinal tumor. The left atrium is invaded by a large plug of tumor (arrow), but flowing (black) blood is seen to surround the tumor mass. Peripheral collapse is seen in the midzone of the right lung.

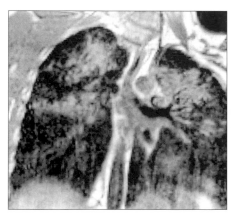

Figure 2.4 Kaposi's sarcoma. Coronal, T1-weighted scan through the chest shows tumor extending along the bronchovascular tree. Tumor is in the tracheal wall, surrounding the main bronchi and extending more peripherally into the lungs. Several smaller intrapulmonary nodules are apparent.

Pulmonary nodules

The role of MRI in the assessment of pulmonary nodules is limited because CT is easier to perform and interpret. With MRI, however, nodules may be easier to differentiate from blood vessels than with unenhanced CT, as they appear as soft-tissue nodules against a virtually signal-free, black background. Some preliminary evidence suggests that dynamic, enhanced MRI may improve the specificity of diagnosis of nodules[5].

Chronic lung disease

It is clear that CT, in particular high-resolution CT, generally images interstitial lung diseases better than MRI. However, it is possible that MRI gives slightly different information. It has been used to determine the water content of abnormal lung and from this the activity of the disease inferred since, in general, more active inflammatory disease has higher water content. This technique has been used for a number of chronic lung disorders, which include sarcoid, bronchiectasis, cystic fibrosis, bronchopulmonary aspergillosis, and aspergillomas (Fig. 2.5). In interstitial lung disease, a macromolecular gadolinium contrast agent has been used experimentally to differentiate between the active alveolitic and late fibrotic phases of disease[6].

A further use of MRI in chronic lung disease is for patients in whom multiple studies are required. To avoid excessive radiation, CT and MRI can be performed as baseline studies and the disease followed with MRI.

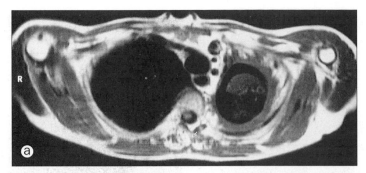

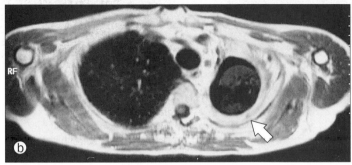

Figure 2.5 Intrapulmonary aspergilloma. Transverse T1-weighted scans made (a) before and (b) after contrast enhancement show a heterogeneous mass caused by an aspergilloma within the thick-walled cavity. The fungus ball does not enhance, whereas the inflammatory wall of the cavity shows strong enhancement (arrow).

Pulmonary emboli and infarction

Pulmonary MRA can now show fifth-order pulmonary vessels and large proximal emboli are seen[7]. First-pass, contrast-enhanced scans and fast-scan techniques (including echoplanar imaging) have been used to examine lung perfusion[8]. Smaller pulmonary emboli can be inferred by the lack of segmental and subsegmental perfusion. Three-dimensional MRA data sets can be acquired and displayed on workstations as moving projections, which helps to show areas of deficient perfusion.

Another area of intense interest has been in the use of polarized gases (helium-3 and xenon-129) to show pulmonary ventilation[9]. With this technique, a process of heating and irradiating with polarized light produces polarized gases. The gases (which have a short half-life) are inhaled and imaged using optimized sequences. The use of dual-frequency probes allows gas and proton images to be acquired and registered, which enables function and anatomy to be correlated.

The opaque lung

The opaque lung, which can result from any combination of collapsed and/or consolidated lung, pleural fluid, or thickening and masses (inflammatory or tumor), may be difficult to assess on CT because the X-ray attenuation of the different tissues may be too similar to differentiate. On MRI, the signal from the tissues is often different, and, coupled with the facility to image in the coronal plane, analysis of the pathology may be considerably easier.

Vascular malformations and congenital anomalies

Increasing evidence shows that MRI can clearly define a number of vascular and developmental anomalies of the lungs by combining anatomic and flow imaging, including the scimitar syndrome,

hypogenetic lung syndrome, pulmonary artery agenesis, bronchopulmonary sequestration, and vascular malformations[10].

Magnetic resonance of the mediastinum
Mediastinal masses

Mediastinal masses are generally well shown on MRI. By using multiple imaging planes, their anatomy is frequently shown better than on CT. As there is no artifact from bone, the involvement of the spine and spinal canal by paravertebral masses can be seen clearly (see Figs 2.2 & 2.6). By using flow-sensitive sequences, MRI can be used to differentiate enhancing masses from aneurysms.

The assessment of mediastinal nodes in such diseases as lung cancer and esophageal tumors generally depends on the size of nodes. Although MRI can show abnormal signal in nodes, this is nonspecific and occurs with reactive nodes and those involved by tumor. Consequently, CT, which is much faster, is the technique of choice in these cases. The facility of MRI to differentiate soft tissue from flowing blood without the use of contrast media can be extremely helpful when children need to be imaged (see Fig. 2.7). Obtaining venous access and delivering a sufficiently large bolus of contrast to opacify the great vessels through small cannulas may be difficult in small children and neonates. Paraspinal tumors, thymic masses, and mediastinal hemangiomas are all well shown on MRI.

Cardiovascular imaging

MRI is regarded as the definitive technique for imaging the aorta for dissection, some aneurysms, and coarctation, and it is widely used for the assessment of congenital heart disease. It can be used to assess cardiac anatomy and function, as well as pericardial disease, and is being used experimentally in some units to image the coronary arteries.

Mediastinal infection

There is little published experience of MRI in mediastinal infection, and this is mainly limited to tuberculous mediastinitis.

Magnetic resonance imaging of the chest wall and associated structures

As invasion is frequently better shown than on CT, MRI is effective for imaging the chest wall in malignant disease (see Figs 2.2 & 2.8). It is particularly useful for showing brachial plexus involvement in patients who have Pancoast tumors (see Fig. 2.9).

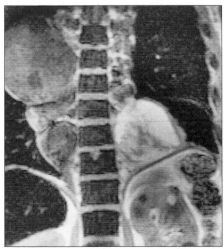

Figure 2.6 Extramedullary hemopoiesis in thalassemia intermedia. The coronal, T1-weighted image shows massive, lobulated, paravertebral masses caused by extramedullary hemopoiesis. The left-sided mass has a very high signal because of hemorrhage within the tumor. The very low signal in the vertebrae and liver results from iron deposition.

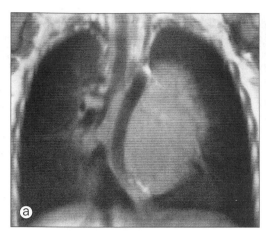

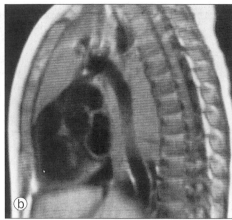

Figure 2.7 Mediastinal neuroblastoma. (a) Coronal and (b) sagittal, T1-weighted images of a 3-year-old child show a large mediastinal mass encasing and displacing the thoracic aorta. The aorta is clearly seen without the use of contrast because of flow void within the vessel.

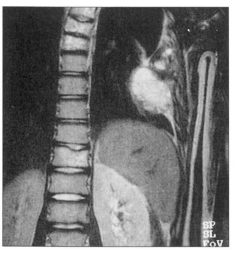

Figure 2.8 Primary, primitive neuroectodermal tumor of the chest wall. Coronal, T2-weighted, turbospin echo image. A large tumor arises from the left chest wall. Several of the thoracic vertebrae have abnormally increased signal and are partially collapsed, which indicates bony metastatic disease.

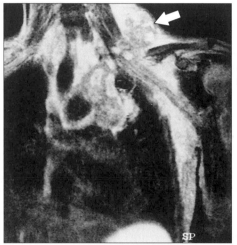

Figure 2.9 Pancoast tumor with invasion of the brachial plexus. Coronal, T2-weighted images show a high-signal mass in the left apex, which has invaded the base of the neck (arrow) to encase the subclavian vessels and infiltrate the left brachial plexus.

Imaging of the diaphragm is difficult on CT as it is a structure best seen in the coronal plane. Diaphragmatic defects and masses are often shown well by coronal MRI scans, but frequently ultrasound imaging from an abdominal approach gives the same information more cheaply and quickly.

RESEARCH

A considerable amount of research is underway on the use of MRI to assess pulmonary perfusion and ventilation, and to guide interventional procedures. The advantages MRI offers to such interventions are the lack of ionizing radiation to the patient and operator, multiplanar imaging, and temperature-sensitive sequences that potentially can show the efficacy of thermally active treatments (laser and radiofrequency therapies). Preliminary reports are emerging of the use of MRI to guide laser thermal ablation of lung tumor and pleural masses.

In conclusion, MRI has a restricted but complementary role to other imaging techniques for imaging the chest, but time and cost constraints limit its widespread use in general practice.

REFERENCES

1. Hanson JA, Armstrong P. Staging intrathoracic non-small-cell lung cancer. Eur Radiol. 1997;7:161–72.
2. Pugatch RD. Radiologic evaluation in chest malignancies. A review of imaging modalities. Chest. 1995;107(6 Suppl.):294S–7S.
3. Bonomo L, Ciccotosto C, Guidotti A, Storto ML. Lung cancer staging: the role of computed tomography and magnetic resonance imaging. Eur J Radiol. 1996;23:35–45.
4. Grover FL. The role of CT and MRI in staging of the mediastinum. Chest. 1994;106(6 Suppl.):391S–6S.
5. Hittmair K, Eckersberger F, Klepetko W, Helbich T, Herold CJ. Evaluation of solitary pulmonary nodules with dynamic contrast-enhanced MR imaging – a promising technique. Magn Reson Imaging. 1995;13:923–33.
6. Berthezene Y, Vexler V, Kuwatsuru R, et al. Differentiation of alveolitis and pulmonary fibrosis with a macromolecular MR imaging contrast agent. Radiology. 1992;185:97–103.
7. Amundsen T, Kvaerness J, Jones RA, et al. Pulmonary embolism: detection with MR perfusion imaging of the lung – a feasibility study. Radiology. 1997;203:181–5.
8. Hatabu H, Gaa J, Kim D, Li W, Prasad PV, Edelman RR. Pulmonary perfusion: qualitative assessment with dynamic contrast-enhanced MRI using ultra-short TE and inversion recovery turbo FLASH. Magn Reson Med. 1996;36:503–8.
9. Gao JH, Lemen L, Xiong J, Patyal B, Fox PT. Magnetization and diffusion effects in NMR imaging of hyperpolarized substances. Magn Reson Med. 1997;37:153–8.
10. Silverman JM, Julien PJ, Herfkens RJ, Pelc NJ. Magnetic resonance imaging evaluation of pulmonary vascular malformations. Chest. 1994;106:1333–8.

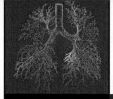

Chapter 3

Radionuclide Scanning

Michael M Graham

In the lung, radioactive tracers are most commonly used to determine the distribution of perfusion and ventilation. However, this approach can also be used to measure permeability, mucociliary clearance, receptor density, and the presence or absence of inflammation, infection, aspiration, or right-to-left shunting. In each of these studies the amount of tracer used is microscopic. Thus, there is essentially no risk of allergic reactions and no risk of changing the parameter of interest by the test itself. The most common radiolabeled tracers used in studies of the lung are listed in Figure 3.1.

PERFUSION

Relative pulmonary perfusion via the pulmonary artery can be determined from images following the injection of technetium-99m (^{99m}Tc) macroaggregated albumin (MAA). The average diameter of the particles is 20–40mm, with 3–4% small enough to pass through the pulmonary capillaries, and the remainder are trapped in a distribution proportional to regional blood flow. The relative counts over the left and right lungs equate to the relative perfusion to the two lungs, a ratio that is useful in predicting postoperative pulmonary function in patients planned for pneumonectomy[1] and in predicting the effect of radiation injury to the

lung. Gamma camera imaging does not yield measures of absolute perfusion, but it is used to determine relative perfusion in different regions and to compare ventilation and perfusion with single photon emission computed tomographic imaging[2].

The most common use of pulmonary perfusion imaging is in patients who have suspected pulmonary embolus (Figs 3.2–3.5)[3].

Common radiotracers used in pulmonary nuclear medicine studies	
Agent	**Use**
Technetium-99m macroaggregated albumin	Perfusion
Technetium-99m pentetate	Ventilation, permeability
Technetium-99m albumin microcolloid	Ventilation, mucociliary clearance
Technetium-99m red blood cells	Bleeding, blood volume
Indium-111 white blood cells	Infection
Xenon-133	Ventilation
Krypton-81m	Ventilation
Gallium-67	Inflammation

Figure 3.1 Common radiotracers used in pulmonary nuclear medicine studies.

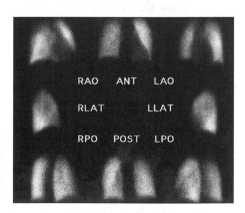

Figure 3.2 Lung perfusion in a normal subject. Technetium-99m macroaggregated albumin was injected intravenously. The gamma camera images were acquired, beginning 1–2 minutes later. The images were acquired at 45° increments to yield eight images. The cardiac impression on the left is the only significant asymmetry seen. (RAO/LAO, right/left anterior oblique; ANT, anterior view; RLAT/LLAT, right/left lateral view; RPO/LPO, right/left posterior oblique; POST, posterior view.)

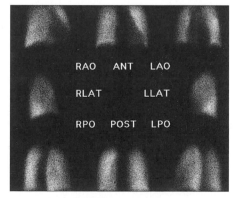

Figure 3.3 Ventilation in the same normal subject as shown in Figure 3.2. Technetium-99m albumin microcolloid was administered via a nebulizer for 2–3 minutes. Albumin microcolloid clears very slowly from the lung over many days. The gamma camera images were acquired immediately after inhalation. (RAO/LAO, right/left anterior oblique; ANT, anterior view; RLAT/LLAT, right/left lateral view; RPO/LPO, right/left posterior oblique; POST, posterior view.)

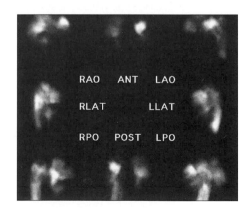

Figure 3.4 Lung perfusion in a subject who has multiple pulmonary emboli. Multiple defects of perfusion are seen. The posterior–basal and anterior–medial–basal segments of the left lower lobe are completely missing. Numerous other subsegmental defects are present throughout both lungs. (RAO/LAO, right/left anterior oblique; ANT, anterior view; RLAT/LLAT, right/left lateral view; RPO/LPO, right/left posterior oblique; POST, posterior view.)

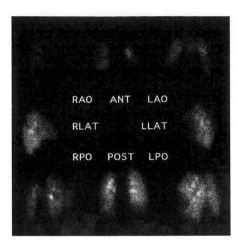

Figure 3.5 Ventilation in the same subject as shown in Figure 3.4. Technetium-99m pentetic acid was administered via a nebulizer for 2–3 minutes, and the gamma camera images acquired immediately thereafter. The images show good ventilation to all segments, which is important in concluding that the patient probably has pulmonary emboli. If the ventilation images looked similar to the perfusion images in Figure 3.3, then the cause of the defects might be other problems such as airways obstruction. The increased activity seen in the medial part of the lung results from deposition of aerosol on the large airways and is usually associated with excessive secretions and airway narrowing. It can also be caused by large aerosol particles. Note that the activity is lower in the top row of images, particularly in the RAO view. This is because pentetic acid is cleared from the lung into the bloodstream and these images were acquired last. Rapid clearance, as seen in this patient, implies increased pulmonary epithelial permeability. (RAO/LAO, right/left anterior oblique; ANT, anterior view; RLAT/LLAT, right/left lateral view; RPO/LPO, right/left posterior oblique; POST, posterior view.)

	Amended Prospective Investigation of Pulmonary Embolism Diagnosis interpretation criteria for ventilation–perfusion lung scans
Probability	**Interpretation**
High	Two or more large (>75% of a segment) segmental perfusion defects without corresponding ventilation or chest radiograph abnormality
	One large segmental perfusion defect and two or more moderate (25–75% of a segment) segmental perfusion defects without corresponding ventilation or chest radiograph abnormalities
	Four or more moderate segmental perfusion defects without corresponding ventilation or chest radiograph abnormalities
Intermediate	Two moderate or one large segmental perfusion defects without corresponding ventilation or chest radiograph abnormality
	One moderate, matched ventilation–perfusion defect with normal chest radiograph
	Corresponding ventilation–perfusion defects and chest radiograph parenchymal opacity in lower lung zone
	Corresponding ventilation–perfusion defects and small pleural effusion
	Difficult to categorize as normal, low, or high probability
Low	Multiple, matched ventilation–perfusion defects regardless of size, with normal chest radiograph
	Corresponding ventilation–perfusion defects and chest radiograph parenchymal opacity in upper or middle lung zones
	Corresponding ventilation–perfusion defects and large pleural effusion
	Any perfusion defects with substantially larger chest radiograph abnormality
	Defects surrounded by normally perfused lung (stripe sign)
	Four or more small (<25% of a segment) segmental perfusion defects with normal chest radiograph
	Nonsegmental perfusion defects (cardiomegaly, aortic impression, enlarged hila)
Very low	Three or fewer small segmental perfusion defects with normal chest radiograph
Normal	No perfusion defects and perfusion outlines the shape of the lung as seen on chest radiograph

Figure 3.6 Amended Prospective Investigation of Pulmonary Embolism Diagnosis interpretation criteria for ventilation–perfusion lung scans. (Adapted from Worsley and Alavi.[4])

The accuracy of ventilation–perfusion ($\dot{V}/\dot{Q}$) scintigraphy in the diagnosis of pulmonary embolism was evaluated in a large clinical trial, the Prospective Investigation of Pulmonary Embolism Diagnosis (PIOPED)[4]. Retrospectively, following examination of the results of the study, the modified PIOPED criteria (Fig. 3.6) for interpretation of $\dot{V}/\dot{Q}$ studies were developed and are currently the most widely used criteria for interpretation; further refinements are continuing[5].

An alternative approach for quantitative determination of regional pulmonary blood flow is to use a bolus injection of oxygen-15 water (half-life of 2 minutes) with rapid positron emission tomography imaging, while rapidly sampling blood from the pulmonary artery[6]. Immediately after injection, oxygen-15 water distributes proportionally to blood flow. The major advantage of this approach is that repeated studies can be undertaken at 10–15 minute intervals to observe changes in blood flow.

VENTILATION

Xenon-133

Radioactive xenon is administered using a specialized rebreathing apparatus. Imaging is usually performed from the posterior view (Fig. 3.7). The initial first breath image is one of relative ventilation (i.e. high count areas are well ventilated and low count areas are poorly ventilated). During equilibration, the patient rebreathes radioactive xenon at constant concentration. A carbon dioxide absorber is usually in the circuit, as well as the capability to add oxygen. During the equilibrium phase of the procedure, all regions of the lung approach the same level of radioactivity, such that poorly ventilated regions have the same activity as well-ventilated regions. Equilibration takes some time – at least 3 minutes, and preferably 5 minutes to ensure that very poorly ventilated regions equilibrate. The washout images show residual increased activity in regions of poor ventilation (Fig. 3.8).

Krypton-81m

Krypton-81m (^{81m}Kr) is the other radioactive gas commonly used for ventilation imaging; it has a half-life of 13 seconds, and is produced from a generator that contains rubidium-81 (^{81}Rb). The ^{81}Rb half-life is 4.6 hours, which limits the use of the ^{81m}Kr generator to 1 day. The ^{81m}Kr is delivered directly to the patient via nasal prongs or a mask, and when inhaled it rapidly

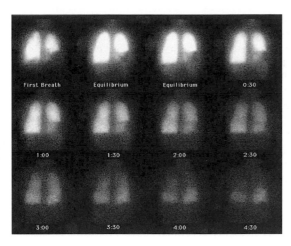

Figure 3.7 Xenon-133 images of ventilation. The images are in the posterior view. The first breath image is acquired immediately after the subject inhales the bolus of xenon-133 in air, image duration is typically 20–30 seconds. The equilibration images are taken while the subject rebreathes the xenon-133 at constant concentration. During this phase, all portions of the lung approach the same concentration of activity. The washout images are labeled with the starting time of their acquisition, and each image is of 30 seconds duration. The first breath image shows impaired ventilation of the right lower lung. This area fills in during the equilibration period and shows persistent activity during the washout phase.

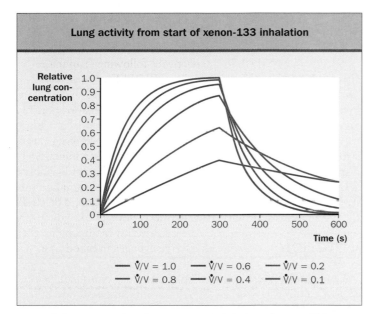

Figure 3.8 Lung activity after beginning inhalation of xenon-133 at a constant concentration. Ventilation per unit lung volume ($\dot{V}/V$, L/min per liter lung volume) varies from normal levels at around 1.0 to quite low values of 0.1. At normal levels of ventilation, lung activity reaches the concentration of the inhaled gas. At lower levels of ventilation, equilibration is reached much more slowly such that, for a $\dot{V}/V$ of 0.1L/min at 5 minutes, lung concentration is only about 40% of the inspired concentration. In these plots, at 5 minutes the inspired concentration is suddenly set equal to zero and the xenon begins to wash out. Note that washout is much slower from the poorly ventilated lung, such that at relatively long times after the start of washout, the more poorly ventilated portions of the lung show greater amounts of activity. This illustrates how xenon-133 ventilation imaging is quite sensitive for identifying regions of the lung with poor ventilation or air trapping.

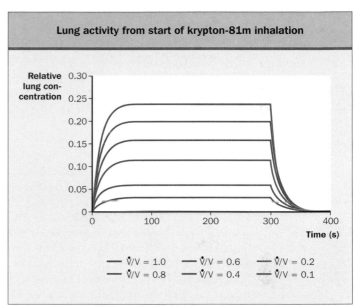

Figure 3.9 Lung activity after beginning inhalation of krypton-81m at a constant concentration. Krypton-81m has a half-life of 13 seconds. After a few half-lives the system equilibrates, such that krypton decays away as fast as it is delivered to the lung. At normal and low levels of ventilation, lung activity is directly proportional to the degree of ventilation, so a lung image accurately reflects regional ventilation. In these plots, at 5 minutes the inspired concentration is suddenly set equal to zero and the krypton begins to washout as well as decay. By 6 minutes most of the activity has disappeared. ($\dot{V}/V$, ventilation per unit lung volume.)

Aerosol imaging of ventilation

Aerosol particles deposit at different levels in the lung, depending on the size of the particles. Most research on the distribution of aerosol particles in the lung is with radiolabeled aerosols. When the particles have diameters of around 1 µm, most of the deposition occurs in distal airways and alveoli. If the particles are labeled with ^{99m}Tc, the resultant gamma camera images give a reasonable approximation of the distribution of ventilation[7]. Although ^{99m}Tc aerosol images can be used to determine roughly the ratio of ventilation between the two lungs, a more detailed quantitation is usually not useful because of variable deposition of the aerosol particles in larger airways. This is particularly

distributes through the air spaces within the lung. After several half-lives (i.e. about 1 minute), an equilibrium state is reached, in which the ^{81m}Kr decays as rapidly as it is replenished. A well-ventilated area has a relatively high concentration of ^{81m}Kr, while a poorly ventilated region contains relatively little activity. Over the range of normal ventilation of the lung, the relationship between ^{81m}Kr concentration and ventilation is approximately linear (Fig. 3.9).

1

3.3

prominent in patients who suffer bronchiectasis, but many patients who have obstructive airways disease show a pattern of increased central deposition.

The major principle behind aerosol ventilation imaging is that no radioactive deposition ocurrs in an unventilated lung. Thus, aerosol ventilation images can be compared with Tc MAA images to determine whether an area with absent perfusion also has absent ventilation (see Figs 3.4 & 3.5). The main advantage of aerosol ventilation imaging over xenon is that images can be obtained in all views and can easily be compared with the perfusion images.

The most commonly used agent for aerosol imaging is ^{99m}Tc DTPA [diethylenetriaminepenta-acetic acid (pentetic acid); see Fig. 3.5]. It is uncharged and can diffuse freely across the pulmonary epithelium into the vascular space, and is cleared from the body via glomerular filtration. Immediately after inhalation, the DTPA aerosol distribution gives a good picture of the distribution of ventilation. Over the next few minutes, it slowly clears from the lung, the speed depending on epithelial permeability. This can be used to measure permeability (see below), but it can be a problem in that delayed images may show little activity remaining in peripheral lung. Another approach is to use a nonabsorbable tracer such as albumin, albumin microcolloid (see Fig. 3.3), or sulfur colloid. These can all be labeled with ^{99m}Tc and can be easily nebulized.

Technegas and Pertechnegas

Technegas and Pertechnegas are very fine aerosol particles with diameters of less than 0.1μm. Technegas is produced by placing pertechnetate in a carbon crucible and rapidly heating it to 2500°C in an argon atmosphere. The particles are insoluble and clear very slowly from the lungs. Pertechnegas is prepared in the same way as Technegas, except in an atmosphere of 3% oxygen and 97% argon[8]. The resultant particles are dry pertechnetate, which is soluble and rapidly clears from the lungs. The quality of the initial images taken immediately after inhalation is excellent, similar to those obtained with Technegas. However, because the agent washes out rapidly, later images are of lower quality.

PERMEABILITY

The primary mechanism of clearance of small, water-soluble molecules from the lung is via diffusion into tissue and then into the bloodstream. The most commonly used tracer for studying the clearance of small molecules is ^{99m}Tc DTPA, an approach used in many studies to investigate lung permeability in smokers[9], infection[10], radiation injury[11], and adult respiratory distress syndrome[12]. The studies are relatively easy to perform and analyze. An important consideration is that the results are very dependent on the type of nebulizer used and the placement of the regions of interest during analysis. As a consequence of this strong effect, it is necessary to establish normal values and to standardize the methods.

The other aspect of lung permeability that can be investigated with tracer techniques is vascular permeability using labeled macromolecules. Studies have been carried out with labeled albumin (iodine-131 or -125) and transferrin, which is labeled *in vivo* by injecting gallium-67 (^{67}Ga), ^{68}Ga, indium-111 (^{111}In), or iron-59[13]. In all studies with labeled macromolecules, the study takes at least 30–60 minutes. Dynamic images are acquired to determine the rate of increase of activity over the

lungs, which indicates leakage of activity out of the plasma into the interstitial space.

MUCOCILIARY CLEARANCE

Aerosol particles of approximately 5μm diameter deposit mainly onto the walls of bronchi, where they are slowly cleared from the lung by mucociliary clearance. The tracer used must be nonabsorbable so that changes in activity only relate to physical clearance, not diffusion into the bloodstream. Agents used include ^{99m}Tc labeled albumin, albumin microcolloid, MAA, and sulfur colloid. The most critical aspect of these studies is standardization of the nebulizer particle size to ensure consistent, reproducible studies. The studies are conducted much like those of lung epithelial permeability described above. Following inhalation of the appropriate aerosol, dynamic images are acquired and then analyzed with a central region of interest. These studies have been used to evaluate patients who have cystic fibrosis[14], bronchiolitis and bronchiectasis[15], and in comparisons of smokers with normal subjects[16].

INFLAMMATION

When injected intravenously, ^{67}Ga binds to transferrin and is taken up by inflammation, infection, and tumors. In the lung, ^{67}Ga has been useful in the evaluation of patients who have interstitial fibrosis[17], sarcoidosis[18], radiation injury[13], and infections associated with acquired immunodeficiency syndrome. A grading scheme has been developed (0 = background, 4 = uptake similar to liver) that correlates with disease severity and also provides a way to monitor response to therapy[19].

INFECTION

White blood cells (WBC) labeled with ^{111}In accumulate in areas of acute infection. Studies with this agent can be used to detect empyema and pneumonia[20]. In the case of pneumonia, activity is often seen at the site of the infection and in the gastrointestinal tract because of swallowed sputum. An alternative approach for labeling WBCs is to use ^{99m}Tc hexamethylpropyleneamine oxide (HMPAO). This agent, which is usually used for cerebral perfusion imaging, is highly lipophilic and labels cells *in vitro* very readily. Since the image quality of WBCs labeled with ^{99m}Tc HMPAO is far higher than that with ^{111}In, they can be imaged within 1–2 hours of injection.

ASPIRATION

Sulfur colloid labeled with ^{99m}Tc and suspended in water has been used to study swallowing, esophageal reflux, and gastric emptying. It can also be used to document reflux with aspiration by demonstrating activity in the lungs following oral administration of the radioactive tracer.

RIGHT-TO-LEFT SHUNTS

A convenient way to demonstrate and quantitate right-to-left shunting is to inject ^{99m}Tc MAA intravenously and obtain a whole body image. If there is no shunt, then >96% of the injected activity should be in the lungs. Usually a small amount of physiologic shunting occurs, as well as a small amount of breakdown of the MAA, which results in up to 4% of the injected activity not being trapped by the lungs. If a right-to-left shunt is present, a larger fraction of the injected activity will not be trapped and is deposited in systemic arterioles. If a shunt is present, the whole body images show obvious activity, particularly in high-flow organs such as the brain and kidneys.

RECEPTORS

The lung contains large numbers of receptor sites responsible for many functions. Many of these receptor systems can be studied using radiolabeled ligands to define receptor density, distribution, and affinity. The systems studied include the β-adrenergic, muscarinic, and angiotensin II receptors[21]. Most of these studies have been carried out using positron-emitting radionuclides and positron tomographs.

PHARMACOKINETICS

Radionuclide tracer methodology is a natural approach to determining the distribution of pharmaceuticals by labeling a drug and following its activity after injection or inhalation[22]. This approach has been used for several different drugs and will continue to be a powerful tool in pharmacokinetics.

CONCLUSION

Nuclear medicine techniques are an important clinical tool and provide a powerful, noninvasive method to study the physiology of the lung in many ways. The methodology is available in virtually every hospital and is quite easily applied. Whenever physiologic studies of the lung are proposed in humans, it is important to consider the use of nuclear medicine as the techniques can often directly measure the parameter of interest.

REFERENCES

1. Larsen KR, Lund JO, Svendsen UG, Milman N, Petersen BN. Prediction of post-operative cardiopulmonary function using perfusion scintigraphy in patients with bronchogenic carcinoma. Clin Physiol. 1997;17:257–67.
2. Lamm WJ, Graham MM, Albert RK. Mechanism by which the prone position improves oxygenation in acute lung injury. Am J Respir Crit Care Med. 1994;150:184–93.
3. Stein PD. Diagnosis and management of pulmonary embolism. Curr Opin Cardiol. 1996;11:543–9.
4. Worsley DF, Alavi A. Comprehensive analysis of the results of the Prospective Investigation of Pulmonary Embolism Diagnosis Study. J Nucl Med. 1995;36:2380–7.
5. Freitas JE, Sarosi MG, Nagle CC, et al. Modified PIOPED criteria used in clinical practice. J Nucl Med. 1995;36:1573–8.
6. Mintun MA, Ter-Pogossian MM, Green MA, Lich LL, Schuster DP. Quantitative measurement of regional pulmonary blood flow with positron emission tomography. J Appl Physiol. 1986;60:317–26.
7. Brain JD, Valberg PA. Deposition of aerosol in the respiratory tract. Am Rev Respir Dis. 1979;120:1325–73.
8. Scalzetti EM, Gagne GM. The transition from technegas to pertechnegas. J Nucl Med. 1995;36:267–9.
9. Effros RM, Mason GR, Mena I. ^{99m}Tc-DTPA aerosol deposition and clearance in COPD, interstitial disease, and smokers. J Thorac Imaging. 1986;1:54–60.
10. Mason GR, Duane GB, Mena I, Effros RM. Accelerated solute clearance in *Pneumocystis carinii* pneumonia. Am Rev Respir Dis. 1987;135:864–8.
11. Susskind H, Weber DA, Lau YH, et al. Impaired permeability in radiation-induced lung injury detected by technetium-99m-DTPA lung clearance. J Nucl Med. 1997;38:966–71.
12. Braude S, Nolop KB, Hughes JM, Barnes PJ, Royston D. Comparison of lung vascular and epithelial permeability indices in the adult respiratory distress syndrome. Am Rev Respir Dis. 1986;133:1002–5.
13. Otsuki N, Brunetti A, Owens ES, Finn RD, Blasberg RG. Comparison of iron-59, indium-111, and gallium-69 transferrin as a macromolecular tracer of vascular permeability and the transferrin receptor. J Nucl Med. 1989;30:1676–85.

14. Regnis JA, Robinson M, Bailey DL, et al. Mucociliary clearance in patients with cystic fibrosis and in normal subjects. Am J Respir Crit Care Med. 1994;150:66–71.

15. Imai T, Sasaki Y, Ohishi H, et al. Clinical aerosol inhalation cine-scintigraphy to evaluate mucociliary transport system in diffuse pan-bronchiolitis. J Nucl Med. 1995;36:1355–62.

16. Chinet T, Collignon MA, Lemarchand P, Barritault L, Huchon G. Effects of smoking on bronchial clearance of technetium-99m-DTPA and indium-113m-DTPA. J Nucl Med. 1995;36:1569–72.

17. Neumann RD, Sostman HD. [67]Ga scintigraphy of the thorax. Chest. 1984;86:253–6.

18. Alberts C, van-der-Schoot JB. Standardized quantitative ^{67}Ga scintigraphy in pulmonary sarcoidosis. Sarcoidosis. 1988;5:111–18.

19. Line BR, Fulmer JD, Reynolds HY, et al. Gallium-67 citrate scanning in the staging of idiopathic pulmonary fibrosis: correlation and physiologic and morphologic features and bronchoalveolar lavage. Am Rev Respir Dis. 1978;118:355–65.

20. Oates E, Ramberg K. Imaging of intrathoracic disease with indium 111-labeled leukocytes. J Thorac Imaging. 1990;5:78–88.

21. Markham J, McCarthy TJ, Welch MJ, Schuster DP. In vivo measurements of pulmonary angiotensin-converting enzyme kinetics. I. Theory and error analysis. J Appl Physiol. 1995;78:1158–68.

22. Rhodes CG, Hughes JM. Pulmonary studies using positron emission tomography. Eur Respir J. 1995;8:1001–17.

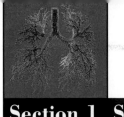

Physiology

Bruce H Culver

Units in this chapter are expressed in mmHg, Torr, or cmH₂O. Conversion into SI units is excluded because the resultant excessive numbers would interrupt the flow of the text. This chapter explains the principles of respiratory physiology, and the reader can follow these without continuously converting into the SI system. Should the reader need SI units at any point, the main conversion factors are:

- 1kPa = 7.6mmHg or Torr;
- 1kPa = 10cmH₂0;
- 1kPa = 1% concentration of gas in the atmosphere; and
- 1mmol/min/kPa = 1mL/min/Hg.

INTRODUCTION

The physiology of respiration includes all the processes involved in the uptake of oxygen and the release of carbon dioxide in support of whole-body metabolism. The lungs, blood, heart, and circulation are inseparably related in this function, but the focus of this chapter is limited to the role of the lungs and their exchange of gases with the blood. The processes involved can be subdivided into the mechanics of the lungs and thorax, the steps of gas exchange from atmosphere to alveoli and from alveoli to blood, and the transport of gases in the blood. It is also necessary to consider the circulations of the lung, the control of ventilation, and the interactions of ventilation with the acid–base status of the blood. Clinical assessment of patients who have pulmonary symptoms is aided by physiologic measurements of pulmonary function at rest and with exercise.

STRUCTURE OF THE THORAX AND LUNGS

The physiology of the respiratory system cannot be considered independently of its structure, particularly those features that affect the mechanical function of the lungs.

Thorax

The bony thorax provides protection for the lungs, heart, and great vessels, but also allows the lungs to change volume from a minimum of 1.5–2.0L to a maximum of 6–8L. Such an expansion is accomplished by the articulation of the ribs, the arrangement of the muscles, and the motion of the diaphragm. The ribs articulate with the transverse processes of the thoracic vertebrae, and have flexible cartilaginous connections with the sternum. The ribs angle down, both from back to front and from midline to side, so that as they are elevated both the anteroposterior and transverse dimensions of the thorax increase (Fig. 4.1). The external intercostal muscles that angle down from posterior to anterior (Fig. 4.2) are well situated to elevate the ribs. With deep

inspiratory efforts, the first and second ribs are elevated and stabilized by the accessory muscles of respiration in the neck – the scaleni and sternocleidomastoids. Muscles of the back attached to the spine and scapulae also act to straighten and stabilize the back. If the scapulae and upper extremities are fixed, the pectoralis muscles can act to raise the ribs (e.g. holding onto a chair back or leaning against a wall when out of breath).

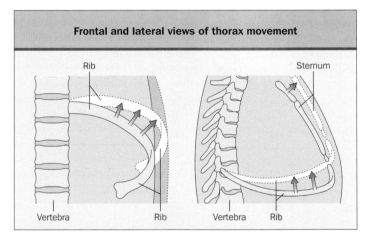

Figure 4.1 Frontal and lateral views of thorax movement. With rib elevation, both the transverse and anteroposterior dimensions increase.

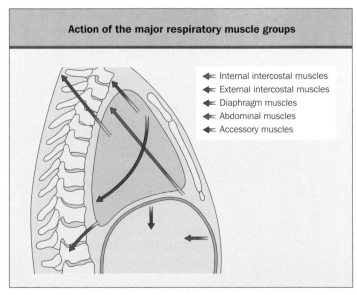

Figure 4.2 Action of the major respiratory muscle groups (intercostals, accessories, diaphragm, and abdominal).

Expiration is normally passive because of the elastic recoil of the lung, but can be assisted by the internal intercostal muscles once the eleventh and twelfth ribs are fixed by the quadratus lumborum to act as a base. Forced expiration (or coughing) requires the abdominal muscles to force the diaphragm upward.

The diaphragm is dome shaped in its relaxed position and can be pulled flatter by muscle contraction. It has a central, tendinous portion with muscular attachments anteriorly and laterally to the xiphoid and the lower ribs and tendinous attachments posteriorly. The diaphragm is most often described as fixed at the periphery so that its action pulls down the center of the dome (Fig. 4.3). However, if it is fixed centrally by the pressure of the abdominal contents, its action is to elevate the ribs. As a result of their articulation, the ribs have to swing outward when elevated, which increases the transverse diameter of the chest. The actual action of the diaphragm is a combination of these two mechanisms, in a proportion that varies with position and abdominal wall tension.

The intercostal muscles are innervated from the thoracic spine at their own level and the abdominal muscles are innervated from the lower thoracic and lumbar levels, but the diaphragm is served by the phrenic nerve, which originates at the cervical level (C3–C5). Thus, the diaphragm remains functional in patients who have spinal injuries below the midcervical level. However, the long course of each phrenic nerve along the mediastinum makes it vulnerable to both transient and permanent interruptions by disease, injury, or surgery. (Occasionally, irritation of a phrenic nerve leads to intractable hiccups.)

Pleural space

The lungs are covered by a thin visceral pleura, which is invaginated into the lobar fissures. The inner aspect of each hemithorax (and top of the diaphragm) is lined with the parietal pleura, which also covers the mediastinum and joins the visceral pleura on each side at the lung hilum. The pleural space between these two layers is a potential space that normally contains only a few milliliters of lubricating fluid. The pleural space extends deeply into the posterior and lateral costophrenic recesses.

The inspiratory force of the chest wall and diaphragm is transmitted to the lung by the creation of a more negative pressure in this potential space. In pathologic states, pleural effusions may form and necessarily make the lung volume smaller by occupying part of the intrathoracic space. Penetration of the chest wall or rupture of the lung surface can allow air to enter the pleural space and create a pneumothorax.

The airways

The upper respiratory passages (nasal cavities and pharynx) serve to conduct the air and to warm and moisten it on the way to the lungs. The respiratory system develops as an offshoot from the digestive system and, like the digestive system, has an absorptive function. It is exposed to particulate and infective agents and is protected by a well-developed lymphoid barrier and, more superficially, a mucous barrier. The upper respiratory passages contain the olfactory areas and conduct and help shape the sounds that produce speech.

The larynx opens off the lowest part of the pharynx and during swallowing is closed off from both the pharynx above and the esophagus posteriorly by the epiglottis. The trachea begins at the lower border of the cricoid cartilage of the larynx, at the level of the sixth cervical vertebra.

The lumen of the trachea is held open by incomplete, C-shaped cartilaginous rings. The posterior membranous portion contains smooth muscle. When the intrathoracic pressure exceeds the intraluminal pressure, the membranous portion is invaginated, the ends of the rings may overlap, and the lumen is greatly narrowed. Smooth muscle contraction narrows the lumen, but increases its rigidity. With deep inspiration the trachea enlarges and lengthens.

The trachea bifurcates into the main bronchi, which in turn become lobar, segmental, and subsegmental bronchi, and end in bronchioles that lack cartilage and are about 1mm in diameter.

Beyond the segmental and subsegmental bronchi and the bronchioles are the respiratory bronchioles, alveolar ducts, sacs, and alveoli that make up the respiratory zone in which gas exchange takes place. Smooth muscle, wound in clockwise and counterclockwise helical bands that overlap, increases proportionately in the smaller bronchioles to occupy about 20% of the wall thickness.

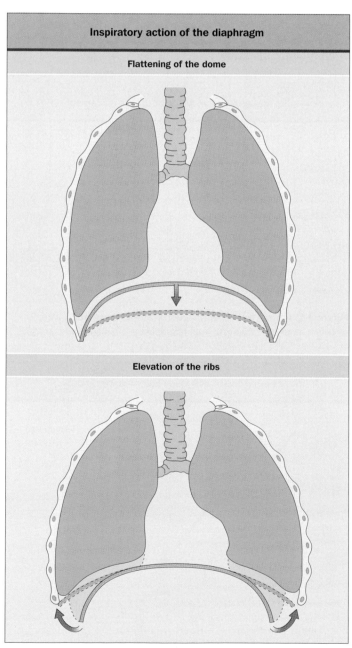

Inspiratory action of the diaphragm

Flattening of the dome

Elevation of the ribs

Figure 4.3 Action of the diaphragm. Inspiratory action includes both flattening the dome and elevation of the ribs.

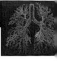

Elastic fibers are a well-developed component at every level of the respiratory system. They stretch when the lungs are expanded in inspiration and their elastic recoil helps to return the lungs to their unexpanded volume. In the smaller bronchi and in the bronchioles, the elastic tissue is a rich component of the connective tissue. While the smooth muscle stops at the portals of the respiratory zone, elastic and collagen fibers contribute to the alveolar wall, and form an irregular, wide-meshed net of delicate, interlacing fibers.

The number of airway generations required to reach the respiratory zone varies with pathway length, so that areas near the hilum may be reached in 15 generations while those in peripheral areas may require 25. Although the size of individual airways becomes smaller, the number of airways approximately doubles with each new generation, so that the total cross-sectional area of the combined air path increases. This is especially so in the smaller bronchi and bronchioles, for which the 'daughters' of each division are only slightly smaller than the 'parent'. The rapidly increasing total cross-sectional area of small airways, shown diagrammatically in Figure 4.4, means that their contribution to air-flow resistance in the lungs is small. Thus, diseases that affect these peripheral airways may be functionally 'silent' until an advanced state.

Interdependence in the lung

Since the lung parenchyma is made up of interconnected alveolar walls, interstitial tissues, and fibers, a local distortion is opposed by the surrounding tissue. That is, if a small zone of alveoli within a lobe begins to collapse, the surrounding tissue is stretched and thus tends to pull the zone back open. This property is termed structural interdependence. It, along with surfactant and the presence of collateral air pathways, helps to prevent the collapse of alveoli (atelectasis), even when small bronchioles become plugged[3]. Since the bronchi and blood vessels travel through the lung parenchyma, they too are affected by the surrounding tissue. As the lung expands, the caliber of these channels also increases.

RESPIRATORY MECHANICS

The properties of the lung and chest that affect and effect the movement of air in and out of the lungs are considered the 'mechanics' of ventilation and are central to understanding both normal and abnormal lung function. Many of the laboratory tests used clinically to assess lung disease are measurements of these static and dynamic mechanical properties.

Lung volumes

The total gas-containing capacity of the lungs can be divided into a series of volumes, as shown in Figure 4.5, which in combination give lung capacities[4]. The largest amount of air that can be held in the lungs at full inspiration is the total lung capacity (TLC). After a complete forced exhalation, the lungs are not empty but contain a residual volume (RV). The difference between TLC and RV, and thus the greatest volume of air that can be inhaled or exhaled, is the vital capacity (VC). This important clinical measurement of lung function can be affected by factors that limit either expansion of the lung or its emptying.

A normal breath has a tidal volume (V_T) that is only a small portion of VC (about 10%), and even during strenuous exercise V_T increases to only 50–60% of VC. Increases in V_T occur by utilizing parts of the inspiratory reserve volume and expiratory reserve volume shown in Figure 4.5. At the end of a relaxed tidal exhalation, the lungs return to a resting position, which is normally about 50% of TLC. The volume contained in the lungs at this end-tidal position is the functional residual capacity (FRC), and the volume that can be inhaled from this point is the inspiratory capacity (IC).

The lung–chest wall system

To understand the process of normal breathing, special maneuvers such as coughing, and the effects of positive pressure ventilators

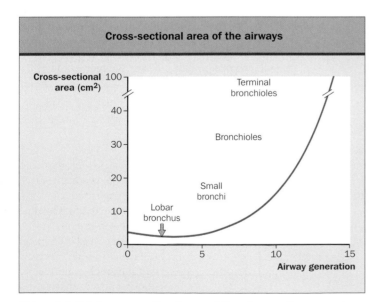

Figure 4.4 Total cross-sectional area of the airways. The aggregate luminal area increases greatly from about 2.5cm² in the trachea and major airways to over 100cm² at the level of the terminal bronchioles. (Modified with permission from Culver[1], data from Weibel[2].)

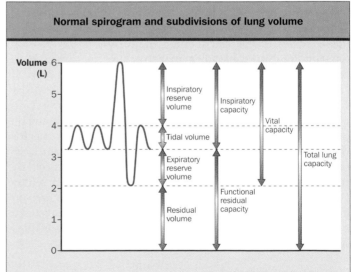

Figure 4.5 Normal spirogram and subdivisions of lung volume. By convention, 'volume' is used to describe the smallest subdivisions that do not overlap (residual volume, expiratory reserve volume, tidal volume, and inspiratory reserve volume), and 'capacity' is used to describe combinations of these volumes (functional residual capacity, inspiratory capacity, vital capacity, and total lung capacity)[4].

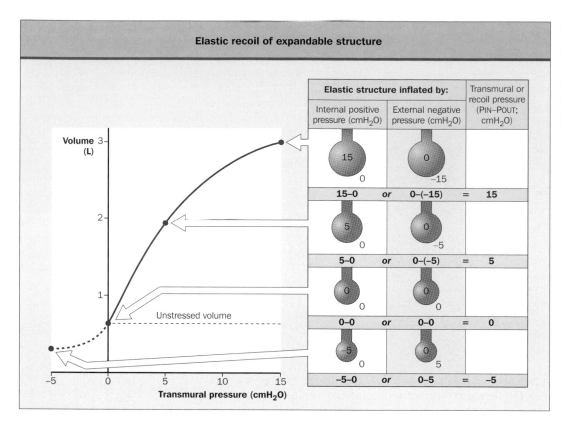

Elastic recoil of expandable structure

	Elastic structure inflated by:		Transmural or recoil pressure (P$_{IN}$–P$_{OUT}$; cmH$_2$O)
	Internal positive pressure (cmH$_2$O)	External negative pressure (cmH$_2$O)	
	15 / 0	0 / −15	
	15–0 *or*	**0–(−15)**	**=** **15**
	5 / 0	0 / −5	
	5–0 *or*	**0–(−5)**	**=** **5**
	0 / 0	0 / 0	
	0–0 *or*	**0–0**	**=** **0**
	−5 / 0	0 / 5	
	−5–0 *or*	**0–5**	**=** **−5**

Figure 4.6 Elastic recoil of an expandable structure. The transmural pressure (P$_{IN}$ – P$_{OUT}$) associated with each volume indicates the tendency to return to the unstressed volume. Positive pressure and negative pressure inflation are equivalent.

requires knowledge of the mechanical properties of the thorax. Three primary forces are involved:
- elastic recoil properties of the lung;
- elastic recoil properties of the chest; and
- muscular efforts of chest wall, diaphragm, and abdomen.

These result in changes in lung (and thorax) volume, in alveolar pressure, and in intrapleural pressure.

Elastic structures

The recoil tendency of a spring can be expressed in terms of an unstressed or resting length and a length–tension relationship. Similarly, for expandable volumetric structures the relevant properties are the unstressed volume and the relationship between volume and the transmural pressure required to achieve that volume (Fig. 4.6). By convention, transmural pressures are expressed as the difference between the pressure inside and the pressure outside the structure (P$_{IN}$ – P$_{OUT}$). It is convenient to think of this as the 'distending pressure' required to achieve a certain volume, but it is also the 'recoil pressure' that reflects the tendency of the structure to return to its unstressed volume (where transmural pressure is zero). A positive recoil pressure indicates a tendency to become smaller. A structure distorted to a volume below its unstressed volume has a negative recoil pressure, which indicates its tendency to become larger.

Elastic properties of the lung

The lungs are elastic structures with a tendency to recoil to a small 'unstressed volume' (usually slightly less than RV). To maintain any lung volume larger than this requires the presence of a force that distends the lungs; this force is the difference between the alveolar pressure (P$_A$) and that surrounding the lungs, the intrapleural pressure, often more simply referred to as pleural

pressure (P$_{PL}$). The elastic properties of the lungs and their tendency to recoil can be represented by plotting lung volume against the transmural pressure (Fig. 4.7). Such graphs apply to an excised lung being inflated by a pump, an in-vivo lung inflated by a ventilator, or the more physiologic normal lung inflated by expanding the chest (to create a more negative pleural pressure); in each case the curve of volume versus the pressure difference (P$_A$ – P$_{PL}$) is the same.

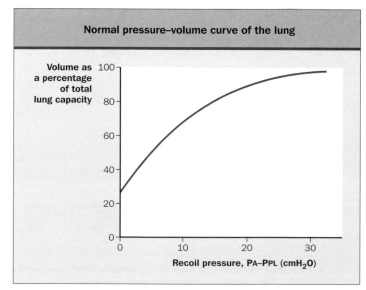

Normal pressure–volume curve of the lung

Figure 4.7 Normal 'pressure–volume' curve of the lung. The elastic recoil pressure of the lung as obtained during a very slow expiration from total lung capacity (the curve on inspiration is somewhat different). (Modified with permission from Culver[1].)

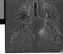

The slope of this pressure–volume curve represents the compliance of the lungs (C_L), equation (4.1).

■ EQUATION 4.1

$$C_L = \Delta V / \Delta P$$

The C_L decreases as the lungs near the limit of their distensibility at TLC. Usually, C_L is measured just above FRC in the tidal breathing range. Since it is normally expressed in absolute volume units (e.g. L/cmH_2O), C_L is strongly dependent on the lung size. A single lung, for example, only has 50% of the volume change for the same pressure change as two lungs. A small child's normal C_L is considerably lower than that of an adult's. For this reason, C_L is often divided by lung volume to give the volume-independent 'specific compliance'.

Elastic properties of the chest wall
The chest wall has elastic properties that can be expressed in the same way as those of the lung (Fig. 4.8). The chest wall differs from many common elastic structures in that its unstressed volume (where recoil pressure = 0) is normally quite high. When expanded above its unstressed volume, it recoils inward, but if the chest wall is 'distorted' to a smaller volume its tendency is to recoil outward. Recoil pressure for the relaxed chest wall is P_{PL} – atmospheric pressure (P_{ATM}), or simply P_{PL} since P_{ATM} is taken to be zero (Fig. 4.9). The compliance of the chest wall is similar to that of the lungs in the mid-volume range, but note that at TLC the chest remains as distensible as it is at FRC.

Lung and chest wall: the respiratory system
In the intact thorax, the lungs and chest wall must move together. The muscular effort required to inspire a volume of air or the pressure that must be developed by a ventilator to achieve the same volume change is determined by the pressure–volume curve of the combined respiratory system, shown by the orange line in Figure 4.8[5]. The lungs and chest wall normally contain the same volume of air, so that only points on the same horizontal line in Figure 4.8 can coexist. Since both the lungs and the chest wall are expanded together, the distending pressure for the respiratory system is the sum of the distending pressures required by the lungs and chest wall. The transmural pressure for the respiratory system is P_A – P_{ATM} (Fig. 4.9). Figure 4.8 shows that a greater pressure change is required to add volume to the respiratory system than to either of its components alone, and thus the compliance of the respiratory system is lower than that of either lungs or chest wall at the same volume. (This may at first seem paradoxic, as the tendency of the chest wall to expand might be thought to help lung expansion; however, as the system volume is increased the outward recoil of the chest wall decreases and this force must be replaced by additional work.)

The third mechanical factor, muscle force, is not considered in Figure 4.8. Thus, the pressure difference across the lung, which has no muscle, can always be taken from its curve, but the pressure across the chest wall (and diaphragm) may reflect muscle tension and is only described by this curve during complete relaxation. Similarly, the curve for the respiratory system shows the pressure that would be measured by a manometer held tightly in

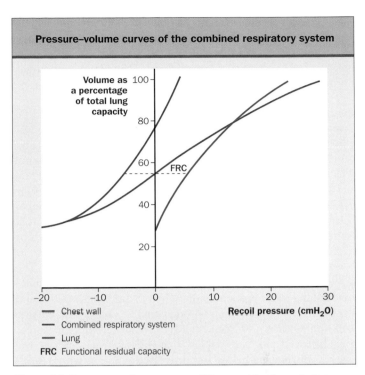

Pressure–volume curves of the combined respiratory system

Volume as a percentage of total lung capacity

Recoil pressure (cmH_2O)

— Chest wall
— Combined respiratory system
— Lung
FRC Functional residual capacity

Figure 4.8 Pressure–volume curves of the combined respiratory system. The relaxed chest wall has a relatively high unstressed volume. The recoil of the combined respiratory system is the sum of the recoil of the chest wall plus lung. (Modified with permission from Culver[1].)

Recoil pressures

Transmural pressure	Pressure inside – pressure outside
Lungs	Alveolar pressure (P_A) – pleural pressure (P_{PL})
Chest wall	P_{PL} – atmospheric pressure (P_{ATM}), or simply P_{PL}
Respiratory system	(P_A – P_{PL}) + (P_{PL} – P_{ATM}) = P_A – P_{ATM}

Figure 4.9 Recoil pressures of the lungs, chest wall, and respiratory system. Measured as the transmural pressure difference (inside – outside).

the mouth after a subject has inhaled or exhaled to a particular volume, and then relaxed all muscle effort.

At the resting end-tidal position of the respiratory system (FRC), no active muscular forces are applied and $P_A = P_{ATM}$ (distending pressure = 0). The lung is distended above its unstressed volume and the chest wall is held below its unstressed volume. The relaxed FRC is the volume at which the opposing tendencies of the lungs to recoil inward and the chest wall to recoil outward are evenly balanced. Any change in the unstressed volume or the compliance of either lungs or chest wall results in a new FRC. For example, obesity reduces the unstressed volume of the chest wall and thus reduces the FRC (and expiratory reserve volume; see Chapter 73). Emphysema increases compliance and unstressed volume of the lung, which results in a higher FRC and a 'shift to the left' of the respiratory system pressure–volume curve.

The opposing forces of lung and chest wall result in a subatmospheric (negative) pressure in the intrapleural space at the

FRC (Fig. 4.10). Since the lungs and chest wall are not directly linked, it is actually the intrapleural pressure that opposes lung recoil and chest wall recoil. It must therefore have the same magnitude as each of these recoil forces. The pleural pressure is normally about $-5cmH_2O$ at FRC.

Events of the respiratory cycle

Inspiration is an active process. Contraction of the inspiratory muscles (primarily the intercostals and the diaphragm) tends to expand the thorax, which creates a more negative intrapleural pressure, which in turn causes PA to become negative with respect to PATM and air is drawn into the lungs. This process continues until the lung volume increases to a point where its recoil pressure is increased to balance the combined muscular and elastic forces of the chest wall. At this point, PA becomes zero and the inspiratory flow stops because a pressure gradient no longer exists along the airways.

During normal breathing, expiration is a passive process. The inspiratory muscles begin to relax and the balance of forces shifts so that lung recoil predominates. Then PA becomes positive and the air moves from alveoli through the airways to the outside atmosphere until FRC conditions are reached, with the forces again balanced and PA zero. Note that with a typical small VT, the chest wall remains below its unstressed volume, with a small outward recoil force, and PPL can be negative throughout the cycle. During active expiration, this process can be assisted by contraction of the expiratory muscles (intercostal and abdominal wall muscles), which makes PPL positive.

Respiratory muscle effort

The maximum inspiratory and expiratory pressures measure the maximal efforts of the respiratory muscles (Fig. 4.11)[6]. That is, if one were to try to inhale against a closed pressure manometer, the negative pressure that can be generated at the mouth is about $100cmH_2O$ at a low lung volume. At TLC, no negative pressure can be generated and thus no more air can be drawn into the chest. Maximum expiratory pressures are somewhat greater, $150–200cmH_2O$ at high lung volume, and fall to zero at RV.

Surface tension

At the surface of a liquid, the intramolecular forces are not balanced by the more widely spaced molecules of the gas phase, which creates a surface tension. The surface tension of the air–liquid interface that lines the alveoli contributes an important part of the elastic properties of the lung shown by the pressure–volume curve. If a lung is filled with liquid, these surface forces are abolished and the resultant pressure–volume curve (Fig. 4.12) reflects only the tissue properties of the lung. This liquid-filled curve is shifted to the left, which shows that the lung can be distended with much less pressure. The air-filled lung, in addition to requiring greater pressures, demonstrates marked hysteresis; that is, the pressure–volume curve during inflation is different from that during deflation[7].

However, the surface tension in the lung is much less and behaves differently than would be expected from an air-filled lung that had a saline-covered surface. The air-filled deflation curve approaches the liquid-filled curve at low lung volume, which shows that the pressure from surface tension becomes small, but given no other parameters, the prediction would be that pressure from surface forces should increase as alveoli become smaller. Laplace's law relates the pressure within a sphere

to wall tension (T) and radius (r), $P = 2T/r$. If the surface tension remains constant as 'r' decreases (smaller alveoli), the pressure from the surface tension should rise. This situation is avoided in the lung by the presence of a unique surface-lining material, surfactant, that not only reduces surface tension (as would a detergent), but does so in a volume-dependent manner. As lung volume and surface area decrease, the lining layer compresses and surface tension decreases until it is nearly abolished at RV. This has three important consequences in the lung:

- work needed to expand the lungs is greatly reduced;
- stability of small alveoli is maintained [if pressure increased in smaller alveoli, they would quickly empty into larger (lower pressure) alveoli, and would require great forces to reopen; surfactant allows interconnecting alveoli of different sizes to coexist at the same pressure];

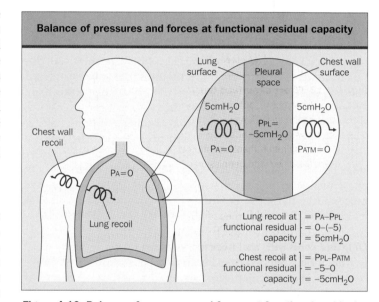

Balance of pressures and forces at functional residual capacity

Figure 4.10 Balance of pressures and forces at functional residual capacity. The opposing recoils of lung and chest wall creates a negative intrapleural pressure. (Modified with permission from Culver[1].)

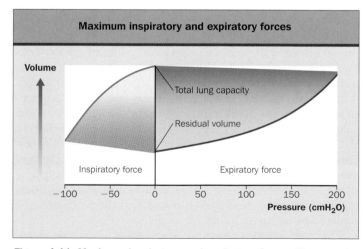

Maximum inspiratory and expiratory forces

Figure 4.11 Maximum inspiratory and expiratory forces. The normal maximum force generated by inspiratory muscles is greatest at low lung volume and the expiratory force is greatest at high lung volume. With occluded efforts, the actual lung volume increases or decreases a small amount due to gas expansion or compression. (Modified with permission from Culver[1].)

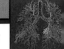

Effect of surface tension on recoil force

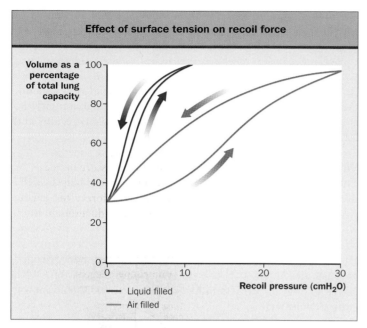

Volume as a percentage of total lung capacity

Recoil pressure (cmH$_2$O)

— Liquid filled
— Air filled

Figure 4.12 Effect of surface tension on recoil force.
Pressure–volume curves obtained on inflation and deflation of a normal air-filled lung and the same lung when filled with saline. The horizontal difference between the curves reflects the effect of surface tension, which is greater on inspiration than expiration and abolished when the lung is liquid filled. (Modified with permission from Culver[1].)

- inwardly directed forces of surface tension in the 'corners' of alveoli act to draw fluid from the capillaries and interstitium into the alveoli, so lowering surface tension helps prevent alveolar edema (discussed later under Circulation).

Flow resistance

Air flow between the atmosphere and alveolar gas is dependent on driving pressure and airway resistance, equation (4.2).

■ EQUATION 4.2

$$\text{Flow} = \dot{V} = \Delta P/R = (P_A - P_{ATM})/R_{AW}$$

The normal airway resistance (R$_{AW}$) during quiet breathing (or a panting maneuver, as it is usually clinically measured) is <2cmH$_2$O/L per second. Air-flow resistance is affected by:
- viscosity of air;
- length of airways (R$_{AW}$ is directly proportional to length); and
- caliber and length of airways (R$_{AW}$ is proportional to $1/r^4$).

Thus, a doubling of length doubles resistance, but a halving of caliber causes a 16-fold increase in resistance. Caliber of airways is affected by:
- position in the bronchial tree;
- lung volume;
- bronchial muscle contraction;
- mucous secretions; and
- pressure across the airway wall.

All of these factors are similar during both inspiration and expiration, except the last. During inspiration, the intrathoracic pressure that surrounds airways is more negative than the intra-airway pressure, so airways tend to be distended (Fig. 4.13). With active

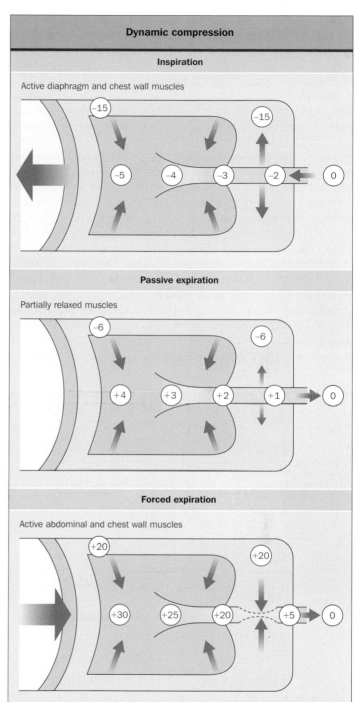

Dynamic compression

Inspiration

Active diaphragm and chest wall muscles

-15   -15
-5   -4   -3   -2   0

Passive expiration

Partially relaxed muscles

-6   -6
+4   +3   +2   +1   0

Forced expiration

Active abdominal and chest wall muscles

+20   +20
+30   +25   +20   +5   0

Figure 4.13 Dynamic compression. Comparison of intrathoracic and intraluminal pressures (in circles; cmH$_2$O) during inspiration, passive expiration, and forced expiration. In each case the lung volume is the same, with a recoil pressure of 10cmH$_2$O. During inspiration, the intrathoracic airways tend to be distended, which lowers airway resistance. In passive expiration, although intrapleural pressure may remain negative (due to chest wall recoil and initial incomplete relaxation of inspiratory muscles), a positive alveolar pressure is generated by lung elastic recoil. Central airways are less distended than during inspiration. In forced expiration, high intrapleural pressure, plus lung recoil, creates a large, positive alveolar pressure to drive flow, but also compresses central airways. Flow is limited once dynamic compression begins downstream from the point where intraluminal pressure falls below pleural pressure (equal pressure point). Further effort increases alveolar driving pressure, but also increases compression. Airway resistance becomes high and varies with the degree of effort.

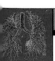

expiratory efforts, the pleural pressure becomes positive and greater than intra-airway pressure. Since their cartilaginous structure is incomplete, airways are compressed under such forces, which reduces the caliber of the lumen. This dynamic compression of airways is a cause of flow limitation during forced expiration[8,9].

Maximum air-flow rates are evaluated by having the subject take a full inspiration (to TLC), and blow the air out as forcefully and completely (to RV) as possible. Using a spirometer, this forced vital capacity (FVC) is recorded as an expiratory spirogram (volume versus time) or, if the flow rate is also measured, the same information can be recorded as a maximum expiratory flow versus volume curve (Fig. 4.14). A remarkable feature of this maneuver is that the maximum flow rate for any volume, except the highest lung volumes near the beginning of the exhalation, is achieved with submaximal effort and cannot be exceeded with further effort. This is demonstrated in Figure 4.15, and is a consequence of the dynamic compression noted above. Since this compression begins when intra-airway pressure falls below PPL pressure, the effective driving pressure becomes $P_A - P_{PL}$ (30 – $20cmH_2O = 10cmH_2O$ in Figure 4.13, forced expiration). This is the same as the elastic recoil pressure of the lung and is a function of lung volume, not effort. For example, in Figure 4.13 if a greater expiratory effort is made, and the PPL is raised to

$40cmH_2O$ at the same lung volume, the P_A becomes $50cmH_2O$ and the effective driving pressure = $50 - 40cmH_2O = 10cmH_2O$, so resultant flow rate remains unchanged.

This mechanism may have its major physiologic significance in normal individuals during a cough. Although overall air-flow rate (L/s) out of the lungs is not increased by the high PPL generated, the air-flow velocity (m/s) through the narrowed major airways is greatly increased, which aids the removal of secretions and foreign material.

Work of breathing

The muscle effort required to raise lung volume above the FRC during inspiration is a form of work. Part of this is the elastic work used to stretch the tissues and surface lining of the lung, while another part is the frictional work required to overcome air-flow resistance in the airways. The elastic work stored in stretched fibers on inspiration then provides the energy needed to push air out on the subsequent passive exhalation. With active expiratory efforts, additional muscle work is done on expiration as well.

The elastic and frictional components of respiratory work are affected differently by lung volume. At low lung volume, airways are narrower and resistance (and thus frictional work) increases rapidly (R is proportional to $1/r^4$). At higher lung volumes the muscles must do more elastic work to keep the lungs stretched. The relaxed FRC is the volume at which the static recoil forces of the lung and chest wall are balanced. Figure 4.16 shows that FRC is also the volume at which work of breathing is least. If either the elastic or frictional contributions to work of breathing change, FRC may change rapidly, or chronically.

The narrowed airways in obstructive disease increase frictional work and the volume for least work shifts up. The accompanying shift of the tidal breathing range to a higher volume may occur quite suddenly in an asthma attack or develop slowly with chronic obstructive disease. When air-flow rates increase, frictional work

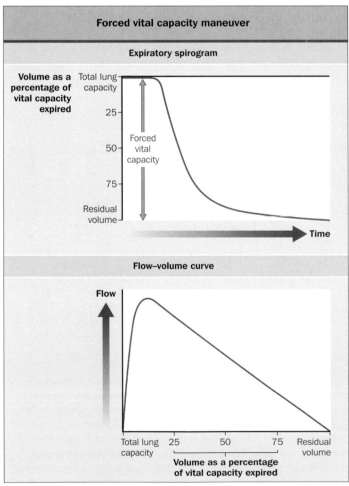

Figure 4.14 Forced vital capacity maneuver. This common breathing test can be displayed as an expiratory spirogram or as a flow–volume curve. Volume axes show percentage of vital capacity expired. (Modified with permission from Culver[1].)

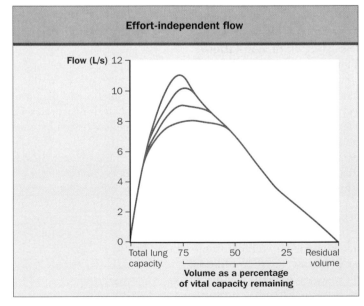

Figure 4.15 Effort-independent flow. The top curve represents a maximum expiratory effort and the lower curves show the flow that results from progressively less effort. At lower lung volumes the maximum flow rate is relatively independent of effort. (Modified with permission from Bates et al[10].)

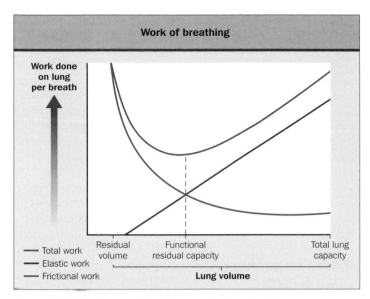

Figure 4.16 Work of breathing. The combined work of lung expansion (elastic) and air-flow resistance (frictional) is normally lowest near functional residual capacity. (Modified with permission from Culver[1].)

becomes relatively more important, so that patients who have obstructive disease may shift to a higher end-expiratory volume during exercise or voluntary hyperventilation.

Restrictive disease processes reduce C_L, which requires the muscles to generate more force to stretch the lung. The elastic work required to breathe at any lung volume is higher and this shifts the volume for least work lower. Increased C_L, as with emphysema, has the opposite effect. Figure 4.8 shows that the static forces predict the same changes in FRC (greater lung recoil results in lower FRC volume and vice versa).

Normally, the energy consumed by breathing is very small. In metabolic terms it requires <1mL/min of oxygen consumption for each liter per minute of ventilation, or only 1–2% of a person's total body oxygen consumption at rest. With severe airway obstruction, the energy cost of breathing becomes much higher.

Distribution of ventilation
The incoming air of each tidal breath is not distributed evenly to all alveoli in the lung. Pleural pressure is not the same throughout the chest, but has a vertical gradient of several centimeters of water because of gravity and the configuration of the chest and diaphragm. At FRC, $-5cmH_2O$ is an average value at mid-level, but near the apices the pressure outside the lung might be $-8cmH_2O$, while near the bases only $-2cmH_2O$. Since alveoli throughout the lung probably have similar maximum volume and similar pressure–volume relationships, and since P_A is the same everywhere, those alveoli near the top of the lung are held at larger volume (distending pressure of $8cmH_2O$) than those near the bottom (distending pressure of $2cmH_2O$). This places the lower alveoli on a steeper (more compliant) portion of their pressure–volume curve. In addition, the proximity of the basal alveoli to the motion of the diaphragm exposes them to a greater increase in distending pressure with inspiration. These two factors combine to give the lower portion of the normal lung a relatively greater proportion of the tidal ventilation than the apices.

A second consequence of the higher P_{PL} (i.e. less negative) in the basal portions of the lung is that the distending pressure of the small airways is also less. At RV, airways may become closed and the basal portions of the lung reach this 'closing volume' first, while higher portions of the lung are still partially distended. Thus, a patient who breathes at very low lung volumes, near RV (e.g. obese patients), may have basal airway closure and consequently little ventilation to the lung bases[11,12].

In summary, respiratory units in the basal portion of the lung contain less gas, but receive more ventilation as long as they remain open. However, they are more susceptible to airway closure and loss of ventilation at low lung volume.

ALVEOLAR GAS EXCHANGE

The primary function of the lung is to provide adequate oxygenation of the blood and to remove carbon dioxide, as first described by Lavoisier in 1777[13]:

> *Eminently respirable air that enters the lung, leaves it in the form of chalky aeriform acids [carbon dioxide] … in almost equal volume … Respiration acts only on the portion of pure air that is eminently respirable [which he later named 'oxygine'] …, the excess [nitrogen], is a purely passive medium which enters and leaves the lung … without change or alteration. The respirable portion of air has the property to combine with blood and its combination results in its red color.*

This gas exchange process can be considered in three parts:
- ventilation of the lungs, which determines the alveolar levels of oxygen and carbon dioxide;
- storage and transport of these gases in the blood; and
- interaction between the two in the process of equilibration between alveolar gas and arterial blood.

The terminology and abbreviations particular to gas exchange are introduced in Figure 4.17.

Gas exchange terminology and abbreviations		
Symbol	**Definition**	**Units**
P	Pressure or partial pressure; e.g. PO_2 = partial pressure of oxygen	mmHg (millimeters of mercury) or Torr (1Torr = 1mmHg under standard gravitational conditions, i.e. sea level)
		kPa (kiloPascal; 1kPa = 7.6mmHg or Torr)
		cmH_2O (centimeters of water; 1mmHg = 1.3cmH_2O)
F	Fraction of a given gas present in a mixture (F × 100 = percentage concentration)	–
V	Volume of gas	L (liters) or mL (milliliters)
V̇	Flow (volume per time)	mL/min (milliliters per minute; e.g. oxygen consumption, $\dot{V}O_2$)
		L/min (e.g. ventilation, $\dot{V}E$)
		L/s (e.g. air-flow rates)

Figure 4.17 Gas exchange terminology and abbreviations. The symbols and modifiers used herein are based on those recommended in the American Medical Association Manual of Style. Main symbols are in capitals and modifiers, usually to indicate location, in small capitals (e.g. I, inspired; E, expired; A, alveolar; often given as subscripts). When two alternative modifiers are possible, the other is given in lower case herein (again, subscripts often used) and usually indicates vascular location (e.g. a, arterial; v, venous; c, capillary).

Functional anatomy of gas exchange

The lung can be functionally divided into a conducting zone of air-ways, and a respiratory zone that consists of the last few branches of air passages and alveoli, in which gas exchange with blood takes place. In the conducting zone, from the upper respiratory tract to the terminal bronchioles, essentially no exchange of respiratory gases with the atmosphere occurs. These airways warm and humidify the incoming air and can remove some gaseous and particulate pollutants.

The terminal bronchioles are succeeded by 2–5 generations of respiratory bronchioles (Fig. 4.18), which have increasing numbers of alveoli in their walls. The next branches are alveolar ducts, which are completely alveolarized with no ciliated epithelium remaining, and terminate in alveolar sacs and individual alveoli. Helical bands of smooth muscle extend to the alveolar ducts and may aid control of the distribution of ventilation. The entire respiratory unit served by one terminal bronchiole is an acinus. Several adjacent acini make up a pulmonary lobule, which has incomplete connective tissue septae that separate it from adjacent lobules. The collateral communication of both air flow and blood flow is better within a lobule than between lobules, although canals of Lambert apparently connect bronchioles of adjacent lobules.

Alveoli are irregular polyhedrons approximately $250\mu m$ in diameter. They increase in number in early childhood to the average adult number of 300 million (it varies with body size). The total alveolar surface area is 85–90% covered with capillaries, which provides an impressive surface area of $70m^2$ for gas exchange. Adjacent alveoli are connected by pores of Kohn that provide routes for collateral air flow, fluid movement, phagocyte mobility, and bacterial spread.

Most of the alveolar surface is covered by epithelial cells that have very attenuated cytoplasm sitting directly on a basement membrane. The capillary endothelial cells are also very thin (except where their nuclei bulge) and again sit directly on a basement membrane. Over much of the area where gas exchange takes place, these basement membranes are fused into one with no intervening interstitial space (Fig. 4.19). Thus, the diffusion distance from alveolar gas to plasma may be $<0.5\mu m$. The distance to a red cell or even within a red cell (about $8\mu m$) may be much greater than that between the alveolar and capillary membrane itself.

Despite the anatomic complexity of the lung, its gas exchange function can be well described by simple models that consist of a conducting zone (branched tube) and a respiratory zone (usually depicted as one or more giant alveoli) with blood flow.

Ambient gas partial pressures (tensions)

Atmospheric or barometric pressure is the total pressure exerted by the kinetic energy of all the molecules in the atmospheric mixture. It varies with altitude, but at sea level it raises a column of mercury in an evacuated tube to a height of 760mm (equivalent to 29.9 inches of mercury and 100kPa) and varies slightly from day to day.

In discussing lung mechanics, the pressure in the chest or lungs is measured relative to PATM, which is therefore set at zero. This is termed gauge pressure and is commonly used, for example, to measure blood pressure or tire pressure. However, gas pressures in the atmosphere, alveoli, and blood are reported in absolute pressure terms, expressed as millimeters of mercury (mmHg) or Torr. A PA value of $13cmH_2O$, or 10mmHg (gauge), is equivalent to 770mmHg in absolute pressure.

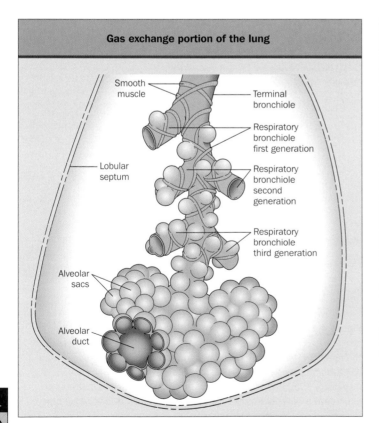

Figure 4.18 Gas exchange portion of the lung.

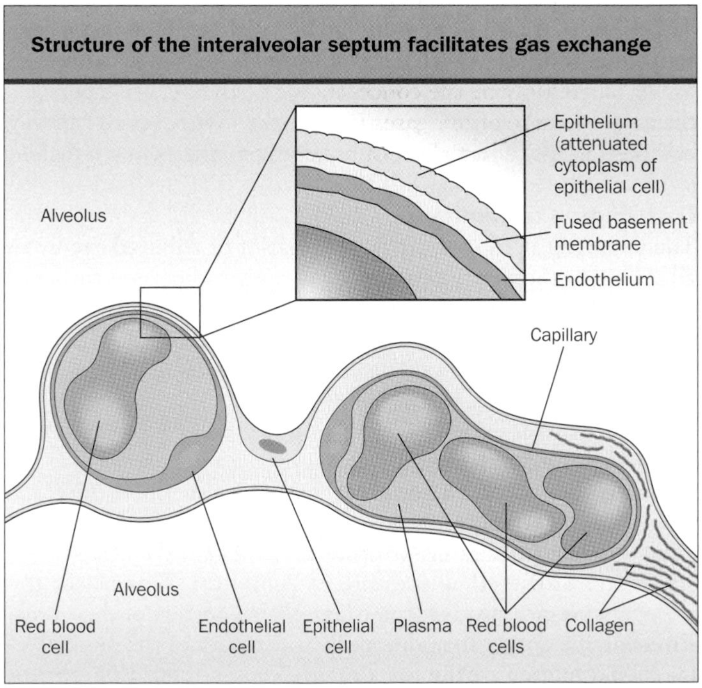

Structure of the interalveolar septum facilitates gas exchange

Figure 4.19 Structure of the interalveolar septum facilitates gas exchange. Capillaries tend to lie asymmetrically within the septum, with most of the interstitial space, structural elements, and cell nuclei on a 'thick side' while the 'thin side' presents a very short path for gas diffusion. (Based on information from Siegwart et al.[14])

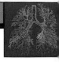

Atmospheric air is a mixture that consists of oxygen (20.95%), nitrogen (78.09%), argon (0.93%), and carbon dioxide (0.03%), with water vapor that varies from 0 to 2% and dilutes the other gases accordingly. For practical purposes, oxygen is taken to be 21%, nitrogen 79%, and carbon dioxide and other trace gases are ignored. Water vapor requires special consideration (see below).

Concept of partial pressure

In a mixture of gases, the pressure exerted by the kinetic energy of each separate gas is referred to as its partial pressure. If the mixture is enclosed in a sealed container, it develops a pressure on the walls of the container by the mechanism of collisions between the gas molecules and the container walls. The force or pressure developed by all the molecules of the mixture as they bounce off the container walls is the total pressure developed by the gas. The partial pressure of any component is the pressure developed by the molecules of that component acting alone. Since the random motion that causes collisions is the same motion that allows diffusion to take place, the partial pressure of a gas is a measure of its tendency to diffuse through either gas or fluid media.

The total pressure of a mixture of gases is equal to the sum of the partial pressures of each gas in the mixture (Dalton's law). Since the alveoli and airways are open to the atmosphere, the sum of the partial pressures in the lung must add up to P_{ATM} (the small variations in P_A during the respiratory cycle are ignored), equation (4.3).

■ EQUATION 4.3

$$P_{ATM} = P_{CO_2} + P_{O_2} + P_{N_2} + P_{H_2O}$$

In the gas phase, partial pressure is proportional to concentration. By convention, gas fractions are measured after water vapor has been removed ('dry' gas). Thus, the partial pressure of a gas is found by multiplying the concentration or fraction of the gas by the total pressure of dry gases (i.e. all but water vapor).

The concept of partial pressure also applies to gases in a liquid, including plasma or blood. When a gas-free liquid is in contact with air, gas molecules move into the liquid by diffusion until the partial pressure in the liquid and air are the same. The relationship of partial pressure of a gas in a liquid to the content of that gas depends on solubility and any chemical binding that takes place. For example, nitrogen and oxygen are both poorly soluble, but large amounts of oxygen are bound to hemoglobin (Hb).

Water vapor

Water vapor requires special consideration, because water is present as both a gas and a liquid in the body. When a gas mixture is in contact with liquid and is saturated with the vapor of that liquid, the partial pressure of that vapor is a function of temperature (Fig. 4.20).

Atmospheric gas is cooler than body temperature and, although it contains some water, it is rarely 100% saturated. Inspired gas that enters the upper portion of the respiratory system is rapidly warmed to body temperature and becomes fully saturated with water vapor. [The small volume change associated with warming and added water vapor can be calculated from gas laws if necessary (Fig. 4.21).] At 37°C, water vapor has a partial pressure of 47mmHg. This pressure does not vary with changes in P_{ATM} or changes in the other components in the gas mixture. Thus, if P_{ATM} is 760mmHg, and P_{H_2O} is 47mmHg, the difference, 713mmHg, is the partial pressure of the remaining dry, inspired gases. Of this total, 21% is oxygen and 79% is nitrogen, so $P_{IO_2} = 0.21 \times 713 = 150mmHg$ and $P_{IN_2} = 0.79 \times 713 = 563mmHg$.

Air has the same relative concentration of gases, even when P_{ATM} is lowered. For example, at the top of Mt. Everest (altitude about 29,000ft), $P_{ATM} = 253mmHg$ and the atmospheric $P_{O_2} = 0.21 \times 253 = 53mmHg$.

Ventilation

The total ventilation per minute ($\dot{V}_E$ = volume exhaled per minute) can be determined by collecting exhaled gas for a measured time. The volume of gas exhaled during one normal respiratory cycle is V_T (see above). The total ventilation is equal to V_T multiplied by the breathing frequency, f ($\dot{V}_E = V_T \times f$).

Alveolar ventilation and dead space

Gas exchange occurs in alveoli when freshly inspired air comes in contact with capillary blood. However, not all the air inspired reaches the alveoli to participate in gas exchange. It must first pass through the conducting airways, from the nose to the distal bronchioles, which contain no alveoli and do not participate in gas exchange. At the end of inspiration, the volume of air that remains in the conducting airways and therefore does not participate in gas exchange is the anatomic dead space. The effect of the conducting airways on ventilation and gas exchange can be considered in two ways. After inspiration, atmospheric air (plus a little water vapor) remains in these airways and leaves as the

Water vapor pressure		
Temperature (°C)	Water vapor pressure	
	mmHg	kPa
0	4.6	0.6
20	17.5	2.3
37	47.0	6.2
100	760.0	100

Figure 4.20 Water vapor pressure. The partial pressure due to water vapor at full saturation varies with temperature.

Gas conditions and corrections
The volume occupied by an amount of gas is directly proportional to its absolute temperature (°Kelvin), is inversely proportional to its total pressure, and is further affected by the volume of water vapor present.
Exhaled gas collected in a spirometer or bag is saturated at ambient temperature and pressure (ATPS).
Lung and ventilatory volumes are conventionally converted into body temperature and pressure, saturated (BTPS) conditions, a volume expansion of 9–10%.
Gas transfer quantities ($\dot{V}_{O_2}$, $\dot{V}_{CO_2}$, and diffusing capacity) are conventionally expressed at standard temperature (273°K), pressure (760mmHg), and dry (STPD) conditions.
While necessary for quantitative calculations, these conversions can be largely ignored for conceptual understanding.

Figure 4.21 Gas law corrections. For quantitative calculations, gas volumes must be corrected for changes in temperature and added water vapor.

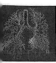

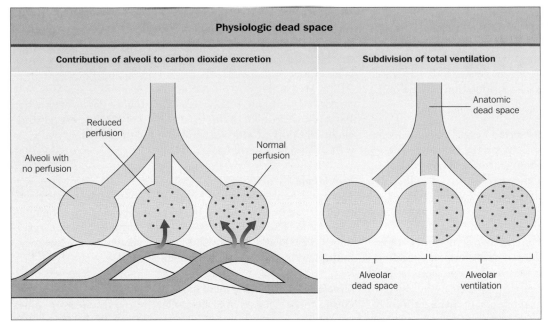

Figure 4.22 **Physiologic dead space.** Alveoli with no perfusion, reduced perfusion, and normal perfusion, and their contribution to carbon dioxide excretion. Subdivision of the total ventilation into anatomic dead space, alveolar dead space with no perfusion, and alveolar ventilation with ideal perfusion. (Modified with permission from Culver[1].)

first gas out on the subsequent exhalation. After expiration, alveolar gas (with carbon dioxide added and oxygen partially removed) fills the anatomic dead space and re-enters the alveoli with the next breath. Thus, a tidal breath may inspire 500mL of air and cause a 500mL expansion of the alveolar volume followed by the expiration of 500mL, but the volume of fresh air delivered to the alveoli and the volume of alveolar air exhaled to the atmosphere are each less than 500mL by an amount equal to the volume of the anatomic dead space.

In addition to the conducting airways, any alveoli that are ventilated with air but not perfused with blood cannot participate in gas exchange. The volume of ventilation that goes to these alveoli is also wasted and is called alveolar dead space. Ventilation to areas of lung that have reduced, but not absent, perfusion can be treated as if a portion were going to alveoli with normal perfusion and a portion to alveoli with no perfusion. This latter portion is also part of the alveolar dead space (Fig. 4.22). The sum of anatomic and alveolar dead space make up the physiologic dead space[15].

The volume of the anatomic dead space in a normal adult male is approximately equal to the lean body weight in pounds (150–180mL). In a young normal individual, the volume of the physiologic dead space (VD) is only slightly greater than this or about 25–35% of an average VT (referred to as the VD/VT ratio). The anatomic dead space is not fixed, but increases at higher lung volumes, because the intrapulmonary airways increase in size along with the surrounding lung tissue via interdependence. Thus, breathing with a large VT, and the accompanying larger end-inspiratory lung volume, is associated with a modest decrease in VD/VT ratio. With exercise, VT may increase to 2.5–3.0L and VD/VT normally falls to 15% or less, but an important additional factor is the increase in pulmonary blood flow, which tends to eliminate any poorly perfused alveolar dead space. At the other extreme, it would seem that as VT became small, approaching the anatomic dead space, alveolar ventilation should fall to zero and gas exchange become impossible. However, it has been demonstrated that gas exchange can be maintained even with VTs equal

to or smaller than the measured anatomic dead space. Some fresh gas reaches alveoli because some path lengths are shorter than others and because airway gas may exchange with alveolar gas by diffusion and by physical mixing induced by the heartbeat.

The physiologic dead space and wasted ventilation may be considerably increased with diseases of the air spaces and vasculature, primarily because of an increase in the alveolar component. (Importantly, increases in the 'physiologic' dead space are almost always abnormal, i.e. pathologic.) The fraction of ventilation 'wasted' by going to physiologic dead space can be calculated from arterial and expired gas values. Dead space has the effect of diluting the carbon dioxide partial pressure of mixed expired gas (P_{ECO_2}) below the alveolar level, and the equation derived in Figure 4.23 is simply a calculation of this dilution. Since the body needs to eliminate a certain volume of carbon dioxide per minute, the effect of a low P_{ECO_2} is to require more total ventilation to maintain homeostasis.

The volume of air that does participate in gas exchange because it is in contact with perfused alveoli is termed the alveolar ventilation ($\dot{V}_A = \dot{V}_E - V_D$). The volume per minute of alveolar ventilation is critical, as it determines the amount of air presented to alveoli into which carbon dioxide can be excreted and from which oxygen can be removed. Note that 'alveolar ventilation' as defined here and widely used in respiratory physiology is a conceptual term and might better be called 'gas exchange ventilation'. It is not the same as the volume of gas that enters or leaves alveoli each minute.

Carbon dioxide elimination

Since the body's carbon dioxide production ($\dot{V}_{CO_2}$) is only eliminated by ventilation, it must equal the volume of carbon dioxide exhaled per minute minus the volume of carbon dioxide inhaled, which is negligible and can be disregarded. All of the carbon dioxide expired must come from alveolar ventilation and is equal to the volume of this ventilation times the concentration of carbon dioxide in the effective gas-exchanging space (F_{ACO_2}), equation (4.8).

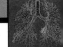

Physiologic dead space calculation

The physiologic dead space, made up of ventilation to anatomic dead space plus that to unperfused alveoli and a portion of that to poorly perfused alveoli, is not an anatomically identifiable volume, but an 'as if' volume may be obtained by calculation from a collection of exhaled gas over 1–3 minutes.

Using a 'conservation of mass' concept, the total expired volume of gas per minute is considered to have two sources:

  ideal alveoli with equal alveolar and arterial partial pressures of carbon dioxide (P_{ACO_2} = Pa_{CO_2}); and

  unperfused areas (conducting airways or alveolar dead space) with P_{ACO_2} = inspired P_{CO_2} = 0.

The total expired volume of carbon dioxide comes entirely from the effective (nondead-space) alveolar ventilation ($\dot{V}E$ – $\dot{V}D$), equation (4.4).

■ EQUATION 4.4

$$\dot{V}_{CO_2} = \dot{V}_E \times F_{ECO_2} = (\dot{V}_E - \dot{V}_D) \times F_{ACO_2}$$

Algebraic manipulation yields equation (4.5).

■ EQUATION 4.5

$$\dot{V}_D \times F_{ACO_2} = \dot{V}_E \times F_{ACO_2} - \dot{V}_E \times F_{ECO_2}$$
$$\dot{V}_D/\dot{V}_E = (F_{ACO_2} - F_{ECO_2})/F_{ACO_2}$$

Multiplying top and bottom by (P_{ATM} – 47) converts fraction to partial pressure, equation (4.6).

■ EQUATION 4.6

$$\dot{V}_D/\dot{V}_E = (P_{ACO_2} - P_{ECO_2})/P_{ACO_2}$$

P_{ACO_2} cannot be readily measured, but in these assumed ideal alveoli P_{ACO_2} = Pa_{CO_2}, so the measured arterial blood gas value can be substituted. P_{ECO_2} is obtained from a collection of expired gas.

By convention, the results are reported as the $\dot{V}D/\dot{V}T$ or wasted fraction of each tidal breath, equation (4.7), but actually they are measured as the average wasted ventilation over 1–3 minutes.

■ EQUATION 4.7

$$\dot{V}_D/\dot{V}_T = \dot{V}_D/\dot{V}_E = (Pa_{CO_2} - P_{ECO_2})/Pa_{CO_2}$$

Multiplying this fraction by the tidal volume or minute ventilation gives the volume of physiologic dead space or wasted ventilation. [In carrying out this measurement, it must be remembered that the volume of air in mouthpiece, connections, and valve (mechanical dead space) also contribute air free of carbon dioxide to the expired collection.]

Figure 4.23 **The fraction of wasted ventilation can be calculated from the relationship of carbon dioxide partial pressure in exhaled gas to the arterial level.**

■ EQUATION 4.8

$$\dot{V}_{CO_2} = \dot{V}_A \times F_{ACO_2}$$

Rearranging equation (4.8) demonstrates that for a given level of metabolic carbon dioxide production, a reciprocal relationship exists between alveolar ventilation and the level of alveolar carbon dioxide, equation (4.9).

■ EQUATION 4.9

$$F_{ACO_2} = \dot{V}_{CO_2}/\dot{V}_A$$

Multiplying both sides of equation (4.9) by the total pressure of dry gases in the alveoli (P_{ATM} – 47) converts the fraction into partial pressure units in which carbon dioxide is commonly measured and yields the useful relationship in equation (4.10), which states that alveolar P_{CO_2} is directly related to the production of carbon dioxide and inversely related to alveolar ventilation ($\dot{V}A$).

■ EQUATION 4.10

$$P_{ACO_2} = (\dot{V}_{CO_2}/\dot{V}_A) \times (P_{ATM}-47)$$

The body maintains a normal alveolar (and arterial) P_{CO_2} of 40mmHg by adjusting ventilation appropriately for the $\dot{V}_{CO_2}$ dictated by metabolic demand.

Hyperventilation is defined as ventilation in excess of metabolic needs. Therefore, a P_{ACO_2} below normal indicates alveolar hyperventilation. Conversely, a P_{ACO_2} greater than normal indicates alveolar hypoventilation.

Any depression in central nervous system (CNS) function can change $\dot{V}E$, and therefore $\dot{V}A$; for example, many drugs such as narcotics and sedatives can reduce $\dot{V}E$. Any increase in $\dot{V}D$ will reduce $\dot{V}A$ unless $\dot{V}E$ increases proportionally. Many disease processes increase physiologic dead space, which is a contributory cause of ventilatory failure when the patient can no longer increase total ventilation.

The alveolar P_{CO_2} level reflects a balance between carbon dioxide that enters the alveolar spaces from the blood, and that which leaves with exhaled gas. In a steady state, production and excretion must be the same. Under resting conditions $\dot{V}_{CO_2}$ is relatively constant at approximately 200mL/min for an individual of normal size. If a person hyperventilates, initially carbon dioxide is exhaled at a greater rate than carbon dioxide production; P_{ACO_2} falls [and with it arterial P_{CO_2} (Pa_{CO_2})]. As P_{ACO_2} falls, the carbon dioxide exhaled per minute decreases, since less is loaded into exhaled air, until carbon dioxide elimination is again equal to carbon dioxide production and a new steady state is established. In hypoventilation, the rate of carbon dioxide exhalation initially falls, and P_{ACO_2} (and Pa_{CO_2}) rises until a new steady state is reached at which excretion again equals production with less ventilation, but each liter of gas that leaves the alveoli carries more carbon dioxide. This mechanism allows patients who have severe lung disease and high work of breathing to excrete their carbon dioxide production at less energy cost.

Alveolar oxygen
The level of alveolar oxygen also reflects a balance of two processes:
- oxygen delivery to the alveoli by ventilation; and
- oxygen removal from the alveoli by capillary blood.

Oxygen delivery to alveoli is determined by their ventilation ($\dot{V}A$) and the fraction of inspired oxygen (F_{IO_2}), but oxygen is also carried away in exhaled air. The gas that leaves alveoli has the alveolar oxygen concentration (F_{AO_2}). So the net oxygen taken up from alveoli is given by $\dot{V}A \times (F_{IO_2} - F_{AO_2})$, which can be written as a conservation of mass equation (4.11) stating that the oxygen consumed to meet metabolic demand ($\dot{V}_{O_2}$) equals that removed from the alveolar ventilation (none is removed from dead space ventilation).

■ EQUATION 4.11

$$\dot{V}_{O_2} = \dot{V}_A \times (F_{IO_2}-F_{AO_2})$$

Rearranging this equation demonstrates that for a given level of metabolic oxygen consumption, a reciprocal relationship exists between alveolar ventilation and the fraction of oxygen removed from the incoming air. That is, when alveolar ventilation is decreased, more oxygen must be extracted from each unit of that incoming ventilation, which results in a lower residual level of alveolar oxygen, equation (4.12).

■ EQUATION 4.12

$$F_{IO_2} - F_{AO_2} = \dot{V}_{O_2}/\dot{V}_A$$

Conversion of equation (4.12) into partial pressure by multiplying both sides by ($P_{ATM} - 47$) gives equation (4.13).

■ EQUATION 4.13

$$P_{IO_2} - P_{AO_2} = (\dot{V}_{O_2}/\dot{V}_A) \times (P_{ATM} - 47)$$

Equation (4.13) shows that P_{AO_2} is determined by P_{IO_2}, $\dot{V}_A$, and $\dot{V}_{O_2}$. If P_{IO_2} and $\dot{V}_{O_2}$ are constant and $\dot{V}_A$ increases, P_{AO_2} must also increase, and if $\dot{V}_A$ decreases, P_{AO_2} must also decrease. Oxygen removal from inspired air is governed by tissue oxygen consumption and varies with activity, but under resting conditions it is approximately 250mL/min for a person of average size. In a steady state, P_{AO_2} does not change, so the removal of oxygen from inspired air just matches the transfer of oxygen to the blood. In hyperventilation, initially alveolar oxygen is added at a greater rate than it is consumed and P_{AO_2} rises. As P_{AO_2} rises, the amount of oxygen given up by inspired air decreases, until a new steady state is established at a higher P_{AO_2}. In hypoventilation, the rate of oxygen delivery to the alveoli initially falls, and P_{AO_2} falls until a new steady state is reached with less ventilation, but each liter of gas that leaves the alveoli has given up more oxygen.

Estimating the alveolar partial pressure of oxygen

Abnormalities in oxygenation often cause a wide disparity between the level of alveolar oxygen and that measured in the arterial blood. To understand fully the clinical arterial blood gas values, it is necessary to estimate quantitatively the P_{AO_2}, but this cannot be readily obtained from equation (4.13) because neither $\dot{V}_{O_2}$ nor $\dot{V}_A$ are easily measured. However, since carbon dioxide production is the metabolic product of oxygen consumption, the quantities $\dot{V}_{CO_2}$ and $\dot{V}_{O_2}$ are tightly linked and their ratio, $\dot{V}_{CO_2}/\dot{V}_{O_2}$, is the respiratory exchange ratio (R). If these values are identical (R = 1), the solutions to equations (4.10) and (4.13) are identical and show that the fall in P_{O_2} from inspired to alveolar air is exactly the same as the rise in P_{CO_2} from zero to the alveolar level. With a more typical R of 0.8, the production of four molecules of carbon dioxide results from the consumption of five molecules of oxygen, and it follows that in the lung the addition of carbon dioxide to a level of 40mmHg in alveolar air would be associated with a P_{AO_2} that showed a 50mmHg reduction from the inspired air, equation (4.14).

■ EQUATION 4.14

$$P_{AO_2} = P_{IO_2} - (P_{ACO_2}/R)$$

Since the measured P_{aCO_2} is very close to P_{ACO_2}, this simplified version of the alveolar gas equation can be rewritten as equation (4.15).

■ EQUATION 4.15

$$P_{AO_2} = P_{IO_2} - (P_{aCO_2}/R)$$

For typical normal values, R = 0.8, $P_{IO_2} = 0.21(760-47)$, and $P_{aCO_2} = 40$, equation (4.16).

■ EQUATION 4.16

$$P_{AO_2} = 150 - (40/0.8) = 100mmHg$$

The alveolar gas equation is often misinterpreted as indicating that alveolar oxygen is displaced by carbon dioxide. This is incorrect, as the removal of oxygen and addition of carbon dioxide proceed as independent processes in the lung, but since the normal respiratory quotient (RQ; see below) in the tissues is typically 0.8–1.0, loss of oxygen from the inspired air to the blood is approximately equal to the gain in carbon dioxide.

Appropriate interpretation of arterial blood gas values always requires thinking through the alveolar gas equation. This helps, for example, to establish whether a low P_{aO_2} is explained by hypoventilation, or if the P_{aO_2} is appropriate for the F_{IO_2}. Figure 4.24 gives examples of the use of the alveolar gas equation.

Metabolism and the respiratory exchange ratio

Energy necessary for life processes is produced by oxidation of carbohydrates, protein, and fats, which produces principally carbon dioxide and water as breakdown products. The quotient RQ is the ratio of metabolic carbon dioxide production to the oxygen consumption of the tissues ($\dot{V}_{CO_2}/\dot{V}_{O_2}$). When metabolizing carbohydrate RQ = 1.0, when metabolizing fat RQ = 0.7, and the RQ of protein has an average value of 0.8. Thus, the RQ for the entire body varies with the percentages of carbohydrate, fat, and protein being oxidized at any given time. The ratio R relates the volume of carbon dioxide eliminated and the net volume of oxygen taken up. In a steady state or over a long period of time, R must equal RQ, but R may vary transiently with factors other than metabolism. For example, if an individual suddenly increases ventilation, R rises because carbon dioxide is 'blown off' from blood and tissue stores (but little oxygen can be added). During exercise, R may reach 1.4 because of hyperventilation and continued excretion of carbon dioxide while an oxygen debt is contracted.

Applying the alveolar gas equation			
	Normal ventilation	Hyper-ventilation	Hypo-ventilation
$P_{IO_2} = (0.21 \times 713)$ (mmHg)	150	150	150
P_{aCO_2} (mmHg)	40	20	64
R	0.8	0.8	0.8
$P_{AO_2} = P_{IO_2} - (P_{aCO_2}/R)$ (mmHg)	150–50 = 100	150–25 = 125	150–80 = 70

Figure 4.24 The alveolar gas equation demonstrates the effect of changes in ventilation on alveolar P$_{O_2}$ (P$_{AO_2}$). The degree of ventilation markedly affects the P$_{AO_2}$ required to equilibrate with capillary blood; this can be estimated utilizing the alveolar gas equation. The P$_{AO_2}$ calculated, which ranges from 70 to 125mmHg in these examples, is a somewhat theoretic value for the average alveoli; some areas of the lung may have higher or lower values.

TRANSPORT OF GASES IN THE BLOOD

Oxygen transport

Respiratory gases are carried in blood in physical solution, by binding proteins, and (for carbon dioxide) through chemical conversion. The small quantities carried in physical solution are calculated in Figure 4.25. For oxygen, with only 3mL of oxygen per liter in physical solution at a normal arterial PO_2, it is impossible to pump enough blood to meet tissue demands without the large additional transport provided by Hb.

Hemoglobin

A complex protein, Hb consists of four polypeptide chains (two α-chains and two β-chains), with four heme groups to bind oxygen. One mole of Hb can carry four moles of oxygen, so the theoretic maximum oxygen carrying capacity is calculated as 1.39mL/g of Hb (but the actual maximum appears to be slightly less because some sites are not available). Normal blood has a Hb concentration of 15g/100mL blood and thus can potentially carry about 20mL oxygen per 100mL of blood as oxyhemoglobin.

The Hb sites fill with oxygen in relation to its partial pressure in solution; the percentage of saturation of Hb indicates the portion of the total oxygen-binding sites actually occupied[16]. The relation between PO_2 and Hb oxygen content or percentage saturation is nonlinear (Fig. 4.26). The curve is S-shaped, which has particular physiologic advantages. In the normal arterial range, the curve is fairly flat, so that moderate decreases in arterial PO_2 cause only small decrements in arterial oxygen saturation (SaO_2) and content. A normal saturation of 97.5% occurs at a PO_2 of 100mmHg. A decrease in PO_2 to 60mmHg still allows the Hb to be 90% saturated. The curve is fairly steep in the normal range of systemic venous PO_2 (PvO_2), which allows further unloading of oxygen to active tissues, with only a small reduction in the partial pressure that drives oxygen diffusion to the cells. A normal resting venous saturation of 75% is associated with a PvO_2 of 40mmHg.

Factors that affect the affinity of hemoglobin for oxygen

The relative affinity of Hb for oxygen is described by the parameter P_{50} (the PO_2 at 50% saturation). Decreased P_{50} or a curve shift to the left means increased affinity or more oxygen bound for any PO_2; increased P_{50} or a curve shift to the right means decreased affinity (Fig. 4.27). Physiologic factors that affect the affinity of Hb for

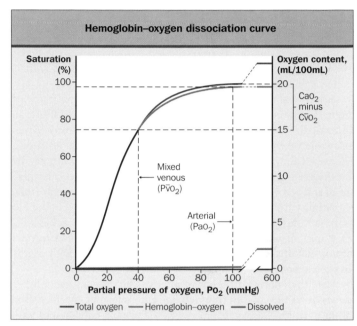

Figure 4.26 Hemoglobin–oxygen (Hb–O₂) dissociation curve shows the percentage saturation of hemoglobin at each PO₂. When the hemoglobin concentration is known, the content of oxygen can be calculated. The total content includes the small additional content of oxygen in solution, which becomes significant at high levels of Po₂. The saturation scale on the left applies only to the Hb–O₂ line. The scale on the right shows content values for a normal hemoglobin level of 15g/100mL blood. (Modified with permission from Hlastala[17].)

Figure 4.25 Content of gases in physical solution in the blood.

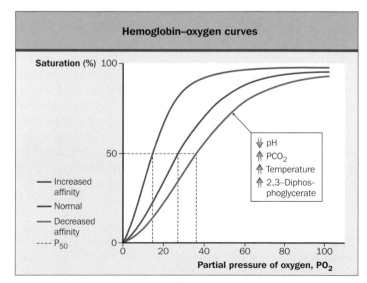

Figure 4.27 Normal, increased affinity (left shift), and decreased affinity (right shift) Hb–O₂ curves. Inset shows factors decreasing Hb-O₂ affinity. Note that decreased affinity means a higher Po₂ at a given saturation (e.g. P₅₀) or a lower saturation at a given Po₂. (Modified with permission from Hlastala[17].)

oxygen, include pH, P_{CO_2}, and temperature. Increases in all of these, as seen in an exercising muscle, shift the curve to the right, which decreases affinity and helps to unload oxygen at the tissues.

The effect of P_{CO_2} is particularly important as the loading of carbon dioxide in tissues produces a right shift of the dissociation curve and enhances the simultaneous unloading of oxygen. Part of this shift is caused by the associated pH change and part results from the binding of carbon dioxide with Hb to form carbamino compounds which have lower affinity for oxygen. The reverse occurs in the lungs as the unloading of carbon dioxide shifts the dissociation curve to the left, which enables the blood to load more oxygen at a given PaO_2. This bidirectional shift is called the Bohr effect.

Additional regulation of Hb–O_2 affinity over a time frame of hours to days occurs via 2,3-diphosphoglycerate (2,3-DPG), an intermediate metabolite in the red-cell metabolic pathway. When upregulated by a stimulus like chronic hypoxia (e.g. altitude), increased 2,3-DPG concentration decreases oxygen affinity by binding to the Hb molecule. Changes in 2,3-DPG level also play an adaptive role during acid–base abnormalities and with anemia.

Affinity for oxygen can also be affected by variation in the Hb polypeptides. At 37°C and pH 7.4 , normal adult Hb A has a P_{50} of 27mmHg, while human fetal Hb has a P_{50} of 20mmHg. Several abnormal Hbs have been identified that have either high or low oxygen affinity.

The physiologic advantage of a curve shift for oxygen delivery depends on the conditions of loading and unloading. An increased affinity means the blood that leaves the alveoli, equilibrated with the alveolar P_{O_2}, has a slightly higher oxygen content, but when required to give up 5mL/100mL or more of its content to metabolically active tissue, the P_{O_2} at the delivery point has to fall to a lower than normal value (see Fig. 4.27). A decreased affinity means that the blood leaving alveoli has a slightly lower content, but not very much lower because of the nearly flat top of the Hb–O_2 curve. This blood can give up the same amount (5mL/100mL) to the tissues and still maintain a higher P_{O_2} at the delivery point. Thus, at near-normal levels of alveolar P_{O_2} a right shift is usually advantageous, but when loading at a markedly reduced P_{O_2} (e.g. via placental exchange or at extreme altitude), a left shift is more helpful.

Carbon monoxide

Carbon monoxide is a particularly dangerous gas because its affinity for Hb is 200–250 times that of oxygen and thus it can fully saturate Hb at a very low ambient concentration. The presence of carbon monoxide decreases the oxygen-carrying capacity by functionally 'removing' Hb sites available for oxygen binding. It also causes an effective increase in oxygen affinity of the remaining Hb. Carbon monoxide poisoning can create a marked disparity between a normal measured PaO_2 and a severely reduced oxygen content.

Arterial blood oxygen content

The equilibration of blood with alveolar gas in the pulmonary capillaries determines the partial pressure of oxygen in plasma, and would do so even if Hb was totally absent. The P_{O_2} is in equilibrium with the Hb, which yields an oxygen saturation determined by the shape and position of the Hb–O_2 curve. The arterial oxygen content (CaO_2) is determined by this saturation and the concentration of Hb present plus a small contribution of dissolved oxygen. With a normal Hb concentration of 15g/100mL, the normal arterial oxygen content is about 20.5mL/100mL

(Fig. 4.28). Blood with decreased Hb concentration (anemia) holds less oxygen, while that with an increased Hb concentration (polycythemia) holds an increased amount of oxygen.

Venous blood oxygen content

A portion of the oxygen carried in arterial blood is given up to the tissues to meet metabolic needs, which leaves a lower oxygen content in the venous blood that returns to the right heart and lungs. This mixed venous oxygen content depends on arterial oxygen content and the balance between tissue oxygen consumption ($\dot{V}O_2$) and blood flow ($\dot{Q}$). It is described by the Fick equation [equation (4.20)], which says that the volume of oxygen consumed per minute is equal to the cardiac output times the content of oxygen removed from each unit volume of blood (Fig. 4.29).

■ EQUATION 4.20

$$\dot{V}O_2 = \dot{Q} \times (CaO_2 - C\bar{v}O_2)$$

An increased oxygen demand in the face of a constant blood flow requires an increased arterial–venous (a–v) oxygen difference. Alternatively, an increased blood flow in the face of a constant metabolic demand yields a decreased a–v oxygen difference.

Normal arterial oxygen content	
Parameter	**Value**
Arterial partial pressure of O_2	90–100mmHg
Arterial saturation of O_2	97%
Hemoglobin (Hb) content	15g/100mL
O_2-carrying capacity of Hb	1.39mL/g Hb
Arterial O_2 content	O_2 bound to Hb plus dissolved O_2 = $(15 \times 1.39 \times 0.97) + (0.003 \times 100)$ = 20.2 + 0.3mL/100mL = 20.5mL/100mL

Figure 4.28 Arterial oxygen content at normal arterial partial pressure and hemoglobin levels.

The Fick equation, $\dot{V}O_2 = \dot{Q} \times (CaO_2 - C\bar{v}O_2)$		
Parameter	**Symbol**	**Typical normal values at rest**
Oxygen consumption	$\dot{V}O_2$	250mL/min
Cardiac output	$\dot{Q}$	5L/minute
Difference between alveolar and mixed venous oxygen content	$CaO_2 - C\bar{v}O_2$	50mL/L blood (or 5mL/100mL blood)
Arterial oxygen content	CaO_2	200mL/L blood (or 20mL/100mL blood)
Mixed venous oxygen content	$C\bar{v}O_2$	150mL/L blood (or 15mL/100L blood)
Mixed venous partial pressure of oxygen	$P\bar{v}O_2$	~40mmHg

Figure 4.29 The Fick equation relates oxygen consumption to cardiac output and the extraction of oxygen at the tissues. If the ventilation of oxygen ($\dot{V}O_2$), and arterial and venous content (CaO_2 and $C\bar{v}O_2$) are measured, cardiac output can be calculated from the Fick equation. The bar in $C\bar{v}O_2$ indicates mixed venous blood, which must be sampled beyond the right atrium after all systemic venous return has mixed, and thus requires a catheter in the right ventricle or pulmonary artery.

The mixed venous partial pressure of oxygen ($P\bar{v}O_2$) is determined by the venous oxygen content and the oxygen dissociation curve. The venous oxygen content and PO_2 varies in the blood that returns from different capillary beds, depending on the matching of blood flow to metabolic demand. For example, blood that leaves exercising muscle may have a very low venous oxygen content, whereas the kidneys have high blood flow and relatively little oxygen extraction. After these flows combine in the right heart, the mixed venous content reflects total body oxygen extraction.

Carbon dioxide transport

As the blood passes through the lung, carbon dioxide equilibrates with the alveolar gas so the arterial PCO_2 is very close to alveolar PCO_2. The alveolar PCO_2, and hence arterial PCO_2, is determined by the balance between alveolar ventilation and carbon dioxide production. Under normal conditions, arterial PCO_2 is regulated near 40mmHg with an arterial carbon dioxide content, related to partial pressure in a nonlinear fashion, normally 47mL/100mL.

The venous carbon dioxide is determined by the arterial carbon dioxide content and the relationship between blood flow and carbon dioxide production, again described by the Fick principle. With a typical RQ of 0.8, a resting oxygen consumption of 250mL/minute is associated with a carbon dioxide production of 200mL/minute and, at a cardiac output of 5L/minute, requires the loading of an additional 4mL/100mL of carbon dioxide into the systemic venous blood. This increase to a venous carbon dioxide content of 51mL/100mL occurs with only a modest rise in mixed venous partial pressure to a $P\bar{v}CO_2$ of 46mmHg.

Carbon dioxide dissociation curve

The overall relationship between carbon dioxide content (CcO_2) and PCO_2 is curvilinear, as indicated in Figure 4.30, but the curve is essentially linear over the limited range between arterial and venous PCO_2 (40–46mmHg)[18]. Although the quantity of carbon dioxide exchanged is similar to that of oxygen (as governed by the RQ), this narrow range of arterial-to-venous PCO_2 is made possible by the steepness of the carbon dioxide dissociation curve. Oxygenation of Hb decreases its ability to carry carbon dioxide, which facilitates the unloading of carbon dioxide at the lung, while the opposite effect occurs at tissues, which increases the 'physiologic' slope of the carbon dioxide curve (as shown in the inset in Figure 4.30). The ability to load or unload carbon dioxide with minimal change in PCO_2 helps to minimize the change in pH between arterial and venous blood.

Carbon dioxide storage in blood

Carbon dioxide is stored in physical solution and in chemical combination with Hb, but in addition a major portion of the carbon dioxide is stored in the blood as bicarbonate (HCO_3^-). The blood stores of carbon dioxide are greater than those of oxygen and, since bicarbonate is also present in the extravascular interstitial fluid, the body stores of carbon dioxide are much greater than those of oxygen. Thus, with a change in ventilation or if breathing ceases (apnea or asphyxia), the carbon dioxide level changes much more slowly than does that of the oxygen.

Since the solubility of carbon dioxide is over 20 times that of oxygen, a greater content of carbon dioxide is carried in physical solution at physiologic partial pressures (see Fig. 4.25) – 2.9mL/100mL

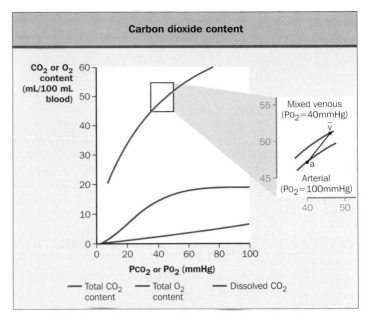

Figure 4.30 Curve of carbon dioxide content versus PCO_2 is steeper than the oxygen content curve, shown for comparison. It includes carbon dioxide bound to hemoglobin and bicarbonate (the largest fraction), and dissolved carbon dioxide. Inset: increasing the PO_2 decreases the carbon dioxide content for any PCO_2 (Haldane effect). As the blood shifts between the oxygenated and the deoxygenated curves, the functional steepness (i.e. $\Delta CcO_2/\Delta PcO_2$) between the arterial point (a) and mixed venous point ($\bar{v}$) increases. (Modified with permission from Hlastala[17].)

represents about 6% of the total amount of carbon dioxide carried in arterial blood.

Carbon dioxide binds with Hb to form carbamino compounds and also, to a small extent, it binds with other proteins. At a normal arterial PCO_2, carbamino binding of carbon dioxide amounts to around 2.1mL/100mL blood, or about 4% of the total carbon dioxide content. Formation of carbamino compounds tends to weaken the Hb–oxygen affinity (the Bohr effect). Conversely, as Hb binds oxygen, carbamino compound formation decreases (the Haldane effect). These interactions assist in the appropriate loading and unloading of oxygen and carbon dioxide in the lungs and tissues. Even though carbamino binding makes up a small part of the blood carbon dioxide storage, it undergoes a relatively large change between venous and arterial blood, so that it accounts for over 25% of the carbon dioxide loaded in tissue and unloaded at the lung.

By far the major storage of carbon dioxide in blood is in the form of HCO_3^-. In blood, carbon dioxide rapidly combines with water to form carbonic acid, which then dissociates to form H^+ and HCO_3^-. The first reaction is catalyzed by carbonic anhydrase (CA) in the red cell, equation (4.21).

■ EQUATION 4.21

$$CO_2 + H_2O \overset{CA}{\rightleftharpoons} H_2CO_3 \rightleftharpoons H^+ + HCO_3^-$$

The whole-blood HCO_3^- concentration of carbon dioxide is equivalent to approximately 42mL/100mL at a normal arterial PCO_2, with most of that in the plasma. This is roughly 90% of the total amount of carbon dioxide stored in the arterial blood.

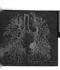

As shown in Figure 4.31, carbon dioxide is carried in plasma as dissolved carbon dioxide or as HCO_3^-, and is carried inside red cells as dissolved carbon dioxide, HCO_3^-, or carbamino compounds. The formation of HCO_3^- in the red cell is extremely rapid because of the presence of CA. Hydrogen ions formed are buffered by Hb, which shifts the Hb–O_2 curve to the right, and thus enhances oxygen release. As a result of the high concentration of HCO_3^- formed, some bicarbonate diffuses out into the plasma and, to maintain charge neutrality, chloride diffuses into the cell. The uncatalyzed HCO_3^- formation extracellularly is extremely slow. Thus, even though the majority of blood carbon dioxide content is in plasma HCO_3^-, the red cell plays a very important role in facilitating its interconversion to and from diffusible gas and in buffering the associated hydrogen ions.

ALVEOLAR–ARTERIAL OXYGEN EQUILIBRATION

In the discussion of alveolar ventilation, the factors that determine the average alveolar PO_2 of the lung were shown to be the inspired PO_2 and the relationship of alveolar ventilation to oxygen consumption. In an ideal cardiorespiratory system, the arterial blood would be perfectly equilibrated with the alveolar PO_2, but even normal individuals fall somewhat short of this; thus, an alveolar–arterial difference in PO_2 ($PAO_2 - PaO_2$) occurs. With lung disease or circulatory abnormalities, $PAO_2 - PaO_2$ may become quite wide. The three factors involved in alveolar–arterial equilibration are diffusion, shunt, and ventilation–perfusion matching.

Diffusion

Oxygen moves from alveolar gas to arterial blood by a passive process of diffusion from higher to lower partial pressure. The flux of a gas across a membrane is equal to a coefficient called the diffusion capacity (DL) times the partial pressure gradient, which in the case of the lung is between alveolar gas and capillary blood.

In the gas phase, diffusion is proportional to the inverse of the square root of the molecular mass. In a liquid, diffusion is proportional to solubility divided by the square root of the molecular mass. In the lung, diffusion is also dependent upon the nature and length of the diffusion pathway and the total surface area available for diffusion, which reflects the effective alveolar capillary bed. The total DL of the lung is made up of two components, that of the diffusion process through the alveolar membrane itself and that attributable to the effective resistance of the red cell plus the process of chemical combination with Hb.

It can be estimated that the average red blood cell spends about 0.75 seconds in the alveolar capillaries (its capillary transit time). With a normal DL, enough oxygen crosses the membrane to bring the red cell Hb to equilibrium with the alveolar PO_2 in 0.25 seconds or less[19]. A diffusion abnormality slows the rate at which oxygen crosses, but usually sufficient time reserve is available for the red cell to be fully oxygenated before it leaves the capillary (Fig. 4.32). Only when the DL is severely limited (e.g. <0.25 normal) or the transit time is markedly shortened is it possible for the blood that leaves the alveolar capillaries to have a lower PO_2 than that of the alveolar gas. Thus, a diffusion abnormality, although present in many diseases, is very rarely the physiologic cause of a low PaO_2 at rest. If diffusion limitation for oxygen exists when breathing air, it may be virtually eliminated by breathing oxygen, because the very high driving pressure of oxygen in alveolar gas increases the rate of equilibration. Thus, on 100% oxygen ($PAO_2 \approx 670mmHg$) it can be arbitrarily stated that diffusion limitation makes no contribution to any $PAO_2 - PaO_2$.

Although it may not indicate the physiologic reason for hypoxemia, it is often useful to measure the DL of the lung to help establish the condition of the alveolar–capillary membrane (surface area and capillary volume, as well as thickness, all contribute and are not separated by the measurement). As it is technically difficult to estimate the back pressure of capillary PO_2 (it is

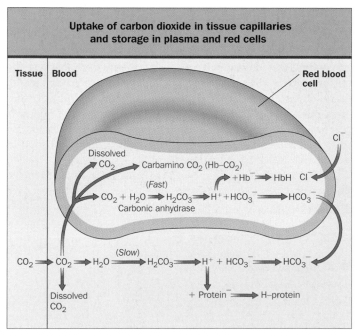

Figure 4.31 Uptake of carbon dioxide in tissue capillaries and storage in plasma and red cells. In the pulmonary capillaries, all the reactions and diffusions are reversed. (Modified with permission from Hlastala[17].)

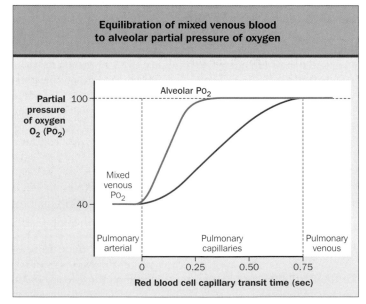

Figure 4.32 Mixed venous blood equilibrates to the alveolar partial pressure of oxygen level by diffusion during transit through the pulmonary capillaries. Even when the diffusion rate is abnormally slow (blue line), the blood may be fully oxygenated within the normal transit time.

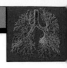

changing, of course, from $P\bar{v}O_2$ to PaO_2), the clinical measurement of DL is established with carbon monoxide. The test is described in the section on Pulmonary Function Testing.

Carbon dioxide also moves from blood to alveolus by diffusion. Although it is a larger molecule, diffusion in a liquid is proportional to solubility, so carbon dioxide diffuses through the alveolar wall more readily than oxygen by a factor of 20. However, the transfer of carbon dioxide out of the blood also depends on chemical reaction rates (remember that much carbon dioxide is carried as HCO_3^-, which must be converted, again via CA, into carbon dioxide). As a result of this, and because the driving pressure difference for carbon dioxide starts much lower, the equilibration rates between blood and alveolus are similar for carbon dioxide and oxygen.

Alveolar–arterial oxygen difference

Since the lung is not a single unit, but consists of approximately 300 million alveoli, one might expect differences from one region to the next. All alveoli do not receive the same amount of ventilation ($\dot{V}A$) or perfusion ($\dot{Q}$), and neither is the matching of ventilation to blood flow ($\dot{V}A/\dot{Q}$) the same for each alveolus; because of this, gas partial pressures vary from one alveolus to the next. A diffusion limitation, if it exists, would create a difference between the alveolar gas partial pressure and that in the capillary leaving it, which would lead directly to a measured alveolar–arterial oxygen difference. In considering ventilation–perfusion abnormalities and shunt it is assumed that each capillary is in complete equilibrium with the alveolus that it passes, but the subsequent mixture of blood from different areas of the lung results in an arterial PO_2 less than the value calculated for alveolar PO_2, that is, a positive $PAO_2 - PaO_2$.

Shunt

Shunt (i.e. R → L shunt) refers to blood that passes from the systemic venous to arterial system without going through gas-exchange areas of the lung. Some normal shunting of blood always occurs, and includes some of the bronchial arterial blood that drains to the pulmonary veins after having perfused and given up oxygen to the bronchial tissues; also included is a small amount of coronary venous blood, which drains directly into the cavity of the left ventricle through the thebesian veins. An abnormal shunt may occur through congenital defects in the heart or blood vessels, or more commonly through areas of atelectasis or consolidation in the lung. For example, if one lung collapses but continues to receive half the cardiac output, deoxygenated blood mixes with oxygenated blood (Fig. 4.33) to cause a marked reduction in the oxygenation of the arterial blood. Note that because of the shape of the Hb–O_2 dissociation curve, the final PO_2 is much closer to that of the shunted blood than to that leaving well-ventilated units.

If a patient who has a 50% shunt breathes 100% oxygen, the alveolar gas equation shows that the PAO_2 in well-ventilated units increases to about 670mmHg, but this causes only a small increase in the content of oxygen in the blood that leaves them. The shunt blood continues to have the mixed venous content (which will be slightly higher if $CaO_2 - C\bar{v}O_2$ remains constant). The mixed arterial blood remains somewhat hypoxemic, with a very large $PAO_2 - PaO_2$.

The effect of shunt can also be visualized graphically from the Hb–O_2 dissociation curve (Fig. 4.34). Since Hb is fully saturated above a PaO_2 of 150mmHg, the additional content results from dissolved oxygen and is linearly related to PO_2. Thus, a

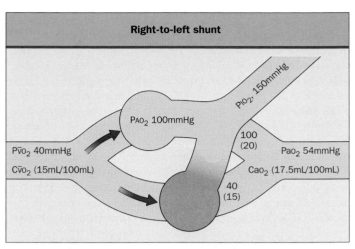

Figure 4.33 Shunt is blood flow not exposed to alveolar gas. To find the PO_2 of the mixed arterial blood (PaO_2), the relative blood flow (50:50 in this example) and oxygen (CaO_2) content contributed by each side must be considered; that is CaO_2 = (shunt fraction × mixed venous content) + (nonshunt fraction × ventilated capillary content). After determining the content (or percentage saturation) of the mixture, the resultant PaO_2 can be found from the hemoglobin–oxygen dissociation curve. (In this example, $CaO_2 - C\bar{v}O_2$ has narrowed to 2.5mL/100mL, which implies an increase in cardiac output. If this does not occur then $C\bar{v}O_2$ drops below 15 and the final PaO_2 will be lower than shown.)

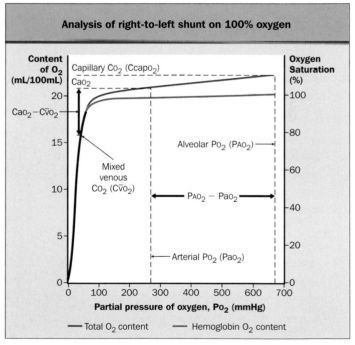

Figure 4.34 Analysis of R → L shunt in a patient who is breathing 100% oxygen. In this example, shunt fraction is 20% of cardiac output, so the arterial oxygen content (CaO_2) represents the mixture of one part venous blood and four parts fully oxygenated blood from alveolar capillaries. Breathing 100% oxygen, the PO_2 of well-ventilated alveoli is about 670mmHg; the content in capillary blood leaving them is shown as $CcapO_2$. A normal $CaO_2 - C\bar{v}O_2$ difference gives the mixed venous content shown. With a 20% shunt, the arterial blood content (CaO_2) is one-fifth of the distance from $CcapO_2$ to $C\bar{v}O_2$ on the vertical axis. Projecting horizontally gives the PaO_2 associated with this content. (Modified with permission from Culver[1].)

fixed relationship exists in this range between an increasing shunt fraction (movement of Ca toward Cv̄ on the vertical axis) and a decreasing Pao_2. For a normal $Cao_2 - Cv̄o_2$ value of 5mL/100mL, this calculates as a fall in Po_2 of about 20mmHg below the alveolar value for each 1% shunt. This rule of thumb is useful to estimate shunt fraction from arterial blood gas values obtained while breathing 100% oxygen. Plotting the appropriate points on Figure 4.34 also shows why the same normal shunt of about 5% causes an $Pao_2 - Pao_2$ of 10–15mmHg while breathing air, but one of about 100mmHg on 100% oxygen.

If $Cv̄o_2$ is measured directly, the shunt fraction can be more accurately calculated from the shunt equation (Fig. 4.35). The impact of any given shunt fraction on arterial oxygenation is greater if $Cv̄o_2$ is abnormally low, as in a low cardiac output state.

Ventilation–perfusion abnormalities

The average $V̇a/Q̇$ is about (4.0L/min)/(5.0L/min), that is 0.8, but this average derives from alveoli with $V̇a/Q̇$ ranging from near 'zero' (unventilated) to nearly infinity (unperfused). In the normal lung the blood flow, influenced by the vascular branching pattern, gravity, and by other factors, is greater at the bottom and less at the top of the lung. In addition, several mechanical factors also cause ventilation to be greater near the bottom than the top of the lung. However, the difference in perfusion from bottom to top of the lung is greater than the difference in ventilation. Accordingly, the ratio of ventilation to perfusion is low in the bottom of the lung and high at the top of the lung. Since the matching of ventilation and perfusion varies, the Pao_2 and $Paco_2$ are different in different areas of the lung. In lung diseases, the scatter of $V̇a/Q̇$ around the mean may be much greater than normal.

For alveolar gas partial pressures in individual alveoli, groups of alveoli, or regions of lung, the same analysis applies as for the lung as a whole. Again, the gas partial pressures in the alveoli are determined by the balance of influx and efflux. However, in place of the $V̇o_2$ of the body, the uptake of oxygen from a small group of alveoli is determined by their blood perfusion and by the change in oxygen content of that blood. Thus, with a decrease in ventilation (or an increase in perfusion) the $V̇/Q̇$ ratio is decreased, which causes Pao_2 to fall. That is, when ventilation is low relative to the blood flow that carries oxygen away, more oxygen molecules must be removed from each unit of incoming air. Thus, the local Pao_2 falls, and as it does, less oxygen is loaded onto the perfusing blood until a new local steady state is reached.

The normal balance of ventilation and oxygen uptake causes the Po_2 to fall from 150mmHg in inspired air to 100mmHg in ideally ventilated and perfused alveoli. As the $V̇/Q̇$ ratio falls toward 0 (near shunt), Pao_2 falls toward the mixed venous value (about 40mmHg), and $Paco_2$ rises toward its mixed venous value (about 46mmHg). Thus, with $V̇/Q̇$ ratios below normal, any Pao_2 from 100 down to 40mmHg is possible ($Paco_2$ values are in the range 40–46mmHg). The range of possible values can be displayed on a Po_2–Pco_2 graph (Fig. 4.36).[20] The specific $V̇/Q̇$ ratio and the rise in capillary oxygen content determine the magnitude of the drop in Po_2 from inspired air to alveolar air. When the blood that perfuses these alveoli, and is in equilibrium with these lowered Pao_2 values, mixes with that from normal alveoli, the mixture of contents results in arterial hypoxemia (Fig. 4.37).

Figure 4.38 shows that, unlike shunt, if the inspired Po_2 is raised even moderately, Pao_2 in these poorly ventilated alveoli rises sufficiently that the hypoxemia is eliminated (although Pao_2 – Pao_2 is still large). If a patient with a $V̇/Q̇$ abnormality is placed on 100% oxygen, the inert gas nitrogen is washed out of the alveoli and

---

Shunt calculation

The oxygen transported in arterial blood is considered to come from two sources – shunt flow ($Q̇s$) with mixed venous oxygen content (Cvo_2) and nonshunt flow (total flow minus shunt flow, or $Q̇t - Q̇s$), with an oxygen content in equilibrium with well-ventilated alveoli ($Ccapo_2$ for capillary oxygen content), hence equation (4.22).

■ **EQUATION 4.22**

$$Q̇tCao_2 = Q̇sCv̄o_2 + (Q̇t - Q̇s)Ccapo_2$$

Algebraic manipulations yield equation (4.23):

■ **EQUATION 4.23**

$$Q̇tCao_2 = Q̇sCv̄o_2 + Q̇tCcapo_2 - Q̇sCcapo_2$$

$$Q̇sCcapo_2 - Q̇sCv̄o_2 = Q̇tCcapo_2 - Q̇tCao_2$$

$$Q̇s(Ccapo_2 - Cv̄o_2) = Q̇t(Ccapo_2 - Cao_2)$$

$$Q̇s/Q̇t = (Ccapo_2 - Cao_2)/(Ccapo_2 - Cv̄o_2)$$

Cao_2 and $Cv̄o_2$ are measured from appropriate blood samples; $Ccapo_2$ is obtained by assuming that $Pcapo_2 = Pao_2$ calculated from the alveolar gas equation ($Pio_2 - Pco_2/R$) or, if the subject is breathing 100% oxygen, only ($Pio_2 - Pco_2$).

To truly calculate shunt fraction the subject must be breathing 100% oxygen. If the measurements are made breathing air or any fraction of inspired oxygen other than 1.0, the 'shunt' calculated is termed venous admixture (or 'physiologic shunt') because it includes any contribution of low $V̇/Q̇$ areas as well as diffusion limitation. The calculation answers the question: if the observed reduction in Pao_2 were entirely caused by shunt, how large would that shunt have to be? Thus, for example, a calculation of 10% venous admixture in a patient breathing air might be caused by a 10% true shunt, or to a larger volume of blood flowing through low $V̇/Q̇$ areas, or to some combination of true shunt, low, and high $V̇/Q̇$ areas.

Figure 4.35 The shunt equation. With appropriate blood sampling, it is possible to calculate the fraction of blood flow 'shunted' from right to left using an equation developed from the concept of conservation of mass.

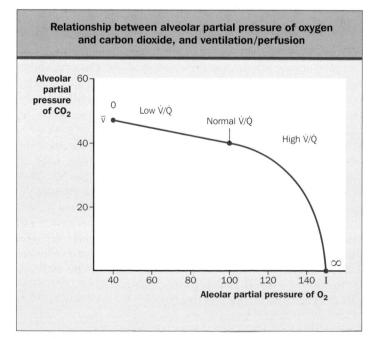

Relationship between alveolar partial pressure of oxygen and carbon dioxide, and ventilation/perfusion

Figure 4.36 Spectrum of alveolar Po_2 and Pco_2 values possible as ventilation/perfusion ($V̇/Q̇$) ranges from zero to infinity. The values follow a line from the mixed venous point (v̄) to that representing inspired gas (I).

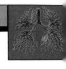
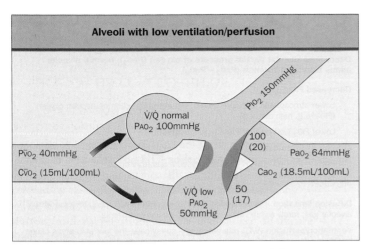

Figure 4.37 In alveoli of low ventilation/perfusion ($\dot{V}/\dot{Q}$), the alveolar P_{O_2} (PA_{O_2}) is low, as more oxygen is removed from the incoming air. In this example, the $\dot{V}/\dot{Q}$ ratio has been arbitrarily chosen to result in a PA_{O_2} of 50mmHg and blood flow is equally divided. The mixture of contents (shown in parentheses) yields a PA_{O_2} well below normal.

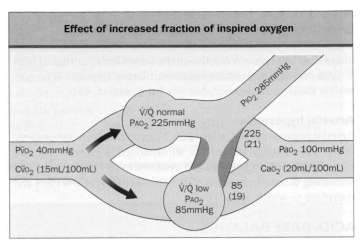

Figure 4.38 Effect of increased fraction of inspired oxygen (F_{IO_2}) when low ventilation/perfusion ($\dot{V}/\dot{Q}$) alveoli are present. Ventilation and perfusion are identical to the example in Figure 4.37, but the F_{IO_2} has been increased to 0.4, which results in a normal arterial P_{O_2}. Unlike the case with shunt, the added oxygen increases the P_{O_2} in both low and normal $\dot{V}/\dot{Q}$ areas. [The drop in P_{O_2} from inspired to alveolar air on the obstructed side (285 – 85 = 200mmHg) is now twice as large as it was on room air, because it takes twice as much oxygen to raise the blood content from 15 to 17 versus 15 to 17mL/100mL; this is also seen to a smaller extent on the normal side.]

blood. (Even if alveoli are very poorly ventilated, the nitrogen is washed out via the blood perfusing them and subsequently eliminated via more functional units.) Once this occurs, oxygen, carbon dioxide, and water are the only gases left in the lung and their partial pressure must add up to P_{ATM} (if not, more gas is drawn in from the airways, or the alveolus shrinks). [If the uptake of oxygen by blood is faster than the inflow of oxygen through a severely obstructed bronchiole ($\dot{V}/\dot{Q} < 0.1$), the alveoli do shrink and eventually collapse in a process known as 'absorption atelectasis'[21], and behave as shunt – one reason to avoid the use of 100% oxygen.) Since PA_{H_2O} is fixed at 47mmHg and PA_{CO_2} cannot exceed $P\bar{v}_{CO_2}$, the Pa_{O_2} of any alveolus is over 650mmHg no matter how low its $\dot{V}/\dot{Q}$ ratio falls. Thus, on 100% oxygen the effect of abnormal $\dot{V}A/\dot{Q}$ ratios on the equilibration of mixed arterial blood with alveolar P_{O_2} is completely eliminated, that is $\dot{V}/\dot{Q}$ mismatching no longer contributes to the observed $PA_{O_2}-Pa_{O_2}$.

If an alveolus is unperfused (e.g. vessels blocked by an embolus), no oxygen can be removed or carbon dioxide added to it. With less severe underperfusion (or overventilation), the $\dot{V}A/\dot{Q}$ ratio rises toward infinity and the alveolar gas values approach that of inspired gas ($P_{O_2} = 150$mmHg, $P_{CO_2} = 0$mmHg; see Fig. 4.36). Note that a high $\dot{V}A/\dot{Q}$ abnormality (Fig. 4.39) does not cause hypoxemia; in fact, it would tend to increase Pa_{O_2} (but not very much, since the oxygen content is only slightly increased and the reduced blood flow from these alveoli is greatly outweighed by that from an equal number of normal alveoli). Carbon dioxide excretion from the high $\dot{V}/\dot{Q}$ portion of the blood flow is increased, which gives a lower end-capillary P_{CO_2} (and a proportionately lower content), but again, since blood flow is small, this has only a modest effect on the overall Pa_{CO_2}. In terms of the ventilation, this is inefficient gas exchange, since each unit of ventilation going to the high $\dot{V}/\dot{Q}$ units carries away less carbon dioxide and thus the overall ventilation has to be increased to maintain homeostasis. These alveoli then contribute to physiologic dead space or 'wasted ventilation'.

Disease processes may cause both low and high $\dot{V}A/\dot{Q}$ areas simultaneously, possibly with a normal overall 'mean $\dot{V}A/\dot{Q}$'. However, the shape of the Hb–O_2 curve shows that little oxygen

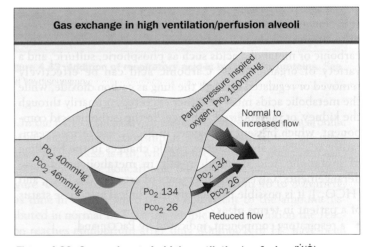

Figure 4.39 Gas exchange in high ventilation/perfusion ($\dot{V}/\dot{Q}$) alveoli. In this example, blood flow is reduced to about one fourth normal. (The missing blood flow must be shifted elsewhere, which affects the $\dot{V}/\dot{Q}$ ratio of 'normal' alveoli.) In the high $\dot{V}/\dot{Q}$ alveoli, P_{O_2} is increased and alveolar P_{CO_2} decreased. (The specific values are for illustration only; as a result of the interaction of $\dot{V}/\dot{Q}$ and blood gas contents, these values are most easily obtained from tables or nomograms.)

content is added as the P_{O_2} increases above 100mmHg. Thus, the blood from these high $\dot{V}/\dot{Q}$ units is unable to compensate for the drop in oxygen content because of the low $\dot{V}/\dot{Q}$ areas. In addition, by definition less blood comes from high $\dot{V}/\dot{Q}$ units than from an equal volume of low $\dot{V}/\dot{Q}$ units. Thus, even a process that results in both high and low $\dot{V}/\dot{Q}$ areas results in arterial hypoxemia.

Abnormal $\dot{V}A/\dot{Q}$ relationships also interfere with the elimination of carbon dioxide, but an elevation of Pa_{CO_2} is not commonly seen in such patients because the normal response to a rising Pa_{CO_2} is to increase overall ventilation. This increases the body, however, the blood and its plasma are in equilibrium for these ions with the extravascular interstitial fluid (but not necessarily with the intracellular fluid). Interstitial fluid contains no Hb and very little protein, so contributes little to the noncarbonic buffering, but as H^+ are buffered in the blood and HCO_3^- levels altered, these ions come into diffusional equilibrium with the interstitial fluid over a time frame of 10–30 minutes. In effect, the buffering capacity of the blood is diluted by the interstitial fluid and, because blood volume is about one third the total ECF volume, the buffering capacity of ECF is about one third that for blood. For total ECF, $b \approx 1/3 \times 30 \approx 10sl$.

Primary acid–base disorders

Understanding acid–base abnormalities first requires the presence and extent of the four primary disorders to be recognized.

- Respiratory acidosis results from a high P_{CO_2}, which reflects hypoventilation and is present by definition whenever P_{CO_2} is >43mmHg. It is associated with a small increase in HCO_3^-, predictable as $\Delta[HCO_3^-] \approx -10 \times \Delta pH$, or 1mmol/L per 0.1 pH unit fall.
- Respiratory alkalosis results from a low P_{CO_2}, which reflects hyperventilation and is present by definition whenever P_{CO_2} <37mmHg. It is associated with a small decrease in HCO_3^-, predictable as $\Delta[HCO_3^-] \approx -10 \times \Delta pH$, or 1mmol/L per 0.1 pH unit rise.
- Metabolic acidosis is recognized by a decrement in HCO_3^- greater than that expected for the pH effect alone and can be quantitated as a decrease in base excess (BE).
- Metabolic alkalosis is recognized by a rise in HCO_3^- greater than that expected for the pH effect alone and can be quantitated as an increase in BE.

Note that the terms acidosis and alkalosis are applied to the pathophysiologic processes that tend to cause an excess or deficit of H^+. It is possible, indeed common, to have processes of both acidosis and alkalosis present simultaneously (e.g. respiratory acidosis plus metabolic alkalosis), with a pH that is low, high, or normal, depending on their relative magnitude. Acidemia and alkalemia are more precise terms used when blood pH is referred to.

As a first approximation, metabolic abnormalities are recognized by a deviation of $[HCO_3^-]$ from the normal value of 24mmol/L, but it must be remembered that, because of the action of the noncarbonic buffers, even a pure respiratory abnormality is associated with changes in $[HCO_3^-]$ of ±3mmol/L over the pH range 7.1–7.7. The BE or base deficit (usually expressed as a negative BE) of the ECF is a better quantification of any metabolic component present. At a pH of 7.4, the noncarbonic buffers hold only their normal complement of H^+ ions and thus do not contribute to buffering. The BE calculates any deviation of $[HCO_3^-]$ from 24mmol/L that would exist at a pH of 7.4 and thus is equal in magnitude to the amount of excess metabolic acid or base added to the system, just as in a simple HCO_3^- solution. Many laboratories report this value along with the blood gas measurements, but it can be estimated with a simple mental calculation (Fig. 4.44) or obtained from a graphic display, as described below.

Compensation for acid–base disorders

If the underlying pathology prevents the body from correcting a primary acid–base disorder (e.g. by restoring hypoventilation to normal), mechanisms come into play to minimize the deviation of pH from normal. The immediate effects of buffering are aided

by a second type of homeostatic mechanism, termed physiologic compensation. The Henderson–Hasselbalch equation shows that pH is a function of the ratio of $[HCO_3^-]$ to P_{CO_2}, so pH is improved if this ratio is restored toward normal. If, for example, the primary disorder is a metabolic acidosis, HCO_3^- is low and the physiologic compensation is to increase ventilation and lower P_{CO_2}. This restores the HCO_3^-/P_{CO_2} ratio closer to normal, even though the absolute values of both HCO_3^- and P_{CO_2} are now abnormal. This response, and the opposite in the case of a metabolic alkalosis, demonstrates ventilatory compensation for a primary metabolic acid–base disorder.

If the primary derangement is ventilatory in origin (e.g. respiratory acidosis with a high P_{CO_2}), the body responds by increasing

---

Base excess calculation

Base excess (BE) is defined as the difference between the patient's $[HCO_3^-]$ after correction to pH 7.40 by change of P_{CO_2} and the normal $[HCO_3^-]$ at pH 7.40 of 24.0mmol/L.

Since the blood gas sample is usually not measured at a pH of 7.4, it is necessary to calculate an adjustment to this pH, which must be done by manipulation of P_{CO_2} so that the metabolic component of interest is not altered. As P_{CO_2} is hypothetically moved up or down to adjust the pH, the hypothetic $[HCO_3^-]$ changes from its measured value as determined by the noncarbonic buffer slope:

$\Delta[HCO_3^-] \approx -10 \times \Delta pH$, or −1mmol/L per 0.1 pH unit rise.

Example 1

Consider the situation in Figure 4.42 where 12mmol/L of excess acid was added to a patient's extracellular fluid and ventilation was maintained normal. The resultant blood gas measurements include pH, 7.2; P_{CO_2}, 40mmHg; $[HCO_3^-]$, 14mmol/L.

The pH must be adjusted up 0.2 units to 7.4, which requires a decrease in P_{CO_2}.

At pH = 7.4, the hypothetic $[HCO_3^-]$ is adjusted by $\Delta[HCO_3^-] \approx -10 \times 0.2 = -2$

The hypothetic $[HCO_3^-]$ equals the measured value of 14−2 = 12

BE = $[HCO_3^-]$ at 7.4−24 = 12−24 = −12mmol/L

The negative base excess of 12mmol/L is equal to the excess acid load added.

Example 2

Consider a patient with the measured values: pH, 7.1; P_{CO_2}, 95mmHg; and $[HCO_3^-]$, 29mmol/L.

The pH is adjusted up 0.3 units to 7.4.

$\Delta[HCO_3^-]$	$\approx -10 \times 0.3 = -3$
Hypothetic $[HCO_3^-]$	= 29−3 = 26
BE	=26−24 = 2mmol/L

While at first this patient may appear to have a significant metabolic alkalosis, which suggests partial compensation for the respiratory acidosis and therefore some chronicity, BE is small and within the normal limit of ±2, so this suggests acute hypoventilation.

Note that as the pH is hypothetically corrected to 7.4, P_{CO_2} or $[HCO_3^-]$ may move in an abnormal direction. It is convenient to remember that, consistent with the hydration reaction for CO_2, the $[HCO_3^-]$ adjustment is always in the same direction as the P_{CO_2} change.

In the examples above, the measured HCO_3^- is hypothetically adjusted to a pH of 7.4 and compared with the normal value of 24mmol/L. Alternatively, the same relationship can be used to adjust the normal HCO_3^- to the normal value expected at the measured pH and subtract the measured HCO_3^-. In Example 2, a 'normal' HCO_3^- is calculated at pH 7.1 to be 27mmol/L and the BE to be 29 − 27 = 2mmol/L. This is what happens visually on the Davenport diagram when the vertical distance of a point above or below the 10sl line is assessed.

Figure 4.44 Metabolic derangements are quantified by a simple calculation of base excess or deficit.

HCO_3^-, and restoring the $[HCO_3^-]/P_{CO_2}$ ratio and pH toward normal. This metabolic compensation for primary respiratory disorders involves both renal retention or excretion of HCO_3^- and physicochemical binding, which occurs in bone and intracellular proteins. The time course of these mechanisms of metabolic compensation is over hours to days, as opposed to the ventilatory compensations that are immediate. Thus, respiratory acid–base disturbances can be subdivided into those that are uncompensated and therefore likely to be of short duration (i.e. acute) and those that are compensated (chronic) processes. This is not possible for metabolic acid–base disturbances, as their normal ventilatory compensation develops concurrently.

In general, compensations for primary acid–base alterations do not completely return pH to 7.40. The primary acid–base disorders and their mechanisms and limits of compensation can be displayed in one of several graphic formats.

Davenport diagram

The Davenport diagram is a commonly used visual display of acid–base relationships (Fig. 4.45), and is a graphic representation of the Henderson–Hasselbalch equation, in which any point shows a potentially coexisting combination of the three variables[24].

Respiratory disorders are shown by moving from the normal central point to higher or lower values of P_{CO_2}. The sloping line that passes through the center shows the 10sl buffer value of the noncarbonic buffers and thus indicates the expected values for pH and HCO_3^- as P_{CO_2} rises or falls in a pure respiratory acidosis

or alkalosis. Vertical displacements above or below this line indicate that a metabolic disorder (either primary or compensatory) has caused an excess or deficit of base in the ECF. If no compensation occurred for a primary metabolic disorder, the values would follow the line that represents $P_{CO_2} = 40$. The Davenport diagram is a convenient way to visualize the paths of primary disorders and their compensation. Figure 4.46 shows, for example, the development of an acute respiratory acidosis with subsequent metabolic compensation. Figure 4.47 shows the range of values seen in common acid–base disorders and illustrates the usual limits of compensation.

Clinical acid–base disorders

Respiratory acidosis

Hypoventilation is defined as alveolar ventilation inadequate for metabolic demand and is indicated by an elevation of arterial P_{CO_2} above the normal $40 \pm 3 mmHg$. It results from inadequate drive to breathe, from mechanical impairments of the chest wall or lung parenchyma, or (most commonly) from severe air-flow limitation [e.g. asthma or chronic obstructive pulmonary disease (COPD)].

An elevated $PaCO_2$ defines the presence of a component of respiratory acidosis regardless of the arterial pH.

Acute respiratory acidosis

Acute respiratory acidosis is identified by high $PaCO_2$, fall in pH, and an increase in $[HCO_3^-]$ that approximates 1mmol/L for each 0.1 decrement in pH (i.e. BE $\approx$ 0). On the Davenport diagram, the values follow the 10sl line to the left (see Fig. 4.45).

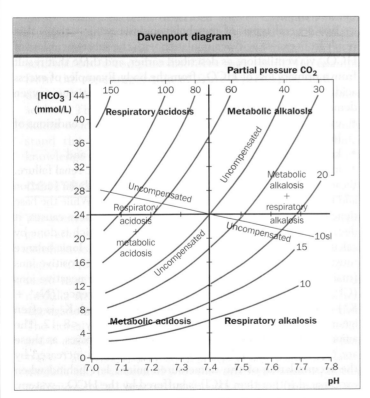

Figure 4.45 Davenport diagram. This graphic display plots plasma HCO_3^- against plasma pH with lines of equal carbon dioxide partial pressure (P_{CO_2}) curving across the graph (intermediate values of P_{CO_2} can be interpolated along vertical lines).

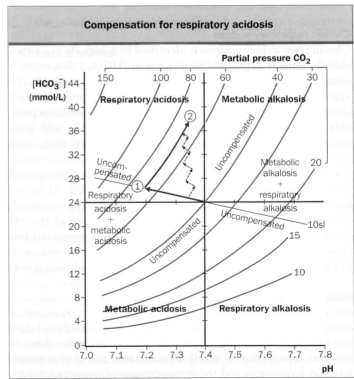

Figure 4.46 Compensation for a respiratory acidosis. Rapid development of hypoventilation, in which carbon dioxide partial pressure rises from 40 to 70mmHg, would follow the 10sl line of acute respiratory acidosis to point 1. If this level of hypoventilation were maintained for days, metabolic compensation would increase HCO_3^-, and improve the pH toward point 2. More likely, a progressive decline in ventilation over days might follow the stuttering, dotted path to the same end point.

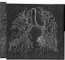

associated with a decrease in resistance[30]. Total cross-sectional area increases at a branching point if the number of daughter branches (n) is greater than the ratio of the parent-to-daughter radii squared, $(a/b)^2$, but resistance decreases only if $n > (a/b)^4$. The latter case occurs in the peripheral airways but not in the vessels, so while peripheral airways contribute little to normal airflow resistance, pulmonary microvessels make up a substantial portion of vascular resistance. Efforts to partition the pressure drop longitudinally suggest that about 25–30% is in the arterial portion (including arterioles), 50–60% in the microvascular portion, and the remainder in the veins[31]. With increases in flow, recruitment occurs mainly at the microvascular level, so their relative contribution to resistance becomes less.

Pulmonary vascular resistance, R, is calculated as intravascular driving pressure, ΔP (mean upstream PPA minus mean downstream PLA), divided by flow rate, $R = \Delta P/\dot{Q}$. The calculated resistance must be interpreted in the context of flow as the relation of driving pressure to flow is usually not linear and does not pass through zero. As shown in Figure 4.51, pulmonary vascular resistance decreases as flow and pressure increase with the attendant recruitment and distention of vessels.

The resistance to flow through a vessel increases with its length, with the viscosity of the fluid, and (most importantly) with the inverse of the radius to the fourth power. In addition to muscle activity in the wall, the caliber of a distensible vessel depends passively on the transmural pressure difference between intravascular and extravascular pressure. This is particularly important in the lungs, where the vessels are embedded in expandable parenchyma. It is convenient to consider separately the effect of lung expansion on the extra-alveolar arterial and venous vessels, which differs from that on the microvessels of the alveolar zone. With lung volume increase, extra-alveolar vessels are distended as the pressure is lowered in the expanding perivascular space around them (Fig. 4.52), and elongated as the lung expands.

By contrast, the alveolar microvessels in the alveolar walls are elongated, but partially collapsed by lung inflation since the alveolar pressure that surrounds them tends to increase relative to the intravascular pressure. This is easy to recognize with positive pressure ventilation, but also occurs with spontaneous inspiration, since intravascular pressures fall relative to atmospheric and alveolar pressure. The sheets of capillaries in the alveolar walls are protected from the full compressive force of the alveolar pressure by the surface tension of the curved layer of fluid that lines the alveolar surface. Microvessels in the corners, where alveolar walls meet, are more fully protected from compression by the sharper curvature of the surface film and perhaps by local distending forces, analogous to the extra-alveolar vessels (Fig. 4.53). The pulmonary vascular resistance is the sum of that through alveolar and extra-alveolar vessels and thus has a complex relationship with lung volume. It is lowest at about the normal (FRC) lung volume, but increases at higher and lower volumes.

Blood flow distribution

Anatomy and gravity influence the distribution of blood flow within the lung. If the upright lung is viewed as a stacked series of slices, a vertical gradient occurs in which the average flow rises progressively down the lung, largely influenced by gravity. However, within each slice a marked variability of blood flow is found between regions, which tends to be higher dorsally and presumably reflects local anatomic branching patterns[32].

The gravitational effect has been conceptualized by dividing the lung into three zones, one above another, based upon the relationship of vascular and alveolar pressures (Fig. 4.54). Intravascular pressures are higher at the bottom than the top of the lung by an amount equal to a vertical hydrostatic column as high as the lung. Near the lung apex, zone I, the pressure in the alveoli (PA) exceeds that in both the pulmonary arteries (PPA) and pulmonary vein (PPV), and collapses the alveolar vessels (except those in the alveolar corners which remain patent, and allow flow

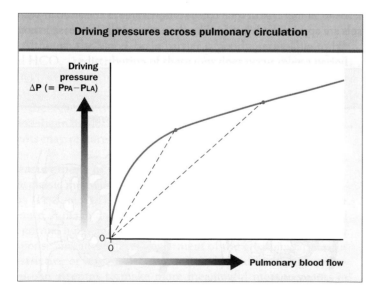

Figure 4.51 Driving pressure across pulmonary circulation [mean pulmonary artery (PPA) minus mean left atrial pressure (PLA)] increases nonlinearly with cardiac output. Resistance, represented by the slope from the origin to any point on the line, decreases with increased pulmonary blood flow, which reflects recruitment and distention of vessels.

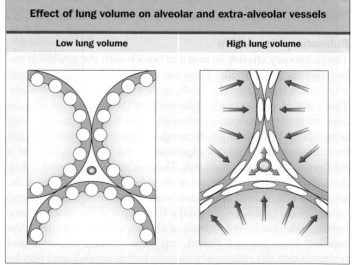

Figure 4.52 Lung volume affects alveolar and extra-alveolar vessels differently. At high lung volume, alveolar microvessels are stretched and compressed as vascular pressures fall relative to alveolar pressure. Extra-alveolar vessels, however, tend to be expanded as the pressure surrounding them decreases. (Modified with permission from Butler[28].)

Alveolar 'corner' at the junction of three, alveolar walls

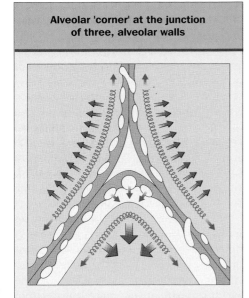

Figure 4.53 Alveolar 'corner' at the junction of three alveolar walls. Surface tension (depicted by springs) holds vessels open, particularly in corners, and promotes fluid transudation by lowering pressure around vessels. (Modified with permission from Butler[28].)

Perfusion in the lungs and arterial, venous, and alveolar pressures

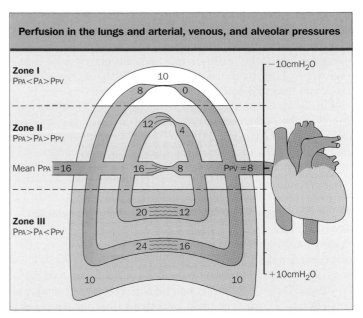

Figure 4.54 Perfusion in the lungs is influenced by the relationship of arterial and venous to alveolar pressures. In this example, the alveolar pressure is $10cmH_2O$, as might be found in a patient who receives positive pressure ventilation. (Modified with permission from Culver[33].)

to continue by a siphon effect). Below this, in zone II, PPA exceeds PA, but PA is greater than PPV, so flow depends on the pressure difference between PPA and PA. The vessels remain open, but are critically narrowed at the downstream end where venous pressure is lower than alveolar pressure. This creates independence of flow from the downstream venous pressure, analogous to a waterfall in which a stream that flows over a precipice is unaffected by a rising level in the pool below, until it rises above the level of the lip. In the mid to lower portion of the lung, zone III, both PPA and PPV exceed PA, the vessels are distended, and blood flow is the highest.

While the three-zone concept can explain the average increase in flow down the lung, it does not explain the observed variability in flow within an isogravitational slice, which implies that other anatomic or vasoregulatory factors are important at this level.

Regulation of pulmonary blood flow

Besides their response to passive mechanisms (anatomy, gravity, lung volume, alveolar pressure), the pulmonary vessels show vasomotor activity as a result of both neural and non-neural factors. Motor efferents from three autonomic networks are anatomically closely related to the vasculature – sympathetic, parasympathetic, and nonadrenergic noncholinergic (NANC) fibers. The sympathetic efferents probably have little effect, while parasympathetic stimulation dilates constricted vessels. Acetylcholine is a potent pulmonary vasodilator. The NANC system is inhibitory and constantly releases small peptides (like vasoactive intestinal peptide) at the ganglia and postganglionic ends of its unique network. Its vasodilator function is augmented on exercise.

Vasoregulation by alveolar gas concentration is most important in matching regional perfusion with ventilation. The arterioles constrict when the PO_2 in the alveoli they serve fall, and additional vasoconstriction results if alveolar PCO_2 rises (Fig. 4.55). This hypoxic vasoconstriction is a response to a low PO_2 in the air spaces rather than the intraluminal blood, which is normally desaturated in these prealveolar vessels. The site and mechanism of this local signal pathway is unclear, but the microvascular endothelium seems to be necessary to signal for the constriction of the more proximal vascular smooth muscle. When ventilation

Hypoxic vasoconstriction serves to reduce blood flow to poorly ventilated areas

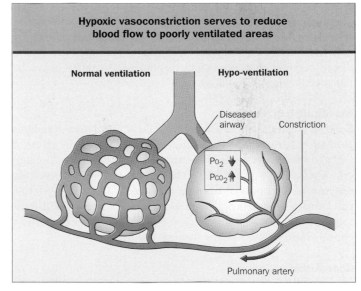

Figure 4.55 Hypoxic vasoconstriction serves to reduce blood flow to poorly ventilated areas. This improves V̇/Q̇ matching and oxygenation, but if generalized it contributes to pulmonary hypertension. (Modified with permission from Butler[28].)

is decreased by an obstructed airway or other injury, local hypoxic pulmonary vasoregulation decreases local blood flow, which tends to restore the local V̇/Q̇ ratio toward normal and thereby improve the PO_2 of the blood that leaves that area.

The blood flow diverted away can serve better ventilated regions, which further contributes to an improvement in overall V̇/Q̇ matching. Considerable individual variability is found in this response, which may be diminished by vasodilating drugs. Diversion of blood flow is most effective in atelectatic lung, in which hypoxic vasoconstriction is unopposed by the radial traction of surrounding expanded lung tissue. A reciprocal reflex in

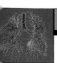

the airways also contributes to better matching, as small airways constrict when intraluminal P_{CO_2} falls and dilate when it rises. Hypoxic vasoconstriction is a helpful, adaptive response to local or regional lung abnormalities, but when alveolar hypoxia is generalized (e.g. hypoventilation or altitude), the increased resistance can lead to pulmonary hypertension.

Finally, locally produced and locally inactivated mediators are found in the pulmonary circulation. For instance, the vasoconstrictive and edemagenic actions of one group of arachidonic acid metabolites released in small amounts by the local endothelium are normally balanced by the vasodilator and membrane stabilizing properties of another group.

Nonrespiratory functions of the pulmonary circulation
Filtering

Aggregates of blood elements and emboli of various types (fat, air) carried in the systemic venous return are continually filtered out, dissolved, or engulfed by the cells of the pulmonary capillary bed. This is a vital protection for the cerebral, coronary, and other systemic beds. The small, potentially ischemic regions that may occur if larger emboli are present may receive limited perfusion by the bronchial circulation via bronchopulmonary anastomoses, and may be exposed to pulmonary venous blood that flows retrogradely into the circulation during lung volume changes. Thus, ischemic damage to the alveoli is prevented while a thrombus is lysed and the pulmonary flow restored.

Large numbers of white cells (mainly leukocytes) are sequestered in and around the small vessels of the pulmonary bed. Many reticuloendothelial cells occur in the lung and now evidence suggests that the vascular endothelial cell itself can be phagocytic when stimulated.

Modification of mediators

Some mediators in the blood, which have regulatory functions throughout the body, are secreted, taken up, or inactivated through specific receptors and enzyme systems in the pulmonary endothelial cells. Best known is the angiotensin-converting enzyme, which converts inactive angiotensin 1 into the systemic vasoconstrictor angiotensin 2. Histamine, bradykinin, and serotonin are, like acetylcholine, largely inactivated by the pulmonary endothelium in one passage through the lungs.

Coagulation

When local injury is present, pulmonary endothelial cells can be a source of thromboplastin and tissue plasminogen activator. In spite of vascular stasis and closure of vessels when flow decreases, clots do not form in pulmonary vessels because of the structure of the endothelial surface and because the secretion of anticlotting substances bathes the surface and prevents the adherence of platelets and cells. Embolic thrombi are dissolved remarkably quickly by local thrombolytic secretions.

Fluid exchange in the pulmonary circulation

The fluid flux across the pulmonary vascular endothelium (F) is influenced by the same pressure relationship as in the systemic capillaries, summarized in the modified Starling equation (Fig. 4.56). The hydrostatic pressure in the pulmonary microvessels (Pmv) exceeds the interstitial hydrostatic pressure (Ppmv) outside the microvessels. This effect favors filtration. The interstitial tissue fluid protein osmotic pressure (πt) is probably about

two thirds that in the vessel (πv); thus, the net osmotic force is absorptive and inward. Fluid flux is sensitive to small intravascular or perivascular pressure changes. Intravascular pressure rises may originate downstream (left heart failure), or may follow overall vascular volume increments (overhydration) or displacement of blood from the systemic to the pulmonary vessels. Fluid exchanges across the capillary walls, but the interstitial space around alveolar microvessels is tightly restricted by the collagen network between the alveolar walls. The two alveolar epithelial layers and the contained capillary bed form an inexpansible sandwich, so leakage is limited. The extra-alveolar arterioles and venules, which are not so confined and are also very thin walled, may be an additional site of fluid leakage.

Surface tension in the fluid film that lines the alveoli opposes alveolar pressure and tends to lower the interstitial pressure around pulmonary microvessels (see Fig. 4.53). An increase in surface tension may contribute to edema when surfactant is lost in an injured lung. Interstitial pressure around the extra-alveolar vessels is close to intrathoracic (pleural) pressure and falls as the lungs are distended, which favors relatively more leakage from them at high rather than at low lung volumes (see Fig. 4.52).

Interstitial edema

Normally, a net outflow of fluid from the upstream capillaries is reabsorbed into the downstream capillaries, where the intravascular pressure is lower. Several factors tend to keep the lung from becoming edematous. Fluid leakage causes local perivascular pressures to rise, particularly in the 'sandwich' between the alveolar walls, which reduces the outward fluid flux. It may also compress the vessels, which leads to a reduction of the total surface available for leakage. Since the fluid that leaks through intact endothelium is largely protein free, it dilutes and washes out the interstitial protein. This reduces perivascular πt, and thus increases the inward osmotic pressure difference and reduces the local fluid leak. If excess leakage does occur, the fluid moves from the alveolar walls, where it could interfere with gas exchange, into the low-pressure interstitial zones around the bronchovascular bundles, where it forms relatively innocuous venous, arterial, and peribronchial cuffs. This fluid is absorbed by the rich bronchial vascular network and by the many lymphatics in the adventitia of the airways and vessels. Edema fluid may also reach the pleural space, where it is absorbed by the pleural lymphatic and blood vessels.

Starling equation	

■ EQUATION 4.28

$F = Kf[(Pmv - Ppmv) - \sigma(\pi v - \pi t)]$

Symbol	Description
F	Net fluid flux out of vessels
Kf	Permeability factor
σ	Reflection coefficient to oncotic agents
Pmv	Pressure in microvessels
Ppmv	Perimicrovascular pressure
πv	Osmotic pressure in vessels
πt	Osmotic pressure of tissues

Figure 4.56 The Starling equation for fluid flux.

When the capillary endothelium is injured, locally or through the effect of circulating mediators, the vascular permeability to fluids and solutes is increased so that even a modest, outward pressure gradient causes a large fluid leak. The ability to retain large molecules is lost, protein-rich plasma leaks out, and πt approaches πv, so that the osmotic force opposing intravascular hydrostatic pressure is lost. This high permeability or 'leaky capillary' edema can be a fulminant process and lead to severe abnormalities of gas exchange.

Alveolar edema

The epithelial membrane that lines the air spaces is normally much less permeable than the endothelial membrane but, finally, underlying interstitial pulmonary edema fluid spills through it into the alveoli. This is thought to be because epithelial cell junctions split apart as the membrane is stretched. Fluid is initially seen only in the corners of the alveoli, where the pressure below the curved fluid film is lowest. As further fluid accumulates, the alveoli tend to rapidly become completely filled, again because of surface tension effects. As alveoli fill, the radius of the curvature of the surface of the fluid in the spheric alveoli becomes shorter and the effect of surface tension greater (Laplace's law), which pulls fluid in more strongly (Fig. 4.57).

Fluid and ions normally exchange across the bronchial and alveolar epithelial surfaces to regulate the character of the mucous blanket and maintain the subphase film beneath the surfactant that lines the alveoli. The epithelial cells have an impressive ability to secrete and reabsorb fluid actively from the alveoli against both hydrostatic and osmotic gradients. Alveolar edema fluid and that passing up into the airways by cilial action is actively reabsorbed. Thus, the sequence of edema development progresses from the perimicrovascular interstitium to the peribronchovascular 'sump' to patchy alveolar flooding.

Respiratory–circulatory interactions

The phasic changes of intrathoracic pressure and lung volume of the respiratory cycle alter the preload and afterload of the right and left heart, which interact to vary cardiac output and blood pressure with the respiratory cycle. The changes are modest during normal tidal breathing, but can be more notable in pathologic states. During inhalation, the decrease in intrathoracic pressure enhances systemic venous return to the chest. The right atrium and ventricle fill and right heart output to the pulmonary vessels increases as the alveoli fill with air. Lung expansion dilates the extra-alveolar pulmonary arterial vessels, which reduces their resistance and helps to accommodate the increased flow. Pulmonary artery pressure stays almost constant relative to alveolar pressure. This surge of blood flow reaches the left heart after 2–3 beats, so that systemic output and blood pressure begins to rise in late inspiration or early expiration. This preload effect is normally dominant, but the inspiratory drop in intrathoracic pressure can also add effective afterload to the left ventricle. When the pressure outside the heart is lower, the myocardium must generate a greater transmural pressure difference to maintain the same blood pressure. Or, more commonly, the systemic blood pressure falls a few millimeters of mercury coincident with inspiration and rises during exhalation. Depending on the respiratory rate, this direct pressure effect may be enhanced or countered by the arrival at the left ventricle of the inspiratory surge of flow.

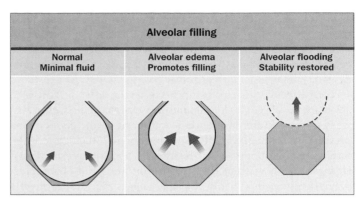

Figure 4.57 Alveoli tend to fill with fluid in an 'all or none' fashion. In the normal alveolus, a small amount of fluid rounds off the corners. Alveolar edema decreases the radius, which increases the inward force of surface tension and pulls in more fluid. When the alveolus is filled, the radius of surface increases so stability is regained.

When intrathoracic pressure swings are exaggerated, as in an asthmatic attack, the inspiratory dip in blood pressure can be 20–30mmHg and creates the clinical finding of 'pulsus paradoxus'. Interestingly, markedly negative inspiratory pressures such as this do not generate a proportionate further increase in systemic venous return because of a flow-limiting, or waterfall, mechanism. When the intraluminal pressure falls in the central veins, the vessels collapse at the point where they are first exposed to atmospheric pressure, in the neck, axillae, and abdomen, and their flow becomes independent of the increasingly negative downstream right atrial pressure.

When the pericardial space is limited (e.g. effusion or constrictive pericarditis) or the pleural surfaces of the cardiac fossa become tense at high lung volume (e.g. positive end expiratory pressure ventilation and large lung volumes, as in emphysema), an additional interaction may become important. Inspiratory filling of the right heart limits the diastolic expansion of the left heart. This 'ventricular interdependence' contributes to an inspiratory decrease in systemic outflow and blood pressure and allows them to increase when the right heart is less full during expiration.

PULMONARY FUNCTION TESTING

Pulmonary function testing encompasses a range of measurements from those that can be obtained readily at the bedside or in the home, to complex physiologic assessments made in a referral laboratory.

Spirometry should be easily available (office outpatient clinics) to screen for abnormalities of air flow or lung volume, to test bronchodilator responsiveness, and for interval assessment of patients who have asthma or COPD. Testing in the pulmonary function laboratory allows further classification and quantification of lung disease by adding data from the measurement of lung volumes and assessment of gas exchange through measurement of diffusing capacity, arterial blood gases, and tests of gas distribution. Special testing is available to assess exercise response, prethoracotomy evaluation, measurement of upper airway obstruction, and bronchoprovocation challenge testing.

Assessments of VC and air flow are based on the forced expiratory volume maneuver in which the subject inhales maximally, and then exhales forcefully and completely to RV. The expiratory air-flow rate at any point during this maneuver is determined by the driving pressure for air flow and the airway resistance. During a forceful exhalation the intrathoracic pressure that surrounds the central airways exceeds the intraluminal pressure, which allows dynamic compression of the airway (see Fig. 4.13). As a result of this, the effective driving pressure becomes the difference between alveolar pressure and the pleural pressure that compresses airways. This pressure difference is equivalent to the elastic recoil pressure of the lung tissue. Thus, even during a forceful effort, the intrinsic elastic properties of the lung are a major determinant of air flow. Airway resistance upstream from the point of compression is determined primarily by airway caliber, which varies directly with lung volume. Throughout exhalation from TLC, both recoil pressure and airway caliber progressively decrease, so that air-flow rates, after an early peak, also progressively decrease.

Spirometry

To obtain a satisfactory spirogram, the preceding inspiration must be maximal and the forced expiratory volume maneuver must be continued to cessation of flow or, when emptying is slowed, for at least 10 seconds[34,35]. The resultant information is commonly displayed in one of two formats. The traditional spirogram (Fig. 4.58) plots volume versus time, with flow rate indicated by the steepness of the plot. The orientation of the axes varies with equipment, with time moving either left or right and exhaled volume either up or down. In the flow–volume display (Fig. 4.59) the flow rate is measured and directly plotted on the vertical axis with volume on the horizontal axis. Time is not shown on this plot, but may be indicated by tick marks. With this display the reproducibility of successive efforts and some patterns of abnormality may be more easily seen. It is important to recognize that both the traditional spirogram and the expiratory flow–volume display are obtained from the same maneuver, but emphasize different aspects of the same information.

Expiratory flow measurements

Basic measurements from the forced expiratory volume maneuver include FVC, the forced expiratory volume in 1 second (FEV_1), and the ratio of FEV_1 to FVC. The FVC or total volume exhaled is equivalent in normal individuals to a 'slow' VC obtained with a complete, but not forceful, exhalation. Patients who have advanced obstructive airway disease often manifest exaggerated dynamic compression (narrowing airways with forceful efforts), so that the FVC is smaller than the slow VC. A reduction in VC reflects a reduction in TLC, an increase in RV, or a combination of both. The FEV_1 is readily obtained from the traditional spirogram by observing the volume exhaled in the first 1 second of effort. This measurement cannot be seen on the flow–volume display, but can be calculated by the microprocessors involved in most modern equipment that uses this display. The FEV_1/FVC ratio is easily obtained from simple equipment and provides the best index of air-flow limitation. This ratio is commonly expressed as a percentage and is sometimes referred to as the percent FEV_1; however, this terminology may cause confusion as the FEV_1 itself is expressed as a percentage of its predicted value.

An additional flow measurement widely reported from the spirogram is the average forced expiratory flow rate between 25 and 75% of the exhaled VC (FEF_{25-75}), formerly referred to as the maximum midexpiratory flow rate. This measurement shows wider variability than does FEV_1 or the FEV_1/FVC ratio, both within and between individuals. When this is appropriately accounted for, it shows a sensitivity for the detection of air-flow limitation very similar to that of the FEV_1/FVC ratio.

Numerous other flow measurements can be obtained from the forced expiratory volume maneuver, but they are highly interdependent with those above and add little new information. The $FEV_{0.5}$ may be used to assess the initiation of effort, but adds little diagnostic information. The FEV_3 and particularly the FEV_3/FVC

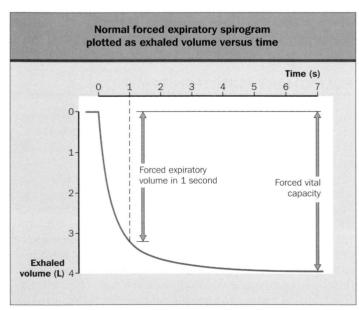

Figure 4.58 Normal forced expiratory spirogram plotted as exhaled volume versus time. The forced expiratory volume in 1 second (FEV_1) and forced vital capacity (FVC) are indicated by arrows. In this example, FEV_1 is 3.35L, FVC is 4L, and the FEV_1/FVC ratio is 84%. (Modified with permission from Culver[36].)

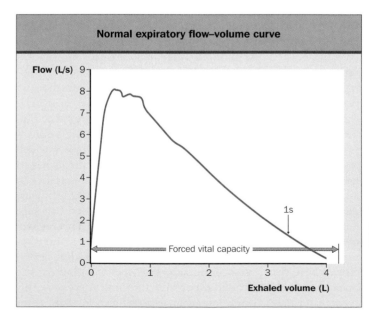

Figure 4.59 Normal expiratory flow–volume curve. The same forced expiratory volume maneuver shown in Figure 4.58 is plotted here as a flow–volume curve. The air-flow rate reaches a peak early in the exhalation, then decreases progressively until air flow ceases at residual volume. (Modified with permission from Culver[36].)

ratio has been shown to be slightly more sensitive than the FEV_1/FVC ratio for the detection of early air-flow obstruction. This is because the measurement is extended later in the spirogram and is thus influenced more by flow at low lung volumes, at which early airway disease is first manifest.

The peak expiratory flow rate achieved during the FVC maneuver cannot be accurately calculated from a spirogram display, but is readily seen on the flow–volume display and can be calculated by microprocessors. It can show considerable effort-to-effort variability, even when FEV_1 and FVC measurements are nearly identical. A peak flow measurement can also be obtained by simple hand-held devices, which are useful for interval follow-up and for home management of patients who have reactive airways disease, but are less sensitive than spirometry for screening.

Whereas spirographic flow measurements are obtained over a time interval or volume interval, measurements from the flow–volume display or current microprocessors can be reported at specific lung volumes. Maximum flow rates at 50% and 75% of exhaled volume are commonly reported, but nomenclature varies and the latter is often designated as the flow rate at 25% of remaining VC.

The maximum voluntary ventilation (MVV) is measurable on some office spirometers, but is primarily a laboratory measurement. The subject is instructed to breathe deeply and rapidly, typically 60–70 breaths per minute, and the total volume of ventilation over a 12–15 second period is extrapolated to liters per minute. Historically, this was the primary dynamic test for obstructive disease but has now been supplanted by the forced expiratory maneuver for the diagnosis of air-flow limitation. It is used as a global assessment of ventilatory capacity in the evaluation of dyspnea, in the interpretation of exercise limitation, in disability assessment, in some preoperative testing, and to evaluate neuromuscular disease of the chest wall and diaphragm.

Prediction equations and limits of normality

Numerous prediction equations have been derived from spirometric surveys of normal populations. Currently accepted studies exclude all smokers as well as individuals who have any thoracic or cardiopulmonary disease[37–39]. Most studies have found that spirometric parameters can be predicted on the basis of gender, age, and height, and that the addition of other body-size measurements does not improve the accuracy of the equations.

The prediction equations give the midpoint of the normal range, which is unfortunately wide for most spirometric measurements. The lower limit of normal (LLN) must be established from the variability among individuals who have the same prediction parameters. For each test, the LLN is best determined by subtracting a fixed quantity, the confidence interval, from the predicted value. For most spirometric measurements this quantity is different for males and females, but does not vary with height, age, or magnitude of the predicted value.

Use of a percentage of the predicted value as a lower limit is convenient, but less accurate as it causes the normal range to vary with the magnitude of the predicted value. A lower limit value equal to 80% of the predicted value has been widely used in spirometric interpretation. While this is a reasonable approximation for FEV_1 and FVC in young individuals, it is overly sensitive for older or smaller individuals. An 80% lower limit is quite inappropriate for FEF_{25-75}, where the normal range may reach 50–60% of the predicted value. The predicted value for the

FEV_1/FVC ratio varies little with body size, but does decline progressively with age (e.g. from 87 to 77% in females, 84 to 74% in males, from the third to the eighth decade). The LLN is approximately 8–10 percentage points below the predicted percentage. Since the ratio is typically expressed as a percentage, to report this value as a percent of the predicted value is confusing and should be avoided.

The lower limit values are chosen to exclude 5% of a normal population, that is 5% will be mislabeled as having disease. In screening a generally healthy population for a rare disease, a borderline low result is more likely to represent this mislabeling than true identification of disease. However, as spirometry is often used to test symptomatic individuals for a common disease, the probability that a borderline result reflects a true abnormality is much higher.

Interpretation of spirometric abnormalities
Obstructive

Air-flow limitation is the hallmark of the obstructive diseases; this physiologic diagnosis rests primarily on the demonstration of an FEV_1/FVC ratio below the LLN. Typically, FVC is normal early in the course of disease, but is reduced in more severe disease as the RV is increased because of trapped air. The severity of air-flow limitation is quantified by the decrement in FEV_1.

Restrictive

A restrictive defect is defined by a reduction in TLC, but restriction in lung volume can be inferred from spirometry when a decrement occurs in FVC and FEV_1 while the FEV_1/FVC ratio is normal or high. A decrement in FVC because of the increased RV of obstruction should not be classified as a restrictive defect, since lung volumes are large. When FVC and the FEV_1/FVC ratio are both decreased, restriction can only be determined by an assessment of TLC.

Reversibility

The usefulness of spirometry in the office or clinic is often enhanced by the assessment of bronchodilator response. Spirometry is repeated after the administration of an inhaled bronchodilator, waiting 15 minutes after a β-agonist or 30 minutes after ipratropium bromide. An increase in the absolute value of FEV_1 by 12–15% represents a significant response in an individual who has near-normal spirometry. With more severe obstructive disease, the improvement should also be at least 200mL to differentiate the pharmacologic response from test-to-test variability. Often FVC improves in parallel with FEV_1. An improvement in FVC by more than 15% in the absence of a change in FEV_1 may reflect either an improvement in flow rates after the first second or simply a longer duration of effort.

Although the FEV_1/FVC ratio is the most useful test for the diagnosis of air-flow limitation, it may remain the same or even decrease postbronchodilator, depending upon the relative change in its two components, and is thus not a useful index of reversibility. Because of its large intraindividual variability, FEF_{25-75} must show an increase of 30–40% to represent a significant bronchodilator effect. Occasionally, this parameter changes little or even decreases despite a clear improvement in FEV_1 or (particularly) FVC. This is because the bronchodilator has allowed exhalation to continue to a lower RV so that the 25–75% increment is now measured at a lower lung volume with consequent lower flow rates.

Lung volumes

Spirometry can measure only those subdivisions of lung volume that lie within the VC range (see Fig. 4.5). Measurement of TLC or of the volume of gas in the chest at FRC requires a method of measuring the gas that remains in the lungs at RV. Typically, the gas volume contained in the lungs at FRC is measured, with TLC and RV determined by adding or subtracting the appropriate increments from an accompanying spirogram.

Methods of measurement

The methods used most widely to measure lung volumes include helium dilution, nitrogen washout, and body plethysmography. Also, TLC can be quite accurately determined from calculations based upon planimetry of posteroanterior and lateral chest radiographs, using one of several geometric models.

Helium dilution

A spirometer is prepared that contains a known volume and concentration of an inert gas, typically 10% helium. The patient or subject is connected to this closed system, breathing through a mouthpiece with nose clipped, and continues doing normal tidal breathing. Over the course of a few minutes the gas in the patient's lung equilibrates with gas in the spirometer and the helium concentration, which is continuously monitored, falls to a new, lower, steady-state level. Carbon dioxide is removed from the closed system by soda lime absorption and a low flow of oxygen is added to compensate for the patient's ongoing oxygen consumption by keeping the mixing chamber or spirometer volume constant. The ratio of the initial to the final concentration of helium allows calculation of the unknown volume (FRC) present in the system.

Nitrogen washout

Nitrogen washout is also based upon the principle of conservation of mass of an inert gas, in this case the nitrogen normally resident within the lungs. The patient breathes on a mouthpiece and, at the end of a relaxed tidal exhalation, is connected to an inspiratory source of 100% oxygen. The patient exhales through one-way valves into a collection bag previously flushed with oxygen so that it contains no nitrogen. The resident nitrogen is washed out of the lungs progressively and monitored with continuous analysis. When the exhaled nitrogen concentration falls to <2%, the test is terminated and the volume of nitrogen collected is measured. The FRC can be calculated on the basis that this nitrogen volume represents 80% of the lung gas contained at the beginning of the test. Instead of the collection bag, current microprocessors use a calculation based upon instantaneous, breath-by-breath measurement of exhaled volume times nitrogen concentration. Washout can be completed in 3–4 minutes in normal subjects, but may require over 15 minutes with severe obstructive airway disease so that the gas volume in slowly mixing spaces can be measured.

Body plethysmography

The volume of gas within the thorax, whether in communication with airways or not, can be measured by this technique, based upon the physical principles of gas compression described by Boyle's law. The subject sits within a fully enclosed rigid box and breathes through a mouthpiece connected through a shutter to the internal volume of the box. Sensitive manometers monitor the pressure at the airway and inside the chamber. The apparatus is electronically calibrated with the subject in place, so that the addition of a known small volume of gas to the inside of the chamber raises the chamber pressure by $1 cmH_2O$. At the end of a tidal exhalation, the airway shutter is closed and the subject asked to make panting efforts with the glottis open. An effort to expand the chest decompresses intrathoracic gas and reciprocally compresses that in the chamber.

Under conditions of constant temperature, well maintained by the high blood flow through the lungs, the product of airway pressure and lung gas volume is a constant. The slope of the relationship between the change in airway pressure and the change in thoracic volume, which can be calculated continuously or plotted on an oscilloscope, is inversely related to the intrathoracic volume. As this technique is sensitive to gas volume not in free communication with the airways, such as that in bullae or even a pneumothorax, the measurement is often called thoracic gas volume, and may exceed the FRC measured by gas dilution techniques. Advantages of this method, besides its inclusion of 'trapped' gas, are that several measurements can be repeated rapidly and that airway resistance can be measured with the same apparatus when panting is continued with the shutter open.

Interpretation of lung volume abnormalities

Inspiration is limited at TLC when the maximum inspiratory force that can be applied by the chest muscles and diaphragm is opposed equally by the increasing recoil force of the lungs as they are distended to higher volumes. Usually, TLC is limited primarily by the elastic properties of the lungs, as variations in muscle strength have only a small effect on total chest expansion until weakness becomes quite marked. Parenchymal restrictive diseases reduce CL, so greater distending pressure is required to achieve any volume change, resulting in a lower TLC. The displacement of intrathoracic gas volume by effusions, edema, intravascular volume, and inflammatory cells also contributes to a reduction in measured lung gas volumes. Except for pleural effusions, these quantities are relatively small and outweighed by the frequently associated changes in lung elastic properties.

The minimum lung volume, or RV, is determined by a combination of two factors. The smallest volume to which the expiratory muscles can raise the diaphragm and squeeze chest wall is the dominant factor in youth. With progressive age and the normal loss of tissue elastic recoil forces, the lung volume at which small airways close and trap remaining gas behind them increases and becomes the dominant factor to determine RV.

Restrictive lung diseases

Restrictive lung diseases are defined as those that cause a significant decrease in TLC. In most parenchymal infiltrative processes, this is accompanied by parallel decrements in FRC, RV, and VC, although early disease may preferentially affect RV. Obesity shows a different pattern in that the primary effect is on the relaxed end expiratory volume or FRC. The large abdomen and heavy chest wall reduce the outward recoil of the thoracic cage, which opposes the inward recoil of the lung parenchyma, resulting in a lower FRC. However, RV is determined by airway closure and is little affected, and the TLC achievable using maximum inspiratory force is only minimally reduced until obesity becomes extreme. Thus, the typical spirogram in obesity shows an FRC that approaches RV, but with a relatively large inspiratory capacity and a near normal TLC and VC.

Obstructive diseases

Obstructive diseases cause airway closure that limits exhalation at higher lung volume because of the combined effects on luminal caliber of airway inflammation and loss of tissue recoil. This results in a progressive increase in RV (Fig. 4.60), as increasing amounts of gas are trapped behind closed airways. These patients breathe at an increased FRC because of the combined effects of a decrease in lung recoil force from emphysema and the need to increase luminal caliber to minimize the resistive work of air flow. The TLC is normal to high, which again reflects the loss of lung recoil forces. Since RV increases to a greater extent than does TLC, the VC decreases with severe airway obstruction.

Diffusion capacity

The diffusion capacity (DL) test, also called transfer factor, measures the capacity to transfer gas from alveolar spaces into the alveolar capillary blood. This process occurs by passive diffusion and is a function of the pressure difference that drives gas, the surface area over which exchange takes place, and the resistive properties to gas movement through the membrane and into chemical combination with the blood. The units are milliliters per minute per millimeter mercury of driving pressure (mL/min per mmHg). Carbon monoxide is used as the test gas (DLCO), because its extreme avidity for Hb allows the back pressure to diffusion to be considered negligible.

In the most widely used, single-breath method the subject exhales to RV, and takes a VC inhalation of the test gas, which contains a low level of carbon monoxide (0.3%) and an inert gas (e.g. 10% helium). After holding inspiration for 8–10 seconds, the subject exhales quickly. The initial portion of the expirate, which includes anatomic dead space, is discarded and a sample of alveolar gas is collected. The reduction in helium concentration in the collected sample allows calculation of the alveolar volume at

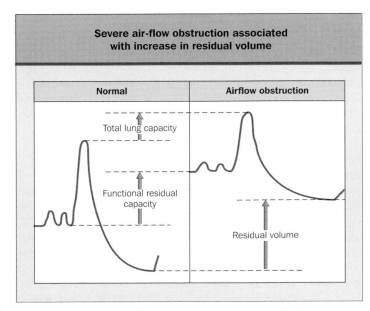

Severe air-flow obstruction associated with increase in residual volume

Figure 4.60 Severe air-flow obstruction is associated with an increase in residual volume. Prolonged expiratory air flow may continue until the subsequent inhalation, and alveolar gas is trapped behind narrowed and closed airways. The functional residual capacity at which tidal breathing occurs is also increased and total lung capacity may be high as well. (Modified with permission from Culver[36].)

TLC into which carbon monoxide was distributed and of the initial carbon monoxide concentration after its dilution by the resident RV. The final concentration of carbon monoxide in the exhaled sample allows calculation of the volume of carbon monoxide transferred out of alveoli and a calculation, for which an exponential decline is assumed, of the mean carbon monoxide driving pressure during the breath-holding period. An effective residence time is calculated from the breath-hold period plus a portion of the time of inspiration and sample collection.

A significant problem with the diffusing capacity measurement is that numerous variations in the handling of small correction factors (for gas conditions, apparatus dead space, timing measurement, etc.) can cumulatively cause the calculated value to vary substantially. Although reproducibility within a laboratory can be quite acceptable, the accuracy of comparisons between laboratories or to published normal standards is much less consistent, as reflected by published predicted values that vary by 20% or more. It is essential that each laboratory choose prediction equations that are appropriate to the nuances of its equipment and technique.

Although diffusion is often thought of as a function of alveolar membrane thickness, the dominant factor is usually the capillary blood volume, which influences both the surface area available for exchange and the volume of blood and Hb available to accept carbon monoxide. The influence of Hb concentration can be accounted for by theoretic or empiric correction factors. The rate of blood flow is not important as carbon monoxide is taken up even by stagnant blood (or extravasated blood in the case of pulmonary hemorrhage), but the recruitment of capillaries during high flow conditions such as exercise or with congenital left-to-right shunt increases the measured diffusing capacity. The LLN needs to be determined according to the same principles as described above for spirometry.

Many laboratories also report the diffusing capacity as a ratio to the alveolar volume (DL/VA). This is called the transfer coefficient (KCO). The implication is that loss of lung volume because of mechanical abnormalities is accompanied by a parallel loss of DL. This, however, is not the case with a voluntary limitation of inspiration, in which capillaries remain perfused and DL/VA rises, or with pneumonectomy, in which capillaries are recruited in the remaining lung and DL/VA is again high. Diffusing capacity is commonly reduced in parenchymal inflammatory diseases, primarily because of the loss of available capillaries. The most common pattern in diseases such as sarcoidosis and interstitial fibrosis is for DL to be reduced and DL/VA to be slightly low or 'normal', as volume is also lost. Both DL and DL/VA are low with the loss of capillary surface area and blood volume in emphysema and in diseases that are primarily vascular, such as vasculitis, recurrent emboli, and pulmonary hypertension.

Tests of gas distribution

Abnormalities of spirometry and air-flow rate reflect overall narrowing of airways, but most lung diseases affect airways irregularly, which leads to abnormalities of gas distribution that may be more sensitive indicators of early airway disease.

Closing volume

As lung volume decreases, the smaller, intraparenchymal airways decrease in caliber until they close at low lung volume and ventilation to or from alveoli beyond them ceases. As there is a vertical gradient in the pleural pressure that surrounds the lungs, the lung tissue is less distended in dependent regions than higher in the thorax. In late exhalation, dependent airways close (and these areas reach their regional RV), while air flow continues from the upper portions of the lung until they too close, and overall RV is reached. The beginning of this wave of ascending airway closure can be detected by physiologic tests and is termed closing volume. Closing volume is usually expressed as a percentage of VC. That is, a closing volume of 20% means that airway closure can be detected during a slow exhalation when 20% of the VC remains before reaching RV (Fig. 4.61). Alternatively, when RV is measured this can be added to closing volume and the sum, termed closing capacity, is expressed as a percentage of TLC.

Both of these measures have been used as tests of early airway dysfunction in the natural history of COPD. Abnormalities can be detected in a high percentage of smokers, including many who do not go on to develop progressive airway limitation. On an individual patient basis, the closing volume is most helpful in its relationship to the lung volume at which tidal breathing occurs. When airway closure occurs at a volume below FRC, the airways are open throughout the lungs during tidal breathing, but when airway closure occurs above FRC, the affected alveoli are underventilated. Since the dependent regions are well perfused, this creates a low $\dot{V}/\dot{Q}$ region, which contributes to hypoxemia. This occurs when the closing volume is increased by normal aging, COPD, and by the effect of peribronchial edema in left ventricular failure. Similar consequences follow when FRC is reduced by recumbent posture or by obesity[11,12].

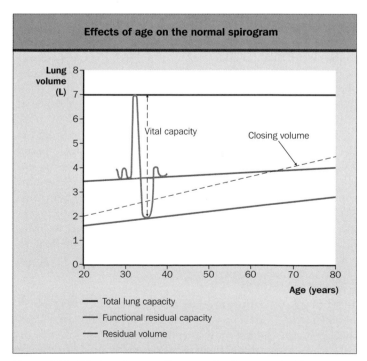

Effects of age on the normal spirogram

Legend:
— Total lung capacity
— Functional residual capacity
— Residual volume

Figure 4.61 Effects of age on the normal spirogram. Residual volume progressively increases with an associated small reduction in vital capacity. The functional residual capacity increases slightly, but the closing volume, at which dependent airways cease to ventilate, increases more steeply and exceeds the normal functional residual capacity in older ages. (Modified from Culver and Butler[40] with permission of The McGraw-Hill Companies.)

Arterial blood gas measurement

Measurement of pH, P_{CO_2}, and P_{O_2} in arterial blood is commonly included in the complete pulmonary function assessment of patients suspected to have significant lung disease. pH and P_{CO_2} are directly measured and the accompanying HCO_3^- concentration is calculated from the Henderson–Hasselbalch equation. (Since this relationship is not in question, the value of this 'calculated' data must not be discounted; it is every bit as accurate as the pH and P_{CO_2} measurements from which it is derived.)

An increase in arterial P_{CO_2} means that alveolar ventilation is low relative to carbon dioxide production, because total ventilation is low, the effective alveolar ventilation is reduced by excessive wasted ventilation, or the carbon dioxide production level has increased without a concomitant increase in ventilation. The matching of ventilation to need is a function of both mechanical capabilities and ventilatory drive. Most patients who suffer hypercapnia have severe mechanical impairments, but those who are affected by relatively low drive are more likely to retain carbon dioxide. Patients who have an FEV_1 >1L rarely retain carbon dioxide unless lack of drive is a major factor. Despite the air-flow obstruction present during an acute asthmatic attack, multiple stimuli tend to increase drive and ventilation. However, when obstruction becomes extreme, again with an FEV_1 in the region of 1L or below for an adult, the development of acute hypercapnia is likely. Most parenchymal restrictive diseases tend to be associated with mild hyperventilation, presumably from mechanical stimuli to the respiratory centers, until the functional abnormalities become very severe.

The normal P_{CO_2} remains in a narrow range around 40mmHg throughout life, but the normal P_{O_2} diminishes progressively with age. This decline is more marked when measured in the supine position and, in both cases, reflects the progressive increase in closing volume with age (see Fig. 4.61). Abnormal reductions in P_{O_2} are caused by hypoventilation, as reflected by an increase in P_{CO_2}, or to the combined effects of pulmonary blood flow to poorly ventilated areas (low $\dot{V}/\dot{Q}$ ratio) and right-to-left shunting. Diffusion abnormalities, unless extremely severe, rarely contribute to a low P_{O_2} among patients at rest. The low P_{O_2} commonly seen in patients who have diffusion abnormalities reflects the concomitant presence of $\dot{V}/\dot{Q}$ abnormalities associated with their disease. Diffusion limitation may make a small contribution to a reduction in P_{O_2} observed during exercise, but again the major component is a worsened effect of the $\dot{V}/\dot{Q}$ abnormalities.

Special testing

Upper airway obstruction

Obstruction in the central airways (e.g. tracheal tumor or stenosis) affects the expiratory flow–volume relationship in a different way than does the more common distal airway obstruction of COPD. The latter has its predominant effect late in expiration, with slowing of terminal flow rates, so that peak flow tends to be relatively maintained while the remaining flow–volume curve becomes progressively convex toward the horizontal axis (Fig. 4.62). Central obstructions have their primary effect early, which results in a truncated, flat-topped flow–volume curve (Fig. 4.63) that reflects a steady effort against a constant resistance. In the latter portion of the expiration, the decreasing lung volume and airway caliber shift the site of major resistance to the more peripheral airways, so that the latter portion of the flow–volume curve is normal.

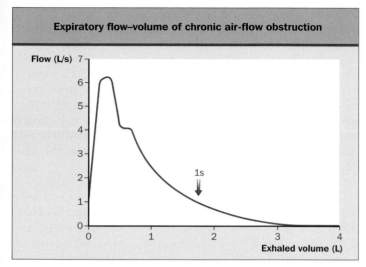

Figure 4.62 Expiratory flow–volume curve of chronic air-flow obstruction. Air-flow rates are markedly reduced at mid-to-lower lung volumes, with a curve that is convex to the horizontal axis. In this example, just under 50% of the vital capacity has been exhaled in 1 second. (Modified with permission from Culver[36].)

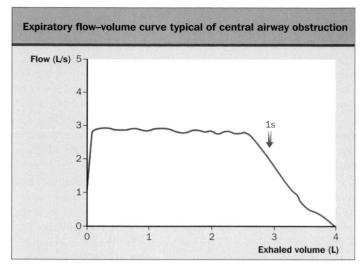

Figure 4.63 Expiratory flow–volume curve showing the pattern typical of central airway obstruction. Peak flow is markedly truncated, but flow rates at low lung volume are unaffected. Despite the dramatic effect on the flow–volume curve, the ratio of forced expiratory curve in 1 second to forced vital capacity is only modestly affected, 71% in this example. (Modified with permission from Culver[36].)

When a central obstruction is in the extrathoracic airway and has some flexibility (e.g. vocal cord paralysis), its effect is much greater during inspiratory flow than expiratory flow. The negative intraluminal pressure generated during inspiration narrows the airway, which exacerbates the obstruction, while during expiration the positive airway pressure below the site of obstruction tends to distend the airway, which reduces the abnormality. These lesions are assessed by recording on the flow–volume display the maximum effort inspiratory flow pattern, as well as that during expiration, to complete a flow–volume 'loop'. The normal inspiratory flow pattern has a hemicircular shape with peak inspiratory flow at midvolume that consistently exceeds midvolume expiratory flow (Fig. 4.64).

Bronchoprovocation testing

Patients who have suspected reactive airways disease frequently have normal spirometry when asymptomatic. When the diagnosis is unclear, provocation testing may be employed in an attempt to explain symptoms or predict future risks. A common clinical provocation of asthma is the airway mucosal cooling and drying effect of exercise hyperpnea, or cold-air inhalation. Provocation testing with exercise can utilize free running, treadmill running, or bicycle pedaling, with the yield of abnormal tests being in that order. Exercise needs to be to approximately two thirds of maximal capability and sustained for 5 minutes or more to have a high yield of abnormal results. Spirometry is done prior to exercise and repeated following exercise, with the most marked decrease in flow rates noted at 5–10 minutes after exercise. A reduction in FEV_1 of 20% is considered significant. Cold-air hyperventilation is less widely available as a provocation test. Spirometry is done before and after isocapneic hyperventilation of air, which has been dehumidified and cooled to 4°C.

Methacholine responsiveness is a nonspecific indicator of airway reactivity. Starting with a single inhalation at a very low concentration, patients are tested after progressively increasing inhaled doses until either a predetermined maximum dose has been achieved or the FEV_1 has been observed to fall by 20%.

Normal individuals do not respond to the maximum dose, whereas patients who suffer asthma respond to low-to-intermediate doses. Subjects who have a family history of asthma or hay fever symptoms may show intermediate responses, as do some patients in the recovery period after viral respiratory infections.

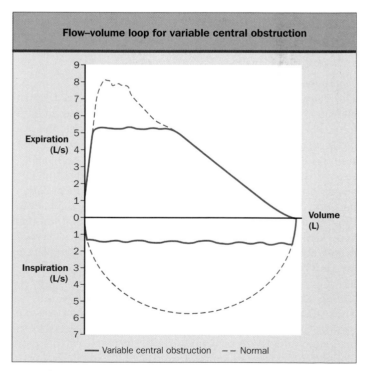

Figure 4.64 Flow–volume loop showing both forced expiratory and inspiratory air flows. The expiratory peak flow is somewhat truncated, consistent with a variable central obstruction during exhalation, while inspiratory flow is markedly reduced compared with the normal curve. This pattern is typical of a flexible, extrathoracic obstruction such as that caused by paralyzed vocal cords. (Modified with permission from Culver[36].)

In selected circumstances, provocation testing may be carried out with suspected specific allergens or occupational exposures. Dose preparation needs to be very careful to avoid an excessive and dangerous response. Studies may be designed to mimic the circumstances of the patient's clinical or occupational exposure. Testing may need to be continued for several hours to seek a late phase reaction.

Respiratory and cardiac response to exercise

Cardiopulmonary exercise testing is carried out to assess a patient's exercise capacity objectively, to observe the response of the components of the oxygen delivery system to this stress, and to determine, if possible, the factor(s) that limit exercise capacity or cause exertional dyspnea[41–43]. Testing procedures can range from very simple measurements, such as the distance walked in 6 minutes, to a complex array of continuously monitored parameters during an incremental work protocol programmed on a calibrated ergometer or treadmill.

Normal exercise

The work of exercise requires additional oxygen delivery to and uptake by muscles, which in turn produces more carbon dioxide. This requires higher levels of alveolar ventilation, cardiac output, and muscle blood flow, and additional oxygen extraction from the blood. When the capacity of aerobic glycolysis approaches limits, additional adenosine triphosphate can be generated, albeit much less efficiently, through anaerobic pathways that result in lactate production and metabolic acidosis. As these additional H^+ ions are buffered, HCO_3^- is consumed and additional carbon dioxide is produced, so that the rate of carbon dioxide output to oxygen uptake, the respiratory exchange ratio (R), rises. In addition, stimulation by the metabolic acidosis drives ventilation further up near maximum exercise, and the resultant washout of carbon dioxide from the blood contributes to a further increase in R.

Ventilatory response

The ventilatory response to exercise is characterized by an increase in minute ventilation ($\dot{V}E$) caused by increases in both frequency and V_T ($\dot{V}E = f \times V_T$). At maximal exercise, the respiratory rate is about 40–50 breaths per minute and V_T approaches about 60% of VC. The effective, gas exchanging, alveolar ventilation increases further as the increased pulmonary blood flow recruits vessels, which allows less wasted ventilation in poorly perfused regions. The V_D/V_T ratio typically falls from about 30% to 15–20% with exercise. Ventilation is not limiting in normal subjects, as the minute ventilation at maximal exercise is only about two thirds of the maximal voluntary ventilation measured during pulmonary testing or estimated from FEV_1.

Cardiac response

The cardiac response to exercise is dominated by a progressive increase in heart rate, as stroke volume increases modestly to a maximum value quite early in exercise. Heart rate can increase 3–4 fold to a maximum approximated as (220 – age). The lower resting heart rate of a well-conditioned individual, which reflects a larger stroke volume, allows a greater relative increase over resting output. Oxygen delivery to active tissues is further increased by a progressively greater extraction, from a resting value of 25% of arterial content to >80%. The venous P_{O_2} levels that leave maximally exercising muscle may be <10mmHg,

with tissue mitochondrial levels probably <1mmHg. Effective redistribution of blood flow to exercising muscle is an important, but not readily measurable, aspect of the cardiovascular response. The need for heat dissipation through increased skin blood flow compromises maximal oxygen uptake when exercise is prolonged or in a hot environment. Exercise capacity in normal subjects is limited by the maximum blood flow that can be delivered to the active muscle and ultimately by cellular hypoxia and acidosis. The resultant drive to ventilation may cause the sensation of dyspnea, which makes it appear that respiratory function is limiting.

Blood gas response

The blood gas response to exercise in a normal subject typically shows mild hyperventilation with a late increase caused by acidosis, and well maintained oxygenation. Arterial P_{O_2} remains normal or may increase as a consequence of alveolar hyperventilation, especially late in exercise. (Small decrements in P_{O_2} have been noted at extreme levels of exercise in athletic subjects, which perhaps reflects the very low mixed venous oxygen that passes through the normal small 'physiologic shunt', or possibly a limit to diffusion of oxygen.) Early in exercise, arterial P_{CO_2} is slightly lower than normal, which reflects an increased drive that may originate from muscle receptors. As anaerobic metabolism develops, metabolic acidosis initially becomes apparent because the Pa_{CO_2} drops without a corresponding increase in pH. As the heart rate and cardiac output limitation is reached, a marked increase in release of lactate occurs. The capacity of a subject to continue past this point is largely a function of training and determination, perhaps enhanced by inherently low ventilatory drive. It is not unusual for a well-motivated subject to exercise to a pH of 7.15.

Exercise testing

Clinical cardiopulmonary exercise testing is most commonly carried out using a progressive work protocol, performed on either a treadmill with increasing speeds and slope, or a stationary bicycle pedaled at a constant rate with a variable resistance to apply an increasing load. Load is increased in a continuous ramp or at intervals ranging from 20 to 180 seconds. In simple screening tests, the electrocardiogram is monitored for heart rate, rhythm, and ischemia, and oxygenation is monitored by pulse oximetry. In more complete testing, the subject breathes through a mouthpiece with measurement of respiratory rate, V_T, and minute ventilation and gases are analyzed either by interval collections or by continuous monitoring with integration over time. For blood gas information beyond oximetry, arterial blood gases can be sampled at end exercise or a radial artery catheter is placed for sequential measurement.

The standard measurement of exercise capacity is the oxygen uptake per minute, $\dot{V}_{O_2}$, and the maximum value that can be achieved during a progressive work test. The value depends to some extent upon the volume of muscle active so that bicycle tests yield maximums about 10% lower than the treadmill tests, in which more upper body activity is required. As the relationships between heart rate and both cardiac output and oxygen consumption are quite linear, some information can be projected from submaximal responses, but the maximum $\dot{V}_{O_2}$ and limits to exercise are best determined by continuing the test until the patient can no longer maintain the pace or is limited by symptoms.

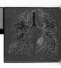

The elements typically reported in the interpretation of exercise testing are given in Figure 4.65.

Patterns of abnormal exercise performance
Cardiac
Patients who have valvular cardiac impairment can reach a normal maximum heart rate, but do so at low levels of work. A low $\dot{V}O_2$max and, at any given level of oxygen consumption, high heart rate means the oxygen pulse is low, which suggests a small forward stroke volume. The minute ventilation is also somewhat higher than normal, particularly toward the end of exercise, consistent with the early onset of anaerobic threshold because of poor oxygen delivery. Patients who have ischemic heart disease or cardiomyopathy similarly have low $\dot{V}O_2$ and oxygen pulse, but also often fail to reach their predicted heart rate.

Obstructive pulmonary disease
Patients who suffer air-flow obstruction commonly have their exercise performance limited by ventilatory mechanics. Minute ventilation is high for the level of activity (increased ventilatory equivalent), which reflects excess wasted ventilation. At maximal exercise, the minute ventilation approaches or even exceeds the maximum level expected for the degree of obstruction (MVV or $35 \times FEV_1$). The heart rate increases appropriately for the work level, but maximum exercise is reached well below the predicted maximum for age. If ventilatory limitation is severe, the anaerobic threshold may not be reached. Arterial blood gases may show a normal or elevated PCO_2, but rarely the low value expected at maximum exercise.

Restrictive pulmonary diseases
Patients who have severe restrictive disease may also be limited by ventilatory mechanics and have similar responses to those described above. With restrictive parenchymal lung disease, $\dot{V}E$max may be higher than the $FEV_1 \times 35$ rule predicts, and the ventilatory response is more likely to be characterized by a rapid rate with low VT. Many restrictive disorders also involve a component of pulmonary vascular disease, as described below.

Pulmonary vascular disease
Patients who have loss of pulmonary vasculature are less able to recruit additional vascular capacity to handle the increased

Cardiopulmonary exercise testing	
Parameter	**Discussion**
Oxygen consumption, $\dot{V}O_2$max (L/min or mL/min) or $\dot{V}O_2$/kg (mL/kg/min)	Reference data show an increase with body size and decline with age, but vary quite markedly from sedentary to regularly exercising 'normal subjects'
	The expected capacity of obese subjects is better predicted from height than weight
Heart rate (beats/min)	Compare maximum value with 220 – age
	Lower values may reflect chronotropic insufficiency (sometimes drug related), incomplete effort, or noncardiac limitation
	Electrocardiogram is also analyzed for arrhythmias and ischemic change
Oxygen pulse, $\dot{V}O_2$/beat (mL)	Reflects the product of stroke volume times arterial – venous O_2 content difference
	Its progressive increase during exercise results mainly from increasing extraction, but as maximum extraction is similar among individuals the maximum O_2 pulse is a surrogate for stroke volume
Blood pressure (mmHg)	Systolic pressure normally increases with exercise
	A failure to increase, or especially a decrease, reflects failure of the right ventricle (pulmonary hypertension) or left ventricle (ischemia) to meet the output demand and is an indication to stop the test
Ventilation, $\dot{V}E$max (L/min)	Compare with measured maximum voluntary ventilation or with $35 \times FEV_1$
	Ventilatory limitation is suggested if exercise $\dot{V}E$ approaches these benchmarks
	The pattern of increase of respiratory rate and tidal volume is quite variable
Ventilatory equivalent, $\dot{V}E/\dot{V}O_2$ (L/L)	Normally about 30–35
	High values suggest either hyperventilation or excessive wasted ventilation
Anaerobic threshold, AT (mL/min or percentage of $\dot{V}O_2$max)	Inferred from an increase in the slope of $\dot{V}E$ versus $\dot{V}O_2$ or from an increase in $R > 1$
	Failure to demonstrate an AT may reflect submaximal effort
	An early AT suggests cardiac disease or poor conditioning
Wasted ventilation, $\dot{V}DS/\dot{V}T$ (%)	Calculated from $PaCO_2$ or less accurately from end-tidal PCO_2
	A failure to decrease normally with exercise shows lack of recruitability and suggests pulmonary vascular disease with a reduction in available capillary bed
Arterial blood gases: $PaCO_2$	Low values throughout exercise suggest anxiety or excessive drive to ventilate
	A rising value above 40mmHg at end exercise is good evidence for ventilatory limitation
PaO_2	A significant decrease with exercise usually reflects low $\dot{V}/\dot{Q}$ areas contributing increasingly desaturated blood as extraction increases and mixed venous content falls
	Flow may be redistributed to low $\dot{V}/\dot{Q}$ areas during exercise as hypoxic vasoconstriction is opposed by higher pulmonary artery pressure
	With pulmonary hypertension, shunt may develop via the foramen ovale
	Diffusion limitation probably plays a minor role, if any

Figure 4.65 Multiple parameters are measured and calculated during cardiopulmonary exercise testing.

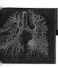
blood flow of exercise. Pulmonary artery pressure increases more than normal and, if pulmonary hypertension is severe, the capacity of the right heart to maintain cardiac output may be the limiting factor. Heart rate is higher than normal for the work level, but does not reach the predicted maximum for age. Likewise, minute ventilation is higher than predicted at all levels, but $\dot{V}E$max is still well below that predicted by MVV. The

VD/VT ratio remains increased with progressive exercise, which reflects the lack of significant recruitment of vessels. Exercise blood gases usually show hypocapnia and progressive hypoxemia as the significant elevation in pulmonary artery pressure may overcome the hypoxic vasoconstriction in poorly ventilated areas of the lung, which increases the venous admixture to the arterial blood.

REFERENCES

1.   Culver BH, ed. The respiratory system. Seattle: ASUW Publications; 1997.

2.   Weibel ER. Morphometry of the human lung. Berlin and New York: Springer-Verlag; 1963.

3.   Hoppin FG Jr, Hildebrandt J. Mechanical properties of the lung. In: West JB, ed. Bioengineering aspects of the lung, Vol. 3 of Lenfant C, exec ed. Lung biology in health and disease. New York: Marcel Dekker; 1977.

4.   Pappenheimer JR, Comroe JH, Cournand A, et al. Standardization of definitions and symbols in respiratory physiology. Fed Proc. 1950;9:602–15.

5.   Rahn H, Otis AB, Chadwich LE, Fenn WO. The pressure–volume diagram of the thorax and lung. Am J Physiol. 1946;146:161–78.

6.   Fenn WO. Mechanics of respiration. Am J Med. 1951;10:77–90.

7.   Bachofen H, Hildebrandt J, Bachofen M. Pressure-volume curves of air- and liquid-filled excised lungs – surface tension in situ. J Appl Physiol. 1970;29:422–31.

8.   Mead J, Turner JM, Macklem PT, Little JB. Significance of the relationship between lung recoil and maximum expiratory flow. J Appl Physiol. 1967;22:95–108.

9.   Pride NB, Permutt S, Riley RL, Bromberger-Barnea B. Determinants of maximum expiratory flow. J Appl Physiol. 1967;23:646–62.

10.   Bates DV, Macklem PT, Christie RV. Respiratory function in disease, 2nd edn. Philadelphia: WB Saunders; 1971:10–95.

11.   Leblanc P, Ruff F, Milic-Emili J. Effects of age and body position on airway closure in man. J Appl Physiol. 1970;28:448–51.

12.   Craig DB, Wahba WN, Don HF, et al. Closing volume: and its relationship to gas exchange in seated and supine position. J Appl Physiol. 1971;31:717–21.

13.   Lavoisier A. As quoted in West JB, ed. Pulmonary gas exchange, Vol. 1. Ventilation, blood flow, and diffusion. New York: Academic Press; 1980.

14.   Siegwart B, Gehr P, Gil J, Weibel E. Morphometric estimation of pulmonary diffusing capacity. IV. The normal dog lung. Respir Physiol. 1971;13:141–59.

15.   Anthonisen NR, Fleetham JA. Ventilation: total, alveolar and dead space. In: Fahri LE, Tenney SM, eds. Gas exchange, handbook of physiology, section 3. The respiratory system, Vol. 4. Bethesda: American Physiologic Society; 1987:113–30.

16.   Baumann R, Bartels H, Bauer C. Blood oxygen transport. In: Fahri LE, Tenney SM, eds. Gas exchange, handbook of physiology, section 3. The respiratory system, Vol. 4. Bethesda: American Physiologic Society; 1987:147–72.

17.   Hlastala MP. Blood gas transport. In: Culver BH, ed. The respiratory system. Seattle: ASUW Publications; 1997:43–52.

18.   Klocke RA. Carbon dioxide transport. In: Fahri LE, Tenney SM, eds. Gas exchange, handbook of physiology, section 3. The respiratory system, Vol. 4. Bethesda: American Physiologic Society; 1987:173–97.

19.   Wagner PD, West JB. Effects of diffusion impairment on O_2 and CO_2 time courses in pulmonary capillaries. J Appl Physiol. 1972;33:62–71.

20.   Rahn H, Fahri LE. Ventilation, perfusion and gas exchange – The $\dot{V}/\dot{Q}$ concept. In: Fenn WO, Rahn H, eds. Handbook of physiology, section 3. Respiration, Vol. 1. Washington: American Physiological Society; 1964.

21.   Wagner PD, Laravuso RB, Uhl RR, West JB. Continuous distribution of ventilation–perfusion ratios in normal subjects breathing air and 100% O_2. J Clin Invest. 1974;54:54–68.

22.   Hornbein TF. Acid–base balance. In: Culver BH, ed. The respiratory system. Seattle: ASUW Publications; 1997:71–93.

23.   Woodbury JW. Body acid–base state and its regulation. In: Ruch TC, Patton H, eds. Physiology and biophysics, 20th edn. Philadelphia, WB Saunders; 1974.

24.   Davenport HW. The ABC of acid–base chemistry, 6th edn. Chicago: The University of Chicago Press; 1974.

25.   Goldberg M, Greene SB, Moss ML, Marbach CB, Garfinkel D. Computer based instruction and diagnosis of acid–base disorders. JAMA. 1973;223:269–75.

26.   Berger AJ, Hornbein TF. Control of breathing. In: Patton HD, Fuchs AF, Hille B, Scher AM, Steiner R., eds. Textbook of physiology, Vol. 2. Circulation, respiration, body fluids, metabolism, and endocrinology, 21st edn. Saunders;1989: 1026–45.

27.   Hlastala MP, Berger AJ. Physiology of respiration. New York: Oxford University Press; 1996:176–95.

28.   Butler J. The circulation of the lung. In: Culver BH, ed. The respiratory system. Seattle: ASUW Publications; 1997:111–22.

29.   Butler J, ed. The bronchial circulation, Vol. 57 of Lenfant C, exec ed. Lung biology in health and disease. New York: Marcel Dekker; 1992.

30.   Culver BH, Butler J. Mechanical influences on the pulmonary circulation. Ann Rev Physiol. 1980;42:187–98.

31.   Bhattacharya J. Physiological basis of pulmonary edema. In: Matthay M, Ingbar D, eds. Pulmonary edema, Vol. 116 of Lenfant C, exec ed. Lung biology in health and disease. New York: Marcel Dekker; 1998.

32.   Glenny RW. State of the art: Blood flow distribution in the lung. Chest. 1998;114:8S–16S.

33.   Culver BH. Hemodynamic monitoring: physiologic problems in interpretation. In: Fallat RJ, Luce JM, eds. Cardiopulmonary critical care management. New York: Churchill Livingstone; 1988.

34.   American Thoracic Society. Standardization of spirometry – 1987 update. Am Rev Respir Dis. 1987;136:1285–98.

35.   Morris AH, Kanner RE, Crapo RO, Gardner RM. Clinical pulmonary function testing: A manual of uniform laboratory procedures, 2nd edn. Salt L:ake City: Intermountain Thoracic Society; 1984.

36.   Culver BH. Pulmonary function testing. In: Kelley WN, ed. Textbook of internal medicine. Philadelphia: JB Lippincott; 1988.

37.   Crapo RO, Morris AH, Gardner RM. Reference spirometric values using techniques and equipment that meet ATS recommendations. Am Rev Respir Dis. 1981;123:659–64.

38.   Knudson RJ, Lebowitz MD, Holberg CJ, Burrows B. Changes in the normal expiratory flow–volume curve with growth and aging. Am Rev Respir Dis. 1983;127:725–34.

39.   Miller A. Pulmonary function tests in clinical and occupational lung disease. Orlando: Grune & Stratton; 1986.

40.   Culver BH, Butler J. Alterations in pulmonary function. In: Andres R, Bierman E, Hazzard W, eds. Principles of geriatric medicine. New York: McGraw-Hill; 1985.

41.   Spiro SG. Exercise testing in clinical medicine. Br J Dis Chest. 1977;71:145–72.

42.   Jones NL. Clinical exercise testing, 4th edn. Philadelphia: Saunders; 1997.

43.   Wasserman K, Hansen JE, Sue DY, Whipp BJ. Principles of exercise testing and interpretation. Philadelphia: Lea & Febiger; 1987.

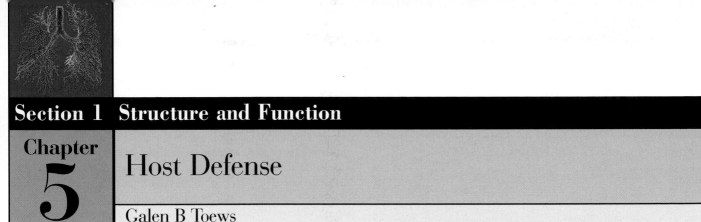

Chapter 5

Host Defense

Galen B Toews

INTRODUCTION

The exchange of gases to support tissue metabolism is the primary function of the lung. This function requires that each day the lungs exchange gases between approximately 10,000L of inhaled ambient air and its immense vasculature. The inhalation of airborne particulates and microbes is an unavoidable consequence of respiration. Elaborate host defenses have evolved to eliminate deposited microorganisms before their multiplication and invasion have deleterious effects on the host. The processes involved in microbial elimination are able to injure the delicate respiratory apparatus; accordingly, antimicrobial responses must be tightly regulated locally to balance the interests of efficient gas exchange and host defense. Pulmonary host defenses are distributed throughout the respiratory tract. The coordinated interactions of cells or cells and soluble factors are involved in most components of pulmonary host defenses. Pulmonary host defenses can be divided into four components:

- structural defenses;
- innate immunity;
- inflammatory responses; and
- specific immunity.

STRUCTURAL DEFENSES

Nasopharyngeal airways

The nose almost completely traps all particulates >10μm diameter and is a relatively effective filter for particles >5μm diameter. The nasopharynx also absorbs both soluble and reactive gases. Sulfur dioxide, a very soluble gas, is almost completely absorbed by the nose under normal breathing conditions. Rapid changes in direction of airflow in the posterior nasopharynx favor inertial deposition of large particulates. Impacted particulates are removed from the nasopharyngeal airways by sneezing, coughing, or swallowing.

Ciliated mucosa is present on the nasal septum and turbinates. Mucociliary action sweeps mucus toward the posterior pharynx, where secretions are swallowed or cleared from the throat.

Conducting airways
Mucociliary escalator

Airway epithelial cells form a continuous lining of the airways (Fig. 5.1). Particulates >2μm in diameter impact in the conducting airway and become trapped in mucus. Mucociliary clearance and cough are the principal means of clearing particulates and microbes from the conducting airway[1]. The removal of an inhaled microbe that encounters the mucus blanket covering the larger airways depends on the coordinated beating of cilia. Cough alone cannot remove mucus efficiently.

The respiratory secretions in the conducting airway contain two distinct layers (see Fig. 5.2)[2]. An upper viscous layer is formed by mucins, a group of highly glycosylated proteins synthesized by epithelial cells. Mucin synthesizing cells include goblet cells in the surface epithelium and mucous cells in the submucosal glands. A watery sublayer underlies the upper viscous layer. The underlying watery layer provides a minimally resistant material that allows the underlying cilia to beat. The ciliary tip of beating cilia just catches the lower edge of the viscous phase, which propels the mucus forward. Mucins give the upper viscous layer its stickiness to trap particulates, and also present potential carbohydrate receptors for more specific

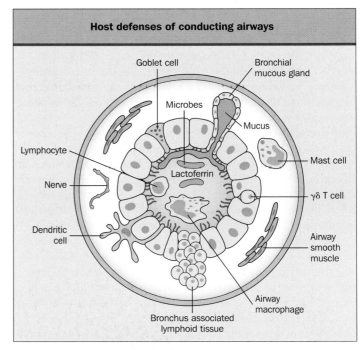

Figure 5.1 Host defenses of conducting airways. The conducting airways of the lung are complex structures composed of approximately 50 different cell types. Ciliated pseudostratified columnar epithelium lines the conducting airways and moves mucus generated by goblet cells and bronchial glands toward the mouth where it is expectorated or swallowed. Airway macrophages, moving across the epithelium recognise, ingest, and kill deposited airborne bacteria. The initiation of specific immune responses requires dendritic cells, which are present beneath and between airway epithelial cells. Lymphocytes are present within the airway, throughout the submucosa and lamina propria, and within lymphoid nodules and bronchus associated lymphoid tissue. Lymphocytes are present between epithelial cells of the bronchial mucosa and intra-epithelial lymphocytes bear γ δ T cell receptors.

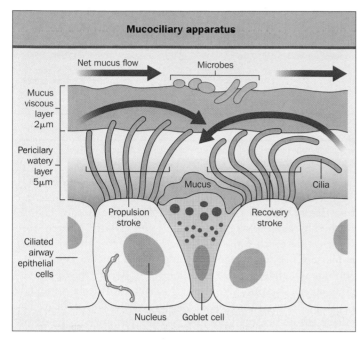

Figure 5.2 Mucociliary apparatus. The mucus blanket that coats the airways consists of two phases: an upper viscous layer and a watery sublayer. The viscous upper layer is moved cephelad by the force of the effective stroke of cilia which just penetrate beyond the lower edge of the viscous phase. The recovery stroke of cilia takes place in a thin, watery, layer in which cilia beat in an energy conserving fashion.

interactions. *Haemophilus influenzae*, *Streptococcus pneumoniae*, and *Staphylococcus aureus* bind avidly to mucins. Bacterial binding probably enhances bacterial clearance in the presence of a normal mucociliary escalator. Conversely, it provides a foot hold that allows bacterial growth and colonization in the absence of normal, efficient mucociliary clearance.

Mucus is propelled up the respiratory tract by pseudostratified, ciliated epithelium. Each ciliated cell possesses approximately 200 cilia, with a ciliary beat frequency of 12–14 beats per second. Microbes can be cleared from the trachea with a half-time of 30 minutes and from distal airways with a half-time of hours.

Abnormal cilia are noted in certain patients. The primary ciliary dyskinesia syndrome is characterized by bronchiectasis sinusitis, otitis media, and male infertility. In 50% of the cases, this syndrome is associated with situs inversus and is then designated Kartagener's syndrome. The cilia of these patients have typical structural defects in the axonemes. The absence of the outer dynein arms is the commonest defect, but missing radial spokes and translocation of the outer doublet microtubules are also seen. Mucociliary clearance is greatly reduced in these patients compared with patients with cystic fibrosis. Patients with primary cilia dyskinesia, although less symptomatic, have more severely impaired mucociliary clearance.

Mucociliary clearance can also be impaired during bacterial infections by several mechanisms. *Mycoplasma* and viruses destroy airway epithelium and cause a temporary decrease in mucociliary clearance. *Haem. influenzae* and *Pseudomonas aeruginosa* have been reported to increase directly or indirectly ciliary beat frequency.

The products of immune effector cells play an important role in altering and regulating mucociliary clearance. Oxidants, which

include hydrogen peroxide and superoxide, impair ciliary function, and proteases, such as elastase, damage cilia and decrease mucociliary activity. Platelet-activating factor also impairs ciliary motility and decreases mucociliary clearance. Factors released from inflammatory cells can also increase ciliary activity. Interferon-γ (IFN-γ), tumor necrosis factor-α (TNF-α), and interleukin-1 (IL-1) increase ciliary beating by a mechanism dependent on nitric oxide. Neural and hormonal mediators upregulate ciliary beat frequency.

Airway secretions

Airway epithelial cells secrete a variety of nonmucin constituents that are important in host defense. These include iron-binding proteins, antioxidants, and antiproteases[2].

Most microbes require iron for their survival – the iron is normally sequestered in cells or firmly complexed to transport proteins. Microbes compete for iron with their own transport proteins known as siderophores. Lactoferrin, which is released by serous cells, avidly binds iron. At mucosal surfaces, this property is used both to inhibit the iron-dependent growth of bacteria and to protect tissues from injury induced by hydroxyl radicals.

Lysozyme is an enzyme that catalyzes the hydrolysis of bonds between constituents of the cell walls of most bacteria, and is secreted in large quantities in human airways (10–20mg/day) where it helps to defend against bacterial and fungal infection. Lysozyme lyses *Strep. pneumoniae* and is toxic to *Cryptococcus neoformans* and *Coccidioides immitis*. Lysozyme can reduce the tissue damaging effects of inflammation by inhibiting chemotaxis and the production of toxic oxygen radicals by stimulated neutrophils.

Conducting airways must be protected from degradation. Leukocytes and bacteria are the major sources of proteases in human airway secretions. Neutrophil elastase can degrade a wide range of extracellular matrix components, including elastin, laminin, fibronectin, and collagen. *Ps. aeruginosa*, *Staph. aureus*, *Haem. influenzae*, and *Strep. pneumoniae* all produce bacterial proteases, which degrade elastin, immunoglobulins, lysozyme, basement membrane, and complement components. To counteract the potentially damaging effects of these proteases, the airway secretions contain both serum derived (α_1-antitrypsin, α_2-antichymotrypsin, and α_2-macroglobulin) and airway epithelial cell-derived antiproteases (secretory leukoprotease inhibitor, elafin). Secretory leukoprotease inhibitor is derived entirely from the pulmonary epithelium. Elafin is produced by Clara cell lines and may also contribute to the antiprotease defenses of the airway.

INNATE IMMUNITY

Two systems of immunity have been selected as a result of host microbe interactions, innate immunity, and specific immunity[3,4]. The essential difference between the two systems is the means by which they recognize microbes. Innate immunity uses proteins encoded in the germ line to identify potentially noxious substances. These proteins, which are both cell surface receptors and soluble substances, usually recognize carbohydrate structures. Thus, innate immunity divides the universe into innocuous and noxious substances according to their particular carbohydrates. Recognition of carbohydrates probably evolved because these microbial cell wall constituents have functions and structures distinct from those of carbohydrates present on the cell surfaces of eukaryotes.

Clearance of microbes from the alveoli depends entirely on cellular and humoral factors. These components include alveolar macrophages, natural killer (NK) cells, complement factors, defensins, collectins, and surfactant.

Alveolar macrophages

Resident pulmonary macrophages constitute the first line of defense against microbes that reach the alveolar surface[5,6]. Resident pulmonary macrophages can be found within the interstitium, lining the alveoli, and within the airways, both in the lumen and within the lining epithelium, and have two origins. Pulmonary macrophages differentiate from monocytes that enter the lung from the circulation. Alveolar macrophages are also derived from proliferating macrophage precursors within the interstitium of the lung. Alveolar macrophage microbicidal function is dependent on four critical attributes (Fig. 5.3) – signal recognition, migration in response to stimuli, microbe ingestion, and secretion of mediators. Macrophages recognize signals in their microenvironment via surface receptors that usually recognize carbohydrate structures[7]. The mannose receptor, a C-type lectin with broad carbohydrate specificity, is effective in mediating phagocytosis of yeasts, mycobacteria, and *Pneumocystis carinii*. Macrophages also have a receptor for lipopolysaccharide (LPS), a common constituent of Gram-negative bacterial outer membranes that signals the presence of infection by binding to CD14. Scavenger receptors [type 1, type 2, macrophage receptor with a collagenous structure (MARCO)] bind a range of polyanionic ligands, including LPS and modified proteins. These receptors mediate phagocytosis of a wide variety of foreign particulates. Macrophages also express two distinct receptors for the third component of complement (the major soluble protein effector of innate immunity). Complement receptor 1 (CR1) preferentially binds C3b, but also binds C3bi and C4b. Complement receptor 3 (CR3, CD11b/18, MAC-1, Mo-1) is a member of the β_2 integrin family and is a receptor for C3bi, but also recognizes LPS and fibrinogen. *Histoplasma capsulatum* binds directly to CR3. Direct binding of microbes to CR3 is an important recognition mechanism of microbes before the onset of specific immunity. Patients who have a genetic deficiency in the CD18 complex have recurrent life-threatening infections, which documents the critical role of CR3 in host defenses against infectious agents.

Phagocytosis occurs following recognition of the microbe. Particle engulfment requires receptor–ligand interactions, which guide pseudopod extensions of macrophages from points of initial local contact to circumferencial envelopment (zipper hypothesis). Phagocytosis thus requires engagement of specific receptors and the generation of transmembrane signals.

Following phagocytosis, the microbe is initially contained within a phagosome that subsequently fuses with one or more lysosomes. Resident alveolar macrophages are not fully activated for microbicidal killing. Four major sources provide activation stimuli for resident alveolar macrophages:

- microorganism itself;
- responding macrophages;
- secreted products of other innate immune cells; and
- plasma proteins.

A cell wall component of bacteria, LPS is a potent macrophage activating signal (Fig. 5.4). Peptidoglycans, lipoarabinomannan, and lipomannan also cause activation. Interaction of the macrophage with LPS can occur either during engulfment of a

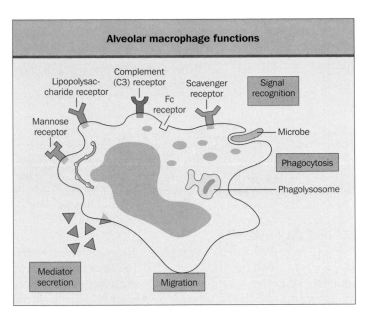

Figure 5.3 Alveolar macrophage functions. Macrophage functions are dependent on their ability to recognise signals, migrate in response to stimuli, ingest microbes, and secrete mediators.

microorganism or after such components have been released by intracellular killing and/or digestion. Macrophage activating stimuli are produced by macrophages themselves. The release of IFN-α and/or IFN-β, induced by LPS, provides the priming signal to augment macrophage microbicidal activity. Similarly, granulocyte–macrophage colony-stimulating factor (GM/CSF) can be a potent stimulator of macrophage activation. Cell types other than macrophages provide important activating stimuli. Interactions with microbes leads to the nonimmune production of IFN-γ by NK cells.

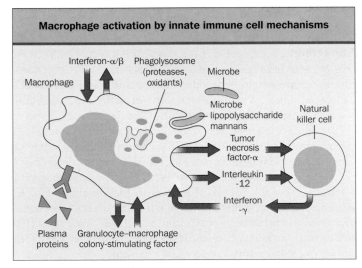

Figure 5.4 Macrophage activation by innate immune cell mechanisms. Resident macrophages that ingest microbes or interact with microbial products via cell surface receptors produce a number of activating cytokines [interferon α/β, granulocyte–macrophage colony-stimulating factor, tumour necrosis factor-α (TNF-α), interleukin-12 (IL-12)]. Some cytokines function in an autocrine or paracrine fashion to activate macrophages. TNF-α and IL-12 induce natural killer cells to produce interferon-γ, a potent activator of macrophage microbicidal activity.

Oxidative and nonoxidative processes are used by alveolar macrophages to kill ingested microbes. Resident macrophages have considerably less antimicrobial activity than monocytes. A decrease in the magnitude of the respiratory burst and the loss of granule peroxidase accounts for the decline. As resident alveolar macrophages contain minimal myeloperoxidase (MPO), their MPO–hydrogen peroxide–halide system is defective.

Microbes can also be killed by macrophage-dependent nonoxidative mechanisms. Defensins are a multiple-member family of cytotoxic peptides that kill many Gram-positive organisms (*Staph. aureus*) and Gram-negative species (*Escherichia coli, Klebsiella pneumoniae, Ps. aeruginosa*). Defensins also kill fungi and inactivate certain viruses.

Natural killer cells

The lung contains NK cells. Macrophage–NK cell interactions are probably critical to the activation of macrophages during innate immune responses[8]. The interaction of macrophages with microbes produces IL-12, which together with TNF-α induces IFN-γ production by NK cells. Early IFN-γ activates macrophages and enhances their microbicidal activity.

Complement

Complement is the major soluble protein effector of innate immunity. Complement is activated when either its alternative pathway interacts with carbohydrate-rich particles that lack sialic acid, or its classic pathway is triggered by the binding of collectin to certain carbohydrates. Normal alveolar lavage fluids contain a functional alternative complement pathway. Complement activation generates C3b, an opsonin that promotes receptor-mediated phagocytosis of microbes by macrophages. Also, complement activation produces C5a, which is an important chemoattractant for polymorphonuclear leukocytes (PMNs). Activation of the entire complement pathway results in the assembly of the C5b–C9 complex on microbial membrane surfaces. Assembly of this membrane attack complex on the surface of a microbe results in its lysis and killing.

Surfactant

Alveolar epithelial cells secrete proteins which play important roles in innate immune responses. Surfactant proteins A (SP-A) and D (SP-D) are members of a group of molecules called collectins. Although SP-A may not function as a true opsonin, SP-A facilitates the uptake of microbes trapped in lipid–SP-A complexes that are cleared by alveolar macrophages and type II alveolar epithelial cells. *In-vitro* exposure of alveolar macrophages to SP-A results in enhanced phagocytosis of *Staph. aureus* and *Ps. aeruginosa*. Also, SP-A directly binds to and opsonizes *Haem. influenzae* type A, promotes chemotaxis of alveolar macrophages, increases secretion of GM/CSF and IL-3, and modifies macrophage production of oxidants. Type II alveolar epithelial cells and nonciliated bronchiolar Clara cells produce SP-D, which mediates agglutination of Gram-negative bacteria. Surfactant also has role in extracellular killing of microbes through its detergent effect.

INFLAMMATORY RESPONSES

The clearance of most bacteria requires a dual phagocytic system that involves both resident alveolar macrophages and recruited PMNs. In the setting of a low bacterial burden, or exposure to minimally virulent organisms, alveolar macrophages can effectively phagocytose and kill invading organisms. However, when the bacterial burden is large, or when more virulent, encapsulated Gram-negative organisms such as *Ps. aeruginosa* or *K. pneumoniae* gain access to the lower air spaces, the recruitment of neutrophils is essential for effective containment and clearance of bacteria.

Recruitment of PMNs into the alveoli is initiated by the generation of chemotaxins within the alveolar space (Fig. 5.5). Complement activation occurs early via the alternative complement pathway, which can be activated by a wide variety of substances that including complex polysaccharides, LPS (bacterial endotoxins), and surface components of certain bacteria and fungi.

Alternative complement pathway activation leads to cleavage of C5. The cleavage fragments of the C5 molecule are important chemotaxins during the early phases of pulmonary host defenses against bacterial microbes. C5-deficient mice have reduced PMN recruitment to the lung after intratracheal inoculation of *Strep. pneumoniae, Ps. aeruginosa*, and *Haem. influenzae* compared with congenic C5-sufficient mice.

Complement fragments possess chemotaxic activity for both PMNs and macrophages. Thus, complement fragments lack the specificity to account for the dominant recruitment of PMNs noted in the acute inflammatory response to bacteria. A supergene family of chemotaxic cytokines, chemokines, possesses relatively high degrees of specificity for PMNs and mononuclear cells. Accordingly, they provide a potential mechanism for the selective recruitment of peripheral-blood leukocytes to specific sites of inflammation.

Four closely related families of chemotaxic cytokines, referred to as CXC, CC, C, and CXXXC chemokines, have been characterized[9]. The CXC chemokine family, which includes (IL)-8, macrophage inflammatory protein (MIP)-2, growth-related protein, epithelial cell-derived neutrophil activator-78, and neutrophil-activating peptide-2, has predominant PMN stimulatory and chemotactic activity. The CC family, which includes monocyte chemoattractant protein (MCP)-1, MCP-2, MCP-3, RANTES, MIP-1α, and MIP-1β, exerts chemotaxic and/or activating effects on macrophages, lymphocytes, eosinophils, basophils, and mast cells. Lymphotactin is the only identified C chemokine and fractalkine is the only identified CXXXC chemokine.

Macrophages are crucially involved in the initiation of chemokine-induced inflammatory responses. Bacterial products stimulate alveolar macrophage production of CXC chemokines. Additionally, bacterial products stimulate the production of TNF-α and IL-1, both of which induce gene expression and secretion of CXC chemokines from endothelial cells, pulmonary epithelial cells, and fibroblasts. Thus, the alveolar capillary membrane is viewed as a dynamic assembly of immune and nonimmune cells that, in aggregate, generates the quantities of CXC chemokines required to recruit specific inflammatory cells.

It has been demonstrated that CXC chemokines are important in pulmonary host defenses in both patients and animal models. Respiratory secretions from patients who have acute pulmonary bacterial infections contain increased amounts of IL-8. Both TNF-α and MIP-2 are rapidly induced in murine lungs following *K. pneumoniae* pulmonary infections. Treatment of infected mice with anti-MIP-2 antibodies results in decreased clearance of *K. pneumoniae*.

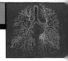

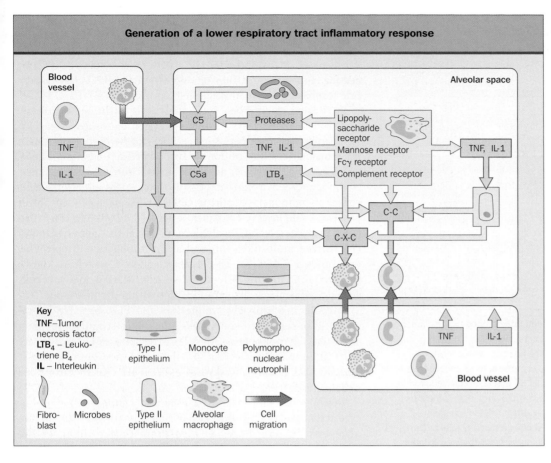

Generation of a lower respiratory tract inflammatory response

Key
TNF–Tumor necrosis factor
LTB$_4$ – Leukotriene B$_4$
IL – Interleukin

Fibroblast · Microbes · Type II epithelium · Alveolar macrophage · Cell migration

Type I epithelium · Monocyte · Polymorphonuclear neutrophil

Figure 5.5 Generation of a lower respiratory tract inflammatory response. Bacteria or bacterial products which enter the alveolus are recognised by alveolar macrophages. Complement activation occurs early and generates C5a. Microbial products stimulate alveolar macrophage production of tumour necrosis factor (TNF)-α, interleukin (IL)-1, IL-8, and leukotrienes (LTs). TNF-α and IL-1β induce chemokine gene expression and chemokine production by epithelial cells and fibroblasts present in the lower respiratory tract. The entire alveolar capillary wall is engaged in the tightly regulated recruitment of inflammatory cells.

When contact is established between a neutrophil and a microbe, the particle is ingested by phagocytosis. Whereas the acidic environment within phagocytic vacuoles can limit the growth of some bacteria, effective killing requires products of molecular oxygen, granule constituents, or both. Hydrogen peroxide is produced by PMNs, as well as highly reactive unstable intermediates such as superoxide and ion radicals, hydroxyl radicals, and singlet oxygen. Although it is not entirely clear how products of the MPO–hydrogen peroxide–halide system alter the viability of bacteria and fungi, it is well established that this system participates in oxygen-dependent killing by neutrophils.

Phagocytes are able to kill some microorganisms effectively by oxygen- and MPO-independent systems. A variety of microbicidal products are stored in cytoplasmic plasmic granules. Lactoferrin limits proliferation of bacteria by virtue of its ability to chelate iron, an essential growth factor for many microbial species. Lysozyme, found in both specific and azurophil granules of human neutrophils, efficiently hydrolyzes certain bacterial cell walls. Elastase, cathepsin G, and other cationic proteins found in neutrophil azurophil granules are capable of killing bacteria. Finally, human neutrophils contain defensins, which kill fungal organisms in a wide variety of Gram-positive and Gram-negative bacteria.

SPECIFIC IMMUNE RESPONSES

Specific immune responses consist functionally of two major effector systems, antibody- and cell-mediated immunity, which are effected by B and T lymphocytes, respectively. Using products of the RAG1 and RAG2 genes, B and T lymphocytes rearrange their immunoglobulin and T cell receptor (TCR) genes to create approximately 10^{11} different clones of B and T lymphocytes that express distinct antigen receptors. The receptors on B lymphocytes recognize native antigens, which may be simple chemical groups, carbohydrates, or proteins. Receptors of T lymphocytes recognize only peptides that are derived from protein antigens. These peptide antigens are bound to cell surface proteins termed major histocompatibility complex (MHC) classes I and II. Clones of lymphocytes that have receptors of adequate affinity are triggered by antigen-presenting cells (APCs) to proliferate and develop into effector cells. After elimination of an infection, antigen-specific clones remain expanded as 'memory' lymphocytes that provide a more rapid response to a second exposure to the antigen.

Selection of antigens for specific immune responses

T helper (T$_H$) lymphocytes orchestrate specific immune responses by promoting intracellular killing of microbes by macrophages, antibody production by B lymphocytes, and clonal expansion of cytotoxic T lymphocytes. The interaction between antigenic peptides presented in association with MHC class II membrane proteins on the surface of APCs and the TCRs of T cells triggers cellular activation (see Fig. 5.6). The peptides are generated from exogenous antigens (bacteria, mycobacteria, fungi) that have been ingested by phagocytosis or pinocytosis. Proteins are proteolytically digested into polypeptide fragments 10–20 amino acids in length. Polypeptides that contain immunodominant epitopes are bound to the antigen-binding groove of the MHC glycoprotein complex and delivered to the surface of the APC. The MHC–antigen–TCR interaction provides specificity for T-lymphocyte activation. A

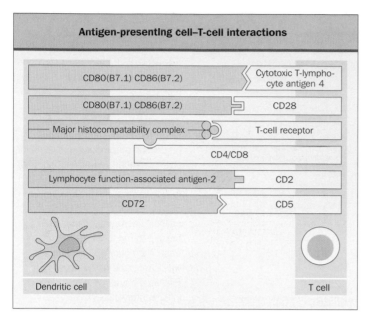

Figure 5.6 Antigen-presenting cell–T cell interactions. A wide variety of cell surface molecules on dendritic cells interact with cell surface molecules on T cells. These include antigen-presenting and antigen recognition structures such as major histocompability complex II, the T-cell receptor and CD4/CD8. Costimulatory molecules such as B7 and CD28 are required to activate T lymphocytes. Adhesion molecules (CD2/lymphocyte function-associated antigen-2, CD5, CD72) play important roles in maintaining cell–cell contact. Antigen-presenting cell–T-cell interactions take place within an 'immunologic synapse' formed by close cell contact between antigen-presenting cells and T cells.

second costimulatory signal is required to activate T lymphocytes to produce cytokines. The costimulatory signal is delivered by CD28, a membrane protein of TH cells that, together with TCRs, costimulates the transcription of the gene encoding IL-2 and stabilizes IL-2 messenger RNA (mRNA). The second signal is provided by the expression of the CD28 ligands B7.1 (CD80) and B7.2 (CD86) on the APC[10]. Cell–cell contact and transmembrane signaling are also promoted by the interaction of lymphocyte function-associated antigen (LFA) molecules on T lymphocytes with intercellular adhesion molecules (ICAMs) on the APC. CD2 interacts with LFA-3 and CD4 interacts with MHC class II molecules. The processes that select proteins for endocytosis by APC augment the expression of B7.1 or B7.2, and augment the expression of adherence molecules, thus determining which antigens activate TH cells[11].

Dendritic cells are the most potent APCs for TH cells. Found in the interstitium, in alveolar septae, and throughout the columnar epithelium of the bronchi, dendritic cells are ideally situated to function as sentinel antigen-detecting cells. After their development in the bone marrow, dendritic cells take up residence in the lung. At the mucosal interface, they have a sentinel role, surveying for and capturing antigens that penetrate beyond the physical and functional barriers of the air–epithelial interface. Proteins internalized by macropinocytosis are degraded and the resultant peptides associate with newly synthesized MHC class II molecules to form complexes that are expressed at the plasma membrane. Dendritic cells select potential T cell antigens by taking up microbial glycoconjugates through specialized receptors. A mannose receptor on dendritic cells mediates the endocytosis of

$>10^5$ molecules per cell per hour. This process increases by 100-fold the efficiency of antigen presentation to TH cells. Following exposure to antigen (activation), sentinel dendritic cells migrate to T cell zones of lymph nodes and mature into effective APCs by ceasing endocytosis, stabilizing expression of MHC class II–peptide complexes, and increasing their expression of B7.1 and B7.2[12].

Activation of pulmonary dendritic cells might occur through two different pathways following antigen exposure (Fig. 5.7). First, microbial products such as LPS might bind to common microbial pattern recognition receptors present on both epithelial cells and macrophages, and lead to the release of cytokines. Second, microenvironmental tissue injury might initiate the activation of pulmonary dendritic cells. The signaling in this latter pathway could involve cytokines, low molecular weight mediators (such as oxygen-free radicals), or changes in the glycosylation of cell surface molecules. Interstitial macrophages and epithelial cells produce GM-CSF, TNF-α, IL-4, and IL-1, which are known to be required for this differentiative step. Mature dendritic cells activate antigen-reactive lymphocytes within the hilar node.

Alveolar macrophages are ineffective APCs for naive T lymphocytes or resting memory cells, but can re-stimulate recently activated T lymphocytes. Alveolar macrophages fail to activate CD4 T lymphocytes effectively because they bind resting T lymphocytes poorly and do not express B7 costimulatory cell surface molecules.

Resident alveolar macrophages actively suppress T lymphocyte activation and proliferation induced by antigens. Depletion of alveolar macrophages *in vivo* dramatically enhances the capacity of experimental animals to mount an immune response. The potential value of such a steady state downregulatory control mechanism in the lung is self-evident, as the lung is frequently exposed to antigens. Immune responses must be restricted and downregulated within the pulmonary parenchyma, since immune reactions inevitably result in significant damage to gas exchange surfaces. Conversely, unchecked microbial growth can also result in significant damage to gas exchange surfaces. Accordingly, alveolar macrophage suppressive activity can be reversed. Both GM-CSF and TNF-α significantly lessen alveolar macrophage suppressive activity and increase dendritic cell maturation. Thus, microbial stimuli (LPS) lessen the downregulatory tone of alveolar macrophages by inducing GM-CSF production by macrophages and/or alveolar and airway epithelial cells and TNF production by macrophages, and simultaneously enhance the immunostimulatory activity of dendritic cells. In aggregate, these LPS-induced changes in APCs allow local T-cell activation in the face of microbial challenges[13].

Selection of the type of specific immune response
Different microbes require different types of responses for their elimination. Type I responses are mediated primarily by activated macrophages and involve the phagocytosis and intracellular killing of microorganisms. Type II responses are mediated by noncytotoxic antibodies, mast cells, and eosinophils. Type I immune responses are mediated by TH1 cells, which secrete IL-2, IFN-γ, TNF-α, and GM-CSF. Type II responses are mediated by TH2 cells, which produce IL-4, IL-5, IL-6, and IL-10[14].

Both TH1 and TH2 cells develop in response to signals derived from the innate immune system[11] (see Fig. 5.8). Activation of tissue macrophages through cell surface carbohydrate pattern

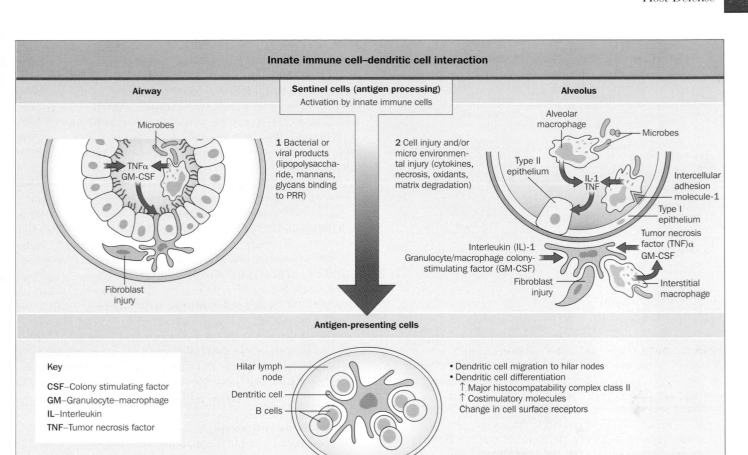

Figure 5.7 Innate immune cell–dendritic cell interaction. Generation of pulmonary immune responses requires maturation and/or activation of pulmonary dendritic cells. Precursor dendritic cells are located in the periphery of the lung in contact with either airway epithelial cells or alveolar epithelial cells. These 'sentinel' cells are efficient antigen-processing cells but are inefficient antigen-presenting cells. Dendritic cells become activated as a result of interaction with microbial products or as a result of interaction with products of cell or microenvironmental tissue injury. Dendritic cell activation/maturation leads to dendritic cell migration to hilar nodes and the differentiation of dendritic cells into potent antigen-presenting cells. Pulmonary epithelial cells and pulmonary macrophages are an essential regulatory link in the generation of microbe-specific T-cell immunity.

receptors or by CD14, to which LPS has been bound, causes secretion of IL-12 and TNF-α. The differentiation of naive TH cells to the TH1 phenotype is induced by IL-12 through its ability to maximize IFN-γ and curtail IL-4 production by T cells[15]. Also, LPS causes macrophages to produce IFN-γ-inducing factor that has similar effects. Both IL-12 and TNF-α synergize with IL-2 from T cells or with IL-15 from activated macrophages to induce production of IFN-γ by NK cells. In turn, IFN-γ augments IL-12 secretion and activity through its capacity to activate both IL-12 production by macrophages and the expression of IL-12 receptor on T and NK cells. Thus, IFN-γ and IL-12 comprise an autocrine positive feedback system that amplifies the levels of IFN-γ for macrophage activation and IL-12 for the proliferation and activation of NK and TH1 cells.

The development of TH2 cells requires IL-4 during the priming of naive T cells. Basophils and mast cells produce IL-4 after exposure to certain antigens. A subpopulation of T cells that express NK 1.1 markers and are CD4+ rapidly produce large amounts of IL-4.

Cytokines produced by the developing TH1 and/or TH2 cells contribute to the control of polarized responses. The development of TH2 cells is suppressed by IFN-γ produced by TH1 cells. Both IL-10 and IL-4 produced by TH2 cells suppresses

the development of TH1 cells. Chronic exposure to antigen is required to produce highly segregated TH1 or TH2 responses.

Lower respiratory tract immune responses mediated by T cells

Immunity mediated by T cells appears to be especially important for host defense against fungi, mycobacteria, and viruses. The kinetics of immune responses mediated by T lymphocytes in the lower respiratory tract have been defined almost exclusively from serial studies of murine models of these infections (see Fig. 5.9).

Cryptococcus neoformans
Host defenses against *Crypt. neoformans* are dependent upon CD4+ and CD8+ T cells. Mice depleted of CD4+ T cells have earlier dissemination of *Crypt. neoformans* from the lung and their burden of *Crypt. neoformans* is greater in extrapulmonary organs. Survival of mice depleted of CD4+ cells is reduced. Mice depleted of CD8+ lymphocytes have both reduced survival and impaired pulmonary clearance. Cellular recruitment of macrophages to the lung is significantly reduced in both CD4+ and CD8+ T cell-deficient mice. Depletion of both CD4+ and CD8+ T cells ablates inflammation and completely abrogates pulmonary clearance.

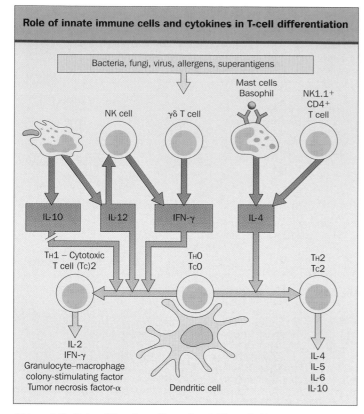

Role of innate immune cells and cytokines in T-cell differentiation

Figure 5.8 Role of innate cells and cytokines in T-cell differentiation. Innate immune cells are a major source of cytokines which control the development of T-helper (TH)1 and TH2 cells. After ingestion of microbes, macrophages produce interleukin (IL)-12 which powerfully induces the development of TH1 cells from naive CD4+ cells following their interaction with antigen bearing dendritic cells. IL-12 also induces interferon (IFN)-γ secretion by natural killer (NK) cells. γδ T lymphocytes also secrete IFN-γ following interactions with microbes. IFN-γ enhances IL-12 production and suppresses the development of TH2 cells. IL-4 is required for the development of the TH2 cells. Following interaction of naive CD4+ cells with antigen bearing dendritic cells, basophils, mast cells, γδ T lymphocytes, and NK1.1+, CD4+ T lymphocytes found in lymphoid tissues produce IL-4. IL-10 and IL-4 suppress the development of TH1 cells.

The molecular signals required for the recruitment of mononuclear phagocytes to the lung after *Crypt. neoformans* infection have been defined. The recruitment of monocytes during *Crypt. neoformans* infection is dependent on both MCP-1 and MIP-1α. Specific T lymphocytes generate GM/CSF, IFN-γ, and TNF-α, all of which activate monocytes, endothelial cells, fibroblasts, and epithelial cells to produce MCP-1. Additionally, activated T lymphocytes produce MIP-1α and RANTES. Studies carried out using neutralizing anti-MCP-1 or anti-MCP-1a-specific antiserum document the importance of these two molecules in mononuclear cell recruitment. A functional network of multiple chemokines is required for effective clearance of *Crypt. neoformans*. MCP-1 plays an important role in the initial recruitment of cells (CD4+ and CD8+ T lymphocytes and a small number of monocytes) that produce MIP-1α. In turn, MIP-1α mediates the bulk of monocyte recruitment into the lungs[16].

Fungi (*Blastomyces dermatidis, Candida albicans, Crypt. neoformans, Hist. capsulatum*) continue to grow within resident pulmonary macrophages. Macrophage-activating cytokines are required to increase the antimicrobial activity of pulmonary macrophages to allow these phagocytes to kill intracellular microbes. Macrophages treated with the T-cell cytokines IFN-γ or GM/CSF exhibit significant fungicidal activity. Of these two, GM/CSF increases complement-dependent phagocytosis with cryptococci. Depletion of CD4+ T cells *in vivo* inhibits multinucleated giant cell formation, which is one mechanism for containing *Crypt. neoformans* in the lung.

Participation of CD8+ T cells in antimicrobial activity against *Crypt. neoformans* could be by three mechanisms:
- CD8+ T cells can act directly on the microbe to inhibit or kill it;
- cytotoxic CD8+ T lymphocytes can lyse infected target cells; and/or
- CD8+ cells enhance the antimicrobial activity of immune cells, particularly monocytes and macrophages, by producing cytokines.

Development of delayed-type hypersensitivity to live or heat-killed *Crypt. neoformans* organisms depends on CD8+ T cells. In the absence of CD8+ T cells, CD4+ T cells produce predominantly TH2 cytokines (IL-4, IL-5, and IL-10) *in vitro*. The mechanism for the switch of CD4+ T cells to TH2 cytokines likely involves CD8+ T cell production of IFN-γ. It is known that CD8+ T cells are potent producers of MCP-1, MIP-1α, and IFN-γ.

Mycobacterium tuberculosis
Antigen-specific CD4+ T lymphocytes isolated from mice infected by *M. tuberculosis* produce IL-2, IFN-γ, and small amounts of IL-4. A combination of TH1, TH2, and/or TH0 cells is involved in pulmonary host responses to *M. tuberculosis*. Class I restricted CD8+ lymphocytes also participate in the immune response to mycobacteria – CD8+ lymphocytes are present in the outer mantle of many granulomatous lesions.

γδ-T lymphocytes are also involved in immune responses to mycobacteria. Mice immunized with *M. tuberculosis* have γδ-T lymphocytes that respond vigorously to *M. tuberculosis* antigens. Interestingly, an extraordinarily high percentage of murine γδ-T cell hybridomas thus far generated react with purified protein derivative. γδ-T lymphocytes can be expanded by *in-vitro* stimulation of peripheral blood cells from patients infected with *M. tuberculosis*. Mycobacteria-stimulated γδ-T lymphocytes have various functions that are relevant to defense against intracellular microbes, which include secretion of TNF-α and IFN-γ and the ability to lyse mycobacterial infected target cells[13].

The recruitment of monocytes and lymphocyte populations to the site of infection is required for granuloma formation. Infection of murine macrophages *in vitro* with several strains of *M. tuberculosis* induced rapid expression of genes that encoded for murine chemokines, MIP-1α, MIP-2, IP-10, and MCP-1. Induction of these chemokine mRNAs was also found in the lungs of mice after aerosol infection. Purified protein derivative, *M. tuberculosis* culture filtrates, and whole bacilli also stimulate TNF-α production from human monocytes and alveolar macrophages *in vitro*. An important immunoprotective role is played by TNF-α in tuberculosis infection in mice via mechanisms that appear to be related to nitric oxide production and granuloma formation. Anti-TNF-α antibody inhibits granuloma formation following Bacille Calmette–Guérin (BCG) challenge and results in a progressive, lethal BCG infection. Thus, proinflammatory cytokines and chemokines secreted during mycobacterial infections play an

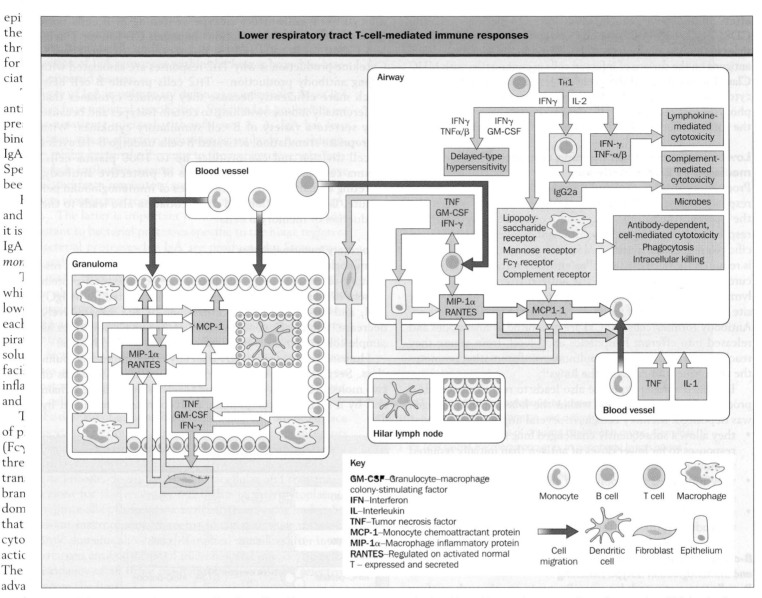

Lower respiratory tract T-cell-mediated immune responses

Key

GM-CSF–Granulocyte–macrophage colony-stimulating factor
IFN–Interferon
IL–Interleukin
TNF–Tumor necrosis factor
MCP-1–Monocyte chemoattractant protein
MIP-1α–Macrophage inflammatory protein
RANTES–Regulated on activated normal T – expressed and secreted

Monocyte   B cell   T cell   Macrophage

Cell migration   Dendritic cell   Fibroblast   Epithelium

Figure 5.9 Lower respiratory tract T-cell mediated immune responses. T cell activation occurs in draining hilar lymph nodes. Activated T lymphocytes recirculate from hilar nodes to sites of microbial multiplication in the lower respiratory tract via a series of highly regulated events involving adherence molecule expression by both lymphocytes and endothelial cells and cell recruitment events in response to cytokines. T helper (TH)1 lymphocytes are stimulated by resident antigen presenting cells to produce high levels of tumour necrosis factor (TNF), granulocyte–macrophage colony-stimulating factor (GM-CSF), and interferon (IFN-γ). C-C chemokines (MCP-1, MIP-1α) produced in response to microbial products and TNF secretion recruit mononuclear phagocytes, which are crucial to granuloma formation and to the clearance of certain pathogens.

important role in mobilizing and activating cellular immune responses and contribute to granuloma formation.

Following phagocytosis of *M. tuberculosis* by mononuclear phagocytes, the bacteria reside in a membrane-bound phagosome. Survival of *M. tuberculosis* within mononuclear phagocytes is partially related to the absence of phagosome–lysosome fusion. The ability of *M. tuberculosis* to reside within endosomes allows macrophages eventually to present *M. tuberculosis* antigens, but also enables the acquisition of nutrients by *M. tuberculosis*[17].

A central role is played by IFN-γ in activating antimicrobial activity in mycobacterium-containing macrophages. Studies of mice that have IFN-γ deletions (IFN-γ-/–) and IFN-γ receptor deletions (IFN-γ-R-/–) demonstrate the crucial role of IFN-γ. *M. tuberculosis*-infected IFN-γ-/– mice develop granulomas with caseous necrosis, widespread tissue destruction, and widespread

dissemination of infection. Both IFN-γ-/– and IFN-γ-R-/– animals fail to produce nitric oxide, which is essential for antimicrobial killing in mice. Both IFN-γ and TNF-α are synergistic in activating the tuberculostatic capacities of murine phagocytes. Both TNF-α and GM/CSF can also cooperate to induce significant intracellular destruction of mycobacteria. Mechanisms for growth inhibition of mycobacteria in murine macrophages have been shown to involve nitric oxide. The mechanisms for killing or growth inhibition of *M. tuberculosis* in human mononuclear phagocytes remain elusive.

Viruses

Antigen-specific, CD8+ cytotoxic T lymphocytes are crucial to the defense of the lung against viral infections. Specific cytotoxic CD8+ T cells appear in the parenchyma of the lung within 1 week

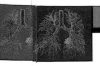

Prebronchoscopy checklist	
1.	Is there an appropriate indication for bronchoscopy?
2.	Has there been a previous bronchoscopy?
3.	If the answer to the above question is yes, were there any problems or complications?
4.	Does the patient [and close relative(s) if patient is unable to communicate] fully understand the goals, risks, and complications of bronchoscopy?
5.	Does the patient's past medical history (allergy to medications or topical anesthesia) and present clinical condition pose special problems or predispose to complications?
6.	Are all the appropriate tests completed and the results available?
7.	Are the premedications appropriate and the dosages correct?
8.	Does the patient require special consideration before bronchoscopy (e.g. corticosteroids for asthma, insulin for diabetes mellitus, or prophylaxis against endocarditis) or during bronchoscopy (e.g. supplemental oxygen, extra sedation)?
9.	Is the plan for postbronchoscopy care appropriate?
10.	Are all the appropriate instruments and personnel available to assist during the procedure and to handle the potential complications?

Figure 6.7 Prebronchoscopy checklist. (Adapted by permission of Mayo Foundation from Prakash UBS, Cortese DA, Stubbs SE. Technical solutions to common problems in bronchoscopy. In: Prakash UBS, ed. Bronchoscopy. New York: Raven Press; 1994:111–33.)

Measurement of prothrombin time, activated partial thromboplastin time, bleeding time, and platelet count should be performed only on patients who are receiving anticoagulant therapy and those with active bleeding, known or clinically suspected bleeding disorders, liver disease, renal dysfunction, malabsorption, malnutrition, or other circumstances identified with acquired coagulopathies. Bronchoscopy for simple visualization of the airways, bronchial washings, diagnostic BAL, and therapeutic bronchoscopy for removal of secretions and mucous plugs can be performed safely even in patients with severe coagulation problems. A prothrombin time <1.6 seconds, creatinine <309μmol/L (3.5mg/dL), and blood urea <5.8mmol/L (35mg/dL) are recommended if bronchoscopic biopsies and other interventional procedures are planned.

Routine analysis of arterial blood gas tensions and pulmonary function testing are also unnecessary before bronchoscopy. Even the severe impairment of pulmonary function encountered in immunosuppressed patients with diffuse pulmonary infiltrates is only a relative contraindication to bronchoscopy. Noninvasive techniques such as sphygmomanometry, electrocardiographic monitoring, and pulse oximetry provide adequate information regarding the patient's cardiopulmonary status during the procedure. If a patient is scheduled to undergo both bronchoscopy and pulmonary function testing within a period of 72 hours, it is recommended that pulmonary function tests be performed first because bronchoscopy can cause bronchial mucosal edema and lead to falsely abnormal results of pulmonary function tests. Preparation for bronchoscopy includes instructions to patients to fast for at least 6 hours beforehand.

Premedication, sedation, and anesthesia

Premedication, consisting of an antisialogogue and an anxiolytic drug, is commonly administered 30–40 minutes before the procedure. An anticholinergic drug such as atropine or glycopyrrolate (0.3–0.5mg intramuscularly for each agent) is advocated to lessen secretions that may hinder proper visualization and examination. Presently, midazolam is the drug of choice for almost all flexible bronchoscopies. Preoperative and intraoperative administration of a sedative aims at achieving antegrade amnesia, relaxation, and cooperation. The dose of midazolam for conscious sedation is 0.07mg/kg, but titration is required in each patient. Males require about 1.0mg more than females. Elderly patients are especially sensitive to midazolam. The choice and dosage of sedation should be tailored for each patient, acknowledging the potential for complications with oversedation. Propofol is another agent that is being used more frequently for rigid bronchoscopy and invasive procedures. Intravenous administration of propofol provides excellent sedation and minimal respiratory depression. Quick recovery from propofol is usual.

The vast majority of the flexible bronchoscopic procedures can be performed with topical anesthesia; lidocaine being the most common agent for this purpose. Lidocaine (lignocaine) is used to anesthetize the upper airways, using an ultrasonic nebulizer, a hand-held atomizer, or a syringe with a long curved cannula, before the insertion of the bronchoscope; it is also given through the working channel of the bronchoscope during the procedure. The total amount of lidocaine used should not be exceed 200mg. General anesthesia may be required for rigid bronchoscopy and complicated and lengthy flexible bronchoscopic procedures, in cases of intense patient anxiety, and for most pediatric bronchoscopies.

Hypoxia is a common phenomenon during bronchoscopy, even in those without pre-existing hypoxemia. Patients with pre-existing hypoxia should be given supplemental oxygen during bronchoscopy. The routine use of pulse oximetry is valuable for assessing the adequacy of oxygenation during bronchoscopy. Other prebronchoscopy precautions, such as prophylactic administration of antibiotics against bacterial endocarditis, should be individualized.

Technique

Flexible bronchoscopy can be performed with the patient seated or supine and in the intensive care unit or in the outpatient setting. Outpatient examinations should be performed in an operating room or in a procedure room dedicated to that purpose. The use of fluoroscopy or bronchoscopic lung biopsy, the need for general anesthesia, therapeutic bronchoscopies in critical care units, and urgent bronchoscopies will require special preparation and locations.

Adequate training in bronchoscopy, the availability of proper equipment, and the ability to manage complications will enable the bronchoscopist to perform a successful procedure irrespective of the location. Equipment and drugs should be readily available to deal with emergencies that may arise, including cardiopulmonary resuscitation if necessary. In the supine position, it is desirable to cover the eyes with protective pads that may be secured with a towel wrapped around the eyes and secured with a towel clip. At this point, a bite block should be inserted into the mouth, primarily to protect the flexible bronchoscope.

The flexible bronchoscope can be inserted transnasally or transorally, with or without an endotracheal tube, through a tracheostomy stoma or a rigid bronchoscope. Nasal prongs or a mask can provide supplemental oxygen for the transnasal approach. An adapter attached to an oxygen supply works well for providing supplemental oxygen if an endotracheal tube or

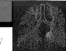

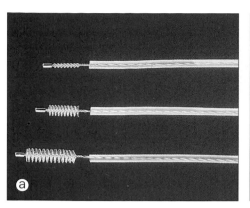
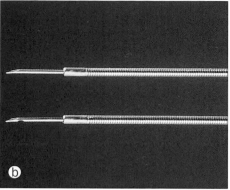
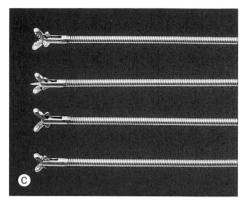

Figure 6.8 Instruments for use in bronchoscopy. (a) Brushes, (b) needles, and (c) biopsy forceps are available in various sizes and types. (Courtesy of Olympus Corporation.)

nasotracheal tube are used. Once the bite block is in place, a brief inspection of the airways might also be accomplished without the use of an endotracheal tube. One may pass an endotracheal tube before insertion of the flexible bronchoscope using indirect laryngoscopy and an endotracheal tube with a stylet.

Whether oral or nasal insertion of the flexible bronchoscope is preferred depends on the individual bronchoscopist's initial training. Every bronchoscopist should be able to perform bronchoscopy by both routes because each technique has its own definite advantages. The oral route via a bite-block or using an endotracheal tube allows the bronchoscopist to remove and reinsert the instrument easily in order to clean the lens and remove mucous plugs from the channel. Moreover, the bronchoscope can be withdrawn and reinserted quickly if bleeding and clots become obstacles; with hemorrhage, one has command of the airway from the outset if an endotracheal tube is employed.

On the other hand, the nasal route is slightly easier to master. The nasal passage itself serves as a stent for the passage of the instrument, allowing leisurely examination of the upper airways and inspection of the glottis and trachea under dynamic or static conditions. The nasal route is also suitable for a short examination when manipulation of the airway is not contemplated, such as a postoperative scrutiny after a bronchoplasty procedure, placement of brachytherapy catheters, or assessment of results of treatment for major airway obstruction.

A normal flexible bronchoscopic examination includes a thorough evaluation of the supraglottic airways as well as the laryngeal structures and their function during phonation. The examination proceeds with the evaluation of the trachea and its movements during phases of respiration and coughing. Then each side is examined so that all segmental bronchi and their branches are inspected for abnormalities of the mucosa, luminal narrowing, and bronchial obstruction. If abnormalities require brushings and biopsies, these are withheld until both sides have been visualized. Depending on the type of abnormality encountered, appropriate procedures and instruments (brushes, needles, or forceps) are selected for obtaining the specimens.

Endobronchial lesions can be sampled with cytology brushes, needles of various sizes, and biopsy forceps with or without teeth or an impaler needle. Each of these instruments is available in different sizes; the bronchoscopist can choose the appropriate equipment from various manufacturers (Fig. 6.8). Repeated performance of these procedures is essential to attain proficiency

and maintain competence in these procedures. Equally important is the processing of the specimens obtained using these techniques. Communication among bronchoscopist, pathologist, microbiologist, and the patient's physician is also crucial to maximize the yield from bronchoscopy.

Bronchoscopic lung biopsy is usually obtained via the flexible bronchoscope (Fig. 6.9). Fluoroscopic guidance to obtain bronchoscopic lung biopsy gives to the bronchoscopist a higher level of confidence in selecting the maximally abnormal areas for biopsies. Fluoroscopic guidance allows accurate placement of the forceps in the periphery of the lung for bronchoscopic lung biopsy near the pleura and for biopsy of smaller parenchymal lesions such as lung nodules (see Fig. 6.10).

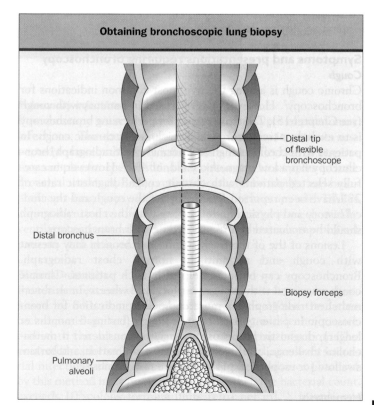

Obtaining bronchoscopic lung biopsy

Distal tip of flexible bronchoscope

Distal bronchus

Biopsy forceps

Pulmonary alveoli

Figure 6.9 The mechanism for obtaining bronchoscopic lung biopsy. The biopsy forceps pinches off the lung tissue located between two branches of terminal bronchi.

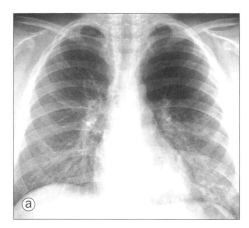

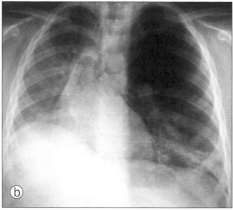

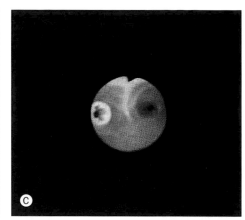

Figure 6.20 Chest radiographs and bronchoscopy of an 8-year-old boy who had cough and wheeze of 7 weeks' duration. (a) Radiograph obtained during full inspiration shows good expansion of both lungs. (b) Image obtained after full expiration reveals hyperinflation of left lung caused by 'check-valve' obstruction of the left main stem bronchus. (c) This pathology was caused by a piece of a toy that the boy had previously aspirated; the piece was seen in bronchoscopic examination, and extracted by bronchoscopy.

stenoses, clinical information should point towards the diagnosis, although an incorrect diagnosis of asthma is not uncommon. The cause of luminal narrowing can be intrinsic or extrinsic.

The commonest etiology of both intrinsic and extrinsic narrowing of the tracheobronchial tree is malignant disease, and bronchoscopy is helpful in establishing the diagnosis in these cases.

Benign strictures (Fig. 6.21) result from diverse processes, including:

- injury from tracheal intubation;
- crush injury of the neck;
- infectious diseases such as histoplasmosis and tuberculosis;
- mediastinal granulomatosis;
- Wegener's granulomatosis; and
- relapsing polychondritis.

In benign strictures, the bronchoscopy may show atrophic mucosa, mucosal edema, or granularity. In all newly suspected benign airway strictures, multiple biopsies should be obtained to exclude malignancy. The presence of granulomas in biopsy specimens may indicate an infectious process or sarcoidosis. Often, the etiology of benign strictures cannot be established.

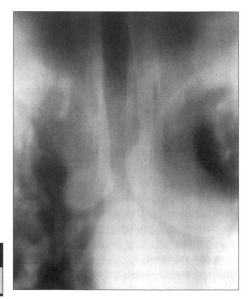

Figure 6.21 Plain tomography of distal tracheal narrowing and significant stenosis of left main stem bronchus and moderate stenosis of right main stem bronchus. The patient had relapsing polychondritis and required bronchoscopic dilatation and placement of a silicone stent.

Chemical and thermal burns

Inhalation of certain chemicals, gases, and superheated air can produce acute, subacute, and chronic pulmonary complications. These include acute severe edema and erythema of the tracheobronchial mucosa and mucosal elevation with sloughing. Smoke inhalation may result in diffuse soot deposition in the tracheobronchial tree. Unconsciousness in victims of inhalation poses the threat of pulmonary aspiration of orogastric contents. Diagnostic bronchoscopy, if performed to assess the extent of mucosal damage, should also exclude an aspirated foreign body.

Bronchoscopy in the subacute stage may reveal necrosis of the tracheobronchial mucosa and hemorrhagic tracheobronchitis. Bronchoscopy in the chronic phase may reveal scarring and stenoses of tracheobronchial tree, bronchiectasis, formation of granulation tissue, and bronchiolitis obliterans if a bronchoscopic lung biopsy is obtained.

Thoracic trauma

Diagnostic bronchoscopy is often indicated in cases of major thoracic trauma. The main reason for performing diagnostic bronchoscopy in patients with recent chest trauma is to exclude serious airway injury, such as fracture of the tracheobronchial tree. Bronchoscopy is useful in the assessment and management of other trauma-related problems, such as atelectasis of a lung, lobe, or segment. Bronchoscopy may also reveal aspirated material or thick secretions and mucous plugging, which can be removed at the time of diagnostic bronchoscopy. Unsuspected foreign bodies in the airways are occasionally encountered in victims of trauma.

Bronchoscopy for evaluation of hemoptysis following chest trauma may reveal pulmonary contusion and hemorrhage. Occasionally, bronchoscopy may fail to reveal signs of traumatic airway lesions and because of the possibility that a lesion might be overlooked by initial bronchoscopy, repeat bronchoscopic examination should be performed if the clinical situation suggests such a lesion.

Paralysis of the vocal cords and diaphragm

The anatomic course of the recurrent laryngeal nerve takes it around the left hilar structures and, therefore, pathologic

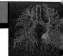

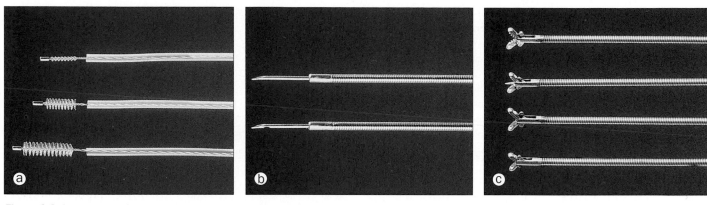

Figure 6.8 Instruments for use in bronchoscopy. (a) Brushes, (b) needles, and (c) biopsy forceps are available in various sizes and types. (Courtesy of Olympus Corporation.)

nasotracheal tube are used. Once the bite block is in place, a brief inspection of the airways might also be accomplished without the use of an endotracheal tube. One may pass an endotracheal tube before insertion of the flexible bronchoscope using indirect laryngoscopy and an endotracheal tube with a stylet.

Whether oral or nasal insertion of the flexible bronchoscope is preferred depends on the individual bronchoscopist's initial training. Every bronchoscopist should be able to perform bronchoscopy by both routes because each technique has its own definite advantages. The oral route via a bite-block or using an endotracheal tube allows the bronchoscopist to remove and reinsert the instrument easily in order to clean the lens and remove mucous plugs from the channel. Moreover, the bronchoscope can be withdrawn and reinserted quickly if bleeding and clots become obstacles; with hemorrhage, one has command of the airway from the outset if an endotracheal tube is employed.

On the other hand, the nasal route is slightly easier to master. The nasal passage itself serves as a stent for the passage of the instrument, allowing leisurely examination of the upper airways and inspection of the glottis and trachea under dynamic or static conditions. The nasal route is also suitable for a short examination when manipulation of the airway is not contemplated, such as a postoperative scrutiny after a bronchoplasty procedure, placement of brachytherapy catheters, or assessment of results of treatment for major airway obstruction.

A normal flexible bronchoscopic examination includes a thorough evaluation of the supraglottic airways as well as the laryngeal structures and their function during phonation. The examination proceeds with the evaluation of the trachea and its movements during phases of respiration and coughing. Then each side is examined so that all segmental bronchi and their branches are inspected for abnormalities of the mucosa, luminal narrowing, and bronchial obstruction. If abnormalities require brushings and biopsies, these are withheld until both sides have been visualized. Depending on the type of abnormality encountered, appropriate procedures and instruments (brushes, needles, or forceps) are selected for obtaining the specimens.

Endobronchial lesions can be sampled with cytology brushes, needles of various sizes, and biopsy forceps with or without teeth or an impaler needle. Each of these instruments is available in different sizes; the bronchoscopist can choose the appropriate equipment from various manufacturers (Fig. 6.8). Repeated performance of these procedures is essential to attain proficiency

and maintain competence in these procedures. Equally important is the processing of the specimens obtained using these techniques. Communication among bronchoscopist, pathologist, microbiologist, and the patient's physician is also crucial to maximize the yield from bronchoscopy.

Bronchoscopic lung biopsy is usually obtained via the flexible bronchoscope (Fig. 6.9). Fluoroscopic guidance to obtain bronchoscopic lung biopsy gives to the bronchoscopist a higher level of confidence in selecting the maximally abnormal areas for biopsies. Fluoroscopic guidance allows accurate placement of the forceps in the periphery of the lung for bronchoscopic lung biopsy near the pleura and for biopsy of smaller parenchymal lesions such as lung nodules (see Fig. 6.10).

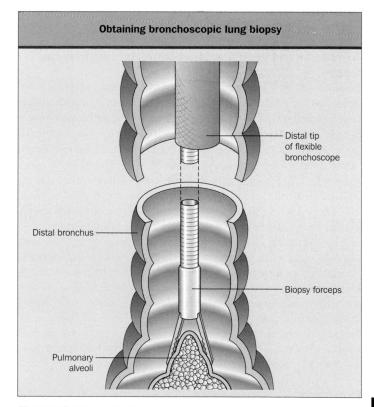

Obtaining bronchoscopic lung biopsy

Distal tip of flexible bronchoscope

Distal bronchus

Biopsy forceps

Pulmonary alveoli

Figure 6.9 The mechanism for obtaining bronchoscopic lung biopsy. The biopsy forceps pinches off the lung tissue located between two branches of terminal bronchi.

Except in unusual cases, the use of fluoroscopy should obviate the need to obtain routine chest radiographs after bronchoscopic lung biopsy[8,9]. A mail survey of 231 bronchoscopists in the UK reported that the incidence of pneumothorax following bronchoscopic lung biopsy was 1.8% when fluoroscopy was used; the incidence increased significantly to 2.9% when it was not used[10]. As to the number of lung biopsies, four to five biopsies seem optimal, although a smaller number of biopsies in sarcoidosis and a larger number (up to eight) in lung transplant patients may be necessary[11]. Bronchoalveolar lavage, if indicated, is obtained before bronchoscopic lung biopsy.

Special procedures such as laser application, bronchoscopic dilatation of airway strictures, stent placement, brachytherapy, electrocoagulation, bronchoscopic needle aspiration, bronchoscopic ultrasound, and other procedures require specialized training and equipment. Each of these has to be individualized. The indications for these procedures are discussed below.

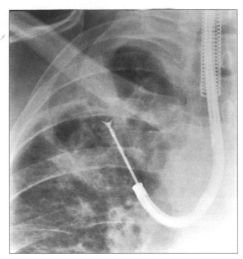

Figure 6.10 Bronchoscopic lung biopsy under fluoroscopic guidance. This technique ensures that the tissue sample obtained is truly representative of the disease process depicted on chest radiograph or computed tomography scan. Fluoroscopic technique significantly reduces the risk of pneumothorax.

Postbronchoscopy care

Most adult patients tolerate bronchoscopy well and are able to care for themselves within a short period after bronchoscopy, provided no general anesthesia is used. A brief period of observation in an adjoining suite next to bronchoscopy suite should suffice is most cases. The bronchoscopist should watch out for complications such as pneumothorax and for delayed bleeding. The patient should be advised not to drink or eat until normal sensation returns to oropharynx. Driving soon after bronchoscopy should be avoided if substantial amounts of sedative have been used.

Routine hospitalization following bronchoscopic lung biopsy is not indicated unless complications such as significant postbronchoscopic lung biopsy bleeding (Fig. 6.11), pneumothorax, and respiratory distress are encountered.

Symptoms and presentations requiring bronchoscopy
Cough

Chronic cough is among the five most common indications for bronchoscopy[2]. However, it is overused in patients with cough (see Chapter 15). The main reason for performing bronchoscopy is to exclude a tracheobronchial etiology for chronic cough. In patients with chronic cough and normal chest radiograph, bronchoscopy has a low diagnostic yield, of 4%[12]. However, in carefully selected patients with chronic cough, diagnostic rates of 28% have been reported. The nature of the cough and the clinical history and physical findings along with the chest radiograph should be evaluated before proceeding with bronchoscopy.

Lesions of the of the trachea and main bronchi may present with cough and an initially normal chest radiograph. Bronchoscopy can be most helpful in such patients. Chronic cough associated with hemoptysis, localized wheeze, or an abnormal chest radiograph is a more compelling indication for bronchoscopy. In patients with chronic cough (lasting 6 months or longer), diagnostic bronchoscopy may be considered if methacholine challenge, otorhinolaryngologic examination, and barium swallow (or esophageal pH study) are not diagnostic.

Hemoptysis

Hemoptysis can arise from various sources within the pulmonary system: bronchial arteries, pulmonary arteries, pulmonary veins, pulmonary capillaries, submucosal tracheobronchial varicose veins

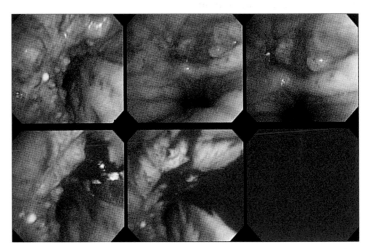

Figure 6.11 Postbiopsy bleeding. This is a consecutive series (from top left to bottom right) of bronchoscopic images obtained before and soon after biopsy of a mucosal lesion in a patient with small cell carcinoma. Continued bleeding required laser coagulation and overnight hospitalization for observation.

and venous anomalies, or new vascular channels that develop after surgery or radiation therapy. Important causes of massive hemoptysis include tuberculous cavities, neoplasms of the tracheobronchial tree, pulmonary mycetomas, bronchiectasis, pulmonary alveolar hemorrhage syndromes, and cystic fibrosis.

Chronic or intermittent streaky hemoptysis is common in patients with chronic bronchitis and may not require bronchoscopy. In contrast, any significant or new hemoptysis requires bronchoscopic evaluation. Bronchoscopy in the presence of a localizing chest radiograph abnormality is more likely to provide helpful information than when the radiograph is normal. The bronchoscopic examination in such cases is often not diagnostic and the only finding may be a 'streak of blood' in the airways. The bronchoscopist should trace this distally as far as possible, preferably to a segmental bronchus, to ensure that an endobronchial lesion is not missed (Fig. 6.12). Using a small-caliber flexible bronchoscope may add to the diagnostic yield by allowing the examination of the distal bronchial tree. Bronchoscopy should be performed as soon as possible after the patient presents with hemoptysis because examination during active hemoptysis is more likely to yield a diagnosis than after it has ceased. The bronchoscopist should also pay special attention to the mucosa and the visible vessels. Obvious vascular abnormalities such as prominent submucosal capillaries, bronchial inflammation, and subtle mucosal abnormalities are valuable findings. Bronchoscopic specimens should be collected for appropriate investigations depending on the underlying clinical situation.

Wheeze and stridor

Generalized wheeze, as encountered in asthmatic patients, is not an indication for bronchoscopy. Diagnostic or therapeutic bronchoscopy should be considered after excluding asthma and other causes of generalized wheezing. If an asthmatic wheeze is difficult to differentiate from a wheeze caused by localized narrowing of a bronchus, a diagnostic bronchoscopy should be considered (Fig. 6.13). A localized wheezing may indicate an obstructing bronchial lesion.

Stridor usually denotes urgency, and emergency laryngoscopy and bronchoscopy may be required. If the stridor is caused by a foreign body or a significant lesion in the large airway, a combined diagnostic and therapeutic bronchoscopy should be planned. Acute stridor is more common in children than in adults. The most common etiologies in children include epiglottitis, croup, rapidly progressive laryngomalacia, laryngeal papillomas, and foreign bodies in the trachea. Acute stridor in adults is caused by acute bilateral vocal cord paralysis, rapidly growing tracheal lesions, and acute extrinsic compression of the trachea by mediastinal and esophageal lesions. In some patients, emergency endotracheal intubation may be needed to secure an optimal airway and adequate ventilation before bronchoscopic examination is undertaken.

Acute tracheal obstruction, which can be fatal, has occurred in patients with large anterior mediastinal masses who have been subjected to general anesthesia. The tracheal obstruction is caused by severe extrinsic compression after induction of general anesthesia. Therapeutic intervention in the form of bronchoscopic intubation under awake anesthesia prevents this serious complication.

Abnormality on chest radiography

Not all patients with an abnormal chest radiograph require diagnostic bronchoscopy. For instance, an otherwise healthy person who develops community acquired pneumonia does not require bronchoscopy. Likewise, the majority of the acute infectious and other inflammatory processes that produce pneumonic infiltrates do not initially require bronchoscopy. In contrast, rapidly progressive pulmonary processes, particularly in immunocompromised patients, may require emergency bronchoscopy with diagnostic BAL to identify potential pathogenic organisms.

Characteristic chest radiograph abnormalities that may indicate diagnostic bronchoscopy include:
- acute or subacute atelectasis of a lung, lobe, or segment;
- enlarging or suspicious pulmonary parenchymal nodules;
- cavitated pulmonary lesions;
- mediastinal masses;
- diffuse parenchymal processes without an established diagnosis;
- rapidly progressive pulmonary infiltrates in immunosuppressed patients; and
- sudden disruption of tracheobronchial air bronchogram.

Hilar, mediastinal, and subcarinal lymphadenopathy in close proximity to the airways is another indication for diagnostic bronchoscopy with needle aspiration.

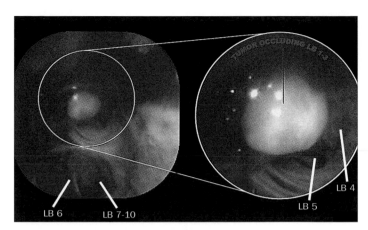

Figure 6.12 Subacute hemoptysis. Images obtained at bronchoscopy in a patient with subacute hemoptysis of 3 months' duration. The initial bronchoscopy showed mucosal inflammation. Later examination revealed the source – metastatic cancer (primary thyroid cancer) in the left upper lobe. (LB, left bronchus.)

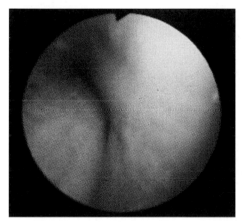

Figure 6.13 Tracheal buckling. Bronchoscopic examination revealed localized upper tracheal buckling on hyperflexion of the neck. The patient's symptoms cleared after three tracheal rings were resected. Pathologic analysis showed localized tracheomalacia.

Pulmonary infections

Bronchoscopy is useful in the diagnosis of all types of pulmonary infections. The main purpose of bronchoscopy in patients suspected to have pulmonary infections is the collection of respiratory samples for special stains and cultures. The samples include bronchial washings, BAL, protected-catheter brushings, and bronchoscopic lung biopsy (see Fig. 6.14). Bronchoscopy with BAL is commonly used to identify infectious organisms in mechanically ventilated patients with pneumonia and in immunocompromised patients with pulmonary infiltrates.

Bacterial infections

Bacterial infections of the lower respiratory tract can be diagnosed by BAL or protected-catheter brush. When the latter technique is applied, appropriate indication and technique are crucial to the accurate diagnosis of underlying infection. The protected-catheter brush is employed in the diagnosis of bacterial infections of the lower respiratory tract; cultures obtained by this method indicate active infection when the bacterial count exceeds 10^3 colony-forming units (cfu) per mL[13]. In patients with ventilator-associated pneumonia, identification of $<10^3$ cfu/mL indicates that pneumonia is unlikely. When $>10^3$ cfu/mL organisms are identified, more than 75% of patients are

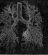

Bronchoscopic techniques and applications in respiratory infections	
Bronchoscopic technique	**Clinical application**
Bronchoscopy (visualization)	1. Assessment of mucosal, intraluminal, and extraluminal pathology 2. Evaluation of endobronchial tuberculosis, mycoses, viral vesicles (in AIDS) 3. Invasive tracheobronchial aspergillosis, candidiasis, and others. 4. Follow-up of endobronchial disease (tuberculosis, etc.)
Bronchial washings	Culture of mycobacteria, fungi, and viruses, and *Pneumocystis* smears
Bronchoalveolar lavage	Culture of all organisms, especially for identification of mycobacteria, fungi, cytomegalovirus, and other viruses, and *Pneumocystis* smears
Protected specimen brushing	Culture of aerobic and anaerobic bacteria
Nonprotected bronchial brushing	Stains and culture for mycobacteria, fungi, *Pneumocystis carinii*, and viruses
Endobronchial biopsy	1. Mucosal lesions caused by mycobacteria, fungi, protozoa, etc. 2. Removal of obstructing lesions responsible for infection (tumor, foreign body, etc.) 3. Drainage of lung abscess, piecemeal removal of mycetomas (aspergillomas and other fungus balls)
Bronchoscopic needle aspiration	1. Stains and culture of extrabronchial lymph nodes for identification of mycobacteria and fungi 2. Drainage of bronchogenic cyst and instillation of sclerosing agent
Bronchoscopic lung biopsy	Stains and culture of all organisms, especially for identification of *Pneumocystis carinii*, mycobacteria, and fungi; also detection of parasitic lung infections
Rigid or flexible bronchoscope	Insertion tracheobronchial prosthesis (stent) to overcome airway obstruction caused by intrinsic stenosis (post-tuberculous or fungal), extrinsic compression caused by mediastinal fibrosis due to histoplasmosis

Figure 6.14 Bronchoscopic techniques and applications in respiratory infections. (AIDS, acquired immunodeficiency syndrome.)

likely to have pneumonia. In patients who are on antibiotics for a previous infection at the time of suspicion of ventilator-associated pneumonia, and in those patients on antibiotic therapy for suspected ventilator-associated pneumonia less than 24 hours before bronchoscopy, the BAL intracellular organism count (>5% cells) and cultures of protected specimen brush (>10^3 cfu/mL) and BAL (>10^5 cfu/mL) are reliable[14].

The protected-catheter brush is also useful in identifying multiple bacteria in patients in whom polymicrobial bacterial pneumonia is likely. Limitations of the protected-catheter brush technique include the fact that this method does not sample a large area of the tracheobronchial tree. Furthermore, culture results from this technique in patients who are already on multiple wide-spectrum antibiotics may not alter the clinical management. Pneumothorax has occurred in up to 8% of mechanically ventilated patients in whom a protected-catheter brush was employed. Mild procedure-induced hemorrhage occurs but has not proven to be a significant problem, even though significant bleeding can ensue in patients with coagulation disorders. Presently, most bronchoscopists have abandoned routine use of protected catheter brush in favor of BAL.

This is because both provide similar diagnostic results but BAL is less expensive and safer even in patients with severe coagulation problems.

Mycobacterial infections

Tuberculosis of the lungs can be diagnosed by bronchoscopic techniques, including brushings, washings, and bronchoscopic lung biopsy. Diagnostic rates ranging from 58 to 96%, with an average rate of 72%, can be expected. Bronchoscopy is the only procedure to provide the diagnosis in 20–45% of patients with active tuberculosis[15]. On the other hand, routine culture of bronchoscopic specimens carries a diagnostic yield of 6% and, when routinely performed, bronchoscopy is likely to be the only procedure to yield the diagnosis in only 5% of patients with tuberculosis. It is, therefore, not the first choice investigation: sputum examination should always be first. In patients with miliary tuberculosis, in whom sputum smears are frequently negative, bronchoscopic brushings, washings, and bronchoscopic lung biopsy are diagnostic in up to 80% of patients, and bronchoscopy is the only procedure to provide the diagnosis in up to 9%[16].

In endobronchial tuberculosis, bronchoscopic examination may reveal mucosal and submucosal granulomas, mucosal ulcerations, endobronchial polyps, bronchial stenosis, and bronchial erosion by a mediastinal lymph node, which may mimic a neoplasm.

Mycotic infections

Bronchoscopy plays a major role in the diagnosis of mycotic infections of the lung. Bronchoscopic identification of fungal organisms responsible for histoplasmosis, coccidioidomycosis, blastomycosis, cryptococcosis, and mucormycosis is highly indicative of respiratory infection. In contrast, growth of *Aspergillus* and *Candida* spp. from bronchoscopic washings does not establish the diagnosis of respiratory aspergillosis or candidiasis because these organisms frequently colonize the respiratory tract. Therefore, the presence of hyphae in bronchoscopic specimens should be correlated with clinical findings. In patients with invasive aspergillosis, however, culture of bronchoscopic specimens are positive for *Aspergillus* spp. in only 23% of patients[17]. Negative results do not exclude the diagnosis and further procedures or empiric therapy may be necessary in the appropriate clinical setting. In patients with hemoptysis caused by an aspergilloma, bronchoscopy helps in identifying the site of bleeding so that appropriate definitive steps are taken to treat the underlying cause.

Histoplasmosis of the respiratory system can involve the lung parenchyma as well as the airways. Bronchoscopy is useful in documenting the diagnosis in patients with cavitated lesions, localized infiltrates, and miliary disease caused by histoplasmosis. In one series of patients undergoing bronchoscopic examination, bronchoscopy was the only technique that diagnosed histoplasmosis in 11% of patients[18]. However, in patients with pulmonary nodules caused by histoplasmosis, bronchoscopy was not helpful.

In patients with histoplasmosis, the bronchoscopic appearance may include bronchial stenosis, mucosal granulomas, increased mucosal vascularity, and extrinsic compression caused by mediastinal fibrosis. In patients with acquired immunodeficiency syndrome (AIDS), endobronchial obstructing lesions secondary to aspergillosis have been described. In patients with severe neutropenia, tracheobronchial invasive aspergillosis has been reported to produce airway obstruction and respiratory distress.

Immunocompromised patients

Bronchoscopy is the most commonly used invasive diagnostic procedure in the diagnosis of pulmonary infiltrates in immuno-compromised patients. The overall sensitivity of bronchoscopic procedures in the identification of infections in this group of patients is 90%. If results of bronchoscopy are negative for an infectious cause of respiratory illness, the probability that infection is not present may be as high as 94% (negative predictive value). As discussed above, BAL is the most helpful and frequently used technique in this group of patients.

Human immunodeficiency virus infection

In patients who have AIDS, caused by human immunodeficiency virus (HIV), suspicion of *Pneumocystis carinii* pneumonia is a common indication for bronchoscopy. Bronchoalveolar lavage and bronchoscopic lung biopsy have about equal sensitivity (over 85%) when used alone for diagnosing *P. carinii* pneumonia. In some studies, BAL alone has provided 95% sensitivity when cytologic examination and special stains were carried out. Bronchoscopic lung biopsy alone is sensitive in more than 94% of patients with *P. carinii* pneumonia. Bronchoalveolar lavage with bronchoscopic lung biopsy has been reported to provide 100% sensitivity when good specimens are obtained. Since empiric therapy prior to bronchoscopy may significantly impair the diagnostic yield of BAL in detecting common pathogens in HIV-infected patients with respiratory symptoms, some physicians recommend bronchoscopy with BAL as soon as possible[19].

Bronchoscopy is also helpful in identifying respiratory infections caused by cytomegalovirus, *Mycobacterium avium–intracellulare*, *Cryptococcus neoformans*, *Mycobacterium tuberculosis*, *Coccidioides immitis*, *Histoplasma capsulatum*, and *Blastomyces dermatides*. Cultures of alveolar lavage fluid is particularly helpful in diagnosing cytomegalovirus and mycobacteria with little added benefit from bronchoscopic lung biopsy.

Lung abscess

The indications for bronchoscopy in patients with lung abscess include collection of culture specimens, exclusion of an endobronchial obstruction (either neoplasm or foreign body) that is responsible for the abscess, and, in some patients, bronchoscopic drainage of the abscess. Bronchoscopic drainage is not uniformly successful.

Diffuse lung disease

Bronchoscopy is frequently used in the diagnosis of diffuse lung diseases. The most commonly employed bronchoscopic procedures are BAL and bronchoscopic lung biopsy (see Figs 6.9 & 6.10).

Bronchoalveolar lavage permits collection of both cellular and noncellular components from the alveolar and epithelial surfaces of the lower respiratory tract. The procedures for BAL and analysis of the effluent vary, since there has been no standardization. Even in the same patient, the cell counts vary between different lung segments. The BAL of a normal adult with 100mL saline yields 40–60mL effluent containing $5–10\times10^6$ cells and 1–10mg protein. It is a relatively safe procedure that adds about 15 minutes to a routine flexible bronchoscopic examination.

Bronchoalveolar lavage has been employed to diagnose various interstitial lung diseases, pulmonary malignancies, and pulmonary infections. Bronchoalveolar lavage has been used to analyze cellular constituents at the alveolar level and thus follow the status of the alveolitis and its response to therapy. However, the role of the procedure in altering the cause of the disease remains in doubt. In summary, it is clear that, at present, BAL has a limited role in the diagnosis and treatment of idiopathic pulmonary fibrosis, lung disease associated with collagen diseases, and other nonmalignant and noninfectious interstitial lung diseases. In many interstitial lung diseases, such as interstitial pulmonary fibrosis, pulmonary lymphangioleiomyomatosis, and pulmonary Langerhans cell granuloma, high-resolution computed tomography (CT) scanning of the chest has supplanted bronchoscopic techniques as the diagnostic tool.

Bronchoalveolar lavage provides the histologic diagnostic information in pulmonary Langerhans cell granuloma (histiocytosis-X), pulmonary alveolar (phospholipo)proteinosis, chronic eosinophilic pneumonia, occult pulmonary hemorrhage, fat embolism syndrome, and pulmonary malignancies including lymphangitic pulmonary metastasis (Fig. 6.15). The ratio of helper (CD4) to suppressor (CD8) T lymphocytes may help in distinguishing sarcoidosis from hypersensitivity pneumonitis; in sarcoidosis, the CD4:CD8 ratio may be as high as 10:1 or 20:1, and in hypersensitivity pneumonitis, the ratio is decreased or reversed. Similar reversal in the normal CD4:CD8 ratio is seen in patients who have AIDS and lymphocytic interstitial pneumonitis.

Bronchoalveolar lavage is very helpful in the diagnosis of lymphangitic pulmonary metastasis. The procedure is particularly valuable in the evaluation of radiographic evidence of metastatic or lymphangitic pulmonary malignancy. Diagnostic BAL with lipid-specific staining technique is valuable in establishing the diagnosis of fat embolism in 60% of adult patients with acute chest syndrome caused by sickle cell disease.

Bronchoscopic lung biopsy provides adequate lung tissue and thus precludes the need for open lung biopsy in many patients. Even though BAL has supplanted this procedure in many instances, bronchoscopic lung biopsy should be considered when a diffuse or localized interstitial, alveolar, miliary, or fine nodular pattern of disease is present on the chest radiograph, and when the diagnosis cannot be established by a BAL, a high-resolution CT scan of the chest, or other less invasive diagnostic techniques. Bronchoscopic lung biopsy in certain diffuse pulmonary disorders is more likely to provide diagnostic information (see Fig. 6.16).

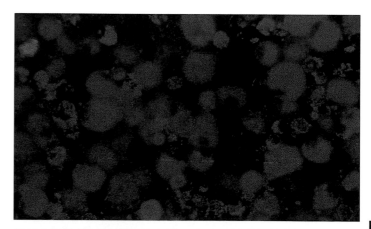

Figure 6.15 Bronchoalveolar effluent stained with CD1a. Numerous CD1a staining cells (orange-colored cells) in a patient with Langerhans cell granuloma of the lung (histiocytosis-X) are shown.

Pulmonary diseases in which bronchoscopic lung biopsy provides high diagnostic yield	
Sarcoidosis	Pneumocystis carinii infection
Hypersensitivity pneumonitis	Mycobacterioses
Eosinophilic granuloma (histiocytosis-X)	Mycoses
Alveolar proteinosis	Cytomegalovirus infection
Lymphangitic metastasis	Pneumoconioses
Diffuse pulmonary lymphoma	Rejection process in lung transplant recipients
Diffuse alveolar cell carcinoma	

Figure 6.16 Pulmonary diseases in which bronchoscopic lung biopsy provides high diagnostic yield. In each of these diseases the diagnostic yield is over 70%. The addition of bronchoalveolar lavage may increase the diagnostic yield in most of these conditions.

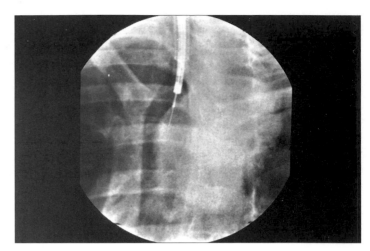

Figure 6.17 Bronchoscopic needle aspiration of a right paratracheal lymph node. An oblique fluoroscopic view documents bronchoscopic needle aspiration of a right paratracheal lymph node in a patient with squamous cell lung cancer and right paratracheal lymphadenopathy. The aspirate was positive for squamous cell carcinoma.

A stronger indication for biopsy is when histologic diagnosis is imperative. Lymphangitic carcinomatosis, miliary tuberculosis, diffuse pulmonary mycoses, sarcoidosis, cytotoxic pulmonary disease, and Langerhans cell granuloma of the lung are some of the entities that can be diagnosed by bronchoscopic lung biopsy.

The diagnosis of idiopathic pulmonary fibrosis by bronchoscopic lung biopsy is controversial because a histologic diagnosis consistent with idiopathic pulmonary fibrosis is present in many pulmonary diseases. The usefulness of bronchoscopic lung biopsy in immunocompromised patients, including those with *P. carinii* pneumonia, and fungal lung infections is discussed above.

Intrathoracic lymphadenopathy and mass

Bronchoscopy is indicated in patients with radiologic diagnosis of intrathoracic lymphadenopathy or mass who have symptoms of tracheobronchial involvement. Bronchoscopy in such patients will ascertain the presence of extrinsic compression of the airways or mucosal involvement of the airway mucosa. In such cases, many surgeons routinely request or perform diagnostic bronchoscopy prior to mediastinoscopy. A bronchoscopic diagnosis of malignancy may obviate the need for mediastinoscopy or thoracotomy.

The flexible bronchoscope is used to obtain needle aspiration of paratracheal or mediastinal lymph nodes (Fig. 6.17). Multiple needle aspirations can be safely obtained from the same site. With a 19-gauge needle, a core of tissue may be obtained for histologic preparation. The overall yield from bronchoscopic needle aspiration in malignant disease is about 75%. The diagnostic accuracy of a positive cytology is very high, but a few false-positive cases have been described[20]. The predictive value of a negative cytology is quite low. A negative needle aspiration of mediastinal lymph nodes does not rule out the possibility of nodal metastasis even when the nodes are of normal size on CT. The diagnostic sensitivity of bronchoscopic needle aspiration is 80–89%, especially if a 19-gauge needle is used (see Chapter 43). Bronchoscopic needle aspiration may be useful in establishing a benign diagnosis.

In patients with suspected sarcoidosis, bronchoscopic needle aspiration biopsies have revealed noncaseating granulomas in 66% of the patients; when combined with mucosal biopsy, the diagnosis of sarcoidosis has increased to 78%[21].

The safety of the bronchoscopic needle aspiration and biopsy and the low incidence of complications have been established. Negligible bleeding is seen at the site of needle puncture. Hemomediastinum, pneumothorax, pneumomediastinum, and bacteremia have occurred in sporadic cases.

Bronchogenic carcinoma

Bronchoscopy is probably the most important diagnostic procedure in the diagnosis of bronchogenic carcinoma. It is also helpful in the staging, early detection, and follow up of patients treated for lung cancer (Fig. 6.18). In patients with chest radiograph and clinical findings suggestive of lung cancer, bronchoscopy is extremely helpful in obtaining biopsies from the abnormal tracheobronchial mucosa and mass lesions in the lung parenchyma. Additionally, cytologic brushings and bronchial washings add to the diagnostic yield from the procedure. Diligent examination of the tracheobronchial mucosa is imperative before biopsy specimens are obtained. If overt changes are absent, subtle abnormalities should be sought. Multiple biopsies and brushings may be needed in some patients and various types of brushes and biopsy forceps are available to the bronchoscopist to accomplish optimal diagnostic bronchoscopy.

Bronchoscopy plays a major role in the staging of primary pulmonary carcinoma (Fig. 6.19). In addition to the visual staging of tracheobronchial involvement by the tumor, bronchoscopy may also help in identifying clinically unsuspected abnormalities, such as vocal cord paralysis due to primary lung cancer and the presence of another neoplastic (multicentric) process or other abnormalities of the tracheobronchial tree. Such findings may alter management options. Bronchoscopic visualization of a bronchogenic cancer will help in deciding the extent of surgical resection feasible. For instance, the involvement of the main carina may place a patient in 'T4' category or stage IIIB (Fig. 6.19). Similarly, the bronchoscopic identification of an occult vocal cord paralysis denotes a worse prognosis. If the biopsy obtained by bronchoscopy establishes the diagnosis of small cell cancer, the option of treatment by surgery can usually be excluded. A bronchoscopic biopsy may indicate the possibility of a metastatic cancer in the bronchus or lung, and this information may drastically alter the therapeutic approach. The role of transcarinal and transbronchial needle aspiration or biopsy in the staging of primary lung cancer is discussed above.

Early detection, localization, and aggressive treatment of preinvasive stages of lung cancer results in 5-year survival rates of

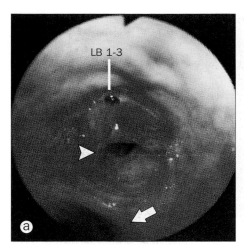
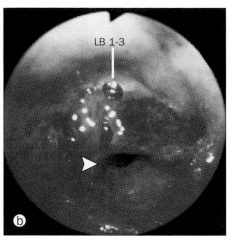
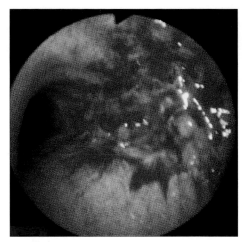

Figure 6.18 Bronchoscopic views of a squamous cell carcinoma of the left upper lobe. Partial obstruction to the bronchus leading to anterior and apical-posterior segments can be seen. (a) The bronchus seen at the 7 o'clock position (arrow) leads to the left lower lobe. (b) A close-up view; the lower bronchus [arrowhead in (a) and (b)] is the bronchus to the lingular segments. (LB, left bronchus.)

Figure 6.19 Bronchoscopic view of an adenocarcinoma. The tumor was completely obstructing the right main stem bronchus and involved the main carina, placing the patient into the 'T4' category or stage IIIB.

70–80%. Once a radiologically occult cancer is suspected, on the basis of positive cytology, cancer of the oropharynx and larynx should be excluded by a thorough examination. In the majority of patients who have positive sputum cytology and a normal chest radiograph (so-called occult cancer), localization of lung cancer can usually be accomplished by direct visualization of the tracheobronchial tree using the flexible bronchoscope. Over 50% of radiologically occult cancers demonstrate mucosal abnormalities at the first bronchoscopic inspection.

In patients with occult lung cancer, localization is difficult because the tumor may not produce obvious mucosal abnormalities. These patients require repeated bronchoscopic examinations over several months before localization is established. Fluorescent compounds such as hematoporphyrin derivative and dihemato-porphyrin ether, when injected intravenously, accumulate in malignant tissue at higher concentrations than normal tissue. When exposed to light of appropriate wavelength, the abnormal tissues containing the fluorescent material emit a characteristic salmon-red fluorescence. Bronchoscopic application of light following intravenous administration of these compounds has provided another method in the diagnosis of early lung cancer. Bronchoscopic detection of mucosal autofluorescence has been used to detect mucosal abnormalities. The results from this technique are still preliminary.

Follow up of patients who have undergone various types of treatments often requires bronchoscopic examination to ascertain the effectiveness of therapy. In such patients, repeat brushings and biopsies will be required to document recurrence or persistence of malignancy. Surgical treatment involving complicated procedures, such as tracheoplasty and reanastomosis, often require intraoperative or immediate postoperative bronchoscopy to assess the technical results of the surgical procedure.

Metastatic cancer in the thoracic cage
Intrathoracic metastases from cancers originating in extrapulmonary organs present with varying respiratory manifestations. Four clinical presentations that often require bronchoscopy are:
- extrinsic compression of the tracheobronchial tree;
- endobronchial metastasis;
- pulmonary parenchymal nodule; and
- interstitial infiltration secondary to lymphangitic spread.

The bronchoscopic diagnostic approaches are similar to those in primary lung cancer. Endobronchial metastasis is more likely from Hodgkin's lymphoma, hypernephroma, and cancers of the breast and colon. Endobronchial hypernephroma tends to bleed more with biopsy. The role of BAL in the diagnosis of lymphangitic metastasis is discussed below.

Esophageal and mediastinal tumors may produce extrinsic compression or directly extend into the tracheobronchial tree. Another complication of these tumors is the occasional occurrence of tracheoesophageal or tracheomediastinal fistula. Because of these possibilities, it is advisable to perform bronchoscopy before extensive surgical resections are undertaken.

Tracheobronchial foreign body
Foreign body aspiration should always be suspected in children with acute or subacute pulmonary symptoms. It is, however, rarely considered in adults with subacute or chronic respiratory symptoms unless a clear history of aspiration is evident. The single diagnostic factor leading to consideration of foreign body aspiration is a high clinical index of suspicion[4]. The diagnosis can be verified by visualizing the foreign body by chest radiography or via bronchoscopy. A nonradiopaque foreign body may be easily missed on a routine chest radiograph but may be suggested by associated atelectasis, infiltration in the postobstructive region, or air trapping and hyperinflation on the postexhalation chest film (see Fig. 6.20).

The site of lodgement of the foreign body is dependent on the anatomic structure of the tracheobronchial tree and the body posture of the patient at the time of aspiration. The most common area for aspiration is the right lower lobe. The common types of foreign body include vegetable matter, dental fragments, straight pins, and safety pins. The treatment of tracheobronchial foreign bodies is discussed under therapeutic bronchoscopy (below).

Tracheobronchial strictures and stenoses
Tracheobronchial strictures and stenoses are caused by benign and malignant diseases. In the majority of patients with significant

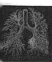
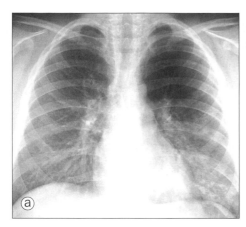

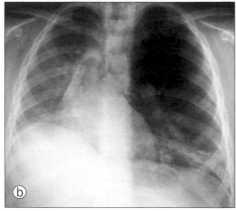

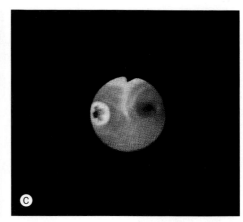

Figure 6.20 Chest radiographs and bronchoscopy of an 8-year-old boy who had cough and wheeze of 7 weeks' duration. (a) Radiograph obtained during full inspiration shows good expansion of both lungs. (b) Image obtained after full expiration reveals hyperinflation of left lung caused by 'check-valve' obstruction of the left main stem bronchus. (c) This pathology was caused by a piece of a toy that the boy had previously aspirated; the piece was seen in bronchoscopic examination, and extracted by bronchoscopy.

stenoses, clinical information should point towards the diagnosis, although an incorrect diagnosis of asthma is not uncommon. The cause of luminal narrowing can be intrinsic or extrinsic.

The commonest etiology of both intrinsic and extrinsic narrowing of the tracheobronchial tree is malignant disease, and bronchoscopy is helpful in establishing the diagnosis in these cases.

Benign strictures (Fig. 6.21) result from diverse processes, including:
- injury from tracheal intubation;
- crush injury of the neck;
- infectious diseases such as histoplasmosis and tuberculosis;
- mediastinal granulomatosis;
- Wegener's granulomatosis; and
- relapsing polychondritis.

In benign strictures, the bronchoscopy may show atrophic mucosa, mucosal edema, or granularity. In all newly suspected benign airway strictures, multiple biopsies should be obtained to exclude malignancy. The presence of granulomas in biopsy specimens may indicate an infectious process or sarcoidosis. Often, the etiology of benign strictures cannot be established.

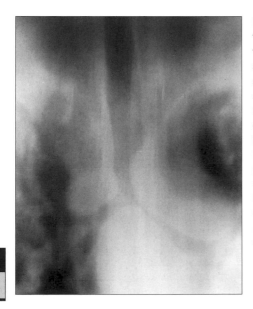

Figure 6.21 Plain tomography of distal tracheal narrowing and significant stenosis of left main stem bronchus and moderate stenosis of right main stem bronchus. The patient had relapsing polychondritis and required bronchoscopic dilatation and placement of a silicone stent.

Chemical and thermal burns

Inhalation of certain chemicals, gases, and superheated air can produce acute, subacute, and chronic pulmonary complications. These include acute severe edema and erythema of the tracheobronchial mucosa and mucosal elevation with sloughing. Smoke inhalation may result in diffuse soot deposition in the tracheobronchial tree. Unconsciousness in victims of inhalation poses the threat of pulmonary aspiration of orogastric contents. Diagnostic bronchoscopy, if performed to assess the extent of mucosal damage, should also exclude an aspirated foreign body.

Bronchoscopy in the subacute stage may reveal necrosis of the tracheobronchial mucosa and hemorrhagic tracheobronchitis. Bronchoscopy in the chronic phase may reveal scarring and stenoses of tracheobronchial tree, bronchiectasis, formation of granulation tissue, and bronchiolitis obliterans if a bronchoscopic lung biopsy is obtained.

Thoracic trauma

Diagnostic bronchoscopy is often indicated in cases of major thoracic trauma. The main reason for performing diagnostic bronchoscopy in patients with recent chest trauma is to exclude serious airway injury, such as fracture of the tracheobronchial tree. Bronchoscopy is useful in the assessment and management of other trauma-related problems, such as atelectasis of a lung, lobe, or segment. Bronchoscopy may also reveal aspirated material or thick secretions and mucous plugging, which can be removed at the time of diagnostic bronchoscopy. Unsuspected foreign bodies in the airways are occasionally encountered in victims of trauma.

Bronchoscopy for evaluation of hemoptysis following chest trauma may reveal pulmonary contusion and hemorrhage. Occasionally, bronchoscopy may fail to reveal signs of traumatic airway lesions and because of the possibility that a lesion might be overlooked by initial bronchoscopy, repeat bronchoscopic examination should be performed if the clinical situation suggests such a lesion.

Paralysis of the vocal cords and diaphragm

The anatomic course of the recurrent laryngeal nerve takes it around the left hilar structures and, therefore, pathologic

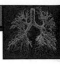

lesions of left hilar structures have the potential to compress or destroy the nerve and cause paralysis of the left vocal cord. Paralysis of the right vocal cord by an intrathoracic process is rare unless the pathologic process extends toward the right side of the neck. Diagnostic bronchoscopy may be indicated if vocal cord paralysis is associated with respiratory symptoms and a suspicious chest radiograph.

Neoplastic involvement of hilar or mediastinal lymph nodes or lymph nodes in the path of the phrenic nerves should be considered in evaluating diaphragmatic paralysis. Tumors that cause diaphragmatic paralysis are usually large enough to be seen on the plain chest radiograph. Computed tomography of the chest may aid in the detection of subtle hilar lymphadenopathy. Bronchoscopy together with transbronchial needle aspiration or biopsy of the perihilar lymph nodes, or both, is a diagnostic option in these patients.

Pleural effusion and persistent pneumothorax

Pleural effusion has been used as an indication for diagnostic bronchoscopy even though the diagnostic yield from bronchoscopy in such cases is low. An occult endobronchial obstructing lesion may contribute to the persistence of pneumothorax or continued air leak following placement of a chest tube. Bronchoscopy is occasionally done to exclude an inapparent bronchial lesion. Bronchoscopy in these patients seldom reveals an endobronchial abnormality. The role of bronchoscopy in treatment of air leaks is discussed below.

Miscellaneous

In patients with bronchiectasis, bronchoscopy has been used to obtain culture specimens (see above). In cases of suspected bronchiectasis, bronchography has often been used to confirm the diagnosis and to assist in planning medical or surgical management. A water-soluble contrast can be instilled via a flexible bronchoscope to obtain a bronchogram in order to detect bronchiectasis. The advent of conventional and high-resolution CT scanning has essentially replaced the need for bronchography.

Therapeutic bronchoscopy

Therapeutic aspects of bronchoscopy are as important as the diagnostic indications. Of the 871 bronchoscopists in North America who participated in the survey on bronchoscopy carried out by the American College of Chest Physicians, 56% indicated that therapeutic bronchoscopy for lobar and segmental atelectasis was one of the five most common indications for bronchoscopy[2]. Among patients in critical care units, up to 75% of bronchoscopies were performed for therapeutic purposes[7,22]. The indications for therapeutic bronchoscopy are listed in Figure 6.5. In clinical practice it is common to perform bronchoscopy for both diagnostic and therapeutic purposes simultaneously.

Retained secretions, mucous plugs, and clots

Retained secretions and mucous plugs together are the most common indication for therapeutic bronchoscopy in adults. The retention of secretions and mucous plugs is a common clinical problem in patients with impaired cough and clearance mechanisms caused by an altered level of consciousness, in those with poor pulmonary function or weakness, recurrent aspiration, ventilator dependence, and in those in the post-thoracotomy state. Inspissated mucus becomes a thick plug and may cause segmental or lobar

atelectasis. Blood clots secondary to bleeding from intrinsic pulmonary lesions or after performance of complicated thoracic surgical procedures pose special problems. Such clots are usually tenacious and more difficult to remove than the mucoid plugs. Therapeutic bronchoscopy is also indicated in patients who develop a pseudomembrane in the tracheobronchial tree following photodynamic therapy of tracheobronchial neoplasms and in patients who develop necrotic debris following chemical or thermal burns of the tracheobronchial mucosa.

The immediate performance of therapeutic bronchoscopy is indicated if atelectasis is responsible for respiratory distress. In less urgent cases, it is sound clinical practice to attempt other means of dislodging the retained secretions before proceeding with bronchoscopy. Each patient should first be carefully evaluated because not all patients with segmental or even lobar atelectasis benefit from therapeutic bronchoscopy. In a study of 31 patients with acute lobar atelectasis, those patients who were randomly allocated to flexible bronchoscopy followed by respiratory therapy for 48 hours did no better than those allocated to respiratory therapy alone. The presence of an air bronchogram proved to be a predictor of delayed resolution for both groups[23].

When the flexible bronchoscope is used for removal of secretions and mucous plugs, a large-channel instrument should be chosen so that thick and tenacious material can be aspirated quickly. An endotracheal tube also helps by allowing the bronchoscopist to remove the instrument from the tracheobronchial tree and clean the bronchoscope if the secretions totally block the suction channel. The patient's coughing during the bronchoscopic suction also helps move the mucus secretions and plugs proximally. Occasionally, very thick and tenacious secretions and mucus plugs require removal by means of a biopsy forceps. Forceps may also be required to remove necrotic mucosa, pseudomembrane, and necrotic debris.

In hypoxemic patients who require vigorous suctioning, the oxygenation should be carefully monitored by pulse oximetry so that the pre-existing hypoxia is not worsened. Large-channel flexible bronchoscopes are more likely to aggravate this problem by virtue of their ability to suck large volumes of gas. Supplemental oxygenation as indicated by pulse oximetry will generally allow safe performance of therapeutic bronchoscopy.

In patients with refractory atelectasis, bronchoscopic bronchial balloon occlusion with application of positive-pressure ventilation delivered through the balloon catheter lumen has resulted in the re-expansion of atelectatic segments. Bronchial tamponade via the bronchoscope is aimed at isolating a pulmonary segment or subsegment distal to the location of the tamponade. The bronchial tamponade technique has been used for the bronchoscopic treatment of bronchial or pulmonary hemorrhage, refractory pneumothorax, persistent air leaks following thoracotomy, and bronchopleural fistula.

Hemoptysis

Hemoptysis is a commonly encountered symptom. However, less than 5% of patients present with massive bleeding, and asphyxiation rather than exsanguination is the cause of death in these cases. As soon as the hemodynamic status and adequate oxygenation is assured, immediate bronchoscopic examination should proceed with the aim of not only localizing the site of bleeding but also of treating it. An instrument with a large working channel passed through an endotracheal tube is recommended. Uncontrollable or excessive bleeding may require the use of the rigid bronchoscope. If the bleeding is originating in a distal segment, every attempt should be made to tamponade the bronchus with the bronchoscope. Iced saline irrigation, instillation of 1 in 20,000 epinephrine or 1 in 10,000 adrenaline solution through the bronchoscope, and broncho-scopic balloon tamponade are some of the methods used in the control of hemoptysis. It is imperative that the rest of the bronchial tree be cleared of aspirated blood and blood clots. If the bleeding is from a visible tumor or an area where tampon-ade technique is not feasible, bronchoscopic coagulation may be necessary. Smaller lesions can be coagulated and cut with the laser; low power (approximately 15 watt) is suitable for coagulation. Often, it is impossible to see the supplying vessel and to distinguish between tumor and blood clot. An alterna-tive technique is the application of electrocautery.

If all other measures fail, endobronchial tamponade through a rigid bronchoscope is required to prevent asphyxiation. In the absence of facilities for rigid bronchoscopy, intubation with a double lumen tube should be considered (Fig. 6.22). It should be noted that the regular flexible bronchoscopes cannot pass through the double lumen endotracheal tube and a smaller cal-iber flexible bronchoscope will be needed to ascertain the posi-tioning of the endotracheal tube. Attempts have been made to use fibrin glue to treat hemoptysis. In patients with massive hemoptysis, the continuous stream of blood tends to flush away the fibrin glue before a stable clot forms. Use of further treat-ments such as bronchial artery embolization and surgical resec-tion of bleeding segment will depend on the therapeutic effectiveness of bronchoscopy.

Tracheobronchial foreign body

Rigid bronchoscopy is the instrument of choice for extracting a tracheobronchial foreign body, particularly in children. In a recent report on 60 foreign body problems in adults, flexible bron-choscopy was effective in 61%, and rigid bronchoscopy in 98%, with an overall efficacy of 95% for both bronchoscopes[4]. Flexible bronchoscopy is helpful in cases in which the foreign body has impacted in airways too distal for access with the rigid broncho-scope. Many large foreign bodies in the proximal airways can also be extracted with the flexible bronchoscope (Fig. 6.23).

Additionally, the flexible bronchoscope has also proved useful in cases in which severe cervicofacial trauma precludes the neck hyperextension that is necessary for rigid bronchoscopic exami-nation. Acute complications from foreign body extraction are uncommon. Bleeding due to bronchoscopy may be noted in patients with large and sharp tracheobronchial foreign bodies.

Tracheobronchial neoplasms

Bronchoscopic resection

The role of the rigid bronchoscope in the bronchoscopic removal of obstructing tracheobronchial tumors is discussed above. This treatment is purely palliative in patients who require immediate relief of airway obstruction secondary to large neo-plasms in the trachea or main stem bronchi. The ability to deploy large biopsy forceps through the rigid bronchoscope permits the removal of large masses of neoplastic tissue that obstruct the major airways. If significant bleeding follows the removal of tumor mass, the suction apparatus available for use through the rigid bronchoscope is helpful in keeping the airways

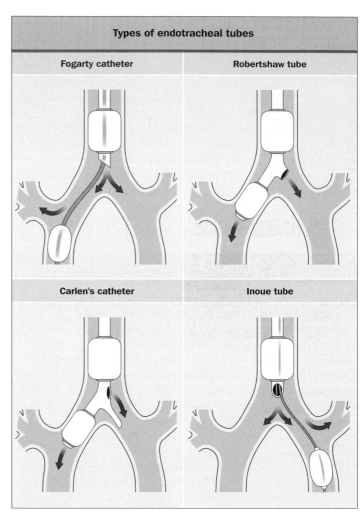

Figure 6.22 Types of endotracheal tubes that can simultaneously control massive hemoptysis and provide adequate ventilation. If a Fogarty catheter is used through an endotracheal tube of size 8 or greater, or if an Inoue tube is used, a standard flexible bronchoscope can be passed easily. Only an ultrathin flexible bronchoscope can pass through a Carlen's tube or a Robertshaw tube.

cleared of blood. The flexible bronchoscope is ill-suited for this purpose because of its small working channel and its inability to remove large pieces of tumor and large volumes of blood. Various types of bronchoscopic therapies employed in the treat-ment of airway stenoses, both benign and malignant, are listed in Figure 6.24.

Laser bronchoscopy

The laser energy causes cell death by intense heat, coagulation, and evaporation of tissue. Assorted types of lasers are available for the treatment of tracheobronchial neoplasms through both the flexible and rigid bronchoscopes. The majority of broncho-scopic laser procedures utilize neodymium yttrium–alu-minum–garnet (Nd:YAG) laser for the treatment of airway neoplasms. As noted above, the rigid bronchoscope is better suited for laser bronchoscopy. Special training in the use of the laser is required. Almost all laser therapies are palliative and are indicated for the relief of the obstruction caused by tumors of trachea and major bronchi. Laser therapy, however, has been used to cure both benign and malignant airway tumors[24]. Laser

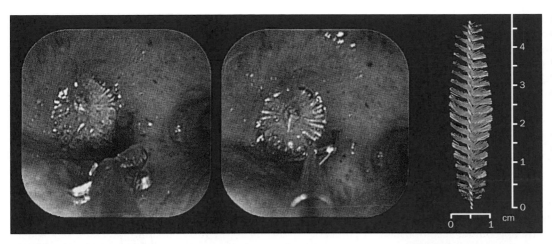

Figure 6.23 Bronchoscopic view of a foreign body lodged in the right bronchus intermedius. The foreign body was a fractured tracheostomy cleaning brush; it was extracted using a flexible bronchoscope and a long-toothed ureteral stone forceps passed through the biopsy channel of the flexible bronchoscope.

Bronchoscopic therapies

Therapy	Type of lesion	Type of bronchoscope	Rapidity of positive result	Repeatability of therapy
Mechanical debridement	Endoluminal or submucosal	Rigid or flexible (rigid preferable)	++++	+++
Laser	Endoluminal	Rigid or flexible (rigid preferable)	++++	++++
Brachytherapy	Endoluminal or submucosal	Flexible	+	+
Cryotherapy	Endoluminal	Rigid or flexible	++	+++
Balloon dilatation	Endoluminal or submucosal with extraluminal compression	Rigid or flexible (rigid preferable)	++++	++++
Photodynamic therapy	Endoluminal	Flexible	++	+++
Electrocautery	Endoluminal	Rigid or flexible	+++	++++
Stent	Endoluminal with extraluminal compression	Rigid or flexible (Dumon stent requires rigid bronchoscope; Wall stents and Gianturco stents require fluoroscopy)	++++	+++

Figure 6.24 Bronchoscopic therapies. ++++, most rapid or repeatable. (Adapted with permission from Ramser ER, Beamis JF Jr. Laser bronchoscopy. Clin Chest Med. 1995;16:415–26.)

therapy provides immediate relief of airway occlusion in over 90% of patients. In a series of 1585 patients who underwent 2253 Nd:YAG laser therapies over an 11-year period, 78% had malignancies that were not small cell lung cancer, 6% had small cell lung cancer, 7% had metastatic tumors, and 5% had unclassifiable tumors; almost all cases were performed under general anesthesia utilizing rigid bronchoscopy. More than 93% showed immediate good results. Complications included 18 hemorrhages, 6 pneumothoraces, and 10 deaths[20]. Peripheral bronchial tumors rarely require laser therapy unless relief of postobstructive pneumonia is necessary in a patient who is not a candidate for surgical resection.

Phototherapy

The use of fluorescent compounds in bronchoscopic phototherapy of tracheobronchial cancers is a therapeutic alternative to surgery in patients deemed unsuitable for surgical treatment. Chemicals such as hematoporphyrin derivative and dihematoporphyrin ether fluoresce when exposed to the light of the proper wavelength and mediate photodynamic chemical reactions that lead to cellular death through the production of toxic radicals, including singlet oxygen and the hydroxyl ion. This method has demonstrated at least a 50% complete response in tumors that measured less than 3cm^2 in largest surface area. Phototherapy has been used as an alternative to

surgery in patients who cannot undergo surgery; complete response lasting longer than 12 months has been noted in up to 50% of patients[25].

Complications from photodynamic therapy are infrequent and include sunburn involving the face and hands, hemoptysis, and expectoration of gray necrotic material. Repeat therapeutic bronchoscopies may be needed to extract the necrotic pseudomembrane.

Brachytherapy

Brachytherapy is defined as the delivery of ionizing radiation therapy from a source of ionizing radiation placed within the tissue being treated or very near it. The bronchoscope has been used to deliver brachytherapy to palliate malignant airway lesions in patients who cannot receive external beam radiation or other types of treatment. Brachytherapy is usually preceded by laser ablation or stent placement[26]. The most commonly used technique for endobronchial brachytherapy employs ^{192}iridium. Other radioactive sources used include ^{137}cesium, ^{60}cobalt, ^{198}gold, and ^{125}iodine. For further information, see Chapter 43.

Airway stenosis

Strictures and stenoses of the tracheobronchial tree often require surgical treatment for the relief of symptoms. The role of rigid bronchoscopy, laser therapy, phototherapy, and brachytherapy

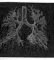

in the treatment of malignant airway disease is discussed above. Laser therapy has been tried in a small number of patients with benign strictures. It is efficient in strictures that are caused by membranous or web-like lesions involving a very short length of the trachea. Thick transmural strictures and long strictures are least likely to respond to laser ablation.

Bronchoscopic dilatation

Bronchoscopic dilatation is an alternative therapy in patients whose airway strictures cannot be treated surgically. Both benign and malignant airway lesions can be treated by bronchoscopic techniques. In benign strictures, the passage of rigid bronchoscopes of gradually increasing diameters may dilate the trachea and main stem bronchi. Balloon dilatation through either the flexible or rigid bronchoscope can be accomplished if the stenosis is limited to a short segment of the airway. Repeated dilatations are often required because of the recurrence of airway stenosis. Bronchoscopic dilatation is more likely to be effective if the stenosis is intrinsic rather than extrinsic. In most patients who require stent placement, preliminary dilatation is necessary.

Airway stents

Placement of airway stents is another therapeutic option in patients who have malignant or benign disease, and who have severe airway narrowing from intrinsic or extrinsic processes. Clinical experience thus far has shown that the stents work best in the trachea and main stem bronchi (Fig. 6.25). They are not suited for lobar and distal bronchial stenoses. In any case, stent placement is seldom indicated for distal airway lesions. Many types of tracheobronchial stents are available and include products of expandable metal wire, molded silicone, or combinations of both[27].

Rigid bronchoscopy is essential for the insertion, manipulation, and removal of most stents. Flexible bronchoscopy and fluoroscopic guidance without bronchoscopy has been used. Special training in the technique of these procedures is necessary. Complications from tracheobronchial stents include migration of the stent, and increased mucous secretions with somewhat decreased clearing by cough, and growth of granulation tissue.

Bronchopleural fistula and pneumothorax

Bronchopleural fistulas and persistent pneumothoraces are challenging problems in the ventilated patient. Definitive therapy of the bronchopleural fistula by the bronchoscopic application of a sealing agent to occlude the fistula site has been tried. The tamponade procedures are time consuming and require deep sedation and general anesthesia. Successful application of the technique requires an accurate determination of the segmental location of the air leak. Balloon tamponade can be accomplished with either the flexible or the rigid bronchoscope. If performed properly, the tamponade will either stop or decrease the air leak through the chest tube. Once the segmental bronchus is identified, further treatment, such as fibrin glue injection or surgery, can be undertaken.

Bronchogenic cysts and mediastinal cysts

Bronchogenic cysts and mediastinal cysts occasionally become filled with liquid, secondary to infection, and compress the tracheobronchial lumen. Bronchoscopic drainage of these cysts has been performed to relieve the airway compression. The bronchoscope has also been used to drain lung abscesses, fluid-filled cysts, and other lesions in the mediastinum and the lung. Such procedures are usually unsuccessful in rapidly emptying the contents of the abscess cavity or the cyst. Patients who undergo bronchoscopic attempts to empty the contents of an abscess cavity may slowly expectorate the contents over a period of hours or days.

Endotracheal tube placement

Patients with endotracheal tubes often require bronchoscopy to facilitate proper placement of the tube. The flexible bronchoscope is helpful in intubating patients with cervical spine trauma or massive facial injuries, and for replacing or changing of such tubes. The flexible bronchoscope has been used to assess the pathogenic factors leading to laryngotracheal injury caused by tracheal intubation in critically ill patients, and in replacing endotracheal tubes in patients on mechanical ventilation who require change of tube.

Therapeutic lavage

Alveolar proteinosis is a condition in which a diffuse intra-alveolar deposition of lipoproteinaceous material leads to progressive respiratory distress. The treatment for this rare disorder has been the insertion of the double-lumen endotracheal tube followed by instillation of several liters of normal saline to wash out the intra-alveolar material. This requires general anesthesia and special equipment and personnel. Several reports have described the use of flexible bronchoscope to carry out therapeutic washing of individual segments. Such procedures are time consuming and may also require deep sedation or general anesthesia.

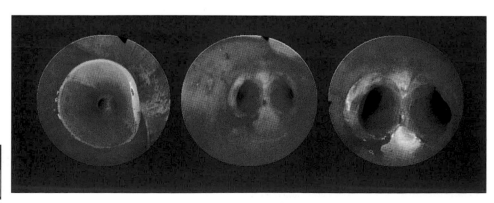

Figure 6.25 Rigid bronchoscopic placement of a silicone Y stent over the main carina. This was done to provide ventilation of both main stem bronchi in a patient with squamous cell carcinoma involving the main carina and proximal main stem bronchi.

MISCELLANEOUS

Bronchoscopic ultrasound is a relatively new technique that is being investigated in the diagnosis and staging of lung cancer as well as certain extrabronchial abnormalities. The major advantage of endobronchial ultrasonography is the ability to discern bronchomediastinal anatomy, including vascular structures and lymph nodes[28].

Virtual bronchoscopy refers to the three-dimensional visualization of tracheobronchial tree derived from special CT techniques. The advantage of virtual bronchoscopy is the ability to visualize the endobronchial anatomy without performing bronchoscopy. This technique may help in identifying lymph nodes and other structures located extraluminally. Irrespective of the information gathered from this technique, standard bronchoscopy is required to obtain tissue samples. For now, virtual bronchoscopy remains an investigational tool.

Light-induced fluorescence endoscopy is a technique that detects early mucosal cancer by differentiating autofluorescence in normal and abnormal mucosa. Early reports show that that this technique, when used as an adjunct to standard bronchoscopy, may enhance the ability to localize small neoplastic lesions, especially intraepithelial lesions[29].

REFERENCES

1. Ikeda S. Flexible bronchofiberscope. Ann Otol Rhinol Laryngol. 1970;79:916–23.

2. Prakash UBS, Offord KP, Stubbs SE. Bronchoscopy in North America: the ACCP survey. Chest. 1991;100:1668–75.

3. Hetzel MR, Smith SGT. Endoscopic palliation of tracheobronchial malignancies. Thorax. 1991;46:325–33.

4. Limper AH, Prakash UBS. Tracheobronchial foreign bodies in adults. Ann Intern Med. 1990;112:604–9.

5. Suratt PM, Smiddy JF, Gruber B. Deaths and complications associated with fiberoptic bronchoscopy. Chest. 1976;69:747–51.

6. Pereira W Jr, Kovnat DM, Snider GL. A prospective cooperative study of complications following flexible fiberoptic bronchoscopy. Chest. 1978;73:813–16.

7. Prakash UBS. Bronchoscopy in the critically ill patient. Semin Respir Med. 1997;18:583–91.

8. Ahmad M, Livingston DR, Golish JA, et al. The safety of outpatient transbronchial biopsy. Chest 1986;90:403–5.

9. Frazier WD, Pope TL Jr, Findley LJ. Pneumothorax following transbronchial lung biopsy: low diagnostic yield with routine chest roentgenograms. Chest. 1990;97:539–40.

10. Simpson FG, Arnold AG, Purvis A, et al. Postal survey of bronchoscopic practice by physicians in the United Kingdom. Thorax. 1986;41:311–17.

11. Roethe RA, Fuller PB, Byrd RB, et al. Transbronchoscopic lung biopsy in sarcoidosis: optimal number and sites for diagnosis. Chest. 1980;77:400–2.

12. Poe RH, Harder RV, Israel RH, et al. Chronic persistent cough: experience in diagnosis and outcome using an anatomic diagnostic protocol. Chest. 1989;95:723–8.

13. Gerbeaux P, Ledoray V, Boussuges A, et al. Diagnosis of nosocomial pneumonia in mechanically ventilated patients: repeatability of the bronchoalveolar lavage. Am J Resp Crit Care Med. 1998;157:76–80.

14. Souweine B, Benoit V, Bedos JP, et al. Diagnostic accuracy of protected specimen brush and bronchoalveolar lavage in nosocomial pneumonia: impact of previous antimicrobial treatments. Crit Care Med. 1998;26:236–24.

15. Russell MD, Torrington KG, Tenholder MF. A ten year experience with fiberoptic bronchoscopy for mycobacterial isolation: impact on the Bactec system. Am Rev Respir Dis. 1986;133:1069–71.

16. Willcox PA, Potgieter PD, Bateman ED, et al. Rapid diagnosis of sputum negative miliary tuberculosis using the flexible fibreoptic bronchoscope. Thorax. 1986;41:681–4.

17. Kahn FW, Jones JM, England DM. The role of bronchoalveolar lavage in the diagnosis of invasive pulmonary aspergillosis. Am J Clin Pathol. 1986; 86:518–23.

18. Prechter GC, Prakash UBS. Bronchoscopy in the diagnosis of pulmonary histoplasmosis. Chest. 1989;95:1033–6.

19. De Gracia J, Miravitlles M, Mayordomo C, et al. Empiric treatments impair the diagnostic yield of BAL in HIV-positive patients. Chest. 1997;111:1180–6.

20. Cavaliere S, Foccoli P, Toninelli C, Feijo S. Nd:YAG laser therapy in lung cancer: an 11-year experience with 2,253 applications in 1,585 patients. J Bronchol. 1994;1:105–11.

21. Pauli G, Pelletier A, Bohner C, et al. Transbronchial needle aspiration in the diagnosis of sarcoidosis. Chest. 1984;85:482–4.

22. Olopade CO, Prakash UBS. Bronchoscopy in the critical care unit. Mayo Clin Proc. 1989;64:1255–63.

23. Marini JJ, Pierson DJ, Hudson LD. Acute lobar atelectasis: a prospective comparison of fiberoptic bronchoscopy and respiratory therapy. Am Rev Respir Dis. 1979;119:971–8.

24. Shah H, Garbe L, Nussbaum E, et al. Benign tumors of the tracheobronchial tree. Endoscopic characteristics and role of laser resection. Chest. 1995;107:1744–51.

25. Cortese DA, Edell ES, Kinsey JH. Photodynamic therapy for early stage squamous cell carcinoma of the lung. Mayo Clinic Proc. 1997;72:595–602.

26. Cavaliere S, Venuta F, Foccoli P, Toninelli C, La Face B. Endoscopic treatment of malignant airway obstructions in 2,008 patients. Chest. 1996;110:1536–42.

27. Bolliger CT, Heitz M, Hauser R, Probst R, Perruchoud AP. An airway Wallstent for the treatment of tracheobronchial malignancies. Thorax. 1996;51:1127–9.

28. Shannon JJ, Bude RO, Orens JB, et al. Endobronchial ultrasound guided needle aspiration of mediastinal adenopathy. Am J Respir Crit Care Med. 1996;153:1424–30.

29. Lam S, Kennedy T, Unger M, et al. Localization of bronchial intraepithelial neoplastic lesions by fluorescence bronchoscopy. Chest. 1998;113:696–702.

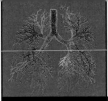

Section 2 Techniques and Indications

Chapter 7

Closed Pleural Biopsy

Stephen Spiro

INTRODUCTION

Pleural effusions are most commonly caused by malignancy and infection, and may need to be investigated by closed pleural biopsy if an initial aspirated sample is negative for malignant cytology or an obvious infection. Most malignant causes are diagnosed on the cytologic examination of a 20mL aliquot of the effusion, which can be aspirated by inserting a needle through the chest wall under local anesthesia. In cases of tuberculosis, the fluid rarely yields acid-fast bacilli when direct smears are examined, but is predominantly lymphocytic and usually has a reduced glucose content. Pyogenic infection or parapneumonia effusions may be milky in color and appear purulent, show a lesser shade of turbidity, or may even be clear but contain neutrophils. Empyemas tend to appear creamy and sometimes have a fecal smell. The rare chylous effusion is paler and more milky in appearance.

INDICATIONS AND CONTRA-INDICATIONS

If the initial pleural aspiration is not diagnostic, it should be repeated, and a closed pleural biopsy performed at the same time. The biopsy is especially useful in cases of suspected tuberculosis, as the pleural histology may yield granulomata in up to 50% of cases. Pleural biopsy adds 2–10% to the yield of cytology for malignancy, particularly in cases of mesothelioma.

TECHNIQUE

A variety of needles are available. The Cope's needle was introduced in 1958, but Abrams' needle remains the most popular. The Raja needle is a modification of Abrams' needle and was introduced in 1993. Tru-Cut biopsy needles are used under ultrasound control by radiologists to produce a core of tissue for histology from obviously thickened pleural tissues. Finally, biopsies can be taken from the parietal pleura using forceps during the course of a thoracoscopy.

Positioning the patient

The patient should sit upright, leaning forward with arms folded across the bed onto a pillow which rests on the bed-table. Position the patient's head on the pillow for several minutes, to allow comfortable breathing. The patient's folded arms will lift the scapula upward and outward and prevent them impeding the procedure.

Anesthesia

After cleaning the skin, introduce 1% plain lidocaine (lignocaine) in the posterior axillary line with as small a needle as possible. Once the skin is anesthetized, a longer, No. 1 needle is advanced.

Push out lidocaine continuously and aim to advance beneath the rib until the pleura is penetrated and fluid can be drawn back into the attached syringe (Fig. 7.1). At this stage, use a second syringe that contains 1% lidocaine to widen the area of anesthesia, keeping the skin entry site as the apex of an imagined pyramid of anesthesia. Always withdraw the needle back to just under the skin before advancing it to a new angle. Best practice is to use a new syringe of lidocaine once the pleural cavity has been entered, as malignant pleural effusions can seed along the needle track from the pleura. A total of 10mL of 1% lidocaine should be sufficient to anesthetize the chest wall of most subjects.

Incision

Next, make a stab incision with a No. 11 scalpel blade along the intended biopsy track. This can easily be widened and extended down to the pleural surface by blunt dissection with a pair of straight Spencer–Wells forceps (Fig. 7.2).

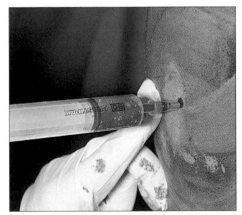

Figure 7.1 Infiltration of chest wall with local anesthetic. The needle penetrates the pleura and fluid is aspirated back into the syringe.

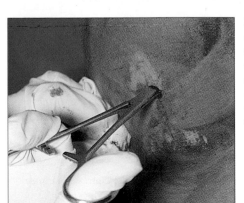

Figure 7.2 A blunt dissection down to and into the pleural cavity. The forceps are opened gently and pushed forward to tease apart the muscle fibers.

Use of Abrams' needle

Abrams' needle contains an inner stylus, which is removed and not used. The inner of the two remaining cylinders has a cutting edge which, when pulled back, opens a triangular aperture on the outer sheath of the needle and allows fluid to enter the inner cannula (Fig. 7.3). To open or close the window in the outer sheath, the ferrule is rotated clockwise or anticlockwise, respectively (Fig. 7.4). The ferrule lies in line with the closed aperture when turned clockwise as far as it can go. The hub of the needle is attached to a three-way tap with a hose to drain fluid for collection, and to a large syringe with a Luer lock fitting.

The knob on the ferrule of the inner sheath must be in line with the needle aperture. With the aperture closed, gently push the needle by a rotating action through the chest wall into the pleural cavity (Fig. 7.5). Blunt dissection (see above) enables the needle to pass easily and prevents it from bursting into the pleural cavity, thus avoiding the risk of trauma. The needle point is blunt, which also limits potential damage, for example a pneumothorax.

Once in the pleural cavity, open the needle and withdraw fluid (Fig. 7.6). Collect samples of 20mL and eject them into specimen containers using a three-way tap. After collecting the pleural fluid samples, attach the needle directly to a 20mL syringe

and then tilt it so that the aperture is felt snagging the pleural surface. By exerting lateral pressure as the needle is slowly pulled back, the pleura is pushed into the aperture (Fig 7.7). While tension is maintained, twist the ferrule closed (Fig. 7.8) and pull the needle out of the chest cavity sharply. Then open the needle over either saline or formal saline (saline plus formaldehyde) and squirt the biopsy into a container or tease it off using a needle. Perform several biopsies around a 24-hour clock, apart from between 10 p.m. and 2 a.m. to avoid damaging an intercostal nerve or vessel lying in the bed of the rib above. One biopsy should be placed into saline for culture for *Mycobacterium tuberculosis* and the others into formal saline.

Abrams' system is relatively easy to use and is recommended as the most effective method of obtaining pleural fluid drawn via the needle and three-way tap, as well as for biopsy specimens.

The Raja needle

The Raja needle is a modification of Abrams' system; it has a biopsy flap that opens once the pleural cavity is entered and the inner sheath is pulled back. The flap fixes onto the parietal pleural surface and, when closed, cuts off a piece of pleura (Fig. 7.9). Comparisons with the more readily available Abrams' needle have suggested a higher diagnostic yield.

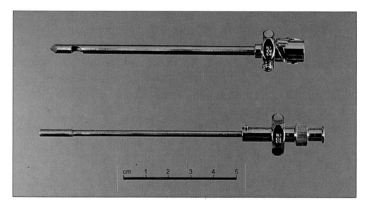

Figure 7.3 The inner and outer sheaths of Abrams' needle showing the aperture in the outer sheath. The tip of the inner sheath cuts the biopsy.

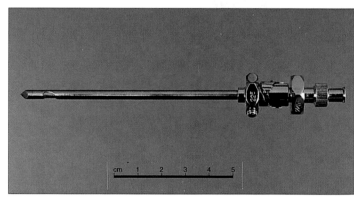

Figure 7.4 Needle assembled showing the ferrule that is rotated to cut the specimen.

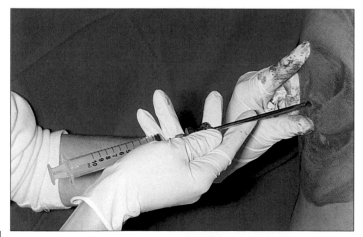

Figure 7.5 Gentle insertion of the closed needle into the pleural cavity. The needle, with aperture closed, should enter the pleural space with only gentle, rotating pressure by the hand of the operator.

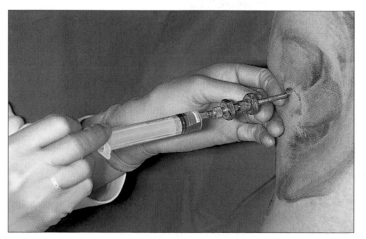

Figure 7.6 Fluid is withdrawn into the syringe with the needle aperture open. A three-way tap system can be added if fluid is to be collected for laboratory testing.

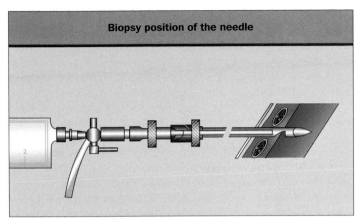

Figure 7.7 Biopsy position of the needle.

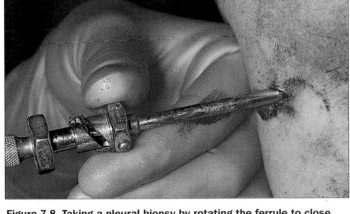

Figure 7.8 Taking a pleural biopsy by rotating the ferrule to close the aperture. Pull the whole apparatus sharply out of the chest.

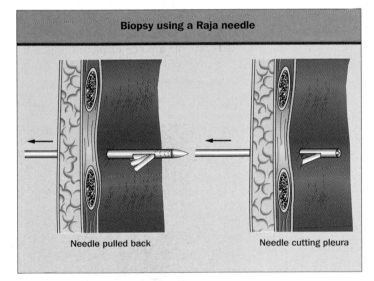

Needle pulled back   Needle cutting pleura

Figure 7.9 Method of biopsy using a Raja needle. The flap impinges on the pleura as the needle is pulled back and cuts off a piece of pleura on closure.

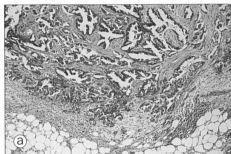

Figure 7.10 Pleural biopsy.
(a) Adenocarcinoma and (b) AUA1 immuno staining positive for adenocarcinoma.

SPECIMEN HANDLING

Always take important biopsy specimens directly to the laboratories. To prevent contamination of the fluid by additional bleeding, remove it for investigation before taking a biopsy. Send the fluid for routine bacterial culture, direct smear and culture for tuberculosis, cytology, protein and glucose estimation (together with a serum glucose sample). Pleural fluid amylase and rheumatoid factor should be requested if they are judged necessary.

Between four and six biopsies are usually taken, and sent for histology in formal saline and culture in normal saline.

Pleural biopsy is very successful in the identification of tuberculosis, but less so for malignancy (Fig. 7.10). Needle biopsies increase the yield for finding tuberculosis, especially if the biopsy is also sent for culture. In malignancy, needle biopsy has a 50% sensitivity compared with pleural fluid cytology, but adds a little to the overall yield. Needle biopsy is, however, very useful for mesothelioma.

CHOICE OF TECHNIQUE

Few studies have compared the different methods for closed pleural biopsy. Abrams' needle remains the most popular, and if an average of five biopsies are taken, the yield (usually tumor or tuberculosis) is 60%[1]. A comparison of the Raja and Abrams needles in 31 patients gave a diagnosis in 82 and 52% of biopsies, respectively[2]. Comparing the Abrams' needle with the Tru-Cut biopsy needle gives similar results[3], and using a fiberoptic thoracoscope for biopsies in general is superior to using Abrams' needle. Rigid thoracoscopy may be even better.

COMPLICATIONS

Very few complications of closed needle biopsy have been reported. Pneumothorax is uncommon as the needle point is blunt and only a small amount of fluid need be present for a biopsy to be taken. Provided the two pleural surfaces part easily, a biopsy can be performed, even in a 'dry' pleural cavity.

Hemorrhage can occur if the intercostal artery or vein is damaged by taking a biopsy at 12 o'clock and pushing up against the inferior surface of a rib. A hematoma of the chest wall can develop rapidly, but usually requires no specific action.

Longer-term complications include seeding of malignant cells along the needle track, which is relatively common in malignant effusions. Should this occur, a single fraction of radiotherapy controls the developing nodule in most cases.

PITFALLS

The aim in pleural disease is to make a diagnosis without emptying the effusion. It is becoming common to insert intercostal tubes into large effusions and then drain them completely. In these cases, pleural fluid samples may have been sent to the laboratory without any biopsy having been taken. Although further fluid can easily be obtained from the chest tube if the fluid examinations are negative, a new incision will have to be made for a closed pleural biopsy. Furthermore, once an intercostal drain is inserted, the patient may need to remain in hospital awaiting results in discomfort for some days and may then need further interventions across the chest wall.

A preferred course is to aspirate 1L of fluid from a large effusion, and send samples to the laboratories. The patient may then be able to go home and await results. If all results are negative, the procedure should be repeated and a closed pleural biopsy performed. If results are still negative and there is no systemic or other obvious cause for the effusion, a thoracoscopy should be performed with biopsies taken from the parietal pleura under direct vision. Even this may not provide a diagnosis but, in experienced hands, thoracoscopy adds about 10% to the overall yield of closed biopsy and cytology diagnoses.

REFERENCES

1. Mungall IPF, Cowen PN, Cooke NT, Roach TC, Cooke NJ. Multiple pleural biopsy with the Abrams needle. Thorax. 1980;35:600–2.
2. Ogirala RG, Agarwal V, Vizioli LD, Pinsker KL, Aldrich TK. Comparison of the Raja and the Abrams pleural biopsy needles in patients with pleural effusions. Am Rev Respir Dis. 1993;47:1291–4.
3. McLeod DT, Ternouth I, Nkanza N. Comparison of the Tru-cut biopsy needle with the Abrams punch for pleural biopsy. Thorax. 1989;44:794–6.

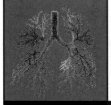

Chapter 8

Other Biopsy Procedures

Penny Shaw

BIOPSY OF INTRAPULMONARY LESIONS

Introduction

In this section the equipment and techniques available to obtain diagnostic tissue from predominantly solid lesions within the lung parenchyma are described. The common lesions and the biopsy equipment used are summarized in Figures 8.1 & 8.2, respectively. It is usual to obtain adequate tissue samples from these types of lesions by needle, and the technique and its indications are quite separate from those required to diagnose more diffuse intrapulmonary disease. The latter, which includes conditions such as idiopathic pulmonary fibrosis, requires an open lung biopsy via a mini-thoracotomy or video-assisted thoracoscopy.

Imaging plays an important role in the confirmation and identification of the site of the lesion, its size, and the quality of surrounding lung tissue. It is also used to assess the extent of the pathology and the presence of other diseases. The radiologist determines whether the lesion is suitable for transthoracic biopsy, and identifies the optimum site for biopsy and under which imaging modality the biopsy should be performed. The choice of needle depends on the patient's safety, whether histology or cytology is required, and the preference of the radiologist.

Indications and contraindications

Transthoracic needle biopsy is an established and accepted technique for the diagnosis of malignant masses or nodules, with a sensitivity of 90–95%[1]. Until recently the technique was limited by the low specificity for benign diseases[2], but this is improving with needle placement under computed tomography (CT) guidance, and by the use of coaxial, transthoracic needle biopsy with an automated cutting needle[3]. The main indication is in cancer to establish the cell type in inoperable, advanced disease with both negative sputum cytology and bronchoscopy. It is also widely used when solitary or multiple masses are present with a known extrathoracic primary malignancy to confirm metastatic disease. During staging of a thoracic malignancy, a contralateral pulmonary nodule, mediastinal, hepatic, or adrenal mass may be identified. To assess operability, it is then of paramount importance to biopsy such lesions. It is also an established technique for confirming a Pancoast tumor. However, the place of biopsy of a solitary mass or nodule is more controversial. If there is a high clinical and radiologic index of suspicion that the lesion is malignant, and the patient is otherwise operable, then the patient may go straight to surgery. However, if a solitary mass is thought clinically and radiologically to be benign a biopsy (preferably a core biopsy) is the next useful step. Fine needle aspiration or biopsy for microorganisms is increasingly used in areas of consolidation or masses, especially in immunocompromised patients[4]. More recently, hilar

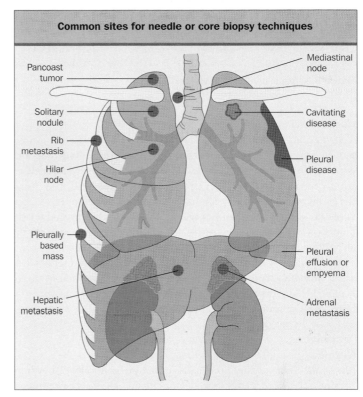

Figure 8.1 Common sites for needle or core biopsy techniques.

Common sites for needle or core biopsy techniques

- Pancoast tumor
- Solitary nodule
- Rib metastasis
- Hilar node
- Pleurally based mass
- Hepatic metastasis
- Mediastinal node
- Cavitating disease
- Pleural disease
- Pleural effusion or empyema
- Adrenal metastasis

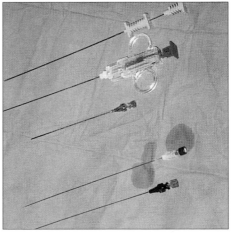

Figure 8.2 Commonly used needles for percutaneous biopsy. Fine aspirating needles provide cytology (bottom), and cutting needles provide cores for histology (top three).

and mediastinal lesions have been biopsied percutaneously, which may be particularly valuable either as an alternative to transbronchial biopsy or mediastinoscopy, or when the lesion is inaccessible to the latter approach[5].

Contraindications to needle biopsy	
Type of contraindication	Comment
Relative	Uncooperative patient: uncontrollable cough inability to lie prone or supine
	Poor lung function/chronic obstructive pulmonary disease (forced expiratory volume in 1 second <1L or multiple bullae)
	Pneumonectomy
	Bleeding disorder
	Pulmonary hypertension
	Very small nodules, less than 5mm diameter
	Hydatid disease (because the risk of anaphylactic reaction)
Absolute	Arteriovenous malformation with high pulmonary artery pressure

Figure 8.3 Contraindications to needle biopsy.

Contraindications

The contraindications are largely relative and summarized in Figure 8.3. Biopsy of a lesion in patients who have very poor lung function is possible, provided the lesion is peripheral and a 'safe' route is identified (usually with CT), that does not traverse the lung parenchyma. The biopsy should avoid a pneumothorax, which could be life threatening. A coagulation screen is performed if risk factors are present, for example hepatic metastases, a history of alcohol ingestion, or if the patient is on warfarin or aspirin. A prothrombin time <15–16s and an international normalized ratio <1.4 are acceptable. Some hydatid lesions have been biopsied but there is still an increased and probably unacceptable risk of an anaphylactic reaction in this group of patients.

Technique
Needles

Many different needles are available, but are generally either fine needles for aspiration for cytology or cutting needles to produce a core for histology (see Fig. 8.2). Fine needles that can be used for aspiration include the Westcott needle, Chiba, Franseen, or those that have a corkscrew appearance such as the Rotex needle. They are usually 20–23-gauge and provide a specimen for cytology or culture. Fine needles have the advantage of fewer complications, but are more flexible and can be difficult to position within a central lesion. The Westcott needle has the advantage that small fragments of tissue are frequently obtained in addition to the aspirate, in the small 'notch' or slotted opening just proximal to the needle tip. This provides small cores in approximately 50% of biopsies.

Aspirates should only be obtained if there is local cytopathologic expertise available. Ideally, the cytologist attends the biopsy to ensure that an adequate specimen is obtained. Larger cutting needles (18- or 20-gauge) provide a core for histology, and have greater rigidity, which allows greater control in placement, but have a higher incidence of complications, particularly hemorrhage[7]. Commonly used cutting needles have a spring-loaded mechanism that fires the inner notched stylet and outer cutting cannula by pushing a button; for example the Bard Biopty Biopsy System (Fig. 8.4) or Bauer Temno biopsy device (Fig. 8.5). The 'gun' or handle of the Bard System is reusable and the needle is disposable. Various sizes are available (14-gauge, 18-gauge, or 20-gauge) and a core of tissue is consistently produced. The 'throw' of the gun is usually 11mm or 23mm and so lesions ideally need to be at least this size. The 23mm 'throw' produces better cores.

The pneumothorax rate is related to the number of pleural passes made, which can be reduced by using a coaxial system that has an introducer needle (18- or 19-gauge thin-walled) through which a fine needle can be passed (Fig. 8.6) or by a fine needle core biopsy (a more recent development)[2]. Fluid introduced into the pleural space can also be used to provide a safer route in some patients. The choice of needle must be made primarily on the basis of safety of the patient, but also according to the approach and choice of the radiologist.

Image guidance

Fluoroscopy is the preferred method of imaging for percutaneous biopsy, as it is quick, cheap, and easily available, but the lesion has to be visible on both frontal and lateral screening (Fig. 8.7). Small lesions may be difficult to visualize, especially on lateral screening, and CT prior to fluoroscopy may provide useful information

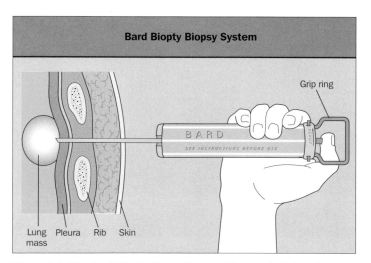

Bard Biopty Biopsy System

Grip ring

BARD
SEE INSTRUCTIONS BEFORE USE

Lung mass — Pleura — Rib — Skin

Figure 8.4 The Bard Biopty Biopsy System. The needle is introduced into the patient so that the tip reaches the area to be biopsied.

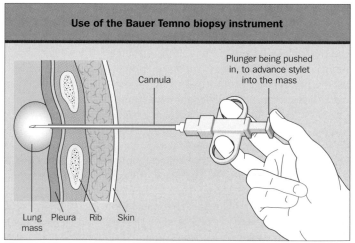

Use of the Bauer Temno biopsy instrument

Plunger being pushed in, to advance stylet into the mass

Cannula

Lung mass — Pleura — Rib — Skin

Figure 8.5 Use of the Bauer Temno biopsy instrument. The stylet is positioned within the lesion to be biopsied, by pushing the plunger. The advantages are that the instrument requires one hand only, is light, easy to use under computed tomography, and produces a 2cm diameter core.

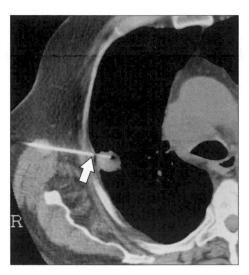

Figure 8.6 Coaxial systems. The arrow marks the distal end of the 18-gauge introducer needle, through which a 20-gauge needle has been passed into the nodule.

oximeter are necessary if sedation is used. The procedure is undertaken in full sterile conditions. Lidocaine (lignocaine) 1% (10mL) (or 5ml of lidocaine 2%) should be administered, taking care that the lung parenchyma and visceral pleura are not punctured, but that the pleura is anesthetized. The patient must be warned that it is not always possible to anesthetize the pleura fully because of the risk of a pneumothorax from the anesthetic needle.

A slight 'give' occurs when the biopsy needle enters the pleural space. The needle is advanced in either suspended respiration or in small, rapid movements during the same phase of gentle respiration to reduce trauma to the parenchyma. Accurate placement of the needle tip is essential and may take time with small nodules. If the lesion is cavitating or has central necrosis, then the specimen must be taken from the periphery. The number of passes varies, but on average is between one and three (less if the patient is at high risk). The aim is to obtain a diagnosis, but the safety of the patient is obviously paramount. Once in position, the central stylet is removed and a finger placed over the hub to prevent air embolism. A syringe is attached and gentle to-and-fro movements are made to obtain an aspirate, aiming the needle in slightly different directions. Pressure is released before withdrawing the needle, or the specimen will be pulled back into the syringe. Saline (2–5mL) can be injected into and aspirated from a localized infiltrate to attempt to identify micro-organisms. The specimen is dealt with immediately.

If the patient is dyspneic at the end of the procedure, a chest radiograph is performed immediately, otherwise at 1 hour. A further chest radiograph is taken approximately 4 hours after the procedure. If the radiograph is satisfactory or if the patient is well but there is a small or static pneumothorax (<30%) at 4 hours, the patient can go home with instructions to return if he/she becomes symptomatic, as a delayed or expanding pneumothorax is a rare complication. If the patient is symptomatic or has a progressive pneumothorax, observation in the hospital is necessary, and the decision to aspirate or drain the pneumothorax taken. If the mass is large and pleurally based, and the patient remains well, no chest radiograph is required. Hemoptysis is a worrying complication but rarely requires treatment.

that helps to localize the lesion relative to fixed structures (e.g. the vertebrae). The pneumothorax rate is lower, which is thought to be related to the speed of the procedure. Ultrasound guidance is useful if the lesion is peripheral, pleurally based, and easily identified, and it has the added advantage that no radiation is involved.

Increasingly, CT is being used for nodules not seen at fluoroscopy, and for lesions adjacent to or in the mediastinum, which allows more precise positioning of the needle within the lesion and avoids vascular structures. The disadvantages are that the procedure takes longer, which can lead to a higher rate of complications. This occurs when a small lesion is biopsied, especially if the lesion is central or in the lower lobes, when slight differences in inspiration alter the position of the nodule.

Procedure
The patient should be fasted and informed consent taken by the person who is going to perform the biopsy. The patient must be informed that following the procedure they may have a pneumothorax or hemoptysis, and (rarely) may need to stay in hospital overnight. The radiologist should explain that more than one pass is usually needed. If the biopsy is performed under fluoroscopy, the skin is marked with a metallic disc that overlies the lesion and an approach above a rib is chosen to avoid the intercostal vessels. A posterior approach is preferable because movement of posterior ribs with respiration is smaller. If the patient is anxious, or at slightly higher risk, intravenous access should be obtained prior to the procedure. An electrocardiogram and pulse

Specimen handling
The aspirated material is smeared on slides, with some fixed in alcohol and the rest air dried. A saline wash of the needle is also taken. Larger cores of tissue are placed in formalin unless fresh tissue is required (if lymphoma or infections are suspected). Advances in cytology such as flow cytometry for lymphoma, estrogen receptors for metastatic breast carcinoma, and

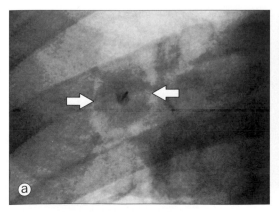
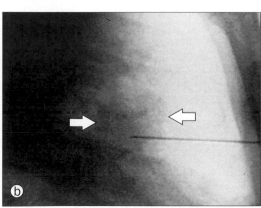

Figure 8.7 Aspiration biopsy under fluoroscopy in an asymptomatic patient. (a) The needle tip is centered over the small lesion on anteroposterior screening (arrows). (b) Lateral screening confirms the needle tip lying within the lesion (arrows). Small cell carcinoma was diagnosed.

immunocytochemistry for prostate malignancies are useful[8]. The specimen is valuable, and it is essential that it reaches the laboratory directly. A cytologist present ensures appropriate handling of this valuable specimen.

Complications

The risk to the patient should always be weighed against the benefits from the procedure (Fig. 8.8). Deaths after aspiration are rare (1/5000–10,000 biopsies) and result from cardiac arrest, air embolism, tension pneumothorax, or hemorrhage. The pneumothorax rate with fine needle aspirates and cutting needle biopsies is similar. Patients may experience sharp chest pain as an indication that it has occurred. Most pneumothoraces are small, but about one in six need treatment. Lying the patient with the puncture site dependent can reduce the rate of pneumothorax development. Drainage through a one-way valve (Heimlich valve) is useful in the emergency situation, and also on recovery, as it allows the patient to remain ambulatory. Aspiration with an 18-gauge catheter attached to a three-way tap also reduces the need for chest tube placement in 70% of patients[9]. Tension pneumothorax occurs within minutes and is a medical emergency. They are rare, but occur in patients who have emphysema.

Hemorrhage is more common with pulmonary hypertension or when cutting needles are used. Any hemoptysis is often preceded by a cough, and usually resolves rapidly. If massive it is potentially life threatening. An air embolism is rare, but should be considered if the patient breathes deeply and collapses. Coughing at the time of needle insertion suggests this possibility. Needles should always be removed during uncontrollable coughing, to reduce this complication and hemorrhage. Treatment includes administration of 100% oxygen, placing the patient head down in a left lateral decubitus position, and transfer to a hyperbaric unit if one is available.

Pitfalls and controversies

The yield in malignant disease is high (sensitivity 90–95%), with fine needle aspirates or cutting needles and even if the nodules are small[6]. If no specific diagnosis is made, the biopsy should be repeated. This enables a further 5–10% of patients who have

undiagnosed but potentially curable malignancy to be identified[10]. The technique of fine needle aspiration was limited by a low yield for specific benign diseases (sensitivity 20–50%), which has been improved (over 70%) by obtaining core biopsies for histology using coaxial systems and cutting needles. The complication rate is higher, but unnecessary surgery is avoided.

Diagnostic difficulties occur in lesions that have a high level of fibrosis, for example metastatic breast carcinoma and Hodgkin's disease. Excessive mucus production, as in bronchoalveolar carcinoma, can also interfere with the diagnosis.

Small needle core biopsies hold promise in benign disease, as they have an improved yield. Certain benign conditions, for example bronchiolitis obliterans organizing pneumonia, Wegener's granulomatosis, and some infections, require cores.

Biopsy of a solitary mass with suspected malignancy in a patient who is potentially operable remains controversial. The argument against is that the patient still requires surgery and therefore management has not been altered. The advantages are that the patient is better informed, the operation is better planned and faster as frozen sections are avoided, and small cell carcinomas are not operated on.

MEDIASTINAL BIOPSIES

Aspiration and cutting needles have been used, but core biopsies are usually necessary for primary mediastinal tumors, in lymphomas, thymomas, and benign diseases. A safe route, with alternative approaches to avoid the transparenchymal route, must be found (Fig. 8.9). This may involve a transpleural approach, through an existing effusion or pneumothorax, or the patient can be positioned in the lateral decubitus position, which causes a slight shift of the mediastinum and can help to avoid the transpulmonary route[11]. An approach through an effusion can be created by injecting saline into the pleural space. This alternative approach reduces the incidence of complications. Biopsy is preferably carried out under CT when vascular structures are more easily identified and avoided.

More recently, fine needle aspiration of only moderately enlarged lymph nodes has been performed and found to be a safe and useful diagnostic procedure with 85–95% sensitivity for malignant disease[4]. An enlarged lymph node is taken to have a short axis >10mm or a long axis >15–20mm. Fine needle aspiration may prove to be an alternative to mediastinoscopy, especially for staging lung cancers. Diagnostic difficulties occur in patients who have

Complications of needle biopsy	
Type	**Complication**
Early complications	Pneumothorax, 5–50%
	Hemoptysis, 5–10%
	Hemorrhage, 10–40%
	Air embolism, rare
Late complications	Tumor seedling, extremely rare
	Empyema
	Bronchopleural fistula
Increased risk of pneumothorax	If the patient has: chronic obstructive pulmonary disease/bullae uncontrollable coughing during the procedure a difficult small central lesion Or if: multiple pleural passes are made fissure is crossed procedure is prolonged

Figure 8.8 Complications of needle biopsy.

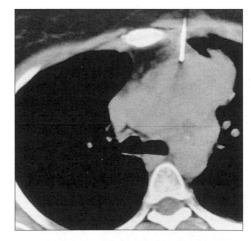

**Figure 8.9
Mediastinal biopsy.**
The needle passes through a small area of contact of the mass with the chest wall to avoid the lung parenchyma.

bronchogenic carcinoma, obstructive pneumonia, or distal atelectasis, who commonly have associated reactive lymphadenopathy.

Mediastinal collections

Aspiration or catheter drainage of mediastinal abscesses secondary to esophageal perforation may be a useful alternative to surgery. It is valuable with advanced collections in patients unfit for surgery, and may be life saving.

PLEURAL AND CHEST WALL BIOPSIES

Pleural and chest wall biopsies are performed under ultrasound (Fig. 8.10) or CT guidance (Fig. 8.11). These peripheral lesions enable core biopsies that are essential to differentiate mesothelioma from metastatic adenocarcinoma to be taken easily and safely. Usually, at least three cores are desirable. If the pleura is not very thickened, multiple passes may be necessary. The optimum route is a course that runs along the main axis of the pathology, which allows more of the lesion to be sampled, but with less risk of a pneumothorax (Fig. 8.12). Radiologists favor

the 18-gauge Bard Biopty biopsy system or Temno cutting needles over the Abrams' needle. Specimens should be sent for microbiology, including acid-fast bacilli, as well as for histology. Fresh specimens may be useful if a lymphoma is suspected.

EXTRATHORACIC BIOPSY

Lesions may be identified in the liver, adrenal glands, or ribs while staging patients who have bronchogenic carcinoma. If appearances suggest metastases, it is essential to biopsy them to confirm this in an otherwise operable patient. Biopsies of hepatic lesions are preferably performed under ultrasound, where they are easily imaged and biopsy is rapid (Fig. 8.13). Adrenal lesions are usually biopsied under CT. It may be necessary even then to traverse the hepatic or pulmonary parenchyma to enter the adrenal mass. If the mass is on the opposite side to the primary carcinoma, the pulmonary parenchymal route should be avoided as a pneumothorax could delay surgery. A coaxial system is useful, as several aspirates or cores can be obtained with a single pass of the introducer needle.

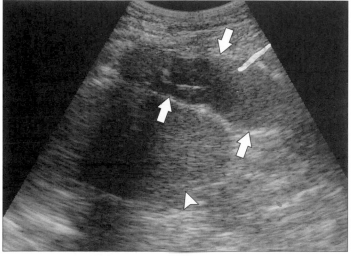

Figure 8.10 Core biopsy of grossly thickened pleura under ultrasound. Squamous carcinoma metastasizing from a previous primary laryngeal tumor was identified. (The arrowhead indicates the spleen, and the arrows the thickened pleura.)

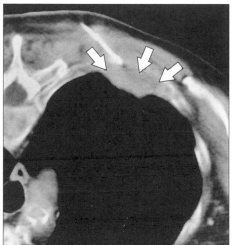

Figure 8.11 Biopsy of a rib metastasis. Nonsmall-cell carcinoma was confirmed (arrows) on this 'safe' biopsy under computed tomography control.

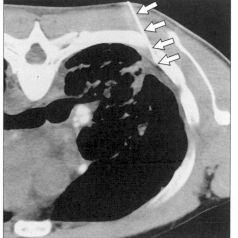

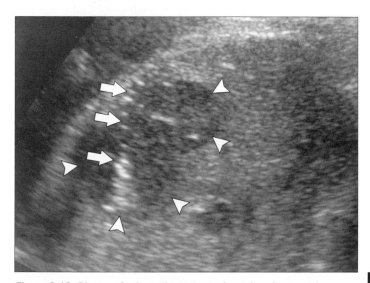

Figure 8.12 Oblique route of biopsy under computed tomography guidance. Granulomatous disease was confirmed from a Biopty gun biopsy without complications.

Figure 8.13 Biopsy of a hepatic metastasis under ultrasound guidance. Inoperability was confirmed from this extrathoracic metastasis. (Arrows indicate the needle, and short arrowheads the metastasis.)

PLEURAL DRAINAGE

Introduction
The most common indications are a malignant effusion or an empyema. Of patients who have community acquired pneumonia, 40% develop a parapneumonic effusion. The majority resolve spontaneously, but they can progress to form an empyema. Early and rapid drainage of an empyema is essential to prevent fibrin deposition, which leads to pleural fibrosis and possibly a restrictive defect. An esophageal rupture or endobronchial lesion should always be considered in a patient who has an empyema with no obvious predisposing cause.

Indications and contraindications
A pleural effusion can be tapped for diagnostic purposes, and a pleural biopsy may be usefully performed at the same time. A pleural effusion can be drained for therapeutic purposes if it is large and the patient is symptomatic (usually with a malignant effusion), if it is infected or is an empyema (if the glucose is low, or if the pH is <7.2), or if a hemothorax (usually following trauma) is present. A bleeding disorder is a relative contraindication, as it predisposes to a hematoma formation.

Technique
Image guidance
Ultrasound is the easiest and quickest way to confirm pleural fluid and indicates the volume present. Echogenic fluid is almost diagnostic of an empyema. Ultrasound also demonstrates the presence of septae and multiple locules, which may hinder drainage and necessitate multiple drainage tubes or streptokinase.

CT has an advantage in evaluating any underlying lung or mediastinal pathology. In empyemas, the pleura is characteristically smooth, diffusely thickened, and enhances after contrast.

Procedure
A large effusion can be drained without image guidance, but smaller or multiloculated effusions are better drained under ultrasound or CT guidance. The patient sits down and leans forward, 'hugging' a pillow against the chest to bring the arms forward to clear the scapulae off the back. A small stool under the feet makes the patient more comfortable, and the optimum skin position is marked. A sterile technique with local anesthetic is again used. The catheter used varies between small, pig-tail catheters or larger catheters for empyemas.

The depth of the effusion can be judged by both ultrasound and using the local anesthetic needle. The catheter can be positioned with a cannula and guide-wire technique or by a single-step procedure. The latter is more commonly used. The catheter and needle are advanced into the pleural space. Once it has been entered, the catheter is advanced into the effusion, simultaneously withdrawing the central stylet. The catheter is connected rapidly to a drainage bag with a three-way tap. Samples for cytology, microbiology, and chemical analysis can be taken. If drainage is for a short time (24–48h), a bag normally suffices. If drainage is required for longer (normal with empyemas) or if the effusion is large – presumably because of active fluid production – the catheter is connected to an underwater drain system.

If aspiration is carried out, no more than 1.5L is taken off at a time because of the risk of pulmonary edema. Larger catheters can be used, but smaller catheters are usually adequate and more comfortable for the patient. The catheters are securely fastened to the skin and regular irrigated with saline to maintain patency (20mL of saline every 4–6h). Fibrinolytics (for example, streptokinase) given early for empyemas have been shown to increase drainage, with faster radiographic improvement and with fewer patients who require surgery[12].

Pleural fluid is sent for cytology, microbiology, and chemical analysis.

Complications
Complications are few, providing no bleeding disorder is present. Pneumothorax occurs in less than 5% of cases. Puncture of other viscera can be avoided by ultrasound guidance and using blunt dissection through the chest wall to avoid traumatizing the catheter. Pain may occur at the site of insertion, but this is eased by inserting the catheter laterally for patient comfort. Reactions caused by streptokinase occur less often when the purified form is used, but previously included anaphylaxis and bleeding both intrapleurally and systemically with large doses.

Pitfalls and controversies
Both chest physicians and radiologists insert catheters for pleural drainage. Image guidance and the radiologist are used for multiloculated, multiple, or small collections. The routine use of streptokinase has not been widely adopted, because of expense and complications with the less purified form, with occasional large hemorrhages, and with using larger doses.

REFERENCES

1. Westcott JL. Direct percutaneous needle aspiration of localised pulmonary lesions: results in 422 patients. Radiology. 1980;137:31–5.
2. Tarver RD, Conios DJ. Interventional chest radiology. Advances in chest radiology. Radiol Clin North Am. 1994;32:689–709.
3. Klein J S, Satoman G, Stewart EA. Transthoracic needle biopsy with a coaxially placed 20-gauge automated cutting needle: results in 122 patients. Radiology. 1996;198:715–20.
4. McLoud TC. Pulmonary infections in the immunocompromised host. Radiol Clin North Am. 1989;27:1059–66.
5. Protopas Z, Westcott JL. Transthoracic needle biopsy of mediastinal lymph nodes for staging lung and other cancers. Radiology. 1996;199:489–96.
6. Westcott JL, Rao N, Colley DP. Transthoracic needle biopsy of small pulmonary nodules. Radiology. 1997;202:97–103.
7. Arakawa H, Nakayima Y, Kurihara Y, et al. CT guided transthoracic needle biopsy: a comparison between automated biopsy gun and fine needle aspiration. Clin Radiol. 1996;51:503–6.
8. Saleh H, Masood, S. Value of ancillary studies in fine needle aspiration biopsy. Diagn Cytopathol. 1995; 13:310–5.
9. Yankelevitz DF, Davis SD, Henschike CI. Aspiration of a large pneumothorax resulting from transthoracic needle biopsy. Radiology. 1996;200:695–7.
10. Allison DJ, Pinet F, Allison HJ. Interventional techniques in the thorax pulmonary radiology. Philadelphia:WB Saunders. 1993;340–60.
11. Bressler EL, Kirkhan JA. Mediastinal masses: alternative approaches to CT guided needle biopsy. Radiology. 1994;191:391–6.
12. Davies RJ, Traill ZC, Gleeson FV. Randomised controlled trial of intrapleural streptokinase in community acquired pleural infection. Thorax. 1997;52:416–21.

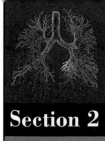

Section 2 Techniques and Indications

Chapter 9 Intercostal Drainage

William S Walker

INTRODUCTION

Intercostal drain insertion is required to remove intrapleural gas and/or fluid. This common minor surgical intervention is usually of high therapeutic value and frequently required on an urgent or emergency basis, and it may be life saving. It is, however, often performed both incorrectly and inadequately, with complication rates of up to 25%[1,2], which is particularly unfortunate as the procedure is unpleasant for the patient and the initial drain insertion provides the best opportunity to achieve a good result. Significant surgical skill is not necessary, but it is important to apply common sense, to follow sound surgical principles when inserting a drain, to possess a good working knowledge of underwater seal drainage, and to have a systematic approach to subsequent management.

INDICATIONS AND CONTRAINDICATIONS

The few absolute indications for chest drainage are either trauma related[3] or concerned with situations that present the potential for acute and severe respiratory embarrassment (Fig. 9.1). Relative indications involve a judgment as to which of alternative strategies (including aspiration, pigtail catheter insertion, or observation) represents the best choice for the patient. Specific examples of common conditions that present such dilemmas are pleural effusion, empyema, and thoracic trauma without pneumothorax or hemothorax.

Extreme caution is required when low drain placement is considered in patients who have obscured diaphragms, as it is easy to misplace a drain in the liver or viscera (the author has even seen intracardiac placement of a drain in a postpneumonectomy patient). Intrapulmonary placement is not uncommon in patients who have pleural adhesions (Figs 9.2 & 9.3) or bullous lung disease. In such circumstances and when operator experience is limited, it may be safer to refer the patient for thoracic surgical management. Except for tension pneumothorax, for which needle decompression is necessary as the least possible first-aid measure, no condition requires immediate placement of a drain.

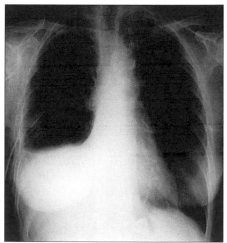

Figure 9.2 Chest radiograph of postsurgical patient who has a drain inserted for 'effusion'. The drain lies in an apparently satisfactory position, but continuous and copious air leakage occurred.

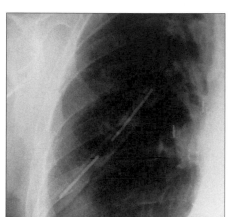

Figure 9.3 Chest radiograph showing close up view of same case as in Figure 9.2. Note the shadow around the drain, which suggests intrapulmonary placement.

Indications, cautionary circumstances, and contraindications for chest drain insertion	
Implication	**Condition**
Indications	
Absolute	Tension pneumothorax
	Large pneumothorax (if aspiration fails)
	Traumatic hemothorax
	Major thoracic surgery
Relative	Large effusion (>30% of hemithorax)
	Empyema
	Intrapulmonary abscess (rarely)
	'Prophylactic' drainage in trauma
Cautionary circumstances	Coagulopathy
	Intrapleural adhesions
	Intrathoracic viscera
	Ipsilateral pneumonectomy
	Bullous lung disease
Contraindications	Inadequate operator experience
	Fused pleura

Figure 9.1 Indications, cautionary circumstances, and contraindications for chest drain insertion.

TECHNIQUE

Many excellent descriptions of chest drain insertion are published[4–6], but all vary somewhat and omit certain points of value. Additional problems occur when dealing with intercostal drainage in special circumstances, and in some situations the operator simply has to rely on basic principles. For example, drain insertion in an emergency department often has to be accomplished with the patient supine and in conjunction with other procedures. Therefore, positioning and consequently access to the chest may be restricted. Similarly, although a more leisurely approach should be possible in an intensive care unit and so positioning is less of an issue, other considerations may apply[7].

Selection of the drain catheters

Two basic types of intercostal drainage catheters are available – silastic tube catheters (Fig. 9.4) and rubber catheters of the Malecot or Foley type. Rubber catheters are of historic interest only and should not now be used. Silastic tube catheters come with or without a central trochar. While a trochar is considered by some operators to facilitate insertion, it is a potentially dangerous instrument and presents an unnecessary risk of inadvertent injury to central thoracic structures. A further problem with some of these tubes can be that, as they have few holes, blockage is frequent. A multiholed trocharless catheter is, therefore, preferable. The size of the catheter depends on the reason for insertion and the size of the patient, but larger drains are generally more painful and more difficult to insert under local anesthetic. As an approximate guide, a simple pneumothorax in an adult is adequately drained with a size 24 French Gauge (FG), while a large air leak or fluid collection benefits from a size 28 FG device. Smaller individuals require appropriately smaller tubes.

Selection of the drain insertion site

Occasionally, drainage of a loculated collection through a specific point of entry determined by radiologic or ultrasound investigation may be indicated. In general, however, the intention is to drain either a pneumothorax (best achieved with a drain placed to the apex of the thoracic cavity) or a fluid collection (in which case a lower drain position is indicated). In either case, access to

the thoracic cavity is best gained through a convenient intercostal space in the mid or anterior axillary line (Fig. 9.5). This typically is the fourth or fifth interspace, but the actual level is less important than being certain that the interspace is easily palpated and that the intended site of entry is posterior to the lateral border of pectoralis major. When inserted, the drain can be directed superiorly in the case of a pneumothorax or inferiorly in the case of a fluid collection. It is incorrect to insert electively a drain directly through the anterior upper chest. This cosmetically poor approach traverses the pectoral muscles and risks injury to the internal mammary artery and other structures. Furthermore, the drain lies perpendicularly in a portion of the chest where the anteroposterior diameter is much reduced, which results in impaired drainage of both air and fluid, greater discomfort, and further problems with nursing care.

Positioning the patient

Elective drain insertion may take up to 20 or 30 minutes from start to finish, so the patient must be placed in a comfortable position that can be sustained easily. An erect sitting position with the patient hunched over a bed table is often recommended, but this can be tiring and patients often slump. Conversely, a supine position may be difficult for dyspneic patients to tolerate. A useful compromise is provided by a semi-upright position in which the patient lies semi supine in bed with the trunk elevated on pillows to a 30° angle. The operative side is rotated forward by about 45° (Fig. 9.6). The upper arm can be positioned over the patient's neck and the hands clasped in a semipraying position, so as to support the upper arm, or they may be placed above the head depending upon which is more comfortable. It helps to place a pillow under the dependent chest, as this arches the chest toward the operated side and thereby opens the interspaces and facilitates drain insertion. The operator should stand at the patient's back.

Preparation, anesthetization, and incision

The chest wall is cleaned with an antiseptic solution and wound drapes applied to produce an operative field of about 20×20cm. Local anesthetic [lidocaine (lignocaine) 1%, 20ml] is infiltrated using a thin (21G) needle, initially under the skin and then through the intercostal layers and directly over a rib until the

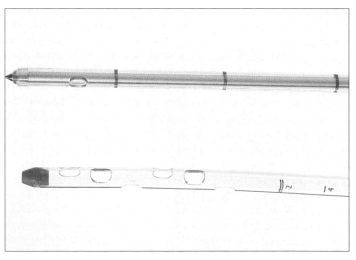

Figure 9.4 Silastic drain catheters. End holed with a central trochar (upper) and multiholed without a trochar (lower).

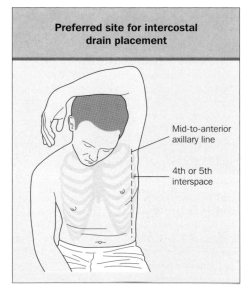

Preferred site for intercostal drain placement

Mid-to-anterior axillary line

4th or 5th interspace

Figure 9.5 Preferred site for intercostal drain placement – mid-to-anterior axillary line, fourth or fifth interspace.

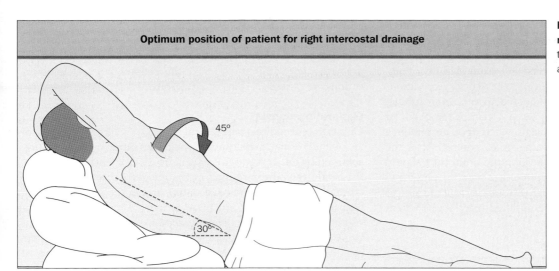

Optimum position of patient for right intercostal drainage

45°

30°

Figure 9.6 Patient positioned for right intercostal drainage. The trunk is elevated on pillows to a 30° angle and rotated by 45°.

pleural cavity is entered and either air or fluid is aspirated. The pleura is especially sensitive and must be thoroughly anesthetized. While the anesthetic takes effect (approximately 10 minutes), the drain and tubing are checked to ensure that all connections fit, the underwater seal set is primed with sterile water in accordance with the manufacturer's instructions, and the tubing is connected to it. The end of the tubing to be connected to the drain can be secured to the sterile drapes for easy access by the operator once the drain is *in situ*. The length of drain to be inserted into the chest is judged by placing it against the sterile field in the manner in which it is intended to lie.

A 2cm skin crease incision is made over the interspace selected for entry. This relatively large incision is necessary for surgical drain insertion and heals cleanly. The drain retention and wound closure sutures are then inserted. It is conventional to employ a purse string suture, but this is bad practice as it results in ischemia of the wound edges, prolonged healing, and greater scarring. The author utilizes two separate sutures. A simple suture serves both to seal the wound beside the drain and to retain the drain, and a loose vertical mattress suture is placed for subsequent wound closure when the drain is removed (Fig. 9.7). These various procedures ensure that the delay between inserting the drain and

having it correctly positioned, connected, and secured (i.e. operational) is minimized.

Drain insertion and connection
Slight variations in the placement of the incision aid drain location. If an apical drain is to be inserted, the incision can usefully be made about 1cm lower, thereby creating an oblique track to reach the upper border of the rib and so angling the drain toward the upper chest. If the drain is designed to remove fluid in the lower chest, a more direct path allows easier orientation toward the base. In either case, the track is created by blunt dissection, preferably with artery forceps rather than scissors, and the pleura is entered over the upper border of a rib to avoid injury to the intercostal bundle. Pleural entry is indicated by air release or fluid leakage. The operator must then insert an index finger (see Fig. 9.8) and palpate to detect:
• entry into the chest and not abdomen;
• freedom from adherent lung; and
• possible pleural lesions.
Once it is established that the pleural cavity has been entered correctly and the lung will not be damaged, the drain is grasped in artery forceps, passed along the dissection track, and inserted

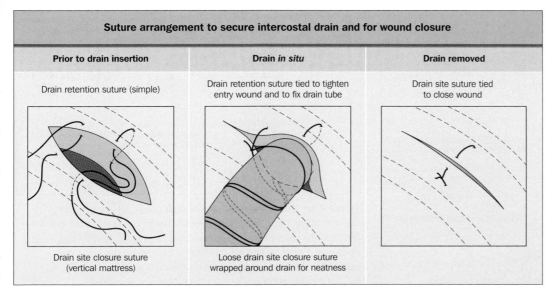

Suture arrangement to secure intercostal drain and for wound closure

Prior to drain insertion	Drain *in situ*	Drain removed
Drain retention suture (simple)	Drain retention suture tied to tighten entry wound and to fix drain tube	Drain site suture tied to close wound
Drain site closure suture (vertical mattress)	Loose drain site closure suture wrapped around drain for neatness	

Figure 9.7 Suggested suture arrangement to secure intercostal drain and for subsequent wound closure.

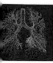

(Fig. 9.9) in accordance with the previously determined length and direction. Patients often cough when the drain is inserted, so to prevent spillage it is a good idea to have a clamp on the end of the tube to drain fluid. This is also an extremely uncomfortable phase for the patient and it is important to be as expeditious as possible. The drain is then connected to the drain tubing, secured with the retention suture, and any clamps removed. At this stage the patient is asked to cough, whereupon air bubbling or a gush of fluid through the drain becomes evident. After the initial burst of drainage, the fluid level in the drain tube should rise and fall slightly with gentle respiration, a process sometimes referred to as 'swinging' (although at this stage continued air loss or fluid drainage may obscure the air–fluid interface). A light dressing is applied to the drain site.

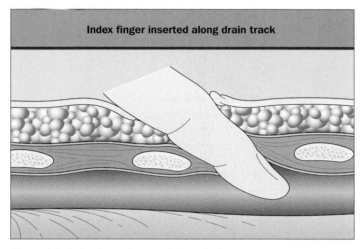

Figure 9.8 Index finger inserted along drain track to exclude adhesions and confirm entry into chest cavity. Note that the track has been created over the upper surface of a rib.

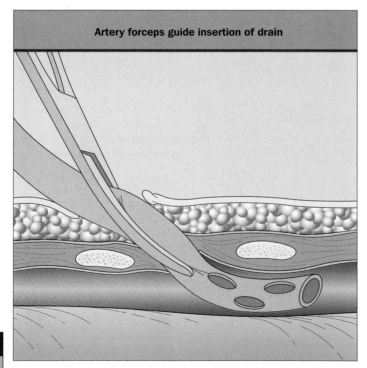

Figure 9.9 Use of artery forceps to guide insertion of drain.

SUBSEQUENT MANAGEMENT

The specific management of various conditions that require chest drainage is not within the scope of this chapter, but certain observations are pertinent to most situations.

General principles

Chest drains require a valvular mechanism to allow the egress of air or fluid while maintaining a negative intrapleural pressure, achieved by either a water seal (Fig. 9.10) or a flutter valve (Fig. 9.11). Flutter valves are used in trauma cases that require intercostal drainage at the place of injury, and in the management of transfer, ambulant, or domiciliary patients. They have the advantages of simplicity and portability, but are less suitable for situations in which fluid loss is likely and are less versatile than underwater seal systems. Most hospital patients can be managed adequately and economically with a simple, single-chamber underwater seal drain. Progress is monitored by observing drain losses and serial chest films, and patency of the drain system is confirmed by the swinging motion of fluid at the end of the drain tubing.

If this system is used for a patient who has an air leak and fluid drainage, however, care must be taken because as fluid accumulates in the drain bottle it increases the distance from the tip of the drain tube to the surface of the drain bottle fluid, which effectively increases the intrathoracic pressure required to expel air through the drain system. Patients who have a blowing pneumothorax must, therefore, either have a trap system that collects fluid prior to the underwater seal chamber or have the drain bottle changed frequently. If gross air loss is present, indicating a significant parenchymal air leak such as may occur in patients who suffer bullous emphysema, the fluid in the drain bottle may froth, which impairs drainage and obscures and distorts the drain fluid level. This problem is improved by adding a small amount of defoaming agent to the drain bottle fluid.

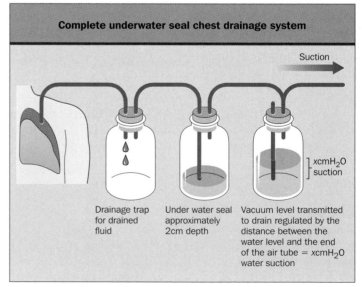

Figure 9.10 Complete underwater seal chest drainage system. In the most basic form, both the trap and vacuum regulation chambers are omitted. The latter is clearly irrelevant if suction is not applied and is not necessary if external suction is reliably controlled. Commercial drain assemblies can incorporate all three chambers in one casing and may include a manometer to measure the pressure at the patient.

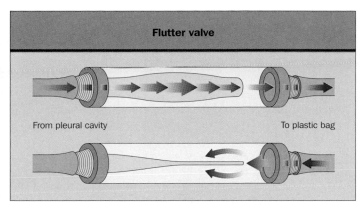

Figure 9.11 Flutter valve. Air expelled from the pleural cavity opens the flutter valve (upper); when the initial pleural pressure falls below atmospheric the flutter value is compressed and sealed (lower).

Suction

In some situations – typically moderate but continuous air leakage – it helps to apply suction to the chest drain according to the principal that to scavenge air from the pleural cavity faster than it leaks from the lung encourages pulmonary expansion. The lung should then adhere to the chest wall, causing the leaking point to seal off. This is not appropriate in patients who have a substantial air leak, as air is effectively pulled out of the airways and respiration impaired.

Suction is commenced only after other avenues have been explored, which include checking the drain system for patency and correct fitting, and inserting a larger or second drain. Suction can be unpleasant for the patient, as it results in pain (probably from mediastinal deviation), cough, and dyspnea. It is, therefore, introduced at a minimal level of 5cmH$_2$O and gradually increased to 15–20cmH$_2$O as tolerated. Commercial drain units are available that combine an underwater seal, trap, and suction regulator in one casing.

Occlusion of drain tubing

In general, drain tubing is not occluded, exceptions being:
- when the bottle or tubing is being changed;
- when the drain is elevated above the patient;
- during staged release of a fluid collection
- during assessment of whether a blowing drain can be removed (see drain removal); and
- at removal.

The decision to occlude the tubing deliberately when the drain is blowing must be taken with great care and with a high level of alertness to the possibility that a tension pneumothorax may occur.

Drain removal

Drain removal is indicated when air leakage or fluid loss ceases and chest radiography shows the lung to be well expanded. It is not necessary to wait until the drain air–fluid interface is static before advising removal. Technique varies, but a common approach utilizes two attendants. The drain retention suture is cut and the patient is then asked to breathe in as deeply as possible. At maximal inspiration one attendant removes the drain while the other ties the preplaced closure suture. A check chest radiograph is obtained after drain removal to ensure that the lung position is preserved.

Sometimes an air leak shows no signs of stopping. In such cases, the lung eventually adheres to the parietal pleura, at which stage the drain may be removed as adhesions maintain the position of the lung. This point is determined by clamping the drain tubing and observing the patient's condition. If this is stable, a radiograph can be obtained and, if the lung position appears unchanged, the clamp can be left in place and a further radiograph obtained on the following day. If this is still unchanged the drain may be removed. In some cases, typically younger individuals who have a prolonged but low-level air leakage, clamping results in slow deflation of the lung; in such cases a flutter valve system may be considered so that the patient can go home and have the drain removed as an outpatient when it stops blowing.

COMPLICATIONS

Insertion difficulties

Negative aspiration
It is essential to be confident that the drain will enter the chest in a region where either a pneumothorax or fluid will be encountered. If aspiration reveals neither, further attempts need to be made through higher and lower interspaces. If neither air nor fluid (as appropriate) is found, the procedure must be abandoned and the situation reconsidered. Either further imaging or a more experienced hand may be required. Failure to observe this precaution may convert a minor difficulty into an emergency with inadvertent insertion of a drain into the lung or other viscera.

Obese patient/marked subcutaneous emphysema
Obesity or marked subcutaneous emphysema makes it difficult to palpate the ribs and, therefore, hinders drain insertion. It may be possible to squash subcutaneous emphysema and displace it from the operative field, and so allow the ribs to be palpated, but this may not work. In either case, the best approach is usually to make a more generous skin incision such that the index finger can be used to break through fat or emphysematous tissue until the chest wall is reached. Drain insertion then proceeds as normal, and a few extra skin sutures repair the access wound.

Intrapleural adhesions
Intrapleural adhesions are detected by palpation. If flimsy, they can often be swept away sufficiently to allow the drain to be inserted safely. Once the drain is in the chest, it is advanced gently as it may have to find its own way around various areas of adhesion.

Abdominal entry
Abdominal entry results from attempts to place a basal drain or, occasionally, when the diaphragm is elevated unexpectedly. It is not a disaster provided digital exploration has been performed and the mistake is appreciated so that the entry site may simply be sealed. The postinsertion chest radiograph demonstrates any air under the diaphragm and the patient requires careful monitoring in case abdominal viscera have been injured.

Impaled structure
An impaled structure requires urgent surgical referral. Clues include drainage of gastrointestinal content (which suggests bowel entry), continuous blowing and bleeding from lung penetration, and major blood loss from hepatic or splenic injury. Cardiac or great vessel injury produces catastrophic bleeding that is likely to

be immediately fatal. If blood does pour out of the drain do not retract it. Apply a clamp to the end and summon help. The situation may be irretrievable, but if all the holes are within the structure the seal around the drain may be sufficient to buy time for surgical rescue if the drain is occluded.

Management problems
Continuous blowing
Continuous blowing usually indicates a source of pulmonary parenchymal injury, either iatrogenic or from a pathologic source such as a ruptured bulla. Occasionally, however, the problem stems from the drain. The drain catheter can sometimes slip so that one or two holes lie outside the pleural cavity – a situation evident from the chest radiograph (Fig. 9.12). Also, the drain track may widen so that air is sucked in from the outside atmosphere and expelled down the drain; this can be tested by squeezing the wound closed around the drain and asking the patient to cough. If the leakage is from air passing around the drain, the rate of loss decreases considerably after several coughs, whereas it remains unchanged if a parenchymal source exists.

Subcutaneous emphysema
Subcutaneous emphysema is caused by air that leaks from the lung under pressure, such as occurs from the air-trapped parenchyma of patients who have chronic obstructive pulmonary disease. Weakening of the soft tissues as a result of corticosteroid therapy may also contribute. A minor degree of subcutaneous emphysema is commonly seen after chest drain insertion for pneumothorax, but when this develops to a massive extent it is a distressing condition that causes uncomfortable crackling in the subcutaneous tissues and may extend to the neck and face. More importantly, the subcutaneous air may track into the laryngeal region and cause difficulty with breathing. The drain system must be inspected to ensure that the drain is not evidently in the lung, the catheter is patent, the tubing is not kinked, and the drainage bottle is connected correctly. Assuming these checks are satisfactory, the rate of air removal is increased by applying suction or inserting a second or larger drain. Surgical referral is also considered, as head and neck swelling can be improved by inserting suction drains into the subcutaneous tissues of the upper anterior thoracic wall under local anesthetic.

Failure of the lung to re-expand
Failure of pulmonary re-expansion after institution of chest drainage for pneumothorax or fluid collection is caused by inadequate drainage in relation to the rate of air or fluid accumulation, bronchial obstruction, or secondary pulmonary changes. Vigorous air loss or copious fluid production are obvious and may require referral for surgical management; other potential causes require

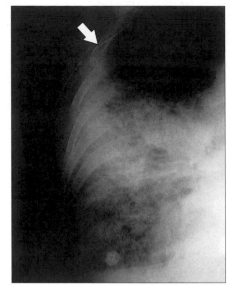

Figure 9.12 Chest radiograph showing slipped drain.

further investigation. Patency of the drainage system can be confirmed by swinging of the fluid column, and if the drain appears to be blocked it must be replaced. If the drain is patent, consider bronchoscopy to exclude an obstruction such as tumor or mucous plugging, and evaluate the history to determine the likelihood of secondary pulmonary changes. Long-standing bronchial obstruction may, for example, result in secondary bronchiectasis, consolidation, and mucous inspissation that obliterates the airways. Hemothorax or empyema may have lead to cortex formation around the lung and external restriction to re-expansion.

Drain blockage
Whether milking or 'stripping' drains[8] is of much value when the drain is blocked is unclear. Although commonly used after surgery to encourage clots to move down the tubing, a risk is that transient, high negative pressures are created at the end of the tube. This can lead to portions of lung being sucked into the holes of the drain tube. It is better to either resite or remove the drain, as clinically appropriate.

Re-expansion pulmonary edema
Re-expansion pulmonary edema, a rare phenomenon[9], is characterized by the onset of noncardiogenic ipsilateral pulmonary edema some hours after the rapid drainage of a large effusion. The exact mechanism is unclear, but the problem appears to be associated with moderately long-standing effusions. It may be avoided by employing a staged approach to the drainage of all large chronic collections.

REFERENCES

1. Hyde J, Sykes T, Graham T. Reducing morbidity from chest drains. Br Med J. 1997;314:914–15.
2. Chan L, Reilly KM, Henderson C, Kahn F, Salluzzo RF. Complication rates of tube thoracostomy. Am J Emerg Med. 1997;15:368–70.
3. American College of Surgeons Committee on Trauma. Thoracic trauma. In: Advanced trauma life support programs for physicians instructor manual. Chicago: American College of Surgeons; 1995.
4. Tomlinson MA, Treasure T. Insertion of a chest drain: how to do it. Br J Hosp Med. 1997;58:248–52.
5. Wells F, Milstein BB. Insertion of a chest drain. In: Wells F, Milstein BB, eds. Thoracic surgical techniques. London: Balliere Tindall; 1990:15–17.
6. Hood RM. Chest tube insertion. In: General thoracic surgery, 2nd edn. Pennsylvania: Lea & Febiger; 1993:41–4.
7. Iberti TJ, Stern PM. Chest tube thoracostomy. Crit Care Clin. 1992;8:879–95.
8. Teplitz L. Update: are milking and stripping chest tubes necessary? Focus Crit Care. 1991;18:506–11.
9. Janocik SE, Roy TM, Killeen TR. Re-expansion pulmonary edema: a preventable complication. J Ky Med Assoc. 1993;91:143–8.

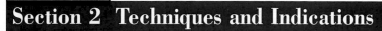
INTRODUCTION

Surgical intervention can contribute to the diagnostic process by providing or refining a tissue diagnosis and by complementing the assessment of tumor stage and operability. The techniques employed include, in order of invasiveness: bronchoscopic, cervical, and supraclavicular node, pleural, mediastinal, and pulmonary biopsy procedures that involve endoscopic, thoracoscopic, or open surgical techniques. Thus, a patient typically enters an investigational ladder at the extreme end of which lies, in theory at least, an exploratory thoracotomy. The choice of procedure and method of access are determined by the reason for investigation and the required success rate. In general, the procedures involved offer a high diagnostic yield with low morbidity and mortality rates, but adverse outcomes do occur and are particularly difficult for patients and their relatives to accept as these procedures are diagnostic and not therapeutic. It is important, therefore, that a referring physician possesses a good understanding of the degree of invasiveness and the risk and benefit implications that relate to each diagnostic surgical procedure.

BASIC CONSIDERATIONS

Fitness for surgical intervention

All diagnostic surgical interventions require a general anesthetic and incur some degree of operative risk. Intervention is not appropriate when:
- no useful therapeutic purpose can be served by acquiring more information; or
- operative risk is excessive.

The former situation typically arises in those patients who are unfit for any treatment. Such patients may include those who have poor respiratory reserve and who could not tolerate thoracotomy, chemotherapy, or radiotherapy. Examples of the second situation would include patients for whom the operative element of the procedure is excessively dangerous, such as those patients who have untreated superior vena cava (SVC) obstruction (for whom the risk of operative hemorrhage may be significant) and those people who are primarily unfit, perhaps from cardiac disease.

An extension of the requirement of a reasonable risk–benefit ratio is that for some patients a lesser procedure, such as a mediastinoscopy, is acceptable, whereas a more significant one, such as a video-assisted thoracic surgery (VATS) assessment, is not.

Preoperative preparation

Preoperative preparation is designed to prepare the patient mentally and physically for the procedure. Important steps include:
- optimizing preoperative medical status;
- obtaining adequate three-dimensional information [chest radiographs, computed tomography (CT), and magnetic resonance imaging scans];
- checking histology requirements;
- counseling regarding the possibility of a negative outcome;
- obtaining consent for conversion to open thoracotomy; and
- ensuring operating room provision and blood transfusion availability.

While consent and operating-room arrangements are surgical issues, the other points can usefully be covered prior to referral for a surgical opinion. Preoperative medical status is checked by reviewing the patient's physical condition and by obtaining specialist advice as necessary. Adequate three-dimensional information must be given to the surgical team, as this aids their decision making and may guide operative strategy. If a biopsy that requires special analyses is requested to facilitate medical management, the team that makes the request must cooperate with the appropriate laboratory, provide simple instructions to the surgical team, and make suitable specimen transport arrangements.

INVESTIGATIVE SURGICAL PROCEDURES AND APPLICATIONS

Surgical diagnostic procedures vary in their application and all have relative merits and limitaions when compared with non-surgical approaches (see Fig. 10.1). They are most commonly utilized in three broad areas:
- assessment of bronchogenic carcinoma;
- diagnosis of interstitial lung disease; and
- sampling of indeterminate pleural, pulmonary, and mediastinal lesions.

The choice of procedure is influenced by risk–benefit considerations, the clinical circumstances, the location of the area to be investigated, and the questions that need to be answered after medical assessment. This process must be individualized for patients who have undiagnosed mass lesions, but for other patients, notably those who suffer lung cancer, the surgical investigative sequence is fairly predictable (see Fig. 10.2).

Rigid bronchoscopy

Rigid bronchoscopy offers several advantages over fiberoptic endoscopy, principally because of the ability to take large biopsy samples (and thereby increase the amount of tissue available for analysis) and the facility to clear an obstructed airway easily by aspirating blood or pus. Other advantages are largely related to the relative ease with which the airways can be instrumented for a variety of purposes, which include dilatation or stenting of tracheobronchial stenosis, debulking of tumor, cauterization of a bleeding point, and extraction of foreign material.

Features of surgical investigative procedures

Procedure	Application	Advantages	Disadvantages
Rigid bronchoscopy	Diagnosis of carcinoma Clear airway obstruction	Removal of secretions/blood Large biopsy specimen may reveal submucosal tumor Opportunity to debulk inoperable tumors or excise benign lesions Assessment of carinal fixation	Poor view of secondary bronchial divisions
Cervical and scalene lymph node biopsy	Diagnosis of enlarged nodes	Safer technique than fine-needle aspiration (FNA) for deeper nodes Large tissue sample	Operative procedure Occasional technical difficulty
Mediastinoscopy	Diagnosis of middle mediastinal pathology (node/mass)	Direct access to mediastinal abnormality Much larger tissue sample than FNA	Operative field restricted to paratracheal and subcarinal areas
Mediastinotomy	Diagnosis of anterior mediastinal pathology (node/mass)	Reaches areas of anterior mediastinum not accessible to mediastinoscopy Useful for subaortic node sampling May be safer to use than mediastinoscopy in patients who have superior vena cava obstruction Much larger tissue sample than in FNA	Operative field restricted to upper anterior mediastinum More complex operative procedure
Thoracoscopy	Pleural biopsy Biopsy of visceral pleura deposits	Can be effected through single puncture Visually directed biopsy	Limited to small biopsies Dependent on pleural cavity being free of adhesions
Video assisted thoracic surgery	Any ipsilateral biopsy or sampling procedure	Complementary to mediastinoscopy and mediastinotomy Excellent view and full operative intervention possible (e.g. wedge excision of pulmonary nodule or dissection of mediastinal mass)	Dependent on pleural cavity being free or adhesions Significant surgical expertise required

Figure 10.1 Features of surgical investigative procedures.

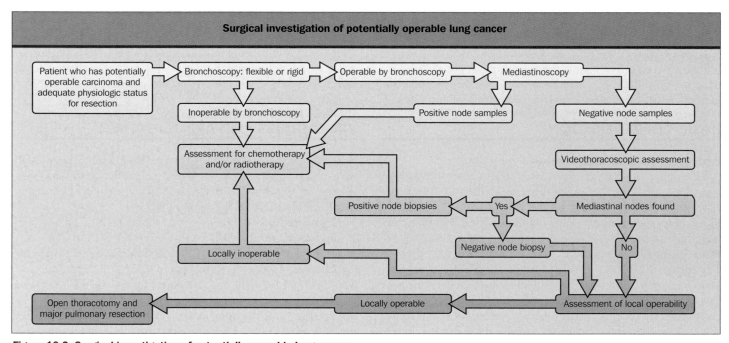

Figure 10.2 Surgical investigation of potentially operable lung cancer.

Technique

Although it is possible to perform rigid bronchoscopy under sedation and local anesthetic, this is largely unacceptable and general anesthetic is required. The patient is paralyzed and positioned supine with about 45° of flexion at the waist. The neck is hyperextended and the rigid bronchoscope inserted and passed under the epiglottis. The cords are visualized and the instrument (Fig. 10.3) is then rotated through 90° so that the beaked lip passes easily between the cords. When it is within the trachea, the anesthetist uses an oxygen jet venturi to maintain ventilation. Telescopes with 0 and 90° lenses are used to view the trachea and bronchi.

Rigid bronchoscopy is a valuable adjunct to flexible bronchoscopy in surgical units, with both therapeutic and diagnostic uses as noted above. It may be combined with mediastinoscopy in the surgical assessment of bronchogenic carcinoma, in which case it allows the surgeon rapidly to assess whether lobectomy or pneumonectomy is required. Carinal involvement by tumor can be judged to some extent by moving the bronchoscope against the distal trachea and gauging the degree of fixation present. The disadvantages are the relatively limited opportunity to assess the distal bronchi (as the view is restricted to the lobar bronchi) and limited opportunity to biopsy lesions within the upper lobes or distal segmental bronchi.

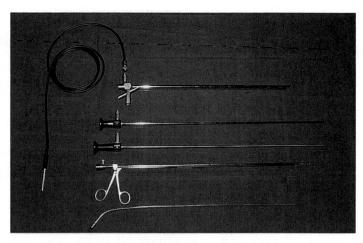

Figure 10.3 Rigid bronchoscopy equipment. Bronchoscope with light cable (top), straight and right-angle surgical telescopes, biopsy forceps, suction cannula (bottom).

Cervical and supraclavicular lymph node biopsy

Thoracic inlet and cervical lymph nodes may become involved by spread of tumor from bronchogenic or esophageal carcinoma, for which they are often the first detectable extrathoracic sites of spread. Indeed, routine excision of the scalene lymph node group (which lies in a fat pad on the scalenus anterior muscle) was once advised as part of the standard staging of bronchogenic carcinoma cases. While routine use of this procedure is no longer regarded as of benefit, it is not uncommon to undertake cervical or scalene lymph node biopsy if any palpable nodes are discovered. Fine-needle aspiration is a valuable alternative, but may not be safe with deep-seated nodes in view of the risk of pneumothorax or great vessel injury, and the greater sample size obtained with open biopsy may be preferable in some instances.

Technique

A 3–4cm long skin crease incision is made about 2cm above the medial half of the clavicle. The underlying sternomastoid is reflected medially to expose the scalene or deep cervical lymph nodes, which are sampled either as an excisional node biopsy or simply by taking a bite out of the node.

There is often pressure to undertake this procedure under local anesthetic as it is usually technically straightforward, but difficult bleeding can occur so it is wiser to work under the more controlled circumstances of general anesthetic. Inpatient stay is usually <1 day. Significant complications are very rare and, apart from pneumothorax, include hemorrhage and lymphatic duct injury, with a distant possibility of air embolism.

Mediastinoscopy

Mediastinoscopy allows the surgeon to reach the paratracheal, pretracheal, anterior carinal, and subcarinal areas. It is principally used to sample mediastinal lymph nodes in the surgical staging of bronchogenic carcinoma[1], but it can also be used to diagnose mediastinal lymphadenopathy of any cause and to biopsy mass lesions, provided that the intended biopsy target is located beside the trachea. Contrary to opinions expressed by some investigators, mediastinoscopy has not been supplanted by CT in the evaluation of lung cancer patients – CT merely identifies the size and location of a node; only histologic examination can determine whether the node is positive or negative for disease[2].

Technique

The surgeon makes a 3cm long transverse skin incision about 1cm above the sternal notch and splits the strap muscles in the mid line. The mediastinoscope is introduced into the pretracheal plane and advanced along the front of the trachea while a long, thin sucker is used to displace tissues and search systematically for lymphatic or tumor tissue. The procedure requires a reasonable level of surgical skill and care as many major structures occur in this region of the mediastinum, notably the aortic arch anterior to the path of the mediastinoscope (Fig. 10.4).

Mediastinoscopy has proved a highly effective strategy in the surgical staging of lung cancer (see Chapter 43, Fig. 43.27), but in this context it requires an experienced and interested surgical team as it is a pointless exercise unless all node stations are systematically examined. In experienced centers diagnostic accuracy rates of over 98% are obtained for all accessible node stations[1,3]. Sensitivity rates (i.e. the likelihood of successful determination of lymph node status) are somewhat lower at 83% or better for all node stations with the exception of subcarinal lymphadenopathy, which is technically more difficult to access and consequently is associated with correspondingly lower sensitivity rates of about 64%.

The procedure requires an inpatient stay of <12 hours postoperatively and for suitable candidates can be undertaken on a day-patient basis. Relative contraindications include untreated SVC obstruction because of the risk of hemorrhage, bleeding disorders and anticoagulation, severe kyphosis, and cervical spine instability. Repeat mediastinoscopy is possible, but as a result of fusion of the mediastinal tissue planes is undoubtedly more difficult than a first procedure. The most significant risk is of hemorrhage that results from injury to a major vessel. Other reported complications include air embolism and mediastinal infection. Although some surgeons disagree, many do not exclude patients who have SVC syndrome from mediastinoscopy provided an intravascular stent has been placed within the SVC in order to decompress the venous system. It is highly desirable to have a tissue diagnosis before initiating therapy for SVC syndrome.

Anterior mediastinotomy

Anterior mediastinotomy is a technique that provides access to the anterior mediastinum and allows the surgeon to sample

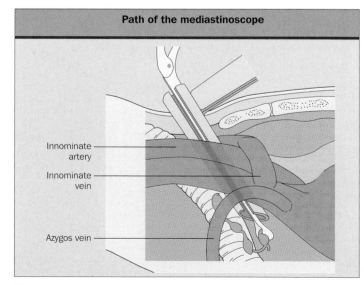

Path of the mediastinoscope

Innominate artery

Innominate vein

Azygos vein

Figure 10.4 Path of the mediastinoscope.

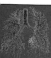
anterior mediastinal masses. It has been used extensively in the past for the assessment of subaortic and anterior aortic lymph nodes (stations L5 and L6), particularly in patients who have left upper lobe tumors in view of the propensity of these lesions to spread directly to these node stations. More recently, sampling of these node stations has been described via extended mediastinoscopy[4] and videothoracoscopic approaches[5].

Technique

A 5cm long incision is made in an appropriate interspace (typically the second) and adjacent to the sternum. It is deepened through the intercostal muscles, the internal mammary vessels may need to be ligated and divided, and the costal cartilages are retracted (occasionally one is excised). The pleura is reflected away from the mediastinum and dissection carried out within the mediastinal tissues until the mass or nodes are reached and biopsied (Fig. 10.5). The surgeon may deliberately choose to enter the pleural cavity to assess the pulmonary hilum.

Mediastinotomy is carried out less commonly than mediastinoscopy and its role in the assessment of bronchogenic carcinoma is probably being overtaken by video-assisted thoracoscopic techniques. It is, however, very useful for obtaining large tissue samples from inoperable anterior mediastinal lesions. Complications and contraindications are similar to those of mediastinoscopy, but the surgical conditions are less demanding so that a moderate degree of venous congestion is acceptable. The

procedure is significantly more invasive than mediastinoscopy and pain is therefore increased because of rib retraction and opening the pleura. Consequently, the inpatient stay can be increased to 2–3 postoperative days, depending on the extent of the procedure and the general condition of the patient.

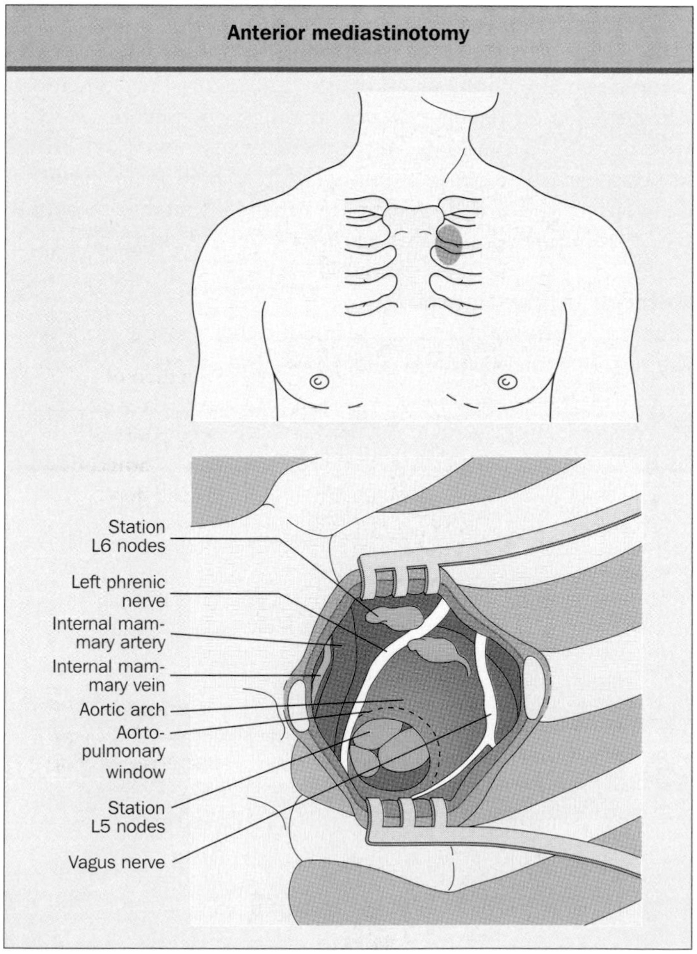

Videothoracoscopy

Thoracoscopy involves the insertion of a surgical telescope into the chest through a stab incision. This provides the opportunity to inspect the pleural cavity and allows visually directed biopsies to be taken from any intrapleural abnormality. The biopsy forceps are introduced either through a channel present in the instrument or occasionally via a separate entry site. This technique had been used for many years for pleural biopsy, in which it offers a good surgical approach to clarify the diagnosis in patients who have a negative transthoracic pleural biopsy – particularly when mesothelioma is suspected. It is usually carried out in a surgical unit under general anesthetic, but several medical centers in Europe and North America report satisfactory experience with thoracoscopy under local anesthetic and sedation[6].

The advent of video imaging systems lead to videothoracoscopy, which provides a far superior view of the thoracic cavity that is displayed on a video monitor, and the availability of surgical instruments designed for use in minimal access abdominal procedures enabled the development of invasive videothoracoscopic surgical procedures. This technique is known as VATS and has revolutionized many aspects of thoracic surgical practice, including diagnostic intervention (Fig. 10.6)[7].

Technique

Videothoracoscopic surgical procedures are performed under general anesthetic and require selective lung ventilation so that the ipsilateral lung can be collapsed. This maneuver provides for operating room within the hemithorax. Three entry sites about 2–3cm long are created into which operating cannulae or ports are inserted. The videothoracoscope and operating instruments are passed through these ports (Fig. 10.7), which serve to maintain an open passage into the chest and also to protect the wounds from seeding of malignant cells.

A target lesion on the pleura (Fig. 10.8) or within the mediastinum (Fig. 10.9) is relatively easy to identify and biopsy, although some dissection may be required to expose mediastinal lesions. Indeterminate pulmonary nodules are more difficult to locate at videothoracoscopic surgery as they are typically less than 1.5cm in diameter. A variety of strategies[8–10] have been utilized to aid identification of these lesions, including preoperative percutaneous insertion of a hook wire or marker injection of methylene blue to identify the location of the lesion. Intraoperative approaches include the use of ultrasound or palpation probes. Ultimately, however, the surgeon's finger (Fig. 10.10) remains the most sensitive detector and can be used to assess most of the lung if endoscopic instruments are used to push the lung forward toward the palpating finger. Once the nodule has been located it can be sampled with a surgically directed needle biopsy (Fig. 10.11) or an excisional biopsy can be performed using an endoscopic stapler (Fig. 10.12), provided that the lesion is located peripherally. Pulmonary wedge biopsy for interstitial lung disease can be taken from any lobe or lobes using an endoscopic stapler. The VATS approach offers the specific advantage of allowing the surgeon to select the best portion of lung to

---

Anterior mediastinotomy

Station
L6 nodes

Left phrenic
nerve

Internal mam-
mary artery

Internal mam-
mary vein

Aortic arch

Aorto-
pulmonary
window

Station
L5 nodes

Vagus nerve

Figure 10.5 Anterior mediastinotomy.

Video-assisted thoracic surgery techniques for diagnostic intervention

Pleural biopsy
Mediastinal biopsy
Indeterminate pulmonary nodule
Interstitial lung disease
Assessment of operability in bronchogenic carcinoma patients

Figure 10.6 Video-assisted thoracic surgery for diagnostic intervention.

biopsy, whereas an open biopsy performed through a limited thoracotomy may commit the surgeon to take a biopsy from the lung immediately beneath the incision.

The use of VATS to augment staging and operability assessment of patients who have bronchogenic carcinoma has been discussed by several authors[11-13]. Although VATS is complementary to mediastinoscopy, which is a better technique for paratracheal node biopsy, it can be used to determine local inoperability and to assess the lower and posterior mediastinum, which are not accessible to mediastinoscopy. These additional assessments prior to open thoracotomy can reduce the risk of open and shut thoracotomy to 2–4%. Also, VATS is useful in establishing the nature of contralateral nodules in patients who have lung cancer.

As the VATS procedure is of relatively limited severity, the delay to definitive surgery is minimized in those who prove not to have bilateral disease.

Recent series confirm that VATS pulmonary biopsy techniques are reliable when compared with open surgery[14] and show that postoperative pain and inpatient stay are reduced[14,15]. These procedures can, however, consume a significant amount of operating room time, which may be a consideration when operating lists are scheduled, and a VATS biopsy must not be requested simply for completeness or if other, simpler solutions are available.

Contraindications specific to VATS techniques include pleural adhesions that make it impossible to work within the chest, gross obesity for which it may not be possible to find a port cannula long enough to reach into the chest, and patients who are not able to tolerate single lung ventilation.

Complications are the same as those that apply to open thoracotomy (no complications are specific to VATS), but a certain proportion of VATS cases require conversion to open thoracotomy either to deal with intraoperative complications or to enable the procedure to be performed because of technical difficulties. This conversion rate varies between 5 and 25% and is usually higher with more complex cases. Port-site implantation of cancer has been a cause for concern, but the incidence of this problem is low and at the time of writing only 30 cases have been described in the literature, of which approximately half are cases associated with

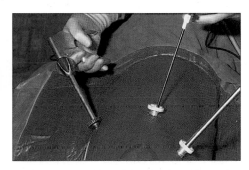

Figure 10.7 Operative ports at videothoracoscopic surgery.

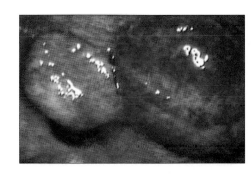

Figure 10.8 Pleural deposit of adenocarcinoma.

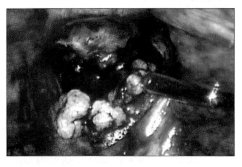

Figure 10.9 Mediastinal tumor deposit in an enlarged azygos node.

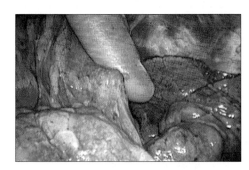

Figure 10.10 Palpation of intrapulmonary nodule during videothoracoscopic assessment.

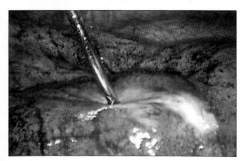

Figure 10.11 Videothoracoscopic needle biopsy.

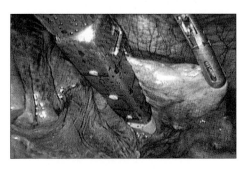

Figure 10.12 Use of endoscopic stapler instrument during video-assisted thoracic surgery biopsy.

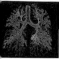
disseminated intrapleural malignancy, notably mesothelioma. Many thousands of VATS procedures have now been performed so the true incidence of such cancer must therefore be extremely low (one author suggests a likely incidence of 0.005%[16]).

Open thoracotomy

Open thoracotomy is an option of last resort, but in some cases no alternative exists. Particular examples include patients in whom fusion of the pleural space has occurred (for whom VATS is not possible), those who have central hilar lesions that require assessment and biopsy under direct vision, and those in whom any other approach is frankly dangerous, such as patients who have lesions in close proximity to the great vessels or heart. Open thoracotomy may be linked with a frozen section so that the surgeon can proceed to definitive resection, as in the case of an undiagnosed hilar mass that is diagnosed at thoracotomy and deemed resectable.

Technique

In most instances the surgeon is likely to attempt a limited thoracotomy, but this is a relative term that has more bearing on the surgeon's view of the situation than that of the patient, for whom it will certainly be a major and disabling procedure. In general, access is gained through the 4th or 5th intercostal space using a 10–20cm thoracotomy incision and a significant degree of rib retraction. The operative view can be surprisingly poor, but this approach carries the great advantage of allowing bimanual palpation, direct tactile and visual guidance, and (if necessary) manual control of the major structures. The chest is closed with pericostal absorbable sutures and one or two intercostal drains remain *in situ* until drainage ceases.

Occasionally, a much more limited approach is adequate – usually because the lesion of interest lies immediately inside the chest wall. A good example of such a situation is in the diagnosis of mesothelioma that has evaded transthoracic biopsy and is associated with pleural fusion. In this case, a 4 or 5cm long incision with resection of 2cm of the underlying rib allows the surgeon to excise a cube of thickened pleura for histologic examination. Clearly, such a limited procedure is entirely different to an open thoracotomy.

The complications relevant to a major open thoracotomy are chiefly respiratory infection, pulmonary embolism, myocardial infarction, bronchopleural fistula, empyema, and pain. Considerable attention to pain relief is required to ensure adequate cooperation with physical therapists and thereby reduce the risk of pulmonary complications. Pain represents a major cause of short- and long-term morbidity after thoracotomy – between 8 and 13% of patients experience permanent, life-impeding symptoms[17].

Mortality after standard thoracotomy is 2–4%, but this is significantly higher in patients deemed inoperable as postoperative pulmonary complications are higher in this group and motivation may be reduced.

CONCLUSION

Surgical techniques provide an array of investigative procedures of varying invasiveness. Most patients can withstand all forms of investigation, so it is always possible to obtain tissue and to make a diagnosis, even to the extent of proceeding to thoracotomy if necessary. The skill of the surgical team lies in obtaining the answer using the least destructive approach possible and in knowing when to stop the investigation. All concerned with the patient's management must recognize that in some instances the cost to the patient of acquiring the information may exceed the value of the information obtained.

REFERENCES

1. Shields TW. Presentation, diagnosis and staging of bronchogenic carcinoma. In: Shields TW. General thoracic surgery, 4th edn. Pennsylvania: Williams & Wilkins; 1994.

2. Kerr KM, Lamb D, Wathen CG, Walker WS, Douglas NJ. Pathological assessment of mediastinal lymph nodes in lung cancer: implications for non-invasive mediastinal staging. Thorax. 1992;47:337–41.

3. Funatsu T, Matsubara Y, Hatakenaka R, Kosaba S, Yasuda Y, Ikeda S. The role of mediastinoscopic biopsy in the preoperative assessement of lung cancer. J Thorac Cardiovasc Surg. 1992;104:1688–95.

4. Ginsberg RJ, Rice TW, Goldberg M, Waters PF, Schmocker BJ. Extended cervical medistinoscopy – a single staging procedure for bronchogenic carcinoma of the left upper lobe. J Thorac Cardiovasc Surg. 1987;94:673–8.

5. Rendina EA, Venuta F, Giacomo TD, et al. Comparative merits of thoracoscopy, mediastinoscopy, and mediastinotomy for mediastinal biopsy. Ann Thorac Surg. 1994;57:992–5.

6. Loddenkemper R. Thoracoscopy – state of the art. Eur Respir J. 1998;11:213–21.

7. Walker WS, Craig SR. Video-assisted thoracoscopic pulmonary surgery – current status and potential evolution. Eur J Cardiothorac Surg. 1996;10:161–7.

8. Lenglinger FX, Schwartz CD, Artmann W. Localization of pulmonary nodules before thoracoscopic surgery: Value of percutaneous staining with methylene blue. Am J Roentgen. 1994;163:297–300.

9. Mack MJ, Shennib H, Landreneau RJ, Hazelrigg SR. Techniques for localization of pulmonary nodules for thoracoscopic resection. J Thorac Cardiovasc Surg. 1993;106:550–3.

10. Shennib H, Bret P. Intraoperative transthoracic ultrasonographic localization of occult lung lesions. Ann Thorac Surg. 1993;55:767–9.

11. Champion JK, McKernan JB. Comparison of minimally invasive thoracoscopy versus open thoracotomy for staging lung cancer. Int Surg. 1996;81:235–6.

12. Roviaro G, Varoli F, Rebuffat C, et al. Videothoracoscopic operative staging for lung cancer. Int Surg. 1996;81:252–4.

13. Waller D, Clarke S, Tsang G, Rajesh P. Is there a role for video-assisted thoracoscopy in the staging of non-small cell lung cancer? Eur J Cardiothorac Surg. 1997;12:214–17

14. Ravini M, Ferraro G, Barbieri B, Colombo P, Rizzato G. Changing strategies of lung biopsies in diffuse lung diseases: The impact of video-assisted thoracoscopy. Eur Respir J. 1998;11:99–103.

15. Landreneau RJ, Mack MJ, Hazelrigg SR, et al. Prevalence of chronic pain after pulmonary resection by thoracoctomy or video-assisted thoracic surgery. J Thorac Cardiovasc Surg. 1995;107:1079–86.

16. Lewis RJ, Caccavale RJ, Sisler GE, Bocage J-P. Does VATS favor seeding of carcinoma of the lung more than a conventional operation? Int Surg. 1997;82:127–30.

17. Dajczman E, Gordon A, Kreisman H, Wolkove N. Long term post-thoracotomy pain. Chest. 1991;99:270–4.

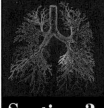

Section 3 Principles of Respiratory Care

Chapter 11 Invasive Mechanical Ventilation

David J Pierson

INTRODUCTION

Although mechanical ventilation is a key component of intensive care, unfamiliar jargon and technical detail render it confusing and formidably difficult for many clinicians. The rapidity and complexity of change in this area of respiratory medicine in recent years adds to the problem.

Figure 11.1 lists a number of factors that are central to a rational approach to mechanical ventilation in acute illness. It is also important that the fundamental goals and objectives of mechanical ventilation (Fig. 11.2)[1,2] be understood, both in general and relative to the individual patient.

INDICATIONS AND CONTRAINDICATIONS

In the absence of a contraindication, mechanical ventilation is indicated whenever any of the circumstances listed under 'clinical objectives' in Figure 11.2 exist to a degree that threatens the life of the patient. Apart from apnea, few individual symptoms, signs, or laboratory findings by themselves always mandate the initiation of ventilatory support. Rather, this therapy becomes

necessary in the presence of the right combination of clinical setting, severity of abnormality, and rapidity of development or worsening of physiologic abnormality.

A summary of the main categories of indications for ventilatory support according to the physiologic mechanism involved is given in Figure 11.3[3].

Inadequate alveolar ventilation

Inadequate alveolar ventilation indicates augmentation of the patient's own ventilatory efforts when its severity indicates an acute threat to life. Alveolar ventilation is most accurately assessed by measuring the arterial partial pressure of carbon dioxide ($PaCO_2$); when the value is higher than normal (e.g. hypercapnia),

Important factors in invasive mechanical ventilation
Clinical setting
Postoperative or other 'routine' mechanical ventilation in patients who have normal lungs
Obstructive lung disease (chronic obstructive pulmonary disease, asthma)
Acute lung injury, acute respiratory distress syndrome
Asymmetric or unilateral pulmonary disease
Neuromuscular disease
Acute brain injury
Flail chest
Patient's underlying pulmonary status
No known pulmonary disease
Obstructive lung disease (chronic obstructive pulmonary disease, asthma)
Restrictive pulmonary disease
Chronic ventilatory failure (underlying carbon dioxide retention)
Volume- versus pressure-targeted ventilation
Volume-targeted: delivered tidal volume fixed, peak airway pressure variable
Pressure-targeted: peak airway pressure fixed, delivered tidal volume variable
Full versus partial ventilatory support
Full ventilatory support: ventilator does all the required work of breathing
Partial ventilatory support: patient must provide at least a portion of required work of breathing

Figure 11.1 Key clinical factors in mechanical ventilation. Primary factors that affect the understanding and successful clinical application of invasive mechanical ventilation.

Goals and objectives of mechanical ventilation
Goals
To replace in whole or in part the gas exchanging functions of the lungs and ventilatory pump in patients whose ability to maintain these functions is temporarily or permanently impaired
To provide these functions with as little disruption of homeostasis and with as few complications as possible
Physiologic objectives
To improve alveolar ventilation, as indicated by arterial pressure of carbon dioxide ($PaCO_2$) and pH
To improve arterial oxygenation, as indicated by PaO_2, saturation, and/or oxygen content
To increase end-inspiratory lung inflation
To increase end-expiratory lung volume (functional residual capacity)
To reduce the work of breathing (i.e. to unload the ventilatory muscles)
Clinical objectives
To reverse acute respiratory acidosis – relief of immediately life-threatening acidemia, rather than necessarily to make $PaCO_2$ and/or pH normal
To reverse hypoxemia – increase PaO_2 [generally such that arterial saturation is 90% or more, e.g. to ≥8kPa (≥60mmHg)] to reverse or prevent clinically important tissue hypoxia
To relieve respiratory distress – improve patient comfort while the primary disease process resolves or improves
To prevent or reverse atelectasis – avoid or correct adverse consequences of incomplete lung inflation
To reverse ventilatory muscle fatigue – unload the ventilatory muscles and allow them to rest while the causes of increased work load are reversed or improved
To permit sedation and/or neuromuscular blockade – render the patient unable to breathe spontaneously, as during surgery or certain intensive care unit procedures
To decrease systemic or myocardial oxygen consumption in certain settings (e.g. severe acute respiratory distress syndrome, cardiogenic shock), when spontaneous breathing or other muscular activity impairs systemic or cardiac oxygenation
To stabilize the chest wall, as in chest wall resection or massive flail chest

Figure 11.2 Goals and objectives of mechanical ventilation. Specific indications and practical application of invasive mechanical ventilation are logical outgrowths of these goals and objectives[1].

Indications for mechanical ventilation

Process	Best available clinical indicators
Inadequate alveolar ventilation	Arterial pressure of carbon dioxide ($PaCO_2$) and pH, considered together
Inadequate lung expansion	Vital capacity, tidal volume, respiratory rate
Inadequate ventilatory muscle strength	Maximum inspiratory pressure, vital capacity, maximum voluntary ventilation
Excessive work of breathing	Minute ventilation required to maintain normal $PaCO_2$, physiologic dead space, respiratory rate
Insufficient or unstable ventilatory drive	Breathing pattern, clinical setting
Severe hypoxemia	[Alveolar PO_2 (PAO_2) – PaO_2]/fraction of inspired oxygen, PAO_2/PaO_2, shunt fraction, venous admixture

Figure 11.3 Indications for mechanical ventilation. Indications for initiation of mechanical ventilation classified according to physiologic process and means of clinical assessment

alveolar hypoventilation is present by definition. However, the severity of acute derangement in alveolar ventilation is judged by arterial pH, and not by the alveolar PCO_2 ($PaCO_2$) *per se*, as many patients who have established ventilatory insufficiency tolerate chronic hypercapnia with no ill effects. In general, an acute rise in $PaCO_2$ such that pH falls below 7.25–7.30 indicates acute ventilatory failure. Patients who suffer acute-on-chronic ventilatory failure, however, such as those who have exacerbations of chronic obstructive pulmonary disease (COPD), can usually be managed without intubation. In such patients, inadequate alveolar ventilation becomes an indication for invasive mechanical ventilation if it is progressive despite aggressive therapy, or if the patient becomes obtunded or unmanageably agitated.

Inadequate lung expansion

Inadequate lung expansion during acute illness may lead to the development of atelectasis or pneumonia, even if alveolar ventilation is adequate as assessed by $PaCO_2$. Inadequate lung expansion may occur during general anesthesia, after upper abdominal operations, following trauma, or in the setting of acute restrictive pulmonary disease. Spontaneous vital capacity (VC) is probably the most practical method of assessment. Rapid shallow breathing, as commonly assessed by the ratio of spontaneous respiratory rate to spontaneous tidal volume (VT) during assessment for weaning (see subsequent section), is also a good indicator of inadequate pulmonary expansion.

Inadequate ventilatory muscle function

Inadequate ventilatory muscle function can lead to inadequate lung expansion, loss of lung compliance, atelectasis, and pneumonia. When severe, inadequate alveolar ventilation results, although ideally ventilatory support is initiated before this late stage occurs. Maximum voluntary ventilation is a useful measure of ventilatory muscle function, although VC and maximum inspiratory pressure (PImax) are more readily assessed. Sequential determinations of these functions can be extremely helpful in following the progression of ventilatory muscle weakness in acute neuromuscular disorders such as Guillain–Barré syndrome. In this setting, mechanical ventilation is initiated when the VC falls to 10–15mL/kg, or the PImax to 20–25cmH$_2$O (2–2.5kPa), rather than waiting for acute respiratory acidosis to develop.

Excessive work of breathing

Excessive work of breathing is manifested by rapid shallow breathing. A respiratory rate in the mid-thirties per minute or higher in an acutely ill patient suggests that the work of breathing may exceed that which is sustainable by the patient. While otherwise healthy individuals can maintain a minute ventilation twice that of normal indefinitely, when the resting ventilation required to maintain a normal $PaCO_2$ exceeds 10–15L/min in the setting of severe acute illness or underlying pulmonary disease, acute respiratory acidosis or inadequate lung expansion may develop. The minute ventilation required to maintain a normal $PaCO_2$ is determined by CO_2 production, which reflects metabolic needs, and dead space ventilation, an index of the efficiency of ventilation. While these factors are rarely measured directly in patients who are not already intubated, consideration should be given to factors that might be expected to increase one or both of them in the acutely ill patient.

Diminished ventilatory drive

Diminished ventilatory drive in relation to metabolic needs is manifested by a decreased respiratory rate or even apnea. It is an independent indication for mechanical ventilation if its cause cannot immediately be reversed. While hypoxic or hypercapnic drive cannot readily be measured at the bedside, the finding of respiratory acidosis in the absence of airway or neuromuscular disease suggests that one or both of these may be impaired. In addition, a risk exists for sudden apnea or life-threatening hypoventilation in the initial hours following closed head injury, drug overdose, or massive cerebrovascular accident, and so ventilatory support may be appropriate in such circumstances, even in the absence of hypercapnia.

Severe hypoxemia by itself is seldom an indication for invasive mechanical ventilation. For example, isolated hypoxemia in patients who have diffuse pneumonia or pulmonary edema can often be managed with high-flow oxygen by mask, with or without continuous positive airway pressure (CPAP). Typically, patients who demonstrate severe hypoxemia in the setting of severe acute illness have other indications for ventilatory support, such as excessive work of breathing or diminished ventilatory drive.

The indications for noninvasive positive-pressure ventilation are discussed in Chapter 12. In general, ventilation via an endotracheal tube rather than a nasal or full-face mask should be selected in cases of acute respiratory failure when:
- patients are unresponsive or sufficiently agitated to preclude cooperation;
- patients' ability to protect their airways from aspiration is impaired;
- excessive respiratory tract secretions are present;
- the cause for acute decompensation is likely to take a number of days to resolve; or
- staff who are properly trained and experienced in noninvasive ventilation are not continuously available.

Contraindications to invasive mechanical ventilation are summarized in Figure 11.4.

TECHNIQUE

Types and modes of mechanical ventilation

A confusing array of possible ways to ventilate a patient's lungs mechanically are available to the clinician, and these are distinguished by numerous variables. Phase variables are used to initiate one of the three phases (trigger, limit, and cycle) of the ventilatory

Contraindications to invasive mechanical ventilation
No indication for ventilatory support exists (see Fig. 11.3)
Noninvasive ventilation is indicated in preference to invasive mechanical ventilation
Intubation and mechanical ventilation are contrary to the patient's expressed wishes
Life-support interventions, including mechanical ventilation, constitute medically futile therapy

Figure 11.4 Contraindications to invasive mechanical ventilation.

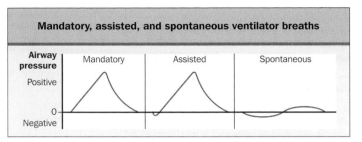

Figure 11.5 Mandatory, assisted, and spontaneous ventilator breaths. Pressures generated at the proximal airway during mandatory, assisted, and spontaneous breaths in a patient who receives mechanical ventilation. In a mandatory breath, all pressure change is positive and all work done on the respiratory system is by the ventilator. An assisted breath involves work by both ventilator and patient – it is delivered by the ventilator under positive pressure, but is initiated (triggered) by the patient's muscular effort, which produces an initially negative pressure deflection. A spontaneous breath reflects only the patient's work, and airway pressure becomes positive only during exhalation as the tidal breath is expelled.

cycle. The trigger variable, which causes inspiration to begin, can be a preset pressure (pressure triggering), a preset volume (volume triggering), a designated flow (flow triggering), or an elapsed time (time triggering). The limit variable is the pressure, volume, or flow target that cannot be exceeded during inspiration. An inspiration may thus be limited when a preset peak airway pressure is reached (pressure limiting), when a preset volume is delivered (volume limiting), or when a preset peak flow is attained (flow limiting). Cycling refers to the factors that terminate inspiration. A breath may be pressure-, volume-, or time-cycled when a preset pressure, volume, flow, or time interval has been reached.

Three different types of breath can be provided during mechanical ventilation, depending upon whether the ventilator or the patient does the work and whether the ventilator or the patient initiates (triggers) the breath. These types are mandatory, assisted, and spontaneous breaths (Fig. 11.5). Mandatory breaths are machine cycled, and are triggered, limited, and cycled by the ventilator. The patient is entirely passive, and the ventilator performs the work of

breathing. Assisted breaths are like mandatory breaths in that they are limited and cycled by the ventilator, but are triggered by the patient. Breathing work is thus partly provided by the ventilator and partly by the patient. Spontaneous breaths are triggered, limited, and cycled by the patient, who performs all the work of breathing.

The relationship between the various possible types of breath and the inspiratory phase variables just discussed is called a mode of ventilation. Figure 11.6 lists and describes the modes currently available for positive-pressure ventilatory support[4].

Types and modes of positive-pressure ventilation		
Type	**Mode**	**Description**
Conventional positive pressure ventilation: tidal volume (VT) preset (volume or time cycled)	Assisted mechanical ventilation or assist/control	All breaths machine delivered at preset VT Patient can increase rate (and thus minute ventilation) by triggering additional machine breaths if desired
	Controlled mechanical ventilation (CMV)	All breaths machine delivered at preset VT Fixed rate (and minute ventilation) cannot be increased by patient effort
	Intermittent mandatory ventilation (IMV)	Fixed rate of machine-delivered, set VT breaths Patient can also breathe spontaneously between machine-delivered breaths if desired
	Synchronized intermittent mandatory ventilation	As in IMV, except that machine-delivered breaths are initiated only after the patient exhales, which prevents 'stacking' on spontaneous breaths
Conventional positive-pressure ventilation: peak pressure preset (flow or time cycled)	Pressure support ventilation	Patient breathes spontaneously and determines rate VT is determined by inflation pressure used and patient's lung–thorax compliance Minute ventilation varies, depending on inflation pressure used
	Pressure control ventilation	Inflation pressure, inspiratory time, and rate are fixed, with VT (and thus minute ventilation) determined by patient's lung–thorax compliance
	Airway pressure release ventilation	Patient breathes spontaneously at high level of continuous positive airway pressure (CPAP), which is intermittently dropped to a lower level to allow brief passive exhalation to a lower lung volume Minute ventilation determined by patient's spontaneous rate and inspiratory effort plus CPAP levels used and frequency of pressure release
High-frequency ventilation	High-frequency positive-pressure ventilation	Preset (usually small) VT, as with assisted mechanical ventilation, CMV, or IMV, at cycling frequencies of 60–110 breaths/minute
	High-frequency jet ventilation	Bursts of high-pressure (jet) gas flow directly into patient's trachea at rates of 60–150 bursts/minute Delivered VT augmented by entrainment from a second, humidified gas source VT and minute ventilation are unknown
	High-frequency oscillatory ventilation	Oscillation of gas in the respiratory tract at 600–1200 cycles/minute (10–20Hz) with both inspiration and expiration active

Figure 11.6 Types and modes of positive-pressure ventilation. Available general types and modes of positive-pressure ventilation, with brief conceptual descriptions of each mode. (Adapted from Pierson[4]).

The distinction between volume-targeted and pressure-targeted ventilation is clinically important. Volume-targeted modes deliver a fixed VT with each breath. This means that airway pressure during a given breath can vary depending on the resistance to air flow during inspiration and on the patient's lung and chest wall compliance. As shown in Figure 11.7, the pressure profile of a volume-targeted breath has several components. Once the breath has been delivered, an end-inspiratory hold maneuver can be performed to measure the static or plateau pressure (PPLAT). The latter is a reflection of lung distention and is used to calculate the static compliance of the respiratory system (equals $\Delta V/\Delta P$). During inspiration, airway pressure reflects the resistance to flow as well as the compliance of the system. Thus, an increase in inspiratory flow, bronchospasm, or airway secretions increases PIMAX, but does not affect PPLAT.

Volume-targeted modes

The most commonly used volume-targeted ventilator modes are shown in Figure 11.8. These are controlled mechanical ventilation (CMV), assist/control (A/C) ventilation, and synchronized intermittent mandatory ventilation (SIMV). With CMV, the patient receives a preset number of fixed-volume breaths and cannot increase minute ventilation by triggering more machine breaths or by breathing spontaneously between them. The difference between A/C ventilation and CMV is that the patient may trigger additional fixed-volume machine breaths if desired. With intermittent mandatory ventilation (IMV), a fixed number of preset-volume breaths is delivered by the ventilator and, if desired (and capable), the patient can also breathe spontaneously from the ventilator circuit. Conceptually, IMV is therefore somewhat like being on both CMV and a T-piece at the same time. The theoretic risk of 'stacking' a mandatory breath on top of a large spontaneous breath, which would produce barotrauma, means that most ventilators deliver IMV in such a way that mandatory breaths can only be delivered after expiration is sensed, called SIMV.

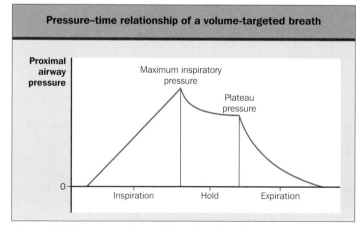

Figure 11.7 Pressure–time relationship of a volume-targeted breath. A single positive-pressure breath, starting from zero end-expiratory pressure. An end-inspiratory hold maneuver is performed to determine static or plateau pressure (PPLAT). Maximum inspiratory pressure (PIMAX) reflects airway resistance during inspiration, and is higher than PPLAT in this volume-targeted breath. Increased inspiratory flow or a narrowing of the airway increases PIMAX, but does not affect PPLAT.

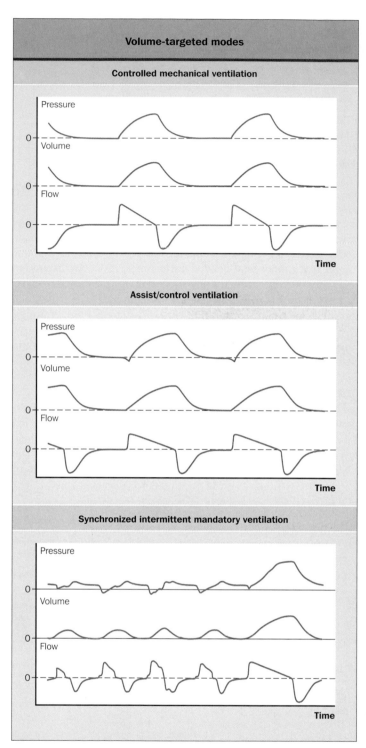

Figure 11.8 Volume-targeted modes. Changes in pressure at the airway opening, lung volume, and flow during controlled mechanical ventilation (CMV), assist/control (A/C) ventilation, and synchronized intermittent mandatory ventilation (SIMV). With CMV, all breaths are machine-triggered mandatory breaths, and the patient is passive throughout the cycle. Essentially, A/C ventilation is the same as CMV, except that the patient may, if desired, trigger the set-volume machine breaths at a more rapid rate. With SIMV, a set number of machine-triggered, mandatory breaths are delivered, as with CMV. However, in SIMV the patient can also breathe spontaneously between mandatory breaths if desired. When the mandatory rate in SIMV is sufficient to provide all the ventilation the patient needs, this mode is effectively the same as CMV.

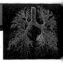

Full ventilatory support is provided by CMV, which means that all work performed on the respiratory system during ventilation is provided by the ventilator (the patient is passive). In A/C ventilation, full ventilatory support is provided when the patient is not triggering, but partial ventilatory support when the patient breathes at a rate greater than the fixed backup rate. In SIMV, full ventilatory support is provided when the patient is not attempting to breathe above the mandatory rate, and partial ventilatory support when any spontaneous ventilation is present.

Pressure-targeted modes

A number of modes are available that preset the maximum inflation pressure rather than a fixed VT. Most widely used among these are pressure support ventilation (PSV) and pressure control ventilation (PCV), illustrated in Figure 11.9.

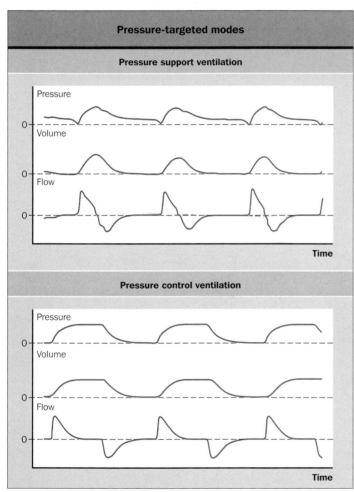

Pressure-targeted modes

Pressure support ventilation

Pressure

0

Volume

0

Flow

0

Time

Pressure control ventilation

Pressure

0

Volume

0

Flow

0

Time

Figure 11.9 Pressure-targeted modes. Changes in pressure at the airway opening, lung volume, and flow during pressure support ventilation (PSV) and pressure control ventilation (PCV). The former is essentially spontaneous breathing with a preset positive pressure that boosts each inspiration. Patients on PSV receive no ventilation if apnea occurs. In that the rate is fixed and the patient cannot trigger additional breaths or breathe spontaneously between mandatory breaths, PCV is analogous to controlled mechanical ventilation (CMV, Fig. 11.8); it differs from CMV in that maximum inspiratory pressure rather than tidal volume is fixed, and both tidal volume and minute ventilation can vary if the patient's lung–thorax compliance or airway resistance changes.

With PSV, the patient breathes spontaneously and is assisted with every breath to a preset inspiratory pressure target. This is conceptually the same as intermittent positive-pressure breathing, although the technical aspects of its delivery are different. Pressure support can be combined with SIMV, so that when the patient takes a spontaneous breath, over and above the set frequency of mandatory volume-targeted breaths, inspiration is assisted to the set pressure support level.

Similar to CMV, in PCV the rate is fixed and cannot be increased by patient effort, but a difference is that it is the peak inflation pressure rather than the VT that is set (Fig. 11.9). Technically, the term for this mode is pressure-controlled continuous mandatory ventilation. On some ventilators it is also possible to deliver pressure-controlled A/C ventilation and SIMV. Pressure-controlled inverse ratio ventilation is not a separate mode, but rather PCV with the inspiratory phase longer than expiration. This variant of PCV has been used in patients who have severe hypoxemic respiratory failure in an attempt to improve oxygenation, but its popularity has waned because of the high incidence of hemodynamic compromise and barotrauma.

A key distinction between volume- and pressure-targeted modes relates to what happens when the mechanics of the patient–ventilator system change. When a patient who receives volume-targeted ventilation develops a pneumothorax or partial airway obstruction by inspissated secretions, the same VT is delivered, but at higher peak and static airway pressures. However, with pressure-targeted ventilation, maximal airway pressure is preset and cannot increase under these circumstances. Instead, with obstruction in the airway or a decrease in compliance, the pressure stays the same and the delivered VT decreases. Thus, the clinician needs to be aware that complications may be manifested differently in the different modes. When managing a patient whose pulmonary process may improve rapidly, as in acute asthma or pulmonary edema, the clinician needs to be prepared to make frequent ventilator adjustments when pressure ventilation is used.

Combined modes

Some ventilators of recent manufacture offer hybrid modes that combine features of volume-targeted and pressure-targeted ventilation, in an attempt to avoid the high peak airway pressures of volume ventilation and also the varying VTs that may occur with pressure ventilation[5]. Manufacturers have attempted to make these combinations unique to their own machines in a competitive market, and as a result several apparently new modes have appeared on the scene. Essentially, these combinations consist either of volume ventilation with high inspiratory flow and a limitation on peak pressure, or pressure ventilation regulated to provide a preset minute ventilation. For example, the Siemens Servo 300 ventilator offers pressure-regulated volume control, in which all breaths are mandatory, the rate is fixed, and the inspiratory pressure is varied to maintain a preset VT. That same ventilator also offers volume support, a combined mode that consists of PSV with a preset target VT or minute volume, which the ventilator achieves by adding mandatory breaths, the inspiratory pressures of which are varied as necessary to achieve the set volume goal.

In Figure 11.10, a comparison is given of the most commonly used volume- and pressure-targeted ventilator modes in terms of their relative advantages and disadvantages.

Advantages and disadvantages of the different commonly used ventilator modes				
Mode	**Advantages**	**Disadvantages**	**Appropriate clinical circumstances**	**Inappropriate clinical circumstances**
Assisted mechanical ventilation (AMV) or assist/control ventilation	Can respond to increased need for ventilation by increasing machine rate Decreased oxygen consumption in patients who have high work of breathing as compared with low-rate intermittent mandatory ventilation (IMV) or spontaneous breathing	Higher mean intrathoracic pressure than with modes that provide partial ventilatory support Respiratory alkalosis in dyspneic or agitated patients if inspiratory flows and/or sedation insufficient	Any patient who requires mechanical ventilation Increased work of spontaneous breathing, as in high minute ventilation or small endotracheal tube Depressed or fluctuating ventilatory drive	Respiratory alkalosis unresponsive to ventilator adjustment and/or sedation Use with Siemens Servo 900C ventilator in dyspneic patient who has normal or low minute ventilation (insufficient flow during inspiration)
Controlled mechanical ventilation (CMV)	Decreased oxygen consumption in patients who have high spontaneous work of breathing Rests ventilatory muscles Least complicated and least expensive mode for long-term ventilation	Cannot respond to increased need for ventilation by either machine-delivered or spontaneous breaths Patient distress if alert and dyspneic Usually requires heavy sedation with or without paralysis	Paralysis or neurologic injury rendering patient incapable of any spontaneous ventilation Deliberate hyperventilation to reduce intracranial pressure	Any patient who is capable of triggering a ventilator breath
Intermittent mandatory ventilation (IMV); synchronized IMV	May reduce patient–ventilator asynchrony Lower mean intrathoracic pressure than with AMV if used for partial ventilatory support Can provide periodic deep breaths to prevent atelectasis in intubated patients who have very low spontaneous tidal volumes (VTS)	Cannot respond to increased patient demand with increased ventilator minute volume Increased work of breathing for patient as compared with AMV when used for partial ventilatory support May decrease total time on ventilator when used for gradual weaning	Any patient who requires invasive mechanical ventilation, provided inappropriate circumstances (next column) are not present Use for partial ventilatory support in patients who have hypovolemia and hypotension on AMV As an alternative volume-targeted mode when patients do not tolerate AMV	Use as partial ventilatory support in patients who have depressed or fluctuating ventilatory drive, ventilatory muscle paralysis or weakness, or in the presence of a small-diameter endotracheal tube
Pressure support ventilation	Increased peak inspiratory flow as compared with volume modes Lower mean intrathoracic pressure than with AMV or IMV Less distressing than volume-preset modes for some patients Can provide smooth transition to spontaneous ventilation during weaning	VT and minute ventilation are not assured Hypoventilation or apnea if patient's ventilatory drive fluctuates Requires closer monitoring of gas exchange and mechanics in critically ill patients than do AMV or IMV Repeated triggering of apnea alarm in patients who have Cheyne–Stokes respiration	As a stand-alone mode for patients who have intact ventilatory drive and who require modest inflation pressures As a transitional mode during recovery from severe acute respiratory distress syndrome (ARDS) or other acute respiratory failure During weaning in any patient in whom decreasing the level of ventilatory support is appropriate	Absent or fluctuating ventilatory drive Rapidly changing lung or chest wall mechanics (e.g. bronchospasm; pulmonary edema) because of need for repeated pressure adjustments
Pressure control ventilation	Increased peak inspiratory flow as compared with volume modes Improved distribution of ventilation in some patients who have severe oxygenation failure, and results in improved oxygenation and/or decreased alveolar pressure in comparison with AMV or IMV	VT and minute ventilation are not assured Requires closer monitoring of gas exchange and mechanics than AMV or IMV Need to switch to another mode for weaning	Critically ill patients who have ARDS or other severe acute respiratory failure when appropriately skilled personnel are continuously available	Use for routine ventilatory support Use in any patient when personnel experienced with its use are not available on a continuous basis

Figure 11.10 Advantages and disadvantages of different ventilator modes. A comparison of the commonly used volume and pressure preset modes of mechanical ventilation, which shows the relative advantages and disadvantages of each, along with clinical circumstances considered appropriate and inappropriate for their use.

Positive end-expiratory pressure

Manipulation of inspiration by means of the phase variables and modes just discussed is one of the two main processes involved in mechanical ventilation. The other is manipulation of end-expiratory pressure, which may be kept equal to that of the atmosphere or deliberately raised to produce positive end-expiratory pressure (PEEP). The application of PEEP has two primary purposes:

* to increase lung volume in patients who have acute lung restriction that produces hypoxemia; and
* to reduce the effort required for patients to trigger the ventilator or breathe spontaneously in the presence of dynamic hyperinflation and auto-PEEP (see below).

When PEEP is applied to the breathing circuit connected to the closed respiratory system of an intubated patient, all breaths start and end at a pressure above ambient. Continuous pressurization of the system from which a patient breathes spontaneously is referred to as CPAP, a term applicable only during spontaneous breathing. Whenever positive pressure above the end-expiratory level is applied during inspiration, the term PEEP is used.

As end-expiratory, end-inspiratory, and mean airway pressures are all increased in the presence of PEEP, the potential exists for a fall in cardiac output because of diminished venous return to the right side of the heart. Regional or generalized lung overdistention can also stretch pulmonary vessels, which reduces their caliber and increases pulmonary vascular resistance. In the presence of a reduced cardiac output secondary to either or both of these mechanisms, any gain in arterial oxygenation may be offset, and tissue oxygen delivery may actually fall. In addition, the application of

Protocol for systematic positive end-expiratory pressure trial	
Protocol	**Comments**
1. Obtain baseline respiratory and hemodynamic data before initiating positive end-expiratory pressure (PEEP) and at each level employed in trial	Respiratory data (all patients) – fraction of inspired oxygen (FIO_2), PEEP level, corrected tidal volume, respiratory rate (mandatory, total), peak inspiratory pressure, end-inspiratory plateau pressure, partial pressure of arterial blood gases (PaO_2, $PaCO_2$), and pH
	Additional respiratory data (in extremely ill or unstable patients, or for more aggressive management approach) – mixed venous PO_2 and saturation, arterial and mixed venous O_2 contents
	Hemodynamic data (all patients) – heart rate, blood pressure, continuous electrocardiographic monitoring
	Cardiac output measurement – recommended for use of PEEP >15cmH$_2$O, suspected hypovolemia (unexplained tachycardia), or coexistent cardiac disease
2. Change only one variable at a time (i.e. PEEP level)	Keep tidal volume, FIO_2, and other ventilator settings the same at each level
	Avoid transfusion, position changes, changes in pressor infusions during trial if possible
3. Keep time intervals between PEEP increments short (e.g. 15–20 minutes)	To minimize confounding data from changes in patient's underlying condition
4. Apply PEEP in sequential increments (e.g. 5cmH$_2$O)	Smaller increments may prolong trial
	Larger increments increase likelihood of adverse effects
5. Monitor for immediate adverse effects at each new PEEP level (e.g. after 3–5 minutes)	Hypotension or >20% fall in cardiac output
	Fall in respiratory system compliance
	Cardiac arrhythmias or increased intracranial pressure, where appropriate
6. Assess arterial oxygenation and other respiratory data collection as in step 1 above once patient has stabilized at each new PEEP level (e.g. 15 minutes)	–
7. Evaluate overall cardiorespiratory response at each PEEP level used	Favorable – improved oxygenation, improved compliance
	Unfavorable – hypotension, decreased cardiac output, decreased compliance, decreased oxygenation
8. Assess results in light of overall goals for PEEP therapy	If O_2 delivery has improved without adverse effects, leave patient on current PEEP level, reduce FIO_2 if possible, and reevaluate frequently as indicated
	If oxygenation is still inadequate or FIO_2 is still unacceptably high, and no adverse effects have occurred, increase PEEP sequentially, applying steps 4–7 above.
	If O_2 delivery has decreased or compliance has fallen significantly at new PEEP level, return patient to previous PEEP level and re-evaluate if:
	Deterioration results from decreased PO_2, reassess indications for PEEP
	Deterioration results from decreased cardiac output, consider volume loading or administration of pressor drugs
	Compliance has fallen but O_2 delivery has not decreased, consider reducing tidal volume to reduce risk of alveolar rupture and ventilator-induced lung injury

Figure 11.11 Protocol for systematic trial of positive end-expiratory pressure (PEEP) in acute respiratory distress syndrome (ARDS) or other acute hypoxemic respiratory failure. Depending upon the goals and overall therapeutic approach being employed, arterial oxygenation and systemic oxygen delivery are optimal at some point between 10 and 20cmH$_2$O of PEEP in most patients who have ARDS. 10cmH$_2$O = 1kPa.

PEEP may increase end-inspiratory lung volume to the point at which individual lung units become overdistended and rupture alveolar membranes, which leads to clinical barotrauma.

The positive end-expiratory pressure trial

Whenever feasible a systematic, incremental 'PEEP trial' should be performed in as controlled a manner as possible (Fig. 11.11). Ideally, only one variable – the amount of PEEP – is altered during the trial, with VT, fraction of inspired oxygen (FIO_2), position, and other factors that might affect oxygenation unchanged. An assessment for both favorable and adverse PEEP effects is made at each level as PEEP increased. As the condition of the patient may change over time, to determine the effects of PEEP most clearly the intervals at each level must be kept short.

As PEEP is increased, the occurrence of cardiac impairment becomes progressively more likely. Direct measurement of cardiac output during the trial is recommended if any of the following circumstances exist:

- levels of PEEP are to be used that are likely to impair cardiac function [e.g. 15cmH$_2$O (1.5kPa) or more];

- unexplained tachycardia or other manifestations of possible hypovolemia are present; or
- the patient has underlying cardiac disease.

Changes in cardiac output and lung compliance are likely to occur rapidly following an increase in PEEP, and should be sought within the first 3–5 minutes at each level.

As PEEP is increased, PaO_2 is measured sequentially as the primary index of a favorable response. If a substantial increase in PaO_2 occurs with no evidence of either cardiac impairment or alveolar overdistention (as assessed using static compliance), that PEEP level can be maintained and the FIO_2 titrated downward to maintain the target PaO_2. Improvement in PaO_2 tends to occur more slowly than changes in cardiac function or compliance as PEEP is increased, and arterial blood gas specimens should be drawn 10–20 minutes after each change. Suggested guidelines are given in Figure 11.11.

Weaning positive end-expiratory pressure

If PEEP is reduced prematurely, some alveoli may remain sufficiently unstable to collapse, which worsens oxygenation. If this

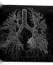
happens, PEEP higher than the previous baseline level may be required to reopen the collapsed alveoli and, conceivably, the patient's requirement for mechanical ventilation may be unnecessarily prolonged. It is thus important to be able to predict when patients are 'ready' for PEEP weaning. The protocol given in Figure 11.12 is designed to facilitate PEEP withdrawal while protecting the patient from possible worsening of hypoxemia[6].

For patients whose arterial oxygenation has previously been shown to be 'PEEP responsive', the following criteria should be met before PEEP is reduced:

- hemodynamic stability with no changes in PEEP during the previous 6–12 hours;
- no signs of sepsis present; and
- adequate arterial oxygenation, as shown by a ratio of PaO_2 to FIO_2 of 26.6kPa (200mmHg) or more.

Using the protocol in Figure 11.12, maximum protection from unintended hypoxemia caused by premature PEEP weaning can be achieved if a 3-minute trial of PEEP reduction is carried out.

Guidelines for ventilator management according to clinical setting

Guidelines for ventilator management according to clinical setting are given in Figure 11.13.

Routine ventilatory support

Most patients who require a period of invasive mechanical ventilation have relatively normal underlying lung function. What may be referred to as 'routine ventilatory support' is encountered most frequently in the postoperative period or in the setting of short-term loss of spontaneous ventilation, such as with a drug overdose. In such settings, a volume-targeted mode such as A/C ventilation is simplest and most reliable, and usually requires fewer adjustments than does pressure-targeted ventilation. Some clinicians prefer to add 5cmH$_2$O (0.5kPa) of PEEP routinely in order to counteract the modest drop in functional residual capacity (FRC) that has been shown to occur with endotracheal intubation, although this is probably unnecessary in most patients.

Healthy individuals normally breathe with a VT of 5–7mL/kg. However, diffuse microatelectasis and an increased difference in alveolar and arterial PO_2 (PAO_2 – PaO_2) soon develops because of decreased surfactant function if these individuals do not more fully expand their lungs several times per hour by sighing. The same problem exists with intubated patients who have normal lungs and who are ventilated with 'normal' VTs in the absence of sigh breaths. The need for sighs, which in the presence of pulmonary disease might overdistend and rupture alveoli, can be obviated if a larger VT (10–12mL/kg) is used.

The cycling rate and hence minute ventilation are adjusted to provide normal arterial pH and PCO_2 values [e.g. 7.40 ± 0.05 units and 5.3 ± 0.6kPa (40 ± 5mmHg), respectively]. Enough supplemental oxygen is used to prevent hypoxemia, although maintaining PaO_2 >13.3kPa (>100mmHg) is unnecessary.

Obstructive lung disease

Compared with individuals who do not have chronic lung disease, patients who have severe COPD or asthma are at increased risk for circulatory impairment and barotrauma when subjected to invasive mechanical ventilation, and a number of modifications of the routine approach are required to avoid these[7].

The most common problem is pulmonary hyperinflation, which patients who suffer obstructive lung disease typically have at baseline, and which worsens during times of acute exacerbation. The three main goals of invasive mechanical ventilation in patients who have acutely exacerbated COPD or acute severe asthma are to:

Protocol for reduction of positive end-expiratory pressure in acute respiratory distress syndrome	
Protocol	**Comment**
1. Patient meets the following criteria for a reduction in positive end-expiratory pressure (PEEP):	
Hemodynamic stability and no changes in PEEP	For at least 6–12h
No clinical signs of sepsis	Features that suggest sepsis include tachycardia, fever or hypothermia, leukocytosis or leukopenia, high cardiac output, and low systemic vascular resistance, with or without positive blood cultures
Oxygenation acceptable on acceptable fraction of inspired oxygen (FIO$_2$)	Arterial partial pressure of oxygen (PaO$_2$) 10.6kPa (80mmHg) or higher on FIO$_2$ 0.40 or less
2. Obtain baseline respiratory and hemodynamic data, including arterial blood gases (as described in Figure 11.11 and as clinically indicated)	Arterial saturation as measured by pulse oximetry is a poor estimate of the change in arterial oxygenation with PEEP reduction unless the PaO$_2$ falls below 8.5–9.3kPa (65–70mmHg); however, pulse oximetry may afford an additional element of safety during PEEP weaning if the initial PaO$_2$ is about 10.6kPa (80mmHg) or less
3. Reduce PEEP level by 5cmH$_2$O	Smaller decrements (e.g. 2.5cmH$_2$O) may be appropriate in pediatric patients or in unstable adults, although this slows the PEEP reduction process unnecessarily for the majority of patients
4. After 3 minutes, obtain a second specimen for arterial blood gas analysis and return PEEP to previous level while awaiting results	As in step 2
5. Compare prereduction and 3-minute PaO$_2$ values	A substantial fall in PaO$_2$ (e.g. more than 20%) suggests that the patient's oxygenation may deteriorate and/or be slow to recover if PEEP is reduced at this point; the PEEP level should be maintained at the higher level for another 6–12h before a repeat PEEP wean is considered
	Satisfactory oxygenation (e.g. no change, or <20% drop in PaO$_2$) on the 3-minute specimen indicates that the PEEP may be decreased by 5cmH$_2$O, with repeat assessment, as in step 2 above, as clinically indicated during the next several hours

Figure 11.12 Positive end-expiratory pressure (PEEP) weaning protocol. The criteria and protocol shown here are intended to prevent inadvertent, premature reduction in PEEP, with subsequent clinical deterioration, as occurs frequently when these or similar procedures are not used. 10cmH$_2$O = 1kPa.

- rest the ventilatory muscles;
- avoid further dynamic hyperinflation; and
- avoid overventilation and acute alkalemia.

Resting the ventilatory muscles may be achieved either by providing full ventilatory support using volume-targeted ventilation (with either A/C ventilation or SIMV), so that the patient makes no respiratory effort, or by providing partial ventilatory support using PSV, such that tachypnea and respiratory distress are relieved. The author prefers the former strategy, using V_TS of 5–8mL/kg and rapid inspiratory flow (e.g. 80–100L/min) to maximize expiratory time and avoid air trapping (see subsequent section on auto-PEEP).

This is one of the two clinical settings in which permissive hypercapnia is appropriate, the other being acute lung injury as discussed below. When the degree of air flow limitation is severe, it may not be possible to provide a sufficient minute ventilation (i.e. respiratory rate × V_T) to reduce the $PaCO_2$ enough to produce a normal pH without a resultant worsening hyperinflation. In obstructive lung disease, PEEP serves a different function than in acute lung injury. Its purpose here is not to increase lung volume (which is already excessive), but to decrease the muscular effort required to trigger the ventilator or breathe spontaneously in the presence of dynamic hyperinflation and auto-PEEP.

Acute lung injury

The goals of mechanical ventilation in acute lung injury and the acute respiratory distress syndrome (ARDS) are to:

- support oxygenation;
- avoid circulatory compromise; and
- avoid ventilator-induced lung injury.

The first of these goals is accomplished through manipulations of FIO_2 and PEEP, the aim of which is to balance the risks of pulmonary oxygen toxicity with those of raised intrathoracic

Guidelines for ventilator settings according to diagnosis and clinical circumstances							
Clinical setting (examples)	Clinical objectives	Mode	Tidal volume	Target pH/partial pressure of carbon dioxide ($PaCO_2$)	Target PaO_2/Oxygen saturation by pulse oximetry (SpO_2)	Positive end-expiratory pressure (PEEP)	Comments
Routine (postoperative ventilation, drug overdose)	Prevent atelectasis, maintain normal acid–base balance, avoid hypoxemia, avoid O_2 toxicity	Volume	10–12mL/kg	Normal	Normal	0–5cmH$_2$O	These settings are appropriate for the majority of patients who require mechanical ventilation
Obstructive lung disease (chronic obstructive pulmonary disease, asthma)	Unload ventilatory muscles, prevent further hyperinflation, maintain acid–base balance appropriate for patient, facilitate weaning	Either volume or pressure	5–8mL/kg	Permissive hypercapnia and acidemia (avoid acute alkalosis)	Normal	0–5cmH$_2$O; more if auto-PEEP present (see Fig. 11.21)	Noninvasive ventilation is preferable if not contraindicated (see Chapter 12)
Acute lung injury [acute respiratory distress syndrome (ARDS)]	Support oxygenation (fraction of inspired oxygen versus PEEP), preserve circulatory function, avoid worsening lung injury, avoid clinical barotrauma	Either volume or pressure	5–8mL/kg	Permissive hypercapnia and acidemia (if not contraindicated)	Mild to moderate – normal; severe ARDS – PaO_2 6.6–8.0kPa (50–60mmHg); SpO_2 80–90%	At least 8–10cmH$_2$O, sufficient to maintain PO_2 target without decreasing cardiac output or compliance	This 'lung-protective' ventilatory strategy requires appropriate sedation
Focal or unilateral pulmonary disease (lobar pneumonia or atelectasis)	Avoid worsening hypoxemia, avoid clinical barotrauma, avoid circulatory compromise	Volume	10–12mL/kg	Normal	Normal; may not be achievable in presence of large shunt effect	Avoid or use cautiously (see Fig. 11.11)	PEEP may worsen hypoxemia by overdistending uninvolved areas of lung and increasing shunt effect
Acute neuromuscular disease without acute lung injury (Guillain–Barré syndrome, cervical spinal cord injury)	Avoid atelectasis, minimize dyspnea	Volume	12–16mL/kg	Normal or mild acute respiratory alkalosis	Normal (avoid even mild hypoxemia)	0–5cmH$_2$O unless required for oxygenation	Such patients usually prefer high inspiratory flows and large tidal volumes, and often maintain a respiratory alkalosis
Acute brain injury (head trauma)	Avoid compromising cerebral perfusion pressure, decrease intracranial pressure	Volume	10–12mL/kg	Normal or acute respiratory alkalosis [$PaCO_2$ 3.3–4.0kPa (25–30mmHg)]	Normal	Avoid	Value of acute respiratory alkalosis disputed except for emergent, short-term reduction of very high intracranial pressure
Flail chest	Maintain adequate lung inflation and gas exchange	Volume	10–12mL/kg unless acute lung injury also present	Normal	Normal	5cmH$_2$O or as needed for support of oxygenation	Ventilatory support usually unnecessary unless acute lung injury also present

Figure 11.13 Initial ventilator settings. Considerations in choosing initial ventilator settings for patients in different diagnostic categories. For further discussion see text. Acceptable volume modes include assist/control and synchronized intermittent mandatory ventilation; acceptable pressure modes include pressure control or (in patients who have intact ventilatory drive and the ability to initiate breaths) pressure support.

Weaning technique

Different approaches to discontinuing ventilatory support abound. However, the time-honored T-piece method remains the favorite of many experienced clinicians, after both short-term and long-term mechanical ventilation. The traditional weaning method (Fig. 11.15) is to assess the weaning parameters listed in Figure 11.16, and (if they are satisfactory) to give the patient a trial of spontaneous breathing through a T-piece or 'blow-by' circuit, which reduces the resistance to breathing to just that imposed by the endotracheal tube. After an interval, if the patient's clinical condition remains good, an arterial blood gas specimen is analyzed to confirm that gas exchange is adequate, and weaning is complete.

For more difficult cases, as with prolonged mechanical ventilation in acute respiratory failure or in patients who have a serious underlying illness in other organ systems, it is helpful to approach weaning in a systematic fashion, considering possible impediments to success in approximate order of their likelihood, as summarized in Figure 11.17. In most cases of initial weaning failure, the reason becomes apparent on proceeding through the algorithm in a stepwise fashion. Indeed, perhaps the most common reason for inability to wean from mechanical ventilation among patients who have been critically ill for a week or more is that the primary illness has not improved sufficiently for weaning to be achievable.

When patients are unable to be weaned because of a high minute ventilation requirement, as is commonly seen in ARDS, the clinician may be helped by an analysis of the physiologic mechanism responsible. Only three basic mechanisms can account for a higher than normal minute ventilation: hyperventilation (i.e. respiratory alkalosis), increased carbon dioxide production, and increased dead space ventilation [dead space volume $(V_D)/V_T$]. Hyperventilation is readily identified by the presence of hypocapnia. Carbon dioxide production and V_D/V_T can be assessed either by collecting expired gas in a bag or using a metabolic cart (as used for determining nutritional requirements), in conjunction with an arterial blood sample. Making these simple measurements can aid in identifying the reason for a high minute ventilation:

- if increased carbon dioxide production is the cause, the clinical problem is a systemic rather than pulmonary one – perhaps the patient is receiving excessive nutritional support; and
- if increased V_D/V_T is responsible, increased ventilation requirement results from inefficient ventilation, as seen with ARDS, dynamic hyperinflation, or pulmonary thromboembolism.

The main techniques currently in use for gradual weaning from ventilatory support are the T-piece method, SIMV, and PSV. The time-honored T-piece method consists of repetitive periods of spontaneous ventilation (as described in Fig. 11.15) to the patient's tolerance, interspersed with periods of rest with full ventilatory support. Weaning with SIMV consists of gradually reducing the mandatory rate and thus progressively decreasing the ventilator's contribution to the required minute ventilation, using the total respiratory rate (mandatory plus spontaneous breaths) and other clinical signs as indicators of progress. When PSV is used in weaning, the patient is switched from full ventilatory support to PSV at an inspiratory pressure sufficient to provide the same V_T as before; inspiratory pressure is then gradually reduced, using the patient's respiratory rate (usually maintained below 30 breaths/min) as a guide to the adequacy of support.

Traditional weaning protocol	
Criteria	**Comments**
Fulfill predetermined objective criteria	Overall clinical condition improved
	Patient awake and cooperative
	Most or all of the weaning criteria listed in Figure 11.16 met
Choose appropriate time and setting	No concurrent procedures, meals, bathing, family visits, etc.
	Adequate nursing and respiratory care staffing
Eliminate or minimize respiratory depressants	Narcotics, anxiolytics discontinued or reduced
Optimize bronchodilator therapy	If patient has obstructive lung disease
Position patient appropriately	Sitting or semi-upright if possible
	Chest and abdomen unencumbered
Suction airway as appropriate	
Switch patient to spontaneous ventilation	T-piece (blow-by) circuit or through ventilator circuit in continuous positive airway pressure (CPAP) mode
	CPAP 5cmH$_2$O optional
Observe patient for signs of respiratory distress	
Assess adequacy of oxygenation and alveolar ventilation	Arterialblood gas analysis after 20–30 minutes

Figure 11.15 Traditional weaning protocol. This protocol is especially effective after short-term ventilatory support. It is based on a physiologic prediction of the patient's ability to breathe spontaneously, and enables patients who no longer need mechanical ventilation to be weaned quickly without having to proceed through sequential reductions in support. Readiness for weaning is confirmed by arterial blood gas analysis.

Predictors of readiness to wean
Arterial partial pressure of oxygen (PaO$_2$) ≥10.6kPa (≥80mmHg) on inspired oxygen fraction (FIO$_2$) ≤0.40 (PaO$_2$/FIO$_2$ >200)
Vital capacity at least 10mL/kg
Minute ventilation to maintain normal PaCO$_2$ ≤10–12L/min
Ability to generate required minute ventilation spontaneously
Ratio of spontaneous respiratory rate to spontaneous tidal volume (rapid shallow breathing index) 100 or less
Maximum inspiratory force ≥20cmH$_2$O

Figure 11.16 Predictors of readiness to wean.

When a patient fails an attempt at weaning it is tempting to ascribe this to the weaning technique employed, and to assume that a different approach might succeed. However, when appropriately used, the differences in efficacy between the different weaning techniques are very small, if any. Two much-discussed multicenter trials compared T-piece, SIMV, and PSV weaning in difficult-to-wean patients[15,16]. Both found that SIMV was the least successful approach, but one[15] favored PSV weaning while the other[16] found that T-piece weaning was most effective. It is most unlikely that additional studies will reveal a 'best' technique for weaning. Instead, while prolonged SIMV is probably the least desirable approach, whether PSV or the T-piece method is used is up to the individual clinician. With either approach, the factors shown in the algorithm (see Fig. 11.17) must be considered, and care taken not to prolong a level of ventilatory support that fatigues and distresses the patient.

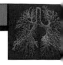

Clinical algorithm for ventilator weaning

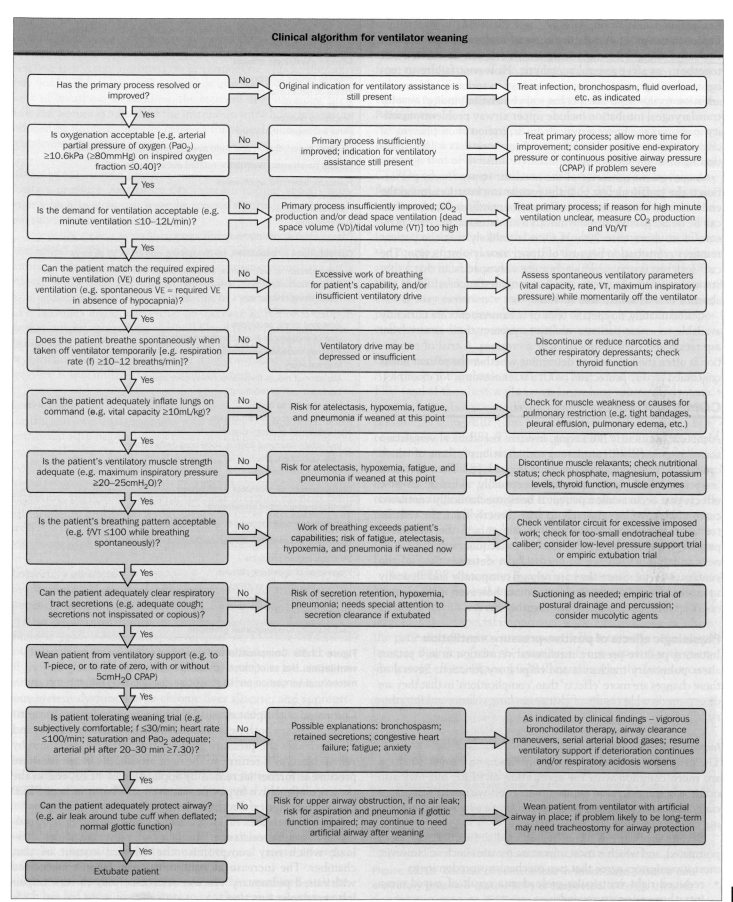

Figure 11.17 Clinical algorithm for weaning patients from mechanical ventilation. This step-by-step approach is especially helpful in cases in which patients have failed previous weaning attempts or are otherwise difficult to wean. $10cmH_2O = 1kPa$.

Prevention of barotrauma
Use small tidal volumes in patients who have obstructive lung disease or other cause for pulmonary hyperinflation
Decrease tidal volume as positive end-expiratory pressure (PEEP) is increased
Use PEEP cautiously in patients at increased risk:
Unilateral, patchy, or cavitary lung disease
Nosocomial pneumonia or sepsis syndrome
Acute respiratory distress syndrome late in clinical course (e.g. after 1–2 weeks)
Chronic obstructive pulmonary disease or asthma
Monitor respiratory system compliance during PEEP trials as a predictor of increased risk for alveolar rupture
Avoid or promptly correct right mainstem bronchus intubation
Avoid end-inspiratory pause
Keep short inspiration:long expiration ratio low
Monitor patient for auto-PEEP; follow steps in Figure 11.21 to reduce it if present

Figure 11.24 Practical steps to minimize the likelihood of barotrauma during mechanical ventilation.

gases and a bedside chest radiograph. On rare occasions, if the patient appears in extremis and tension pneumothorax cannot be excluded at the bedside, empiric measures to drain the chest may be warranted.

Deteriorating oxygenation in the ventilated patient

Deteriorating arterial oxygenation during mechanical ventilation, a common reason for 'fighting the ventilator', should initiate a systematic search for specific mechanisms and therapy rather than simply an increase in F_{IO_2} or level of PEEP. Possible causes for worsening oxygenation fall into several categories[23].

The problem could be with the ventilator and its circuitry. The patient's primary disease process (e.g. pneumonia, ARDS) could be worsening, or a new medical problem may have appeared. Examples of the last include pneumothorax, acute lobar atelectasis, pulmonary edema from fluid overload, nosocomial pneumonia or sepsis, aspiration of gastric contents, retained secretions, and bronchospasm. A fall in cardiac output can also cause worsening oxygenation in a patient who has significant pulmonary venous admixture.

Interventions and procedures can also lead to a decline in oxygenation. Examples include the effects of airway suctioning, chest physical therapy, or even changes in body position, especially in patients affected by heterogeneously distributed pulmonary involvement. Bronchoscopy, thoracentesis, and hemodialysis can also lead to a decline in oxygenation. Finally, a number of drugs administered to patients undergoing mechanical ventilation can interfere with arterial oxygenation. Among these are vasodilators (which can decrease hypoxic vasoconstriction), β-blockers (which can depress cardiac output and induce bronchospasm), and bronchodilators (which can alter ventilation/perfusion ratios).

Effects of suboptimal ventilator management

Some adverse effects of mechanical ventilation are iatrogenic. With increasing complexity of the ventilators and their modes, it becomes more likely that the physician, nurse, or respiratory therapist who adjusts the ventilator may not fully understand the consequences of a given adjustment. Figure 11.25 lists several such iatrogenic problems, the clinical circumstances in which they typically occur, and steps to prevent or correct them.

PITFALLS AND CONTROVERSIES

Few aspects of invasive mechanical ventilation rest on the firm foundation of scientific data. As it is carried out in critically ill patients, in whom controlled trials are exceedingly difficult to conduct, mechanical ventilation remains largely empiric, driven very much by the biases of the individual clinician. In the literature, at conferences, and at the bedside, ongoing debate occurs as to the best mode, the best monitors, and the best end points for the management of mechanical ventilation. In very few instances do good data support a 'best' anything in this field. The approaches offered in this chapter are those of the author, developed through many years of experience in the course of managing thousands of patients, but no pretense is made that these are the only or necessarily the best ways to carry out mechanical ventilation.

Of numerous areas of unresolved controversy, brief discussion is given here of oxygen toxicity and ventilator-induced lung injury.

Oxygen toxicity

After the desire to avoid high peak airway pressures, the drive to prevent pulmonary oxygen toxicity[24] is a dominant force in shaping ventilator management in critically ill patients. In experimental animals and normal human volunteers signs of oxygen toxicity appear within hours of exposure to high F_{IO_2}, and 100% oxygen can be fatal in a day or two. The bountiful data that document these statements have led many intensivists to assume that serious or even fatal oxygen toxicity is a threat to the ventilated patient if the F_{IO_2} cannot be decreased to 0.50 or sometimes considerably less within one to several days.

Yet there is a discrepancy between the results of laboratory studies and observations in the intensive care unit. Although it is difficult to separate the signs of potential oxygen toxicity from those of ARDS or other primary processes that causes respiratory failure, the author is not convinced that any instance of oxygen toxicity has occurred in a critically ill patient, despite administration of 70 or even 100% oxygen, when necessary, for many days. Evidence from animal experiments supports the notion that critical illness, and especially severe hypoxemia, prevents or ameliorates the toxic effects of oxygen on the lung.

Whether high F_{IO_2} is injurious to the lungs or not, the measures used to avoid oxygen toxicity have adverse effects that are unquestioned, frequent, and potentially life threatening.

How one balances the somewhat nebulous threat of oxygen toxicity against the likelihood of adverse effects from high levels of PEEP remains an individual decision. However, several guidelines seem prudent regardless of the philosophic approach used. A PEEP trial must be used to determine the best level for the patient, with adjustments guided by the patient's course. No more oxygen should be used than is necessary to saturate the hemoglobin, and in severe ARDS arterial saturation levels of 80–90% [PaO_2 6.6–8.0kPa (50–60mmHg)] should be accepted. Consideration must be given to erythrocyte transfusion in the presence of anemia, to increase arterial oxygen content. The F_{IO_2} must be adjusted downward as rapidly as possible as the patient improves.

Ventilator-induced lung injury

The 'lung-protective strategy' for ventilatory management described earlier is intended to prevent or reduce ventilator-induced lung injury. Studies that use experimental animals

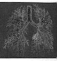

Suboptimal ventilator management that adversely affects patients		
Problem	**Clinical setting**	**Prevention or correction**
Unintended hyperventilation (acute respiratory alkalosis)	'Normalizing' arterial partial pressure of carbon dioxide ($PaCO_2$) in patient with 'acute-on-chronic' carbon dioxide retention	Recognize underlying metabolic alkalosis (high serum bicarbonate) Use arterial pH, not $PaCO_2$, as guide for ventilator adjustments
	Too-rapid ventilator cycling in assist-control mode	Adjust triggering sensitivity to minimum level that prevents spontaneous cycling (e.g. $1–1.5cmH_2O$) Make sure inspiratory flow is sufficient for patient's needs Sedate patient if needed
Unintended hypoventilation (acute respiratory acidosis)	Unstable or fluctuating ventilatory drive in patient on low synchronized intermittent mandatory ventilation (SIMV) rate (potential for variable patient contribution to required minute ventilation)	Increase SIMV rate to meet patient's total minute ventilation requirement Switch to assist/control (A/C) ventilation mode
	Back-up rate set too far below patient's triggering rate in A/C ventilation	Increase back-up rate to 2–3 breaths/min less than patient's stable triggering rate
Excessive patient work of breathing	Low SIMV rate with small-diameter endotracheal tube or weak and/or fatigued patient	Increase SIMV rate to provide all or most of patient's required minute ventilation Switch to A/C mode Add inspiratory pressure support sufficient to overcome tube resistance
	T-piece trial with small-diameter endotracheal tube A/C mode with excessive triggering effort	Add inspiratory pressure support sufficient to overcome tube resistance at patient's required minute ventilation Adjust trigger/assist sensitivity to $1–1.5cmH_2O$
Inappropriate use of neuromuscular blocking agents	Patient who previously was tolerant now 'fighting the ventilator'	Disconnect patient from circuit and ventilate manually to make sure ventilator is functioning normally (volume; pressure; flow pattern) Rapidly assess airway patency, symmetry of chest expansion, vital signs, and other monitoring data Perform more complete patient assessment and adjust ventilator settings as clinically indicated
	Unintended hyperventilation (acute respiratory alkalosis)	Recognize underlying metabolic alkalosis (high serum bicarbonate) – use arterial pH, not $PaCO_2$, as guide for ventilator adjustments Sedate patient with appropriate agent (e.g. benzodiazepine) if above does not apply and assessment of patient and ventilator reveals no acute problem
	Neuromuscular blocking agent used without concomitant sedation	Administer sufficient sedative to calm patient and produce amnesia
Technology gap in patient management	Physician ordering ventilator mode or settings fails to appreciate technical or clinical problem with therapy as ordered	Discussion between physician, nurse, and respiratory therapist before therapy is carried out, initiated by either party (especially important with new or unfamiliar ventilator modes)
	Nurse or respiratory therapist unfamiliar or uncomfortable with ventilator, mode, or settings as ordered	–
Bedside communication failure	Those caring for patient at bedside (nurse, respiratory therapist) do not understand patient's problem or rationale for ordered therapy	Explanation by physician caring for patient about diagnosis, pathophysiology, and/or therapeutic rationale
	Failure on part of nurse or respiratory therapist to communicate concerns about above problem	Discussion with attending physician, initiated by concerned nurse or respiratory therapist

Figure 11.25 Iatrogenic complications of mechanical ventilation. Summary of problems created by the way the clinician sets the ventilator, with suggested remedies.

demonstrate convincingly that high inflation pressures and distending volumes can damage the lung, and produce lesions not too dissimilar from those of human ARDS[25]. Using smaller VTs protects the same animals from injury, even when airway pressure is high. Chest computed tomographic scans and other techniques show that a large proportion of the lungs of patients who have ARDS consolidate or collapse, which substantially reduces the number of alveoli that receive the VT delivered by the ventilator (see Chapter 69). These findings are all consistent with the idea that keeping alveolar distending pressures and volumes low may protect the lungs from ventilator-induced injury.

In addition, repetitive opening and closing of collapsed alveoli and small airways produces large sheer forces that could cause parenchymal lung damage. It is protective to prevent this sequential opening and closing through the use of PEEP to raise FRC and carry out tidal ventilation at a higher lung volume[25].

These findings have led to the current ventilation strategy for ARDS described earlier, which uses a PEEP level titrated on the basis of a respiratory system pressure–volume curve to keep marginal lung units inflated, and small VTs to avoid alveolar overdistension. Several uncontrolled studies and one randomized controlled trial[9] document improved survival in ARDS using this approach, which has prompted some authorities to advocate its routine use in this condition[26]. Other leaders in ARDS management stop short of endorsing the lung-protective strategy for use outside the research setting.

Sedation and paralysis
Use of neuromuscular blocking agents during mechanical ventilation has become more widespread in recent years. In some instances, this is because modes of ventilation, such as pressure control with inverse ratio ventilation, are used that are uncomfortable for patients and result in 'fighting the ventilator' if they are awake and alert. In others, it is part of an attempt to optimize oxygen extraction by reducing peripheral oxygen utilization in the aggressive management of ARDS or sepsis. Sedation and muscle

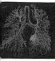
relaxation are necessary for operative surgery, certain diagnostic procedures such as angiography and computed tomographic scanning in uncooperative patients, and various invasive procedures performed in the intensive care unit. In most instances, patients must be paralyzed for the construction of pressure–volume curves to guide the selection of PEEP level and V_T. In general, however, neuromuscular blocking agents are overused in many centers.

Rendering a patient incapable of movement is a hazardous undertaking, associated with increased risks for venous thrombosis, nosocomial pneumonia, and skin breakdown, among other complications. Making sure that the patient is adequately sedated is difficult and often given insufficient attention. Except for the specific settings mentioned above, sedation and paralysis should seldom be necessary in ventilator management.

Should the ventilatory muscles be rested or exercised?

Controversy has existed for more than 25 years as to whether the ventilatory muscles of a patient who receives invasive mechanical ventilation need to be rested or exercised. Advocates of resting the muscles point out that failure of the ventilatory pump is the proximate cause of most cases of acute hypercapnic respiratory failure, especially in patients who have underlying obstructive lung disease. To permit the fatigued ventilatory muscles to recover through rest seems intuitive. However, the opposite camp maintains a 'use it or lose it' stance, pointing to evidence of rapid loss of skeletal muscle mass and functional capability when patients are immobilized. Advocates of exercising the ventilatory muscles often use partial ventilatory support throughout the period of mechanical ventilation, which makes the muscles do at least some of the work of breathing.

Studies that support both positions have been published, and the controversy is unresolved. However, because the work of breathing in relation to a patient's capabilities is a major determinant of dyspnea, it is important to address the issue in the context of patient comfort. Although the rationale behind partial ventilatory support for a patient who has ongoing respiratory failure and who is not yet ready to be weaned is understandable, any benefit to be derived from making that patient struggle to breathe seems questionable. When partial ventilatory support is used at any stage of management, whether via SIMV or PSV, enough support should be provided to keep the total respiratory rate below about 30 breaths per minute. Patients who breathe more rapidly are typically restless, tachycardic, and diaphoretic, and are surely not deriving any benefit from exercising their ventilatory muscles.

Weaning from ventilatory support necessarily involves loading the patient's ventilatory muscles, and hence stressing them. When weaning is not actively being attempted, however, patient comfort should be given a high priority. During weaning, particularly in difficult-to-wean patients who are undergoing a gradual weaning regimen, it is important to provide sufficient support to rest the ventilatory muscles after each episode of spontaneous breathing in which fatigue is induced.

REFERENCES

1. Slutsky AS. American College of Chest Physicians Concensus Conference on Mechanical Ventilation. Chest. 1993;104:1833–59.
2. Nahum A, Marini JJ, eds. Recent advances in mechanical ventilation. Clin Chest Med. 1996;17:355–613.
3. Pierson DJ. Indications for mechanical ventilation in acute respiratory failure. Respir Care. 1983;28:570–8.
4. Pierson DJ. Respiratory therapy techniques. In: Kelley WN, ed. Textbook of internal medicine, 3rd edn. Philadelphia: Lippincott-Raven Publishers; 1997:2127–33.
5. Branson RD, MacIntyre NR. Dual-control modes of mechanical ventilation. Respir Care. 1996;41:294–305.
6. Hudson LD, Weaver LJ, Haisch CE, Carrico CJ. Positive end-expiratory pressure: reduction and withdrawal. Respir Care. 1988;33:613–17.
7. Leatherman JW. Mechanical ventilation in obstructive lung disease. Clin Chest Med. 1996;17:577–90.
8. Stewart TE, Meade MO, Cook DJ, et al. Evaluation of a ventilation strategy to prevent barotrauma in patients at high risk for acute respiratory distress syndrome. N Engl J Med. 1998;338:355–61.
9. Amato MPB, Barbas CSV, Medeiros DM, et al. Effect of a protective-ventilation strategy on mortality in the acute respiratory distress syndrome. N Engl J Med. 1998;338:347–54.
10. Roupie E, Dambrosio M, Servillo G, et al. Titration of tidal volume and induced hypercapnia in acute respiratory distress syndrome. Am J Respir Crit Care Med. 1995;152:121–8.
11. Marik PE, Krikorian J. Pressure-controlled ventilation in ARDS: a practical approach. Chest. 1997;112:1102–6.
12. Sharar SR. Weaning and extubation are not the same thing. Respir Care. 1995;40:239–43.
13. Sahn SA, Lakshminarayan S. Bedside criteria for discontinuation of mechanical ventilation. Chest. 1973;63:1002–5.
14. Yang KL, Tobin MJ. A prospective study of indexes predicting the outcome of trials of weaning from mechanical ventilation. N Engl J Med. 1991;324:1445–50.
15. Brochard L, Rauss A, Benito S, et al. Comparison of three methods of gradual withdrawal from ventilatory support during weaning from mechanical ventilation. Am J Respir Crit Care Med. 1994;150:896–903.
16. Esteban A, Frutos F, Tobin MJ, et al. A comparison of four methods of weaning patients from mechanical ventilation. N Engl J Med. 1995;332:345–50.
17. Marik PE. The cuff-leak test as a predictor of postextubation stridor: a prospective study. Respir Care. 1996;41:509–11.
18. Keith RL, Pierson DJ. Complications of mechanical ventilation. A bedside approach. Clin Chest Med. 1996;17:439–51.
19. Pinsky MR. Effects of mechanical ventilation on the cardiovascular system. Crit Care Clin. 1990;6:663–78.
20. Zwillich CW, Pierson DJ, Creagh CE, Sutton FD Jr, Schatz E, Petty TL. Complications of assisted ventilation: a prospective study of 354 consecutive episodes. Am J Med. 1974;57:161–70.
21. Benson MS, Pierson DJ. Auto-PEEP during mechanical ventilation of adults. Respir Care. 1988;33:557–65.
22. Lodato RF, Tobin MJ. Estimation of auto-PEEP. Chest. 1991;99:520–2.
23. Glauser FL, Polatty RC, Sessler CN. Worsening oxygenation in the mechanically ventilated patient: causes, mechanisms, and early detection. Am Rev Respir Dis. 1988;138:458–65.
24. Durbin CG, Wallace KK. Oxygen toxicity in the critically ill patient. Respir Care. 1993;38:739–50.
25. Dreyfuss D, Saumon G. Ventilator-induced injury. In: Tobin MJ, ed. Principles and practice of mechanical ventilation. New York: McGraw-Hill; 1994:793–811.
26. Kacmarek RM, Chiche JD. Lung protective ventilatory strategies for ARDS – the data are convincing! [Editorial]. Respir Care. 1998;43:724–7.

Chapter 12 Noninvasive Mechanical Ventilation

Nicholas S Hill

INTRODUCTION

Noninvasive ventilation is mechanical ventilation that is administered without an invasive artificial airway. Since the first description of a prototype negative pressure 'tank' ventilator 150 years ago, many types of noninvasive ventilators have been developed[1]. 'Tank' ventilators like the iron lung were the mainstay of mechanical ventilatory assistance during the polio epidemics that occurred from the 1920s to the 1950s. By the 1960s, invasive positive-pressure ventilation became the preferred mode for the treatment of acute respiratory failure. Noninvasive ventilators, mainly of the negative-pressure type, continued to be used sporadically for chronic respiratory failure until the early 1980s, but following the introduction of nasal ventilation during the late 1980s, noninvasive ventilation has seen a resurgence.

RATIONALE FOR THE USE OF NONINVASIVE VENTILATION

Invasive mechanical ventilation has proven to be effective and reliable, but the use of an endotracheal airway may cause complications. These complications have been described in detail[2], and may be categorized in three ways:
- traumatic complications, such as hemorrhage or tracheal laceration;
- complications related to bypassing the airway defense system; and
- discomfort-related complications, including pain and interference with communication and swallowing.

These complications apply to acute translaryngeal intubations as well as to chronic tracheostomies. Furthermore, airway invasion interferes with normal airway clearance mechanisms, such as cough, and serves as a continual irritant, increasing mucus production and necessitating intermittent suctioning. By avoiding these complications, noninvasive ventilation has the potential of enhancing patient satisfaction and reducing the cost of care[3]. However, it must be emphasized that the patients who are to receive noninvasive ventilation must be selected carefully (see below).

TECHNIQUES AND EQUIPMENT FOR NONINVASIVE VENTILATION

Noninvasive positive-pressure ventilation

Noninvasive positive-pressure ventilation (NPPV) consists of a positive-pressure ventilator connected by way of tubing to a mask or 'interface' that applies positive air pressure to the nose or mouth, or both.

Interfaces
Nasal masks

Nasal masks are the most commonly used interfaces for chronic respiratory failure because they are convenient and permit normal speech and swallowing. Manufacturers offer numerous modifications of three basic types of nasal mask:
- standard nasal continuous positive airway pressure (CPAP) masks;
- nasal 'pillows' or 'seals'; and
- custom-fitted masks.

Standard nasal CPAP masks consist of triangular clear plastic domes that fit over the nose (Fig. 12.1). A soft cuff makes contact with the skin around the perimeter of the nose to form an air seal. These masks must be properly fitted in order to minimize pressure over the bridge of the nose, which may cause redness, skin irritation, and occasionally ulceration. Thin plastic flaps over the cuff (to permit air sealing with less mask pressure) and forehead spacers are used to minimize pressure on the bridge of the nose. Strap systems that hold the masks in place are also important for patient comfort. Recently, mini-masks that fit over the tip of the nose and nostrils have been introduced to enhance patient comfort further.

Nasal 'pillows' or 'seals' consist of small rubber cones that are inserted directly into the nostrils (Fig. 12.2). These have been

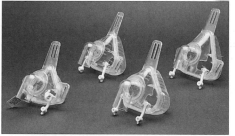

Figure 12.1 Standard nasal masks. Various sizes of standard nasal mask are available, ranging from small (on left) to large (on right).

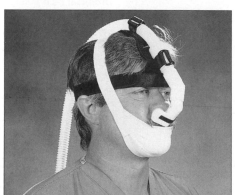

Figure 12.2 Nasal 'pillows'. These avoid placing pressure on the bridge of the nose. The chin strap helps to keep the mouth closed, reducing air leakage.

useful for patients who have nasal bridge irritation or ulceration because they make no contact with the bridge of the nose. Some patients alternate between different types of masks as a way of minimizing discomfort.

Custom-fitted masks use rapidly drying plastics or heat-molded materials. Although kits for custom molding are available commercially, they require skill for successful application and are generally made only at experienced centers.

Oronasal masks

Oronasal masks cover both the nose and mouth (Fig. 12.3) and have the capability of reducing air leaking through the mouth that may limit the efficacy of nasal ventilation. Although they are widely used in the acute setting, oronasal masks interfere with speech and eating more than nasal masks, have more dead space, and may be less acceptable to patients for chronic use. Concerns have been raised about the risk of aspiration if the patient vomits or asphyxiation if the ventilator fails, so recommended masks come with quick-release straps and antiasphyxia (nonrebreathing) valves.

Oral interfaces

Commercially available oral interfaces use a mouthpiece inserted into a lip seal that is strapped tautly around the head to minimize the leakage of air. In my experience, this device is poorly tolerated because it interferes with speech and swallowing. Mouthpieces that are custom fitted by an orthodontist may not require a strap for adequate sealing and can be easily expectorated if necessary, even by patients with severe neuromuscular disease. These devices have been used for round-the-clock ventilatory support in patients with neuromuscular disease, some of whom have little or no measurable vital capacity[4].

Ventilators for noninvasive positive-pressure ventilation

Noninvasive positive-pressure ventilation may be administered using volume-limited or pressure-limited modes on 'critical care ventilators' (designed mainly for invasive ventilation in the acute setting) or portable positive-pressure ventilators (designed mainly for use in the home). The choice of ventilator depends largely on practitioner preference and patient needs. For example, some practitioners prefer simple portable pressure-limited ventilators because they lack sophisticated alarm systems that may needlessly interrupt sleep in patients requiring only nocturnal ventilatory

assistance at home. On the other hand, others prefer the enhanced alarm and monitoring capabilities of critical care ventilators for acute applications. For chronic use in the home, simplicity and portability are important features.

Critical care ventilators

Many of the microprocessor-controlled ventilators currently used in critical care units can be adapted for noninvasive ventilation. Either volume-limited or pressure-limited modes may be selected, although most practitioners prefer pressure support ventilation. The responses of these ventilators to the air leaks that inevitably occur with NPPV may be problematic, sometimes necessitating modifications in masks or disabling of alarms. This should be done only in a closely monitored setting such as a critical care or step-down unit as long as the patient remains acutely ill.

Portable volume-limited ventilators

Portable volume-limited ventilators (Fig. 12.4) are commonly used to administer NPPV to patients with chronic respiratory failure. The ventilators are usually set in the assist–control mode to allow for spontaneous patient triggering, and the back-up rate is usually set at slightly below spontaneous patient breathing rate. Currently available volume-limited ventilators have more alarm and pressure-generating capabilities than most portable pressure-limited ventilators, and they may be better suited to patients in need of continuous ventilation or those who have severe chest wall deformity or obesity who need high inflation pressures.

Portable pressure-limited ventilators

Portable ventilators that deliver pressure assist or pressure support ventilation (often referred to as 'bilevel' devices) have seen increasing use in recent years. These deliver a preset inspiratory positive airway pressure (IPAP) that can be combined with positive end-expiratory pressure (PEEP or EPAP) (Fig. 12.5). The difference between the IPAP and EPAP is the level of inspiratory assistance, or pressure support. Pressure support modes usually provide sensitive inspiratory triggering and expiratory cycling mechanisms, permitting excellent patient–ventilator synchrony, reducing diaphragmatic work, and improving patient comfort[5]. As these devices are lighter (5–10kg), more compact ($<0.025m^3$), and have fewer alarms than critical care

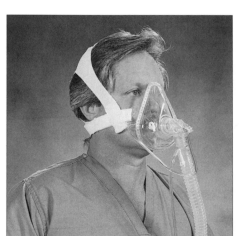

Figure 12.3
Oronasal face mask.
Note the rapid-release strap (suspended over tubing) and the antiasphyxia valve (at the connecting point between the mask and tubing).

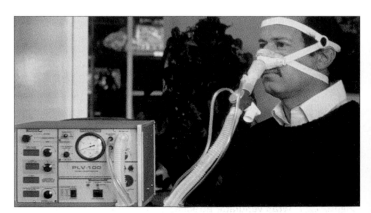

Figure 12.4 Typical volume-limited portable ventilator configured to deliver nasal ventilation.

or portable volume-limited ventilators, they are preferred for patients requiring only nocturnal use in the home. Most have limited IPAP capabilities [up to 2.0–3.5 kPa (20–35cmH$_2$O), depending on the ventilator] and lack battery back-up systems, so unless they are appropriately modified they are not recommended for patients who require high-inflation pressures, who are dependent on continuous mechanical ventilation, or who are receiving invasive ventilation.

Unlike volume-limited ventilators, the 'bilevel' devices are able to adjust inspiratory air flow to compensate for air leaks, thereby potentially providing better support of gas exchange during leakage. However, because they use a single tube with a passive exhalation valve, rebreathing that interferes with the ability to augment alveolar ventilation may occur if the patient exhales nasally. This rebreathing may be minimized by using nonrebreathing exhalation valves or EPAP pressures of 0.4kPa (4cmH$_2$O) or greater, which ensure higher bias flows during exhalation.

Negative-pressure ventilation

Negative-pressure ventilators are used much less now than they were in the past, but they may be effective in patients who fail to adapt to NPPV. Negative-pressure ventilators include tank ventilators (like the iron lung; Fig. 12.6) and the smaller, more portable wrap (or jacket; Fig. 12.7) and cuirass (or shell) ventilators (Fig. 12.8). The wrap ventilator consists of an impermeable nylon jacket suspended by a rigid chest piece that fits over the chest and abdomen. The cuirass ventilator is a rigid plastic or metal dome fitted over the chest and abdomen. Negative-pressure ventilators expand the lungs by intermittently applying a subatmospheric pressure to the chest wall and abdomen, and expiration occurs passively by elastic recoil of the lung and chest wall. The efficiency (tidal volume generated for a given negative pressure) of negative-pressure ventilation is determined by the compliance of the chest wall and abdomen, and the surface area over which the negative pressure is applied. Thus, the tank is the most efficient and the cuirass least efficient of these ventilators.

The tank ventilator is reliable and relatively comfortable, but it is bulky (3m long) and heavy (300kg). It is also intolerable to claustrophobic patients and interferes with nursing care, although it does have portholes on the sides. A more portable fiberglass tank ventilator is available, but it still weighs approximately 50kg. The chest shell and wrap are lightweight, but the negative-pressure generators that are necessary to power them weigh 12–25kg. Furthermore, the tank and wrap ventilators restrict patients to the supine position, often inducing musculoskeletal back and shoulder pain. The chest shell may be used in the sitting position, but it can induce discomfort and pressure sores at points of skin contact, particularly if the fit is suboptimal. Patients with chest wall deformities are poor candidates for negative-pressure ventilators, although they can be managed with custom-fit cuirasses.

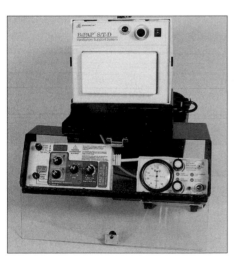

Figure 12.5 Typical 'bilevel' type portable positive pressure-limited ventilator. The control box (lower left) and pressure monitor and alarm (lower right) are for in-hospital use.

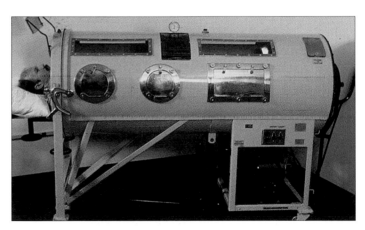

Figure 12.6 'Iron lung'. Tank-type negative-pressure ventilator that was widely used during the polio epidemics.

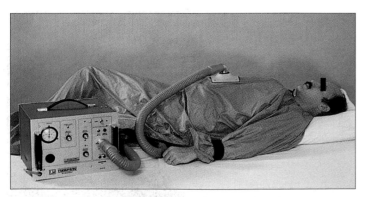

Figure 12.7 Wrap ventilator attached to a negative-pressure generator (on left). Note the contour of the rigid plastic chest piece, which suspends the wrap above the chest and abdomen.

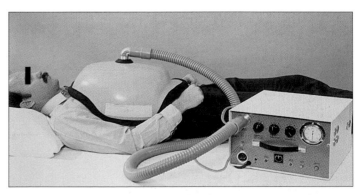

Figure 12.8 Chest cuirass attached to negative-pressure generator.

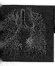

Most of these limitations of negative-pressure ventilation can be overcome with fitting adjustments or nonsteroidal anti-inflammatory drugs. However, obstructive sleep apneas associated with severe oxygen desaturations are common in patients with neuromuscular disease using negative-pressure ventilators and may necessitate a switch to NPPV[6]. The lack of a preinspiratory contraction of pharyngeal muscles to prevent collapse of upper airway structures during a normal patient-initiated breath appears to be responsible for the apneas. Traditional negative-pressure ventilators lack patient-triggered modes, making the upper airway susceptible to collapse before ventilator-triggered breaths. Newer patient-triggered negative-pressure ventilators may alleviate this problem, but this has not been evaluated.

Abdominal displacement ventilators

The rocking bed and the intermittent abdominal pressure respirator or 'pneumobelt' both rely on displacement of the abdominal contents to assist ventilation. The rocking bed (Fig. 12.9) consists of a mattress on a motorized platform that rocks in an arc of approximately 40°[7]. The patient lies supine on the mattress with the head and knees raised slightly to prevent sliding. When the head rocks down, the abdominal viscera and diaphragm slide toward the head, assisting exhalation. As the head rocks up, the viscera and diaphragm slide toward the feet, assisting inhalation. The rocking rate is between 12 and 24 times per minute, adjusted to optimize patient comfort and minute volume as measured with a hand-held spirometer or magnetometer. The chief advantages of the rocking bed are ease of operation, lack of encumbrances, and patient comfort. Disadvantages include bulkiness, noisiness, lack of portability, and limited efficacy.

The pneumobelt[7] uses a corset wrapped around the patient's midsection to hold an inflatable rubber bladder firmly against the anterior abdomen (Fig. 12.10). Intermittent inflation of the rubber bladder by a positive-pressure ventilator compresses the abdomen, forcing the diaphragm upward and actively assisting exhalation. With bladder deflation, gravity returns the diaphragm to its original position, assisting inhalation. Tidal volume is determined by bladder inflation pressure, which is usually between 3.5 and 5.0kPa (35 and 50cmH$_2$O), and the compliance of the patient's abdomen and respiratory system. Desired minute volume can be attained by adjusting the ventilator rate, which is usually between 12 and 22 per minute. The pneumobelt is highly portable, can be mounted on a wheelchair to facilitate mobility, is easily hidden under clothing, and leaves the hands and face unencumbered, facilitating desk work. Because gravity is necessary to pull the diaphragm down during bladder deflation, it is ineffective unless patients sit at an angle of at least 30°. Hence, nocturnal use is limited to patients who can learn to sleep while sitting.

Because their main action is to assist diaphragm motion, both the rocking bed and pneumobelt are well suited to patients who have bilateral diaphragmatic paralysis[7]. However, they are both relatively ineffective ventilators and are of limited use in patients who have acute respiratory decompensations. Furthermore, the efficacy of both depends on abdominal and chest wall compliance, so that patients who have severe kyphoscoliosis, excessive thinness, or obesity may not be adequately ventilated.

Other types of ventilatory assistance

Although not technically forms of 'mechanical' ventilation, diaphragm pacing and glossopharyngeal breathing are ventilatory methods used in selected patients to enhance independence from mechanical ventilation. Diaphragm pacers consist of a radiofrequency transmitter and antenna that signal a surgically implanted receiver and electrode to stimulate the phrenic nerve[8]. An intact phrenic nerve and diaphragm are required for successful application, so use is limited to patients who have quadriplegia caused by high spinal cord lesions or central hypoventilation. Because of a number of limitations, including high cost and the tendency to produce upper airway obstruction necessitating a tracheostomy in up to 90% of users, diaphragm pacers are uncommonly used today except in children who are unable to adapt to noninvasive ventilation.

Glossopharyngeal or 'frog' breathing utilizes intermittent gulping motions of the tongue and pharyngeal muscles to force air into the trachea[9]. The technique can be used to provide freedom from mechanical ventilation for periods of up to several hours, even in severely compromised patients. Use is limited to patients who have intact upper airway musculature, more or less normal lungs and chest walls, and the ability to learn the technique. Good candidates include those who have high spinal cord injuries,

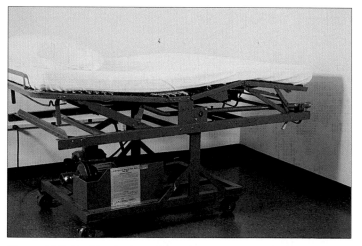

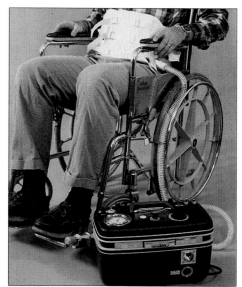

Figure 12.10 Intermittent abdominal pressure respirator or 'pneumobelt'. This consists of a rubber bladder within the corset strapped to the patient's abdomen and attached to a portable-positive pressure ventilator.

Figure 12.9 Rocking bed ventilator. At usual settings, the head rocks down approximately 10° and the feet approximately 27°. Sliding of the abdominal viscera serves to assist diaphragm motion.

those who have postpolio syndrome, and appropriate patients affected by other neuromuscular diseases.

ACUTE APPLICATIONS OF NONINVASIVE VENTILATION

Although negative-pressure ventilation is used to treat acute respiratory failure in some centers in Spain and Italy[10], most of the recent enthusiasm for noninvasive ventilation has been directed at NPPV. Earlier observations that NPPV reduces the work of breathing in patients with respiratory disease led investigators to hypothesize that it would be useful for ventilatory support of patients with acute respiratory deteriorations who were developing respiratory muscle fatigue.

Avoidance of intubation

Evidence suggests that NPPV successfully avoids intubation in selected patients with acute respiratory failure. Many studies have reported success rates of 60–80% in avoiding intubation, although few have been adequately controlled. Among randomized, controlled studies, one enrolled patients with all forms of respiratory failure[11], and a second enrolled only patients with exacerbations of chronic obstructive pulmonary disease (COPD)[12]. Both found nearly identical reductions in the percentage of patients needing intubation, from 73 and 74%, respectively, in controls, to 26% in patients receiving NPPV. In the study that accepted patients with various forms of respiratory failure, intubation was avoided mainly in the subgroup with COPD exacerbations. The efficacy of NPPV in avoiding intubation in patients who have acute respiratory failure from causes other than COPD has been assessed in too few patients to draw firm conclusions, but uncontrolled trials suggest that for patients who have certain diagnoses (Fig. 12.11), success rates may approach those obtained in patients who have COPD. Also, controlled trials have demonstrated that 0.98kPa (10cm H_2O) CPAP administered via a face mask is effective at reducing intubation rates among patients with acute pulmonary edema[13].

Improvements in vital signs and gas exchange

Noninvasive positive-pressure ventilation consistently lowers arterial partial pressure of carbon dioxide ($PaCO_2$) and respiratory and heart rates, improves pH and oxygenation, and reduces the sensation of dyspnea in patients successfully managed with NPPV, usually within the first few hours of initiation. In COPD patients with chronic CO_2 retention, the improvement in $PaCO_2$ may initially be as small as a few mmHg. A stable $PaCO_2$ is no cause for alarm as long as respiratory rate and sternocleidomastoid muscle activity promptly drop and the patient appears comfortable. However, if these improvements do not occur within the first 2 hours of initiation, later success is unlikely[14].

Morbidity, mortality, and duration of stay

Avoidance of intubation and improvements in vital signs, gas exchange, and dyspnea may not justify the routine use of NPPV in patients with acute respiratory failure unless outcomes like morbidity, mortality, and costs are also favorably affected. One controlled trial[15] found a lower mortality among NPPV-treated patients (4%) than controls (30%), although few of the control patients who died received any form of mechanical ventilatory assistance. Thus, this study is most accurately portrayed as showing that NPPV lowers mortality in COPD patients who are not

to be intubated. A multicenter European study[12] found that patients randomized to receive NPPV had lower rates of complications (16 versus 48%) and mortality (9 versus 29%) and shorter hospital stays (23 versus 35 days) than conventionally treated patients. Thus, evidence is accruing to suggest that NPPV therapy of acute respiratory failure, mainly in COPD patients, improves morbidity and mortality in comparison with conventional treatment, and has the potential of reducing costs.

Time demands on medical personnel

The potential advantages of NPPV over conventional therapy for acute respiratory failure will go unrealized if time demands on medical personnel are excessive. Although earlier reports raised this as a potential problem, this may have been related to lack of experience with the technique. More recent studies have found that nurses rate NPPV as no more demanding of care than conventional therapy[15], and spend no more time with patients receiving NPPV than with controls[11]. On the other hand, respiratory therapists tend to spend more time with NPPV than with conventionally treated patients during the first 8 hours of use, although this falls significantly during the second 8 hours[11]. These findings suggest that NPPV initially requires more time to administer, but as patients and medical practitioners become familiar with the technique, time demands rapidly diminish. Alternatively, those not needing continuous (or frequent intermittent) attention may not need any type of external ventilatory assistance.

Determinants of success

Factors that have been found to predict NPPV success are shown in Figure 12.12. In effect, these predictors indicate that patients

Non-COPD causes of acute respiratory failure treated with noninvasive positive-pressure ventilation	
AIDS-related pneumonia	Cystic fibrosis
Adult respiratory distress syndrome	Neuromuscular diseases
	Pneumonia
Asthma	Postoperative complications
Cardiogenic pulmonary edema	Upper airway obstruction

Figure 12.11 Non-chronic obstructive pulmonary disease (COPD) causes of acute respiratory failure treated with noninvasive positive-pressure ventilation. Patients must be selected following guidelines presented in Figure 12.13. AIDS, acquired immunodeficiency syndrome.

Characteristics of patients successfully treated with noninvasive positive-pressure ventilation
Cooperative
Intact neurologic function
Able to coordinate breathing with ventilator
Moderately high (but not very high) APACHE II scores
Intact dentition
Less air leakage through the mouth than in patients in whom treatment fails
Able to control secretions
Hypercapnic, but not severely so
Acidemic, but not severely so (pH >7.10)

Figure 12.12 Characteristics of patients successfully treated with noninvasive positive-pressure ventilation. APACHE, acute physiology and chronic health evaluation.

who are most likely to succeed with NPPV have advanced, but not catastrophic, respiratory failure. They suggest that there is a 'window of opportunity' for implementation of NPPV when success is most likely. Noninvasive positive-pressure ventilation should be started when patients are ill, with evidence of acute respiratory distress and high scores in acute physiology and chronic health evaluation II (APACHE II) scores, but not too late, when patients have very advanced CO_2 retention and acidemia, higher APACHE II scores, and are unable to cooperate.

Selection guidelines for noninvasive positive pressure ventilation in acute respiratory failure

Selection guidelines for the use of NPPV in acute respiratory failure, partly based on studies examining determinants of success, are shown in Figure 12.13. In the two-step process, patients entering the 'window of opportunity' are identified as those at risk of needing ventilatory assistance (and intubation) on the basis of clinical and blood gas indicators. Patients who have mild respiratory distress are excluded, because they should do well without ventilatory assistance.

The second step is to exclude those who would be at higher risk of complications if managed noninvasively. Exclusions are listed in Figure 12.13 and include patients who are too medically unstable or uncooperative, who have frank or imminent cardiopulmonary arrest, or who cannot protect their airway. On the other hand, obtundation is not necessarily an exclusion. Assiduous observation of the guidelines helps to ensure the safe administration of

noninvasive ventilation, but patients are still at risk for deterioration and should be monitored closely until stabilized.

The underlying etiology and potential reversibility of the acute respiratory deterioration are also important considerations in patient selection. In this regard, NPPV may be viewed as a 'crutch' that assists the patient through a critical interval of hours or days, allowing time for other therapies such as bronchodilators, corticosteroids, or diuretics to act. Severe, less reversible forms of respiratory failure that will require prolonged periods of ventilatory support, such as status asthmaticus or adult respiratory distress syndrome requiring controlled hypoventilation, should be managed invasively. It might be argued that there is little to lose in trying noninvasive ventilation in a failing 'do-not-intubate' patient. However, NPPV should probably be used only if there is a reasonable expectation of reversal of the acute process and after the patient and next-of-kin have been informed that NPPV is a form of life support (albeit noninvasive).

Other acute applications of noninvasive positive-pressure ventilation

Evidence is accruing to suggest that NPPV may help in weaning from invasive mechanical ventilation. Recently, NPPV was reported as reducing total length of time on a ventilator and complication and mortality rates when used to extubate patients early after bouts of acute respiratory failure[16]. Others use NPPV to avoid reintubation after unsuccessful extubations or as a way of improving oxygenation and avoiding atelectasis immediately following chest, cardiac, or abdominal surgery. Identifying those in need and determining whether NPPV reduces the need for more invasive interventions remains problematic, however.

LONG-TERM APPLICATIONS OF NONINVASIVE VENTILATION

Uncontrolled studies during the early 1980s on patients with chronic respiratory failure caused by neuromuscular diseases and chest wall deformities showed consistent improvements in gas exchange and symptoms after several months of nocturnal ventilatory assistance using negative pressure ventilation. However, because of greater difficulty of application, limited efficacy, and the tendency to aggravate or even induce upper airway obstructions, negative-pressure and other 'body' ventilators have been relegated to a second-line role in the management of chronic respiratory failure. Hence, the focus of the following is on positive-pressure techniques.

Restrictive thoracic diseases

Numerous uncontrolled studies have shown efficacy of nasal NPPV in treating chronic respiratory failure caused by various neuromuscular and chest wall diseases. These studies consistently show improvements in gas exchange and symptoms after a few weeks' nocturnal nasal ventilation. They also demonstrate reversal of chronic hypoventilation in patients with severe kyphoscoliosis and obstructive sleep apnea who have failed to improve with nasal CPAP alone. In addition, severe nocturnal oxygen desaturations are ameliorated when patients are switched from negative pressure ventilation to NPPV[17]. Although no studies have yet compared nasal and mouthpiece NPPV, Bach et al. have reported that mouthpiece NPPV may be used for long-term ventilatory support in patients with

Selection guidelines for use of noninvasive positive-pressure ventilation in patients with acute respiratory failure
Identify patients at risk of needing ventilatory assistance
Clinical criteria
Moderate to severe respiratory distress
Increased dyspnea
Tachypnea (respiratory rate >24/minute)
Use of accessory muscles
Paradoxic breathing pattern
Blood gas criteria
$PaCO_2 > 45mmHg$ (>6.0kPa) and pH <7.35, or $PaO_2/FiO_2 < 200$
Exclude patients who would be more safely managed invasively
Respiratory arrest
Medically unstable
Shock states
Unstable cardiac status
Acute severe ischemia or infarction
Uncontrolled life-threatening arrhythmias
Active severe upper gastrointestinal bleeding
Uncooperative or agitated
Unable to protect airway
Excessive secretions
Severe cough or swallowing impairment
Severe facial trauma
Appropriate, reversible cause for respiratory failure (as in Fig. 12.11)

Figure 12.13 Selection guidelines for use of noninvasive positive-pressure ventilation in patients with acute respiratory failure. The use of arterial partial pressure of oxygen (PaO_2)/ fraction of inspired oxygen (FiO_2) <200 as a blood gas criterion is a tentative guideline that has not been established in controlled trials.

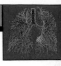

severe neuromuscular diseases who have virtually no measurable vital capacity[4].

Prospective, randomized trials to establish the efficacy of NPPV in patients with restrictive thoracic diseases have not been done, largely for ethical reasons. However, temporary withdrawal of nocturnal nasal ventilation from patients with chronic respiratory failure caused by restrictive thoracic diseases results in worsening nocturnal gas exchange, daytime symptoms, and sleep quality, offering strong evidence that NPPV is effective in reversing nocturnal hypoventilation and improving symptoms in these patients[18]. In addition, long-term follow-up studies on several hundred patients using NPPV for 3–5 years have observed favorable rates for NPPV continuation (and hence survival) among patients with postpolio syndrome, most myopathies, and kyphoscoliosis[19].

Although the long-term efficacy of NPPV for patients who have restrictive thoracic diseases appears to be well established, the optimal time for initiation is unclear. Most authorities recommend waiting for the onset of symptoms or daytime hypoventilation before initiating long-term NPPV. This is partly for pragmatic reasons, because patients comply better if motivated by the desire for symptom relief.

Chronic obstructive pulmonary disease

The most controversial application of noninvasive ventilation has been in patients with severe 'stable' COPD. During the early 1980s, investigators theorized that the respiratory muscles in patients with severe COPD may be chronically fatigued and might benefit from intermittent rest. Early trials found that intermittent daytime sessions using negative-pressure wrap ventilators improved daytime gas exchange and inspiratory and expiratory muscle strength in patients with severe COPD[20]. Unfortunately, longer-term controlled studies failed to demonstrate the same favorable effects of intermittent negative pressure ventilation in patients with severe COPD[21]. In addition, COPD patients tolerated the wrap ventilators poorly, using them for less time daily than recommended, and having trouble sleeping during use.

The disappointing results with negative-pressure ventilators stimulated interest in the use of NPPV for severe COPD, but these studies have yielded conflicting results as well. In a 3-month cross-over trial on 19 patients with severe COPD, only seven of whom completed the trial, improvement was detected only in tests of neuropsychologic function and not in nocturnal or daytime gas exchange, sleep quality, pulmonary functions, exercise tolerance, or symptoms[22]. In contrast, a similar study on 18 patients with severe COPD found that NPPV improved nocturnal and daytime gas exchange, total sleep time, and quality of life scores[23]. The substantial differences in baseline characteristics of patients entering these trials may offer some insight into the conflicting results. Patients entering the favorable study had greater hypercarpnia [$PaCO_2$ 7.6kPa (57mmHg) versus 6.3kPa (47mmHg)] and more nocturnal oxygen desaturations despite having less severe airway obstruction [forced expiratory volume in 1 second (FEV_1 0.81L versus 0.54L)] than patients entering the unfavorable trial. These findings support the hypothesis that the subgroup of patients most likely to benefit from NPPV is that with substantial daytime CO_2 retention [>6.7kPa (>50mmHg)] and nocturnal oxygen desaturations. Further support is provided by anecdotal series of cystic fibrosis patients with severe airway obstruction and CO_2 retention who have been supported using NPPV while awaiting

lung transplantation. Clearly, further studies are needed to determine which COPD patients are appropriate candidates for NPPV, which ventilator modes and settings work best, and whether NPPV enhances quality of life, reduces hospitalization or prolongs survival relative to oxygen therapy alone.

Selection guidelines for long-term noninvasive ventilation

It is possible to identify a number of characteristics that permit selection of appropriate candidates for noninvasive ventilation among patients without COPD (Fig. 12.14). There should be at least mild-to-moderate daytime CO_2 retention (usually an indication of more severe nocturnal CO_2 retention) and symptoms attributable to hypoventilation and associated poor sleep quality. Patients with symptomatic nocturnal hypoventilation but no daytime CO_2 retention may also benefit. Secondary considerations include a history of repeated hospitalizations for bouts of respiratory failure.

Patients should be excluded from consideration if they are unable to protect their airway adequately because of swallowing impairment or excessive secretions, particularly if combined with a weakened cough mechanism. If such patients desire aggressive support, they are usually more safely managed with invasive ventilation.

The patient's diagnosis is also an important consideration. Those with stable or slowly progressive neuromuscular diseases or chest wall deformities are the best candidates. Others, such as those with central hypoventilation or obstructive sleep apnea who have failed a trial of nasal CPAP, are also acceptable candidates. On the other hand, patients with rapidly progressive neuromuscular processes like Guillain–Barre syndrome, particularly if there is upper airway involvement, are poor candidates. Tentative selection guidelines are also listed for patients with

Selection guidelines for long-term noninvasive ventilation
For restrictive thoracic or central respiratory disorders
Gas exchange
Daytime arterial partial pressure of carbon dioxide ($PaCO_2$) >45mmHg (6.0kPa), or nocturnal hypoventilation
Sustained O_2 saturation <88% (without supplemental O_2)
Sustained $PaCO_2$ >50mmHg (6.7kPa; using an arterial line)
and
Symptoms
Hypersomnolence, morning headaches, excessive fatigue, nightmares, enuresis, depression
or
Signs
Cor pulmonale
For chronic obstructive pulmonary disease
Gas exchange
Daytime $PaCO_2$ >50mmHg (6.7kPa), and nocturnal hypoventilation
Sustained O_2 saturation <88% (with supplemental O_2)
Sustained $PaCO_2$ >55mmHg (7.3kPa; using an arterial line)
or
Daytime $PaCO_2$ >55mmHg (7.3kPa)
and
Symptoms or signs as above; dyspnea on exertion alone should not be considered an adequate symptom

Figure 12.14 Selection guidelines for long-term noninvasive ventilation.

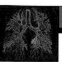
chronic airway obstruction. Because of the numerous studies showing no benefit among COPD patients with daytime CO_2 levels of 5.3–6.0kPa (40–45mmHg), the suggested threshold for CO_2 retention is higher than for restrictive thoracic diseases.

APPLICATION OF NONINVASIVE POSITIVE-PRESSURE VENTILATION

Initiation

Techniques for initiation of NPPV are similar in the acute and long-term settings except that the level of urgency differs. In both settings, initiation must be tailored for each individual patient. In the acute setting, the interface and ventilator must be selected rapidly, so it is advisable to attach an 'interface bag' containing a variety of types and sizes of masks and straps to a noninvasive ventilation cart. This permits rapid sizing and selection of a comfortable interface. In the chronic setting, it is also useful to have a variety of interfaces readily available, but mask interchanges can be made over periods of days to weeks rather than minutes. In both settings, establishment of a relaxed, comfortable setting and implementation by experienced practitioners who can impart a sense of confidence and reassurance are helpful.

The importance of a proper mask fit cannot be overemphasized. The mask that just fits around the perimeter of the nose is best; selection of too large a mask is a common error that necessitates excessive tightening of the straps to minimize air leakage. The type of interface is probably less important than optimizing patient comfort; no study has yet demonstrated superiority of one interface over another. Likewise, the type of ventilator selected is probably not critical to success. Both pressure-limited and volume-limited ventilators have been used to administer NPPV. Success rates (defined as patient tolerance of NPPV and avoidance of intubation) have been similar regardless of the ventilator, ranging from two thirds to three quarters of patients. One direct comparison of pressure-support and volume-limited modes found equivalent success rates with both modes but higher comfort ratings among patients using the pressure support mode[24].

To begin, the mask should be placed on the patient's face and ventilation started. Highly cooperative patients may feel more comfortable if they hold the mask themselves (Fig. 12.15). Initial ventilator settings should be relatively low to enhance patient comfort and acceptance, but inspiratory pressure or tidal volume should be adjusted upward as tolerated to provide adequate ventilatory assistance. Although typical initial settings on pressure-limited ventilators are 0.8–1.2kPa (8–12cmH$_2$O) for inspiratory and 0.2–0.4kPa (2–4cmH$_2$O) for expiratory pressures (pressure support of 0.5–1.0kPa (5–10cmH$_2$O) and PEEP of 0.2–0.4kPa (2–4cmH$_2$O), the well-documented phenomenon of auto-PEEP (or intrinsic PEEP) that accompanies acute exacerbations of COPD implies that more attention should be focused on expiratory pressures. For volume ventilation, initial tidal volumes range from 10 to 15mL/kg. The ventilator is usually set to allow patient triggering (assist–control mode). The ventilator back-up rate is set at the spontaneous breathing rate if the aim is to entrain the patient's breathing and minimize respiratory muscle work, or slightly below this level to encourage spontaneous breathing. Expiratory pressures are usually minimal so that the difference between the inspiratory and expiratory pressures (or pressure support) can be maximized. However, if the patient has obstructive sleep apnea or severe COPD, expiratory pressure are titrated upward to eliminate apneas or counterbalance auto-PEEP. With portable pressure-limited devices, expiratory pressures of 0.4kPa (4cmH$_2$O) or greater are suggested to minimize rebreathing, and in the acute setting, some practitioners increase expiratory pressures to ameliorate hypoxemia.

Once the patient appears to be synchronizing with the ventilator, the head straps can be tightened. These should be adjusted to minimize air leakage, particularly into the eyes, but the practitioner should still be able to slip one or two fingers under the strap. Forehead spacers and thin plastic flaps under the mask are useful in minimizing pressure on the bridge of the nose. Humidification is rarely needed in the acute setting for short-term use, but can be added for long-term applications if the patient complains of dryness. Oxygen is administered via the blender on critical care ventilators, or directly via a cannula connected to the mask or T-connector in the ventilator tubing when using 'bilevel' ventilators.

Initiation of 'body' ventilation follows a similar approach, with initial adjustment of pressures to optimize patient acceptance and later adjustments to achieve gas exchange goals. If the patient can tolerate them, pressures to augment tidal volume by 30–50% over baseline are apt to augment ventilation sufficiently to improve gas exchange. With both NPPV and 'body' ventilators, tidal volume, end-tidal PaCO$_2$ and oximetry monitoring or an arterial blood gas measurement during the initial period of use may help in assessing the need for further adjustments.

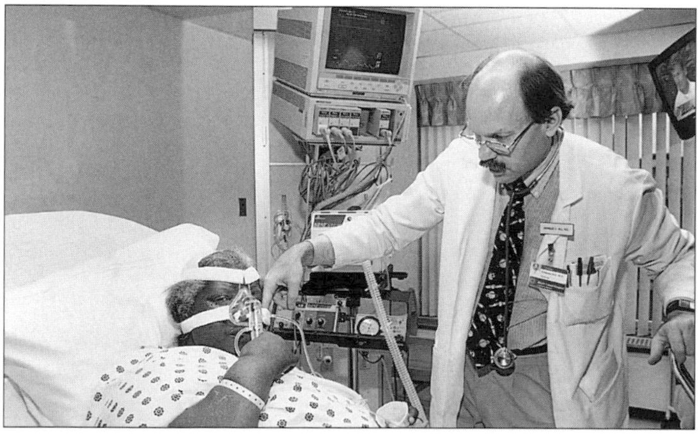

Adaptation and monitoring

In the acute setting, the first hour or two are critical in achieving successful adaptation. Coaching and encouragement are usually required to assist the patient in keeping the mouth shut during nasal ventilation and in adopting a breathing pattern that permits synchronization with the ventilator and reduction of breathing effort. Instructions like 'try to take slow deep breaths and let the machine breathe for you' may be helpful. Also, judicious administration of low doses of sedatives such as midazolam may be helpful in enhancing patient acceptance.

Ventilators designed to administer noninvasive ventilation lack sophisticated monitoring capabilities but even when critical care

Figure 12.15 Initiation of noninvasive positive pressure ventilation. A patient is shown holding the nose mask in place while the practitioner makes certain that strap tension is not excessive by demonstrating that a finger can easily be inserted between the strap and the face.

ventilators are used for noninvasive ventilation in the acute setting, monitoring via the ventilator may be inaccurate or even misleading because of air leaks. Accordingly, close bedside monitoring is essential until the patient's respiratory status stabilizes (raising concerns about the time – and cost-effectiveness). Although NPPV can easily be administered on general medical wards, the acuteness of the patient's illness and need for close monitoring should dictate the site of administration. Acutely ill patients should be treated in an intensive care or step-down unit until their condition stabilizes, regardless of whether they are treated with invasive or noninvasive ventilation.

Achieving patient comfort (or at least minimizing discomfort) is the most important initial goal, so frequent bedside assessments are obligatory. Oxygen saturation is monitored continuously, with oxygen supplementation titrated to achieve a target such as 92% or greater. Patient synchrony with the ventilator, respiratory and heart rates, and steinocleidomastoid muscle activity are monitored closely. Blood gases are also monitored as clinically indicated. Inspiratory pressures or tidal volumes are usually adjusted upward as tolerated to bring about desired improvements in $PaCO_2$.

In the chronic setting, adaptation usually requires a much longer period of time than in the acute setting, mainly because the patient must learn to sleep using the ventilator. The patient is instructed to initiate noninvasive ventilation at home for an hour or two during the daytime, and then to try to fall asleep with the device at bedtime. The patient is encouraged to leave the equipment on as long as tolerated, but is allowed to remove it if desired. During this period, frequent contact with an experienced home respiratory therapist help to assure proper use and adjustment. Some patients successfully sleep through the night within days of initiation, but others require several months. Perhaps 20% of patients are unable to adapt successfully to NPPV, usually because of mask intolerance. In these patients, trials with alternative noninvasive ventilators such as negative pressure or abdominal ventilators may still be successful, as long as the patient has no more than mild obstructive sleep apnea.

Patients should be seen every few weeks by a physician during the initial adaptation period. At the time of office follow-up, symptoms and physical signs should be assessed for evidence of nocturnal hypoventilation or cor pulmonale. Spirometry is indicated, particularly in patients who have progressive neuromuscular syndromes. Daytime arterial blood gases or pulse oximetry and end-tidal $PaCO_2$ levels should be obtained at the time of visits or when symptoms worsen. Although there is no consensus on the ideal target level, values for daytime $PaCO_2$ ranging from about 5.3 to 7.3kPa (40 to 55mmHg) are usually associated with good control of symptoms. Nocturnal monitoring using oximetry, multichannel recorders, or full polysomnography is also useful after adaptation to noninvasive ventilation to assure adequacy of oxygenation and ventilation.

Commonly encountered problems and possible remedies
Noninvasive ventilation is safe and well tolerated in most properly selected patients. With NPPV, either for the acute or chronic settings, the most commonly encountered problems are related to the interface or air pressure or flow (Fig. 12.16). Patients often complain of mask discomfort, which can be alleviated by minimizing strap tension, or trying different mask sizes or types. The most common error is to select a mask that is too large,

necessitating excessive strap tension to minimize leaks. For acute applications, patients may be anxious and experience difficulty in synchronizing their breathing efforts with the ventilator. Adjustments in ventilator mode (to pressure support, which usually enhances synchrony) and in inspiratory and expiratory pressures, plus judicious use of sedation, may help. In patients with severe COPD who have auto-intrinsic PEEP, increases in expiratory pressure may facilitate triggering.

Excessive air pressure leading to sinus or ear pain is another common complaint, alleviated by lowering pressure temporarily, and then gradually raising it again as tolerance improves. Patients may also complain of dryness or congestion of the nose or mouth. For dryness, nasal saline or gels or efforts to reduce air leaking may help. For chronic applications, flow-by humidifiers may also be helpful, particularly in dry climates or during winter. For nasal congestion, inhaled corticosteroids or decongestants or oral antihistamine–decongestant combinations may be used.

Other commonly encountered problems include erythema, pain or ulceration on the bridge of the nose related to nasal mask pressure. This can be ameliorated by minimizing strap tension, using artificial skin, or switching to alternative masks such as nasal 'pillows'. Gastric insufflation is common, but it is usually not severe, probably because inflation pressures are low compared with those used with invasive ventilation.

Air leaking through the mouth (with nasal masks), through the nose (with mouthpieces), or around the mask (with all interfaces) is inevitable during NPPV. Nasal and oronasal masks, particularly if too large, may leak air onto the eyes, causing conjunctival irritation. Refitting or reseating the mask usually alleviates this problem. Pressure-limited devices compensate for air leaks by maintaining inspiratory air flow during leaking; tidal volumes on volume-limited ventilators may be increased by the practitioner to compensate. To reduce air leaking through the mouth, patients are coached to keep the mouth shut or use chin straps or oronasal masks. Air leaking occurs during the majority of sleep in many patients, but fortunately gas exchange is usually well maintained[25]. Leaks may still contribute to arousals and poor sleep quality, however, and ven-

Adverse side effects and complications of noninvasive positive-pressure ventilation	
Mask-related	Discomfort Nasal bridge redness, ulceration Anxiety, claustrophobia Acne-like skin rash
Related to air flow or pressure	Nasal or oral dryness or congestion Eye irritation Sinus or ear pain Gastric insufflation Air leakage Sleep arousals
Related to ventilator type	Asynchrony; inability to sense inspiration or expiration Inability to compensate for leaks Rebreathing
Major complications	Failure to tolerate or ventilate, need for intubation (25–33%) Aspiration pneumonia Pneumothorax

Figure 12.16 Adverse side effects and complications of noninvasive positive-pressure ventilation. Aspiration pneumonia and pneumothorax are unusual in appropriately selected patients.

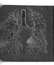
tilatory assistance may occasionally be compromised. In this case, options include trials of alternative interfaces or ventilators, or, if these fail, tracheostomy. Major complications of noninvasive ventilation, such as aspiration or pneumothorax, are unusual if patient selection guidelines are observed[26].

SUMMARY AND CONCLUSIONS

Noninvasive ventilation, mainly in the form of NPPV, is establishing itself as an important ventilator modality. In the acute setting, NPPV may be the preferred alternative to invasive positive-pressure ventilation for selected patients with COPD exacerbations, because of reduced morbidity and mortality, the possibility of reduced costs, and enhanced patient comfort. Noninvasive positive-pressure ventilation is also suitable for initial mechanical ventilatory assistance in patients with a variety of other forms of acute respiratory failure as long as selection guidelines are observed. These are designed to identify patients at risk of needing mechanical ventilatory assistance, while excluding those who are too ill to be safely managed noninvasively. Also, the patient should have an etiology for the respiratory failure that is likely to be reversed within a few days.

Noninvasive positive-pressure ventilation has more definitely been established as the ventilatory modality of first choice for a variety of causes for chronic respiratory failure, including neuromuscular diseases, chest wall restrictive processes, and central hypoventilation. Here, NPPV offers comfort, convenience and cost advantages over invasive positive-pressure ventilation. Ideal candidates should require only intermittent ventilatory assistance and have intact upper airway function, but NPPV has been successfully applied even in patients requiring continuous assistance and those with bulbar dysfunction.

Efficacy of NPPV has not been firmly established in patients who suffer chronic respiratory failure due to COPD, but patients who have substantial hypercarbia and nocturnal oxygen desaturation appear to be the ones most likely to benefit.

If NPPV fails in patients with chronic respiratory failure, alternative forms of noninvasive ventilation, such as negative-pressure ventilators, pneumobelts, or rocking beds, may occasionally be effective.

REFERENCES

1. Woollam CHM. The development of apparatus for intermittent negative pressure respiration. Anaesthesia. 1976;3:666–85.
2. Pingleton SK. Complications of acute respiratory failure. Am Rev Respir Dis. 1988;137:1463–93.
3. Bach JR. A comparison of long-term ventilatory support alternatives from the perspective of the patient and care giver. Chest. 1993;104:1702–6.
4. Bach JR, Alba AS, Saporito LR. Intermittent positive pressure ventilation via the mouth as an alternative to tracheostomy for 257 ventilator users. Chest. 1993;103:174–82.
5. Brochard L, Pluskwa F, Lemaire F. Improved efficacy of spontaneous breathing with inspiratory pressure support. Am Rev Respir Dis. 1987;136:411–15.
6. Hill NS, Redline S, Carskadon MA, et al. Sleep-disordered breathing in patients with Duchenne muscular dystrophy using negative pressure ventilators. Chest. 1992;102:1656–62.
7. Hill NS. Clinical applications of body ventilators. Chest. 1986;90:897–905.
8. Moxham J, Shneerson JM. Diaphragmatic pacing. Am Rev Respir Dis. 1993;148:533–6.
9. Bach JR, Alba AS, Bodofsky E, et al. Glossopharyngeal breathing and noninvasive aids in the management of post-polio respiratory insufficiency. Birth Defects. 1987;23:99–113.
10. Corrado A, Gorini M, Villella G, DePaola E. Negative pressure ventilation in the treatment of acute respiratory failure: an old noninvasive technique reconsidered. Eur Resir J. 1996;9:1531–44.
11. Kramer N, Meyer TJ, Meharg J, et al. Randomized, prospective trial of noninvasive positive pressure ventilation in acute respiratory failure. Am J Respir Crit Care Med. 1995;151:1799–806.
12. Brochard L, Mancebo J, Wysocki M, et al. Noninvasive ventilation for acute exacerbations of chronic obstructive pulmonary disease. N Engl J Med. 1995;333:817–22.
13. Bersten AD, Holt AW, Vedig AE, et al. Treatment of severe cardiogenic pulmonary edema with contiuous positive airway pressure delivered by face mask. N Engl J Med. 1991;325:1825–30.
14. Soo Hoo GW, Santiago S, Williams J. Nasal mechanical ventilation for hypercapnic respiratory failure in chronic obstructive pulmonary disease: Determinants of success and failure. Crit Care Med. 1994;27:417–34.
15. Bott J, Carroll MP, Conway JH, et al. Randomised controlled trial of nasal ventilation in acute ventilatory failure due to chronic obstructive airways disease. Lancet. 1993;341:1555–7.
16. Nava S, Bruschi C, Orlando A, et al. Noninvasive mechanical ventilation (NINMV) facilitates the weaning fof patients with respiratory failure due to chronic obstructive pulmonary disease. Ann Intern Med. 1998;128:721–8.
17. Ellis ER, Bye PT, Bruderer JW, et al. Treatment of respiratory failure during sleep in patients with neuromuscular disease. Positive-pressure ventilation through a nose mask. Am Rev Respir Dis. 1987;135:148–52.
18. Hill NS, Eveloff SE, Carlisle CC, et al. Efficacy of nocturnal nasal ventilation in patients with restrictive thoracic disease. Am Rev Respir Dis. 1992;101:516–21.
19. Leger P, Bedicam JM, Cornette A, et al. Nasal intermittent positive pressure. Long-term follow-up in patients with severe chronic respiratory insufficiency. Chest. 1994;105:100–5.
20. Braun NM, Marino WD. Effect of daily intermittent rest of respiratory muscles in patients with severe chronic airflow limitation (CAL). Chest. 1984;85:59S–60S.
21. Shapiro SH, Ernst P, Gray-Donald K, et al. Effect of negative pressure ventilation in severe chronic obstructive pulmonary disease. Lancet .1992;340:1425–9.
22. Strumpf DA, Millman RP, Carlisle CC, et al. Nocturnal positive-pressure ventilation via nasal mask in patients with severe chronic obstructive pulmonary disease. Am Rev Respir Dis. 1991;144:1234–9.
23. Meecham Jones DJ, Paul EA, Jones PW. Nasal pressure support ventilation plus oxygen compared with oxygen therapy along in hypercapnic COPD. Am J Respir Crit Care Med. 1995;152:538–44.
24. Vitacca M, Clini E, Rubini F, et al. Non-invasive mechanical ventilation in severe chronic obstructive lung disease and acute respiratory falure. Short and long-term prognosis. Intensive Care Med. 1996;22:94–100.
25. Meyer TF, Pressman MR, Benditt J, et al. Mouth leaking during nocturnal nasal ventilation. Effect on sleep quality. Am J Respir Crit Care Med. 1995;151:A423.
26. Hill NS. Complications of noninvasive positive pressure ventilation. Respir Care. 1997;42:432–442.

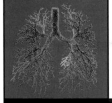

Chapter
13

Hemodynamic Monitoring in the Intensive Care Unit

Jonathan Sevransky and Roy Brower

INTRODUCTION

Many critically ill patients require frequent or continuous assessments to identify potentially life-threatening conditions and to guide the use of life-sustaining treatments. Hemodynamic monitoring devices aid clinicians in the assessment of circulatory function, arterial blood oxygenation, and oxygen delivery to systemic tissues. Devices used frequently in intensive care units (ICUs) include central venous catheters, pulmonary artery catheters (PACs), pulse oximeters, and systemic arterial catheters. The rationale for the use of each of these monitoring devices is reviewed in this chapter. Detailed instructions and illustrations are provided for the placement of indwelling vascular catheters, risks and complications are explained, and fine points and caveats for data interpretation are discussed.

CENTRAL VENOUS CATHETERS

A catheter placed in the superior vena cava (SVC) allows measurement of central venous pressure (CVP), which is usually very similar to right ventricular end-diastolic pressure. It may, therefore, be used to estimate right ventricular end-diastolic volume (preload). Since ventricular end-diastolic volume is a primary determinant of stroke volume and cardiac output, CVP is sometimes useful in the assessment of patients affected by circulatory dysfunction. For example, a low CVP in a patient who suffers hypotension suggests that vascular volume is inadequate and that the administration of intravenous fluids and/or blood products may be appropriate. A high CVP in a patient who has diffuse pulmonary infiltrates and hypoxemia may suggest volume overload or congestive heart failure and the need for diuretics and fluid restriction. Central venous catheters are also frequently necessary for the intravenous administration of vasoactive drugs and caustic infusates.

The most common sites of insertion of central venous catheters are the internal jugular vein and the subclavian vein. Under some circumstances, the external jugular, brachial, cephalic, and femoral sites are used. The best site depends on the specific patient's anatomy, risks of bleeding, and other complications, and the operator's experience with the different approaches.

Techniques for insertion of central venous catheters

Many variations in technique are used, depending on the route of access, but some general principles are followed for all central venous catheterizations. The patient is positioned optimally for the route of access chosen. The skin is extensively prepared with povidone–iodine solution. Local anesthesia may be accomplished with 1% lidocaine (lignocaine) solution injected subcutaneously using a small-bore needle, which avoids intravenous injection.

Maximal barrier precautions decrease the incidence of catheter-associated infections[1,2]. In most instances, these precautions include wearing a cap, mask, gown, and gloves in addition to preparing a large, sterile operating field. With some approaches, a small-bore 'finder needle' may be used to avoid inadvertent arterial puncture with a larger needle.

The preferred technique for catheter placement is the guidewire-assisted method developed by Seldinger[3]. The vein is entered with a needle, and a long, thin wire with a flexible J tip is threaded through the needle into the vein. The needle is removed, leaving the wire in place (Fig. 13.1). If the wire does not

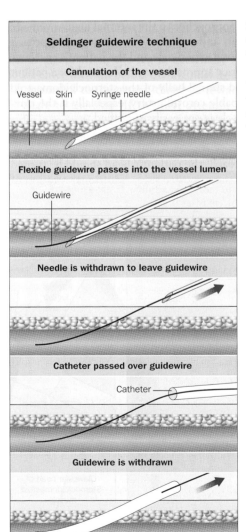

Seldinger guidewire technique

Cannulation of the vessel

Vessel | Skin | Syringe needle

Flexible guidewire passes into the vessel lumen

Guidewire

Needle is withdrawn to leave guidewire

Catheter passed over guidewire

Catheter

Guidewire is withdrawn

Figure 13.1
Seldinger guidewire technique. The vessel is cannulated with a thin gauge needle, and free blood flow is obtained. A thin, flexible guidewire is passed through the needle into the vessel lumen, after which the needle is withdrawn to leave the guidewire in place. The catheter is passed over the guidewire, with care taken to maintain control of the guidewire at all times. A small incision with a number 11 scalpel may be required prior to passage of the catheter. A rigid dilator my be passed over the wire to dilate the tract (not shown). Once the catheter has been threaded into the vessel, the guidewire is removed.

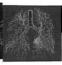
Choice of site for central venous catheterization

The decision as to which vessel to cannulate is made on the basis of the patient's clinical status and anatomy, and the operator's experience. The subclavian vein may be the preferred approach in a patient who is hypovolemic and has normal coagulation parameters. During cardiopulmonary resuscitation, the femoral site might be preferred while the airway is being secured. In patients who have coagulopathies, the cephalic, brachial, and femoral sites may be preferred because they can be compressed to reduce bleeding more easily. If possible, the subclavian vein is avoided in patients who have hyperinflated lungs or bullae because these predispose to pneumothorax. Risks and benefits of the different approaches to central venous access are compared in Figure 13.5.

Complications of central venous catheterization

All catheters represent potential sources of infection. To prevent catheter-related blood stream infections, strict attention to sterile procedures and maintenance techniques must be followed[1,2]. Some reports suggested that the femoral site is more prone to infectious complications and venous thrombosis, but this has not been confirmed in more recent studies[2]. Other complications of central venous catheters are often related to the site of insertion. The most frequent mechanical complications from internal jugular cannulation are carotid artery puncture, hematoma, and pneumothorax. With subclavian vein catheterization, patients are at risk for pneumothorax, subclavian artery puncture, hemothorax, and hematoma. Risks of femoral vein catheterization include femoral artery puncture, which may cause a retroperitoneal hematoma. All central venous catheters can cause venous thrombosis, but the clinical significance of these clots is not clear. Mechanical complications of central vein catheterization are included in Figure 13.5.

The risk of complications, both mechanical and infectious, are directly proportional to the number of attempts at catheterization[7-9]. In some studies, the incidence of complications was substantially higher when the procedures were performed by less experienced operators[7,9]. As a general rule, operators who are unsuccessful in gaining access at a single site with two or three passes should attempt to obtain access from another site or seek assistance from a more experienced operator. When attempts to obtain access via the subclavian or internal jugular route are unsuccessful, a chest radiograph is required to rule out pneumothorax prior to attempting insertion on the contralateral site.

Limitations of central venous pressure monitoring

In many clinical situations, CVP does not accurately reflect left ventricular end-diastolic pressure and therefore cannot be used to estimate left ventricular preload. For example, a patient affected by pulmonary hypertension might have elevated CVP but normal or low left ventricular end-diastolic pressure and volume. In patients who have acute left ventricular myocardial infarction, CVP may be modestly elevated while left atrial and left ventricular end-diastolic pressures are severely increased with radiographic and clinical evidence of pulmonary edema[10]. Moreover, changes in CVP frequently do not predict the changes in left heart pressures[10].

Right atrial pressure is discordant with left atrial pressure in over 25% of patients who have mitral valve disease[7]. In some of these patients, fluid loading caused right and left atrial pressures to diverge, and responses of right atrial pressure and left ventricular end-diastolic pressure to pressor agents were inconsistent[11,12]. Thus, in many critically ill patients, CVP may provide misleading information regarding left heart pressure and preload or responses to therapy. Additional methods to evaluate cardiac filling pressures and function are frequently required.

PULMONARY ARTERY CATHETERS

In 1970, Swan et al.[10] reported the development of a balloon-tipped, flow-directed catheter to measure pulmonary artery pressure and estimate left ventricular end-diastolic pressure (Fig. 13.6). The catheter was introduced through a central vein, such as the subclavian or internal jugular vein, and advanced through the chambers of the right heart into a medium-sized pulmonary artery. The small balloon at the catheter tip caused cessation of blood flow distal to the catheter, which resulted in a stagnant column of blood through the pulmonary capillary bed that extended to a confluence of medium-sized veins. Thus, the pressure measured at the catheter tip immediately distal to the balloon [pulmonary capillary wedge pressure (Pcw)] reflected a pressure close to the left atrium and therefore could be used to estimate left ventricular end-diastolic pressure. Use of Pcw avoids some of the previously described limitations of the use of CVP to assess vascular filling and left ventricular preload.

Several years after the introduction of the balloon-tipped, flow-directed catheter, measurements of cardiac output were developed utilizing a modification of the catheter used by Swan et al. Cooled fluid is injected through a separate channel of the catheter, and exits the channel through a side hole in the right heart. Blood temperature is monitored with a thermistor at the catheter tip. When the change in blood temperature is plotted against time, analysis of the area and shape of the curve allows a calculation of flow (cardiac output) between the sites of cooled fluid injection and the thermistor at the distal catheter tip. With concomitant measurements of blood pressure, right and left atrial pressures, and arterial and mixed venous blood gases, the PAC

Advantages and disadvantages of major routes of access for central line insertion		
Site	**Advantages**	**Disadvantages**
Internal jugular	↓ Risk of pneumothorax	Landmarks may be obscured with intubated patient or patients who have a tracheostomy
	Easily compressible	More difficult in hypovolemic patient
	Higher rate success with inexperienced operators	?↑ Risk of infection
Subclavian	Consistent landmarks	Noncompressible site
	Patient comfort	May be higher risk of complications with inexperienced operators
	Most reliable access in hypovolemic patient	↑ Risk of pneumothorax
Femoral	Easily accessed during cardiopulmonary resuscitation	Difficult access in hypovolemic patient
	Compressible site	?↑ Risk of infection
	No need for Trendelenburg	?↑ Risk of thromboembolism
		May be less effective for monitoring central venous pressure in some patients

Figure 13.5 Advantages and disadvantages of major routes of access for central line insertion.

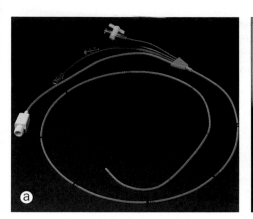
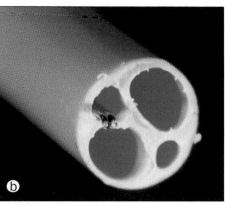

Figure 13.6 Pulmonary artery catheter.
(a) Red = channel for balloon inflation. Blue = channel to proximal port (for right atrial pressure and injectate). Yellow = channel to distal port (for measurement of pulmonary artery pressure and pulmonary capillary wedge pressure). Bright yellow = thermistor connection. (b) Cross-section of pulmonary artery catheter – clockwise from left: thermistor wire, distal port channel, balloon channel, proximal port channel.

allows determinations of systemic and pulmonary vascular resistance, systemic oxygen delivery, and oxygen extraction by systemic tissue. Since its development and introduction to clinical practice, the PAC has become an important part of the hemodynamic monitoring armamentarium of many intensivists.

Insertion of pulmonary artery catheters

Insertion of PACs is technically easiest from the right internal jugular and left subclavian vein sites because of the orientation of these veins in relation to the right heart. The left internal jugular vein is also favorable, but in some patients the catheter does not advance easily into the right heart and pulmonary outflow tract from this site. With the right subclavian site, the introducer tip may lie in, or point directly toward, the left subclavian vein, or its position and orientation may require a sharp turn by the PAC to advance toward the right heart. The femoral vein site can also be used, but PAC insertion from this site is technically more challenging and may require fluoroscopy to navigate the pathway. An antecubital vein was used in earlier reports of PAC insertion, but this approach is rarely used now.

After the vein is entered and the guidewire inserted (as described in the section on central venous cannulation), a small incision is made in the skin with a scalpel to facilitate passage of an introducer catheter. The dilator is inserted completely into an introducer catheter, and both are advanced together over the guidewire using a gentle twisting motion. Once the introducer is advanced into the vein, the dilator and wire are removed simultaneously while holding the introducer firmly in place. The patient is then redraped to create a large sterile field to accommodate the PAC.

The PAC is inserted through a sterile protective sheath covering. The balloon is then checked by injecting 1.5mL air for several seconds. The catheter ports are flushed with infusate (usually 0.9% saline with 1 unit heparin/100mL saline) and an electronic pressure transducer is attached to the channel of the PAC that leads to the port at its tip. Pressure at the distal tip of the PAC is displayed continuously on a monitor in the patient's room. To ensure that the catheter, transducer system, and monitor are working, the catheter tip may be shaken while viewing the monitor screen to confirm the presence of pressure artifacts. Prior to insertion of the catheter into the introducer, the natural curve of the catheter should approximate the curved pathway it must follow through the right heart into the proximal pulmonary artery.

The catheter is inserted into the introducer with the balloon deflated and advanced approximately 15cm, until it is past the distal tip of the introducer. The balloon is then inflated with 1.5mL air and advanced several more centimeters. When the catheter enters the thorax, the pressure tracing should show respiratory variations. As it approaches the right atrium, a, c, and v waves characteristic of atrial activity should become apparent. The catheter is then advanced smoothly with the balloon inflated while observing the pressure waveforms on a monitor screen. When the catheter tip enters the right ventricle (approximately 25–30cm from the right internal jugular entry site), a ventricular waveform is observed, with a relatively high systolic pressure [low normal = 2.0–2.6kPa (15–20mmHg)] and diastolic pressure usually returning to 0–0.7kPa (0–5mmHg; Fig. 13.7). Limiting the time with the catheter tip in the right ventricle reduces the

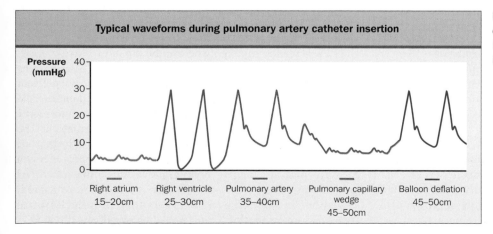

Figure 13.7 Typical waveforms obtained during pulmonary artery catheter insertion. Distances shown are approximate from right internal jugular vein entry site.

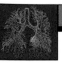

risk of catheter-induced arrhythmias. In patients who have right ventricular dilatation, the catheter may coil in the right ventricle rather than advance into the pulmonary artery. Familiarity with distances from insertion site to right atrium, right ventricle, pulmonary artery, and wedged positions help in recognition of this problem. As the PAC is advanced, a 'step up' of the diastolic pressure to at least 0.7–1.3kPa (5–10mmHg) and the appearance of a dicrotic notch signifies crossing the pulmonic valve and entering the pulmonary artery. The catheter is advanced approximately 5–10cm until the pulmonary artery systolic and diastolic waveforms are replaced by a narrower waveform at a lower mean pressure, which signifies that the balloon has 'wedged' into a medium-sized artery. If the balloon is deflated in this position, the pulmonary artery waveform should reappear (see Fig. 13.7). With the catheter in this position, the sterile sheath is advanced and locked into position on the introducer hub.

If the PCW waveforms are atypical, a sample of blood is withdrawn from the distal port with the balloon inflated, the first 5mL is discarded, and the blood is analyzed for blood gases. If blood does not flow freely back through the PAC, the catheter tip may be clotted or lodged against a vessel wall. The catheter must be withdrawn several centimeters and repositioned. The partial pressure of oxygen (PO_2) of the sample should be similar to the PO_2 of arterial blood. If the PO_2 is similar to values commonly seen in mixed venous blood [4.7–6.0kPa (35–45mmHg)], the balloon probably does not occlude the artery completely, and the pressure waveform may reflect a damped pulmonary artery pressure.

When the PAC is in an apparently satisfactory position, the pressure transducer is checked for appropriate positioning (at the level of the heart), 'zeroing', and calibration. A chest radiograph with the PAC balloon deflated should demonstrate the catheter tip in the main pulmonary artery or the left or right hilum. If the catheter tip is in a mid or peripheral lung zone, the patient is at risk for pulmonary artery rupture during balloon inflation. The radiograph must also be inspected carefully for pneumothorax, which may be more apparent if the film is taken of the patient at end-exhalation.

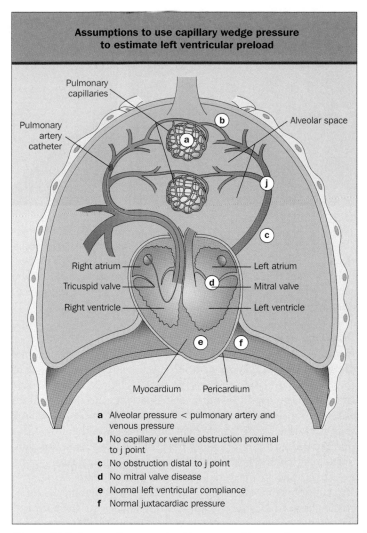

Figure 13.8 Assumptions required to use capillary wedge pressure to estimate left ventricular preload.

Interpretation of pulmonary artery catheter data

Several assumptions are required to use PCW to estimate left ventricular end-diastolic volume (Fig. 13.8). These assumptions pertain to the following two key questions:

- how well does PCW represent left ventricular end-diastolic pressure (Fig. 13.8, assumptions a, b, c and d); and
- how well does left ventricular end-diastolic pressure represent left ventricular end-diastolic volume (Fig. 13.8, assumptions e and f)?

Intensivists must consider these assumptions to avoid errors in reading PCW tracings and interpreting their significance.

Some mechanically ventilated patients require high levels of positive end-expiratory pressure (PEEP) or continuous positive airway pressure (CPAP) to improve oxygenation. This raises juxtacardiac pressure and tends to cause a misleading elevation in PCW (Fig. 13.8, assumption f). To correct for this effect, some workers advocate measuring PCW approximately 1 second after briefly disconnecting the ventilator from the endotracheal tube. However, this may cause hypoxemia from decreased alveolar recruitment or could contribute to lung injury from repeated closing and reopening of small airways. Another approach is to estimate the effect of positive airway pressure on juxtacardiac

pressure and subtract this amount from the measured PCW. As a rule of thumb, this adjustment can be made by subtracting 25% of the PEEP or CPAP value from PCW.

It is important to read the PCW at end expiration, the point in the respiratory cycle when juxtacardiac pressure is closest to atmospheric pressure [regardless of the level of PEEP or CPAP (Fig. 13.8, assumption f)]. Identifying the point of end expiration on the PCW tracing is straightforward in patients who breath spontaneously, without positive pressure ventilatory assistance: the PCW is read immediately before the dip in pressure that signifies the beginning of inspiration (Fig. 13.9). In patients who receive positive pressure ventilation and make no inspiratory efforts of their own, end expiration is easily identified on the PCW tracing as the point immediately before the increase in pressure that signifies the effects of positive pressure inspiration (Fig. 13.9). In patients who continue to make inspiratory efforts while they receive positive pressure ventilation, the appearances of PCW tracings are highly variable and often ambiguous. The patient's inspiratory effort usually causes a dip in PCW, which may or may not be followed by a rise in PCW from the effects of positive pressure inspiration (Fig. 13.9). The size of the dip in PCW

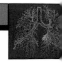

Representative capillary wedge pressure traces

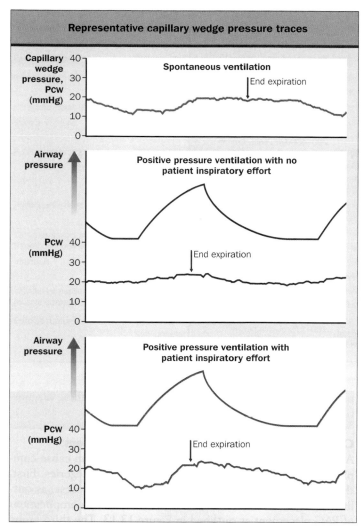

Figure 13.9 Representative capillary wedge pressure traces.
Shown are spontaneous ventilation, positive pressure ventilation with no patient inspiratory effort, and positive pressure ventilation with patient inspiratory effort.

Proximal v-waves in a capillary wedge pressure tracing

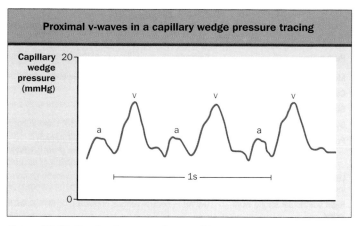

Figure 13.10 ProximaL v-waves in a capillary wedge pressure tracing.

enlarged v-waves (Fig. 13.10), which may also appear in other conditions such as mitral stenosis and hypervolemia. If the mean PCW is read in the presence of large v-waves, left ventricular end-diastolic pressure and diastolic filling may be overestimated. To avoid this error, the PCW tracing must be read immediately prior to the start of the v-wave, as close as possible to end expiration. This usually appears around the time of the T-wave during simultaneous electrocardiograph recordings.

Role of the pulmonary artery catheter

Experienced physicians frequently have difficulty using common clinical and laboratory data in their assessments of circulation in critically ill patients. This is especially true for patients who require mechanical ventilation. In a study of patients in whom PACs were placed, attending intensivists and critical care fellows were correct in just over 50% of their estimations of cardiac index, PCW, and mean pulmonary artery pressure. Changes in therapy were made in 48% of cases based on information subsequently obtained from PACs[13].

In general, a PAC should be considered when two conditions occur together:

• usual clinical observations and laboratory data are ambiguous with respect to the assessment of circulation, particularly in the presence of hypotension; and
• consequences of the wrong treatment decision may worsen the physiologic abnormalities.

As an example of the first condition, a patient may have hypotension and low urine output, which suggests low cardiac output from inadequate vascular volume. However, the same patient may also have edema and diffuse pulmonary infiltrates, which suggest volume overload or cardiac dysfunction.

In this case, the second condition is fulfilled if the patient described was truly hypovolemic, but if a diuretic was prescribed shock would worsen. If the patient was in congestive heart failure, but intravenous fluids and blood products were given, pulmonary edema would worsen. Under some circumstances, it may be prudent to attempt a trial of therapy based on clinical impressions prior to PAC placement. For example, in a young hypotensive patient with apparent sepsis, warm extremities, and marginal urine output, intravenous fluids followed by vasopressors may be prescribed. If improvement is not apparent or if the patient deteriorates over the next several hours, perhaps with worsening azotemia and hypotension, the decision to place a PAC can be reconsidered.

in early inspiration and the subsequent rise in PCW from ventilator pressure depend on the magnitude of patient effort in relation to ventilator flow rate. In patients who make vigorous inspiratory efforts, PCW tracings resemble those in patients who breathe spontaneously without positive pressure assistance: the rise in PCW that results from ventilator assistance may not occur at all. Regardless of the magnitudes of these dips and rises in PCW, it is paramount to read PCW at end expiration. Reading PCW at the wrong point in the cycle can lead to incorrect treatment decisions.

The effect of left ventricular end-diastolic compliance must also be considered when interpreting a PCW value (see Fig. 13.8, assumption e). In a patient who has normal left ventricular end-diastolic compliance, a PCW of 1.6kPa (12mmHg) may reflect ample diastolic filling. In contrast, in a patient who has a reduced diastolic compliance, as in hypertrophic cardiomyopathy, a PCW of 1.6kPa (12mmHg) may reflect inadequate end-diastolic volume.

When there is increased atrial filling during ventricular systole, as in mitral regurgitation, the PCW tracing may show

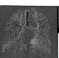
15. Reeves RA. Does this patient have hypertension? How to measure blood pressure. JAMA. 1995;273:1211–18.

16. Seneff M. Arterial line placement and care. In: Rippe JM, Irwin RS, Fink MP, eds. Procedures and techniques in intensive care medicine. Boston: Little, Brown; 1995:36–47.

17. Geddes LA. Cardiovascular devices and their applications. New York: Wiley; 1984.

18. Aoyagi T, Kishi M, Yamaguchi K, Watanabe S. Improvement of the ear-piece oximeter. In: Abstracts of the 13th annual meeting of the Japanese Society of Medical Electronics and Biological Engineering. 1974:90–1.

19. Jubran A. Pulse oximetry. In: Tobin MJ, ed. Principles and practice of intensive care monitoring. New York: McGraw-Hill; 1998:261–87.

20 Eisenberg PR, Jaffe AS, Schuster DP. Clinical evaluation compared to pulmonary artery catheterization in the hemodynamic assessment of critically ill patients. Crit Care Med. 1984;12:549–53.

21. Steingrub JS, Celoria G, Vickers-Lahti M, Teres D, Bria W. Therapeutic impact of pulmonary artery catheterization in a medical/surgical ICU. Chest. 1991;99:1451–5.

22. Connors AF, Dawson NV, Shaw PK, Montenegro HD, Nara AR, Martin L. Hemodynamic status in critically ill patients with and without acute heart disease. Chest. 1990;98:1200–6.

23. Connors AF, Speroff T, Dawson NV, et al. The effectiveness of right heart catheterization in the initial care of critically ill patients. JAMA. 1996;276:889–97.

24. Gore JM, Goldberg RJ, Spodick DH, Alpert JS, Dalen JE. A community-wide assessment of the use of pulmonary artery catheters in patients with acute myocardial infarction. Chest. 1987;92:721–7.

25. Robin ED. The cult of the Swan–Ganz catheter. Ann Intern Med. 1985;103:445–9.

26. Cobb DK, High KP, Sawyer RG, et al. A controlled trial of scheduled replacement central venous and pulmonary-artery catheters. N Engl J Med. 1992;327:1062–8.

Chapter 14 Airway Management

Jeanine P Wiener-Kronish and Thomas E Shaughnessy

INTRODUCTION

The decision to instrument the airway is made in response to one or more of three circumstances: failure of oxygenation, failure of ventilation, or for airway protection. The medical provider responsible for securing the airway must know the problems and advantages of the various available techniques and rapidly utilize these in the patient who needs assistance, as often only limited time is available to correct the problems.

Adverse outcomes occur with failure to restore ventilation, failure to recognize an esophageal intubation, or massive aspiration with peri-intubation[1,2]. Death or hypoxic brain damage can occur when airway management is performed poorly. Closed claim analyses have determined that, in many instances, there is an associated failure to recognize the scope of the clinical problem, and/or a failure to act in a timely manner[3,4].

INDICATIONS AND CONTRAINDICATIONS

The most common indication for airway control is respiratory failure and the need to deliver positive pressure ventilation, which may be manifested by hypoxia, hypercapnia, or an excessive work of breathing. Other indications include protection from aspiration of gastric contents or blood, insurance of airway patency in the setting of facial or airway trauma and/or swelling of upper airway structures, and situations in which neuromuscular paralysis must be administered, intracranial hypertension must be treated, improved airway suctioning is necessary, or alterations in the patient's mental status compromise the ability to protect the airways.

TECHNIQUES

General considerations

The initial approach to management of the airway is to obtain a history of any prior airway problems and to recognize situations that are associated with difficulty in obtaining an airway. Patients who have a restricted oral opening, small pharyngeal space, non-compliant submandibular tissue, limited atlanto-occipital extension, or partial airway obstruction can be difficult to manage[4]. Mask ventilation may be difficult in edentulous patients, those with full beards, or those who have airway restrictions.

Special considerations

A number of special considerations arise. Patients who are at risk of aspiration (bowel obstruction, abdominal problems, vomiting, pregnant, postprandial, obese, diabetic with gastroparesis) require the Sellick maneuver (i.e. applying cricoid pressure) during direct laryngoscopy or they should be intubated awake[5].

Patients who have myocardial ischemia, acute myocardial infarction or failure, or who are hypovolemic or on pressors have a higher incidence of death peri-intubation[6]. These patients do not tolerate significant increases in heart rate or blood pressure. Accordingly, medications and techniques that maintain normal hemodynamics need to be employed.

Patients with aneurysms do not tolerate large variations in their blood pressures, as this increases the risk of rupture; again, medications and techniques that maintain normal hemodynamics must be utilized.

Patients who are chronically hypercapnic or who have severe airflow limitation should be ventilated with small tidal volumes and low respiratory rates. Hypercapnia should be maintained in patients who are chronically hypercapnic[7].

Airway management paradigms

Six broad types of airway management include noninvasive ventilation, awake intubation, anesthetic with spontaneous ventilation, anesthetic with neuromuscular paralysis, transtracheal catheter, and surgical airway management.

Noninvasive ventilation

Patients may maintain adequate oxygenation and ventilation if assisted with continuous positive airway pressure with a mask, or bilevel positive airway pressure (see Chapters 12 and 37). Contraindications to these techniques include ventilatory or hemodynamic instability, a requirement for sedation, inability to handle upper airway secretions, severe hypoxia, risk of aspiration, or inability to wear a tight mask[7].

Awake intubation

When possible, patients should be intubated when awake, but the airway may be difficult to secure such that the patient can continue to ventilate and oxygenate spontaneously. Approaches for awake intubation range from nasal intubation that does not require laryngeal visualization, to awake, direct laryngoscopy that utilizes fiberoptic laryngoscopes or bronchoscopes.

Anesthetic with spontaneous ventilation

Doses of sedative agents administered as a bolus can maintain spontaneous ventilation, yet permit laryngoscopy, the application of a laryngeal mask airway, a transilluminating stylet, or the insertion of a fiberoptic bronchoscope (see Fig. 14.1)[8,9].

Anesthetic with neuromuscular paralysis

Anesthetic with neuromuscular paralysis is the most common method utilized for direct laryngoscopy because relaxation of the masseter muscle facilitates direct visualization of the glottis[1,2].

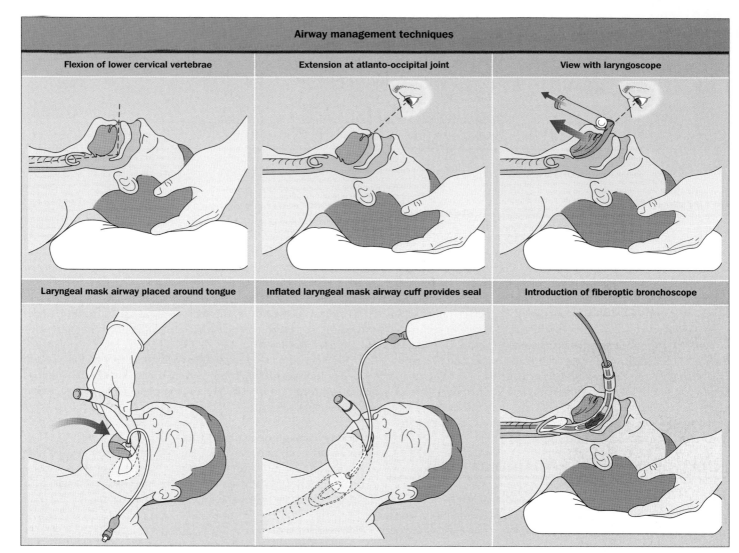

Airway management techniques

Flexion of lower cervical vertebrae	Extension at atlanto-occipital joint	View with laryngoscope

Laryngeal mask airway placed around tongue	Inflated laryngeal mask airway cuff provides seal	Introduction of fiberoptic bronchoscope

Figure 14.1 Airway management techniques. Correct positioning is important to optimize the view during direct laryngoscopy. Flexion of the lower cervical spine brings the trachea in line with the pharynx, while extension at the atlanto-occipital joint aligns the trachea with the oral cavity. The laryngoscope is usually introduced from the right side of the mouth. The tongue is displaced leftward into the mandible by traction in an anterocaudal direction (arrow) to reveal the glottis. The laryngeal mask airway (LMA) is placed manually around the tongue in an unconscious patient. The LMA cuff seats around the glottis and when inflated provides a seal to allow spontaneous or limited positive pressure ventilation. The LMA cuff also lies over the esophagus, which gives the possibility of gastric inflation, regurgitation, and pulmonary aspiration. A fiberoptic bronchoscope may be introduced via the mouth or nose and used to traverse the larynx. (A bronchoscope can also go through the LMA.) An endotracheal tube is then guided over the bronchoscope into the trachea.

Loss of spontaneous respiration means the practitioner must obtain immediate airway control, or assure adequate ventilation by mask. When this option is selected the provider must have an alternative plan, as the larynx is not always visualized.

A rapid sequence approach is undertaken in patients thought to have an airway that can be controlled with little difficulty by laryngoscopy, but are at risk for aspiration of gastric contents[5]. The goal is to secure the airway rapidly. The patient is preoxygenated (no nitrogen measured during exhalation). A sedative agent and a short-acting muscle relaxant are administered in high doses simultaneously (Fig. 14.2). At the same time, an assistant applies pressure to the cricoid cartilage (the only complete ring in the tracheobronchial tree), which occludes the esophagus and decreases the risk of aspiration of gastric contents. This external pressure is maintained until the airway is secured by tracheal intubation (Fig. 14.3)[19–20].

Transtracheal catheter

Transtracheal catheter, a nonsurgical approach, is commonly utilized for urgent situations in which one approach has failed and improvement in oxygenation is imperative. The technique achieves minimally acceptable levels of oxygenation and provides time for more definitive measures to obtain an airway, but ventilation is not possible (see Fig. 14.4).

Surgical airway management

Surgical access is necessary when the mouth cannot be opened, when adequate laryngeal visualization cannot be achieved, or when an obstruction occurs in the oropharynx. A tracheostomy is time consuming and cumbersome in an emergency, while a cricothyroidotomy is technically easier, and may be accomplished quickly, with readily available equipment (see Fig. 14.4).

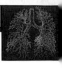

Common agents used for airway control			
Drug		**Dosage (mg/kg)**	**Comments**
Sedative drugs	Thiopental	3–5	Cardiac depression, vasodilatation, can cause severe hypotension during hypovolemic states
	Propofol[10,11]	2	Rapid onset and offset, vasodilates, easily contaminated, affirm sterility
	Etomidate[12]	0.25	Hemodynamic stability, myoclonus, associated adrenal suppression
	Ketamine	1 (i.v.); 4 (i.m.)	Analgesic, sympathetic stimulant, bronchodilator, causes dysphoria
	Midazolam	0.1	Vasodilatation, hypotension, dangerous in hypovolemic states
Neuromuscular blocking agents	Succinylcholine[13,14]	1–2	Most rapid onset, lasts <5 minutes; contraindicated in hyperkalemia, burns, and chronic neural injuries; associated with malignant hyperthermia and masseter spasm in children
	Vecuronium[15]	1–2	Clinical duration 30 minutes; higher dose required for rapid onset; associated with prolonged paralysis in corticosteroid-dependent patients
	Rocuronium[16]	1.2	Rapid onset, but clinical duration 20 minutes; associated with prolonged paralysis in corticosteroid-dependent patients
	Cisatracurium[17,18]	0.2	Slightly delayed onset, clinical duration 30 minutes; metabolism via plasma cholinesterase

Figure 14.2 Common agents used for airway control. A wide array of sedative and/or hypnotic agents and neuromuscular relaxants is available. The choice of agent is based on the drug's unique properties and the demands of a given clinical situation. The suggested doses of sedative drugs are for the induction of healthy adults. Dosage requirements are decreased in patients who have hypovolemia, neonates, elderly, or with concurrent administration of other sedatives or opiates.

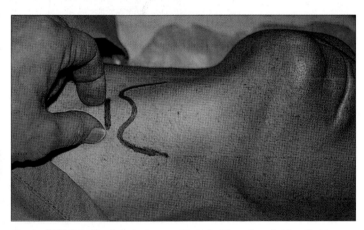

Figure 14.3 The Sellick maneuver. The cricoid cartilage is identified by palpation below the thyroid cartilage. Firm pressure is placed on this structure to occlude the esophagus. Pressure is maintained until after intubation, and airway control is documented by auscultation of the lung fields.

Considerations in the choice of airway control

A number of considerations affect the choice of airway control. Whether all structures are seen by laryngoscopy or by bronchoscopy, any visualization is preferable to blind techniques when placement of the endotracheal tube must be precise (i.e. when oxygenation is low, the patient is unstable, or the patient is soiling the airway).

Techniques that maintain the patient's spontaneous ventilation give the clinician time, and the opportunity to try different approaches. Neuromuscular paralysis commits the practitioner to ventilating the patient. Practitioners must be able to achieve ventilation by mask if paralytic agents are being administered, but the relaxation of glottic structures that occurs with paralysis may make mask ventilation more difficult.

Fiberoptic procedures usually take longer than 3 minutes and, accordingly, should not be utilized in emergency situations. When these approaches are selected, alternative methods, which include laryngeal mask airways, should be available to deal rapidly with acute deteriorations.

New or unfamiliar techniques should not be tried in emergency situations that require immediate action or in critically ill patients who have a limited respiratory or ventilatory reserve.

If the approach selected is unsuccessful, proper judgment dictates abandoning the procedure, aiding the patient with mask ventilation as necessary, and either obtaining help or trying another approach.

The patient must be oxygenated! Remember that only 3 minutes are available to achieve oxygenation when the patient stops breathing. Transtracheal ventilation or cricothyroidotomy should be attempted instead of repeated attempts at laryngoscopy. Clinicians who instrument the airway must practice transtracheal ventilation and/or cricothyroidotomies until they can obtain an emergency airway in 3 minutes or less (see Fig. 14.5).

COMPLICATIONS

The most serious complication is the inability to perform mask ventilation or to oxygenate a patient, and then not be able to instrument and control the airway, but many other complications may occur. Prolonged intervals of hypoxia are caused by poor technique, lack of delivery of oxygen, or poor cardiac output, and peri-intubation aspiration also results from poor technique.

Mucosal damage arises from intubation attempts (e.g. mask ventilation that causes trauma of the eyes, subcutaneous emphysema from airway perforations, aspiration because of insufflation of the stomach). Blades, stylets, and other objects in the airway can damage the airway mucosa and cause life-threatening hemorrhage. These risks are increased in the patient who has a coagulopathy or underlying friable mucosa (e.g. mucositis).

Transtracheal needles or catheters can lead to massive and life-threatening subcutaneous emphysema. Tracheotomy tubes may be misplaced in nontracheal structures, which can result in subcutaneous emphysema or life-threatening hypoxemia. Also, endotracheal tubes may be misplaced in the right mainstem bronchus. The position of all endotracheal and tracheotomy tubes should be confirmed by radiographs or by direct visualization and withdrawn sufficiently to sit above the carina.

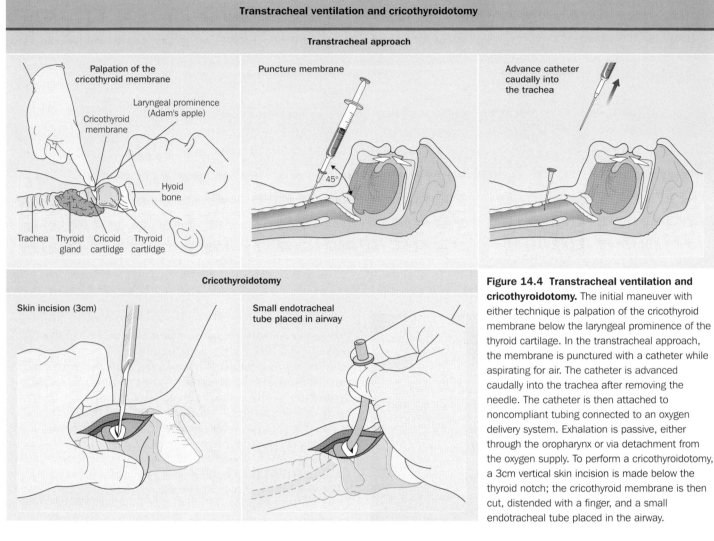

Transtracheal ventilation and cricothyroidotomy

Transtracheal approach

Palpation of the cricothyroid membrane

Laryngeal prominence (Adam's apple)

Cricothyroid membrane

Hyoid bone

Trachea Thyroid gland Cricoid cartlidge Thyroid cartlidge

Puncture membrane

45°

Advance catheter caudally into the trachea

Cricothyroidotomy

Skin incision (3cm)

Small endotracheal tube placed in airway

Figure 14.4 Transtracheal ventilation and cricothyroidotomy. The initial maneuver with either technique is palpation of the cricothyroid membrane below the laryngeal prominence of the thyroid cartilage. In the transtracheal approach, the membrane is punctured with a catheter while aspirating for air. The catheter is advanced caudally into the trachea after removing the needle. The catheter is then attached to noncompliant tubing connected to an oxygen delivery system. Exhalation is passive, either through the oropharynx or via detachment from the oxygen supply. To perform a cricothyroidotomy, a 3cm vertical skin incision is made below the thyroid notch; the cricothyroid membrane is then cut, distended with a finger, and a small endotracheal tube placed in the airway.

Tracheotomies can lead to bilateral pneumothoraces secondary to the surgical site's proximity to the apices of the lungs, as well as to damage to the veins in the neck, with the possibility of life-threatening hemorrhage. Newly placed tracheotomy tubes should not be replaced by inexperienced clinicians because of the difficulty in finding the proper position in the trachea, and the danger of creating a false passage. A reasonable option for the management of a dislodged fresh tracheostomy includes orotracheal intubation for airway control, followed by the elective replacement of the tracheostomy tube as a surgical procedure.

PITFALLS AND CONTROVERSIES

Oral versus nasal intubation
The nasal approach is somewhat easier than the oral because of the broader curve that the oral endotracheal tube must traverse before reaching the glottis, and it also requires smaller tubes and topical application of vasoconstrictors. However, the nasal approach should be avoided in patients who have coagulopathies or in those who have sustained midface-trauma.

Stabilization of the injured cervical spines
The risk of catastrophic neurologic injury makes it imperative that any lateral displacement of the cervical spine be avoided in

patients who have sustained traumatic injuries. While gentle manual stabilization may be all that is available, it must be appreciated that this stabilization does not fully immobilize the head during the atlanto-occipital extension that occurs with direct laryngoscopy[21,22]. The placement of a halo-vest on such a patient fully protects their C-spines[21,22]. Fiberoptic or blind nasal techniques should be utilized for situations in which full neck extension cannot be tolerated.

Ventilation after a failed rapid sequence induction
When the trachea cannot be intubated during a rapid sequence maneuver, the external pressure on the cricoid cartilage should be maintained[19]. Ventilation with small rapid breaths maintains airway pressure at a low level so the pressure that compresses the esophagus is not exceeded.

Management of regurgitation during mask ventilation
Positive pressure in the airway forces gastric contents into the trachea and can cause acute lung injury. Appropriate management includes maintenance of cricoid pressure and rapidly placing the patient in the Trendelenburg position. The bulk of the gastric contents are removed by manual clearance or by suctioning. If conditions warrant, immediate direct laryngoscopy may be performed to inspect the vocal cords and intubate the trachea[2,5].

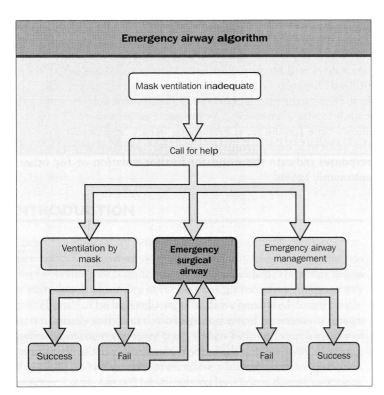

Emergency airway algorithm

- Mask ventilation inadequate
  - Call for help
    - Ventilation by mask
      - Success
      - Fail
    - **Emergency surgical airway**
    - Emergency airway management
      - Fail
      - Success

Figure 14.5 Emergency airway algorithm. If mask ventilation is insufficient, additional assistance from personnel should be obtained to perform a jaw thrust and to place oral airways. If these attempts fail, the provider must obtain an emergent airway (i.e. laryngeal mask airway, retrograde intubation techniques, transtracheal ventilation) or a surgical airway. (Adapted with permission from the American Society of Anesthesiologists.)

If continued mask ventilation is necessary, small, gentle breaths are administered to limit esophageal insufflation and the distal migration of gastric material.

Aspiration prophylaxis

Aspiration prophylaxis is a prudent measure in the high-risk patient (e.g. full stomach, obese patients who have bowel motility dysfunction, patients who have gastroesophageal reflux, parturients). Antacids administered immediately prior to tracheal intubation rapidly increase the gastric pH above 2.5. Aspiration of particulate antacids is associated with the development of severe pneumonitis, and thus nonparticulate antacids, such as 30mL of sodium citrate, are recommended to increase gastric pH. While the administration of this volume of medicine increases the gastric fluid volume, animal studies suggest that pulmonary injury is worse after the aspiration of small quantities of low pH fluid compared with the aspiration of larger quantities of liquid that has a high pH. H_2-receptor antagonists take longer to act and do not affect the pre-existing gastric contents; thus, they are of little value in the management of acute situations[1,2,19].

Size of endotracheal tube

For adults, 7.5–8.0mm internal diameter (ID) tube for men and 7.0–7.5mm ID tube for women are appropriate for the average person. For pediatric patients, tube size selection may be based on age using the formula ID = (age + 16)/4.

Tubes at least one size larger and smaller should always be available to accommodate individual anatomic variations.

Type of blade

Laryngoscope blades come in a variety of styles and sizes. The most commonly used blades include the curved Macintosh and the straight Miller blades. The curved blades are inserted into the vallecula, immediately anterior to the epiglottis, which is then flipped out of the visual axis to expose the larynx. The Miller blade is inserted past the epiglottis, which is simply lifted out of the way of the glottis. Many clinicians feel the Macintosh blade is technically easier because the wider blade prevents intrusion of the tongue into the visual field. However, in difficult situations (i.e. anteriorly situated larynx, large epiglottis), the straight blade frequently affords improved visualization.

Positioning the obese patient

The proper 'sniff' position (neck flexion, head extension) should be achieved prior to attempts at direct laryngoscopy. In the obese patient this sometimes requires elevating and supporting the shoulders (by the placement of towels underneath these structures), in addition to elevating the head to optimize the visual axis. In addition to providing elevation, this maneuver also creates more room for head extension (Fig. 14.6).

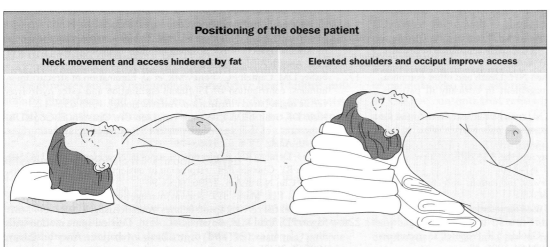

Positioning of the obese patient

Neck movement and access hindered by fat	Elevated shoulders and occiput improve access

Figure 14.6 Positioning the obese patient. With the obese patient in the supine position, neck movement and access with a laryngoscope is hindered by fat. The same patient positioned with shoulders elevated and occiput further elevated so that the head again assumes a 'sniffing' position greatly facilitates access to the airway.

Computed tomography

When compared with conventional chest radiography, CT has clearly been shown to be superior for imaging the peripheral and central airways, mediastinum, and lung parenchyma. In particular, CT often supplies additional information about radiographic findings and allows the detection of unsuspected parenchymal nodules, cavities or infiltrates, endobronchial masses, bronchiectasis, and vascular abnormalities. Therefore, CT should be very useful in patients with unexplained hemoptysis, and this has been confirmed by a number of recent studies[6–9,16].

In the presence of a normal or nonlocalizing chest radiograph, CT detects an unsuspected cause of hemoptysis, most commonly bronchiectasis or a parenchymal nodule or cavity, in approximately 50% of patients (Figs 17.6 & 17.7). When performed

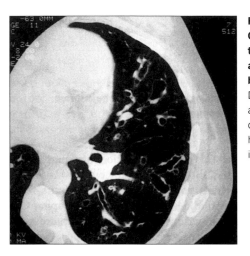

Figure 17.6 Computed tomography (CT) appearance of bronchiectasis. Dilated peripheral airways are clearly demonstrated by this high-resolution CT image.

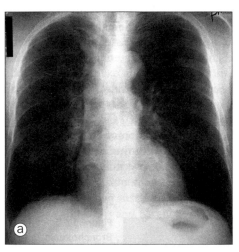

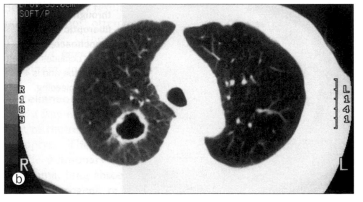

Figure 17.7 Chest radiograph and computed tomography in a patient who has a cavitary, squamous cell carcinoma. The cavitary lesion cannot be seen on the (a) chest radiograph, but is clearly demonstrated by (b) computed tomography.

after a nondiagnostic FOB, CT still identifies a potential bleeding site in about one third of these patients[6–9,16]. Also, CT is useful for over half of all patients who have a localizing chest radiograph[6,7,9], either by identifying a new source of hemoptysis or by providing additional information about a previously recognized abnormality. When performed after FOB, CT identifies an unsuspected cause of hemoptysis in approximately 25% of these patients.

In patients who have neoplasms that involve the central airways, CT has a reported sensitivity >90% (Fig. 17.8), and false-negative results occur primarily in patients who have endobronchial lesions <2mm in diameter[17,18]. In patients with hemoptysis, the sensitivity of CT may be even greater, since it is unlikely that very small tumors would produce clinically apparent bleeding. This is supported by the results of five studies that compared the use of CT and FOB in the evaluation of hemoptysis[6–9,16]. Out of a total of 80 patients with malignancy, CT identified all but one (a patient who had a small endobronchial Kaposi's sarcoma[9]). However, as discussed above, CT often detects a malignancy in patients whose FOB is nondiagnostic. Most commonly, this occurs in those who have a peripheral lesion that cannot be visualized endoscopically. This is of particular importance since many of these tumors are surgically resectable and potentially curable[8]. Finally, CT can define the exact location and extent of disease in patients who have suspected bronchogenic carcinoma, and thereby improves the diagnostic yield of both transbronchial biopsy and transbronchial needle aspiration.

To maximize the ability of CT to detect the cause of hemoptysis, specific imaging techniques have been recommended[9,17]. The central airways are evaluated using contiguous, 5mm thick sections from the level of the carina to the inferior pulmonary veins. Above and below this region, high-resolution scans are obtained using 1–3mm thick sections every 8–10mm.

Diagnostic algorithm

Based on the information discussed above, a suggested approach to the patient who has hemoptysis is shown in Figure 17.9. If the initial evaluation yields a firm diagnosis, appropriate therapy is instituted. Occasionally, the initial evaluation suggests an uncommon cause of hemoptysis that requires one or more specific confirmatory tests. For example, an echocardiogram may reveal the presence of LVF or mitral stenosis, and pulmonary embolism may be diagnosed by means of a ventilation–perfusion lung scan. In virtually all other patients, CT is the most appropriate next step in the diagnostic evaluation. As discussed previously, CT often identifies an unsuspected cause of hemoptysis, even in patients whose chest radiograph is normal or nonlocalizing, and may provide a 'road map' for bronchoscopy, as well as other important information in patients who already have a presumptive diagnosis. If CT suggests a disorder that is amenable to bronchoscopic diagnosis, such as neoplasm, infection, broncholithiasis, or interstitial lung disease, FOB is performed next in the diagnostic evaluation. Additional studies such as mediastinoscopy or surgical lung biopsy may be required if FOB is nondiagnostic. When CT is either normal or suggests another cause of hemoptysis, the role of FOB is less clearly defined. When appropriate imaging techniques are used, the absence of an endobronchial abnormality is associated with a low incidence of malignancy. Available data suggest that FOB may be safely omitted in nonsmokers <40 years of age. As CT occasionally fails to detect a small endobronchial lesion, FOB should probably be performed in all other patients.

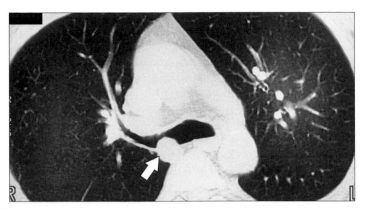

Figure 17.8 Computed tomography appearance of an endobronchial mass. A bronchogenic carcinoma is clearly visible in the right main bronchus.

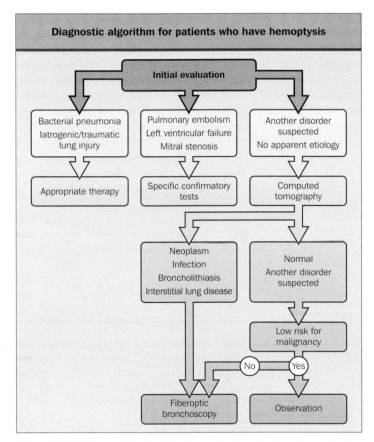

Diagnostic algorithm for patients who have hemoptysis

Figure 17.9 Diagnostic algorithm for patients who have hemoptysis.

TREATMENT

In most cases, hemoptysis requires no specific therapy. Instead, treatment must be directed at its underlying cause, and therapy for most of these disorders is discussed in detail in other chapters of this text. Patients with cryptogenic hemoptysis have an excellent prognosis[12]. Hemoptysis typically resolves within several days, is usually not recurrent, and is very rarely found to be caused by a serious pulmonary disorder.

MASSIVE HEMOPTYSIS

No definition of massive hemoptysis is generally accepted, although the most commonly used criteria require between 200mL and 600mL of blood over 24 hours[19,20]. Any definition is, of course, arbitrary, especially since the amount of blood expectorated is often difficult to quantify. Since morbidity and mortality are dependent not only on the volume of expectorated blood, but also on the rate of bleeding, ability of the patient to clear blood from the airways, and extent and severity of any underlying lung disease, it is evident that a single definition is not applicable to all patients. Instead, for clinical purposes, it is more appropriate to define massive hemoptysis simply as bleeding that leads to impairment of respiratory function and gas exchange and which is, therefore, potentially life-threatening. Overall, the risk of death from massive hemoptysis is approximately 20%, although reported mortality rates vary widely between 0 and 75%. Not surprisingly, the rate at which bleeding occurs appears to be the most important prognostic factor.

Massive hemoptysis is relatively uncommon and occurs in fewer than 5% of patients with lower respiratory tract bleeding. Although any of the disorders listed in Figure 17.1 may potentially give rise to life-threatening hemorrhage, massive hemoptysis is typically caused by only a few. In decreasing order of frequency, these disorders include tuberculosis (either active or inactive), bronchiectasis, mycetoma, bronchogenic carcinoma, lung abscess, and vascular–bronchial fistula.

The associated morbidity and mortality mean that massive hemoptysis is a respiratory emergency and requires rapid evaluation and therapy. Unlike patients with small amounts of bleeding, in whom the emphasis is placed on determining the underlying cause, the primary goals in patients with massive hemoptysis are to maintain a patent airway and to localize and control the bleeding. Patients are closely monitored in an intensive care unit, and elective endotracheal intubation is indicated when patients are unable to clear blood adequately from the airways. Bronchoscopy is performed immediately in an effort to localize the bleeding to a specific segment, lobe, or lung. Localization is usually unsuccessful in the absence of active hemorrhage, and repeated procedures during episodes of recurrent bleeding may be required. Either rigid bronchoscopy or FOB may be used, depending largely on the clinical circumstances. Rigid bronchoscopy, with its large lumen, affords excellent airway control and suctioning capability and is ideally suited for patients with very rapid bleeding. Disadvantages include relatively poor visualization of the segmental and lobar bronchi and the need for general anesthetic. In most patients, FOB is the procedure of choice since it can be performed rapidly, requires only light sedation, and allows excellent airway visualization. All patients with massive hemoptysis should be intubated prior to FOB. This optimizes airway control, allows effective suctioning should the rate of bleeding increase, and permits the bronchoscope to be removed easily and reinserted if the suction channel becomes occluded.

Localization of the bleeding site is important for two reasons. First, it provides a guide for therapy to control ongoing hemorrhage (see below). Second, in the setting of persistent, severe hemoptysis, it allows isolation of the bleeding site, and thereby prevents aspiration of blood throughout the tracheobronchial tree. Guided by the fiberoptic bronchoscope, a balloon catheter may be used to occlude a segmental or lobar airway. When bleeding can only be localized to one lung, a larger balloon may be inflated in a main stem bronchus. Alternatively, the fiberoptic bronchoscope can be used to intubate selectively and ventilate the nonbleeding lung.

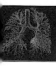
Double-lumen endotracheal tubes also allow unilateral lung ventilation through a cuffed bronchial lumen, which is placed in the left main bronchus, and a tracheal lumen, which is positioned above the carina. These endotracheal tubes have a number of significant drawbacks, however. They are difficult to insert, the correct position is difficult to achieve and maintain, and suction is limited by the small diameter of each lumen.

Once the bleeding site has been localized and a stable airway has been achieved, therapy must be performed to control ongoing hemorrhage. Two options are available – arterial embolization and surgical resection. In over 90% of cases, massive hemoptysis originates from a bronchial artery or, less commonly, from a collateral vessel of the axillary, subclavian, internal mammary, or intercostal arteries. Guided by the results of bronchoscopy, abnormal vessels may be visualized using selective arteriography and occluded with embolized material, most commonly polyvinyl alcohol, a nonabsorbable particulate[18,21]. Arterial embolization is successful for the acute control of hemorrhage in approximately 85% of patients. Although complications are uncommon, unintentional arterial occlusion can have devastating consequences. For example, reflux of material from the bronchial artery into the aorta may lead to systemic embolization, and bronchial artery occlusion proximal to the origin of the anterior spinal artery may result in spinal cord infarction and paralysis. Embolization therapy is ideally suited for patients who have bilateral disease, limited pulmonary reserve, or another contraindication to surgery, and may be repeated as needed to control recurrent hemorrhage. Since surgical resection during active bleeding is accompanied by a mortality rate that approaches 30%, arterial embolization is also the initial procedure of choice in most patients who would otherwise be surgical candidates. Elective surgery can be performed, if necessary, once the patient's condition has been stabilized. Emergency surgery is reserved for patients in immediate danger of asphyxiation and for those in whom arterial embolization is unsuccessful.

Once bleeding has resolved, either spontaneously or following embolization therapy, its cause must be determined using the diagnostic algorithm (see Fig. 17.9). Specific treatment, such as antibacterial or antituberculous therapy, may successfully prevent further episodes of hemoptysis. When effective medical therapy is not available, recurrent bleeding is common[18,19,21]. Approximately 35% of patients in whom bleeding spontaneously resolves have recurrent and often life-threatening hemorrhage within 6 months, and bleeding recurs in 10–20% of patients who have undergone successful embolization therapy. Based on this information, elective surgical resection should be strongly considered in appropriate patients.

REFERENCES

1. Weaver LJ, Solliday N, Cugell DW. Selection of patients with hemoptysis for fiberoptic bronchoscopy. Chest. 1979;76:7–10.
2. Gong H, Salvatierra C. Clinical efficacy of early and delayed fiberoptic bronchoscopy in patients with hemoptysis. Am Rev Respir Dis. 1981;124:221–5.
3. Johnston H, Reisz G. Changing spectrum of hemoptysis. Arch Intern Med. 1989;149:1666–8.
4. O'Neil KM, Lazarus AA. Hemoptysis: indications for bronchoscopy. Arch Intern Med. 1991;151:171–4.
5. Santiago S, Tobias J, Williams AJ. A reappraisal of the causes of hemoptysis. Arch Intern Med. 1991;151:2449–51.
6. Haponik EF, Britt EJ, Smith PL, Bleeker ER. Computed tomography of the chest in the evaluation of hemoptysis. Chest. 1987;91:80–5.
7. Naidich DP, Funt S, Ettenger NA, Arranda C. Hemoptysis: CT-bronchoscopic correlations in 58 cases. Radiology. 1990;177:357–62.
8. Set PA, Flower CD, Smith IE, et al. Hemoptysis: comparative study of the role of CT and fiberoptic bronchoscopy. Radiology. 1993;189:677–80.
9. McGuinness G, Beacher JR, Harkin TJ, et al. Hemoptysis: prospective high-resolution CT/bronchoscopic correlation. Chest. 1994;105:1155–62.
10. Lederle FA, Nichol KL, Parenti CM. Bronchoscopy to evaluate hemoptysis in older men with nonsuspicious chest roentgenograms. Chest. 1989;95:1043–7.
11. Jackson CV, Savage PL, Quinn DL. Role of fiberoptic bronchoscopy in patients with hemoptysis and a normal chest roentgenogram. Chest. 1985;87:142–4.
12. Adelman M, Haponik EF, Bleecker ER, Britt EJ. Cryptogenic hemoptysis: clinical features, bronchoscopic findings, and natural history in 67 patients. Ann Intern Med 1985; 102:829–834.
13. Heimer D, Bar-Ziv J, Scharf SM. Fiberoptic bronchoscopy in patients with hemoptysis and nonlocalizing chest roentgenograms. Arch Intern Med. 1985;145:1427–8.
14. Poe RH, Israel RH, Marin MG, et al. Utility of fiberoptic bronchoscopy in patients with hemoptysis and a nonlocalizing chest roentgenogram. Chest. 1988;92:70–5.
15. Santiago SM, Lehrman S, Williams AJ. Bronchoscopy in patients with haemoptysis and normal chest roentgenograms. Br J Dis Chest. 1987;81:186–8.
16. Millar AB, Boothroyd AE, Edwards D, Hetzel MR. The role of computed tomography in the investigation of unexplained hemoptysis. Respir Med. 1992;86:39–44.
17. Naidich DP, Harkin TJ. Airways and lung: correlation of CT with fiberoptic bronchoscopy. Radiology. 1995;197:1–12.
18. Marshall TJ, Flower CDR, Jackson JE. The role of radiology in the investigation and management of patients with haemoptysis. Clin Radiol. 1996;51:391–400.
19. Cahill BC, Ingbar DH. Massive hemoptysis: assessment and management. Clin Chest Med. 1994;15:147–68.
20. Stoller JK. Diagnosis and management of massive hemoptysis: a review. Respir Care. 1992;37:564–81.
21. Lampmann LEH, Tjan TG. Embolization therapy in haemoptysis. Eur J Radiol. 1994;18:15–9.

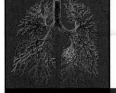

INTRODUCTION

Chest pain is the most frequent new symptom reported by patients referred to outpatient clinics. As it may prefigure a number of potentially life-threatening diseases, chest pain always demands a thorough and careful investigation. Unfortunately, it is a remarkably nonspecific symptom, which can occur as a manifestation of a large and diverse group of conditions (Fig. 18.1).

DIFFERENTIAL DIAGNOSIS

The pathophysiology of chest pain is understood for many, but not all, of the conditions with which it is associated.

Myocardial ischemia

Chest pain associated with myocardial ischemia is attributed to an imbalance between myocardial oxygen supply and demand. For most body organs or tissues, increased oxygen demands can be met by increasing oxygen delivery and/or oxygen extraction. The oxygen content of coronary venous blood is, however, much lower than that of blood flowing from other organs or tissues, which thus limits the ability of the myocardium to increase oxygen extraction (see Fig. 18.2). Thus, the primary mechanism by which the oxygen demands of the myocardium are met is by increased oxygen delivery.

As with flow through any vessel, coronary blood flow is determined by the driving pressure (i.e. the aortic pressure minus the left ventricular end-diastolic pressure) and the resistance of the coronary arteries. The importance of coronary arterial diameter is emphasized by Poiseuille's law, in which resistance is inversely related to the vessel radius taken to the fourth power. Accordingly, chest pain can be caused by conditions that increase myocardial demand (e.g. hypertension, hyperthyroidism), decrease mean aortic pressure (e.g. aortic stenosis), decrease oxygen delivery (e.g. anemia, hypoxemia), increase the downstream pressure for coronary arterial flow (e.g. aortic and mitral valve disease, asymmetric septal hypertrophy), or by anything that might result in even a small change in coronary arterial diameter (e.g. coronary arterial spasm, thrombosis, atherosclerosis).

Pericardial pain

The visceral pericardium has no pain fibers, and the pain fibers in the parietal pericardium are localized to the caudal (i.e. diaphragmatic) region. The paucity of pericardial pain fibers may explain why various noninflammatory causes of pericardial effusions (e.g. myocardial infarction, uremia) are not associated with chest pain. Those effusions of infectious or other inflammatory etiologies may cause pain only when the inflammation spreads to the pleura.

Causes of chest pain
Cardiac system
Myocardial infarction
Myocardial ischemia
Angina pectoris
Variant angina
Syndrome X (microvascular angina in setting of noninsulin-dependent diabetes mellitus, dyslipidemia, and central obesity)
Myocarditis
Aortic dissection
Pericarditis (infections, Dressler's syndrome)
Aortic stenosis
Syphilitic aortitis
Takayasu's aortitis
Myocarditis
Hypertrophic cardiomyopathy
Pulmonary system
Pleurisy
Tracheobronchitis
Tumor
Pneumothorax
Pulmonary embolus (with or without infarction)
Pulmonary hypertension
Gastrointestinal system
Esophageal reflux
Esophageal dysmotility (i.e. spasm, achalasia, hyperactive lower sphincter)
Esophageal rupture
Peptic ulcer disease
Biliary colic
Pancreatitis
Splenic or hepatic flexure syndrome
Musculoskeletal conditions
Costochondritis
Subacromial bursitis
Biceps, supraspinatus, or deltoid tendinitis
Shoulder or spinal arthritis
Intercostal muscle cramps
Hyperabduction or strains of the anterior scalene or rectus abdominus muscles
Fibromyalgia
Slipping rib syndrome (pain at the costochondral junction, generally affecting the eighth, ninth, or tenth rib; may be post-traumatic)
Rib fractures
Sternal marrow pain (with acute leukemia)
Neurologic conditions
Neuritis–radiculitis (cervical compression, herpes zoster infection)
Brachial plexus involvement (cervical rib, spasm of the scalenus anterior, Pancoast's tumors)
Others
Breast inflammation
Chest wall tumors
Mondor's syndrome (thrombophlebitis of the superficial thoracic veins)
Diaphragm spasm
Mediastinal emphysema
Mediastinitis
Panic attacks
Hyperventilation syndrome

Figure 18.1 Causes of chest pain. Classification based on organ system grouping.

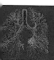

Oxygen extraction at rest and maximum exercise		
Rest	**Body**	**Myocardium**
Arterial oxygen content (mL/100mL blood)	20	20
Venous oxygen content (mL/100mL blood)	15	8
Oxygen extracted (mL/100mL blood)	5	12
Extraction ratio	0.25	0.60
Maximum exercise		
Arterial oxygen content (mL/100mL blood)	20	20
Venous oxygen content (mL/100mL blood)	5	5
Oxygen extracted (mL/100mL blood)	15	15
Extraction ratio	0.75	0.75
Increase in oxygen extraction (%)	300	125

Figure 18.2 Oxygen extraction at rest and maximum exercise. High myocardial oxygen extraction at rest limits the ability to increase oxygen availability in response to exercise.

Mitral valve prolapse

Although this condition has frequently been included as one of the causes of chest pain, recent epidemiologic studies indicate that this might not be the case.

Pulmonary pain

The lung parenchyma and the visceral pleura are insensitive to most painful stimuli. Pain can arise from the parietal pleura, the major airways, the chest wall, the diaphragm, and from mediastinal structures. Inflammatory conditions in the lung periphery or the peripheral portions of both hemidiaphragms cause chest-wall pain when the process extends to the parietal pleura and stimulates the respective intercostal nerves. Stimulation of the parietal pleura lining the central portions of the diaphragm affects the phrenic nerves; thus pain that results from inflammation in this region is referred to the ipsilateral neck or shoulder. The augmentation of pulmonary pain during inhalation is attributed to the stretching of the inflamed pleura.

Pulmonary embolus

The pain associated with pulmonary emboli is poorly understood. Pain that occurs acutely is thought to result from distention of the central pulmonary arteries. That which occurs later is attributed to infarction of a peripheral segment of lung and inflammation of the adjacent pleura.

Pulmonary hypertension

The pain of chronic pulmonary hypertension is attributed to the disparity between oxygen supply and demand in the right ventricular myocardium.

Musculoskeletal pain

Costochondral and chondrosternal articulations are common sites of anterior chest pain. The articulations of the second, third, and fourth ribs are most commonly involved. When accompanied by swelling, redness, and heat, the condition is referred to as Tietze's syndrome. The pain resulting from intercostal neuritis most frequently is due to cervical osteoarthritis. Intercostal neuritis is also seen with herpes zoster infection, in which the onset of pain may antedate the typical rash by 1 or 2 days (Fig. 18.3). Thoracic roots are most commonly involved.

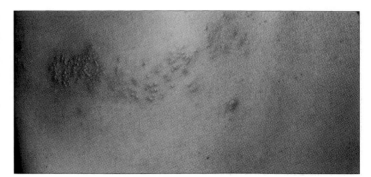

Figure 18.3 Herpes zoster infection affecting an intercostal nerve.

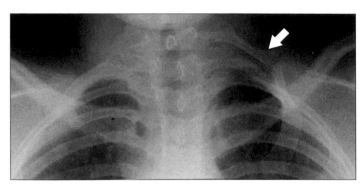

Figure 18.4 Chest radiograph showing a cervical rib. The aberrant rib results in compression of the left cervical nerve roots (arrow).

Subacromial bursitis, biceps or deltoid tendinitis, and arthritis of the shoulder may manifest as chest pain with extension to the shoulder and arm. The brachial plexus and subclavian artery can be compressed by a cervical rib (i.e. the thoracic outlet syndrome) (Fig. 18.4) or by spasm of the scalenus anterior muscle. Pancoast's syndrome (most commonly, but not exclusively, caused by bronchogenic carcinoma) may result from invasion of the C8, T1, and T2 nerve roots (Fig. 18.5).

Esophageal reflux or dysmotility

The chest pain that results from esophageal reflux or dysmotility (i.e. esophageal spasm, achalasia, hyperactive lower sphincter) is caused by acid irritation of the esophageal mucosa. Esophageal reflux or dysmotility explains chest pain in as many as 30% of patients who have chest pain and normal coronary arteriograms.

PATIENT EVALUATION

The approach to patients who complain of chest pain is dictated by the potentially lethal result of overlooking myocardial ischemia or one of the other potentially life-threatening conditions associated with this symptom. Severe pain is more commonly associated with life-threatening causes, but all of these conditions may occur with minimal symptoms. Accordingly, patients are frequently treated as if their chest pain were life-threatening until these more serious conditions have been excluded by studies that are more specific than the information obtained at the time of presentation.

Presentation

If the patient presents acutely and is gravely ill, the diagnoses to be considered include myocardial infarction, pulmonary

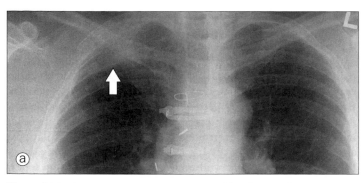
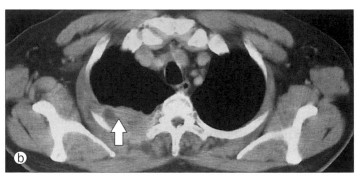

Figure 18.5 Pancoast's tumor invading the C8, T1, and T2 nerve roots. (a) Chest radiograph showing destruction of the posterior portion of the right second rib (arrow). (b) Chest computed tomography scan showing necrotic tumor and rib destruction (arrow).

embolism, pericardial tamponade, dissecting aneurysm, and tension pneumothorax (Fig. 18.6). Occasionally, patients with a ruptured esophagus may also present in this fashion. For others, the approach is governed primarily by the history and physical examination, interpreting these on the basis of actual or estimated probabilities for each of the conditions listed in Figure 18.1. For example, a middle-aged man with known risk factors for coronary artery disease (e.g. hypercholesterolemia, diabetes, hypertension, obesity, smoking) and who presents with exertional chest pain that abates with rest or nitroglycerin has a >90% probability of having myocardial ischemia as the cause of his symptom. A similarly high risk is present for patients who present with exertional pain that occurs with ST depression, cardiac wall motion abnormalities, an increased or decreased blood pressure, an S4 gallop, or a systolic murmur indicative of ischemia-induced mitral regurgitation.

Recent studies have emphasized the importance of chest pain as a presenting manifestation of myocardial ischemia in women[1], and have confirmed that major or intermediate risk factors for coronary artery disease include:
- typical pain;
- being postmenopausal without receiving hormonal replacement;
- smoking;
- diabetes mellitus;
- peripheral vascular disease;
- hypertension or lipoprotein abnormalities.

History
The onset, duration, location, radiation pattern, character, and intensity of the pain should be determined, as should the factors that precipitate or diminish it. Unfortunately, both the sensitivity and specificity of the history are low for many of the conditions that must be considered. For example, most episodes of electrocardiogram (ECG)-documented ischemia in patients with stable angina are asymptomatic. Nonetheless, the information acquired from the history is critical for determining the subsequent approach.

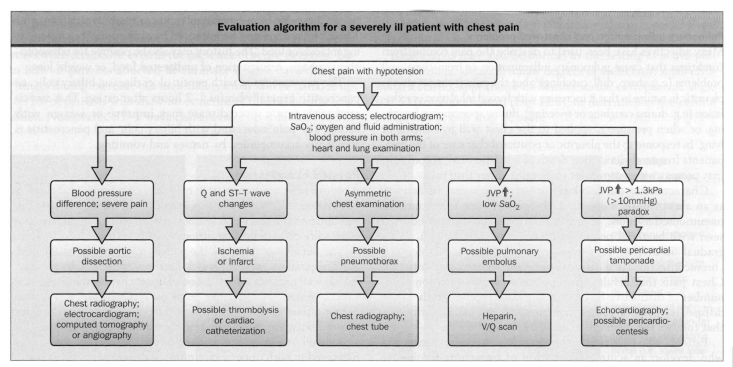

Figure 18.6 Evaluation algorithm for a severely ill patient with chest pain. Therapeutic approach is determined by blood pressure and findings on brief examination of the neck, chest and head. SaO₂, arterial oxygen pressure; JVP, jugular venous pressure.

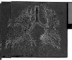

What is the likely pathogen?

A wide range of microbial pathogens can cause pulmonary infection, which potentially makes management difficult. In many patients the cause of the infection is never identified. In those in whom a pathogen is found, a delay always occurs between the patient's presentation and the culture result becoming available. Since therapy should be started immediately, it is helpful to identify markers that may help to predict the etiology and hence to direct therapy. Generally, information obtained at presentation may point to potential groups of pathogens rather than to individual pathogens, since few features are pathogen specific.

Airway infections are often of viral origin. When bacteria are present *Haemophilus influenzae*, *Streptococcus pneumoniae*, and *Moraxella catarrhalis* are most frequently found, although such organisms may simply represent colonization rather than pathogens. Nevertheless, when antibiotics are indicated (see Chapter 38) the initial empiric therapy is directed against these organisms. These bacteria are important in bronchiectasis, in which for some patients *Staph. aureus* and *Ps. aeruginosa* may also be important. The latter two organisms are particularly important in patients who have cystic fibrosis. In all patients who suffer from bronchiectasis, knowledge of previous sputum culture results may be helpful (Chapter 43).

The range of potentially treatable pathogens that may cause pneumonia is much more diverse. Classification of the pneumonia according to the immune status of the patient and the likely origin of the infection (Fig. 19.10) is helpful. Risk factors for unusual exposures (e.g. birds for psittacosis, grazing animals for Q fever), immune compromise (e.g. unsuspected intravenous drug abuse or sexual contact for human immunodeficiency virus risk) must always be sought.

The most frequent identifiable cause of CAP is *Strep. pneumoniae*, but a number of other pathogens are regularly encountered (Fig. 19.10). Clinical and epidemiologic features are rarely specific and should be used with caution (Fig. 19.11). The widespread skin rash of varicella-zoster virus in a patient who has pneumonia is one of the few clinical features specific to a particular pathogen.

In general, the same pathogens are important in different age groups, with the exception of a lower incidence of *Mycoplasma* infection in the elderly. Some studies report a higher frequency of CAP caused by Gram-negative Enterobacteriaceae in the elderly, but these are probably only important organisms in patients who are debilitated or who live in closed communities such as nursing home residents[9-11]. Similarly, all the pathogens encountered in the community can produce illnesses of varying severity, although legionellal, staphylococcal, and Gram-negative enterobacterial infections are more commonly found in severely ill patients.

Combinations of these presenting features have been used and even quantified into scores in an attempt to predict pathogens, but none are accurate. It is common clinical practice to attempt to differentiate 'atypical' from 'typical' pneumonias. Young age, gradual onset, long duration of symptoms, absence of clinical consolidation, diffuse radiographic shadowing, and normal WBC count are features of 'atypical' pneumonia. While statistically more infections are caused by organisms like *Mycoplasma*, *Chlamydia*, and *Coxiella* in the 'atypical' group, and *Strep. pneumoniae* and other conventional bacteria in the 'typical' group, recent studies showed that this distinction may only be helpful for patients at the extreme ends of the spectrum of clinical presentation found in pneumonia – for the majority it does not work.

Classification of the pneumonias according to likely origin and immune status	
Pneumonia group	**Likely pathogens**
Community-acquired	Gram-positive bacteria *Mycoplasma*, *Chlamydia*, *Coxiella* Common viruses (e.g. influenza)
Nosocomial, early	As for community-acquired
Nosocomial, late	Gram-negative enterobacteria *Staphylococcus aureus* Antibiotic-resistant bacteria
Immunocompromised	Opportunist organisms

Figure 19.10 Classification of the pneumonias according to likely origin and immune status. It is usually possible to place a patient into one of these categories at presentation. For each category the range of possible pathogens differs and hence the empiric approach and therapy differ[2-11].

Prediction of microbial etiology in community-acquired pneumonia	
Microorganism	**Features that occur more frequently in community-acquired pneumonia caused by this organism**
Streptococcus pneumoniae	Abrupt illness onset
Haemophilus influenzae	Pre-existing lung disease
Staphylococcus aureus	Concurrent influenza epidemic Radiographic cavitation Severe illness
Legionella spp.	Recent foreign travel Concurrent epidemic Countries that border the Mediterranean
Mycoplasma pneumoniae	Age <65 years Diffuse radiographic shadowing
Chlamydia psittaci	Recent bird contact At-risk occupation
Coxiella burnetii	Animal contact At-risk occupation
Gram-negative Enterobacteriaceae	Nursing home resident South Africa
Pseudomonas pseudomallei	Southeast Asia, northern Australia
Tuberculosis	Nonindustrialized countries

Figure 19.11 Prediction of microbial etiology in community-acquired pneumonia. Given are features that statistically make particular pathogens more likely (remember that no feature is uniquely associated with any individual pathogen).

Legionella pneumonia is often included in the 'atypical' pneumonia group. In fact, the clinical features of this illness have much more in common with severe pneumococcal infection.

Radiographic features also usually do not help to differentiate causative pathogens[12]; however, cavitation (when present) may help since it occurs most commonly in staphylococcal, anaerobic (Fig. 19.12), fungal, and tuberculous infections, and rarely with other pathogens.

It is helpful to distinguish NPs that develop within the first 7 days of hospitalization from those that develop thereafter. In the former group, *Strep. pneumoniae* and *H. influenzae* are common, but these organisms are rarely found after 7 days, after which *Staph. aureus* (both methicillin sensitive and resistant strains) and Gram-negative *Enterobacteriaceae* are seen. No specific clinical

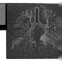

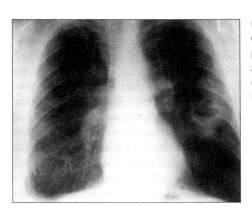

Figure 19.12 Cavitating pneumonia. Left mid-zone consolidation caused by anaerobic infection.

or laboratory features allow an accurate prediction of the causative pathogen in NP; however, *Ps. aeruginosa* is less common in patients who have NP that developed outside the intensive care unit.

Antibiotic resistance is becoming increasingly important in both community-acquired and nosocomial pathogens, although the frequency varies widely geographically and between institutions. In areas where antibiotic resistance is common, a history of prior antibiotic therapy predicts a higher risk of infection with resistant organisms. The clinical value of this information varies between institutions for the above reasons, and it is therefore important to know the local resistance patterns of common pathogens.

The range of pathogens that cause pneumonia in the immunocompromised is very broad and, in addition to routine bacterial and viral infections, also includes infections by opportunistic organisms that are usually nonpathogenic in the immunocompetent host[8]. Polymicrobial infections also occur more commonly in these patients. Prediction of likely pathogens is again imprecise, but attention should be paid to the nature and degree of the immunosuppression, the time course of events, cytomegalovirus (CMV) status of donor and recipient, use of prophylactic therapies, and radiographic features (Fig. 19.13). Symptoms and signs, as in NP, are seldom helpful, although pancytopenia commonly accompanies CMV infections.

Identification of the causative pathogen
Minimally invasive tests
Throat swab
A throat swab may be used to identify some predominantly intracellular pathogens such as viruses, *Mycoplasma*, and *Chlamydia*. Organisms can be identified by direct immunofluorescence (*Chlamydia*, viruses) or cell culture. The yields are low and the methodologies often labor intensive, which means that in adults this is usually impractical, other than for research. In children, detection of respiratory syncytial virus by this method may be helpful (see Fig. 19.14).

Sputum
In many patients who have respiratory infection sputum is easy to obtain. When not available it may be induced in skilled hands by inhalation of nebulized hypertonic saline – this is probably only of value for the detection of *Mycobacterium tuberculosis* or of *Pn. carinii* in immunocompromised patients. The value of examining sputum has been studied exhaustively and its utility remains controversial. The main problems are that airway secretions have to pass through the oropharynx, which may be colonized by a variety of microorganisms, such that organisms identified in sputum may not be representative of what is happening in the lung.

Predicting microbial etiology in pneumonia in an immunocompromised host		
Feature	**Criteria**	**Cause**
Nature of immunosuppression	B-cell dysfunction	Bacterial
	T-cell dysfunction	Opportunist
	Neutropenia	Bacteria Fungi
Severity in HIV infection	CD4 >200	Bacteria Tuberculosis
	CD4 <200	*Pneumocystis carinii* pneumonia (PCP) Other opportunists
Time course of events	0–1 month post-transplant	Bacterial infection
	1–6 months post-transplant	Opportunist
Cytomegalovirus (CMV) status	CMV+ donor to CMV− recipient	CMV
Prophylactic therapy	PCP prophylaxis	PCP less likely + atypical presentations occur
Radiology	Focal consolidation	Bacterial infection
	Nodule	Lung abscess Fungi
	Diffuse shadowing	PCP CMV (transplants only)

Figure 19.13 Predicting microbial etiology in pneumonia in an immunocompromised host. Features that should be considered in the assessment of pneumonia in any patient who is immunocompromised.

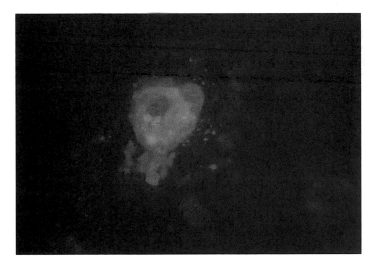

Figure 19.14 Respiratory syncytial virus. Throat swab specimen showing cytoplasmic fluorescent staining by antibody to respiratory syncytial virus.

Second, bacteria may colonize the normally sterile airways when host defenses are compromised (e.g. by chronic bronchitis or intubation). The clinical illness may be attributed to these organisms when found in sputum even though another process (e.g. viral infection) is responsible. Some organisms are always pathogens (e.g. *Mycobacterium*, *Pneumocystis*, *Legionella*), and their identification in sputum is always helpful. For other organisms, determination of the quality of the sputum sample is essential.

Various tests can be performed on sputum, of which Gram-stain and routine culture are the best known (see Fig. 19.15). Visualization of an organism on Gram-stain is more specific than cul-

Bacillus anthracis

Bacillus anthracis is a Gram-positive, large rod that causes anthrax. It is found in the soil, water, and vegetation and infects cows, sheep, and horses, which in turn infect humans after contact with contaminated materials. Fever and malaise usually appear progressively. Three forms of anthrax are found: cutaneous, intestinal, and pneumonic. Inoculation of *Bcl. anthracis* into superficial wounds or skin abrasion causes cutaneous anthrax, which is characterized by a black, crusted pustule on a large area of edema. Intestinal anthrax results from ingestion of contaminated material and is severe. Pneumonic anthrax is caused by inhalation of the contaminated material. Nonproductive cough and chest pain precede dyspnea, stridor, tachypnea, cyanosis, and edema of the neck and anterior chest. Peribronchovascular edema, enlargement of mediastinum, and pleural effusions are usually seen on the chest radiograph.

Brucella species

Brucella species are Gram-negative coccobacilli found in the genitourinary tract of cows, pigs, goats, and dogs. Brucellosis results from contact with infected animals or from ingestion of unpasteurized milk products (e.g. cheese and milk). The pathogen spreads through the body via the bloodstream. General symptoms include fever, malaise, and headache. Hepatic enlargement and splenomegaly are common, as is lower back pain. Respiratory symptoms are less frequent than abnormalities on the chest radiograph, which include nodules, miliary, infiltrates, and lymphadenopathy.

Moraxella catarrhalis

Moraxella catarrhalis, formerly named *Branhamella catarrhalis*, is a Gram-negative diplococcus that is commonly found in the oropharynx of normal subjects. Pneumonia caused by *Mrx. catarrhalis* is seen in patients who have underlying chronic diseases such as COPD, congestive heart disease, or malignancy. Symptoms and radiographic findings are nonspecific. Leukocytosis is usual and the course is usually favorable.

DIAGNOSIS

History

The approach to the diagnosis of patients who have CAP depends almost entirely on a careful history and physical examination, which focus on the possibility that the infection may be the result of unusual pathogens (e.g. exposure to birds or parturient animals, recent foreign travel, lymphadenopathy, splenomegaly). The infection must also be considered in the context of the specific patient (e.g. recent influenza or varicella infection, oropharyngeal colonization with Gram-negative rods in nursing home patients, and occupations or hobbies with animal exposures). Finally, the chest radiograph must be examined for findings that suggest pathogens other than the common ones (e.g. abscesses, effusions, adenopathy, and cavitation). When the clinical presentation suggests an unusual pathogen, every attempt must be made to obtain a bacteriologic diagnosis. In the absence of this suspicion, the value of bacteriologic studies is unclear.

Bacteriology

The reasons for not routinely performing a sputum examination in patients who have LRTI are numerous:
- investigation is difficult to perform in the outpatient setting;
- results are nonspecific and of questionable sensitivity; and

- antibiotic treatment, if needed, has to be started before the results are obtained, based on the pathogens that are likely to be responsible for pneumonia in the community.

In most studies no microorganisms were found in just under 50% of outpatients investigated for CAP, viruses were found in 10%, *Strep. pneumoniae* was found in 25%, *H. influenza* in 7%, *Mycoplasma*, *Legionella*, and *Chlamydia* spp. in 10%, and Gram-negative bacteria and *Staph. aureus* in only 1%. In hospitalized patients who have CAP, Gram-negative bacteria and *Staph. aureus* strains are more frequent (Fig. 20.5).

Specific pathogens

Chest radiography in patients who have *H. influenzae* pneumonia is thought to show a peribronchial distribution of infiltrates (i.e. bronchopneumonia), as opposed to the more peripheral lobar or segmental consolidations seen with streptococcal pneumonia. The sensitivity and specificity of this distinction are low, however.

In *Myc. pneumoniae* infections, the leukocyte count is generally normal, although mild-to-moderate leukocytosis can be seen. Cold agglutinins are frequently present. The diagnosis can be made by acute and convalescent blood serologic testing. Despite a favorable response to therapy, *Myc. pneumoniae* may persist in the oropharynx for 1–3 months during which it may be transmissible to others.

The diagnoses of *Clm. pneumoniae*, *Clm. psittaci*, and Q fever is based on acute and convalescent blood serologies obtained 2–6 weeks apart.

Legionella pneumonia may be diagnosed by direct immunofluorescence studies on respiratory tract specimens (e.g. sputum or tracheobronchial aspirates) or on urine in a few hours; respiratory tract specimens can be analyzed by a DNA probe and cultured. A fourfold increase in the antibody titers can be seen on two samples obtained within 2 months[18].

Bacteriologic diagnosis of anaerobic infections critically depends on the type of specimen and on the quality of the anaerobic transport; various Gram-negative and Gram-positive agents are found, sometimes in conjunction with aerobic pathogens.

The pus in sinus tracts caused by *Actinomyces* spp. contains sulfur granules, which are mineralized, 2mm diameter, yellow

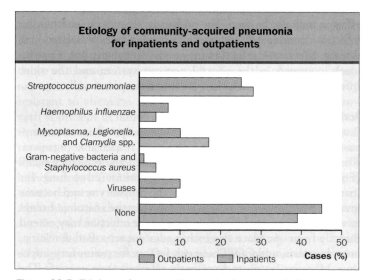

Figure 20.5 Etiology of community-acquired pneumonia for inpatients and outpatients.

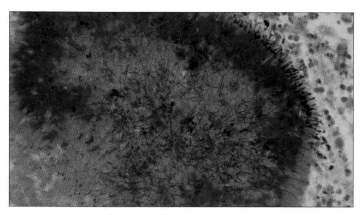

Figure 20.6 Gram stain of an actinomycotic sulfur granule.

granules made of *Actinomyces* or *Arachnia* spp. When examined by Gram stain, these appear as dense aggregates of the organism (Fig. 20.6). Microbiologic diagnosis relies on characterization of the pathogens in a specimen from biopsy, exudate, and/or pus, using histopathologic evaluation and culture in anaerobic conditions.

Tularemia is diagnosed by serologic testing on paired serum specimens.

Microbiologic diagnosis of *Y. pestis* and *Bcl. anthracis* is made on blood, sputum, or lymph node aspirate culture, using routine bacteriologic or fluorescent antibody staining techniques.

A titer of *Brucella* agglutinins ≥ 1/160 indicates active brucellosis.

Diagnosis of *Pseud. pseudomallei* is made when the organism is cultured from respiratory tract secretions, cutaneous lesions, or blood, or when serologic tests are positive.

TREATMENT

Severity and hospitalization
When a diagnosis of pneumonia is suspected, one of the important early questions is whether the patient needs hospitalization. Criteria suggested by the European Respiratory and American Thoracic Societies[3,19] and recently studied by Fine et al. are given in Figure 20.7[20].

Empiric antibiotic therapy
The initial antibiotic choice for CAP is empiric because:
- in at least half of cases, the responsible organism(s) cannot be isolated using even the most sophisticated methods;
- it is inappropriate to delay treatment pending a microbiologic result as this increases the risk of complications and mortality, whereas correctly chosen empiric therapy improves the CAP outcome; and
- studies have shown that clinical data and radiologic findings, together with an assessment of comorbidity, risk factors for complications, and the severity of the episode of CAP, enable appropriate decisions to be made regarding the choice of antibiotics and the necessity for hospitalization.

Many recommendations on the management of patients who present with CAP have been made[19–22]. All suggest that the antibiotic treatment must be started as early as possible, without waiting for microbiologic results (if microbiologic investigations are performed).

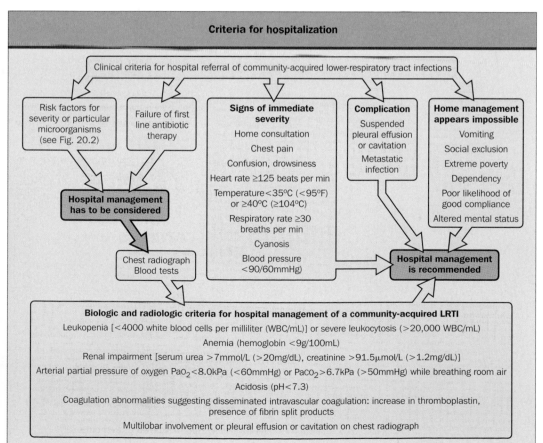

Figure 20.7 Criteria for hospitalization for community-acquired pneumonia. Biologic and radiologic investigations may be performed either in patients referred to the hospital or in outpatients (depending in part on the local health care system and facilities) according to the criteria listed in Figure 20.1. (Adapted with permission from Huchon et al.[3])

Antibiotic selection

Antibiotic activity against the bacteria that cause CAP is summarized in Figure 20.8. For patients who have no risk factors and who do not require hospitalization, an oral β-lactam antibiotic is prescribed when the clinical presentation is consistent with *Strep. pneumoniae* or other bacterial infections associated with typical pneumonias. When the clinical presentation is consistent with an atypical pneumonia, adding a macrolide is recommended. Aminopenicillins have the advantage of being active against most extracellular bacteria, including *Strep. pneumoniae*, and against a few intracellular bacteria.

In patients who have risk factors, an aminopenicillin associated with a β-lactamase inhibitor, or a second-generation cephalosporin, is indicated, possibly in conjunction with a macrolide or a fluoroquinolone (if infection by intracellular agents is a possibility). Newer quinolones (e.g. third-generation quinolones[3]) are likely to be very useful since they are active against most intra- and extracellular pathogens that cause CAP.

Local resistance patterns of microorganisms to antibiotics obviously must be taken into account when choosing the appropriate medications, and studies document that patterns of resistance can vary markedly. A decrease in the sensitivity of *Strep. pneumoniae* to penicillin was found in 32% of strains isolated in France in 1994 and in 33% of strains found in Spain in 1992. Resistance of *Strep. pneumoniae* to macrolides was found in 41% of strains in France in 1994, and 14% of strains in Spain in 1992. The recommended strategy for the choice of first-line antibiotics for other organisms is summarized in Figure 20.9[3].

The recommended duration of the antibiotic treatment of CAP is 1 week when the infection is caused by extracellular organisms and 2 weeks when it is thought to result from intracellular germs. As they have a prolonged effect, new macrolides such as azithromycin could be used for a shorter period of time; however, it is unclear whether shortening the duration of treatment carries any risk.

Severe bacterial pneumonia

Bacterial pneumonia is considered to be severe when is accompanied by extension outside the lung parenchyma, lung necrosis, or septicemia, or when it occurs in patients who have comorbid diseases. In such cases, it becomes much more important to establish a specific bacteriologic diagnosis. Antibiotics are initially administered intravenously and the choice of medication requires consideration of the diffusion of antibiotics into lung parenchyma, iatrogenic risks, and contraindications related to hepatic or renal function. As *L. pneumophila* pneumonias may be

Antibiotics active against bacteria responsible for pneumonia					
Bacteria	**Antibiotics**	**Bacteria**	**Antibiotics**	**Bacteria**	**Antibiotics**
Acinetobacter spp.	Aminoglycosides and piperacillin Aminoglycosides and imipenem	Gram-negative enterobacteria, including *Klebsiella pneumoniae and Haemophilus influenzae*	Aminoglycosides and cephalosporins Aminoglycosides and aminopenicillins Cephalosporins (third generation) Clarithromycin Azithromycin Quinolones Aminopenicillin and penicillinase inhibitor Chloramphenicol Trimethoprim–sulfamethoxazole	*Nocardia*	Trimethoprim–sulfamethoxazole Aminopenicillins Amikacin
Actinomyces spp.	Penicillins			*Pasteurella multocida*	Penicillins Tetracyclines Chloramphenicol
Anaerobes	Clindamycin Penicillin and metronidazole Cefoxitin Aminopenicillin and penicillinase inhibitor Imipenem			*Pseudomonas aeruginosa*	Aminoglycosides and piperacillin Aminoglycosides and ceftazidime Aminoglycosides and aztreonam Aminoglycosides and cefoperazone
Bacillus anthracis	Penicillins Chloramphenicol Erythromycin Tetracyclines			*Pseud. pseudomallei*	Tetracyclines Ceftazidime Sulfonamides Chloramphenicol Kanamycin
Brucella	Streptomycin Trimethoprim–sulfamethoxazole	*Legionella*	Macrolides Trimethoprim–sulfamethoxazole Tetracyclines Quinolones	*Rhodococcus equi*	Vancomycin Erythromycin Chloramphenicol Rifampin (rifampicin)
Chlamydia burnetii	Tetracyclines Chloramphenicol				
Clm. pneumoniae	Tetracyclines Macrolides Quinolones	*Moraxella catarrhalis*	Cephalosporins Aminopenicillin and penicillinase inhibitor Erythromycin Tetracyclines Quinolone Trimethoprim–sulfamethoxazole	*Staphylococcus aureus*	Oxacillin Cephalosporins (first generation) Methicillin Vancomycin and rifampin
Clm. psittaci	Tetracyclines Chloramphenicol			*Streptococcus* spp.	Penicillins Macrolides Cephalosporins (first generation) Vancomycin
Clm. trachomatis	Macrolides Sulfisoxazole				
Coxiella burnetii	Tetracyclines Chloramphenicol	*Mycoplasma pneumoniae*	Macrolides Tetracyclines Quinolones	*Streptococcus pneumoniae*	Penicillins Macrolides Cephalosporins (first generation)
Francisella tularensis	Aminoglycosides Tetracyclines Chloramphenicol	*Neisseria meningitidis*	Penicillin Cephalosporins (third generation) Chloramphenicol	*Yersina pestis*	Streptomycin Tetracyclines

Figure 20.8 Antibiotics active against bacteria responsible for pneumonia.

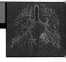

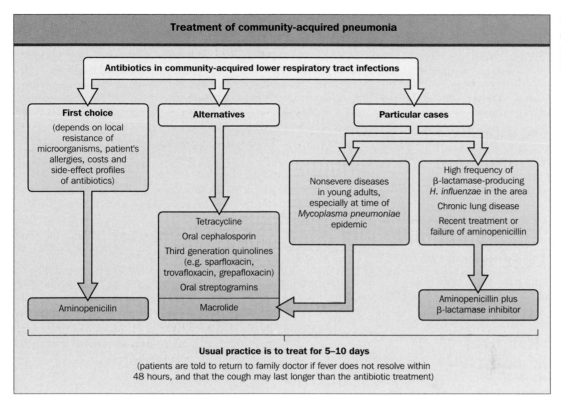

Figure 20.9 Treatment of community-acquired pneumonia. (Adapted with permission from Huchon et al.[3])

severe, and are frequently associated with diarrhea, treatment is with intravenous regimens that provide good intracellular penetration [e.g. erythromycin (3–4g/24h), pefloxacine (800mg/24h), and rifampin (rifampicin; 1200mg/24h)].

Patients who have actinomycetic infections are treated for prolonged periods (e.g. up to 6 months).

The choice of antibiotic(s) to treat *Nocardia* infection is based on in-vitro susceptibility testing; duration of treatment (usually >6 weeks) and drainage of purulent collections are critical factors for the outcome.

CLINICAL COURSE AND PREVENTION

The course of CAP is favorable in the large majority of cases. Fever declines over a few days and the abnormalities seen on the chest radiograph generally begin to resolve within 1–3 weeks. Persistence of fever suggests a resistant organism, a complication such as a cavitation of the infected lung or an empyema, development of a nosocomial pneumonia caused by a resistant organism, and a drug fever. Also, poor resolution may be caused by the presence of another problem such as lung carcinoma, bronchial foreign body, bronchiectasis, or chronic infection of the upper respiratory tract.

Bacterial pneumonia can be prevented in various ways, such as by reducing risk factors like smoking and alcoholism, and by vaccination. Influenza vaccine is used in subjects over 65 years of age, in cases of chronic diseases, and in medical and nursing home employees[23,24]. Pneumococcal vaccine is recommended in subjects older than 65 years of age and in younger patients who have cardiovascular or pulmonary diseases, diabetes mellitus, alcoholism, liver cirrhosis, cerebrospinal fluid leaks, and immunodepression (including human immunodeficiency virus infection, chronic renal failure, organ transplant recipients, hematologic and lymphatic malignancies, asplenia, and sickle cell disease)[25,26].

REFERENCES

1. Woodhead MA, Macfarlane JT, McCracken JS, Rose DH, Finch RG. Prospective study of the aetiology and outcome of pneumonia in the community. Lancet. 1987;i:671–4.
2. Jokinen C, Heiskanen L, Juvonen H, et al. Incidence of community-acquired pneumonia in the population of four municipalities in Eastern Finland. Am J Epidemiol. 1993;137:977–88.
3. Huchon GJ, Woodhead MA, Gialdroni-Grassi G, et al. Guidelines for management of adult community-acquired lower respiratory tract infections. Eur Respir Rev. 1998;11:986–91.
4. Niederman MS, Fein AM. Pneumonia in the elderly. Geriatr Clin North Am. 1986;2:241–68.
5. Marrie TJ. Epidemiology of community-acquired pneumonia in the elderly. Semin Respir Infect. 1990;5:260–8.
6. Gilbert K, Fine MJ. Assessing prognosis and predicting patient outcomes in community-acquired pneumonia. Semin Respir Infect. 1994;9:140–52.
7. Adams HG, Jordan C. Infections in the alcoholic. Med Clin North Am. 1984;68:179–200.

8. Perlino CA, Rimland D. Alcoholism, leukopenia, and pneumococcal sepsis. Am Rev Respir Dis. 1985;132:757–60.

9. Niederman MS. Malnutrition and host lung defenses: implications for the pathogenesis and prevention of pneumonia. In: Ferranti RD, Rampulla C, Fracchia C, Ambrosino N, eds. Nutrition and ventilatory function. Verona: Bi & Gi, 1992:87–98.

10. Ortqvist A, Hedlund J, Grillner L, et al. Aetiology, outcome and prognostic factors in community-acquired pneumonia requiring hospitalization. Eur Respir J. 1990;3:1105–13.

11. Pachón J, Prados MD, Capote F, Cuello JA, Garnacho J, Verano A. Severe community-acquired pneumonia: aetiology, prognosis and treatment. Am Rev Respir Dis. 1990;142:369–73.

12. Fine MJ, Smith DN, Singer DE. Hospitalization decision in patients with community-acquired pneumonia: a prospective cohort study. Am J Med. 1990;89:713–21.

13. Almirall J, Mesalles A, Klamburg J, Parra O, Agudo A. Prognostic factors of pneumonia requiring admission to the intensive care unit. Chest. 1995;107:511–16.

14. Fang GD, Fine M, Orloff J, et al. New and emerging etiologies for community-acquired pneumonia with implications for therapy. A prospective multicenter study of 359 cases. Medicine. 1990;69:307–16.

15. Koivula I, Sten M, Makela PH. Risk factors for pneumonia in the elderly. Am J Med. 1994;96:313–20.

16. Farr BM, Mandell GL. Gram-positive pneumonia. In: Pennington JE, ed. Respiratory infections: diagnosis and management. New York: Raven Press; 1994:349–67.

17. Woodhead MA, Gialdroni-Grassi G, Huchon G, Léophonte P, Manresa F, Schaberg T. Use of investigations of lower respiratory tract infection in the community: a European survey. Eur Respir J. 1996;9:1596–600.

18. Lieberman D, Porath A, Schlaeffer F, Boldur I. Legionella species community-acquired pneumonia. A review of 56 hospitalized adult patients. Chest. 1996;109:1243–9.

19. Niederman MS, Bass JB Jr, Campbell GD, et al. Guidelines for the initial management of adults with community-acquired pneumonia: diagnosis, assessment of severity and initial antimicrobial therapy. Am Rev Respir Dis. 1993;148:1418–26.

20. Fine MJ, Auble TE, Yealy DM, et al. A prediction rule to identify low-risk patients with community-acquired pneumonia. N Engl J Med. 1997;336:243–50.

21. British Thoracic Society. Guidelines for the management of community-acquired pneumonia in adults admitted to hospital. Br J Hosp Med. 1993;49:346–50.

22. Gialdroni-Grassi G, Branchi L. Guidelines for the management of community-acquired pneumonia in adults. Monaldi Arch Chest Dis. 1995;50:21–7.

23. Partriarca PA, Weber JA, Parker RA. Efficacy of influenza vaccine in nursing homes: reduction in illness and complications during influenza A (H3N2) epidemic. JAMA. 1985;253:1136–9.

24. Saah AJ, Neufeld R, Rodstein M, et al. Influenza vaccine and pneumonia mortality in a nursing home population. Arch Intern Med. 1986;146:2353–7.

25. Fedson DS. Influenza and pneumococcal vaccination of the elderly: newer vaccines and prospects for clinical benefits at the margin. Prev Med. 1994;23:751–5.

26. Gable CB, Holzer SS, Engelhart L, et al. Pneumococcal vaccine: efficacy and associated cost savings. JAMA. 1990;264:2910–15.

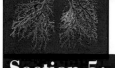

Chapter 21

Viral Pneumonia

Gérard Huchon and Nicolas Roche

INTRODUCTION

Although viral infections of the upper respiratory tract are common, viral pneumonia in nonimmunocompromised patients is rare, except in children and the elderly. Four major groups of viruses account for the large majority of viral pneumonias in immunocompetent children (Fig. 21.1).

EPIDEMIOLOGY AND RISK FACTORS

Pneumonia accounts for 20–40% of viral lower respiratory tract infections in children[1]. In adults, influenza is the most frequent cause of viral pneumonia, although respiratory syncytial virus (RSV) is also seen, and pneumonia may also occur as part of systemic viral infections such as measles, chickenpox, and the hantaviruses.

Influenza virus infection

Three types of influenza virus have been identified (A, B, and C)[2]. Type A is responsible for the most severe and widespread disease and type C does not appear to be pathogenic. Major antigens of the virus envelope are hemagglutinin and neur-aminidase (sialidase). In influenza A viruses, the former undergoes periodic changes, which may be major (resulting in antigenic shifts because of reassortments between strains, and lead to an entirely new gene) or minor (resulting in antigenic drifts because of point mutations). Most of the host immune response is directed against hemagglutinin.

Influenza A and B viruses are responsible for at least 50% of the viral pneumonia encountered in immunocompetent adult subjects. Antigenic shifts are associated with pandemics when antigenic modifications lead to a decrease in the immunity of the community, whereas antigenic drifts are commonly associated with more limited epidemics. Outbreaks of severe disease occur every 10–30 years. During an outbreak, children are usually infected before adults (with attack rates that may reach 50–75%)[3]. The excess mortality because of influenza may be as high as 10,000 patients/year and the economic consequences of outbreaks are considerable.

The host immune response involves both cellular and humoral defenses, as well as local antibody responses because of secretory IgA. The result is mucosal inflammation that consists of hyperemia, edema, and, in severe cases, hemorrhage[4]. Transmission is by respiratory secretions.

Pneumonia may occur directly following the acute illness (termed 'primary pneumonia', which is caused by the virus itself) or it may occur after a period of clinical improvement ('secondary pneumonia', which results from bacterial superinfection, most commonly with *Streptococcus pneumoniae*, *Haemophilus influenzae*, or *Staphylococcus aureus*). Primary pneumonia seems to occur more commonly in association with conditions that result in increased left atrial pressure, whereas secondary pneumonias occur mainly in older adults, or in patients who have comorbid conditions, such as chronic cardiovascular or respiratory disease, diabetes mellitus, or chronic hepatic or renal failure.

Parainfluenza virus infection

Four serotypes are identified, of which types 1, 2, and 3 are responsible for most infections in humans. Parainfluenza viruses are responsible for up to 20% of the respiratory infections that occur in children, but are found infrequently in immunocompetent adults. The epidemiologic and clinical characteristics depend on the serotype and are summarized in Figure 21.2[5].

As with influenza, parainfluenza viruses are transmitted between humans via respiratory secretions. The incubation period lasts 2–6 days, and humoral, local, and cellular immunity generate neutralizing circulating antibodies, local secretory IgA, and cytotoxic and helper T lymphocytes, respectively.

Respiratory syncytial virus

The leading cause of respiratory tract infection in young children, RSV is responsible for 25% of hospital admissions for pneumonia, and 75% of bronchiolitis cases in children younger than 6 months of age. The incubation period lasts 4–6 days; epidemics

	Influenza	Parainfluenza	Respiratory syncytial virus	Adenovirus
Respiratory viruses that cause pneumonias in nonimmunocompromised hosts				
Family	Orthomyxoviridae	Paramyxoviridae	Paramyxoviridae	Adenoviridae
Genome	Single-stranded RNA	Single-stranded RNA	Single-stranded RNA	Double-stranded DNA
Envelope antigens	Hemagglutinin Sialidase	Hemagglutinin Sialidase Fusion Glycoprotein	Fusion Glycoprotein G glycoprotein	250 capsomeres
Serotypes	Three (pathogenic in humans: A and B)	Four (pathogenic in humans: 1, 2, and 3)	Two (A and B)	50
Infected cells	Epithelial cells	Epithelial cells	Epithelial cells	Epithelial cells Lymphoid cells
Frequency among lower respiratory tract infections[1]	Type A: 1–13% Type B: 1–9%	4–41%	6–63%	2–35%

Figure 21.1 Respiratory viruses that cause pneumonias in nonimmunocompromised hosts.

Epidemiologic and clinical characteristics of parainfluenza infection depending on the serotype		
	Serotypes	
	1 and 2	**3**
Epidemiology	Epidemics during the fall	Endemic with increases during fall, winter, or spring
Clinical features	Croup (laryngotracheobronchitis); less severe with type 2	Bronchiolitis Pneumonia

Figure 21.2 Epidemiologic and clinical characteristics of parainfluenza infection depend on the serotype.

occur in the late fall and spring, and usually last 1–5 months. Almost all children older than 5 years have anti-RSV antibodies.

Transmittal of RSV is by contaminated skin followed by autoinoculation in the conjunctiva or nose, or by aerosols produced by coughing or sneezing.

Immunity mainly involves local and serum antibodies, but cell-mediated immunity also develops. Infection by RSV induces IgE production, the magnitude of which predicts the risk of subsequent wheezing episodes.

Adenovirus

Adenoviruses are responsible for up to 5% of respiratory infections in children, but for <2% of those in adults, except in military recruit populations among which epidemics have been reported. Almost all adults have serum antibodies against adenoviruses (usually against several serotypes).

Adenovirus respiratory infection may be the consequence of airborne or of fecal–oral contamination. The incubation period lasts 4–7 days. Latent infection may develop and has even been implicated in the pathogenesis of chronic airways diseases such as asthma or chronic obstructive pulmonary disease.

Measles (rubeola)

Measles virus belongs to the Paramyxoviridae family, and is therefore similar to parainfluenza virus and RSV[6]. Portals of entry are the respiratory tract and conjunctiva. Lower respiratory tract manifestations affect up to 50% of patients who have measles, and include mainly bronchitis and pneumonia (which may be complicated by bacterial superinfection in up to 50% of cases). In the USA, pneumonia is the cause of 60% of measles-related deaths in children.

Varicella

Varicella causes pneumonia in adults, but this complication is unusual in immunocompetent children. Epidemics occur in the winter and spring, with infectivity rates that exceed 90% within the first 2–3 weeks following exposure.

Hantavirus

The hantavirus pulmonary syndrome was first recognized in the USA in 1983, but the disease was retrospectively identified using serologic testing in patients who had a similar illness in 1959. The syndrome can result from several hantaviruses, such as Sin Nombre virus. Almost all cases have been reported in North and South America. Rodents (e.g. field mice, voles, chipmunks) serve as the reservoir, and transmission to humans results from aerosolization of viruses contained in their feces. Person-to-person spread rarely, if ever, occurs.

CLINICAL FEATURES

Influenza virus infection

A typical presentation includes the acute onset of cough, sore throat, conjunctival hyperemia, nasal discharge and congestion, fever, myalgias, headache, and malaise. Symptoms and findings of pneumonia are infrequent and the disease is usually self-limited[2]. Reappearance or worsening of respiratory symptoms and signs suggest pneumonia, but radiographic evidence of pneumonia may be found in the absence of such findings.

The radiographic findings of primary pneumonia generally are diffuse, interstitial, or patchy infiltrates. Secondary pneumonia may have a more segmental or lobar pattern. Primary and secondary pneumonia may occur in the same patient at the same time.

Parainfluenza virus infection

In adults, the disease may be completely asymptomatic or may present as a common upper respiratory tract infection with rhinitis and pharyngitis. Fever is unusual, as is the progression to pneumonia. When pneumonia does occur, the symptoms and signs are nonspecific and the chest radiograph shows diffuse, interstitial infiltrates consistent with any type of atypical or viral pneumonia.

Respiratory syncytial virus

Usually, RSV infection begins in the upper respiratory tract with nasal congestion and pharyngitis, and is associated with fever of variable intensity. The lower respiratory tract rapidly becomes involved in 25–40% of cases, which leads to worsening cough, dyspnea, wheezing, and rhonchi. Hypoxemia is common. Two types of lower respiratory tract involvement occur – pneumonia and bronchiolitis. Both are associated with interstitial infiltrates, the former from lung inflammation and the latter from peripheral atelectasis and/or hyperinflation. In older adults who have chronic cardiopulmonary disease, RSV may cause severe bronchitis, pneumonia, or both[7].

Adenovirus

In children and military recruits, adenoviruses can cause bronchiolitis and pneumonia of variable severity[8].

Measles

Patients who have measles show a typical viral prodrome that consists of fever, rhinitis, malaise, and anorexia, and which lasts for approximately 1 week prior to the onset of the rash. The maculopapular rash begins on the face and neck and progresses to the trunk and extremities. Leukopenia is seen early. Measles pneumonia can cause hilar lymphadenopathy and pleural effusions, in addition to the reticulonodular parenchymal infiltrates. Secondary bacterial pneumonia also occurs.

Varicella

The initial presentation is generally the appearance of a rash on the face and head, with subsequent spread to the thorax, abdomen, and extremities. The rash has a rather orderly progression, initially with erythematous macules that progress to vesicles within hours to days. These subsequently become pustular and finally crust over. Lesions may also be found on mucosal surfaces (e.g. pharynx, vagina). When pneumonia occurs it generally presents within the first 4–5 days after the onset of the rash[9]. Cough is common and pleuritic chest pain and hemoptysis may occur. Other organs such

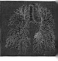

as the liver, kidney, heart and brain may also be involved. Diffuse, small nodular infiltrates are the characteristic radiographic abnormality, and hilar adenopathy and effusions are common. With resolution, the nodules may calcify and persist lifelong (Fig. 21.3).

Hantavirus

The initial presentation is that of a flu-like syndrome of fever, myalgias, nausea, vomiting, and gastrointestinal pain suggestive of gastroenteritis. These are followed by a dry cough, which portends diffuse noncardiogenic pulmonary edema (sometimes associated with bilateral pleural effusion) that may lead to acute respiratory distress syndrome, and shock in severe cases. Hematologic examination usually demonstrates neutrophilic leukocytosis, hemoconcentration, thrombocytopenia, and circulating immunoblasts. Renal failure may occur, but is uncommon.

DIAGNOSIS

Influenza virus infection

Indirect diagnosis is primarily used for epidemiologic purposes, as it requires two serologic assays performed 10–14 days apart. Direct diagnosis can be made by:

- culture of respiratory secretions or lung tissue, a process that takes 2–5 days (but may be less if antigen-detection techniques are used);
- immunofluorescence or enzyme-linked immunosorbent assay (ELISA) techniques on nasal or pharyngeal cells obtained by brushing or washing, a process that takes approximately 15 minutes; and
- antigen detection in respiratory secretions, a less sensitive but more rapid technique.

Parainfluenzavirus infection

Indirect diagnosis requires a rise in antibody titers. Direct diagnosis relies on obtaining positive cultures from respiratory tract secretions, brushings, or washings.

Respiratory syncytial virus

Serologic diagnosis can be made, but the tests may be less reliable in children younger than 4 months of age. Direct diagnosis requires cultures from respiratory secretions, nasopharyngeal washings, or throat swabs; virus detection is possible after 2–7 days. Immunofluorescence techniques are now frequently used, as they allow a reliable and more rapid detection in nasal scrapings or washings[10]. The ELISA assay is less sensitive.

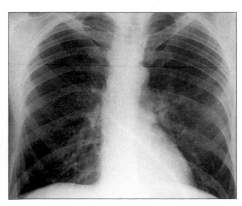

Figure 21.3 Radiograph of calcific varicella nodules. Multiple 3–5mm calcified nodules in the upper and lower lobes of a patient who had varicella pneumonia as a child.

Adenovirus

Rapid diagnosis requires antigen detection or histopathologic examination of biopsy specimens (which show intranuclear basophilic inclusions). Virus isolation requires 3 days to several weeks, and serodiagnosis requires both acute and convalescent sera[10].

Varicella

The infection can be diagnosed by a cytologic examination of scrapings from the lesions (i.e. the Tzanck smear, seeking multinucleated giant cells), although the sensitivity of this test is low. The virus may be cultured or found by polymerase chain reaction. A number of serologic tests are available, which include the fluorescent antibody to membrane antigen test and ELISA.

Hantavirus

The diagnosis can be made by serologic or immunohistochemical techniques.

TREATMENT

Influenza virus infection

In addition to supportive care, specific antiviral therapy with amantadine (100mg/kg per day for 5 days) or rimantadine may be beneficial if administered early in the course of the disease (i.e. within 48 hours following the onset of symptoms)[11,12]. Early inhaled and/or intranasal administration of a new antiviral agent, zanamivir, reduces the duration of symptoms by 1 day (4 versus 5 days)[13].

Antibiotics active against *Strep. pneumoniae*, *Haem. influenzae*, and *Staph. aureus* are needed to treat patients who have secondary pneumoniae.

Parainfluenza virus infection

Although ribavirin (tribavirin) has some *in vitro* activity, in the treatment of patients it is only supportive. Corticosteroids have been reported anecdotally to accelerate recovery in patients who have severe involvement.

Respiratory syncytial virus

Aerosolized ribavirin improves the clinical course and should be administered for 12–18 hours per day to patients who have severe disease, for 2–5 days. Systemic corticosteroids are also given to those who suffer the most severe involvement.

Adenovirus

Treatment is supportive (i.e. analgesics, cough suppressers).

Measles

Treatment is supportive, and antibiotics are required when bacterial secondary infection occurs. No consistent data are available on the effects of corticosteroids.

Varicella

Early administration of acyclovir (10–12.5mg/kg, given intravenously every 8 hours for 7 days) is recommended for immunocompromised hosts who have varicella, and for immunocompetent patients who suffer pneumonia[9,14].

Hantavirus

Treatment is mainly supportive, but the results of controlled trials of intravenous ribavirin are pending. Although *in vitro* effects of ribavirin have been demonstrated, preliminary results from an open-label trial are not impressive.

CLINICAL COURSE AND PREVENTION

Influenza virus infection
The morbidity and mortality of influenza pneumonia are high and patients can deteriorate to the point of developing the acute respiratory distress syndrome. In such cases, the likelihood of developing a secondary pneumonia is high.

Inactivated influenza vaccines are modified each year to follow the antigenic modifications of influenza A strains. They provide 50–80% protection against influenza-related illnesses, and 30–65% protection against influenza-related hospitalizations and deaths in the elderly[15]. Accordingly, vaccination is recommended for all patients over 65 years of age, all patients who have chronic comorbid conditions (regardless of age), patients who reside in chronic care facilities, and health workers (because of their increased risk of contacting patients who have influenza and spreading it to other, noninfected patients). The preventive administration of amantadine or rimantadine during the 2 weeks following vaccination has been recommended in very high-risk patients, to provide protection during the period required to develop an effective immunologic response.

Parainfluenza virus infection
No vaccine is yet available.

Respiratory syncytial virus
Since RSV may spread in hospitalized children and hospital staff, prevention of nosocomial infection is recommended (Fig. 21.4). No vaccine is available.

Adenovirus
Effective, enteric-coated, live vaccines have been developed for military recruits[16], but they are not used in other settings.

Preventive measures against nosocomial respiratory syncytial virus infections

Isolation or cohorting of hospital-admitted infected infants in specific areas

Surface decontamination of objects and furniture

Isolation measures

Handwashing

Use of gowns, gloves, and eye–nose goggles

Figure 21.4 Preventive measures against nosocomial respiratory syncytial virus infections.

Measles
The measles vaccine has reduced the incidence of disease by 98% in developed countries, and has shifted the median age of onset to the teenage years.

Varicella
Preventive administration of oral acyclovir in adults who have varicella may be prudent, especially in elderly subjects, pregnant women, or patients who suffer chronic obstructive pulmonary disease[9]. Zoster immune globulin is recommended to reduce the severity of illness in immunocompromised patients exposed to varicella. A live, attenuated vaccine is in development.

The infection can readily spread in the hospital setting such that strict isolation must be employed until all lesions have become crusted over.

Hantavirus
Avoidance of areas in which infected rodents reside is the only recognized preventive measure.

REFERENCES

1. Henrickson KJ. Lower respiratory viral infections in immunocompetent children. Adv Pediatr Infect Dis. 1994;9:59–96.
2. Piedra PA. Influenza virus pneumonia: pathogenesis, treatment, and prevention. Semin Respir Infect. 1995;10:216–23.
3. Glezen WP. Serious morbidity and mortality associated with influenza epidemics. Epidemiol Rev. 1982;4:25–44.
4. Bender BS, Small PA, Jr. Influenza: pathogenesis and host defense. Semin Respir Infect. 1992;7:38–45.
5. Foy HM, Cooney MK, Maletzky AJ, et al. Incidence and etiology of pneumonia, croup and bronchiolitis in preschool children belonging to a prepaid medical care group over a four year period. Am J Epidemiol. 1973;97:80–92.
6. Yang E, Rubin BK. 'Childhood' viruses as a cause of pneumonia in adults. Semin Respir Infect. 1995;10:232–43.
7. Garvie DG, Greg J. Outbreak of respiratory syncytial virus infections in the elderly. Br Med J. 1980;201:1253–4.
8. Brandt CD, Kim HW, Vargosdo AJ, et al. Infections in 18,000 infants and children in a controlled study of respiratory tract disease. I. Adenovirus pathogenicity in relation to serologic type and illness syndrome. Am J Epidemiol. 1969;90:484–500.
9. Gogos CA, Bassaris HP, Vagenakis AG. Varicella pneumonia in adults. A review of pulmonary manifestations, risk factors and treatment. Respiration. 1992;59:339–43.
10. Leland DS, Emanuel D. Laboratory diagnosis of viral infections of the lung. Semin Respir Infect. 1995;10:189–98.
11. Centers for Disease Control and Prevention. Prevention and control of influenza: recommendations of the Advisory Committee on Immunization Practices (ACIP). MMWR Morb Mortal Wkly Rep. 1998;47:1–26.
12. Hall CB, Dolin R, Gala CL, et al. Children with influenza A infections: treatment with rimantadine. Pediatrics. 1987;80:275–82.
13. Hayden FG, Osterhaus ADME, Treanor JJ, et al. Efficacy and safety of the neuraminidase inhibitor zanamivir in the treatment of influenzavirus infections. N Engl J Med. 1997;337:874–80.
14. Haake DA, Zakowski PC, Haake DL, Bryson YJ. Early treatment with acyclovir for varicella pneumonia in otherwise healthy adults: retrospective controlled study and review. Rev Infect Dis. 1990;12:788–98.
15. Gross PA, Hermogenes AW, Sacks HS, Lau J, Levandowski RA. The efficacy of influenza vaccine in elderly persons. A meta-analysis and review of the literature. Ann Intern Med. 1995;123:518–27.
16. Top FHJ. Control of adenovirus acute respiratory disease in US army trainees. Yale J Biol Med. 1975;48:185–95.

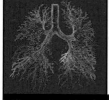

Section 5 Infectious Disease: community-acquired pneumonia

Chapter 22 Aspiration

Gérard Huchon and Nicolas Roche

Problems that result from aspiration vary depending on the nature of the aspirated material. In this chapter, the aspiration of gastric contents, oropharyngeal secretions, and lipoid substances, as well as near drowning, are addressed.

EPIDEMIOLOGY AND RISK FACTORS

The risk factors that predispose to aspiration are summarized in Figure 22.1. Nearly 50% of normal subjects aspirate oropharyngeal secretions during sleep[1]. The prevalence increases to as much as 70% when consciousness is impaired by medications or neurologic disorders, or when patients are intubated or have a tracheostomy[1,2]. In normal subjects, the volume of material aspirated is small, the host is protected by the pulmonary defense mechanisms, and the episodes have no clinically detectable consequence. Even in urgent intubations, clinically apparent aspiration is rare (3.5%)[3].

Aspiration of gastric contents

Aspiration of gastric contents initially causes a chemical pneumonitis as a result of the low pH of the fluid. Pneumonitis may be observed, however, even when the pH is relatively high (≥ 6). When this occurs the lung injury is transient, whereas when the pH is lower (e.g. <2.5) more persistent inflammatory and hemorrhagic bronchial damage may occur. Animal experiments suggest that the volume of material must exceed 1–4ml/kg to cause inflammation[4]. Atelectasis is frequent and occurs early, and likely arises from the deleterious effect of gastric acid on surfactant.

Aspiration pneumonia

The diagnosis of aspiration pneumonia is generally restricted to patients who have a bacterial lung infection that occurs in association with a condition predisposing them to aspiration (see Fig. 22.1). Organisms encountered include a number of anaerobic bacteria (e.g. anaerobic streptococci, *Fusobacterium* and *Bacteroides* spp.) and Gram-negative enteric bacilli[5]. Periodontal disease is found in many of these patients, and these pockets of infection in the gums are thought to be the source of these pathogens.

Lipoid pneumonia

Lipoid pneumonia results from aspiration of exogenous lipids contained in orally administered laxatives or nasal decongestants. The histology is that of giant-cell inflammation with oil-containing vacuoles and phagocytes, type II cell metaplasia, degeneration of arteriolar or bronchial walls, necrosis, and fibrosis. Oil droplets or lipophages may be transported by lymphatics or via the blood to the liver, spleen, kidney, or other organs. Special stains allow exogenous lipoid pneumonia to be distinguished from those that arise from accumulation of endogenous lipids, as occasionally occurs in the setting of chronic primary lung inflammation (Fig. 22.2)[6].

Near drowning

Drowning is the third most common cause of accidental death in the USA[7]. Near drowning is defined as survival after suffocation caused by submersion in water.

Conditions that predispose to aspiration pneumonias		
Cause	Intrinsic	Extrinsic including iatrogenic
Neurologic disorders	Seizures, stroke, trauma, multiple sclerosis, Parkinson's disease, myasthenia gravis, pseudobulbar palsy, amyotrophic lateral sclerosis	Trauma, alcoholism, drug abuse, general anesthesia
Gastrointestinal disorders	Esophageal achalasia, stricture, tumor, diverticula, tracheoesophageal fistula, cardiac sphincter incompetency, protracted vomiting, bowel obstruction, gastric distension or delayed emptying	Upper gastrointestinal endoscopy, nasogastric tube
Respiratory disorders	Larynx incompetency (vocal cord paralysis), impairment of tracheobronchial mucociliary clearance	Endotracheal intubation, tracheostomy, pharyngeal anesthesia

Figure 22.1 Conditions that predispose to aspiration pneumonias.

Histopathologic differences between exogenous and endogenous lipoid pneumonias		
Characteristic	Exogenous lipids	Endogenous lipids
Fat	Large droplets	Small droplets
Foreign body granulomas	Present	Absent
Birefringence under polarized light	Absent	Present
Special stainings		
Periodic acid–Schiff	Negative	Positive
Sudan black	Light blue	Black
Sudan IV	Orange	Red
Oil red O	Orange	Red
Nile blue sulfate	Negative	Light violet
Osmium tetroxide	Negative	Positive

Figure 22.2 Histopathologic differences between exogenous and endogenous lipoid pneumonias[6].

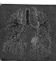

CLINICAL FEATURES

Aspiration of gastric contents

Mendelson originally described the syndrome in 1946 in 61 obstetric patients who developed aspiration pneumonia after ether anesthesia[8]. Manifestations begin very rapidly after the event and include cough (dry, or with pink sputum because of bronchoalveolar hemorrhage), tachypnea, tachycardia, fever, diffuse crackles, cyanosis, and bronchospasm in some cases. Chest radiographs show extensive atelectasis and infiltrates, and arterial blood gases show hypoxemia and normo- or hypocapnia. In the most severe cases, the arterial partial pressure of carbon dioxide may be elevated and metabolic acidosis may be present.

Aspiration pneumonia

A number of clinical features help distinguish aspiration pneumonia from other community-acquired pneumonias. Aspiration pneumonia tends to have a more insidious course, such that the patient frequently has an empyema, a lung abscess, or a necrotizing pneumonia at the time medical care is first sought. The sputum may be putrid because of anaerobic bacteria, and weight loss is common. Chest imaging commonly shows necrotizing infiltrates or abscesses, typically located in dependent regions (Fig. 22.3).

Lipoid pneumonia

Symptoms include cough, dyspnea, fever, chest pain, or hemoptysis. The onset may be acute, but more commonly it is chronic, and is accompanied by weight loss. In 50% of cases, the disease is clinically silent and discovered on a chest radiograph. A number of radiologic presentations may be found (Figs 22.4 & 22.5). Computed tomography or magnetic resonance imaging may be useful when they demonstrate attenuation values of −30 to −150 Hounsfield units, or high-intensity T1 signals with slow decrease on T2-weighed images, respectively, as a result of the low density of fat. Sputum, bronchoalveolar lavage fluid, or transbronchial biopsies can be examined for fat-containing macrophages after the application of special stains.

Near drowning

Clinical presentation may be the result of asphyxia (from acute laryngospasm), water aspiration, and/or changes in blood volume. Asphyxia causes central nervous system anoxia. The extent of damage may be far less than predicted based on the presumed or witnessed duration of anoxia, as cold water immersion decreases the basal metabolic rate, induces bradycardia, causes peripheral vasoconstriction, and redistributes blood toward the heart and brain. Water aspiration results in hypoxemia because of atelectasis and intrapulmonary shunting. Clinically, important blood volume changes are unusual, but large volumes of fluid resuscitation may be needed in the setting of salt-water aspiration.

TREATMENT

Aspiration of gastric contents

The lower airways are suctioned immediately after aspiration. When solid material is aspirated, fiberoptic bronchoscopy is performed in an attempt to remove as much of the material as possible by directed suctioning. Tracheobronchial lavage with buffering solutions has little effect on the course of the disease, since aspirated acids are rapidly neutralized by the outpouring of

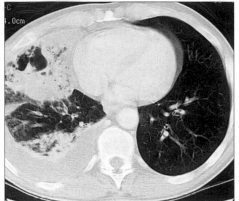

Figure 22.3 Necrotizing aspiration pneumonia. Chest computed tomography demonstrates involvement of the entire right middle lobe (which suggests pulmonary gangrene) and an effusion, which was found to be an empyema.

Findings in exogenous lipoid pneumonia on chest radiography
Dense consolidation with air bronchograms
Ground glass infiltrates
Cavitation
Interstitial infiltrate
Fibrotic infiltrates
Nodules, masses
Atelectasis
Emphysema
Pleural effusion

Figure 22.4 Findings in exogenous lipoid pneumonia on chest radiography.

plasma that occurs as a result of the chemical injury. Intravascular volume support may be needed. Fever, purulent secretions, leukocytosis, and new pulmonary infiltrates may be observed in the course of gastric aspiration in the absence of infection. Accordingly, prophylactic antibiotics are not generally used, as they do not appear to modify the course of the disease and may select for resistant bacteria. The decision as to when to begin antibiotics is, accordingly, based on clinical suspicion that a secondary bacterial infection has developed. Trials of corticosteroids have been disappointing[9].

Aspiration pneumonia

Antibiotics are selected for their activity against anaerobic bacteria. Choices include amoxicillin plus clavulanate (as up to 40% of anaerobic bacteria produce β-lactamase), penicillin or amoxicillin plus metronidazole, or clindamycin. The increased risk of *Clostridium difficile* infection with clindamycin leads some investigators to suggest it should only be given to patients who have evidence of necrotizing pneumonia, as it is in this group that the benefit of clindamycin over other treatments has been demonstrated.

When the areas of necrosis progress to involve the entire lobe, pulmonary gangrene must be considered. This condition is thought to result from thrombosis of the lobar pulmonary artery such that the major blood supply to the lobe is lost. Older literature suggests that pulmonary gangrene should be treated with lobar resection or open drainage, as conservative treatment has been associated with an increased mortality.

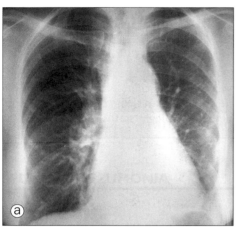
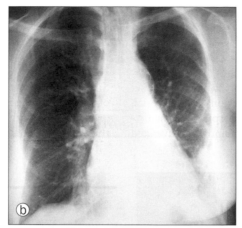
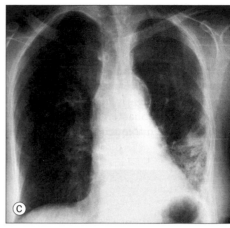

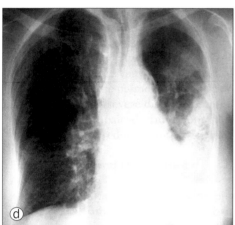
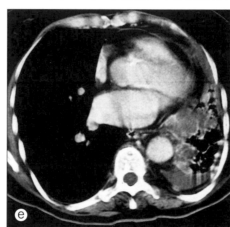

Figure 22.5 Lipoid pneumonia. This series of radiographs demonstrates infiltration of the left lower lobe that slowly progressed over a period of 19 years [from 1974 (a) to 1993 (d)]. The patient liberally applied a mentholatum-containing nasal grease each night before bed and her husband documented that the patient routinely slept on her left side. The CT scan shows low-density consolidation of the left lower lobe and a small left pleural effusion.

Lipoid pneumonia

The most important intervention is to stop the administration of the causative agent. Corticosteroids do not appear to be beneficial.

Near drowning

The first intervention is cardiopulmonary resuscitation and the provision of ventilatory support. Bronchodilators may be helpful. Attempts to remove the aspirated fluid from the lung are unnecessary.

CLINICAL COURSE AND PREVENTION

Aspiration of gastric contents

All of the patients reported by Mendelson recovered rapidly, whereas subsequent studies demonstrated mortality rates as high as 60%[8,9]. The discrepancy likely results because Mendelson's patients were healthy young women, whereas later reports included patients who were older and had numerous comorbid illnesses.

Bynum and Pierce characterized three patterns of response to gastric aspiration[10]:
- rapid recovery (62%);
- rapid deterioration into the adult respiratory distress syndrome (ARDS) with death within 24 hours (12%); and
- initial recovery with subsequent development of fever and new infiltrates (26%), which suggests pulmonary superinfection, which may progress to ARDS.

When bacterial infection is demonstrated, the mortality increases by a factor of three[10].

Preventive measures are summarized in Figure 22.6 and are employed in patients who have predisposing conditions[14]. A number of surgical techniques have been advocated for patients who have anatomic abnormalities in their larynx or hypopharynx, which include tracheostomy, cricopharyngeal myotomy, laryngeal suspension, cricoid resection, and vocal cord medialization[10]. Aspiration of tube-fed patients can be detected by adding a food dye to the feeding formula and seeking evidence of its presence in tracheobronchial secretions, or by measuring the glucose content of the secretions. Neither of these approaches appears to be

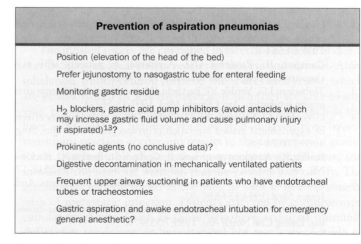

Prevention of aspiration pneumonias

Position (elevation of the head of the bed)

Prefer jejunostomy to nasogastric tube for enteral feeding

Monitoring gastric residue

H_2 blockers, gastric acid pump inhibitors (avoid antacids which may increase gastric fluid volume and cause pulmonary injury if aspirated)[13]?

Prokinetic agents (no conclusive data)?

Digestive decontamination in mechanically ventilated patients

Frequent upper airway suctioning in patients who have endotracheal tubes or tracheostomies

Gastric aspiration and awake endotracheal intubation for emergency general anesthetic?

Figure 22.6 Prevention of aspiration pneumonias[11,12].

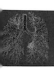

Blastomycosis

Blastomycosis is found in North America (in areas largely overlapping those of histoplasmosis), Mexico, the Middle East, Africa and India, and results from inhalation of *Blastomyces dermatitidis*. The fungus grows in the soil, and the spores become airborne and are inhaled before converting into the yeast form within the lung. *B. dermatitidis* infection may occur sporadically or in epidemics. The initial defense mechanism involves polymorphonuclear cells followed by macrophages and giant cells, and epithelioid granulomas often develop. Depending on the type of the predominant inflammatory response (i.e. pyogenic or granulomatous), the histopathologic pattern can mimic that of a bacterial infection, sarcoidosis, or a mycobacterial disease. After multiplication of the yeast in the lungs, it may spread to the skin, bones, brain, peripheral lymph nodes, or other organs, and extrapulmonary manifestations may occur many years after the initial infection.

Coccidioidomycosis

Coccidioidomycosis results from another soil-dwelling fungus, *Coccidioides immitis*. It is endemic in the southwestern USA and northern Mexico, and occurs mainly during hot, dry summers. Inhalation of airborne spores leads to polymorphonuclear-mediated suppurative and cell-mediated granulomatous inflammatory responses. The incubation period is 10–16 days.

Paracoccidioidomycosis

Paracoccidioidomycosis results from inhalation of a soil fungus that is found mainly in South and Central America, and in Mexico.

Cryptococcosis

The fungus is found throughout the world in bird guano.

Clinical features

Aspergillosis

The clinical presentation of ABPA is that of recurrent exacerbations of asthma coupled with fever, expectoration of brown mucus plugs, radiographic abnormalities (which include infiltrates, mucous impactions in the airways, atelectasis, and central bronchiectasis), and eosinophilia.

Aspergillomas are often asymptomatic, but the most common presentation is hemoptysis, which may be life-threatening.

Histoplasmosis

The large majority of patients who have acute primary infections are undiagnosed because histoplasmosis remains subclinical[2]. Those who inhale larger numbers of spores (frequently as a result of exposure occurring in a closed space) develop a syndrome approximately 14 days later that has an abrupt onset and resembles influenza, bacterial pneumonia, or tuberculosis (Fig. 23.2). When the inoculum is particularly large, patients may develop the acute respiratory distress syndrome (ARDS).

Blastomycosis

The clinical manifestations of blastomycosis differ from one country to another[3]. In North America, acute epidemic blastomycosis mimics bacterial pneumonia with the abrupt onset of fever, chills, arthralgias and myalgias, cough with purulent sputum, and pleuritic chest pain. In milder cases, which are more frequent, the presentation is that of a more chronic disease, resembling tuberculosis, in which low-grade fever, cough, anorexia, and weight loss develop insidiously[4]. Physical examination sometimes demonstrates erythema nodosum or findings of pulmonary consolidation, but it may be normal. The radiographic manifestations are nonspecific and include cavities, infiltrates, rounded densities, consolidation with air bronchograms, perihilar masses, or even a miliary pattern. Mediastinal lymph node involvement is rare (i.e. <10% in most studies)[4], and pleural effusions are quite uncommon. In the most severe cases, infection with *B. dermatitidis* can cause ARDS, even in immunocompetent hosts[5]. Patients who suffer cutaneous blastomycosis frequently have a history of a self-limited pulmonary syndrome that occurred some years in the past.

Coccidioidomycosis

Patients who have coccidioidomycosis can complain of fever, chills, arthralgias, myalgias, and headache in addition to cough, pleuritic chest pain, dyspnea, and, on occasion, hemoptysis (which results from areas of lung necrosis manifested by cavitation). Physical examination may reveal a macular rash, erythema nodosum, or erythema multiforme, as well as rhonchi, wheezes or signs of consolidation and/or pleural effusion. In many patients, the physical examination is normal. Chest radiographs initially show one or more areas of consolidation, which may cavitate. Hilar lymphadenopathy may be found. Cavities and/or multiple calcified nodules may persist lifelong. Occasionally, patients develop progressive primary coccidioidomycosis, a condition in which the

Clinical presentations of acute histoplasmosis			
	Mild acute pneumonitis	**Pneumonic histoplasmosis**	**Progressive disseminating primary infection**
Symptoms and physical signs	None or acute, influenza-like symptoms. Arthralgia–erythema nodosum–erythema multiforme complex	Fever, chills, sweat, anorexia, weakness, cough with mucopurulent sputum, pleuritic chest pain. Sometimes consolidation, rarely pleural effusion	Severe acute illness, often in immunocompromised patients. Weight loss, low-grade fever, abdominal complaints, cough. Sometimes mucosal ulcers, adrenal involvement
Chest radiography	Normal or consolidation ± lymph node enlargement	Infiltrates of varying density, often with hilar lymph node enlargement, sometimes with pericarditis	Normal, or multiple nodules, linear opacities ± lymph node involvement, or miliary aspect
Blood examination	–	–	In severe disease, leukopenia, thrombocytopenia, disseminated intravascular coagulation
Diagnosis	–	–	Few granulomas and many organisms in the most severe disease, the opposite in less severe forms
Clinical course	Spontaneous resolution; residual calcified nodules and lymph nodes	–	–

Figure 23.2 Clinical presentations of acute histoplasmosis.

infiltrates and lymphadenopathy progress in association with fever, cough, and weight loss. Several months following the primary pulmonary infection, disseminated coccidioidomycosis may become manifest (e.g. skin, bones, joints, genitourinary system, meninges), particularly but not exclusively in immunocompromised patients.

Paracoccidioidomycosis

In nonimmunocompromised patients, paracoccidioidomycosis presents as a chronic or subacute lung infection that is usually self limited. In immunocompromised subjects, the clinical manifestations are those of an acute, severe disseminated infection.

Cryptococcosis

Cryptococcosis is a rare infection, and is usually asymptomatic and self-limiting in immunocompetent patients. In those who have impaired, cell-mediated immunity it may cause lung infection and meningitis. Symptoms of pulmonary infection include fever, malaise, cough, and chest pain. The chest radiograph may show large, nonspecific nodules (Fig. 23.3) or infiltrates, sometimes associated with lymphadenopathy.

Diagnosis

Aspergillosis

The diagnosis of ABPA is established using the criteria summarized in Figure 23.4.

Aspergillomas are suggested by finding an air crescent on top of a mass within a pre-existing parenchymal cavity (Fig. 23.5). Serology is usually positive.

Histoplasmosis

The growth of *Histoplasma* spp. is slow, such that one to several weeks are needed for cultures to become positive. Giemsa staining of blood or bone marrow smears may be diagnostic when the fungus load is high, but this is unusual in immunocompetent patients. Tissue samples can demonstrate the organisms with silver or periodic acid–Schiff (PAS) staining. Indirect diagnosis may be provided by several serologic techniques, which include complement fixation, immunodiffusion, or radioimmunoassay, all of which may require several weeks to become positive[2].

Blastomycosis

The diagnosis of blastomycosis is made by microscopic examination of respiratory secretions digested by potassium hydroxide,

or by histopathologic examination of tissue samples after silver or PAS staining[6]. In cultured respiratory samples, detectable growth takes up to 1 week.

Coccidioidomycosis

The diagnosis of coccidioidomycosis may be made by serologic or skin testing, both of which are most useful for epidemiologic purposes. Direct diagnosis can be made by microscopic examination of sputum or pus after potassium hydroxide digestion or Papanicolaou staining, by histopathologic examination of tissue biopsies after silver

Diagnostic criteria of allergic bronchopulmonary aspergillosis	
Major criteria	Asthma
	Central bronchiectasis
	Recurrent pulmonary infiltrates on chest radiographs
	Blood and sputum eosinophilia (>1000/mm^3 in serum)
	Increased total IgE titers (>1000IU/ml)
	Immediate hypersensitivity to *Aspergillus fumigatus* as determined by skin prick tests, or specific anti-*Asp. fumigatus* IgEs in serum
	Precipitins against *Asp. fumigatus* in serum
Minor criteria	Presence of *Asp. fumigatus* in sputum
	Late hypersensitivity to *Asp. fumigatus* as determined by skin prick tests
	Expectoration of plugs

Figure 23.4 Diagnostic criteria of allergic bronchopulmonary aspergillosis. The first six major criteria should be present for the diagnosis to be made.

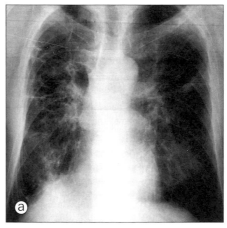
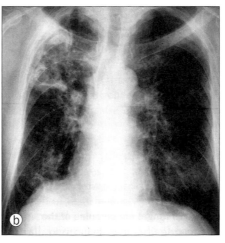

Figure 23.5 Aspergilloma. (a) This patient had lung scarring from diffuse, necrotizing pneumonia, which occurred several years earlier. (b) Note the rim of air on top of the aspergilloma in the right upper lobe.

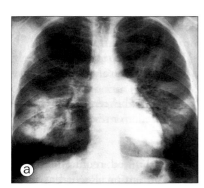
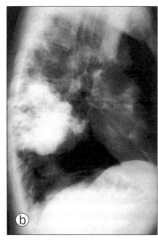

Figure 23.3 Cryptococcal lung infection. Chest radiographs of immunocompetent patient that show bilateral, large nodular densities.

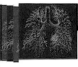
exposure to antiviral therapy, which is potentially hazardous and expensive, and risks the emergence of ganciclovir resistance. Thus, pre-emptive treatment directed by diagnostic tests for CMV has been advocated.

Pre-emptive intravenous ganciclovir therapy in allograft BMT recipients directed by BAL surveillance on day 35 following transplantation improved survival for BAL CMV-positive patients who received antiviral therapy[15]. A second strategy in BMT recipients using peripheral blood culture for CMV also resulted in improved survival, but with this approach, 12% of patients developed CMV disease in advance of being blood-culture positive[16]. BMT recipients who received pre-emptive ganciclovir directed by CMV antigenemia had significantly more CMV infection compared with those who received intravenous ganciclovir prophylaxis[9]. Yet there was no difference in survival between the two groups, possibly because the patients who received ganciclovir prophylaxis had a significantly greater incidence of fungal infection. In heart and lung transplant recipients, pre-emptive treatment directed by CMV antigenemia resulted in a significant reduction in CMV disease[17]. These observations suggest that pre-emptive treatment directed by CMV antigenemia does not eliminate CMV infection, but facilitates control with reduced ganciclovir exposure and fewer complications.

Oral ganciclovir prophylaxis (1g q8h) is an alternative strategy, but randomized studies of oral ganciclovir versus placebo showed no difference in survival, despite less CMV disease with ganciclovir[18].

The role for vaccination in the prevention of CMV and influenza infection is uncertain. In the setting of an influenza outbreak, amantadine or rimantadine (anti-influenza drugs) may be given to high-risk, immunocompromised patients[19].

A variety of strategies are available for the control of viral infection in immunocompromised patients. Optimal control of CMV includes the application of acyclovir or valacyclovir for prophylaxis, with surveillance for CMV infection by CMV antigenemia, or qualitative PCR and ganciclovir for pre-emptive treatment in the presence of an increasing viral load[20].

REFERENCES

1. Grundy JE, Lui SF, Super M, et al. Symptomatic cytomegalovirus infection in seropositive kidney recipients: reinfection with donor virus rather than reactivation of recipient virus. Lancet. 1988;ii:132–5.
2. Cone RW, Hackman RC, Hunang MW, et al. Human herpes virus 6 in lung tissue from patients with pneumonitis after bone marrow transplantation. N Engl J Med. 1993;329:156–61.
3. Sable CA, Hayden FG. Orthomyxoviral and paramyxoviral infections in transplant patients. Infect Dis Clin North Am. 1995;9:987–1003.
4. Wendt CH. Community respiratory viruses: organ transplant recipients. Am J Med. 1997;102(Suppl. 3A):31–6.
5. Van der Meer JT, Drew WL, Bowden RA, et al. Summary of the international consensus symposium on advances in the diagnosis, treatment and prophylaxis of cytomegalovirus infection. Antiviral Res. 1996;32:119–40.
6. Egan JJ, Barber L, Lomax J, et al. Detection of human cytomegalovirus antigenaemia: a rapid diagnostic technique for predicting cytomegalovirus infection/pneumonitis in lung and heart transplant recipients. Thorax. 1995;50:9–13.
7. Barber L, Egan JJ, Lomax J, et al. A comparative study of several PCR assays with antigenaemia and conventional techniques for the diagnosis of HCMV infection in lung and heart transplant recipients. J Med Virol. 1996;49:137–44.
8. Boeckh M, Gooley TA, Myerson D, Cunningham T, Schoch G, Bowden RA. Cytomegalovirus pp65 antigenaemia-guided early treatment with ganciclovir versus ganciclovir at engraftment after allogenic marrow transplantation: a randomised double-blind study. Blood. 1996;88:4063–71.
9. Englund JA, Piedra PA, Jewell A, et al. Rapid diagnosis of respiratory syncytial virus infection in immunocompromised adults. J Clin Microbiol. 1996;34:1649–53.
10. Balfour HH, Fletcher CV, Dunn D. Prevention of cytomegalovirus disease with oral acyclovir. Transplant Proc. 1991;23(Suppl. 1):17–19.
11. Prentice HG, Gluckman E, Powles RL, et al. Impact of long term acyclovir on cytomegalovirus infection and survival after allogenic bone marrow transplantation. Lancet. 1994;343:749–53.
12. Merigan TC, Renlund DG, Keay S, et al. A controlled trial of ganciclovir to prevent cytomegalovirus disease after heart transplantation. N Engl J Med. 1992;326:1182–6.
13. Winston DJ, Ho WG, Bartoni K, et al. Ganciclovir prophylaxis of cytomegalovirus infection and disease in allogenic bone marrow transplant recipients. Results of a placebo-controlled, double blind trial. Ann Intern Med. 1993;118:179–84.
14. Goodrich JM, Bowden RA, Fisher L, Keller C, Schoch G, Meyers JD. Ganciclovir prophylaxis to prevent cytomegalovirus disease after allogenic marrow transplant. Ann Intern Med. 1993;118:173–8.
15. Schmidt GM, Horak DA, Niland JC, et al. A randomised controlled trail of prophylactic ganciclovir for cytomegalovirus infection in recipients of allogenic bone marrow transplants. N Engl J Med. 1991;324:1005–11.
16. Goodrich JM, Mori M, Gleaves CA, et al. Early treatment with ganciclovir to prevent cytomegalovirus disease after allogenic bone marrow transplantation. N Engl J Med. 1991;325:1601–7.
17. Egan JJ, Lomax J, Barber L, et al. Preemptive treatment for the prevention of cytomegalovirus disease in heart and lung transplant recipients. Transplantation. 1998;65:747–52.
18. Gane E, Saliba F, Valdecasas GJC, et al. Randomised trial of efficacy and safety of oral ganciclovir in the prevention of cytomegalovirus disease in liver-transplant recipients. Lancet. 1997;350:1729–33.
19. Wiselka M. Influenza: diagnosis, management, and prophylaxis. Br Med J. 1994;308:1341–5.
20. Griffiths PD. Prophylaxis against CMV infection in transplant patients. J Antimicrob Chemother. 1997;39:299–301.

Section 5 Infectious Diseases: pneumonia in the immunocompromised host

Chapter 26

Fungal Pneumonia

Jim Egan

Fungal infection is a major problem in immunocompromised patients because of the difficulty in establishing a diagnosis and the limitations of treatment. Increasingly sophisticated and intense immunosuppression, in conjunction with interventions that disrupt the host's mucosal integrity, predisposes patients to fungal infection. Inevitably, the lung is the key target organ for invasive fungal disease.

EPIDEMIOLOGY AND RISK FACTORS

Aspergillus fumigatus, an inhaled environmental pathogen, is the most common cause of invasive pulmonary disease and is an ever-increasing problem, with infection rates increasing from 2.2% to 5.1% over a 14-year period in one autopsy study[1]. *Candida albicans* is the most common cause of fungal infection in immunocompromised patients, but it rarely causes invasive pulmonary disease. *Candida* is endogenous in origin, emanating from the gastrointestinal tract, and usually results in mucocutaneous candidiasis. Nevertheless, in the immunocompromised host, candidemia may be a cause of sepsis, and may be a pathogen in conjunction with Gram-positive or Gram-negative organisms that result in pneumonia.

The incidence of fungal infection, including candidemia, approaches 50% in bone marrow transplant (BMT) and 35% in lymphoma patients. The incidence of invasive pulmonary

aspergillosis (IPA) in BMT patients ranges from 6 to 15%[2], with a bimodal incidence, occurring early (<40 days) and late following transplantation (>40 days). In liver transplant recipients, IPA has an incidence of 1–10%. Isolated lung and heart–lung transplant recipients are commonly colonized with *Aspergillus* (25–40%), with an incidence of invasive disease of 15–25%. Heart transplant and renal transplant recipients have a rate of infection <10%[3], but the reported rates of infection, particularly in solid organ transplant recipients, are often influenced by outbreaks associated with local environmental factors. The overall mortality is of the order 80–100%.

Aspergilli have a small spore size with the capacity to be inhaled. Pathogenicity is promoted by the ability to adhere to epithelial cells and also to survive over a wide temperature range, up to 50°C. *Aspergillus* includes a number of species, of which *A. fumigatus* is the most common, causing approximately 80% of invasive infections, while *A. flavus* causes 5–10% and particularly affects the sinuses.

The pathology of IPA results from the spectrum of adherence, destructive invasion, and ultimately infarction of pulmonary tissue with systemic embolization and fungemia. Localization of IPA can be peripheral within the lung parenchyma or central with a tracheobronchial distribution (Fig. 26.1).

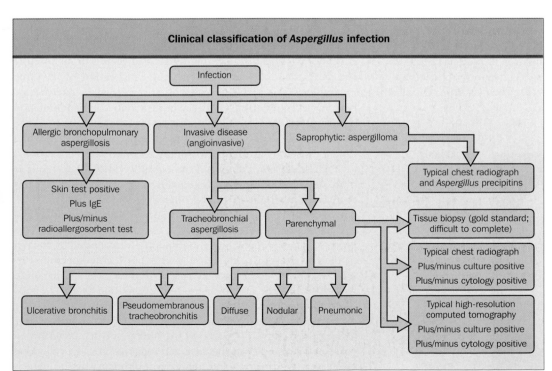

Figure 26.1 Classification of *Aspergillus* infection. Flow chart demonstrating the clinical classification of *Aspergillus* infection and disease.

Some patients, particularly lung transplant recipients with impaired mucociliary clearance and poor cough reflex, develop tracheobronchial aspergillosis[4]. This begins with *Aspergillus* colonization progressing to *Aspergillus*-induced tracheobronchitis, more severe ulceration, and an increasingly severe inflammatory response that culminates in membrane formation with mucous and necrotic tissue (Fig. 26.2).

A number of risk factors are associated with the development of IPA, including neutropenia, corticosteroid exposure, and prior fungal infection, as well as the use of broad-spectrum antibiotics, concurrent cytomegalovirus (CMV) infection, and graft-versus-host disease (GVHD).

Fungi, including *Cryptococcus* and *Mucorales* spp., are uncommon causes of invasive pulmonary disease in immunocompromised patients; mucormycosis carries a worse prognosis than aspergillosis. Other fungi have a particular geographic distribution, such as *Coccidioides* in southwestern areas of North America and in South America, and *Histoplasma* in central North America and in South America. These fungi are associated with acute and chronic illnesses, and their clinical effects mimic acute sarcoidosis and chronic mycobacterial infection, respectively.

Pneumocystis carinii is a widely distributed, eukaryotic pathogen that affects immunocompromised patients. Traditionally, *Pneumocystis* has been classified as a protozoal organism on the basis of its morphologic appearance and its response to antibiotics. Recent taxonomy, however, has shown that it is more closely related genetically to fungi than to protozoal organisms (see Chapter 6.32)[5].

CLINICAL FEATURES

Invasive pulmonary aspergillosis does not have specific clinical features that allow a clinical diagnosis to be made with a high predictive value. Diffuse, nodular, central, and peripheral patterns of infection occur (see Fig. 26.1), and more than one diagnosis may occur at one time. The clinical diagnosis is dependent on a high index of suspicion in susceptible patients.

In febrile, neutropenic patients, pyrexia unresponsive to broad-spectrum antibiotics prompts further investigation and/or empiric treatment. In other immunocompromised patients, fever may not be present. Clinical examination of the respiratory tract is often normal, and other organs subject to metastatic infection by fungi need to be examined, including the eye, skin, central nervous system, and the urinary tract.

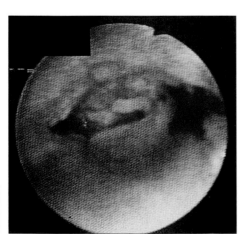

Figure 26.2 Tracheobronchial aspergillosis. Bronchoscopic finding of bronchial aspergillosis with ulceration of the right lower-lobe bronchus with membrane formation.

DIAGNOSIS

Despite the protean, heterogeneous clinical manifestations of invasive aspergillosis a clinical–radiologic classification schema can be applied (see Fig. 26.1), which prompts an ordered strategy of investigation and treatment (Fig. 26.3). The gold standard for diagnosis is based on histopathologic examination of lung tissue. However, this is rarely achieved, particularly in complex, thrombocytopenic, immunocompromised patients. Often the question is posed whether sputum that is culture positive for *Aspergillus* represents colonization or invasive disease. Unfortunately, there is no robust way to discriminate between colonization and invasive infection without microscopic examination of tissue. The diagnosis is dependent on a high index of suspicion in at-risk patients.

The application of surveillance techniques, including antigen detection (galactomannan), for the early diagnosis of invasive disease is limited, because most of the techniques available have low negative-predictive values[6]. The measurement of antibody to *Aspergillus* is often not helpful, especially in profoundly immunosuppressed patients, because the host has a limited capacity to mount an antibody response. In immunocompromised patients who can mount an antibody response, such a response often postdates the clinical infection.

The isolation of fungi from blood in neutropenic patients is rare and often thought to represent contamination. Nevertheless, candidemia, in particular, does occur and, if identified, should prompt further investigation. The sensitivity of blood culture surveillance for fungemia can be increased by collecting a minimum of 20mL for aerobic culture.

Nasal culture specimens have demonstrated encouraging positive-predictive values for invasive aspergillosis in BMT recipients[6].

Sputum culture in neutropenic patients is often limited by insufficient leukocytes to generate sputum. The sensitivity of sputum culture is increased by collecting at least three consecutive samples[7], and sputum from an immunocompromised patient which is *Aspergillus*-culture positive should prompt a high index of suspicion, further cultures, and bronchoalveolar lavage (BAL).

In invasive mycosis, the chest radiograph may be normal or abnormal, and may demonstrate a nodular or diffuse pattern. An abnormal chest radiograph demands targeted bronchoscopy and BAL. Nodular disease is highly suggestive of invasive aspergillosis (Fig. 26.4), as well as of nocardial, *Legionella*, or *Pneumocystis* infection. A diffuse infiltrate also demands a bronchoscopy and BAL, because such a pattern may be due to CMV, *Pneumocystis*, or bacterial infection. Wedge-shaped shadowing can be caused by an *Aspergillus*-induced pulmonary infarction.

High resolution computed tomography (HRCT) scanning is more sensitive and specific than plain radiology for the diagnosis of invasive aspergillosis[8], and is now widely used. Abnormalities on HRCT can be categorized as nodular or diffuse. Nodular disease is highly characteristic of IPA and reflects the pathologic process. In neutropenic patients, a nodule surrounded by an area of increased attenuation (ground glass) is highly specific (Fig. 26.5)[9]. This CT pattern is referred to as the 'halo' sign. Pathologically, the area of increased attenuation that surrounds the nodule represents hemorrhage. HRCT may also identify another characteristic sign of invasive aspergillosis – 'crescent' formation (Fig. 26.5). Infarction of the lung tissue occurs with vascular invasion, and tissue necrosis and repair results in a collection of air between normal and abnormal pulmonary tissue, which

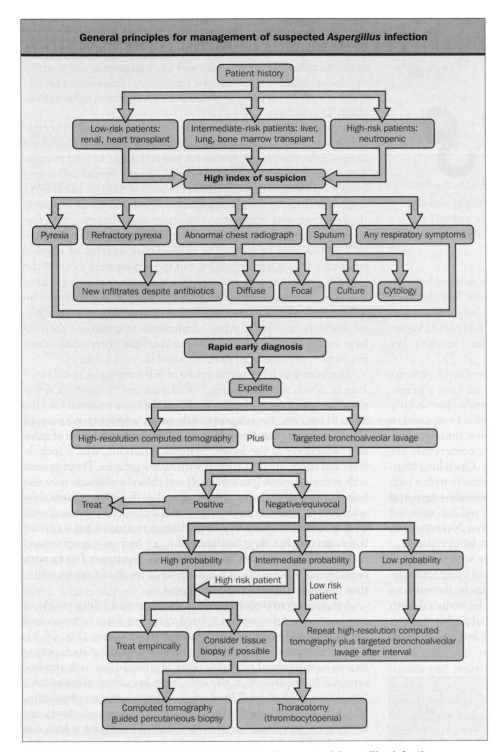

Figure 26.3 General principles for management of suspected *Aspergillus* infection.
A pulmonologist must understand the kinetics of risk factors, prevalence, and level of immunosuppression against the background of prophylaxis duration and timing of empiric therapy.

The flowchart: General principles for management of suspected *Aspergillus* infection

- Patient history
  - Low-risk patients: renal, heart transplant
  - Intermediate-risk patients: liver, lung, bone marrow transplant
  - High-risk patients: neutropenic
- High index of suspicion
  - Pyrexia
  - Refractory pyrexia → New infiltrates despite antibiotics
  - Abnormal chest radiograph → Diffuse / Focal
  - Sputum → Culture
  - Any respiratory symptoms → Cytology
- Rapid early diagnosis
- Expedite
  - High-resolution computed tomography — Plus — Targeted bronchoalveolar lavage
    - Positive → Treat
    - Negative/equivocal
      - High probability
      - Intermediate probability (High risk patient / Low risk patient)
      - Low probability → Repeat high-resolution computed tomography plus targeted bronchoalveolar lavage after interval
        - Treat empirically
        - Consider tissue biopsy if possible
          - Computed tomography guided percutaneous biopsy
          - Thoracotomy (thrombocytopenia)

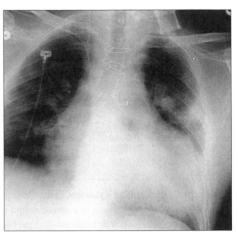

Figure 26.4 Nodular invasive aspergillosis.
Chest radiograph of a heart transplant recipient with refractory cardiac rejection who is receiving high-dose corticosteroids. Cardiomegaly and bilateral nodular infiltration of the lungs is seen, particularly in the left upper zone, which results from invasive pulmonary aspergillosis.

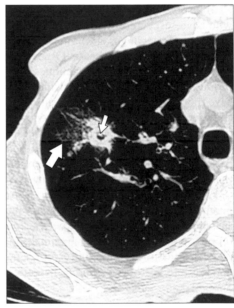

Figure 26.5 High-resolution computed tomography of invasive aspergillosis. This scan of a neutropenic patient who has invasive pulmonary aspergillosis shows a nodule of invasive aspergillosis surrounded by a ground-glass infiltration, 'halo' sign (large arrow). Within the nodule is a crescent of air and an area of opacification, a 'crescent' sign (small arrow).

manifests as a crescent of air. Now HRCT is commonly used to exclude IPA because of the specificity of the 'halo' and 'crescent' signs, although a negative HRCT does not preclude with certainty the need for other investigations for IPA.

Fiberoptic bronchoscopy and BAL are important for the diagnosis of invasive aspergillosis, particularly in *Aspergillus* tracheobronchial disease, in which the chest radiograph is commonly normal (see Fig. 26.2). Here, samples from the area are usually culture positive for *Aspergillus*, and stains of the sample for cytologic examination are also positive (see Fig. 26.6). Nevertheless, in the absence of a coagulopathy, such lesions should be biopsied.

In peripheral, localized, nodular aspergillosis, bronchoscopy is of limited value for diagnosis, and percutaneous, CT-guided biopsy is preferable. With peripheral disease, however, it is important to

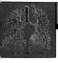

The first step in prophylaxis is the application of high-efficiency, particulate air filters, laminar flow rooms, avoidance of organic, uncooked food, and judicious use of broad-spectrum antibiotics and corticosteroids. Each hospital inevitably has continuing ongoing expansion and/or refurbishment that may release fungal spores. Environmental surveillance by air sampling with fungal culture is important. A single fungal colony of growth in a hospital area with air filtration systems demands further investigation of the environment.

The choice of pharmacologic prophylaxis varies between centers. Local prophylaxis in the form of intranasal or nebulized amphotericin has been used on the basis that the sinuses are an important reservoir for *Aspergillus* in BMT recipients and for augmenting local defenses against an inhaled pathogen in patients who have impaired mucociliary function.

For oral therapy, the imidazoles and triazoles are potentially ideal candidates for prophylaxis. Studied agents include ketoconazole, fluconazole, and itraconazole. Fluconazole, a synthetic triazole active against *Candida*, is widely used as prophylaxis against candidemia. However, in a controlled study of 356 BMT recipients who received 400mg of fluconazole per day during neutropenia, C. *albicans*-related infections were reduced, but no difference in survival was observed[15]. The use of fluconazole as prophylaxis has seen increasing colonization with C. *kruzi* and *Torulopsis glabrata*, yeasts inherently resistant to fluconazole. Similarly, *Aspergillus* resistance to itraconazole has now been described[16].

In allogenic BMT recipients, low-dose (i.e. 20mg/day) intravenous, conventional amphotericin B may be an effective preventive regimen, but this effect has not been reported consistently. A study in autologous BMT recipients failed to show a benefit with low-dose amphotericin B. The use of inexpensive but potentially nephrotoxic prophylaxis has to be balanced against the absolute requirement for other nephrotoxic drugs, which include aminoglycosides, cyclosporin, and/or tacrolimus.

Cost efficacy of prophylaxis is an important issue, particularly because liposomal amphotericin is being used increasingly. The potential advantages of intravenous liposomal formulations of amphotericin have been emphasized by a randomized comparison between liposomal amphotericin (1mg and 3mg/kg per day) versus conventional amphotericin B[17]. This study evaluated the effect of amphotericin in the treatment of antibiotic-resistant, febrile neutropenia. The end point was resolution of the pyrexia during the period of neutropenia. Both doses of liposomal amphotericin were significantly safer than conventional amphotericin B, and 3mg/kg of liposomal amphotericin was significantly more efficacious than 1mg/kg or conventional amphotericin B for lysis of the pyrexia (64 versus 49%).

Amphotericin, and particularly the liposomal preparations may have a role in the management of patients who have suspected fungemia, but these strategies are limited by the absence of clear evidence for improved survival and cost-effective reduction in rates of invasive disease.

REFERENCES

1. Groll AH, Shah PM, Mentzel C, Schneider M, Just-Nuebling G, Huebner K. Trends in the post mortem epidemiology of invasive fungal infections at a university hospital. J Infect. 1996;33:23–32.
2. Jantunen E, Ruutu P, Niskanen L, et al. Incidence and risk factors for invasive fungal infections in allogeneic BMT recipients. Bone Marrow Transplant. 1997;19:801–8.
3. Denning DW. Diagnosis and management of invasive aspergillosis. Curr Clin Top Infect Dis. 1996;16:277–99.
4. Kramer MR, Denning DW, Marshal SE, et al. Ulcerative tracheobronchitis after lung transplantation. Am Rev Respir Dis. 1991;144: 552–6.
5. Edman JC, Kovacs JA, Masur H, et al. Ribosomal RNA sequence shows *Pneumocystis carinii* to be a member of the fungi. Nature. 1988;334:519–22.
6. Denning DW, Evans EG, Kibbler CC, et al. Guidelines for the investigation of invasive fungal infections in haematological malignancy and solid organ transplantation. Eur J Clin Microbiol Infect Dis. 1997;16:424–36.
7. Horvath JA, Dummer S. The use of respiratory-tract cultures in the diagnosis of invasive pulmonary aspergillosis. Am J Med. 1996;100:171–8.
8. Blum U, Windfuhr M, Buitrago-Tellez C, Sigmund G, Herbst EW, Langer M. Invasive pulmonary aspergillosis, MRI, CT and plain radiographic findings and their contribution for early diagnosis. Chest. 1994;106:1156–61.
9. Kuhlman JE, Fishman EK, Burch PA, Karp JF, Zerhouni EA, Siegelman SS. Invasive pulmonary aspergillosis in acute leukaemia. Chest. 1987;92:95–9.
10. Ellis ME, Spence D, Bouchama A, et al. Open lung biopsy provides a higher and more specific diagnostic yields compared to bronchoalveolar lavage in immunocompromised patients. Scand J Infect Dis. 1995;27:157–62.
11. Ng TT, Denning DW. Liposomal amphotericin B (AmBisome) therapy in invasive fungal infections. Evaluation of United Kingdom compassionate use data. Arch Intern Med. 1995;155:1093–8.
12. Hiemenz JW, Walsh TJ. Lipid formulations of amphotericin B: recent progress and future directions. Clin Infect Dis. 1996; 22(Suppl. 2):S133–44.
13. Kramer MR, Marshall SE, Denning DW, et al. Cyclosporin and itraconazole interaction in heart and lung transplant recipients. Ann Intern Med. 1990;113:327–9.
14. Wong K, Waters CM, Walesby RK. Surgical management of invasive pulmonary aspergillosis in immunocompromised patients. Eur J Cardiothorac Surg. 1992;6:138–43.
15. Goodman JL, Winston DJ, Greenfield RA, et al. A controlled trial of fluconazole to prevent fungal infection in patients undergoing bone marrow transplantation. N Engl J Med. 1992;326:845–51.
16. Denning DW, Venkateswarlu K, Oakley KL, et al. Itraconazole resistance in *Aspergillus fumigatus*. Antimicrob Agents Chemother. 1997;41:1364–8.
17. Prentice HG, Hann IM, Herbrecht R, et al. A randomised comparison of liposomal versus conventional amphotericin B for the treatment of pyrexia of unknown origin in neutropenic patients. Br J Haematol. 1997;98:711–18.

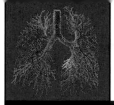
Chapter 27

Bacterial Pneumonia

Antoni Torres and Mustafá El-Ebiary

EPIDEMIOLOGY

After urinary tract infections, pneumonia is the second most common nosocomial infection, accounting for approximately 10–15% of all hospital-acquired infections. The overall incidence of nosocomial pneumonia is approximately 6.0–8.6/1000 admissions, but the risk is greatly increased for all patients in intensive-care units (12–29%), where respiratory infections have been reported to be the most frequent type of nosocomial infections. The risk in patients who receive mechanical ventilation is as high as 25–70%[1].

As many as 15% of all deaths that occur in hospitalized patients are directly related to nosocomial pneumonia. Studies have shown that inadequate initial antibiotic treatment is related to the prognosis.

CLINICAL FEATURES

The clinical features of nosocomial pneumonia include the presence of new and persistent pulmonary infiltrates, fever >38.3°C or hypothermia <36°C, leukocytosis > 12,000/mm³ or leukopenia <4000/mm³, and purulent secretions[2]. Although these criteria are well-accepted for establishing a diagnosis in spontaneously breathing patients, a number of studies suggest that they are less reliable in diagnosing pneumonia in patients who require mechanical ventilation. Clinical criteria result in up to a 29% incidence of misdiagnosis of pneumonia in patients who have acute respiratory distress syndrome when compared with autopsy findings as the gold standard. Radiographic criteria alone have a 32% incidence of misdiagnosis. As a result of these difficulties, a diagnostic scoring system was developed recently. A patient's score can range from 0 to 12, based on the following variables: temperature, blood leukocyte count, macroscopic evaluation of tracheal secretions, oxygenation [(arterial partial pressure of oxygen)/(fraction of inspired oxygen) ratio], chest radiograph, and semiquantitative culture of tracheal aspirates. A score >6 has a good correlation with a diagnosis of pneumonia on the basis of quantitative cultures performed on bronchoalveolar lavage (BAL) fluid (Fig. 27.1).

DIAGNOSIS

Noninvasive methods
Blood cultures
It is obligatory to obtain blood cultures when considering a diagnosis of nosocomial pneumonia. Unfortunately, the sensitivity is low (10–25%), and the specificity is reduced in critically ill patients who are at risk of bacteremia from multiple infectious foci. Accordingly, microorganisms isolated in blood cultures can only be considered as the definitive etiologic cause of

Clinical pulmonary infection score		
Variable	**Criterion**	**Points**
Temperature	≥36.5 to ≤38.4°C	0
	≥38.5 to 38.9°C	1
	≥39 to ≤36°C	2
Leukocyte count	≥4000 to ≤11000	0
	<4000 to >11000	1
	Band forms	2
Tracheal secretions	<14+ aspirations	0
	≥14+ aspirations	1
	Purulent secretions	2
Oxygenation (Pao₂/Flo₂ ratio)	>240 or acute respiratory distress syndrome	0
	≤240	2
Chest radiograph	No infiltrate	0
	Diffuse	1
	Localized	2
Semiquantitative tracheal aspirate cultures (0, 1, 2, or 3+)	Pathogenic bacteria ≤1+ or no growth	0
	Pathogenic bacteria >1+	1
	Same pathogenic bacteria on Gram's stain	2

Figure 27.1 The clinical pulmonary infection score. This score ranges from 0 to 12 and includes six variables. A clinical score higher than 6 has a good correlation with pulmonary infection.

nosocomial pneumonia when they coincide with the microbiologic results of respiratory secretions.

Sampling of the proximal airways
Qualitative culturing of sputum or endotracheal aspirates (in mechanically ventilated patients) is not an accurate way to diagnose nosocomial pneumonia. Although the sensitivity of this technique is high (60–90%), the specificity seems to be very low (0–33%) as the oropharynx and upper airways of intubated patients are frequently contaminated by flora that do not cause pneumonia. In the absence of prior antibiotic treatment, however, the negative predictive value of these techniques (i.e. negative cultures indicating absence of bacteria pneumonia) is high. Recent studies suggest that quantitative cultures of endotracheal aspirates using 10⁵–10⁶ colony-forming units (cfu)/mL as the cutoff point may be diagnostically acceptable when BAL is not available.

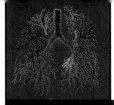

Chapter 29
Tuberculosis and Diseases Caused by Atypical Mycobacteria

William A Broughton and John B Bass, Jr

INTRODUCTION

The term tuberculosis (TB) describes an infectious disease that is believed to have plagued mankind since Neolithic times. It is caused by two species of *Mycobacterium* – *M. tuberculosis* and *M. bovis*. This illness was called phthisis by physicians in ancient Greece, to reflect its wasting character. In developing, urban Europe during the 17th and 18th centuries, as many as 25% of the deaths were caused by TB. Poor understanding of the contagious and progressive nature of the illness lead to widespread fear and played a role in the development of a frightening mythology of revenants and vampires to explain the course of the illness in the community.

A more complete understanding of the illness began with Laennec's uniting of pulmonary and extrapulmonary tuberculous disease. The disease was verified as communicable by Villemin in 1865. When Koch isolated the tubercle bacillus in 1882, and reproduced the disease with the isolate, the microbiologic nature of the disease was established.

Despite this new understanding of the illness, fear and ignorance predominated. Without effective treatment patients were isolated in sanatoria. Interventions such as pneumoperitoneum, therapeutic pneumothorax, plombage and thoracoplasty (Fig. 29.1) were carried out in attempts to decrease lung size and to close open tuberculous cavities. Despite the lack of a truly effective treatment, the use of sanatoria led to a decrease in death rate. It was not until streptomycin therapy for TB was introduced in 1946 and isoniazid became available in 1952 that realistic anti-infective therapy was available.

While there is much concern today about multidrug-resistant TB threatening our 'control' of TB, it is important to recognize that an estimated 3 million people worldwide die from this disease every year. Our progress with TB is relatively recent – the last of the sanatoria in the USA closed in the mid-1970s.

When the term tubercle bacillus is used it refers to two species of the family of Mycobacteriaceae, Actinomycetales: *M. bovis* and *M. tuberculosis*. The former causes illness in cattle that can be transmitted to humans, but this is relatively rare nowadays in developed countries. Currently, the tubercle bacillus and *M. tuberculosis* are considered synonymous for all intents and purposes.

An obligate aerobe, *M. tuberculosis* is rod shaped and slow growing (12–18 hour generation time). Its cell wall has a high mycolic acid (long chain, cross-linked fatty acid) content and it is quite hydrophobic. Thus, *M. tuberculosis* is impermeable to the common bacteriologic stains. The organism absorbs carbolfuchsin dye and maintains the resultant red color despite decolorization with acid alcohol. For this reason, it is referred to as 'acid fast' (Fig. 29.2). However, the term acid-fast bacilli (AFB) refers to mycobacteria in general, even though a few other organisms demonstrate acid-fast staining characteristics (e.g. *Nocardia* and *Cryptosporidium* spp.).

The tubercle bacillus is a quite hearty organism and survives concentration and digestion techniques that would kill lesser organisms. It grows slowly and requires special enriched media. The colony appearance is buff colored and cord-like or heaped up. Since *M. tuberculosis* is the only mycobacterium to produce niacin, the presence of niacin as the product of a bacterial growth confirms identification.

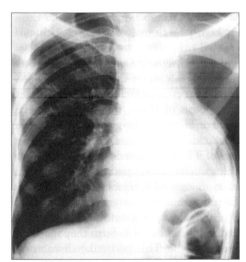

Figure 29.1 Thoracoplasty treatment for tuberculosis. Thoracoplasty was used to limit the size of the diseased lung and hopefully close tuberculous cavities. The procedure could involve only inversion of the upper ribs to close an apical cavity or near-complete obliteration of the hemithorax.

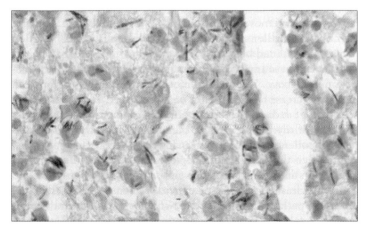

Figure 29.2 Acid-fast bacilli in tissue. Ziehl–Neelsen stain of *Mycobacterium tuberculosis* in a tissue specimen.

with brushing, washing, bronchoalveolar lavage, and transbronchial biopsy specimens. In children who cannot cooperate with sputum induction, samples of the early morning gastric aspirate have been reported positive in as many as 40% of patients. The morning specimen is thought to be valuable on the basis of ongoing swallowing of lower respiratory secretions during the night.

On standard staining, *M. tuberculosis* is weakly Gram-positive or colorless because of the hydrophobic nature of the cross-linked fatty acids in the cell wall, called mycosides. These cell-wall mycolic acids take up carbolfuchsin red dye which cannot be washed out by acid alcohol. Kinyoun and the Ziehl–Neelson stains were used routinely in the relatively recent past to identify AFB on smears. These stains produced a blue background with the classic, beaded, corded-red organisms known as 'red snappers'. Light microscopy of such specimens is still acceptable, but it is time consuming. Current laboratory techniques use florescent staining to speed the process of organism recognition. These fluorescent stains are not specific for *M. tuberculosis*, but are merely modified AFB techniques with a fluorescent moiety. *Nocardia* spp. can stain positive with current fluorescent techniques.

Mycobacterial culture

When a specimen stains positive for AFB, the underlying etiology may represent active TB or infection or colonization by an NTM. For this reason, all specimens are submitted for culture. Since active tuberculous disease is potentially contagious, strong consideration is given to the initiation of antituberculous therapy at the time of culturing.

Clinical specimens should be processed as rapidly as possible. Many specimens require liquefaction of organic components and a decontamination process to remove other microbial flora that might overgrow the slowly dividing tubercle bacillus in the culture. This is usually accomplished by the treatment of specimens with a combination of a mucolytic agent (e.g. *N*-acetylcysteine) and 1–2% sodium hydroxide to limit other bacterial growth. Adding a step that provides concentration of the specimen (e.g. centrifugation) increases culture sensitivity. As previously noted *M. tuberculosis* organisms are reduced in number by the process of liquefaction and decontamination, but the procedure optimizes the likelihood of a positive result. Laboratories look for a culture contamination rate between 2 and 5% to assure that optimum processing is in place. Cultures obtained from normally sterile sites do not require digestion or decontamination.

Quantitative studies that examined the number of organisms necessary to produce positive smears indicate a need for 5000–10,000 organisms per milliliter to be present for an AFB smear to appear positive. Culture is a slower, but more sensitive method that requires only 10–100 organisms per milliliter for a positive result. Of specimens that have a positive smear, <1% have a negative culture when mycobacterial contamination is not present.

After appropriate handling, specimens are placed on or in media for culture. Current culture media include Löwenstein–Jensen media (egg based), Middlebrook 7H10/7H11 (agar based), and selective media. Growth is more rapid on agar media, and specimens grow most rapidly in liquid media. Currently, an automated culture system using carbon-14 based liquid media and radiometric detection methods (the Bactec 460™ system) is commercially available. This system reduces the time necessary for positive culture detection from 3–8 weeks to 1–3 weeks. Cultures are usually held for 8–12 weeks before being reported as negative and discarded. Overall sensitivity of culture has been reported by the American Thoracic Society (ATS) to be 80–85% with a specificity of 98%.

Direct identification of *Mycobacterium* species

Polymerase chain reaction (PCR) is a nucleic acid amplification technique that has proved quite helpful in the detection and identification of *M. tuberculosis*. These techniques split and copy specific portions of an organism's DNA until a target area can be detected by a DNA probe. At present, specificity and sensitivity are quite good for PCR when the AFB smear is positive. In smear-negative cases, the sensitivity and specificity of a positive PCR result drops off rapidly. These techniques are currently considered adjuncts to standard smear and culture. At present, PCR and DNA probe testing is only recommended for smear-positive specimens.

Two new techniques to identify the tubercle bacillus are becoming available, both of which require pure cultures of organism for adequate sensitivity and specificity. High-performance liquid chromatography identifies cell-wall mycolic acid specific to TB, and nucleic acid hybridization utilizes specific molecular probes for mycobacterial species. Monoclonal antibodies, enzyme-linked immunoabsorbent assay, radioimmunoassay, and dot-blot immunoassays are all methods under evaluation for the rapid detection of TB, but are not commercially available.

TREATMENT OF TUBERCULOSIS

Standard therapy for active TB in adults and children consists of a 6-month regimen, the first 2 months with isoniazid, rifampin (rifampicin), and pyrazinamide followed by 4 months of isoniazid and rifampin alone[8]. Ethambutol or streptomycin are added until drug sensitivity is known only if the possibility of drug resistance is high. Streptomycin is chosen as the additive drug in children who are too young for visual acuity testing (required to monitor toxicity of ethambutol). Drug resistance is considered unlikely when the following situations occur:

- <4% primary resistance to isoniazid in the community;
- no prior history of treatment with antituberculous medications;
- patient is not from a country with a high prevalence of drug-resistant TB; and
- no known exposure to a drug-resistant case.

This regimen appears to be effective in both HIV-infected and non-HIV-infected individuals. However, in HIV-infected individuals, the duration of therapy is uncertain, and clinical and bacteriologic assessment is imperative for judging the need for prolonged therapy. An initial drug regimen of isoniazid, rifampin, pyrazinamide, and ethambutol (or streptomycin) is effective, even when the infecting organism is isoniazid resistant.

As an alternative therapeutic regimen in those people who cannot take one of the standard three first-line drugs, therapy for a total of 9 months' duration is necessary with ethambutol or streptomycin added unless the possibility of drug resistance is low. When isoniazid resistance is recognized, rifampin and ethambutol should be combined for no less than 12–18 months.

Some general considerations for effective antituberculous therapy include:

- Multiple drugs are required in an effective therapeutic regimen to reduce the likelihood of the emergence of resistant organisms. The spontaneous occurrence of drug-resistant organisms is well documented, but the likelihood of the spontaneous occurrence of a tubercle bacillus resistant to two medications simultaneously is very low from a statistical standpoint.
- A single drug should not be added to a failing antituberculous regimen.
- Sensitivity testing for *M. tuberculosis* isolates must be performed in every case.
- Directly observed therapy is considered for all cases of active TB if the patient's compliance is in doubt. Compliance with the use of medications is a major determinant of case outcome. Twice or thrice weekly dosing regimens are helpful in assuring compliance in patients who are living far away or just difficult to find.
- Individualized therapy in consultation with a TB expert is recommended in multidrug-resistant cases.
- Children are treated with the same considerations as noted above for adults, with the appropriate adjustment of medication dosing.
- Extrapulmonary TB is treated along the standard treatment guidelines for pulmonary TB, except that children who have miliary TB, tuberculous meningitis, tuberculous arthritis, or tuberculous arthritis and bone disease are treated for at least 12 months.

At times, individuals have an illness that resembles TB in clinical and radiographic appearance. For such individuals, treatment is frequently initiated in the face of negative AFB smears pending culture. The administration of appropriate treatment seems to bring about an improvement in these patients' symptoms and chest radiographic appearance, but the cultures remain negative (Fig. 29.9). It has been demonstrated that 4 months of isoniazid and rifampin therapy is adequate for treatment of this 'culture-negative' TB. Figures 29.10 and 29.11 summarize dosing, activity, and side effects of first- and second-line anti-TB medications.

In pregnancy, the need to treat active TB outweighs the risk of therapy for mother and fetus. Standard therapy includes isoniazid and rifampin, along with ethambutol unless the risk of drug resistance is low (see above). Pyrazinamide is used in pregnant women in many parts of the world, although little data as to its administration and potential teratogenic effects are available. In the USA, at present, pyrazinamide is not recommended. Streptomycin is not recommended in a pregnant woman, since it can cause deafness in the fetus. Also, women on appropriate antituberculous therapy are not discouraged from breast feeding (nursing). Although isoniazid, rifampin, and ethambutol cross the placenta readily, antituberculous therapy is not toxic for the newborn. Supplemental pyridoxine is always recommended in pregnant women.

A summary of antituberculous regimens is given in Figure 29.12.

PREVENTION OF TUBERCULOSIS

Bacille Calmette–Guérin

Bacille Calmette–Guérin (BCG) is named for two French researchers who developed the live, attenuated strain of *M. bovis* in 1921. It is currently used as a vaccination to prevent TB

in areas of the world with high disease prevalence. Despite its use in millions of people globally, the efficacy of this intervention is uncertain. Data suggest that it prevents disseminated TB and tuberculous meningitis in children, but protection against pulmonary TB has not been proven. Numerous trials have given unclear results, from suggestions of up to 80% protection from pulmonary TB with the administration of BCG to an increased susceptibility to active disease in those vaccinated.

In many people who receive the vaccination, BCG produces a positive tuberculin reaction that cannot be distinguished from a tuberculin reaction caused by exposure to other mycobacteria. Since BCG is used in areas of high prevalence of disease, it is best to evaluate every positive PPD skin test for the presence of tuberculous disease.

In the USA, BCG is not recommended. However, it may be useful in children and infants in the following situations[9]:

- continuous exposure to active TB;
- those who are frequently exposed to isoniazid- and rifampin-resistant tubercle bacilli; and
- groups with a new infection rate >1% per year.

Also, BCG is contraindicated in patients infected with HIV and those who might be otherwise immunocompromised.

Antimicrobial prophylaxis of tuberculosis

The only way to reduce and eliminate the occurrence of TB is to prevent the disease with chemoprophylaxis. To date, 6–12 months of therapy with isoniazid has been shown to reduce the future risk

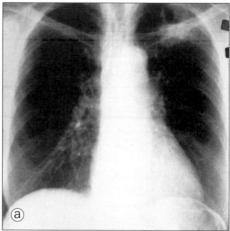

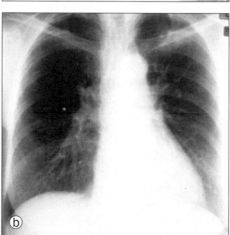

Figure 29.9 Chest radiographs of 'culture-negative tuberculosis'. (a) Left upper-lobe cavitary lesion with appropriate symptomatology in a 64-year-old woman with long history of a 'very positive' purified protein derivative skin test 40 years previously. (b) Same patient 8 weeks later with all smears and cultures negative and appropriate antituberculous therapy. The left upper-lobe cavity and infiltrate have almost resolved.

First-line drugs for the treatment of tuberculosis in adults and children					
First-line drug	Dosage (daily dosing)	Dosage (weekly dosing)	Common side effects	Recommended follow-up tests	Special considerations
Isoniazid	Adults: 5–10mg/kg (p.o. or i.m.), maximum dose 300mg/day Children: 10–20mg/kg, same maximum dose as adults	Adults: 15mg/kg (p.o. or i.m.) Children: 20–40mg/kg in children	Peripheral neuropathy Hepatotoxicity Hypersensitivity Drug interactions	Follow aspartate transaminase and glutamic–pyruvic transaminase (GPT) in patients 35 years of age and older and in those who drink alcohol	Bactericidal Pyridoxine 50mg/day helpful for neuropathy Interacts with some anticonvulsants and ketoconazole
Rifampin	Adults: 10mg/kg (p.o. or i.v.), maximum dose 600mg/day Children: 10–20mg/kg	Adults and children: 10–20mg/kg (p.o.), maximum dose 600mg	Thrombocytopenia Leukopenia Hepatitis Fever Eosinophilia Interference with protease-inhibitor action and metabolism in patients infected by human immunodeficiency virus	In the appropriate situation: aspartate transaminase, GPT, and full blood count and differential	Bactericidal Turns bodily secretions orange Interferes with oral contraceptives, quinidine, oral anticoagulants, and methadone
Pyrazinamide	Adults and children: 15–30mg/kg (p.o.), maximum dose 2g/day (usually used only in the first 2 months of therapy)	Adults and children: 50–70mg/kg (p.o.), maximum dose 4g	Hyperuricemia Hepatotoxicity Hypersensitivity	Uric acid levels Aspartate transaminase, GPT when appropriate	Bactericidal Particularly active against dormant bacilli in the macrophage Not used in pregnancy (in the USA)
Ethambutol	Adults and children: 15–25mg/kg (p.o.), no maximum dose (the lower range of dosing has less optic neuritis)	Adults and children: 50mg/kg	Optic neuritis (usually reverses with discontinuation of drug – first sign often loss of color vision) Gastrointestinal intolerance	Check red–green color discrimination and visual acuity	Renally excreted – may need drug levels checked in those with renal insufficiency May want to avoid ethambutol when eye testing not feasible
Streptomycin	Adults: 15mg/kg (i.m.) for first 2–8 weeks of therapy with maximum dose 1g Children: 20–40mg/kg, same maximum dose as adults	Adults and children: 25–30mg/kg, maximum dose 1.5g (often given in this way after first 2–8 weeks)	Auditory and vestibular dysfunction Nephrotoxicity	Check vestibular function and audiogram Blood urea nitrogen Creatinine	Bactericidal Avoid in elderly and those with renal impairment Not used in pregnancy

Figure 29.10 Summary of first-line antituberculous medications.
Given are the dosages for adults and children (<12 years of age) for daily and weekly therapy, common adverse effects, appropriate clinical testing for adverse effects during therapy, and special considerations for each drug. A chemical derivative of rifampin, rifapentine, has been approved in the USA. It has a longer half-life than rifampin and can be effective in once or twice weekly regimens. No treatment regimen is currently approved.

of active TB in infected individuals by up to 90%. Rifampin alone has been suggested for infected organisms thought to be isoniazid resistant, but few data are available to support this. The indications for isoniazid prophylaxis in individuals positive for the PPD skin test (see above for skin-test positivity parameters) are:

- HIV-infected persons and those suspected to be HIV infected (HIV testing is recommended for all patients who are found to have active TB[10]).
- Close contacts of people with newly diagnosed, infectious TB (in very young children and adolescents, the risk of developing TB is twice that of adults). In this group, PPD-negative patients are recommended to receive 3 months of isoniazid with repeat skin testing at the end of that period. If repeat PPD testing is negative, isoniazid can be stopped. If it is positive, isoniazid therapy is continued for a minimum of 6 months.
- Recent skin test converters – those patients <35 years of age with a ≥ 10mm increase in PPD induration and those ≥ 35 years of age with a 15mm increase in PPD induration within 2 years (the highest risk of disease development is concentrated in the first 2 years after skin test conversion).
- Persons with medical conditions that have been reported to increase the incidence of TB:

- diabetes mellitus;
- treatment with corticosteroids at a dose >15mg/day for >2–3 weeks;
- those on immunosuppressive therapy;
- those with certain hematologic and reticuloendothelial diseases (e.g. leukemia, Hodgkin's disease, etc.);
- HIV-negative intravenous drug abusers;
- end-stage renal disease; and
- any clinical situation associated with rapid weight loss (e.g. postgastric-bypass patients, postgastrectomy patients, alcoholics, those with malabsorption syndrome, etc.).

Also, persons <35 years of age in the following groups are considered appropriate candidates for prophylactic isoniazid therapy in the presence of a positive skin test:

- those born in countries with a high prevalence of TB;
- those who come from medically underserved, low-income populations (in the USA mainly blacks, Hispanics, and native Americans); and
- residents of long term-care facilities (correctional facilities, nursing homes, and mental institutions).

A 10–20% risk is reported for hepatic dysfunction during isoniazid treatment. The reaction is usually subclinical and associated

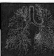

Second-line drugs for the treatment of tuberculosis in adults and children

Second-line drug	Dosage (daily dosing)	Dosage (weekly dosing)	Common side effects	Recommended follow-up tests	Special considerations
Ethionamide	Adults and children: 15–20mg/kg (p.o.), maximum dose 1g	Not recommended	Gastrointestinal intolerance Hepatotoxicity Hypersensitivity Impotence Gynecomastia Metallic taste	None except when in doubt	Bacteriostatic If hepatic enzymes increase, a 5-fold increase is important even in the absence of symptoms
Para-aminosalicylic acid	Adults and children: 150mg/kg (p.o.), maximum dose 12g	Not recommended	Gastrointestinal disturbance Hepatotoxicity (rare) Hypersensitivity Na$^+$ load	Hepatic enzymes	Bacteriostatic Should be given acidic drink like orange juice
Capreomycin	Adults and children: 15–30mg/kg (i.m.), maximum dose 1g	Not recommended	Auditory, vestibular, and renal toxicities	Check vestibular function and audiogram Blood urea nitrates Creatine	High-frequency hearing loss in 3–9% of cases Renal toxicity more common than with streptomycin Avoid in the elderly and those with renal impairment
Kanamycin	Adults and children: 15–30mg/kg (i.m.), maximum dose 1g	Not recommended	Auditory and renal toxicity (vestibular toxicity rare)	Audiogram monthly Blood urea nitrates Creatine	See capreomycin
Cycloserine	Adults and children: 15–20mg/kg (p.o.), maximum dose 1g	Not recommended	Convulsions Psychosis Rash Peripheral neuropathy especially when on isoniazid Interaction with phenytoin	Assessment of mental status	Give with pyridoxine 150mg Avoid in those with history of psychologic difficulties

Figure 29.11 Summary of second-line antituberculous medications for adults and children (<12 years of age). These drugs are reserved for difficult situations in the treatment of tuberculosis (TB) and are more difficult to use than first-line agents. The advice of an expert in the treatment of TB is recommended if these drugs are perceived to be necessary. Fluoroquinolone antibiotics are showing promise in the treatment of multi-drug-resistant TB. Sparfloxacin, so far, shows the greatest activity against *Mycobacterium tuberculosis*, and lovofloxacin shows promise.

Effective treatment regiments for tuberculosis

Indication	Drugs	Duration of therapy (months)
New cases (smear positive, culture positive or suspected)	Isoniazid–rifampin–pyrazinamide (ethambutol or streptomycin added to standard regimens when a high risk of drug-resistance; see text)	6 (2 isoniazid–rifampin–pyrazinamide; 4 isoniazid–rifampin)
New cases in pregnancy	Isoniazid–rifampin (pyrazinamide not approved for pregnancy in the USA)	9
Isoniazid intolerance	Rifampin–pyrazinamide–ethambutol	9 (2 rifampin–pyrazinamide–ethambutol; 7 rifampin–ethambutol)
Rifampin intolerance	Isoniazid–pyrazinamide–ethambutol	18 [2 isoniazid–ethambutol–streptomycin (±pyrazinamide); 16 isoniazid–ethambutol]
Pyrazinamide intolerance	Isoniazid–rifampin	9
Isoniazid and rifampin resistance	Pyrazinamide–ethambutol–streptomycin + ofloxacin	12–18
New 'culture-negative' case	Isoniazid–rifampin–pyrazinamide (ethambutol or streptomycin added to standard regimens when a high risk of drug-resistance; see text)	4 (2 isoniazid–rifampin–pyrazinamide; 2 isoniazid–rifampin)
Retreatment of standard case (while susceptibility studies are pending or are unavailable)	Isoniazid–rifampin–pyrazinamide–ethambutol–streptomycin	8 [2 isoniazid–rifampin–pyrazinamide–ethambutol–streptomycin; 6 isoniazid–rifampin–ethambutol (if/when susceptibility data become available continuation of therapy should be tailored accordingly)]
Resistance to all first-line therapeutic agents	Injectable agent (choices include amikacin, kanamycin, or capreomycin and three of ethionamide, para-aminosalicylic acid, ofloxacin, cycloserine)	24 (2–6 amikacin, kanamycin, or capreomycin based on patient tolerance)

Figure 29.12 Effective treatment regimens for tuberculosis. These regimens are known to be effective for the indications given. In treatment failure or relapse, the opinion of an expert in tuberculosis must be sought. A single drug must not be added to a failing antituberculous regimen.

only with a mild elevation of the transaminase. The primary mechanism of hepatic toxicity is thought to result from a toxic metabolite of isoniazid. Examination of the rate of serious hepatitis occurrence indicates a jump from <1% incidence to 1.2% in the age group 35–49 years. The incidence increases to 2.3% in patients over the age of 50 years. It is for this reason that the 'age 35' restrictions are noted above. Isoniazid prophylaxis should probably be avoided in those who have active hepatic disease and those with a history of hepatic disease. Daily consumers of alcohol are counseled to reduce their alcohol intake and their liver function is followed closely. If a patient older than 35 years of age requests prophylaxis with isoniazid, base-line assessment of the liver function is carried out with monthly follow-up.

It is unclear how to deal with exposures to multidrug-resistant TB. Prophylaxis with isoniazid or rifampin is expected to be ineffective. Recent decision-analysis data suggest preventive therapy with pyrazinamide–ciprofloxacin is a reasonable choice in such situations[11].

Recently, sequencing of the entire genome of *M. tuberculosis* has been achieved, which may be as significant as Koch's isolation of the tubercle bacillus. For the first time we will be able to work toward control of tuberculous disease with full knowledge of the workings of the bacillus. It is hoped that full knowledge of the pathogen's genome will allow future therapeutic options that more effectively target *M. tuberculosis* and more readily control TB in humans.

DISEASES CAUSED BY ATYPICAL MYCOBACTERA

Until the late 1950s, mycobacteria other than *M. tuberculosis* and *M. bovis* represented a heterogeneous group of organisms that were thought to cause disease in humans only occasionally. In 1959, Runyon reported a classification system for these organisms that, for the first time, organized them according to microbiologic characteristics. His categorization has since been referred to as the Runyon Classification (Fig. 29.13), which excluded *M. leprae*. Four groups were included in the schema based on tendencies toward the formation of pigmented colonies in various culture conditions and the speed of bacterial growth. While Runyon's groups brought some order to the consideration of NTM, as more and more species of *Mycobacterium* were recognized the categorization became less useful[12]. Currently, of the more than 50 different species of *Mycobacterium* approximately 40% appear to cause disease in humans. In a recent report on NTM disease gives a classification of disease-causing NTM based on the clinical diseases they produce[13]. The current disease groups presented are NTM pulmonary disease, NTM lymphadenitis, NTM cutaneous disease, and disseminated NTM disease.

Epidemiology
Exposure to NTM primarily arises from the environment, specifically soil and water. It is not thought that transmission from animals or person-to-person spread represents a significant aspect of transmission of the disease to humans. The reservoir for transmission of *M. avium* complex (MAC; a complex of *M. avium* and *M. intracellulare*) to the HIV-infected population is unclear, but MAC is frequently isolated from common tap water, which may be the source. Infections caused by rapidly growing NTM have been associated with exposure to various water sources, which include fish tanks,

swimming pools, and salt and/or fresh water sites. Isolation of NTM from soil has been achieved, but some organisms like *M. kansasii* cannot survive more than about 12 hours in the earth.

Based on the occurrence of geographic and specific clusters of infections, it is likely that certain local conditions favor disease development with particular organisms. Some general statements can be made regarding certain NTM organisms:

- *M. malmoense* has been recovered from waters in Finland and, not surprisingly, has emerged as a pathogen in Northern Europe;
- *M. simiae* disease has been isolated in certain geographic areas and disease has occurred in those pockets, primarily in the southwestern USA, Cuba, and Israel; and
- *M. xenopi*, a thermophilic organism, has been isolated from hot water sources in hospitals where it has been at times associated with the occurrence of cutaneous and pulmonary disease – this organism is now being reported as a common cause of insidious pulmonary disease in Western Europe.

While consideration of the source of infection is important for epidemiologic reasons, geographic location and situation play little role in the diagnosis and management of disease caused by NTM. However, research continues with skin-test surveys and DNA fingerprinting of isolated organisms in the hope of learning more about the geographic tendencies of the disease. At present, the environment is thought to be the primary source of inoculation for NTM that cause disease.

Host factors are important in any infection with NTM organisms. The ATS guidelines list the following as predisposing conditions: alcoholism, bronchiectasis, cyanotic heart disease, cystic fibrosis, prior mycobacterial disease (abnormal anatomy secondary to scarring), pulmonary fibrosis, smoking, chronic obstructive pulmonary disease, immunosuppression (including neoplastic and iatrogenic causes), and HIV-disease with CD4 cell counts <200 per mm^3.

In AIDS patients, *M. avium* is becoming a common presenting diagnosis. Current data suggest that HIV-positive individuals with CD4 cell counts of <100 per mm^3 develop disseminated *M. avium* disease at a rate of about 20%/year. As a result, prophylaxis for a nontuberculous organism is being considered once CD4 cell counts fall to that level.

The Runyon Classification of nontuberculous mycobacteria		
Runyon group	**Pigment production**	**Representative organisms**
I	Photochromogens – develop yellow pigment when exposed to light	*M. kansasii* *M. marinum*
II	Scotochromogens – develop yellow–orange pigment when exposed to light	*M. scrofulaceum* *M. szulgai*
III	Nonchromogens – no pigment develops when exposed to light	*M. gordonae* *M. terrae* *M. gastri*
IV	Rapid growers	*M. chelonae* *M. fortuitum* *M. smegmatis*

Figure 29.13 The Runyon Classification. A classification system for nontuberculous mycobacteria based on the tendency to form pigment in the presence or absence of light, the lack of pigment formation, and speed of growth. The classification was more useful in previous years and newer classification schema are based on the type of disease the organisms cause in humans. The terms continue to be used today.

Clinical features

Since newer classifications deal with the general categorization of diseases caused by the various NTM, here clinical presentation is discussed by disease category in the order: pulmonary disease, lymphadenitis, cutaneous disease, and disseminated disease.

Pulmonary disease caused by nontuberculous mycobacteria

The clinical presentation of pulmonary disease caused by NTM is nonspecific. Historical considerations are routinely unhelpful since common symptomatology consists of routine pulmonary and constitutional symptoms such as cough, production of sputum, and fatigue. Fever, malaise, weight loss, and hemoptysis are infrequently seen. The physical examination also may be unhelpful. While crackles, decreased breath sounds, or amphoric breath sounds may be heard, physical findings are nonspecific with NTM lung infection, and these patients frequently have underlying chronic lung disease.

The chest radiograph may be more helpful since NTM-induced pulmonary disease has a somewhat different appearance to that of pulmonary TB. The cavities formed with NTM-related pulmonary disease tend to have thin walls and little surrounding inflammatory process. Air–liquid interfaces in the cavities and pleural effusions are uncommon. Apical pleural reaction in the area of involvement may be intense, and these chronic, thickened pleural reactions are virtually pathognomonic of NTM infection. In many cases, numerous small pulmonary nodules may also be seen. Bronchiectasis is a frequent finding on high-resolution CT in NTM-related disease (Fig. 29.14).

Mantoux testing for exposure to specific NTM is limited in utility by considerable cross-reactivity with *M. tuberculosis* and other NTM. Therefore, diagnosis usually rests on the demonstration of these atypical mycobacteria from culture of sputum and other fluids or tissue samples. The question of 'colonization' with NTM, in the absence of primary NTM pulmonary disease, remains somewhat controversial. As a result, specific guidelines for the diagnosis of pulmonary disease caused by NTM have been recently published[13] (see below).

Nontuberculous lymphadenitis (scrofula)

While mycobacterial lymphadenitis can occur in all age groups, NTM is most commonly the cause in children between 1 and 5 years of age (95% of mycobacterial lymphadenitis seen in patients outside this age group is caused by *M. tuberculosis*). Insidious onset of nodal enlargement, usually unilateral and non-tender, occurs, primarily in the submandibular, submaxillary, cervical, or preauricular nodes (although any nodal group may be involved). Constitutional symptoms are uncommon. Rapid nodal enlargement is frequently seen and at times the involved nodes can rupture with a purulent discharge and consequent fistula formation. Histopathology, radiographic studies, and PPD skin studies are unhelpful in the younger, high-risk group. Specialized skin studies for specific species of NTM have been developed, but are also unhelpful and are not commercially available.

In contrast to tuberculous lymphadenitis, which requires both surgery and antituberculous chemotherapy, treatment of lymphadenitis caused by NTM is primarily surgical. In most cases, the reason for pursuing a microbiologic diagnosis is the possibility of TB as the potential etiology.

Less invasive diagnostic techniques for lymphadenitis in the group at high risk for NTM are not very helpful. Incision and drainage of these lesions frequently results in the formation of fistulae, and needle aspirate of involved nodes is only positive in about 50% of cases. Although NTM-compatible histopathology (see Fig. 29.15) of excised nodes is common, microbiologic recovery of the organisms occurs in only 50–80% of cases. The most common pathogen varies by geographic region. In the USA, MAC causes the majority of disease with the remaining cases primarily caused by *M. scrofulaceum*. In Northern Europe, Scandinavia, and the UK, MAC is also the most common cause of NTM lymphadenitis, but *M. malmoense* is the second most common cause. In children, only about 10% of lymphadenitis caused by AFB results from *M. tuberculosis*.

Cutaneous and soft-tissue disease caused by nontuberculous mycobacteria

Cutaneous infections caused by NTM usually result from direct inoculation of organisms into the skin. Virtually all atypical mycobacteria have been implicated in cutaneous involvement, but the most common organisms responsible are *M. abscessus*, *M. fortuitum*, *M. marinum*, and *M. ulcerans*. When the site of inoculation occurs where the skin has suffered trauma, *M. chelonae* is the prime suspect.

The most common cutaneous syndrome from NTM is infection with *M. marinum* to give 'fish-tank' or 'swimming-pool' granuloma, which presents as slowly enlarging papules or heaped up lesions that can ulcerate. Healing may be spontaneous, but is quite slow and the use of surgical excision and appropriate antimicrobial agents are recommended.

Skin disease caused by *M. ulcerans* is most commonly seen in Australia, Africa, and Mexico. The lesion it produces is known as the Buruli ulcer, which is progressive and destructive. It can result in severe, deforming changes in the extremities. Surgical excision

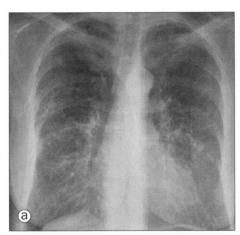

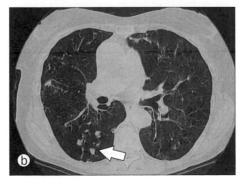

Figure 29.14
***Mycobacterium avium* complex.**
(a) Posteroanterior chest radiograph shows some patchy infiltrates in the mid-lung bilaterally.
(b) Computed tomography scan from a different patient shows the typical nodular lesions (arrow) associated with this organism.

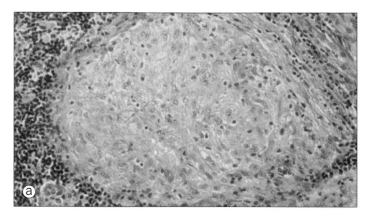

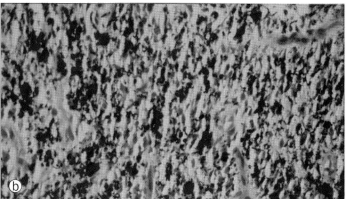

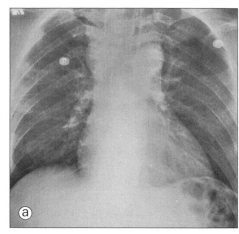

Figure 29.16 *Mycobacterium avium* complex infection in a patient who has acquired immunodeficiency syndrome (AIDS). (a) Chest radiograph and (b) computed tomography scan show mediastinal adenopathy in a patient who has AIDS and active *Mycobacterium avium* complex (MAC) disease. Isolated mediastinal adenopathy is a common manifestation of disseminated MAC in patients who have AIDS.

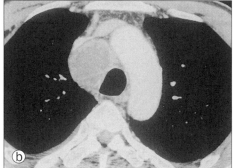

Figure 29.15 Histopathology of infection of lymph node related to *Mycobacterium avium* complex. (a) Lymph node pathology with noncaseating granuloma. (Hematoxylin and eosin.) (b) Ziehl–Neelson stain over hematoxylin and eosin at higher magnification reveals numerous acid-fast (red-staining) organisms.

and skin grafting is most helpful since single drug therapy is of little utility. Cutaneous disease may also be caused by *M. malmoense*.

Bone and joint involvement with NTM can result in very significant illness. After cardiac surgery, *M. abscessus* and *M. fortuitum* have produced sternal wound infections with devastating results. Numerous other atypical mycobacteria can cause infections that involve the joint space, synovium, tendons, and bony tissue and produce a form of indolent chronic disease.

Disseminated infection caused by nontuberculous mycobacteria
In adults who do not have HIV infection the dissemination of atypical mycobacteria is usually associated with some form of immunosuppression. Corticosteroid therapy, use of negative immunomodulating drugs, transplant patients, and those who have reticuloendothelial neoplasms are the most commonly afflicted. Mortality rates depend upon the degree of immunosuppression and clinical involvement. The most frequent offending NTM organisms are MAC, *M. fortuitum*, *M. kansasii*, and *M. chelonae*. Diagnosis requires isolation of the organism from a blood culture or sterile site (e.g. blood culture, bone marrow specimen, etc.).

In the HIV-infected patient, the likelihood of dissemination increases as the CD4 cell count declines; MAC is the common causative organism (Fig. 29.16).

More than 90% of the time disseminated MAC infection in AIDS patients is associated with prolonged fever and night sweats. Diarrhea, abdominal pain, adenopathy, and weight loss are also common. This usually signals profound involvement of the bowel, the site from which dissemination is thought to occur, and the organism can commonly be isolated from stool or sputum specimens in AIDS patients. The diagnosis requires isolation of the organism from cultures of blood or a usually sterile site. When AFB-positive sputum specimens and abnormal chest radiographs are seen in an AIDS patient, the cause is more likely to be *M. tuberculosis* than MAC.

Diagnosis of disease caused by nontuberculous mycobacteria
Handling of specimens, specimen staining, and culture techniques for NTM are similar to the techniques described for *M. tuberculosis*. When the AFB smear is positive, no staining property can reliably distinguish the NTM from *M. tuberculosis*. As noted above (Runyon Classification) certain growth characteristics, such as pigmentation under various culture conditions and speed of growth, suggest a particular group of NTM, but final species identification is still likely to require biochemical testing, DNA probes, or high-pressure liquid chromatography. At present, relatively reliable DNA probes for MAC, *M. kansasii*, and *M. gordonae* are available. Certain species of NTM can be highly suspected on the basis of growth patterns. For *M. genavense*, a quite fastidious organism, growth is often poor, which leads to a somewhat difficult identification process, but its growth characteristics are quite unusual, as it grows well on solid media but not in liquid media. Also, on an AFB stain it has a unique coccobacillary form.

The isolation of NTM in a culture does not in all cases constitute evidence of infection, especially when the culture is from the

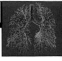

pulmonary system. For some organisms, isolation from cultures obtained on multiple occasions is necessary to establish diagnosis. Isolation of an organism such as *M. kansasii* is usually indicative of disease. A positive culture from a usually sterile site may also be diagnostic. As a consequence of the frequent uncertainty associated with a culture positive for atypical mycobacteria, a new diagnostic system for the diagnosis of pulmonary disease caused by NTM has been proposed. The schema requires the fulfillment of clinical, radiographic, and bacteriologic confirmation of disease (Fig. 29.17).

Treatment of disease caused by nontuberculous mycobacteria

While all the mycobacterial organisms share the same family and genus, their response to antimicrobial therapy is highly variable. Some respond to standard antibiotics while others require specific regimens of antituberculous therapy (see Fig. 29.18). The need for adjunctive treatments, such as surgery, also varies from species to species and even according to the nature of the disease the organism appears to be causing. For this reason, no blanket statement can be made regarding the various treatments for the common causes of NTM disease. A summary of the various disease categories, causative organisms, and appropriate treatment measures is given in Figure 29.18.

Sometimes it is not clear whether the sporadic positive-culture results for NTM organisms in the presence of a questionable pulmonary infiltrate represent identification of the cause of disease. In many cases cautious observation is acceptable, but in the face of clearly progressive illness it may be prudent to initiate treatment regardless of whether or not criteria for the diagnosis are met.

Our understanding of disease related to NTM has progressed rapidly, given the general disregard for the category of organisms up until the 1950s, but we are still learning about the nature of infectious disease caused by the atypical mycobacteria. Medical progress is slowly enabling more rapid diagnosis and providing effective therapy in some NTM illness. In the interim, we continue to make our best efforts to standardize diagnosis and management and to watch carefully when the diagnosis is in doubt.

PITFALLS AND CONTROVERSIES

When dealing with infection from *M. tuberculosis*, a few common errors must be kept in mind. The practitioner seldom makes the diagnosis if tuberculosis is not considered in the differential diagnosis. The presentation of the disease can range from cavitary lung disease to nonspecific constitutional symptoms. To avoid missing a treatable cause of a potentially devastating and contagious illness, always think of the tubercle bacillus as a possible cause and order the appropriate studies. When the clinical situation is suggestive and no other diagnosis comes to light, do not hesitate to institute appropriate therapy, since antituberculous therapy is usually well tolerated.

In HIV-infected individuals, do not expect a 'typical' presentation of the illness. In these patients, any pulmonary infiltrative pattern may be consistent with tuberculosis. Infection with *M. tuberculosis* must be part of the differential diagnosis in any patient who is HIV-infected and has respiratory symptoms.

Once the diagnosis of tuberculosis is made, the task is far from over. It has long been known that the most common cause

Category	Criteria
Criteria for the diagnosis of nontuberculous mycobacterial pulmonary disease	
Clinical	Compatible signs and symptoms (cough, fatigue, fever, weight loss, hemoptysis, or dyspnea with documented deterioration in clinical status of underlying disease)
	Reasonable exclusion of other disease and/or treatment of other underlying diseases
Radiographic	Any of the following radiographic abnormalities:
	Evidence of progression if baseline films >1 year old
	Infiltrates with or without nodules
	Cavitation
	Multiple small nodules as a solitary finding
	Any of the following high-resolution computed tomography findings:
	Multiple small nodules
	Multifocal bronchiectasis with or without nodules
Bacteriologic	At least three sputum/bronchial wash specimens within previous year:
	Three positive cultures with negative acid-fast bacilli (AFB) smears [the presence of general, significant, immunosuppression not related to human immunodeficiency virus (HIV) requires positive culture with 1+ or greater growth; for HIV-infected individuals with CD4 cell count <200, positive culture with 1+ or greater growth is required (excludes *Mycobacterium avium* complex)]
	Two positive cultures and one positive AFB smear
	OR
	Inability to obtain sputum and one available bronchial wash:
	Positive culture with 2–4+ growth, or
	Positive culture with 2–4+ AFB smear
	OR
	Biopsy specimen, any of the following:
	Any growth from bronchopulmonary tissue biopsy
	Granulomata and/or AFB on lung biopsy pathology with at least one positive culture from sputum or bronchial wash
	Any growth from a usually sterile extrapulmonary site

Figure 29.17 Criteria for the diagnosis of pulmonary disease caused by nontuberculous mycobacteria (NTM). To conclusively diagnose pulmonary disease caused by NTM, all three criteria must be satisfied: clinical, radiographic, and bacteriologic[13].

of treatment failure is patient noncompliance with the medical regimen. Also, recent data suggest that the most probable cause of the emergence of multidrug-resistant disease is failure to take prescribed antituberculous therapy appropriately. The doctor must follow-up patients who are infected with the tubercle bacillus carefully, with ongoing smear and culture studies to insure the appropriate progression to culture sterility. If local health department assistance is available, it is always advisable to enlist their help with epidemiologic aspects of care and to ensure compliance with the medical regimen. Directly observed therapy is always a reasonable option.

When dealing with infections caused by NTM, it is important to be certain infection truly exists. Except in cases where the isolates involve *M. kanasii*, MAC (in the appropriate circumstances – i.e., HIV infection), or isolation of an atypical organism from a usually sterile site, multiple repeat isolates are usually necessary to separate transient colonization from true infection. It is also important to monitor therapy and side effects of therapy carefully in this group of patients. At times, the adverse effects of therapy can be worse than the disease.

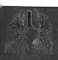
Diseases caused by the nontuberculous mycobacteria and recommended therapy			
Clinical disease	**Common etiologies**	**Recommended antimicrobial therapy**	**Other etiologies**
Pulmonary	*Mycobacterium avium* complex	Patients negative for human immunodeficiency virus: three-drug regimen – clarithromycin 500mg q12h or azithromycin 250–500 three-times weekly, rifabutin 300mg/day or rifampin 600mg/day, and ethambutol 25mg/kg per day for 2 months and then 15mg/kg per day for 8–10 months (add streptomycin 2–3 times weekly for first 2–3 months of therapy); duration 10–12 months	*M. simiae* *M. szulgai* *M. fortuitum* *M. celatum* *M. asiaticum* *M. haemophilum* *M. smegmatis*
	M. kansasii	Isoniazid 900mg/day, rifampin 600mg/day, ethambutol 25mg/kg per day for 2 months followed by 15mg/kg per day for 18 months with at least 12 months of negative sputum cultures (all *M. kansasii* isolates are resistant to pyrazinamide)	
	M. abscessus	4–6 months of low-dose amikacin and high-dose cefoxitin may be curative; unfortunately high cost and morbidity suggest that intermittent suppressive therapy with i.v. antibiotics and oral macrolides may be all that can be done	
	M. xenopi	Clarithromycin + rifampin or rifabutin + ethambutol ± initial streptomycin	
	M. malmoense	As for *M. xenopi*	
Lymphadenitis	*M. avium* complex	Surgical excision of infected lymph nodes	*M. fortuitum* *M. chelonae* *M. abscessus* *M. kansasii* *M. haemophilum*
	M. fortuitum	See *M. avium* complex	
	M. chelonae	See M. *avium* complex	
Cutaneous	*M. marinum*	Observation, excision, and/or antibiotics: ethambutol 15mg/kg per day and any of the following for at least 3 months – clarithromycin 500mg q12h, minocycline or doxycycline 100mg q12h, trimethoprim–sulfamethoxazole 160/800mg q12h, or rifampin 600mg/day	*M. ulcerans* *M. avium* complex *M. kansasii* *M. nonchromogenicum* *M. smegmatis* *M. haemophilum*
	M. fortuitum	Amikacin 5–7.5mg i.v. q12h (decrease dose over 50 years of age) and cefoxitin 12g/day i.v. for the first 2 weeks; surgery is required for extensive disease	
	M. chelonae	Tobramycin i.v. (better activity *in vitro* than amikacin) and cefoxitin (or imipenem when isolate resistant to cefoxitin); sometimes requires surgery	
	M. abscessus	No studies available but *in-vitro* data suggest that clarithromycin, imipenem, cefoxitin, cefmetazole, and amikacin may be effective; for severe disease use clofazamine and clarithromycin, and possibly excision	
Disseminated	*M. avium* complex	Three drugs are recommended: clarithromycin 500mg q12h (or azithromycin), ethambutol 15mg/kg per day (possibly 25mg/kg per day for first 2 months), and rifabutin (depending on use of antiprotease re drug interaction); consider adding amikacin or streptomycin in severe disease.	*M. abscessus* *M. xenopi* *M. malmoense* *M. genavense* *M. simiae* *M. conspicuum* *M. marinum* *M. fortuitum*
	M. kansasii	See *M. kansasii* under Pulmonary above	
	M. chelonae	Resistant to antituberculous drugs; consider combination from tobramycin [sensitivity (sens.) 100%], amikacin (sens. 100%), clarithromycin (sens. 100%), doxycycline (sens. 25%), ciprofloxacin (sens. 20%), and clofazamine	
	M. haemophilum	Suggested drugs: ciprofloxacin, clarithromycin, and rifampin	

Figure 29.18 Diseases caused by the nontuberculous mycobacteria and recommended therapy. These diseases are relatively uncommon and the recommended therapies given are based on data available and expert opinion. If the appropriate regimen is unclear, advice from an expert consultant is necessary[13].

REFERENCES

1. American Thoracic Society. Diagnostic standards and classification of tuberculosis. Am Rev Respir Dis. 1990;142:725–35.
2. Seibert AF, Haynes J, Middleton R, Bass JB. Tuberculous pleural effusion – twenty year experience. Chest. 1991;99:883–6.
3. Light RW. Tuberculous pleural effusions. In: Retford DC, ed. Pleural effusions, 3rd edn. Baltimore; Williams and Wilkins; 1995:154–65.
4. Gelb AF, Leffler C, Brewin A, Mascatello V, Lyons HA. Miliary tuberculosis. Am Rev Respir Dis. 1973;108:1327–33.
5. Weir MR, Thornton GF. Extrapulmonary tuberculosis. Experience of a community hospital and review of the literature. Am J Med. 1985;79:467–78.
6. Schepers GWH. Tuberculous pericarditis. Am J Cardiol. 1962;9:248–76.
7. Thompson NJ, Glassroth JL, Snider DE, Farer LS. The booster phenomenon in serial tuberculin testing. Am Rev Respir Dis. 1979;119:587–97.
8. American Thoracic Society. Treatment of tuberculosis and tuberculosis infection in adults and children. Am J Respir Crit Care Med. 1994;149:1359–74.
9. American Thoracic Society. Control of tuberculosis in the United States. Am Rev Respir Dis. 1992;146:1623–33.
10. Barnes PF, Silva C, Otaya M. Brief communications. Testing for human immunodeficiency virus infection in patients with tuberculosis. Am J Respir Crit Care Med. 1996;153:1448–50.
11. Stevens JP, Daniel TM. Chemoprophylaxis of multidrug-resistant tuberculous infection in HIV-uninfected individuals using ciprofloxacin and pyrazinamide – a decision analysis. Chest. 1995;108:712–17.
12. Wolinsky E. State of the art. Nontuberculous mycobacteria and associated diseases. Am Rev Respir Dis. 1979;119:107–59.
13. American Thoracic Society. Diagnosis and treatment of disease caused by nontuberculous mycobacteria. Am J Respir Crit Care Med. 1997;156(Suppl. 2):S1–25.

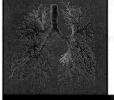

Chapter

30

Complications of Pneumonia

Neil C Barnes

INTRODUCTION

Most cases of pneumonia resolve completely with appropriate antibiotic treatment and supportive care. However, a number of important complications of pneumonia may occur that require specific management. The occurrence of these complications, or failure to manage them appropriately, contributes significantly to the mortality associated with pneumonia, and to both acute and chronic morbidity. The complications of pneumonia can be conveniently divided into acute complications, which cause problems during the initial illness, and long-term or chronic sequelae (Fig. 30.1). Acute presentations usually result from infective complications such as lung abscess and empyema. Such complications may occur during any episode of pneumonia, but are more likely to occur in patients who have an underlying debilitating medical condition, such as diabetes or renal failure, or in the elderly and in those who have underlying lung conditions, such as chronic obstructive pulmonary disease or bronchiectasis. They are also more likely to occur in association with certain pathogens (e.g. lung abscess is more frequent after staphylococcal pneumonia).

CLINICAL FEATURES

Frequently the diagnosis of these complications is delayed. Acute infective complications commonly present with a continuing pyrexia despite appropriate antibiotic therapy. They may present more insidiously, with either a grumbling pyrexia or with no fever at all, but with general ill health and continuing debility. The critical initial investigation is the chest radiograph. It is becoming less common to obtain repeat chest radiographs in patients who have pneumonia, but any patient whose fever does not settle or remains unwell requires a repeat radiograph to rule out one of the complications. If an empyema or lung abscess is discovered, further imaging with computed tomography (CT) scanning and/or ultrasound is often necessary.

Acute and chronic complications of pneumonia	
Acute	**Chronic**
Parapneumonic effusion	Bronchiectasis
Empyema	Fibrosis
Lung abscess	
Bronchopleural fistula	
Organizing pneumonia	

Figure 30.1 Acute and chronic complications of pneumonia.

PARAPNEUMONIC EFFUSIONS AND EMPYEMA

Pneumonias are not infrequently complicated by a pleural effusion, often termed a parapneumonic effusion, which goes through three stages. The first is a serosanginous effusion that is free flowing and without loculations. In the next phase, fibrinous strands cause loculation of the effusion. The effusion is no longer free running, and if a chest drain is inserted the effusion does not drain completely. In the third stage, obvious infection of the pleural space occurs, and is termed an empyema. An empyema may be free running and the insertion of a chest drain may lead to its evacuation, but frequently empyemas are loculated and cannot be managed effectively using tube drainage alone.

The symptoms suggestive of parapneumonic collection are increased breathlessness (particularly if the patient has underlying lung disease or the effusion is large) or continuing pyrexia. Clinical examination reveals dullness to percussion, decreased breath sounds, and decreased vocal fremitus and vocal resonance. If the collection is localized or small, these clinical findings may be subtle and difficult to detect. The most important initial investigation is a chest radiograph, which usually demonstrates the collection of fluid. Sometimes extensive consolidation makes it difficult to be certain that fluid is present and occasionally a posterior collection can be mistaken for consolidation. In such cases a lateral chest radiograph is useful to confirm the presence of fluid. It is vital to perform a diagnostic aspiration of the effusion to determine whether it is clear or whether an empyema is present. The fluid is sent for bacterial examination and, if any suggestion of an underlying carcinoma is present, for cytologic examination. Patients who have these infective complications, and particularly empyema, may have other systemic problems so the urea, electrolytes, and albumin need to be measured.

A small and free flowing parapneumonic effusion often resolves purely with appropriate antibiotic treatment, but the larger the effusion and the more loculated it is, the more likely the need for tube drainage. Tube drainage is essential for empyema. Radiologic features that suggest loculation or empyema formation are a distorted profile of the effusion or an effusion that is localized posteriorly or anteriorly. The presence of loculations can be confirmed by ultrasound of the chest, which delineates the fibrinous strands particularly well. Loculations can also be detected by CT scans, but these tend to be less sensitive. The presence of loculations is inferred by the finding of multiple 'air bubbles' within the fluid, or by multiple discrete air–fluid levels. Loculations are also often discovered when a chest drain is inserted and does not completely drain the effusion.

The initial management of a complicated parapneumonic effusion or an empyema is with a large gauge intercostal tube drainage. Antibiotic therapy needs to be reviewed if there is an empyema. Anaerobic infection is frequently present and so addition of metronidazole to the treatment regimen is advisable. Further antibiotic changes are guided by the bacteriology of the empyema. Failure of the parapneumonic effusion or empyema to drain may arise from incorrect placement of the tube, blockage of the tube, or loculations. Incorrect placement may be diagnosed from a chest radiograph, but in difficult cases visualization with CT scanning can be helpful.

If tube drainage alone is unsuccessful, the treatment of complicated effusions or empyemas has traditionally involved surgical intervention with either decortication or rib resection. Recently, a revival of interest has occurred in a technique that employs fibrinolytic agents, and was first used in the 1930s, but abandoned because the preparations were impure. A number of published series have used intrapleural streptokinase or urokinase for complicated parapneumonic effusions or empyemas[1-4]. These series suggest that the use of fibrinolytic agents can drain collections and effectively prevent the need for surgery (Fig. 30.2). A recent controlled trial indicated a benefit for intrapleural fibrinolytic agents, and their use has been endorsed by recent review articles[1]. Contraindications to the use of streptokinase are an allergy to streptokinase, its previous use for myocardial infarct within 2 years, and coagulation disorders. It must not be used in the presence of bronchopleural fistula and the presence of malignancy is a relative contraindication. Potential complications are of allergic reactions, although these do not seem to be a frequent problem with modern preparations, and hemorrhage, which is again rare.

No comparison has been made of different techniques in the application of streptokinase, but one reported in a number of series is to use 250,000 units mixed in 100mL of normal saline inserted intrapleurally via a chest drain, which is then left clamped for 4 hours, after which it is left on free drainage or negative suction if necessary. More than one application of streptokinase may be required to fully establish drainage. Use of up to eight installations of streptokinase has been reported, the usual reason for stopping being failure of complete drainage of the effusion rather than complications. Use of intrapleural fibrinolytic agents requires close co-operation with the radiology department to assess progress. With the presence of underlying consolidation of the lung and thickening of the pleura it can often be difficult to determine from plain radiographs whether complete drainage has occurred, so CT scanning or ultrasound is often necessary to exclude a significant collection of fluid. Failure of intrapleural fibrinolytic agents to manage empyema is an indication for surgical intervention using either decortication or rib resection and insertion of a large drain.

LUNG ABSCESS

Lung abscess may occur with any bacterial pneumonia, but is most common with staphylococcal pneumonias in which case multiple abscesses may form[5]. A lung abscess may be asymptomatic or can present with a continuing pyrexia or a cough productive of large volumes of often offensive sputum. An abscess may complicate a pre-existing bulla or cyst in the lung. A lung abscess may also complicate carcinoma of the bronchus, particularly squamous cell carcinoma, and surrounding consolidation may make it difficult to decide whether a tumor is present or not. Bronchoscopy can be useful to exclude a bronchial carcinoma

and by removing any secretions may promote drainage of the abscess. It may also provide useful information regarding the presence of an underlying carcinoma or an abscess complicating a pneumonia. Also, abscess formation may follow the inhalation of a foreign body that may only be apparent at bronchoscopy, although removal may require a general anesthetic and a rigid bronchoscopy. Many lung abscesses can be treated conservatively

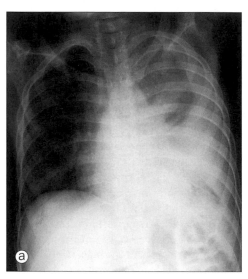
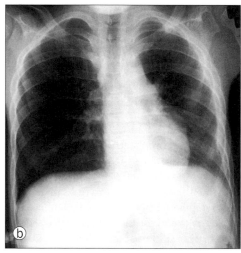
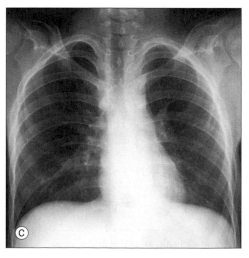

Figure 30.2 Empyema treated with streptokinase. (a) Large left-sided empyema that did not drain with intercostal drainage. (b) Immediately following chest radiograph of empyema treated with intrapleural drainage and intrapleural streptokinase on four occasions showing left-sided pleural thickening. (c) Chest radiograph taken 6 months later showing almost complete resolution of pleural thickening.

with continuation of antibiotics. Mixed aerobic infections are common and it is worth adding metronidazole. If a lung abscess does not resolve with conservative measures, it can be aspirated via a tube drainage (using a pigtail catheter inserted under CT or ultrasound guidance); surgical drainage or resection of the abscess may be necessary. Antibiotic therapy needs to be prolonged: commonly for 6 weeks.

BRONCHOPLEURAL FISTULA

A bronchopleural fistula is caused by a connection between the pleural space and the consolidated lung, and may complicate either an empyema or a lung abscess. The presentation of a bronchopleural fistula is either with a pyopneumothorax (i.e. air above a collection of infected fluid in the pleural space), or that on drainage of an empyema not only pus but also air exits through the chest drain. If confirmation of a bronchopleural fistula is needed, this can be achieved easily by placing a small amount of methylene blue into the pleural space or abscess, which is expectorated, or by inserting (using chest radiograph or CT) a small amount of radiopaque contrast into the pleural space. A bronchopleural fistula does not seal unless infection is controlled. Initial treatment is conservative, with antibiotics and tube drainage, to allow the fistula to seal. If it does not seal, surgery may be necessary, for which a variety of procedures are possible. These include a primary closure of the fistula or closure of the potential space using other living tissues such as muscle flaps. The management of bronchopleural fistulas that do not close with conservative treatment requires specialist thoracic surgical skills.

ORGANIZING PNEUMONIA

Organizing pneumonia, also sometimes known as cryptogenic organizing pneumonia or bronchiolitis obliterans organizing pneumonia, is a condition in which an organizing inflammatory exudate with fibroblast proliferation occurs after an episode of pneumonia[6,7]. The consolidation is often patchy and may be flitting. Organizing pneumonia after a bacterial infection is suggested when residual consolidation, often flitting, remains despite adequate antibiotic treatment. Investigation includes examination of sputum or bronchial washings to exclude infection, and a CT scan may help to visualize the consolidation and exclude other causes. The definitive investigation is an open lung biopsy that shows the typical histologic appearances. If suspicion is great enough and the physician confident enough of the diagnosis, a course of corticosteroids usually leads to resolution, although sometimes when the corticosteroids are stopped a relapse occurs and further treatment for several months may be necessary in these cases (see Chapter 48).

BRONCHIECTASIS

Permanent dilatation of the bronchus can occur after a severe pneumonia and cause localized bronchiectasis (Fig. 30.3). Bronchial dilatation may be shown by CT scanning during or after an episode of acute pneumonia, and so the diagnosis cannot be made with confidence until sometime after the pneumonia has completely resolved. The presence of bronchiectasis is suggested by a continual cough productive of sputum or recurrent infections in one part of the lung. Investigation consists of sputum examination when organisms associated with bronchiectasis, such as

Haemophilus influenzae or *Pseudomonas aeruginosa*, may be isolated. The diagnostic test of choice now is a thin section (1–3mm slices), high resolution CT scan. Management is with postural drainage of the infected lobe, and antibiotic treatment for any acute infections. In patients who have co-existing air-flow obstruction, treatment with bronchodilators or inhaled corticosteroids may be helpful.

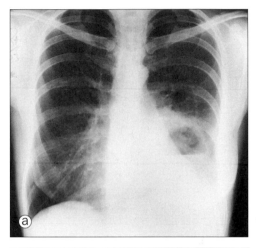

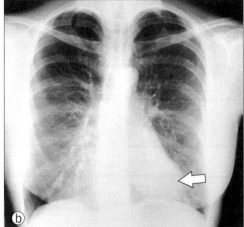

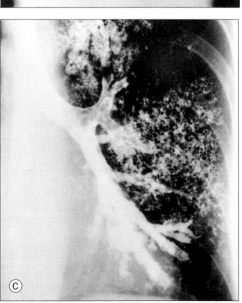

Figure 30.3 Left lower lobe pneumonia.
(a) Lung abscess associated with a left lower lobe pneumonia.
(b) Chest radiograph 3 months after resolution of the lung abscess showing widened airways with thickened walls in the left lower lobe (arrow). These bronchiectatic changes were consequent to the pneumonia. (c) A perbronchoscopic bronchogram of the lower left lobe confirming the gross dilatation of the airways typical in postinfective bronchiectasis.

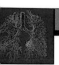

FIBROSIS

Most cases of pneumonia resolve completely and leave no residual problems. Occasionally, particularly with prolonged or severe pneumonia, localized fibrosis with loss of lung volume may occur. Unless there is co-existent lung disease, this is rarely sufficiently severe to cause dyspnea. If fibrosis occurs or is suspected, corticosteroids are sometimes used. It has not been proved, however, that they effectively prevent this condition. The presence of fibrosis may be visible on plain chest radiographs and can be confirmed by CT scanning. Sometimes the differential diagnosis of fibrosis and loss of lung volumes may be a carcinoma of the bronchus and fiberoptic bronchoscopy may be necessary to exclude a bronchial neoplasm.

REFERENCES

1. Deegan PC, Macfarlane JT. Intrapleural streptokinase – the answer to community acquired pleural infection. Thorax. 1997;52:403.
2. Light RW, Girard WM, Jenkinson SG, George RB. Parapneumonic effusions. Am J Med. 1980;69:507–11.
3. Taylor RFM, Rubens MB, Pearson MC, Barnes NC. Intrapleural streptokinase in the management of empyema. Thorax. 1994;49:856–9.
4. Davies RJO, Traill ZC, Gleeson FU. Randomised controlled trial of intrapleural streptokinase in community acquired pleural infection. Thorax. 1997;52:416–21.
5. Moore-Gillon J, Eykyn SJ. Lung abscess. In: Brewis RAL, Gibson GJ, Geddes DM, eds. Respiratory medicine. London: Bailliere Tindall; 1990:974–9.
6. Davison AG, Heard BE, McAllister WAC, Turner-Warwick MEH. Cryptogenic organising pneumonia. Q J Med. 1983;52:382–94.
7. Epler GR, Colby TV, McLeod TC, Carrington CB, Gaensler EA. Bronchiolitis obliterans organising pneumonia. N Engl J Med. 1985;312:152–8.

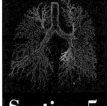
Chapter 31

Rhinitis and Sinusitis

David Mitchell

EPIDEMIOLOGY, RISK FACTORS, AND PATHOPHYSIOLOGY

Rhinitis and sinusitis are terms that refer to inflammatory conditions of the nose and paranasal sinuses caused by:

- allergy;
- infections; and
- other causes or unknown.

As conditions that involve the nose and the sinuses can be regarded as a continuous spectrum, in this chapter rhinitis and sinusitis are discussed under the unifying term of rhinosinusitis. Considerable overlap occurs; for example allergic rhinitis characterized by sneezing, itching, and watery discharge results in extensive mucosal swelling, which may result in reduced sinus drainage and allow secondary infection to occur[1]. Both allergic and infective inflammatory rhinosinusitis may be exacerbated by the presence of anatomic and mechanical defects, such as a deviated nasal septum or enlarged turbinates.

It is also important to consider the possibility of underlying conditions, early recognition of which may be necessary to prevent later damage (e.g. defects of immunity, defects of cilial motility, and vasculitic and granulomatous conditions). Rhinosinusitis is frequently associated with respiratory disease; for example about one third of patients who have bronchiectasis also have chronic sinusitis, and patients who suffer cystic fibrosis invariably have sinusitis and frequently develop nasal polyps. In cystic fibrosis, pneumatization of the frontal sinuses often fails and the presence of opacification in the maxillary sinuses is the norm. Patients affected by asthma frequently have rhinosinusitis. A rare subgroup are aspirin hypersensitive who tend to have late onset asthma, are not atopic, and have nasal polyps.

It is usually possible to make a distinction between an allergic or infective cause. Allergic rhinitis is characterized by sneezes, itching, watery discharge, and intermittent nasal blockage, whereas the common cold has short-lived symptoms of which stuffiness and discomfort predominate. A classification of rhinosinusitis into allergic and nonallergic, with nonallergic being further subdivided into infective and noninfective, has much to recommend it on account of its simplicity (Fig. 31.1). However, the distinction between allergic and infective rhinitis is not always easy, as both may occur together and, indeed, one may precede the other[2,3]. A useful way to classify rhinosinusitis is by the cause or underlying factors, although more than one factor may operate in any particular case.

In the rest of this section, specific features of the causes of rhinosinusitis listed in Figure 31.1 are described.

Allergy
Allergic rhinosinusitis

Apart from the common cold, this is the most common cause of nasal symptoms; it affects 10–16% of the population and results from IgE-mediated immediate hypersensitivity reactions that occur in the mucous membranes of the nasal airways. Allergic rhinitis occurs in atopic individuals who have the genetic predisposition to produce IgE-antibody responses to allergens, which are innocuous to normal individuals. The allergens responsible are usually airborne, so-called aeroallergens, and consist of plant pollen, fungal spores, insect aeroallergens (for example, from the house dust mite), and dander from domestic pets such as cats and dogs. Allergic rhinitis may be divided into seasonal and perennial rhinitis.

In the UK and other North European countries, symptoms in the spring are frequently caused by allergy to tree pollens such as birch, plane, ash, and hazel. In late spring and early summer, the classic hay fever season, allergic rhinitis results from allergy to grasses such as rye, timothy, and coxfoot. In the late summer, weed pollens, such as nettle and mugwurt, are responsible, whereas in autumn the fungi *Cladosporium* spp., *Alternaria* spp., and *Aspergillus* spp. provoke symptoms. In the USA, ragweed

Etiologic classification of rhinosinusitis	
Allergic	Seasonal
	Perennial
	Occupational
	Food
Nonallergic	
Infective	Acute (e.g. coryza, acute bacterial sinusitis)
	Chronic [e.g. bacterial or underlying predisposing condition (either direct cause or contributory conditions): immune defects, human immunodeficiency virus, hypogamma-globulinemia, mucus clearance defects, Kartagener's, Young's syndrome]
Noninfective	Idiopathic (e.g. intrinsic rhinitis, 'autonomic rhinitis', 'vasomotor rhinitis')
	Structural (e.g. deviated septum, tumor)
	Granulomas (e.g. sarcoid)
	Hormones
	Drugs
	Irritants
	Atrophic

Figure 31.1 Etiologic classification of rhinosinusitis.

a pressure gradient with a pneumotachograph and face mask. A more simple test is to measure peak inspiratory nasal flow using a modified peak flow meter, whereas acoustic rhinometry uses a sound pulse to measure the nasal cross-sectional area.

Nasal resistance can change very dramatically within a few minutes. Congestion is produced by engorgement of venous erectile tissue within the nose; the mucous membrane receives dense, autonomic innervation. Nasal resistance falls with epinephrine and other sympathomimetic drugs, but also with exercise, rebreathing, and adoption of the erect posture. Nasal resistance increases in rhinitis and, in some individuals, with alcohol, aspirin, and other drugs, as well as when the supine posture is adopted.

Evaluation of allergic rhinitis

The diagnosis is usually obvious from a careful history and examination. Skin tests using allergen extracts to elicit IgE-mediated immediate hypersensitivity responses can be used to confirm or exclude atopy. If all the skin tests are negative, it is unlikely that the rhinitis is allergic. However, positive tests do not confirm the diagnosis, as many asymptomatic individuals have positive skin tests to common allergens. Skin tests are also of value as occasionally it is possible to identify an allergen that can be avoided. Measurement of total IgE is generally not helpful as only 10% of patients affected by perennial rhinitis of all causes and 50% of seasonal rhinitis patients have an elevated level, whereas 40% of this group have positive skin tests. However, measurement of specific IgE levels to common aeroallergens by means of radioallergosorbant testing may be useful and the results show a good correlation with skin test results. Very occasionally, particularly where occupational rhinitis may be a possibility, nasal challenge and provocation tests (with the offending allergen, histamine, or methacholine) may be required.

Nasal cytology

Discolored nasal secretions may be caused by infection in association with the presence of neutrophils or eosinophils in allergic conditions. It may be of value to perform nasal secretion cytology to determine the presence or absence of eosinophils in patients who have perennial rhinitis, negative skin tests, and who are not atopic. A subset of these patients suffer nasal secretion eosinophilia, and are more likely to have allergic features such as sneezing and congestion; they may also respond to topical corticosteroids.

TREATMENT

Allergic rhinitis

Treatment can be approached in three ways:
- identify and avoid allergens;
- immunotherapy to desensitize the immune response against the allergen; and
- suppression of the allergic inflammatory response.

Identify and avoid allergens

In practice, the identification and avoidance of allergens may be extremely difficult. House dust mites are responsible for much perennial allergic rhinitis. Mites flourish in temperatures around 15°C (59°F) and 60–70% relative humidity, conditions present in many homes that contain central heating. They flourish particularly in soft furnishings, mattresses, pillows, and bed covers, as well as in carpets. Allergen avoidance and measures to reduce the load

(i.e. wooden floors rather than carpets, regular vacuum cleaning, and barrier covers for mattresses and pillows) effectively reduce rhinitic symptoms. Acaricides that kill the mites do not eliminate the antigen, which is present in the fecal pellets. Removal of a pet may not remove symptoms as allergens may persist in rooms for many months, if not years. Avoidance of pollen is difficult, but staying indoors when the pollen count is high, closing windows, and shutting car windows when driving through the country, as well as avoiding open grassy spaces, may all help.

Immunotherapy

Desensitization involves the administration of increasing doses of allergen extract by subcutaneous injection over a period of months and has been shown to effectively diminish symptoms of allergic seasonal rhinitis to grass pollen, ragweed, and birch pollen. Some studies also suggest efficacy to house dust mite and some animal danders. Desensitization has largely been superseded by the success of effective medical therapy in the suppression of allergic inflammation (see below). Desensitization does not work in all cases[5], concerns have been raised regarding occasional anaphylactic reactions to the procedure, and deaths have been recorded.

Medical suppressive therapy

Topical corticosteroids

Topical corticosteroids are very effective for most symptoms of allergic rhinitis. For very severe symptoms with marked nasal blockage, instillation of betamethasone nasal drops in the head-down position for the first 2 weeks of therapy may be more effective than starting with spray or metered dose inhaler. Generally, aqueous nasal sprays are more pleasant than metered dose inhalers. Side effects include local irritation and approximately 5% of patients experience a little local bleeding. Failure of therapy most usually results from failure of compliance. Sodium cromoglycate is less effective than topical corticosteroids for nasal symptoms, but may be suitable for children, whereas severe conjunctival symptoms are best treated with sodium cromoglycate or nedocromil sodium. Corticosteroid eye drops are avoided. For very severe symptoms, a short course of oral prednisolone, starting with 20mg daily, is appropriate.

Antihistamines

Antihistamines provide excellent relief of sneezing, itching, and rhinorrhea, but are not so good for nasal blockage and congestion; they have the advantage of being effective for mouth and eye symptoms. Chlorpheniramine is best taken at night, if this is required, because of its sedating properties. The newer H_1-specific histamine receptor antagonists have the advantage of being nonsedating. Terfenadine is nonsedating, but there have been recent concerns as a result of QT prolongation on the electrocardiogram and ventricular arrhythmia's, although these do not occur with fexofenadine. Astemizole also produces QT prolongation. Loratadine has rapid onset, can be taken once daily, and is nonsedating. Cetirizine also has rapid onset, is taken once daily, but occasional sedation may occur. Azelastine and levocabastine are useful topical antihistamines.

Other agents

Vasoconstrictors are useful in the short-term for marked congestion, but long-term use must be avoided because of the risk of rhinitis medicamentosa. Anticholinergics such as ipratropium bromide may be useful if extensive, watery secretion is a major problem.

Surgical intervention

Where medical treatment is only partially successful, a full otorhinolaryngologic assessment is performed as correction of a deviated nasal septum or reduction of hypertrophied mucosa may improve the symptoms. With coexistent chronic sinus infection, functional endoscopic sinus surgical techniques (FESS) may be necessary to facilitate sinus drainage, aeration. and access for medications.

Infections

Acute coryza – the common cold

Numerous studies have failed to show benefit from a number of therapies in terms of shortening the natural history of the common cold, so that treatment is essentially symptomatic with analgesics, antipyretics, rest, and broad-spectrum antibiotics if secondary infection is present.

Acute sinusitis

Most cases resolve spontaneously. Analgesics and antipyretics provide symptomatic relief, but aspirin must be avoided in those who may be hypersensitive. Acetaminophen (paracetamol) and codeine are satisfactory alternatives. Decongestants such as oxymetazaline and xylometazaline reduce edema and may improve sinus drainage. Broad-spectrum antibiotics are appropriate, but must have activity against the most common pathogens, namely *Strep. pneumoniae*, *H. influenzae*, and *M. catarrhalis*. Amoxicillin, trimethoprim–sulfamethoxazole (co-trimoxazole), or a macrolide such as clarithromycin are appropriate. Amoxicillin–clavulanate has the added advantage of activity against *Staph. aureus* and penicillin-resistant *H. influenzae*. If anaerobic infection is suspected, a combination of amoxicillin–clavulanate and metronidazole or clindamycin is appropriate.

Chronic sinusitis

The aims of treatment are to identify any underlying cause (e.g. immunologic defect, anatomic abnormality that prevents drainage) and to restore the integrity of the mucous membranes to allow normal ventilation of the sinuses and drainage (see Fig. 31.5). As chronic sinusitis frequently follows acute sinusitis, the same measures apply, namely analgesics and antipyretics, antibiotics, and decongestants. Topical corticosteroids may help to reduce mucous membrane swelling and improve drainage. Initially, betamethasone drops taken in the head-down position are used.

Surgical interventions for acute and chronic sinusitis

Major changes have occurred in recent years as a result of the advent of high-resolution CT scans and FESS. Better demonstration of the nasal and sinus anatomy is achieved with CT scans, as well as recognition of the importance of the ostiomeatal complex, the vital region where sinus drainage by mucociliary clearance occurs. Obstruction in this zone is very important in the generation of chronic sinus disease. The main aim of FESS is to restore adequate drainage for the frontal, maxillary, and ethmoidal sinuses with minimal disruption to the normal anatomy (Fig. 31.6). In addition, anatomic variants and abnormalities can predispose to the development of chronic sinusitis and many of

these are appropriate for surgical correction. Where this fails, more radical sinus surgery may be needed, which includes antral washouts, intranasal antrostomy, and the more radical Caldwell–Luc procedure.

Noninfectious causes

Intrinsic rhinitis

Anticholinergics (ipratropium bromide) are useful for troublesome rhinorrhea, particularly when eosinophils are absent from nasal secretions. When eosinophilia is present, a response to topical corticosteroid therapy is usual. α-Agonist decongestants, such as pseudoephedrine and xylometazaline, are used sparingly. Surgical procedures may help if nasal obstruction is predominant.

Structural defects

Occasionally topical corticosteroid therapy may ameliorate structural defects, but normally surgical correction is required.

Immune defects

Therapy of immune defects is directed toward correction of the immunologic defect.

Mucus clearance defect

It is not possible to correct the underlying mucus clearance defect, so therapy relies on, as far as possible, improved drainage and aeration and prevention of secondary infection.

Granulomas

Appropriate, specific antimicrobial therapy is required for infectious causes of granulomatous disease. Sarcoidosis that involves the nose responds to either local or systemic glucocorticoid therapy.

Drug-induced disease

A careful drug history must be taken and the incriminated drug excluded.

Nasal polyps

Treatment is with topical corticosteroids, initially with betamethasone drops twice daily for 1 month (50% of patients improve with this). Failure of medical treatment is an indication for surgery. Unilateral nasal polyps must be referred to exclude transitional cell papilloma, squamous cell carcinoma, encephalocele, or other sinister pathology[6] (Fig 31.7).

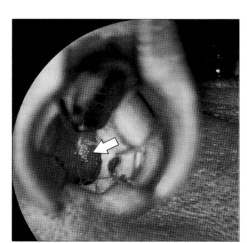

Figure 31.7 Speculum examination of nose shows a pale, watery polyp (arrow) occluding airway. (Courtesy of St Mary's Hospital Audio-Visual Department.)

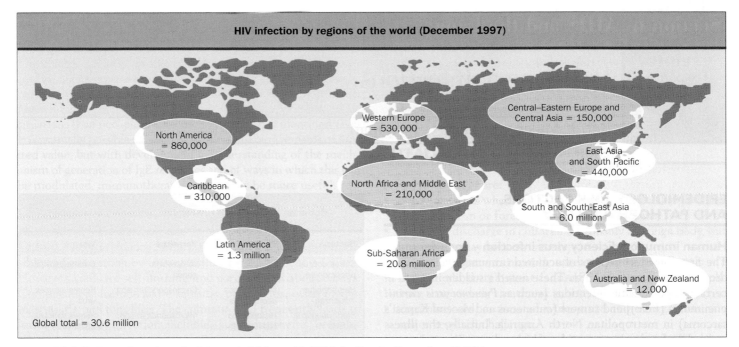

HIV infection by regions of the world (December 1997)

North America = 860,000

Western Europe = 530,000

Central–Eastern Europe and Central Asia = 150,000

East Asia and South Pacific = 440,000

Caribbean = 310,000

North Africa and Middle East = 210,000

South and South-East Asia = 6.0 million

Latin America = 1.3 million

Sub-Saharan Africa = 20.8 million

Australia and New Zealand = 12,000

Global total = 30.6 million

Figure 32.2 Estimated number of adults and children with HIV infection (to December 1997) by regions of the world. (Source: UNAIDS/WHO Working Group on Global HIV/AIDS and STD Surveillance.)

Centers for Disease Control and Prevention classification

Group	Infection
I	Acute primary
II	Asymptomatic
III	Persistent generalized lymphadenopathy
IV	Other disease
Subgroup A	Constitutional disease (e.g. weight loss >10% of body weight or >4.5kg; fevers >38.5°C lasting >1 month; diarrhea lasting >1 month)
Subgroup B	Neurologic disease (e.g. HIV encephalopathy, myelopathy, peripheral neuropathy)
Subgroup C	Secondary infectious diseases
Subgroup C1	AIDS-defining secondary infectious disease (e.g. *Pneumocystis carinii* pneumonia, cerebral toxoplasmosis, cytomegalovirus retinitis)
Subgroup C2	Other specified secondary infectious diseases (e.g. oral candida, multidermatomal varicella zoster)
Subgroup D	Secondary cancers (e.g. Kaposi's sarcoma, non-Hodgkin's lymphoma)
Subgroup E	Other conditions (e.g. lymphoid interstitial pneumonitis)

Figure 32.3 Centers for Disease Control and Prevention (CDC) classification of HIV infection (1985). This descriptive classification system is widely used for disease reporting, but, unlike a staging system, it cannot predict individual outcomes. The CDC classification is based on evidence of HIV infection with clinical indicators of impairment in cell-mediated immunity.

Adult AIDS indicator diseases (1993)

Candidiasis of esophagus, trachea, bronchi, or lungs

Cervical carcinoma, invasive

Coccidioidomycosis, disseminated or extrapulmonary

Cryptococcosis, extrapulmonary

Cryptosporidiosis, with diarrhea for over 1 month

Cytomegalovirus disease (not in liver, spleen, or lymph nodes)

Encephalopathy caused by HIV (AIDS–dementia complex)

Herpes simplex: ulcers for 1 month or pneumonitis, esophagitis

Histoplasmosis, disseminated or extrapulmonary

Isosporiasis, with diarrhea for over 1 month

Kaposi's sarcoma

Lymphoma: Burkitt's or immunoblastic or primary in brain

Mycobacteriosis (including pulmonary tuberculosis)

Pneumocystis carinii pneumonia

Pneumonia recurrent within a 12-month period

Progressive multifocal leukoencephalopathy

Salmonellal (nontyphoid) septicemia, recurrent

Toxoplasmosis of brain

Wasting syndrome caused by HIV

Figure 32.4 Adult AIDS indicator diseases (1993).

Once HIV is inside the cell it can, via the enzyme reverse transcriptase (RNA-dependent DNA polymerase), transcribe its HIV RNA into a DNA copy which may translocate to the nucleus and integrate with host-cell DNA using its viral integrase. The virus (as proviral DNA) remains latent in many cells until the cell itself becomes activated. This may arise from cytokine or antigen stimulation. The viral genetic material is then transcribed into new RNA which, in the form of a newly created virion, buds from the cell surface and is free to infect other CD4-bearing cells.

As has been described, the problem with HIV infection is that it directly attacks the immune system, in particular the T-helper cells that orchestrate the immune response. This leads to pro-

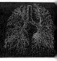

gressive immune dysfunction and an inability to resist opportunistic disease. The pathogenic process is not well defined, although the picture that is emerging suggests that at the time of primary infection HIV spreads to the lymph nodes, circulating immune cells and thymus. At this stage a relatively potent immune response is present in most HIV-infected individuals. However, HIV replication is both very effective and error prone, such that the immune system has to try and control a rapidly moving target. Taken together with the direct cell killing caused by HIV, this ultimately leads in the majority of individuals to progressive immune destruction and dysfunction. The end results of this are seen not only in the clinical diseases, which indicate profound immunosuppression, but also in the gradual reductions in circulating absolute CD4 cells, in percentage of T cells that express CD4 markers, and in CD4 to CD8 T-cell ratio that occur over time.

Natural history of HIV infection

The use of antiretroviral agents, as well as prophylactic therapies for opportunistic infections, is starting to alter the 'natural history' of HIV infection. However, in the absence of such treatments, the median interval between HIV seroconversion and progression to AIDS in the developed world has been estimated to be 10 years. In practice, the course of HIV infection can be divided clinically into certain distinct periods:

- acquisition of the virus;
- seroconversion with or without a clinical illness (primary infection);
- clinically silent period;
- development of symptoms and signs that indicate some degree of immunosuppression;
- AIDS (where the subject has opportunistic disease implying profound immunosuppression, e.g. PCP).

Acute primary HIV infection

The time from primary HIV infection to the development of detectable antibodies (the window period) is usually about 6–8 weeks. Studies suggest that between 30 and 70% of individuals who become infected develop a seroconversion illness. Normally, HIV antibody is detectable within 2–3 weeks of these symptoms.

The nonspecific features of primary HIV infection are almost always self-limiting and typically seroconversion mimics glandular fever. The vast majority of individuals who have primary HIV infection recover from the acute symptoms within 4 weeks. A proportion may have persistent symmetric, generalized lymphadenopathy. There is no difference in prognosis in this group compared with asymptomatic, HIV-positive individuals.

Chronic HIV infection

Although a proportion of individuals remain completely well for an extended period of time (approximately 20% after 10 years), many HIV-infected individuals show minor symptoms and signs that suggest immune dysfunction. Examples of these include new or worsening skin rashes (including herpes simplex), tiredness, cough, and low-grade anemia. Certain clinical symptoms and signs provide important prognostic information. Most studies show that oral thrush and constitutional symptoms (e.g. malaise, idiopathic fever, night sweats, diarrhea, and weight loss) are the strongest clinical predictors of progression to AIDS[2].

Since AIDS itself is a surveillance definition, it has been modified to incorporate the expanding spectrum of diseases recognized

to affect immunosuppressed individuals, such as cervical carcinoma and recurrent bacterial pneumonia (Fig. 32.4). The 1993 Centers for Disease Control and Prevention classification included immunologic criteria for AIDS (CD4 count <200 cells/μL or CD4 percentage <14% of total lymphocytes), irrespective of clinical symptoms (Fig. 32.5). These data are used to define a point at which the risk of severe opportunistic infection rises dramatically. An example of this is seen in the Multicenter AIDS Cohort Study (MACS) of homosexual and bisexual men who do not have AIDS[2], which found that the incidence of PCP in subjects not using prophylaxis rose from 0.5% at 6 months in men with a baseline CD4 count >200 cells/μL to 8.4% in those with a CD4 count <200 cells/μL.

Diseases that indicate AIDS differ little between men and women. In the developed world, differences in sex, racial, and HIV risk-factor survival after an AIDS diagnosis mainly arise from differences in the ease with which medical care can be obtained. Median AIDS survival in 1995 was over 20 months, which represents a doubling since 1981, primarily because of improved survival after PCP and tuberculosis. Long-term survival after AIDS is well documented and will almost certainly become more common over the next few years with the advent of new, highly effective regimens of antiretroviral drugs.

For the same reasons, clinical AIDS may also be occurring later because of primary prophylaxis of opportunistic infection and increasing use of combination antiretroviral therapy. Thus, patients may remain healthier for longer, but when they do become ill they ultimately die more rapidly from 'late-stage' incurable diseases such as lymphoma.

Prognostic markers

Laboratory markers and clinical symptoms (e.g. oral thrush) can independently reflect the immune changes that lead to serious disease[2]. Staging systems have therefore been developed that can predict the risk of progression to AIDS. The fall in absolute blood CD4 T-lymphocyte count is the most widely used prognostic marker, although it should be remembered that CD4 counts can be affected by a number of factors apart from HIV, such as intercurrent infection, smoking, exercise, time of day, and laboratory variation. The percentage of CD4 cells and ratio of

Revised (1993) CDC classification system for HIV infection – clinical categories			
CD4 T-cell categories (cells/μL)	A: Acute (primary) HIV, asymptomatic or persistent generalized lymphadenopathy	B: Symptomatic (not A or C – see caption)	C: AIDS indicator conditions
≥500	A1	B1	C1
200–499	A2	B2	C2
<200	A3	B3	C3

Figure 32.5 Revised (1993) Centers for Disease Control and Prevention classification system for HIV infection. This classification stratifies patients clinically (A–C) and immunologically (1–3). Groups A3 and B3 satisfy immunologic but not clinical criteria for AIDS. Category B consists of symptomatic conditions that are not included in category C, but can be either attributed to, or complicated by, HIV infection. Examples include thrush (oral or persistent vulvovaginal), moderate or severe cervical dysplasia, thrombocytopenia, and peripheral neuropathy.

CD4 to CD8 cells are more stable measures, and may be used if CD4 absolute counts appear to vary widely from visit to visit.

Measurement of plasma HIV RNA viral load is now accepted as a routine, standardized test that provides important prognostic information to both guide therapy and suggest long-term outcome[3]. It has a particular value in subjects who are clinically well and have high CD4 counts, as here it can indicate the expected speed of clinical progression. The use of other prognostic markers (e.g. indicators of cellular activation) has, for the time being, been largely abandoned outside of the research setting.

Risk factors for respiratory disease

An individual's risk for respiratory disease is determined by medical history (e.g. use of effective prophylactic or antiretroviral therapy), place of residence and travel history (e.g. the influence of geography on mycobacterial and fungal disease), and state of host immunity. Falling blood CD4 counts and/or high plasma RNA viral load increase the chance of respiratory infection, with an increased spectrum of potential organisms responsible for infection in the more immunosuppressed individual. For example, HIV-infected individuals with a CD4 count <200 cells/µL are four times more likely to have one episode of bacterial pneumonia per year than those with higher CD4 cell counts. More exotic organisms are found in subjects with very low CD4 counts. These include bacteria such as *Rhodococcus equi* and *Nocardia asteroides* and fungi such as *Aspergillus* spp. and *Penicillium marneffei*. Just as with *Pn. carinii*, this reflects the importance of T-cell depletion and macrophage dysfunction in the loss of host immunity (a process that has been confirmed by animal experiments).

Among HIV-infected patients, intravenous drug users are at greatest risk of developing bacterial pneumonia and tuberculosis. Individuals who have had previous respiratory episodes (PCP or bacterial pneumonia) appear to be at increased risk of further disease. Whether this relates to host or environmental factors is not certain, although it seems likely that structural lung damage and abnormal pulmonary physiology would in part contribute to this. That HIV-infected smokers have higher rates of pneumonia than nonsmokers further strengthens this argument. Smoking has been shown in one study to be associated with a more rapid progression to a first AIDS illness and death, although more recent work has not confirmed this relationship.

CLINICAL FEATURES

Bacterial infection

Bronchitis

Presentation of bronchitis mimics bacterial exacerbations of chronic obstructive lung disease; most patients have a productive cough and fever. The pathogens most commonly identified are similar to those in the general population (*Streptococcus pneumoniae* and *Haemophilus influenzae*). However, patients who have advanced disease may be infected with *Pseudomonas aeruginosa* or *Staphylococcus aureus*. Response to appropriate antibiotic therapy in conventional doses is good, although relapses frequently occur.

Bronchiectasis

Bronchiectasis is increasingly recognized in HIV-infected patients who have advanced HIV disease and low CD4 lymphocyte counts. It probably arises secondary to recurrent bacterial or *Pn. carinii*

infections. The diagnosis is most often made by high-resolution (fine-cut) computed tomography (CT) scanning. Its prevalence has not been accurately determined, although with improved survival from both opportunistic infections and HIV disease it is likely to be encountered increasingly in clinical practice. Pathogens commonly isolated in bronchiectatics are those seen in bronchitis. In addition, *Ps. cepacia* and *Moraxella catarrhalis* have been described.

Pneumonia

Community-acquired bacterial pneumonia occurs more frequently in HIV-infected individuals than in the general population. It is especially common in intravenous drug users who are HIV infected. Recurrent bacterial pneumonia in an HIV-infected patient is an AIDS-defining diagnosis. The spectrum of bacterial pathogens is similar to that in individuals who are not HIV infected (see Fig. 32.1). The commonest cause is *Strep. pneumoniae*, followed by *Ha. influenzae*. Those HIV-infected individuals who have *Strep. pneumoniae* pneumonia are frequently bacteremic, and *Strep. pneumoniae* is also one of the most common causes of invasive bacterial infection in HIV-infected patients. In one study, the rate of pneumococcal bacteremia in HIV-infected patients was 9.4/100 patient years; in contrast, other studies in patients who are not HIV infected give bacteremia rates of 0.07/100 patient years.

Most HIV-infected patients who have bacterial pneumonia present with features similar to those seen in those who are not HIV infected. Chest radiographs are frequently atypical, however, mimicking PCP in up to 50% of cases (Fig. 32.6). In contrast, radiographic lobar or segmental consolidation may also be seen in a wide range of bacterial infecting organisms (Fig. 32.7). A recent retrospective study from London analyzed 53 episodes of community-acquired lobar or segmental pneumonia in patients who had AIDS[5]. A definitive microbiologic diagnosis was made in 35 episodes (66%), 12 had PCP (4 had co-pathogens), and 23 had a bacterial cause, which included *Strep. pneumoniae* in 10, *Ps. aeruginosa* in 2, *Ha. influenzae* in 2, and *Mycobacterium tuberculosis* in 4. Of the 53 patients, 20 had pleural effusion and 8 had intrapulmonary cavities.

In subjects who have more advanced HIV disease and low CD4 lymphocyte counts, *Ps. aeruginosa* and *Staph. aureus* also cause pneumonia. Two patterns of presentation of *Pseudomonas* pulmonary infection have been described:

- Acute pneumonia and 'sepsis', a presentation often nosocomially acquired, and patients are frequently neutropenic, receiving chemotherapy and/or glucocorticoid therapy and may have indwelling intravenous catheters. Bacteremia is a frequent finding and the chest radiograph shows diffuse pulmonary infiltrates, which may mimic PCP. Mortality is high, and in bacteremic patients may be up to 40%.
- Community-acquired indolent infection, in which patients frequently have a subacute presentation without the risk factors listed above. The mortality rate is low, although there is a high rate of relapse following treatment.

Complications of bacterial pneumonia frequently occur, and include empyema and intrapulmonary abscess formation in up to 10% of patients. Inevitably, the mortality rate is high (approximately 10%).

Other bacteria

Nocardia asteroides infection

Nocardia asteroides infection has been reported in patients who have advanced HIV disease and low CD4 lymphocyte counts. The widespread use of trimethoprim–sulfamethoxazole

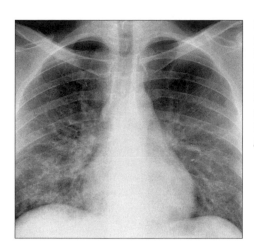

Figure 32.6 Chest radiograph showing bilateral, diffuse, interstitial infiltrates mimicking *Pneumocystis carinii* pneumonia. Etiology is *Streptococcus pneumoniae*.

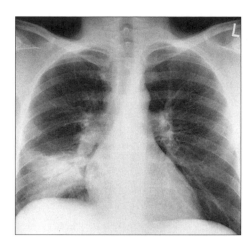

Figure 32.7 Chest radiograph showing lobar consolidation. Etiology is *Salmonella choleraesuis*.

(TMP–SMX) for prophylaxis of PCP may have reduced the incidence of infection. The clinical presentation is often indistinguishable from other bacterial infections. Chest radiographic appearances may mimic tuberculosis (see below), with upper-lobe consolidation, cavitation, interstitial infiltrates, pleural effusion, and hilar lymphadenopathy. The diagnosis is made by identification of the organism in sputum, bronchoalveolar lavage (BAL) or lung tissue.

Rhodococcus equi
Rhodococcus equi usually produces pneumonia in patients who have advanced HIV infection and have been in contact with farm animals or with soil from fields or barns where animals are housed. The presentation is subacute with 2–3 weeks of cough, dyspnea, fever, and pleuritic chest pain. The chest radiograph typically shows consolidation with cavitation.

Pleural effusions are common. The diagnosis is usually made by culture of sputum or blood; fiberoptic bronchoscopy with BAL or pleural aspiration may be necessary in some cases.

Rochalimaea henselae
Rochalimaea henselae is a Gram-negative bacillus that causes bacillary angiomatosis in HIV-infected patients. Clinically, the cutaneous lesions may mimic Kaposi's sarcoma from which they may be differentiated by demonstration of organisms in tissue using Warthin–Starry silver stain. Bacillary angiomatosis may also infect the lungs, where it produces endobronchial red or violet polypoid angiomatous lesions, which again can resemble Kaposi's sarcoma. Biopsy is necessary to confirm a diagnosis.

Mycobacterial infections
Tuberculosis
Tuberculosis is one of the most important diseases associated with HIV infection – worldwide, HIV infection is the most important risk factor for the development of tuberculosis. Tuberculosis has become a major cause of morbidity and mortality in patients who have AIDS.

Many centers in the UK and United States routinely offer HIV-antibody testing to all patients who have tuberculosis, regardless of risk factors for HIV infection. The advantage of such a strategy is that individuals who are found to be HIV infected can be offered highly active, antiretroviral therapy. Furthermore, counseling to modify risk behavior and reduce HIV transmission can be carried out.

Tuberculosis may infect not only the immunosuppressed, but also the immunocompetent. Thus, clinical disease may occur at any stage of HIV infection. In the United States, UK, and most European countries the reporting of tuberculosis in both HIV-infected and non-HIV-infected individuals is mandatory.

Clinical disease in HIV-infected individuals may arise in several different ways – by reactivation of latent tuberculosis, by rapid progression of pulmonary infection, and by reinfection from an exogenous source. Studies using restriction fragment length polymorphisms show that up to 30% of HIV-associated tuberculosis in New York is caused by exogenous reinfection.

Tuberculosis in HIV-infected persons presents as pulmonary disease in over two thirds of cases. The clinical presentation of pulmonary tuberculosis is related to the stage of HIV-induced suppression of cell-mediated immunity; thus, in individuals who have early HIV disease, the clinical features are similar to 'normal' adult postprimary disease (Fig. 32.8). Symptoms typically include weight loss, fever with sweats, cough, dyspnea, hemoptysis, and chest pain[6]. In many patients who have early HIV disease and tuberculosis, no clinical features suggest associated HIV infection. The chest radiograph frequently shows upper-lobe consolidation and cavitary change is common (see Fig. 32.9). Tuberculin skin test (purified protein derivative) is usually positive and the likelihood of spontaneously expectorated sputum or BAL fluid being 'smear positive' is high.

Tuberculosis and HIV infection		
	Stage of HIV disease	
	Early	**Late**
Chest radiograph	Upper-lobe infiltrates and cavities (compare with post primary infection)	Lymphadenopathy, effusions Miliary or diffuse infiltrates (compare with primary infection) Normal
Sputum or bronchoalveolar lavage smear positive	Frequently	Less commonly
Tuberculin test positive	Frequently	Less commonly
Extrapulmonary disease	Less commonly	Frequently

Figure 32.8 Tuberculosis and HIV infection.

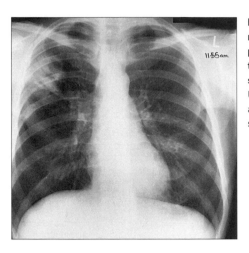

Figure 32.9 Chest radiograph of pulmonary tuberculosis in early-stage HIV infection. Upper-lobe infiltrates and cavities are shown.

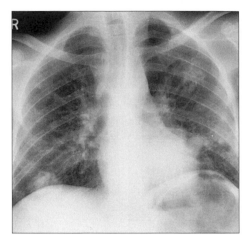

Figure 32.10 Chest radiograph of pulmonary tuberculosis in late-stage HIV infection. Patchy focal infiltrates are shown.

In individuals who have advanced HIV disease with low CD4 lymphocyte counts and clinically apparent immunosuppression, it may be difficult to diagnose tuberculosis[6]. This is because the clinical presentation is often with nonspecific symptoms – fever, weight loss, fatigue, and malaise being mistakenly ascribed to HIV infection itself. In this context, pulmonary tuberculosis is often similar to primary infection, with the chest radiograph showing diffuse or miliary shadowing, hilar or mediastinal lymphadenopathy, or pleural effusion; cavitation is unusual (Fig. 32.10). In some patients the chest radiograph may be normal, in others the pulmonary infiltrate may be bilateral, diffuse, and interstitial in pattern, thus mimicking PCP. Hilar lymphadenopathy and pleural effusion may also be produced by pulmonary Kaposi's sarcoma or lymphoma with which *M. tuberculosis* may co-exist. The tuberculin skin test is usually negative and spontaneously expectorated sputum and BAL fluid are often smear negative (but culture positive).

In addition to pulmonary tuberculosis, extrapulmonary disease occurs in a high proportion of HIV-infected individuals who have low CD4 lymphocyte counts (<150 cells/μL). Mycobacteremia and lymph-node infection are common, but involvement of bone marrow, liver, pericardium, and meninges may also occur. Disseminated tuberculosis is an important factor in the development of 'slim' disease in HIV-infected patients in Africa. This typically presents with fever, marked wasting, and diarrhea.

Evidence of extrapulmonary tuberculosis is sought in any HIV-infected patient who has suspected or confirmed pulmonary tuberculosis, by culture of stool, urine, and blood or bone marrow. Culture and speciation may take 6–10 weeks. Radiometric methods (e.g. Bactec, Becton Dickenson) that detect early growth may provide a diagnosis in only 2–3 weeks. Molecular diagnostic tests using *M. tuberculosis* genome detection by the polymerase chain reaction (PCR) offer the possibility of yet more rapid diagnosis (within hours), but are not yet in widespread clinical use. Until the results of culture and speciation are known, acid-fast bacilli identified in respiratory samples, biopsy tissue, an aspirate, or from blood in an HIV-infected individual, irrespective of the CD4 lymphocyte count, should be regarded as being *M. tuberculosis* and conventional antituberculosis therapy commenced. If culture fails to demonstrate *M. tuberculosis* and instead an atypical mycobacteria (see below) is identified, treatment can be modified.

Drug-resistant tuberculosis

Multiple-drug-resistant (MDR) tuberculosis – that is, *M. tuberculosis* resistant to isoniazid and rifampin (rifampicin), with or without other drugs – is now an important clinical problem in HIV-infected individuals in the United States, where it is responsible for approximately 3% of all tuberculosis in HIV-infected patients. Outbreaks of MDR tuberculosis have occurred in both HIV-infected and non-HIV-infected individuals in the United States in prison facilities, hostels, and hospitals. Similar outbreaks have also been documented among HIV-infected patients in Italy, Spain, and the UK. Inadequate treatment (and supervision of treatment) of tuberculosis and poor patient compliance with antituberculosis therapy are major risk factors for the development of MDR tuberculosis. Other cases have arisen because of exogenous reinfection of profoundly immunosuppressed HIV-infected patients who are already receiving treatment for drug-sensitive disease.

Despite antituberculosis therapy, the median survival in HIV-infected individuals who have MDR tuberculosis is only 2–3 months. The outlook is also poor in patients who are not HIV infected and in health-care workers who acquire MDR tuberculosis.

Mycobacteria other than Mycobacterium tuberculosis
Mycobacterium avium-intracellulare complex
Up to 50% of HIV-infected individuals will develop disseminated *Mycobacterium avium-intracellulare* complex (MAC) infection at some stage before death. Disseminated MAC infection tends to occur in patients who have advanced HIV disease and CD4 lymphocyte counts <100 cells/μL. Clinical presentation is nonspecific and may be confused with the effects of HIV itself. Fever, night sweats, weight loss, anorexia, and malaise are common. Anemia, hepatosplenomegaly, abdominal pain, and chronic diarrhea are frequent findings. The diagnosis of disseminated MAC infection is made by culture of the organism from blood, bone marrow, lymph node, or liver biopsy specimens. Also, MAC is frequently identified in BAL fluid, sputum, stool, and urine, but detection of the organism at these sites is not diagnostic of disseminated infection. Evidence of pulmonary MAC infection is not normally obtained from a chest radiograph, which may be normal or show nonspecific infiltrates. Rarely, focal consolidation, nodular infiltrates, and apical cavitation (resembling *M. tuberculosis*) have been reported.

Mycobacterium kansasii

Mycobacterium kansasii is the second most common nontuberculous, opportunistic mycobacterial infection in HIV-infected individuals, and usually appears late in the course of HIV infection in patients with CD4 lymphocyte counts <100 cells/μL. The most frequent presentation is with fever, cough, and dyspnea. In approximately two thirds of those who have *M. kansasii* infection, the disease is localized to the lungs; the remainder have disseminated disease that affects bone marrow, lymph node, skin, and lungs. The diagnosis is made by culture of the organism from respiratory secretions or from bone marrow, lymph node aspirate, or skin biopsy. Focal upper-lobe infiltrates with diffuse, interstitial infiltrates are the most common radiographic abnormalities; thin-walled cavitary lesions and hilar adenopathy have also been reported.

Pneumocystis carinii pneumonia

The development of PCP is largely related to underlying states of immunosuppression induced by malignancy, treatment thereof, organ transplantation, or HIV infection. In 1998 in the United States, UK, Europe, and Australasia, PCP is only seen in HIV-infected individuals unaware of their serostatus or in those who are intolerant of, or noncompliant with, anti-*Pn. carinii* prophylaxis and highly active antiretroviral therapy.

Until recently, *Pn. carinii* was regarded taxonomically as a protozoan, based on its morphology and the lack of response to antifungal agents such as amphotericin B. Use of molecular biologic techniques suggest, however, that *Pn. carinii* is a fungus. The demonstration of antibodies against *Pn. carinii* in the majority of healthy children and adults is regarded as supportive of the hypothesis that *Pn. carinii* in an immunocompromised individual arises by reactivation of a symptomless, childhood-acquired latent infection. This is challenged by the failure to demonstrate *Pn. carinii* in BAL fluid or autopsy lung tissue of immunocompetent individuals using conventional silver staining, immunofluorescence, or DNA amplification, and by the finding of low levels of detectable *Pn. carinii* DNA in only 20% of HIV-infected individuals who present with respiratory episodes and diagnoses other than *Pn. carinii*[7]. The hypothesis is further eroded by reports of nosocomial case clusters among immunosuppressed patients.

The clinical presentation of *Pn. carinii* is nonspecific, with the onset of progressive exertional dyspnea over days or weeks, together with a dry cough with or without expectoration of minimal quantities of mucoid sputum. Patients often complain of an inability to take a deep breath in, which is not because of pleural pain (Fig. 32.11)[8]. Pyrexia is common, yet patients rarely complain of fever or sweats. In HIV-infected individuals the presentation is generally more insidious than in patients who receive immunosuppressive therapy, with a median time to diagnosis from onset of symptoms of 25 days in those who have AIDS compared with 5 days in the patients who are not HIV infected. In a small proportion of HIV-infected individuals the disease course of PCP is fulminant, with an interval of only 5–7 days between onset of symptoms and progression to development of respiratory failure. In others the presentation is indolent, with respiratory symptoms that worsen almost imperceptively over several months. Rarely, *Pn. carinii* may present without respiratory symptoms as a pyrexia of undetermined origin.

Clinical examination is usually remarkable only for the absence of physical signs; occasionally, fine, basal, end-respiratory crackles are audible. Features atypical for a diagnosis of PCP that suggest

an alternative diagnosis include a cough productive of purulent sputum or hemoptysis, chest pain (particularly pleural pain), and signs of focal consolidation of pleural effusion (Fig. 32.11)[8].

The chest radiograph in PCP is typically normal initially. Later, diffuse reticular shadowing, especially in the perihilar regions, is seen and may progress to diffuse alveolar consolidation that resembles pulmonary edema if untreated or if the patient presents late with their pneumonia. In the late stages the lung may be massively consolidated and almost airless (Fig. 32.12). Up to 20% of chest radiographs are atypical showing lobar consolidation, honeycomb lung, multiple thin-walled cystic air space formation, intrapulmonary nodules, cavitary lesions, pneumothorax, and hilar and mediastinal lymphadenopathy. Predominantly apical change, resembling tuberculosis, may occur in patients who develop PCP

Presentation of *Pneumocystis carinii* pneumonia		
Examination	**Typical presentation**	**Atypical presentation**
Symptoms	Progressive exertional dyspnea over days or weeks	Sudden onset of dyspnea over hours or days
	Dry cough ± mucoid sputum	Cough productive of purulent sputum
	–	Hemoptysis
	Difficulty taking in a deep breath not because of pleuritic pain	Chest pain (pleuritic or crushing)
	Fever ± sweats	–
	Tachypnea	–
Chest	Normal breath sounds or fine end-inspiration basal crackles	Wheeze, signs of focal consolidation or pleural effusion
Chest radiograph	Early: normal, perihilar haze, or bilateral interstitial shadowing	–
	Late: alveolar-interstitial changes or 'white out' (marked alveolar consolidation with sparing of apices and costophrenic angles)	–
Arterial blood gases	PaO_2: early, normal; late, low	–
	$PaCO_2$: early, normal or low; late, normal or low	–

Figure 32.11 Presentation of *Pneumocystis carinii* pneumonia. (Reproduced from Malin and Miller[8], by permission of the publisher Churchill Livingstone.)

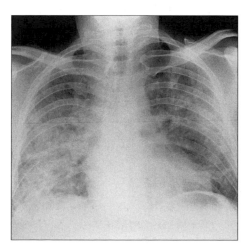

Figure 32.12 Chest radiograph of severe *Pneumocystis carinii* pneumonia. Diffuse bilateral interstitial infiltrates are shown.

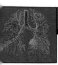

having received anti-*Pn. carinii* prophylaxis with nebulized pentamidine (Fig. 32.13). All these radiographic changes are nonspecific and similar changes occur with other pulmonary pathogens, including pyogenic, bacterial, mycobacterial, and fungal infection, and also with Kaposi's sarcoma and nonspecific interstitial pneumonitis. It is important to remember that respiratory symptoms in an immunosuppressed, HIV-infected individual with a normal chest radiograph should not be discounted, as over an interval of 2–3 days radiographic abnormalities may appear.

The diagnosis of PCP is made by demonstration of the organism in induced sputum, BAL fluid, or lung biopsy material using histochemical or immunofluorescence techniques.

Fungal infections

Many fungal infections of the lung are confined to specific geographic regions, although with widespread travel they may present in patients outside these areas. *Candida*, *Aspergillus*, and *Cryptococcus* spp. are ubiquitous and occur worldwide.

Candidal infection

In contrast to infections of the oropharynx and esophagus, candidal infection of the trachea, bronchi, and lungs is rare in HIV-infected patients, as is candidemia, disseminated candidiasis, and deep, focal candidiasis. The clinical presentation of pulmonary candidal infection has no specific features. Chest radiography is equally nonspecific – it may be normal or show patchy infiltrates. Isolation of *Candida* spp. from sputum may simply represent colonization and does not mean the patient has candidal pneumonia. Indirect evidence may be obtained from positive cultures or rising antibody titers. However, in HIV-infected patients a high antibody titer alone is a less reliable indicator and antibodies may be absent in proved cases of invasive candidal infection. Some correlation occurs between identification of large quantities of *Candida* spp. in BAL fluid and *Candida* spp. as the cause of pneumonia. Definitive diagnosis is made by lung biopsy.

Aspergillar infection

Infection with *Aspergillus* spp. is relatively rare in patients who have AIDS. This is in contrast to patients who are immunosuppressed and made neutropenic by systemic chemotherapy. Of HIV-infected patients who have aspergillosis, over one half are

neutropenic or receive corticosteroids. Neutropenia is commonly induced by drug therapy such as zidovudine or ganciclovir. Fever, cough, and dyspnea are the most common presenting symptoms, but pleuritic chest pain and hemoptysis are found in approximately one third of patients.

Patterns of disease that involve the lung include cavitating upper-lobe disease, focal radiographic opacities that resemble bacterial pneumonia, bilateral opacities that are diffuse and patchy (being nodular or reticular–nodular in pattern), pseudomembranous aspergillosis, which may obstruct the lumen of airways, and tracheobronchitis. The diagnosis of pulmonary aspergillosis is made by identifying fungus in sputum, sputum casts, or BAL fluid and by identifying tissue invasion of the lung or airways by fungus (Fig. 32.14).

Cryptococcal infection

Infection may present in one of two ways – either as primary cryptococcosis or as complicating cryptococcal meningitis as part of disseminated infection with cryptococcemia, pneumonia, and cutaneous disease (umbilicated papules mimicking molluscum contagiosum – Fig. 32.15). Primary pulmonary cryptococcosis presents in a very nonspecific way and is frequently indistinguishable from other pulmonary infections. In disseminated infection, the

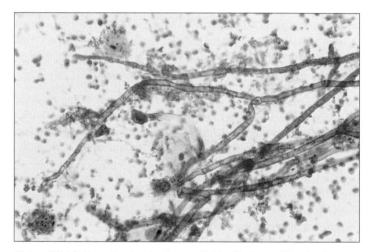

Figure 32.14 Bronchoalveolar lavage fluid with *Aspergillus fumigatus*.

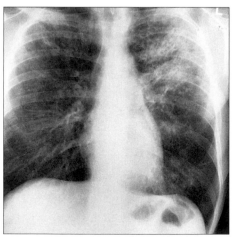

Figure 32.13 Chest radiograph of *Pneumocystis carinii* pneumonia. Upper-lobe infiltrates are seen in this patient who had received nebulized pentamidine.

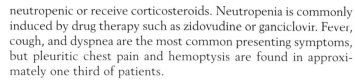

Figure 32.15 Skin in disseminated cryptococcosis. The multiple, umbilicated lesions resemble molluscum contagiosum.

presentation is frequently overshadowed by headache, fever, and malaise (caused by meningitis). The duration of onset may range from only a few days to several weeks. Examination may reveal skin lesions, lymphadenopathy, and meningism. Within the chest, signs may be absent or crackles may be audible. Arterial blood gas tensions may be normal or show hypoxemia. The most common abnormality on the chest radiograph is focal or diffuse interstitial infiltrates. Less frequently, masses, mediastinal or hilar lymphadenopathy, nodules, and effusion are seen.

The diagnosis of cryptococcal pulmonary infection (Fig. 32.16) is made by identification of C. neoformans in sputum, BAL fluid, pleural fluid, or lung biopsy, and by staining with India ink and/or mucicarmine and culture. Cryptococcal antigen may be detected in serum using the cryptococcal latex agglutination test. Titers are usually high, but may be negative in primary pulmonary cryptococcosis, in which case BAL fluid (cryptococcal latex agglutination) will be positive. In patients who have disseminated infection, C. neoformans may also be cultured from blood and cerebrospinal fluid.

Endemic mycoses
The endemic mycoses caused by *Histoplasma capsulatum*, *Coccidioides immitis*, and *Blastomyces dermatitidis* are found in HIV-infected patients living in North America (especially the Mississippi and Ohio river valleys). Histoplasmosis is also found in South-East Asia, the Caribbean Islands, and South America. Coccidioidomycosis is endemic in the south-west of the United States (Southern California, North Mexico) and parts of Argentina and Brazil; blastomycosis has a similar distribution, with an extension north into Canada.

Histoplasmosis
Progressive, disseminated histoplasmosis in patients who have AIDS typically presents with a subacute onset of fever and weight loss; approximately 50% of patients have mild respiratory symptoms with a nonproductive cough and dyspnea. Hepatosplenomegaly is frequently found on examination and a skin rash (similar to that produced by *Cryptococcus* spp.) may be seen. Rarely, the presentation may be atypical, being fulminant with clinical features of the sepsis syndrome, anemia, and/or disseminated intravascular coagulation. The chest radiograph is normal in approximately one third of patients; characteristic abnormalities

are bilateral widespread nodules 2–4mm in diameter. Other radiographic abnormalities are nonspecific and include interstitial infiltrates, reticular nodular shadowing, and alveolar consolidation.

Histoplasmosis may disseminate to the central nervous system and produce meningoencephalitis or mass lesions. The diagnosis is made reliably by identification of the organism by Wright-stained peripheral blood or by Giemsa staining of bone marrow, lymph node, skin, sputum, BAL fluid, or lung tissue. It is essential that identification is confirmed by culture. Detection of *Hi. capsulatum* var *capsulatum* polysaccharide antigen by radioimmunoassay has a high sensitivity. False-positive results may occur in patients with *Blastomycosis* and *Coccidioides* spp. Tests for *Histoplasma* antibodies by complement fixation or immunodiffusion may be negative in immunosuppressed, HIV-positive patients.

Coccidioidomycosis
The clinical presentation of coccidioidomycosis is very variable. The chest radiograph may show focal pulmonary disease with focal alveolar infiltrates, adenopathy, and intrapulmonary cavities, or alternatively diffuse reticular infiltrates. Diagnosis is made by isolation of the organism in sputum or BAL fluid. Disseminated disease is identified by isolating the fungus in blood, urine, or cerebrospinal fluid. Serologic tests may also be used for diagnosis.

Blastomycosis
Blastomycosis presents in patients who have advanced HIV infection when CD4 lymphocyte counts are usually <200 cells/µL. Patients may present late in respiratory failure. The clinical symptoms include cough, fever, dyspnea, and weight loss, and disseminated disease may occur with both pulmonary and extrapulmonary features. There is frequently multiple involvement of the skin, liver, brain, and meninges. Chest radiographic abnormalities include focal pneumonic change, miliary shadowing, and diffuse interstitial infiltrates. Diagnosis is made by culture from BAL, skin, and blood. In this infection cytologic and/or histologic diagnosis is important for early diagnosis, as culture of the organism may take 2–4 weeks. A high mortality occurs in patients who have disseminated infection.

Penicillium marneffei infection
Most HIV-infected patients present with disseminated infection and solitary skin or oral mucosal lesions, or with multiple infiltrates in the liver and/or spleen, or bone marrow (giving rise to presentation with pancytopenia). Pulmonary infection has no specific clinical features and chest radiographs may be normal or show diffuse, small, nodular infiltrates. The diagnosis is made by identifying the organism in bone marrow, skin biopsies, blood films, or BAL fluid.

Viral infections
Community-based respiratory viral infections
Community-based respiratory viral infections occur with equal frequency in HIV-infected and non-HIV-infected patients; however, respiratory complications following influenza infection are increased in patients affected by underlying conditions such as cardiac and/or pulmonary disease and immunosuppression. In prospective studies of HIV-infected patients undergoing bronchoscopy for evaluation of suspected lower respiratory tract disease, the community-acquired respiratory viral infections (i.e. influenza, parainfluenza, respiratory syncytial virus, rhinovirus, and adenovirus) are found only rarely, if at all[9].

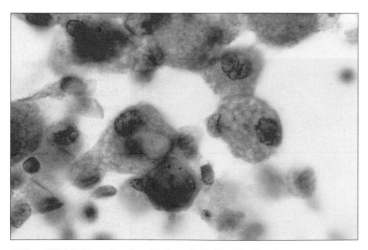

Figure 32.16 Bronchoalveolar lavage fluid with *Cryptococcus neoformans*.

Lung-function testing

Abnormalities of lung function are well documented with HIV infection. However, if those measurements that reflect changes in the conducting airways and those that relate to gas exchange are differentiated, the majority of abnormalities have been documented in the latter group. In general, an overall reduction in diffusing capacity (D_{LCO}) occurs at all stages of HIV infection, with the largest changes found in HIV-infected patients who have PCP (in one large study, the mean D_{LCO} was 49% of predicted)[10]. Thus, patients who have probable PCP can be differentiated and treatment guided. In everyday practice, this requires equipment dedicated to lung-function testing. A normal D_{LCO} in an individual who has symptoms but a normal or unchanged chest radiograph makes the diagnosis of PCP extremely unlikely. Recent data from the North American PSPC cohort study suggest that individuals with rapid rates of decline in D_{LCO} are at an increased risk of developing PCP.

Computed tomography scanning

High-resolution (fine-cut) CT scanning of the chest may be helpful when the chest radiograph is either normal, unchanged, or equivocal. The characteristic appearance of an alveolitis (i.e. areas of ground-glass attenuation through which the pulmonary vessels can be clearly identified) may be present, which indicates active pulmonary disease. This feature is, however, neither sensitive nor specific for PCP; a negative test result implies an alternative diagnosis.

Nuclear medicine

The rate at which inhaled technetium-99 pentetic acid (DTPA) is cleared provides an indication of the permeability of the alveolar and respiratory bronchiolar epithelium. A biphasic curve (i.e. with a rapid initial component) is the hallmark of an alveolitis, and is therefore often taken as evidence for PCP. This finding is nonspecific and may also be seen in other inflammatory or infectious conditions that produce an alveolitis, and also in heavy smokers. A normal chest radiograph together with a normal DTPA scan almost completely excludes active pulmonary disease that requires treatment.

Gallium-67 citrate scanning may be used when a patient has a normal chest radiograph despite symptoms. Apart from PCP, a positive scan may occur in a number of different infectious conditions, as well as in pulmonary lymphoma and lymphocytic interstitial pneumonitis. Focal or diffuse accumulation of gallium-67 is not seen with pulmonary Kaposi's sarcoma if no secondary infection is present. The pattern of tracer distribution within the lung and the rest of the body may provide some clues to the pneumonic etiology. For example CMV disease may also produce focal accumulation in the eyes, adrenals, and esophagus, and persistence in the colon. A major problem with gallium-67 scans is the delay in obtaining results, which take up to 72 hours after injection.

Invasive tests

From the above it is evident that noninvasive tests cannot reliably distinguish the different infecting agents from each other, but may usefully exclude acute opportunistic disease. Thus, the clinician is left with either proceeding to diagnostic sampling of lung fluid or tissue (using either induced sputum collection or bronchoscopy and BAL with or without transbronchial biopsy; Fig. 32.21), or treating an unknown condition empirically.

Induced sputum

Spontaneously expectorated sputum is inadequate for the diagnosis of PCP. Sputum induction by inhalation of ultrasonically nebulized, hypertonic saline for 20–60 minutes may provide a suitable specimen. The technique requires close attention to detail and is much less useful when samples are purulent. The sensitivity of induced sputum varies widely (55–90%), and therefore a negative result for *Pn. carinii* prompts further diagnostic studies.

Bronchoscopy

Fiberoptic bronchoscopy with BAL is commonly used to diagnose HIV-related pulmonary disease. When a good 'wedged' sample is obtained, the test has a sensitivity of over 90% for detection of *Pn. carinii* (Fig. 32.22). Fluorescent staining methods increase the diagnostic yield, which makes it the procedure of choice in most centers. More technically demanding (both of the patient and the operator) than induced-sputum collection, BAL has the advantages that direct inspection of the upper airway and bronchial tree is possible and, if necessary, biopsies can be taken. Transbronchial biopsies may marginally increase the diagnostic yield of the

Induced sputum, bronchoalveolar lavage, and surgical biopsy in the diagnosis of *Pneumocystis carinii* pneumonia				
Technique	Ease of procedure	Diagnostic sensitivity (%)	Cost	Notes
Induced sputum	Simple – once technique established	50–90	Low	Requires dedicated staff and facility Risk to staff from expectorated aerosol
Bronchoalveolar lavage	Moderate	90–>95	Moderate	Risk of deterioration post procedure Risk to staff from coughed secretions Sensitivity may be increased by two-lobe lavage
Surgical biopsy	Complex	>95	High	Requires staff with surgical expertise

Figure 32.21 Comparison of induced sputum, bronchoalveolar lavage, and surgical biopsy in the diagnosis of *Pneumocystis carinii* pneumonia.

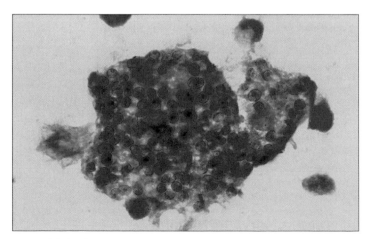

Figure 32.22 Bronchoalveolar lavage fluid with *Pneumocystis carinii*. Grocott's silver staining.

procedure. This is relevant for the diagnosis of mycobacterial disease, although the relatively high complication rate in HIV-infected individuals (pneumothorax in approximately 8%) outweighs the advantages of the technique for routine purposes.

Samples of BAL are examined for bacteria, mycobacteria, viruses, fungi, and protozoa. Inspection of the cellular component may also provide etiologic clues – co-operation of a pathology department with experience in opportunistic infection diagnosis is vital. The drug interactions associated with antiretroviral protease inhibitors mean that special care must be exercised when using either benzodiazepine or opiate sedation during bronchoscopy in patients on these drugs. Prolonged sedation and life-threatening arrhythmias have been reported[6].

A diagnostic strategy therefore includes sputum induction and, if the results are nondiagnostic or if the test is unavailable, bronchoscopy and BAL. If this does not yield a result, consideration is given to either a repeat bronchoscopy and BAL with transbronchial biopsies or surgical biopsy. The latter can be performed as either an open lung or thoracoscopic procedure. Surgical biopsy has a high sensitivity[11].

Empiric diagnosis

Although usually reserved for the management of presumed bacterial pneumonias, and at first sight may appear unwise when dealing with possible opportunistic infection, in reality PCP is almost invariably a diagnosis of exclusion and certain clinical and laboratory features may guide the assessment of an HIV-infected individual's risk for this condition. The likelihood that *Pn. carinii* is the causative organism increases if the subject is not taking effective pneumocystic drug prophylaxis and/or has a previous medical history with clinical or laboratory features that suggest systemic immunosuppression (i.e. recurrent oral thrush, long-standing fever of unknown cause, clinical AIDS, or blood CD4 count <200 cells/μl). Hence some centers advocate that empiric therapy may be used for HIV-infected patients who present with symptoms, chest radiographic, and blood gas abnormalities typical of mild PCP, without the need for bronchoscopy[12]. Invasive measures are reserved for those who have an atypical radiographic presentation, those who fail to respond to empiric therapy by day 5, and those who deteriorate at any stage.

Most clinicians in North America and the UK seek to obtain a confirmed diagnosis in every case of suspected PCP. In practice, both strategies appear to be equally effective, although a number of caveats must be borne in mind when empiric treatment is applied for PCP. Patients who have PCP typically take 4–7 days to show clinical signs of improvement, so a bronchoscopically proved diagnosis ensures that the correct treatment is given to the patient particularly in the first few days of therapy, when it may not be well tolerated. In addition, the diagnosis of PCP has implications for the infected individuals – it may be psychologically important to clarify whether or not they have an AIDS-defining illness and it may also influence their decision over starting either antiretroviral drug therapy or pneumocystic prophylaxis. Finally, empiric therapy requires the patient to be maximally adherent with the treatment, as otherwise nonresolution of the symptoms may be seen as failure of therapy rather than of compliance.

Nucleic acid detection

The techniques of molecular biology (such as PCR) are increasingly used in the diagnosis of respiratory disease. Two examples of this are DNA amplification of loci of the *Pn. carinii* and *M. tuberculosis* genomes[7]. The advantages of molecular methods are that the diagnosis can be made using body fluids more easily obtainable than BAL (i.e. expectorated sputum or nasopharyngeal secretions), and also that these methods are rapid (the answer may be available within a working day, compared with conventional mycobacterial culture, which may take weeks). However, despite encouraging results in the research setting (sensitivity and specificity reported as 60–100% and 70–100%, respectively), problems persist when these techniques are applied to routine diagnostic samples. These include extraction of nucleic acid from clinical material, cross-contamination with the products of previous assays, and clinical interpretation of a test result. It is expected that these difficulties will, within a short time, be overcome and that molecular methods will become a part of the standard diagnostic work-up.

TREATMENT

Individuals infected with HIV, when compared with the general population (i.e. not HIV infected), have an increased likelihood of adverse reactions to therapy, not just to TMP–SMX (see below), but to other drugs, including antimycobacterial agents. In addition, there are complex drug interactions with other medications, particularly the powerful combinations of highly active antiretroviral therapy[13]. Before instituting therapy for any infectious complication in an HIV-infected individual, it is important to consult with a physician experienced in the care of patients who have HIV infection and to seek advice from a specialist pharmacist.

Bacterial pneumonia

The spectrum of organisms that cause pneumonia in HIV-infected individuals is similar to the spectrum that cause community-acquired pneumonia in the general population. Thus, bacterial pneumonia in HIV-infected patients is treated in the same way as in the non-HIV-infected general population, using published American Thoracic Society and British Thoracic Society guidelines. In addition, expert advice on local antibiotic resistance patterns must be sought from infectious disease or microbiologist colleagues, as treatment is usually begun on an empiric basis before the causative organism is identified and the antibiotic sensitivities are known. The same clinical and laboratory prognostic indices that are described for the general population apply to HIV-infected individuals and are sought on presentation.

Response to the appropriate antibiotic therapy is usually rapid and is similar to that seen in the non-HIV-infected individual. Early relapse of infection following successful treatment is well described. Those HIV-infected patients who have presumed PCP, are being treated empirically with high-dose TMP–SMX, and have infection with either *Strep. pneumoniae* or *H. influenzae*, rather than *Pn. carinii*, also improve. In addition, in those patients who are treated with benzylpenicillin for proved *Strep. pneumoniae* pneumonia but do not respond, if penicillin resistance can be discounted as the cause, it is important to consider whether there is a second pathology, such as PCP.

Pneumocystis carinii pneumonia

Before instituting treatment, it is important to make an assessment of the severity of PCP using the history, findings on examination, arterial blood gas estimations, and chest radiographic abnormalities to stratify patients into those who have mild, moderate, or

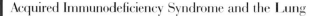

biopsies. Thoracic lymphomas in HIV-positive patients can have a distinctive tracheal or bronchial involvement – exophytic growths in tracheal or bronchial lumen, patchy necrosis of the tracheal or bronchial wall, mucosal thickening, and extrinsic compression. The demonstration of clonal rearrangements confirms the neoplastic origin of the infiltrate.

Hodgkin's lymphoma
Although HD has not been included in AIDS-defining conditions, it is five times more prevalent in patients who have AIDS than in HIV-negative individuals[15]. An interesting association between EBV infection and HD has been demonstrated in HIV-infected patients. The majority of cases are of the mixed cellularity type and most patients show a poor prognosis. Pulmonary involvement by HD is rare in HIV-infected patients[3,4]. It may occur with or without associated hilar and mediastinal lymphoadenopathy.

Lung cancer
The peculiar epidemiologic distribution of lung cancers in some ethnic populations and the demonstration that bronchogenic carcinoma may be documented in young patients (including intravenous drug users) raises the question whether frequency of pulmonary cancer increase during HIV infection[15]. Those HIV patients who develop lung cancers are usually young, male smokers with a history of intravenous drug use. The predominant histologic type of lung tumor in HIV-infected individuals is adenocarcinoma, and an association between pulmonary tuberculosis and lung cancer has been reported in some series of patients. Recently, the occurrence of pseudomesotheliomatous adenocarcinoma was reported in HIV-infected subjects. The usual symptoms include cough, dyspnea, and hemoptysis, as in non-HIV-infected patients. The diagnosis is made using the same diagnostic procedures as for non-HIV-infected patients (see Chapter 43). The prognosis is poor.

TREATMENT

Alveolitis associated with human immunodeficiency virus in asymptomatic patients
Clinical action is not required in subjects who have lymphocytic or macrophagic alveolitis but no symptoms – most cases resolve spontaneously.

Nonspecific interstitial pneumonitis
The patient is followed without therapy to evaluate whether NSIP spontaneously resolves or stabilizes. Corticosteroids may occasionally be used in HIV-infected patients who present with severe symptoms. Therapy with trimethoprim–sulfamethoxazole may have beneficial effects, even if infectious agents are not detected.

Lymphoid interstitial pneumonitis
Corticosteroids represent the treatment of choice for symptomatic patients who have LIP. Other immunosuppressants (chlorambucil) and antiviral therapy have been used in HIV-infected subjects who have LIP, but it is unclear whether immunosuppressive treatments should be used only until the patient shows improvement or whether they should be maintained for a longer period of time to avoid further recurrence of the disease.

Local immunodeficiency induced by human immunodeficiency virus
Chapter 32 describes symptoms, and clinical and radiologic findings observed in the different infectious complications that affect the respiratory tract during HIV disease and their treatment. A new therapy is needed to arrest the progression toward local immunodeficiency using highly active antiretroviral therapy and cytokines to reverse the alteration of the immunoregulatory networks that occurs in the pulmonary tract during HIV disease. However, the therapeutic application of these molecules is not yet determined.

Bronchiolitis obliterans organizing pneumonia
In the majority of patients, glucocorticoid treatment results in a remission or stabilization of the disease. Treatment using macrolides is helpful in cases of cryptogenic organizing pneumonia. Nonetheless, BOOP may rapidly relapse when corticosteroids are withdrawn, often within 1 month, but retreatment using corticosteroids re-establishes control of the condition in most cases.

Pulmonary hypertension related to human immunodeficiency virus
Specific treatments do not exist, but potent antiretroviral therapies may exert a beneficial effect on the pressure gradient.

Kaposi's sarcoma
Curative treatment options have not been clearly documented for KS, in particular for the pulmonary involvement of the disease, which has a life expectancy of less than 1 year[3,4]. While patients who have cutaneous KS may be observed or treated with α-interferon and antiviral therapy, chemotherapy and radiotherapy are the therapeutic modalities employed in patients who have visceral involvement. In general, vincristine and bleomycin are employed both as single agents and in dual-agent chemotherapy. Low-dose, multiagent chemotherapy is also used in advanced KS and involves various combinations of drugs that are active in single-agent chemotherapy [doxorubicin, bleomycin, vinblastine, actinomycin D (dactinomycin), decarbazine, and etoposide]. Liposomal doxorubicin seems to improve survival and quality of life in patients who have disseminated, AIDS-associated KS. Cases of regression of AIDS-associated KS after highly active antiretroviral therapy were reported recently. Unfortunately, concurrent opportunistic infections may be troublesome during chemotherapy. In addition, discontinuation of chemotherapy is associated with a high rate of relapse, and α-interferon does not prolong remission time.

Non-Hodgkin's lymphomas
Overall, the prognosis is poor and the patients are usually managed using chemotherapy. In particular, no chemotherapy regimens are designed specifically for HIV-related NHL in which patients are subdivided into individualized groups according to the presence or absence of prognostic factors. Patients who have a previous history of opportunistic infection and poor performance status are treated using low-dose chemotherapy regimens [e.g. a CHOP-like regimen (cyclophosphamide, vincristine, doxorubicin, and prednisone)] and antiviral therapy. Low-risk patients are eligible for intensive treatment [e.g. MACOP-B (methotrexate, doxorubicin, cyclophosphamide, vincristine, and prednisone) or LNH-84 (doxorubicin, cyclophosphamide, vindesine, bleomycin, and prednisone)]. For all patients, CNS and *P. carinii* prophylaxis are recommended.

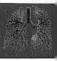

Hodgkin's lymphoma

Combinations of antineoplastic chemotherapy [MOOP (nitrogen mustard, vincristine, procarbazine, and prednisone) or ABVD (doxorubicin, bleomycin, vinblastine, and dacarbazine)] with and without antiretroviral therapy have been used to treat Hodgkin's lymphomas in HIV-infected patients.

Lung cancer

Surgery may be considered for resectable tumors. Chemotherapy is unlikely to help, and palliative measures are more appropriate in patients who have advanced disease.

CLINICAL COURSE AND PREVENTION

The development of a respiratory failure may be observed in most patients who suffer noninfectious, HIV-related pulmonary complications, particularly in severely immunocompromised patients who have a CD4+ T-cell count of <200 cells/mm³. Follow-up studies showed that superimposed opportunistic infections of the respiratory tract are the most important factors in the development of lung function abnormalities in patients who have idiopathic manifestations or lung neoplasms. Thus, preventive therapy for pulmonary infections is an important element in the management of HIV-infected patients who have noninfectious pulmonary complications.

Tuberculosis, P. carinii, and bacterial infections are the main targets of prophylaxis. Trimethoprim–sulfamethoxazole, pentamidine aerosols, and dapsone are used for the prophylaxis of pneumocystosis; specifically, P. carinii prophylaxis is indicated for all patients who receive chemotherapy, regardless of the CD4+ T-cell count. Isoniazid remains the recommended drug to prevent disease progression in HIV-infected patients coinfected with Mycobacterium tuberculosis. While bacterial infections are frequent in HIV-infected patients whose CD4+ T-cell count is <200 cells/mm³, clear guidelines for a preventive strategy of bacterial pneumonia do not exist; uncontrolled trials suggest the use of trimethoprim–sulfamethoxazole to protect against severe bacterial infections.

The frequency of fatal pulmonary complications that affect the clinical course of HIV infection has resulted in attempts to better define candidates for prophylaxis through an improved definition of risk factors for the development of respiratory failure. A number of abnormalities predict the clinical outcome of pulmonary involvement. The presence of gas-exchange abnormalities and the accumulation of neutrophils in BAL may strongly correlate with imminent mortality in HIV-seropositive patients who have pulmonary complications[3,7]. Phenotypic evaluation of BAL cell populations may also help to define the natural history of HIV-associated pulmonary complications – in the multivariate model a low number of BAL CD4+ T cells represents an adverse prognostic factor[7]. The rate of CD4+ T-cell decline in peripheral blood also predicts survival, but only up to a CD4+ T-cell count of 100 cells/mm³.

Recent findings suggest that HIV-infected individuals whose therapy involves potent antiretroviral drugs (double and triple regimens with protease inhibitors) have significantly lower mortality and longer AIDS-free survival. Inhibition of HIV replication using antiretroviral therapy may result in reduced infectiousness of the lung environment and improved local immune function. Indeed, in patients whose therapy involves protease inhibitors, the viral burden progressively reduces and the number of lung CD4+ T cells may increase. Favorable outcomes may result, with reductions in the incidence of infectious and noninfectious pulmonary complications.

PITFALLS AND CONTROVERSIES

Idiopathic and immunologic pulmonary manifestations

The differential diagnosis of pulmonary idiopathic inflammatory manifestations may be difficult in HIV-positive patients. A diagnosis of NSIP should be considered only after a reasonable effort has been made to exclude opportunistic infections in the lung. In particular, P. carinii must be carefully sought in induced sputum and BAL fluid. In addition, a transbronchial lung biopsy through a flexible or rigid bronchoscope is considered a necessary diagnostic step. The appropriate management of this condition is still unclear – the role of trimethoprim–sulfamethoxazole is under review, and probably a prophylaxis strategy using this antibiotic should be initiated in any patient.

A diagnosis that should be considered in children who have respiratory complications is LIP. Clinical experience suggests that LIP is quite uncommon in adults, so adults who have suspected LIP require an open lung biopsy to obtain a definitive diagnosis, inasmuch as the diagnostic yield of the transbronchial lung biopsy is poor. Specific therapies for LIP are limited, and the role of new anti-HIV drugs in the treatment of LIP in children is unclear.

As reported above, BOOP is a nonspecific histopathologic lung lesion. A number of infectious agents can give BOOP as their prevalent morphologic expression in immunocompromised hosts (e.g. Mycoplasma pneumoniae, Chlamydia pneumoniae, Legionella pneumophila, community-acquired pneumonias, P. carinii). Also, BOOP-like lesions occur as a manifestation of drug pulmonary toxicity or in tissues that surround neoplastic infiltration. Serologic tests, enzyme immunoabsorbent assays, immunofluorescence, immunohistochemical, and polymerase chain reaction tests on serum, BAL fluid, or lung tissue are recommended for the diagnosis of pulmonary infections. Exposure to drugs that are potentially toxic to the pulmonary tract or neoplastic involvement of the lung must be excluded. Some clinicians suggest that therapy with macrolides and/or rifampin (rifampicin) be used along with corticosteroids, even if the underlying infectious agents are not identified. Finally, since BOOP is a fairly common lesion in both immunocompetent and immunocompromised individuals, its occurrence may be merely coincidental in an HIV-infected subject.

As HIV-related PH is an incurable disease, clinicians should consider any alternative diagnostic hypothesis in which a specific treatment may help. A search for anticardiolipin and lupus anticoagulant antibodies and deep venous thromboses must be conducted, and a liver-related PH excluded.

The possible use of cytokines to modulate local immune responses is also unclear. The effect of cytokines on HIV viral replication in the pulmonary microenvironment needs to be specified. Several cytokines that could theoretically be used to restore the cell-mediated response in the lung of patients who have pulmonary opportunistic infections have been shown to upregulate viral expression in cells chronically or latently infected with HIV, which operatively prevents their therapeutic use. New biologic modifiers that may potentiate local antiviral mechanisms and avoid the risk of spread of HIV infection are needed.

Acquired Immunodeficiency Syndrome and the Lung

Lung neoplasms

As KS is related to HHV-8, it is important to establish whether detection of this virus in BAL fluid could be a sensitive and specific method to diagnose tracheobronchial KS. Pitfalls in the diagnosis of AIDS-associated KS may arise because the differential diagnosis of granulation tissue in the lung or of bacillary angiomatosis (rarely reported in lung parenchyma of HIV-infected subjects) may be difficult.

A number of clinical trials using different chemotherapeutic agents for pulmonary malignancies linked to HIV infection are underway. However, comparison of the efficacy of the chemotherapeutic regimens being used is fraught with difficulties. Pitfalls present in many clinical trials often reflect the staging systems used to group patient populations. Naturally, partial remission rate differs between patients who belong to better or worse prognostic groups, or between patients who have more or less limited neoplastic disease. Furthermore, it is unclear whether antiviral therapy should be started at the end of the chemotherapy regimen and, if so, which drug to use. The palliative therapy to use in HIV patients who have poor prognosis is also unclear.

Epidemiologically, the significance of lung cancer in young patients who have HIV infection needs to be established.

REFERENCES

1. Agostini C, Zambello R, Trentin L, Semenzato G. HIV and pulmonary immune responses. Immunol Today. 1996;17:359–64.
2. Plata F, Autran B, Martins LP, Wain-Hobson S, Raphael M, Mayaud C. AIDS-virus specific cytotoxic T lymphocytes in lung disorders. Nature. 1987;328:348–51.
3. Semenzato G, ed. AIDS and the lung. Eur Respir Monogr. 1995;2:1–384.
4. White DA, Stover DE, eds. Pulmonary complications of HIV infection. Clin Chest Med. 1996;17:621–822.
5. Pantaleo G, Graziosi C, Demarest JF, et al. Role of lymphoid organs in the pathogenesis of human immunodeficiency virus (HIV) infection. Immunol Rev. 1994;140:105–30.
6. Semenzato G, Agostini C, Ometto L, et al. CD8$^+$ T lymphocytes in the lung of AIDS patients harbor human immunodeficiency virus type 1. Blood. 1995;85:2308–14.
7. Agostini C, Adami F, Poulter LW, et al. Role of bronchoalveolar lavage in predicting survival of patients with HIV-1 infection. Am J Respir Crit Care Med. 1997;156:1501–7.
8. Israel-Biet D, Cadranel J, Beldjord K, Andrieu M, Jeffrey A, Even P.
Tumor necrosis factor production in HIV-seropositive subjects. Relationship with lung opportunistic infections and HIV expression in alveolar macrophages. J Immunol. 1991;147:490–4.
9. Saukkonen JJ, Farber HV. Lymphocytic interstitial pneumonitis. In: Zumla A, Johnson MA, Miller RF, eds. AIDS and respiratory medicine. London:Chapman & Hall; 1997:331–43.
10. Mani S, Smith GJ. HIV and pulmonary hypertension: a review. South Med J. 1994;87:357–62.
11. Mesa RA, Edell ES, Dunn WF, Edwards WD. Human immunodeficiency virus infection and pulmonary hypertension: two new cases and a review of 86 reported case. Mayo Clin Proc. 1998;73:37–45
12. Levine AM. AIDS-related malignancies: the emerging epidemic. J Natl Cancer Inst. 1993;85:1382–97.
13. Biggar R, Rabkin S. The epidemiology of acquired immunodeficiency syndrome-related lymphoma. Curr Opin Oncol. 1992;4:883–93.
14. Levine AM. Acquired immunodeficiency syndrome-related lymphoma. Blood. 1992;80:8–20.
15. Tirelli U, Vaccher E, Spina M. Other cancers in HIV-infected patients. Curr Opin Oncol. 1994;6:508–11.

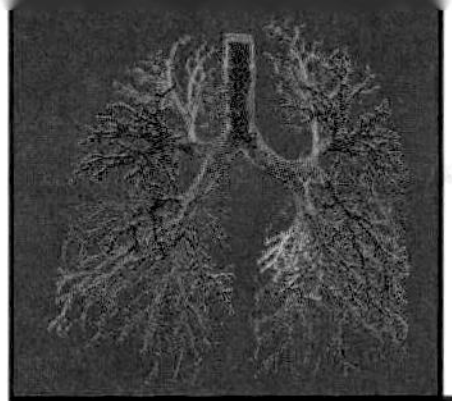

Chapter 34

β-Agonists, Anticholinergics, and Other Nonsteroid Drugs

Peter J Barnes

INTRODUCTION

Asthma therapy can be classified into two main types – bronchodilators (or relievers), which give rapid relief of asthma symptoms, and controllers, which give long-term control of asthma symptoms either by suppression of the chronic inflammatory process (anti-inflammatory drugs), by inhibition of the release of bronchoconstrictors, or by some other mechanism that does not involve a direct relaxant effect on airway smooth muscle (Fig. 34.1)[1]. Chronic obstructive pulmonary disease (COPD) is treated predominantly by bronchodilators, as there is little evidence that controllers influence progression of COPD. In this chapter the mode of action and the clinical use of the main classes of drug used in asthma therapy, apart from corticosteroids (see Chapter 7.35), are reviewed. While drugs are traditionally classified as controllers and relievers, some drugs, such as theophylline and antileukotrienes, appear to have bronchodilator and anti-inflammatory properties.

β₂-AGONISTS

Inhaled β₂-agonists are the most effective bronchodilators and have minimal side effects when used correctly, and so they are the treatment of choice. Short-acting and nonselective β-agonists, such as isoproterenol (isoprenaline) and orciprenaline, have no place.

Mode of action

β-Agonists produce bronchodilatation by directly stimulating β₂-receptors in airway smooth muscle, which leads to relaxation. This can be demonstrated *in vitro* by the relaxant effect of isoproterenol on human bronchi and lung strips (indicating an effect on peripheral airways) and *in vivo* by a rapid decrease in airway resistance. β-Receptors have been demonstrated in airway smooth muscle by direct receptor-binding techniques, and autoradiographic studies indicate that β-receptors are localized to smooth muscle of all airways from the trachea to the terminal bronchioles[2].

Activation of β₂-receptors results in activation of adenylate cyclase and an increase of intracellular cyclic adenosine-3,5-monophosphate (cAMP) (Fig. 34.2). This leads to activation of a specific kinase (protein kinase A) that phosphorylates several target proteins within the cell, resulting in:

- lowering of intracellular calcium ion (Ca^{2+}) concentration by active removal of Ca^{2+} from the cell into intracellular stores;
- inhibitory effect on phoshoinositide hydrolysis;
- direct inhibition of myosin light-chain kinase;
- opening of a large-conductance, calcium-activated potassium channel (K_{Ca}) that repolarizes the smooth muscle cell and may stimulate the sequestration of Ca^{2+} into intracellular stores (β-agonists may be directly coupled to K_{Ca}, and relaxation of airway smooth muscle may therefore occur independently of an increase in cAMP).

Current therapy for asthma

Relievers (bronchodilators)	Controllers (anti-inflammatory treatments)
β₂-Agonists	Corticosteroids
Theophylline	Cromones
Anticholinergics	Antileukotrienes
	Corticosteroid-sparing therapies:
	Methotrexate
	Gold
	Cyclosporin A

Figure 34.1 Current therapy for asthma.

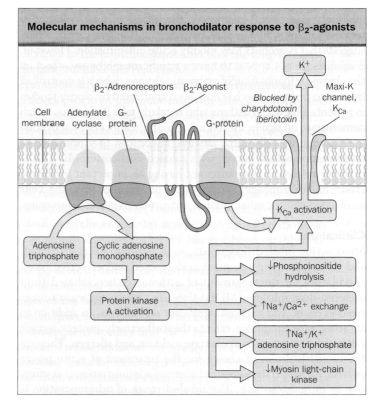

Molecular mechanisms in bronchodilator response to β₂-agonists

Figure 34.2 Molecular mechanisms involved in bronchodilator response to β2-agonists. Activation of β₂-adrenoceptors on airway smooth muscle cells is coupled via a G-protein to adenylyl cyclase, which results in increased intracellular cyclic adenosine monophosphate formation. This activates protein kinase A which phosphorylates a number of substrates, including large-conductance calcium-activated potassium channels (maxi-K, K_{Ca}), which can also be directly coupled to β₂-receptors.

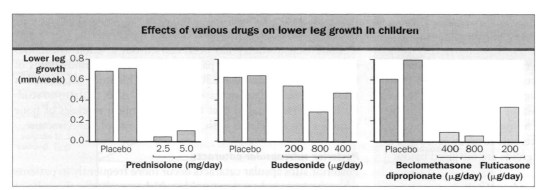

Figure 35.8 Effect of treatment with placebo, prednisone 2.5 or 5.0mg for 1 week, or increasing inhaled doses of budesonide, beclomethasone dipropionate (BDP), or fluticasone on lower leg growth, measured by knemometry, in children. Prednisone and BDP 400 or 800μg/day significantly reduced lower leg growth. (Adapted with permission from Barnes and Pedersen[17] ©American Lung Association.)

Risks of lung infection

Risks of lung infection are not increased in patients who use inhaled glucocorticosteroids. Also, inhaled glucocorticosteroids do not increase the risks of reactivation of pulmonary tuberculosis, and therefore prophylactic isoniazid treatment is not needed when inhaled glucocorticosteroids are used in patients who have inactive pulmonary tuberculosis.

Skin bruising

Skin bruising does occur as a dose-dependent side effect of inhaled corticosteroid use. It is rare at daily doses of <1000μg/day, and its incidence increases with age and duration of treatment. In one study of older patients on high doses of BDP, the prevalence of easy bruising was 47% for those on inhaled glucocorticosteroids and 22% for those who were not[24].

CONCLUSIONS

Corticosteroids are a valuable and widely used treatment for a variety of lung diseases. Inhaled corticosteroids are the mainstay of asthma treatment, and their pharmacokinetics, pharmacodynamics, and systemic unwanted effects have been the focus of extensive research since their introduction in 1972. The availability of topically potent corticosteroids, with effective first-pass metabolism in the liver, has ensured that the efficacy is obtained in almost all patients at doses not associated with clinically relevant unwanted effects.

REFERENCES

1. Gelfand ML. Administration of cortisone by the aerosol method in the treatment of bronchial asthma. N Engl J Med. 1951;245:293–4.
2. Medical Research Council. Controlled trial of effects of cortisone acetate in status asthmaticus. Lancet. 1956;2:803–6.
3. Foulds GS, Greaves DP, Herxheimer H, Kingdom LG. Hydrocortisone in treatment of allergic conjunctivitis, allergic rhinitis, and bronchial asthma. Lancet. 1955;1:234–5.
4. Muller M, Renkawitz R. The glucocorticoid receptor. Biochem Biophys Acta. 1991;1088:171–82.
5. Toogood JH, Baskerville JC, Errington N, Jennings B, Chuang L, Lefcoe NM. Determinants of the response to beclomethasone aerosol at various dosage levels: a multiple regression analysis to identify clinically useful predictors. J Allergy Clin Immunol. 1977;60:367–76.
6. Toogood JH, Baskerville JC, Jennings B, Lefcoe NM, Johansson S-A. Bioequivalent doses of budesonide and prednisone in moderate and severe asthma. J Allergy Clin Immunol. 1989;84:688–700.
7. Ryrfeldt A, Andersson P, Edsbacker S, Tonnesson M, Davies D, Pauwels R. Pharmacokinetics and metabolism of budesonide, a selective glucocorticoid. Eur J Respir Dis. 1982;63:86–95.
8. Brogden RN, McTavish D. Budesonide. An updated review of its pharmacological properties and therapeutic efficacy in asthma and rhinitis. Drugs. 1992;44:375–407.
9. Pedersen S, Steffensen G, Ekman I, Tonnesson M, Borga O. Pharmacokinetics of budesonide in children with asthma. Eur J Clin Pharmacol. 1987;31:579–82.
10. Miller-Larsson A, Mattsson H, Hjertberg E, et al. Reversible fatty acid conjugation of budesonide. Novel mechanism for prolonged retention of topically applied steroid in airway tissue. Drug Metab Dispos. 1998;26:623–30.
11. O'Byrne PM, Cuddy L, Taylor DW, Birch S, Morris J, Syrotiuk J. The clinical efficacy and cost benefit of inhaled corticosteroids as therapy in patients with mild asthma in primary care practice. Can Respir J. 1996;3:169–75.
12. van Essen-Zandvliet EE, Hughes MD, Waalkens HJ, Duiverman EJ, Pocock SJ, Kerrebijn KF. Effect of 22 months of treatment with inhaled corticosteroids and/or β2-agonists on lung function, airway responsiveness and symptoms in patients with asthma. Am Rev Respir Dis. 1992;146:547–54.
13. Pauwels RA, Lofdahl C-G, Postma DS, O'Byrne PM, Barnes PJ, Ullman A. Effect of inhaled formoterol and budesonide on asthma exacerbations. N Engl J Med. 1997;337:1405–11.
14. Busse WW. Chervinsky P, Condemi J, et al. Budesonide delivered by Turbuhaler is effective in a dose-dependent fashion when used in the treatment of adult patients with chronic asthma. J Allergy Clin Immunol.1998;101:457-63.
15. Pedersen S, Hansen OR. Budesonide treatment of moderate and severe asthma in children: a dose–response study. J Allergy Clin Immunol. 1995;95:29–33.
16. Dahl R, Lundback B, Malo J, et al. A dose-ranging study of fluticasone propionate in adult patients with moderate asthma. Chest. 1998;104:352–8.
17. Barnes PJ, Pedersen S. Efficacy and safety of inhaled corticosteroids in asthma. Am Rev Respir Dis. 1993;148:S1–26.
18. Laitinen LA, Laitinen A, Haahtela T. A comparative study of the effects of an inhaled corticosteroid, budesonide, and of an inhaled β2-agonist, terbutaline, on airway inflammation in newly diagnosed asthma. J Allergy Clin Immunol. 1992;90:32–42.
19. Bisgaard H, Damkjaer Nilsen M, Andersen B. Adrenal function in children with bronchial asthma treated with beclomethasone dipropionate or budesonide. J Allergy Clin Immunol. 1988;80:213–17.
20. Birkebaek NH, Esberg G, Andersen K, Wolthers O, Hassager C. Bone and collagen turnover during treatment with inhaled dry powder budesonide and beclomethasone dipropionate. Arch Dis Child. 1995;73:524–7.
21. Wolthers O, Hansen M, Juul A, Niehörster M, Nielsen H, Pedersen S. Knemometry, urine cortisol excretion, and measures of the insulin-like growth factor axis and collagen turnover in children treated with inhaled glucocorticosteroids. Pediatr Res. 1997;41:44–50.
22. Balfour-Lynn L. Effect of asthma on growth and puberty. Pediatrician. 1987;24:237–41.
23. Wolthers OD, Pedersen S. Short term growth during treatment with inhaled fluticasone propionate and beclomethasone dipropionate. Arch Dis Child. 1993;90:517–19.
24. Mak VHF, Melchor R, Spiro SG. Easy bruising as a side-effect of inhaled corticosteroids. Eur Respir J. 1992;5:1068–74.

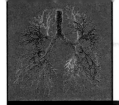

Section 7 Airway Diseases: pharmacology of the airway

Chapter 36

Delivery of Medication to the Lungs

Stephen Spiro and G Mac Cochrane

INTRODUCTION

The value of the inhaled route to carry medication to the lungs has long been realized, as by ancient civilizations in India and China, and by individuals, such as Hippocrates and Galen. Sulfurs, volatile aromatic substances, such as menthol and eucalyptus, and smoke from plant leaves, such as *Atropa belladonna*, were used.

Inhaled therapy has, in principle, several advantages over other routes – aerosol particles have a favorable surface-to-volume ratio, which allows a small dose to disperse widely over airways and alveolar surfaces. The dose can be small, side effects minimal, and (in some lung diseases) the onset of action rapid. However, for the dose to be effective, it needs to be delivered from a simple, readily usable vehicle, to be of the optimal particle size, and to arrive at the correct target within the respiratory system. The available modes for delivery of drug particles to the lung are remarkably inefficient, but the small doses that arrive can invoke dramatic and rapid responses, which make this the preferred mode of delivery of bronchodilators, inhaled corticosteroids (ICS), anticholinergic medication, and also, in special situations, antibiotics, mucolytics, and sometimes just saline.

The most common vehicles for delivery are the pressurized metered-dose inhalers (pMDIs), dry-powder inhaler (DPI) systems, and nebulizers of liquid drug. The main delivery systems are summarized in Figure 36.1.

AEROSOLS

An aerosol is a suspension of fine particles (liquid or solid) in air with a range of particle sizes. A mist is an aerosol made by dispersion of liquid particles (e.g. nebulized), and a dust or smoke is from solids.

The size of the particles and their distribution are expressed as if the aerosol is composed of a suspension of spheres of different diameters. The mass median diameter of the aerosol is the diameter about which 50% of the total particle mass resides. The mass median aerodynamic diameter (MMAD) is the product of the mass median diameter and the square route of the particle density. The MMAD of an aerosol has a profound effect on where the majority of particles that enter the lung land and thereby act. Particle deposition is influenced by inspiratory flow – the higher the entry flow, the more central is the deposition – because of inertial impaction, particularly of large particles (>6μm diameter). Smaller particles (<5μm diameter) reach smaller airways and those of 2–3μm diameter reach the alveoli. Small particles may not settle and are expired. The relationship of site of deposition and particle size is shown in Figure 36.2.

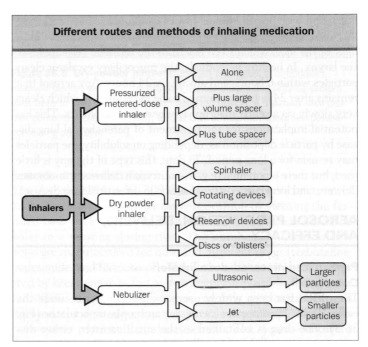

Figure 36.1 Different routes and methods of inhaling medication.

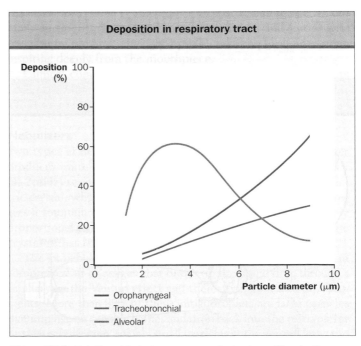

Figure 36.2 Relationship between percentage deposition in the respiratory tract and the diameter of the aerosol particles.

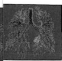
majority. Skin bruising does occur and is related to the duration of use of the ICS, the dose given, and the patient's age[8]. A spacer seems to make no impact on the prevention of skin bruising, which probably results from lung systemic absorption.

In children, no evidence of serious systemic side effects (e.g. growth stunting) has been found if the ICS are taken in moderate doses (<800µg/day). Serum cortisol is, however, affected by ICS within 4 weeks of regular treatment of budesonide or beclomethasone in children who taking 400µg/day[9]. The nocturnal serum cortisol production fell by 35% after 4 weeks of treatment and the urinary cortisol by 48%. However, ACTH and growth hormone values were not affected by treatment with either drug[9]. Nevertheless, other studies report no adrenal suppression, including when children take 800µg/day of budesonide or beclomethasone[10]. However, the lowest possible dose of ICS should always be used.

If the ICS is given through a nebulizer, the patient should inhale via a mouthpiece and not use a face mask, as the latter permits deposition on the face with the risk of thinning of the facial skin.

Anticholinergics

Ipratropium bromide can cause a dry mouth, particularly if given in higher nebulized doses. Care should also be taken to avoid nebulization with a face mask – use a mouthpiece – as the mist can drift into the eyes and occasionally cause acute glaucoma.

Freon effect

The cooling effect of the boiling off of CFCs can cause upper airway bronchoconstriction with cough, wheeze, and breathlessness.

COMPLIANCE

Poor adherence to medication regimens is a well-documented phenomenon and compliance with the prescribed dosage depends on the patient's perception of the risks and benefits of treatment, frequency of dosing, complexity of the regimen, and duration of treatment. Little information is available on the compliance of patients who use inhaled medication – it is almost impossible to check this in individuals. Therapeutic levels are undetectable in the serum. Consultations and prescription collection is a possible way to monitor, but patients may accumulate inhalers, especially the relievers, and keep one in several places (e.g. bathroom, living room, car). Lack of compliance may also involve overuse, particularly of reliever medication, which may be detected by earlier prescription demand than normal, but overuse is less common than failure to take prophylactic medication.

In a 2-year study of pMDI adherence as part of the Lung Health Study, compliance was assessed both by questionnaire and canister weight. At 1 year self-reported satisfactory compliance was confirmed by canister weight in only 48% of participants. At the first 4 months follow-up visit, only 70% of participants reported satisfactory adherence to their prescribed treatment, and this declined to 60% over the next 18 months. The best compliers were those who were married, older, Caucasian, had more severe airways obstruction, less shortage of breath, and fewer hospital admissions, and who had not been confined to bed for respiratory illness[11].

Noncompliance is also associated with a complex mix of psychosocial factors, such as higher-than-average depression and anxiety scores[12].

The other aspect of compliance is proper use (see Fig. 36.4). In a study of 56 subjects who had asthma or COPD, measurements made with an unobtrusive sensing system attached to a pMDI showed that only 25% of inhalations were acceptably performed[13]. Men were better than women, and there were no differences in technique between younger and older subjects, or between those who had asthma or COPD. Thus, most patients of all ages are likely to use a pMDI incorrectly.

Patient education, with regular checks on inhaler technique, is essential to ensure optimal choice and delivery of these extremely effective drug-delivery systems.

REFERENCES

1. Zainuddin BMZ, Biddiscombe M, Tolfree SEJ, Short M, Spiro SG. Comparison of bronchodilator responses and deposition patterns of salbutamol inhaled from a pressurised metered dose inhaler, as a dry powder inhaler, and as a nebulized solution. Thorax. 1990;45:469–73.

2. Chrystyn H. Is total particle dose more important than particle distribution? Respir Med. 1997;91(Suppl. A):17–19.

3. Melchor R, Biddiscombe M, Mak VHF, Short M, Spiro SG. Lung deposition patterns of directly labelled salbutamol in normal subjects and in patients with reversible airways obstruction. Thorax. 1993;48:506–11.

4. Mitchell DM, Soloman MA, Tolfree SEJ, Short M, Spiro SG. Effect of particle size of bronchodilator aerosol on lung distribution and pulmonary function in patients with chronic asthma. Thorax. 1987;42:456–61.

5. Zainuddin BMZ, Tolfree SEJ, Short M, Spiro SG. Influence of breathing pattern on lung deposition and bronchodilator response to nebulized salbutamol in patients with stable asthma. Thorax. 1988;43:987–91.

6. Muers MF. The rational use of nebulizers in clinical practice. Eur Respir Rev. 1997;7:189–97.

7. Cochrane GM. Acute severe asthma: oxygen and high dose beta agonist during transfer for all? Thorax. 1995;50:1–2.

8. Mak VHF, Melchor M, Spiro SG. Easy bruising as a side effect of inhaled corticosteroids. Eur Respir J. 1992;5:1068–74.

9. Nicholaizik WH, Marchant JL, Preece MA, Warner JO. Endocrine and lung function in asthmatic children on inhaled corticosteroids. Am J Respir Crit Care Med. 1994;150;624–8.

10. Goldstein DE, Konig P. Effect of beclomethasone diproprionate on hypothalamic–pituitary–adrenal axis function in children with asthma. Pediatrics. 1983;72:60–4.

11. Rand CS, Nides M, Cowles MK, Wise RA, Connett J for the Lung Health Study Research Group. Long term metered-dose inhaler adherence in a clinical trial. Am J Respir Crit Care Med. 1995;152:580–8.

12. Bosley CM, Fosbury JA, Cochrane GM. The psychological factors associated with poor compliance with treatment in asthma. Eur Respir J. 1995;8:899–904.

13. Goodman DE, Israel E, Rosenberg M, Johnston R, Weiss ST, Drazen JM. The influence of age, diagnosis and gender on proper use of metered-dose inhalers. Am J Respir Crit Care Med. 1994;150:1256–61.

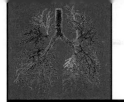

Section 7 Airway Diseases: chronic airflow limitation

Chapter 37

Chronic Obstructive Pulmonary Disease

Bartolome Celli, Joshua Benditt, and Richard K Albert

Chronic obstructive pulmonary disease (COPD) is character-ized by airflow limitation that results from intrinsic airways dis-ease (e.g. chronic bronchitis), bronchospasm, and/or emphysema (e.g. the parenchymal destruction with associated loss of elastic recoil, which leads to a reduction in the tethering, or distending, function of the lung parenchyma on airways). The airflow limi-tation is generally progressive, may be accompanied by airway hyperactivity, and may be potentially reversible to some extent[1,2].

Chronic bronchitis is defined in clinical terms as the presence of chronic cough with sputum production that occurs most days of the week, at least 3 months a year, for more than two con-secutive years, in the absence of other specific causes (e.g. asthma, bronchiectasis, cystic fibrosis). Importantly, most patients who have only chronic bronchitis do not have any substantive air-flow limitation. Those who do not should not be classified as having COPD. Pathologic findings that correlate with a clinical history of chronic bronchitis include mucosal and submucosal edema and inflammation, with an increase in the number and size of the submucosal mucus glands (Fig. 37.1). This aspect is quan-tified by relating it to the thickness of the corresponding bronchial wall (i.e. the Reid index).

Emphysema is defined pathologically as a permanent, abnor-mal air-space enlargement that occurs distal to the terminal bron-chiole, and includes destruction of alveolar septa (Fig. 37.2). When the distribution of the emphysema is limited to the res-piratory bronchioles, as opposed to the more terminal air spaces, the disease is categorized as centriacinar. When both the proxi-mal and distal air spaces are involved the disease is categorized as panacinar. Histologic examination frequently demonstrates that the two distributions coexist.

Asthma is an inflammatory disease of the airways that results in reversible airflow limitation. Figure 37.3 graphically represents the interrelationships of the different components grouped under the COPD heading and depicts the various types of overlap that may be seen clinically. Although the large majority of patients who seek care for COPD have a combination of chronic bronchitis,

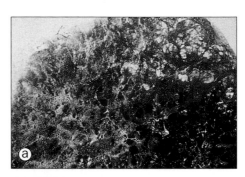

Figure 37.2 Pathologic specimens of (a) panlobular and (b) centrilobular emphysema.

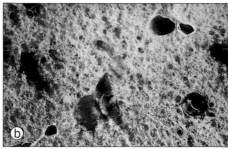
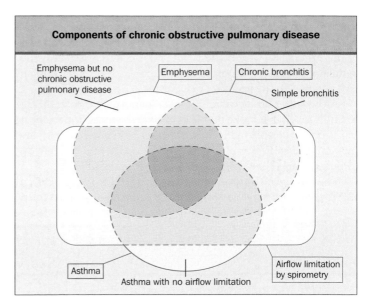

Components of chronic obstructive pulmonary disease

Emphysema but no chronic obstructive pulmonary disease

Emphysema

Chronic bronchitis

Simple bronchitis

Asthma

Asthma with no airflow limitation

Airflow limitation by spirometry

Figure 37.3 Components of chronic obstructive pulmonary disease (COPD). Each circle represents a nosologic entity. The rectangle represents airflow limitation as documented in a forced vital capacity maneuver. The shaded area corresponds to patients diagnosed as having COPD. Notice that a patient may present with emphysema but no COPD (e.g. a patient who has bullae on chest radiography but no airflow limitation). Similarly, a patient may present with sputum production and normal spirometry (with simple bronchitis). Finally, an asthmatic may present with no airflow limitation, and is only diagnosed after a positive bronchoprovocation test.

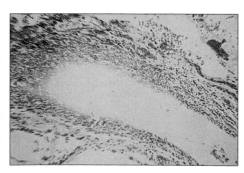

Figure 37.1 Histology of bronchitis.

emphysema, and airflow limitation, importantly many patients can have chronic bronchitis with no airflow limitation, and airflow limitation can occur from conditions that are not associated with COPD or asthma (e.g. upper airway obstruction, tracheomalacia). Most patients who suffer asthma have substantial reversible airways constriction and respond well to inhaled and systemic anti-inflammatory therapy, and therefore do not have COPD. The small minority of asthmatics who develop minimally reversible airflow limitation are considered to have COPD and are treated as such. An additional subgroup that is not depicted in Figure 37.3 are patients who have smoking-related chronic bronchitis and some degree of fixed airflow limitation, and who develop a marked, acute increase in the extent of their airflow limitation in association with episodes of acute bronchitis. These patients are classified as having asthmatic bronchitis, and some investigators suggest that they may have both asthma and COPD.

EPIDEMIOLOGY, RISK FACTORS, AND PATHOPHYSIOLOGY

Approximately 14 million people in the USA have COPD, and the number affected has increased by 42% since 1982. Although the prevalence in adult men varied from 4 to 6% between 1979 and 1986, and from 1 to 3% in adult women, the prevalence has increased more for women than for men over this period.

In 1991, COPD was the fourth leading cause of death in the USA (85,544 people) and was the most rapidly increasing cause of death between 1979 and 1991 (a 33% increase)[3]. The age-adjusted death rate from COPD rose 72% between 1966 and 1986, during which time death from heart and cerebrovascular disease decreased 45 and 85%, respectively.

Although the percentage of the population that smokes has progressively declined in the USA (mostly because of reduced smoking rates in men rather than women), the habit is still practiced by 75 million citizens in that country alone. Assuming the same prevalence worldwide (and evidence suggests that it may actually be higher), an astonishing total of 1.2 billion humans are exposed to the ravages of cigarettes.

Although a number of additional independent risk factors for COPD have been identified (Fig. 37.4), the most important by far is cigarette smoking[4]. The only other risk factor of comparable importance is α_1-antitrypsin (AAT) deficiency, but this disorder accounts for <1% of patients who have COPD.

The only host factor proven to lead to COPD is deficiency of AAT[5] (see Chapter 39). This serum glycoprotein is coded for by

a single gene on chromosome 14, is produced in the liver, and inhibits the activity of neutrophil elastase. The normal range of AAT is 150–350mg/dL (commercial standard) or 20–48mg/dL (laboratory standard). Rare patients who have normal levels of dysfunctional AAT have been reported. Most patients with severe AAT deficiency are homozygous for the Z allele (i.e. PiZZ) and generally have AAT levels <20% of normal. These patients develop premature emphysema, often with chronic bronchitis, nonspecific airway hyperreactivity, and occasionally with bronchitis. The onset of their disease is accelerated by smoking, as symptoms begin at a median age of 50 years in nonsmokers but 40 years in smokers. The threshold protective level of AAT seems to be around 80mg/dL (about 35% of normal) since heterozygous patients (i.e. PiSZ) who have levels in this range rarely develop emphysema. Not all patients who have AAT deficiency develop emphysema, especially if they are not exposed to cigarettes or pollution. Patients should be screened for AAT if they present with a premature onset of COPD (before 50 years of age), predominance of basilar emphysema (on radiography), presence of nonremitting asthma in a young person, or liver cirrhosis with no apparent risk factors.

In some countries where solid fuels are used for indoor temperature control without adequate ventilation, and in other heavily industrialized urban environments, an increased prevalence of COPD has been noted in nonsmokers, suggesting pollutants are involved in the pathogenesis. Variations in the frequency of acute COPD exacerbations have been associated with variations in air pollution, particularly sulfur dioxide concentrations.

Children and adults who are exposed to cigarette smoke passively manifest a higher prevalence of respiratory symptoms and diseases than those who are not. Exposed children also have measurable abnormalities in pulmonary function tests. Although some hypothesize that childhood exposure alone may lead to COPD, this has yet to be established.

The morbidity and mortality of COPD is higher in Caucasians than in non-Caucasians, and is higher in blue-collar than in white-collar workers. Also, COPD aggregates in families independently of AAT deficiency.

Cell biology

A number of neutrophil and macrophage enzymes can destroy various components of the extracellular matrix and cause emphysema (e.g. elastase, cathepsin G, collagenase, gelatinase). The lung parenchyma has a ready source of neutrophils that adhere to the pulmonary microcirculation. Their enzyme-containing granules can be released without the cells having to move across the cellular barriers into the interstitium or alveolus, and the enzymes can degrade matrix even in the presence of high concentrations of inhibitors[6]. Recognition of the importance of proteases in the development of emphysema stems from a number of experimental studies in which inhalation or instillation of various elastases resulted in histologic evidence of emphysema after resolution of an initial inflammatory response. Interaction between various proteases is suggested because elastase-induced emphysema is worse in animals that also receive trypsin or chymotrypsin[7].

Mechanics and gas exchange

Functionally, COPD is characterized by a reduction in airflow that becomes more prominent on maximal exhalation[8]. The distribution of airflow limitation is not uniform, such that the

Risk factors for the development of chronic obstructive pulmonary disease		
Established	**Probable**	**Possible**
Cigarette smoking	Air pollution	Low birth weight
Occupational exposure (wood smoke)	Poverty	Childhood respiratory infections
	Childhood exposure to smoke	Family history
α_1-Antitrypsin deficiency	Alcohol	Atopy
	Hyperreactive airways	IgA nonsecretor
		Blood group A

Figure 37.4 Risk factors for the development of chronic obstructive pulmonary disease.

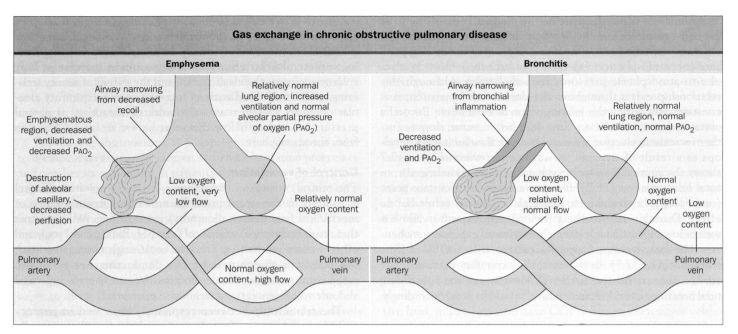

Gas exchange in chronic obstructive pulmonary disease

Figure 37.5 Ventilation/perfusion distribution in emphysema (left) and in bronchitis (right).

distribution of alveolar ventilation is heterogeneous. In patients who have a preponderance of emphysema (as opposed to bronchitis; Fig. 37.5), the heterogeneous distribution of ventilation is matched by a similar heterogeneous distribution of perfusion, as the emphysematous destruction of the terminal lung units includes destruction of the corresponding alveolar capillaries. When this occurs, the volume of blood that perfuses the poorly ventilating alveoli is very low, such that the reduction in pulmonary venous oxygen content may be trivial (Fig 37.5, left panel). If the emphysematous process is more widespread, the degree of capillary destruction can be so extensive that pulmonary arterial pressure can increase and the degree of perfusion through even relatively well-ventilated regions can exceed the degree of ventilation, which results in hypoxemia.

In patients who have a greater extent of bronchitis, the ability to redirect perfusion away from poorly ventilated regions is impaired (perhaps as a result of inflammatory cytokines with vasodilatory capacity that are generated as part of the airway inflammation). The resultant ventilation/perfusion (V̇/Q̇) heterogeneity causes hypoxemia (Fig. 37.5, right panel)[9]. As elastic recoil worsens, physiologic dead space and work of breathing increase, the maximum minute ventilation (V̇E) becomes limited by airflow limitation and approaches the resting V̇E, which eventually decreases the alveolar ventilation and an increase in arterial partial pressure of carbon dioxide ($PaCO_2$) results.

Since the relationship between structure and function in COPD is poorly understood[10–12], correlation between the degree of emphysema or bronchitis, as evaluated by currently available scoring systems, and the degree of airflow limitation is poor. At present, the best predictor of morbidity and mortality is the postbronchodilator forced expiratory volume in 1 second (FEV_1).

During inhalation, the bellows must draw air through the conducting airways into alveoli. The ability to do so depends on the strength of the respiratory muscles, the compliance of the respiratory system (i.e. the lung and chest wall), and the resistance of the airways. Normally, exhalation is passive, and is

governed by elastic recoil. In emphysema, the respiratory system compliance is increased, manifested by a shift of the lung pressure–volume curve up and to the left (Fig. 37.6). Both emphysematous and normal lungs undergo a greater volume change in response to a given change in transpulmonary pressure at lower, compared with higher, lung volumes. As a result of the increased compliance seen in emphysema, however, the disparity is augmented such that areas that are the most overdistended receive the least ventilation.

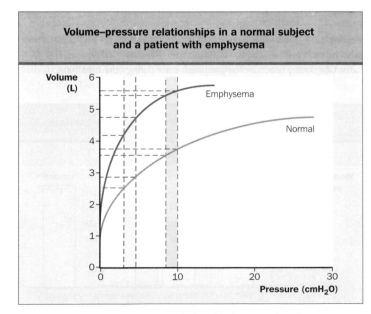

Volume–pressure relationships in a normal subject and a patient with emphysema

Figure 37.6 Volume–pressure relationship in normal and emphysemic lung. At low volume, a small change in pressure results in a larger volume increase in the emphysematous lung. At higher lung volume, a similar change in pressure results in minimal change in volume in the emphysematous lung, which now behaves as a stiff lung (see text for details). ($10cmH_2O = 1kPa$.)

patients under stable conditions as their disease progresses. If this observation is correct, respiratory muscle function could potentially be improved by assisting inhalation mechanically (and/or by reducing the inspiratory load by countering auto-PEEP). Although a number of studies provide evidence to support this idea, other studies give no indication that intermittent, noninvasive ventilatory assistance has this effect.

The respiratory muscles are forced to work at a length that limits their contractile strength in patients who have COPD because of the hyperinflation that develops with the progression of the emphysema. Initial reports of the effect that lung volume reduction surgery (LVRS) has on respiratory muscle function indicate that both the strength and pattern of recruitment improve, presumably because a more normal diaphragmatic curvature and chest wall diameter are restored.

Integrative approach

The numerous components of the respiratory system can be integrated into a comprehensive model, as shown in Figure 37.10. Central to the model are the problems of loss of elastic recoil, airway narrowing, and hyperinflation. To reverse this abnormal physiology in this system, elastic recoil must be increased and the extent of airway narrowing and hyperinflation must be decreased. Each of these objectives is accomplished by LVRS, at least over the short term (i.e. 3–6 months following surgery).

CLINICAL FEATURES

A summary of the clinical evaluation of COPD is given in Figure 37.11.

History

The typical patient who develops COPD has smoked more than 20 pack years before symptoms develop. Those whose smoking history is less extensive should be evaluated for AAT deficiency and/or for asthma. Frequently, COPD patients present in the fifth decade of life and complain of a cough productive of mucoid sputum, or of an acute respiratory illness. Although dyspnea is usually not observed until the sixth or seventh decade, it may become a crippling symptom that leads to markedly decreased physical activity.

During exacerbations, sputum generally increases in volume and becomes purulent. These episodes of acute bronchitis are usually accompanied by increased dyspnea, bronchospasm, and low-grade fever. As the disease progresses, the intervals between exacerbations shorten. Late in the course, the patient may develop hypoxemia, which (if severe) may manifest as cyanosis, which can be accentuated by erythrocythemia. Complaints of morning headache suggest the presence of hypercapnia. Weight loss occurs in some patients (although the mechanism is, as yet, undefined), and cor pulmonale with right ventricular failure and edema may develop in those who have abnormal oxygenation. Hemoptysis may be reported by patients who have bronchitis, raising the concerns for bronchogenic carcinoma. Although such COPD patients are obviously at increased risk for carcinoma, and bronchoscopic evaluation is generally undertaken when hemoptysis occurs, most episodes result from bronchial mucosal inflammation rather than from cancer.

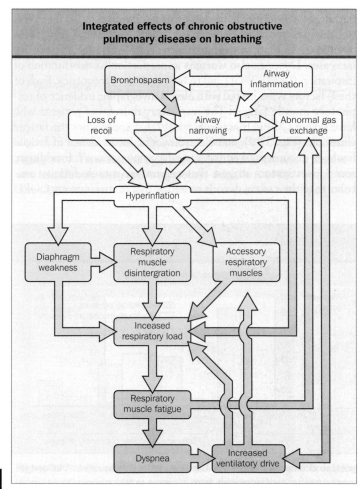

Figure 37.10 Effects of chronic obstructive pulmonary disease on breathing. (See text for details.)

Clinical evaluation of chronic obstructive pulmonary disease	
Evaluation	**Symptom**
History	Positive smoking history
	Family history
	Cough, sputum production
	Dyspnea
	Exercise limitation
Physical	Increased respiratory rate
	Increased anteroposterior diameter of thorax
	Use of accessory respiratory muscles
	Retraction of the lower rib cage
	Prolonged exhalation
	Bronchospasm
	Edema
	Cor pulmonale (increased jugular venous pressure, pedal edema)
Laboratory	Decreased forced expiratory volume in one second (FEV_1) and FEV_1/forced vital capacity
	Radiographic evidence of emphysema
	Decreased diffusing capacity of lung for carbon monoxide
	Hypoxemia and hypercapnia (but arterial blood gases may approach normal)

Figure 37.11 Clinical evaluation of chronic obstructive pulmonary disease.

Physical examination

Initially, the chest examination may only show wheezes on forced exhalation. As airflow limitation progresses, however, hyperinflation becomes evident by inspection as the anteroposterior diameter of the chest increases. The diaphragm flattens and becomes limited in its caudal motion. Breath sounds are decreased at this stage, and heart sounds often become distant with displacement of the point of maximal intensity to the subxiphoid region. Decreases in elastic recoil and/or increases in airway narrowing are demonstrated when forced exhalation continues for >4 seconds, when measured with the stethoscope placed over the trachea. Patients who have COPD breathe at a more rapid rate than normal individuals, but rarely at a rate >30 breaths per minute because of the expiratory flow limitation. Faster rates are indicative of impending ventilatory failure.

The patient who has end-stage COPD may adopt postures that relieve and/or facilitate the function of the accessory respiratory muscles (i.e. leaning forward while standing or sitting with the arms positioned on the knees or table), and thereby reduce dyspnea (Fig. 37.12). Exhalation often occurs through pursed lips, or even through narrowed vocal cords, with an audible, high-pitched expiratory humming. Forced contractions of the abdominal muscles can be seen throughout the expiratory cycle, and these increase at end exhalation. A paradoxical inward movement of the lower chest wall during inhalation is a classic finding, first described by William Stokes in 1837. In the setting of cor pulmonale, neck veins are distended, the liver may be enlarged, patients may have right upper-quadrant tenderness, and bilateral pedal edema occurs. Kussmaul's sign (i.e. increasing jugular venous pressures during inhalation) may be observed in the absence of heart failure, as a result of the compressive effect of lung inflation on cardiac filling. Asterixis may be found with severe hypoxemia or hypercapnia.

DIAGNOSIS

Chest radiography

Since emphysema is defined anatomically, it is reliably diagnosed using standard imaging modalities. Hyperinflation is shown by a flattened diaphragm on the lateral chest film[19], and the volume of retrosternal air space may be enlarged (Fig. 37.13). The posteroanterior view can show large, elongated lungs with a narrow cardiac silhouette. Rapid tapering of the vascular markings accompanied by hyperlucency of the lungs is a characteristic finding, as are emphysematous bullae >1cm in diameter (although bullae have several causes, some of which are not associated with emphysema). Studies that correlate lung structure with chest radiography show that emphysema can only be diagnosed when the disease is severe. Although computed tomography (CT), particularly high-resolution CT, has a greater sensitivity and specificity than standard chest radiography for detecting emphysema (Fig. 37.14)[20], it has little place in the

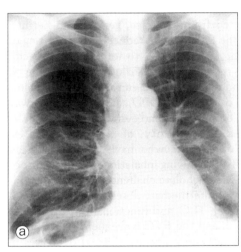
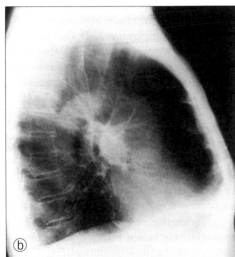

Figure 37.13 Posteroanterior (a) and lateral (b) chest radiographs of a patient who has emphysema.

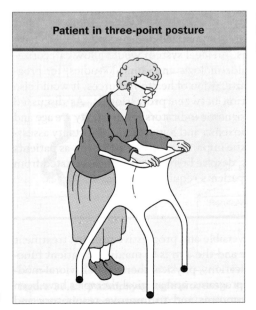

Patient in three-point posture

Figure 37.12 Patient in three-point posture.

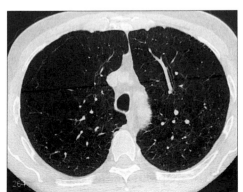

Figure 37.14 High-resolution computed tomography of a patient who has emphysema.

REFERENCES

1. European Respiratory Society. Optimal assessment and management of chronic obstructive pulmonary disease. Eur Respir J. 1995;1398–420.

2. American Thoracic Society. Standards for the diagnosis and care of patients with chronic obstructive pulmonary disease. Am J Respir Crit Care Med. 1995;152:78–121.

3. Feinlieb M, Rosenberg HM, Collins JG, Delozier JE, Pokras R, Chevarley FM. Trends in COPD morbidity and mortality in the United States. Am Rev Respir Dis. 1989;140:S9–18.

4. Buist SA. Smoking and other risk factors. In: Murray JF, Nadel JA, eds. Textbook of respiratory medicine, 2nd edn. Philadelphia: WB Saunders; 1994:1259–87.

5. Snider GL. Pulmonary disease in alpha-1-antitrypsin deficiency. Ann Intern Med. 1989;111:957–9.

6. Lucey EC, Stone PJ, Snider GL. Consequences of proteolytic injury. In: Crystal RG, West JB, eds. The lung: scientific foundations. New York: Raven Press; 1789–801.

7. Osman M, Keller S, Hosannah Y, Canator JO, Turino GM, Mandl I. Impairment of elastin resynthesis in the lungs of hamsters with experimental emphysema induced by sequential administration of elastase and trypsin. J Lab Clin Med. 1985;105:254–8.

8. Bates DV. Respiratory function in disease, 3rd edn. Philadelphia: WB Saunders; 1989;172–87.

9. Wagner PD, Dantzker DR, Dueck R, Clausen JL, West JB. Ventilation–perfusion inequality in chronic obstructive pulmonary disease. J Clin Invest. 1977;59:203–16.

10. Thurlbeck WM. Pathophysiology of chronic obstructive pulmonary disease. Clin Chest Med. 1990;11:389–403.

11. Berend N, Woolcock AJ, Marlin GE. Correlation between the function and the structure of the lung in smokers. Am Rev Respir Dis. 1979;119:695–702.

12. Nagai A, Yamawaki I, Takizawa T, Thurlbeck WM. Alveolar attachments in emphysema of human lungs. Am Rev Respir Dis. 1991;144:888–91.

13. Begin P, Grassino A. Inspiratory muscle dysfunction and chronic hypercarpnia in chronic obstructive pulmonary disease. Am Rev Respir Dis. 1991;143:905–12.

14. Gorini M, Misuri G, Corrado A, et al. Breathing patterns and carbon dioxide retention in severe chronic obstructive pulmonary disease. Thorax 1996;51:677–83.

15. De Troyer A, Estenne M. Functional anatomy of the respiratory muscles. Clin Chest Med. 1988;9:175–93.

16. Martinez FJ, Couser JI, Celli BR. Factors influencing ventilatory muscle recruitment in patients with chronic airflow obstruction. Am Rev Respir Dis. 1990;142:276–82.

17. Killian K, Jones N. Respiratory muscle and dyspnea. Clin Chest Med. 1988;9:237–48.

18. Cohen C, Zagelbaum G, Gross D, Roussos C, Macklem PT. Clinical manifestations of inspiratory muscle fatigue. Am J Med. 1982;73:308–16.

19. Sanders C. The radiographic diagnosis of emphysema. Radiol Clin North Am. 1991;29:1019–30.

20. Klein JS, Gamsu G, Webb WR, Golden JA, Müller NL. High-resolution CT diagnosis of emphysema in symptomatic patients with normal chest radiographs and isolated low diffusing capacity. Radiology. 1992;182:817–21.

21. Auerbach O, Hammond EC, Garfinkel L, Benante C. Relation of smoking and age to emphysema. Whole-lung section study. N Engl J Med. 1972;286:853–7.

22. The Intermittent Positive Pressure Breathing Trial Group. The intermittent positive pressure breathing therapy of chronic obstructive pulmonary disease. A clinical trial. Ann Intern Med. 1983;99:612–20.

23. Lacasse Y, Wong E, Guyatt GH, King D, Cook DJ, Goldstein RS. Meta-analysis of respiratory rehabilitation in chronic obstructive pulmonary disease [see comments]. Lancet. 1996;348:1115–19.

24. Pavia D, Agnew JE, Glassman JM, et al. Effects of iodopropylidene glycerol on tracheobronchial clearance in stable, chronic bronchitic patients. Eur J Respir Dis. 1985;67:177–84.

25. Medical Research Council Working Party. Long term domiciliary oxygen therapy in chronic hypoxic cor pulmonale complicating chronic bronchitis and emphysema. Report of the Medical Research Council Working Party: Skeletal muscle adaptation to endurance training in patients with chronic obstructive pulmonary disease. Lancet. 1981;28:681–6.

26. Nocturnal Oxygen Therapy Trial Group. Continuous or nocturnal oxygen therapy in hypoxemic chronic obstructive lung disease: a clinical trial. Nocturnal Oxygen Therapy Trial Group: Ann Intern Med. 1980;93:391–8.

27. Celli BR. Pulmonary rehabilitation for patients with advanced lung disease. Clin Chest Med. 1997;18:521–34.

28. Wijkstra PJ, Van A-R, Kraan J, Otten V, Postma DS, Koeter GH. Quality of life in patients with chronic obstructive pulmonary disease improves after rehabilitation at home. Eur Respir J. 1994;7:269–73.

29. Celli BR. The clinical use of upper extremity exercise. Clin Chest Med. 1994;15:339–49.

30. Leith DE, Bradley M. Ventilatory muscle strength and endurance training. J Appl Physiol 1976;41:508–16.

31. Ries AL, Kaplan RM, Limberg TM, Prewitt LM. Effects of pulmonary rehabilitation on physiologic and psychosocial outcomes in patients with chronic obstructive pulmonary disease. Am Int Med. 1995;122:823–32.

32. Maltais F, LeBlanc P, Simard C, et al. Skeletal muscle adaptation to endurance training in patients with chronic obstructive pulmonary disease. Am J Respir Crit Care Med. 1996;154:442–7.

33. Benditt JO, Albert RK. Surgical options for patients with advanced emphysema. Clin Chest Med. 1997;18:577–93.

34. Fitzgerald M, Keelan P, Angell D. Long-term results of surgery for bullous emphysema and chronic obstructive pulmonary disease. Surgery. 1974;68:566–82.

35. Brantigan O, Mueller E, Kress M. A surgical approach to pulmonary emphysema. Am Rev Respir Dis. 1959;80:194–201.

36. Cooper JD, Trulock EP, Triantafillou AN, et al. Bilateral pneumectomy (volume reduction) for chronic obstructive pulmonary disease. J Thorac Cardiovasc Surg. 1995;109:106–16 (discussion 116–19).

37. Cooper JD, Pohl MS, Patterson GA. An update on the current status of lung transplantation: report of the St. Louis International Lung Transplant Registry. Clin Transplant. 1993;1993:95–100.

38. Meyer TJ, Hill NS. Noninvasive positive pressure ventilation to treat respiratory failure [see comments]. Ann Intern Med. 1994;120:760–70.

39. Shapiro SH, Macklem PT, Gray D-K, et al. A randomized clinical trial of negative pressure ventilation in severe chronic obstructive pulmonary disease: design and methods. J Clin Epidemiol. 1991;44:483–96.

40. Fletcher EC, Luckett RA, Miller T, Costarangos C, Kutka N, Fletcher JG. Pulmonary vascular hemodynamics in chronic lung disease patients with and without oxyhemoglobin desaturation during sleep. Chest. 1989;95:757–64.

41. Fletcher C, Peto R. The natural history of chronic airflow obstruction. Br Med J. 1977;1:1645–8.

42. Anthonisen NR, Connett JE, Kiley JP, et al., for the Lung Health Study Group. The effects of smoking intervention and the use of an inhaled anticholinergic bronchodilator on the rate of decline of FEV_1: The Lung Health Study. JAMA. 1994;272:1497–505.

43. Smee C. Effect of tobacco advertising on tobacco consumption: a discussion document reviewing the evidence. London: Economic and Operational Research Division, Department of Health; 1992.

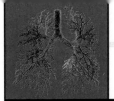

Chapter
38

Management of Acute Exacerbations

Jadwiga A Wedzicha and Peter R Mills

EPIDEMIOLOGY

Exacerbations of chronic obstructive pulmonary disease (COPD) are a major cause of morbidity and mortality. They lead to frequent hospital admissions and contribute greatly to the cost of managing patients who have COPD. Approximately 30,000 deaths result from exacerbations of COPD per year in the UK. In 1986, nearly 2 million Americans were hospitalized for COPD exacerbations, and this represented the fifth most frequent cause of death[1]. Although no long-term, large-scale studies exist, data from smaller ones in which patients were followed for several years after their acute exacerbation indicate that the exacerbation does not adversely affect the decline in forced expiratory volume in 1 second (FEV_1) over time.

Although the pathophysiology and etiology of acute exacerbations are poorly understood, they have been associated with a number of precipitating factors (Fig. 38.1). Exacerbations occur more frequently with increasing severity of COPD. Many seem to be associated with bacterial infection or viruses, particularly rhinovirus and others that cause the common cold. That COPD exacerbations are more common in the winter months has been attributed to an increased seasonal viral load, which causes more airway inflammation[2]. Patients who suffer COPD may have increased airflow obstruction during the winter, and thus may become even more susceptible to those factors that cause acute exacerbations. Environmental factors, such as atmospheric pollutants, may also be important.

The number of past exacerbations is a predictor of exacerbation frequency, which suggests that some patients may have a particular susceptibility. The quality of life scores for the subgroup of COPD patients who suffer frequent acute exacerbations is reduced compared with those affected by similar degrees of airflow limitation who do not[3].

Most patients who have acute exacerbations can be treated as outpatients, and only the most severe ones, associated with arterial blood gas deterioration, are admitted to hospital.

Pathophysiology

Relatively little information is available on the pathologic changes that occur in the airway during a COPD exacerbation. Airway inflammation increases, which produces a variable increase in airflow obstruction as a result of mucosal and submucosal edema, mucus accumulation in the airway, and/or bronchospasm that develops in response to release of a variety of inflammatory mediators (Fig. 38.2). The resultant air-trapping increases the work of breathing, as both chest wall and lung parenchymal compliance are reduced, and the development of autopositive end-expiratory pressure requires that the patient generate a more negative pleural pressure to initiate inspiratory flow. The adverse effects of the increased

work are magnified by the reduction in the mechanical performance of the respiratory muscles as they lengthen in response to the air-trapping, and exceed their optimal length–tension relationship.

Minute ventilation may be normal during an acute exacerbation, but the respiratory rate is generally increased while the tidal volume is decreased. Although this breathing pattern may

Factors that precipitate exacerbations of chronic obstructive pulmonary disease	
Type	**Examples**
Bacterial infection	*Streptococcus pneumoniae*, *Haemophilus influenzae*, *Moraxella catarrhalis*
Viral infections	Rhinovirus, influenza A and B viruses, adenovirus
Atmospheric pollutants	Particulate matter (<10μm diameter and ultrafine particles)
Temperature	Drops in both indoor and outdoor temperatures

Figure 38.1 Factors that precipitate exacerbations of chronic obstructive pulmonary disease.

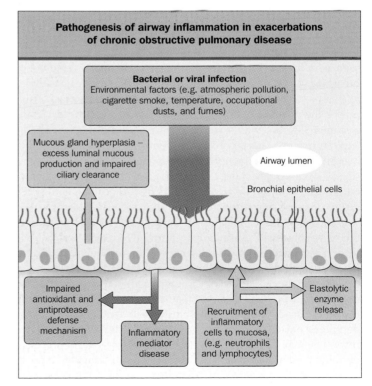

Figure 38.2 Pathogenesis of airway inflammation in exacerbations of chronic obstructive pulmonary disease (COPD). The interplay of different factors involved in the pathogenesis of airway in ammation in exacerbations of COPD.

be optimal with regard to reducing the work of breathing, the associated increase in physiologic dead space impairs carbon dioxide elimination, and the resulting acidemia can further reduce inspiratory muscle function.

The hypoxemia seen in acute COPD exacerbations results from a combination of alveolar hypoventilation and an increase in ventilation–perfusion ($\dot{V}/\dot{Q}$) heterogeneity. The reduction in alveolar ventilation occurs because of the factors summarized above. Increases in $\dot{V}/\dot{Q}$ heterogeneity are attributed to:

- reduction in the efficiency of hypoxic vasoconstriction as a result of an increase in pulmonary artery pressure (which develops in response to the alveolar hypoxia) and/or the release of vasodilating inflammatory mediators;
- inability to redirect perfusion away from poorly ventilating alveoli because of diffuse disease or a reduction in the pulmonary vascular bed, which occurs as part of the emphysematous process.

Acidemia may be an important adverse prognostic factor[4].

CLINICAL FEATURES

Acute exacerbations of COPD most frequently present with increasing cough, increasing or decreasing sputum production, an increase in the purulence and viscosity of the sputum, and a worsening of dyspnea. The effect of this deterioration depends on the severity of the underlying disease. There may be a recent history of upper respiratory tract infection. Patients who have night time hypoxemia and/or carbon dioxide retention may report morning headaches or even confusion. Associated symptoms include an increase in aerophagia, a diminished appetite, orthopnea, and a deterioration in sleep duration and quality. Some patients describe a substernal burning sensation, generally associated with coughing, and others complain of an inability to clear secretions from the throat.

Patients generally appear in distress. Accessory muscle use is seen with increasing severity of the exacerbation and purse-lip breathing may be observed frequently. Wheezing may be audible without a stethoscope. On occasion, patients may spontaneously mimic the effects of purse-lip breathing by using their larynx in a similar fashion, which results in a prolonged, high-pitched, expiratory hum. This is particularly common in those affected by overinflated lungs and emphysematous changes (Fig. 38.3). Vital signs show tachypnea and tachycardia, and blood pressure may be reduced in response to the effects of autopositive end-expiratory pressure. Hypertension also occurs as a function of acute respiratory acidemia. Cyanosis is an insensitive physical finding but, when observed, commonly indicates hypoxemia and/or erythrocythemia. Finger or ear-lobe oxmetry may frequently indicate hypoxemia, but a normal or low–normal oxygen saturation does not exclude the possibility of carbon dioxide retention and acute respiratory acidemia. The vasodilatation associated with hypercapnia causes warm, flushed skin, papilledema, and a strong peripheral pulse. Patients who have severe, acute carbon dioxide retention may present in coma. If cor pulmonale is present, peripheral edema is observed, as is an elevated jugular venous pressure, hepatomegaly, and/or ascites. Cardiac sounds are frequently difficult to hear because of the wheezing and air-trapping, but are most frequently found in the subxiphoid region as a result of lung inflation on the position of the heart. A right ventricular gallop may be heard in the setting of pulmonary hypertension.

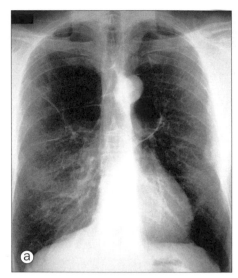

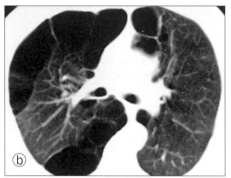

Figure 38.3 Radiograph and computed tomography (CT) scan of a patient who has chronic obstructive pulmonary disease (COPD). (a) Chest radiograph of a patient with COPD. Note the hyperinflated lungs and decrease in pulmonary markings. (b) Chest CT scan of the same patient shows areas of bullous emphysema and consequent pulmonary arterial prominence.

DIAGNOSIS

No additional investigations are required in patients affected by mild-to-moderate exacerbations, and are deemed to be candidates for outpatient therapy. Patients who suffer more severe exacerbations and require admission need a careful evaluation for conditions that might mimic, or be associated with, the acute respiratory decompensation. The decision to admit a patient is made on the basis of a number of factors, which include the patient's living circumstances, mental status, degree of hypoxemia and/or hypercapnia, and routinely taken medications. Those who are too dyspneic to manage the activities of daily living independently or who have confusion or a deterioration of their arterial blood gases require admission, as might those who are already on a maximal outpatient medical regimen that includes systemic corticosteroids.

When respiratory decompensation is observed in the absence of a history of acute bronchitis, and if the patient does not have clinical or radiographic evidence of pneumonia, it is important to search for another cause of such a presentation that may require a completely different therapeutic approach (e.g. pulmonary embolus, pneumothorax, pulmonary edema, noncompliance with medications, any type of problem that results in decreased abdominal compliance, which, in turn, limits the inspiratory excursion of the diaphragm).

Any patient admitted to the hospital with an acute exacerbation of COPD must have arterial blood gases measured, with care taken to record the inspired oxygen concentration at the time the blood is obtained. Hypoxemia should be corrected, but an arterial saturation greater than 90–92% is not needed, and may be detrimental (see below). Some suggest obtaining a daily measurement of airflow

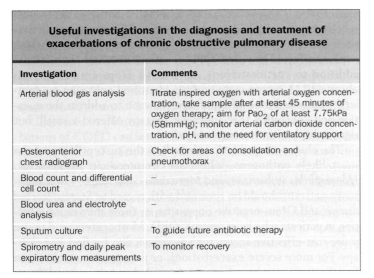

Useful investigations in the diagnosis and treatment of exacerbations of chronic obstructive pulmonary disease	
Investigation	**Comments**
Arterial blood gas analysis	Titrate inspired oxygen with arterial oxygen concentration, take sample after at least 45 minutes of oxygen therapy; aim for PaO_2 of at least 7.75kPa (58mmHg); monitor arterial carbon dioxide concentration, pH, and the need for ventilatory support
Posteroanterior chest radiograph	Check for areas of consolidation and pneumothorax
Blood count and differential cell count	–
Blood urea and electrolyte analysis	–
Sputum culture	To guide future antibiotic therapy
Spirometry and daily peak expiratory flow measurements	To monitor recovery

Figure 38.4 Useful investigations for the diagnosis and treatment of exacerbations of chronic obstructive pulmonary disease.

(e.g. FEV_1 or peak flow), but the utility of this practice has not been established. Other investigations are summarized in Figure 38.4.

TREATMENT

Treatment of exacerbations of COPD is given in Figure 38.5.

Pharmacologic

Inhaled bronchodilator therapy

Both β_2-agonists [e.g. albuterol (salbutamol)] and anticholinergic agents (e.g. ipratropium bromide) are generally administered to patients who suffer an acute exacerbation. Although both have bronchodilating activity, symptomatic improvement can be attained without marked changes in spirometry, probably as a result of reduced air-trapping[5]. Studies in stable COPD have found that anticholinergic agents produce a greater bronchodilator response than that seen with β_2-agonists, presumably because of the excessive, cholinergic, neuronal bronchoconstrictor tone seen in this condition and/or loss or downregulation of β_2-receptors[6]. When the two agents are given in combination there seems to be an additive effect, although this point is still unclear in the setting of acute exacerbations[7–9].

Although many physicians routinely administer bronchodilators via a nebulizer, numerous studies have found no benefit to nebulization over simple, metered dose inhalers (MDIs) – assuming the patients are capable of activating the MDI. Spacers seem to allow patients more freedom regarding the timing of MDI activation and actual inhalation, although studies of efficacy in the setting of acute exacerbations are lacking.

Of far greater importance is the technique used by patients when they administer inhaled agents. Many studies indicate that inhaler technique is frequently suboptimal in stable outpatients who have COPD. The situation is likely to be far worse during acute exacerbations. Clinical experience indicates that the most common problem is that patients begin the inhalation at a lung volume that is far above functional residual capacity or residual volume. Accordingly, the 'vital capacity' is so small that a minimal amount of nebulized medication actually reaches the lower airway. When the medications are delivered by nebulization most patients

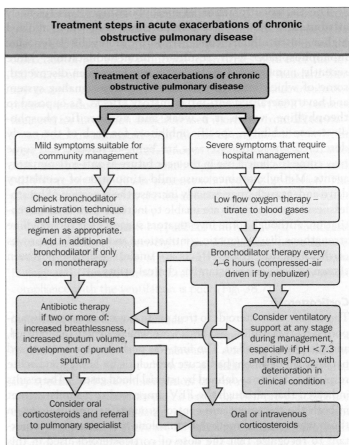

Figure 38.5 Treatment of exacerbations of chronic obstructive pulmonary disease.

simply perform repeated tidal breathing, with no attempt to reach maximum inspiratory capacity. Additional errors frequently encountered include inhaling the medication too rapidly (which results in excess deposition on the posterior pharynx) and failure to hold the inspiration for a few seconds (to allow the medication to deposit on the airway walls). To assure maximum bronchodilator delivery, patients must be carefully coached and prompted to exhale to near maximum prior to triggering the MDI and starting inhalation.

The dose and frequency of bronchodilator administration are also unclear. One end of the spectrum proposes continuous, high-dose nebulization. The other (based on a variety of *in-vitro* studies) suggests that prolonged contact of β_2-agonists with their receptors interferes with intracellular transport of corticosteroids to their upstream regulatory sites on a variety genes, and thereby interferes with anti-inflammatory protein production.

Methylxanthines

Methylxanthines such as theophylline were previously used extensively in the management of both stable COPD and acute exacerbations. Although they do have bronchodilating effects, the degree of response is far less than that seen after inhaled β_2-agonists or anticholinergics. Studies of intravenous aminophylline therapy in acute exacerbations of COPD showed no significant beneficial effect over and above that of conventional therapy[10]. In addition, the propensity of methylxanthines to cause side effects (most commonly nausea and difficulty sleeping) is high, and many medications and acute and chronic illnesses interfere with methylxanthine metabolism, and thereby raise blood levels to toxic concentrations.

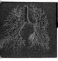
quality of life[23]. A smaller study suggests that patients who die within 2 years of an episode of respiratory failure do so from conditions other than COPD[24].

Influenza and pneumococcal vaccinations are recommended for all patients with COPD. Long-term antibiotic therapy has been used in patients with very frequent exacerbations, although there is little evidence of effectiveness. Recently, the effects of an immunostimulatory agent were reported for patients who had COPD exacerbations, with reduction in severe complications and hospital admissions in the actively treated group[25]. Further studies on the effects of these agents are required.

Increased patient education about detecting and treating exacerbations is necessary. More specific written treatment plans for the at-risk COPD patients may be useful (as are produced for asthmatics), though such an approach requires testing. Following an exacerbation, the COPD patient's condition should be reviewed and attention given to risk factors and compliance with therapy.

PITFALLS AND CONTROVERSIES

Although exacerbations are an important event in the natural history of patients who have COPD, limited information is available on the frequency of exacerbations and their effect on the course of COPD. A recent study showed that patients who suffer COPD tend to under-report exacerbations, and many of the exacerbations in the community are self-limiting[4]. Patients who have COPD accept their chronic disability and may not notice warning symptoms of deterioration in their clinical condition. It is possible that earlier presentation to the doctor with the exacerbation could prevent complications, although this has not been investigated. Not only should COPD patients receive education about their disease, but also instruction on the need to recognize symptoms of exacerbation at an early stage.

A number of randomized trials have shown NIPPV to be effective in the management of acute exacerbations with respiratory failure. However, most of the studies recruited patients with pH levels of <7.35, and few of these studies included patients with pH <7.26, when the prognosis is reduced. It is possible that a number of these patients would have improved spontaneously, and no comparisons have been made of the use of NIPPV in patients with pH levels of 7.27–7.35, as opposed to patients with pH levels <7.26. Administration of NIPPV requires skilled staff, who must be available on a 24-hour basis.

REFERENCES

1. Higgins MW, Thorn T. Incidence, prevalence and mortality: intra and intercountry difference. In Hensley MJ, Saunders NA, eds. Clinical epidemiology of chronic obstructive pulmonary disease. New York: Marcel Dekker; 1989;23–39.
2. Donaldson GC, Seemungal T, Evans C, Paul EA, Wedzicha JA. Effects of outdoor temperature on daily lung function and exacerbations in patients with COPD. Thorax 1996;51:A19.
3. Seemungal TA, Donaldson GC, Paul EA, Bestall JC, Jeffries DJ, Wedzicha JA. Effect of exacerbation on quality of life in patients with chronic obstructive pulmonary disease. Am J Respir Crit Care Med. 1998;157:1418–22.
4. Jeffrey AA, Warren PM, Flenley DC. Acute hypercapnic respiratory failure in patients with chronic obstructive lung disease: risk factors and use of guidelines for management. Thorax. 1992;47:34–40.
5. Belman MJ, Botnick WC, Shin JW. Inhaled bronchodilators reduce dynamic hyperinflation during exercise in patients with chronic obstructive pulmonary disease. Am J Respir Crit Care Med. 1996;153:967–75.
6. Braun SR, McKenzie WN, Copeland C, Knight L, Ellersieck M. A comparison of the effect of ipratropium and albuterol in the treatment of chronic obstructive airway disease. Arch Intern Med. 1989;149:544–7.
7. Combivent Inhalation Aerosol Study Group. In chronic obstructive pulmonary disease, a combination of ipratropium and albuterol is more effective than either agent alone. Chest. 1994;105:1411–19.
8. Rebuck AS, Chapman KR, Abboud R, et al. Nebulized anticholinergic and sympathomimetic treatment of asthma and chronic obstructive airways disease in the emergency room. Am J Med. 1987;82:59–64.
9. Karpel JP. Bronchodilator responses to anticholinergic and beta-adrenergic agents in acute and stable COPD. Chest. 1991;99:871–6.
10. Rice KL, Leatherman JW, Duane PG, et al. Aminophylline for acute exacerbations of chronic obstructive pulmonary disease. A controlled trial. Ann Intern Med. 1987;107:305–9.
11. Albert RK, Martin TR, Lewis SW. Controlled clinical trial of methylprednisolone in patients with chronic bronchitis and acute respiratory insufficiency. Ann Intern Med. 1980;92:753–8.
12. Thompson WH, Nielson CP, Carvalho P, Charan NB, Crowley JJ. Controlled trial of oral prednisolone in outpatients with acute COPD exacerbations. Am J Respir Crit Care Med. 1996;154:407–12.
13. Anthonisen NR, Manfreda J, Warren CPW, Hershfield ES, Harding GKM, Nelson NA. Antibiotic therapy in exacerbations of chronic obstructive pulmonary disease. Ann Intern Med. 1987;106:196–204.
14. Sachs APE, Koeter GH, Groenier KH, Van der Waaij D, Schiphuis J, Meyboom-de Jong B. Changes in symptoms, peak expiratory flow and sputum flora during treatment with antibiotics of exacerbations in patients with chronic obstructive pulmonary disease in general practice. Thorax. 1995;50:758–63.
15. Saint S, Bent S, Vittinghoff E, Grady D. Antibiotics in chronic obstructive pulmonary disease exacerbations. A meta-analysis. JAMA. 1995;273:957–60.
16. Moser KM, Luchsinger PC, Adamson JS, et al. Respiratory stimulation with intravenous doxapram in respiratory failure. N Engl J Med. 1973;288:427–31.
17. Angus RM, Ahmed AA, Fenwick LJ, Peacock AJ. Comparison of the acute effects on gas exchange of nasal ventilation and doxapram in exacerbations of chronic obstructive pulmonary disease. Thorax. 1996;51:1048–50.
18. Bott J, Carroll MP, Conway JH, et al. Randomised controlled trial of nasal ventilation in acute ventilatory failure due to chronic obstructive airways disease. Lancet. 1993;341:1555–7.
19. Brochard L, Mancebo J, Wysocki M, et al. Noninvasive ventilation for acute exacerbations of chronic obstructive pulmonary disease. N Engl J Med. 1995;333:817–22.
20. Kramer N, Meyer TJ, Meharg J, Cece RD, Hill NS. Randomized prospective trial of noninvasive positive pressure ventilation in acute respiratory failure. Am J Respir Crit Care Med. 1995;151:1799–806.
21. Ambrosino N, Foglio K, Rubini F, Clini E, Nava S, Vitacca M. Non-invasive mechanical ventilation in acute respiratory failure due to chronic obstructive pulmonary disease: correlates for success. Thorax. 1995;50:755–7.
22. Brown JS, Meecham Jones DJ, Mikelsons C, Paul EA, Wedzicha JA. Using nasal intermittent positive pressure ventilation on a general respiratory ward. J R Coll Physicians Lond. 1998;32:219–24.
23. Connors AF, Dawson NV, Thomas C, et al. Outcomes following acute exacerbation of severe chronic obstructive pulmonary disease. Am J Respir Crit Care Med. 1996;154:959–67.
24. Martin TR, Lewis SW, Albert RK. The prognosis of patients with chronic obstructive pulmonary disease after hospitalization for acute respiratory failure. Chest. 1992;82:310–14.
25. Collet JP, Shapiro S, Ernst P, et al. Effect of an immunostimulating agent on acute exacerbations and hospitalization in COPD patients. Am J Respir Crit Care Med. 1997;156:1719–24.

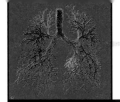
Chapter 39   Other Causes of Emphysema

James K Stoller and Loutfi S Aboussouan

Although cigarette smoking is by far the most common cause of emphysema, other causes must be recognized by the careful clinician, especially when emphysema occurs in a young individual or in a non- or minimal smoker. The purpose of this chapter is to consider these less common etiologies of emphysema (Fig. 39.1).

EPIDEMIOLOGY, RISK FACTORS, AND PATHOPHYSIOLOGY

α_1-Antitrypsin deficiency

α_1-Antitrypsin (AAT) deficiency is a glycoprotein member of the serine protease inhibitor (or serpin) family that is synthesized in the liver and secreted into the bloodstream. The main purpose of this 394 amino acid, single-chain protein is to neutralize neutrophil elastase in the lung interstitium and to protect the lung parenchyma from elastolytic breakdown[1]. Severe deficiency of AAT accordingly predisposes to unopposed lung elastolysis, with the clinical sequelae of early-onset panacinar emphysema (see Fig. 39.2). Deficiency of a α_1-antichymotrypsin may also predispose to early-onset emphysema[2].

Deficiency in AAT is inherited as an autosomal codominant condition and, since its description in 1963[3], over 75 different alleles have been described. The gene is located on the long arm of chromosome 14 and has been sequenced, cloned, and

Condition	Cause of emphysema	Age at onset (years)	Clinical features	Prevalence (%)	Distribution and pathology	Specific therapies	Remaining controversies
Smoking	Promotes elastase-induced injury	>45	'Pink puffer'	10–15	Apical/centriacinar	Smoking cessation	–
Proteinase deficiency	Unchecked elastase-induced injury	35–45	Liver disease Family history of emphysema, liver disease, or panniculitis	48–87	Basilar/panacinar	Pooled human plasma α_1-antitrypsin	Does infused α_1-antitrypsin forestall lung disease? Benefits of population screening
Intravenous drug use	Damage to the capillary bed by insoluble filler Elastolysis	<30	History of intravenous injection drugs	2	Apical/bullae (heroin, cocaine) Basilar/panacinar (methylphenidate, methadone)	Cessation of drug use	–
Human immunodeficiency virus (HIV)	Malnutrition?, local cytokines, cytotoxicity, decreased glutathione	<40	History of risk factors for HIV infection	12 (42 in auto-immune deficiency syndrome)	Apical and cortical/bullae	Antiretroviral therapy	No confirmation of emphysema by pathology
Pneumocystis carinii pneumonia	Leukoelastase from secretions	<40	Subacute cough, fever, dyspnea	10–20	Cysts/no specific location	Treatment for *Pneumocystis carinii* pneumonia reverses cysts	–
Hypocomplementemic urticarial vasculitis syndrome	Humoral autoimmune process?	<30	Female/male: 8/1, urticaria, arthritis, angioedema	68 (80 in smokers)	Panacinar	Cytotoxic drugs and dapsone	Efficacy of drug treatment?
Malnutrition	Unchecked elastase-induced injury	<40	Temporal wasting, sunken eyeballs	14	Peripheral	Refeeding	–
Salla disease	Impaired antiproteolytic function	<35	Mental retardation, ataxia, nystagmus	40	Basilar/centriacinar	–	–
Cutis laxa	Developmental defect of elastin, protease	Neonate	Appearance of premature aging	33–100	Panacinar	–	–
Marfan syndrome	Developmental defect of elastin	Neonate	Skeletal, cardiac, subluxation	10	Apical/bullae	–	–
Down syndrome	Alveolar hypoplasia	Infant	Epicanthal folds	20	Subpleural cysts No alveolar damage	–	–

Causes of emphysema and associated characteristics

Figure 39.1 Causes of emphysema and associated characteristics.

with basilar and panacinar emphysema, similar to that seen in AAT deficiency. Physiologic studies indicate that hyperinflation, air trapping, and a reduction in the diffusing capacity can occur in HIV-positive patients who have no prior history of pulmonary disease[17].

The pulmonary manifestations of Marfan syndrome include spontaneous pneumothorax, emphysema, and bronchiectasis[26].

DIAGNOSIS

Of the approximately 75 different alleles for AAT variants that have been described, 10–15 are associated with serum levels below the protective threshold (see Fig. 39.2)[5]. By far the most common severe variant is the Z allele, which accounts for 95% of the clinically recognized cases of severe AAT deficiency. The diagnosis of severe AAT deficiency is confirmed when the serum levels falls below the protective threshold value – between 3 and $7\mu mol$ can be taken as indicative of the PI*ZZ allele. Specific phenotyping is reserved for instances in which serum levels are between 7 and $11\mu mol$, or when genetic counseling or family analysis is needed.

The defining laboratory features of HUVS are decreased levels of C1q and detectable immunoglobulin G antibodies to C1q. Laboratory evaluation also demonstrates decreased serum complement levels in keeping with the characteristic feature of complement activation. A positive serum antinuclear antibody is observed in 61% of individuals, occasionally with anti-double stranded DNA[18].

TREATMENT

As depicted in Figure 39.2, in treatment strategies for AAT deficiency, the neutrophil elastase burden in the lung is reduced (e.g. primarily by smoking cessation) and levels of AAT are augmented. Available augmentation strategies include pharmacologic attempts to increase endogenous production of AAT by the liver (e.g. danazol, tamoxifen) or, more promisingly, administration of purified AAT by periodic intravenous infusion or by inhalation. Gene therapy represents another augmentation strategy but to date has been confined to animal models.

Although tamoxifen can increase endogenous production of AAT by a limited extent, this increase can have major clinical importance in selected patients who have the PI*SZ phenotype and whose serum levels fall just below the protective threshold. Intravenous augmentation therapy is the only currently available approach that can increase serum levels above the $11\mu mol$ protective threshold. The ability of intravenous AAT augmentation to alter the clinical course of patients who have AAT deficiency has not been demonstrated, but studies have shown that the infusions can maintain serum levels above $11\mu mol$ when replacement is given weekly (60mg/kg), biweekly (120mg/kg), or monthly (250mg/kg)[27], and weekly infusions are associated with decreased urinary excretion of elastin breakdown products[28]. Uncontrolled observations of patients in the National Institutes of Health registry also suggest that the FEV_1 may fall at a slower rate in those patients who receive AAT replacement than in those who are not offered treatment. Intravenous augmentation therapy also ameliorates panniculitis that results from AAT deficiency.

Therapy of the emphysema associated with HUVS generally includes bronchodilators and corticosteroids, which have been reported to relieve bronchospasm, but not to alter disease progression. Cytotoxic therapy (e.g. with cyclophosphamide or azathioprine) has been used with variable success, and dapsone has resulted in improvement in a small number of recipients[29].

CLINICAL COURSE AND PREVENTION

Although not all patients who have the PI*ZZ phenotype develop emphysema, longitudinal studies of selected populations show accelerated rates of FEV_1 decline (e.g. –86mL/year) in non-smoking PI*ZZ individuals, which is even higher in smokers (e.g. –132mL/year)[30]. Data from the Danish registry suggest that non-smoking PI*ZZ individuals who lack symptoms have a survival close to that of the overall Danish population and higher than survival rates for smokers[31]. The mortality rate in the Nationsl Heart, Lung, and Blood Institute Registry was 3% per year over a 7-year follow-up interval.

Since the diagnosis of AAT deficiency has genetic implications for the individual's family, and because early identification can enhance avoidance of smoking and allow intravenous augmentation therapy to be considered, enhanced detection is desirable, and could lead to disease prevention.

PITFALLS AND CONTROVERSIES

The natural history of AAT deficiency is still unknown, and the effect of replacement therapy has not yet been determined in controlled, randomized trials. Although some investigators have argued that the duration and associated cost of controlled studies make such clinical trials impractical, the cost of AAT replacement is enormous and lack of consistent data regarding the course of untreated disease results in considerable skepticism about its efficacy. Whether population screening should be undertaken is also unclear.

REFERENCES

1. Gadek JE, Crystal RG. Alpha 1-antitrypsin deficiency. In: Stanbury JB, Wyngaarden JB, Frederickson DS, et al., eds. The metabolic basis of inherited disease, 5th edn. New York: McGraw-Hill, 1983:1450–67.
2. Lindmark BE, Arborelius M Jr, Eriksson SG. Pulmonary function in middle-aged women with heterozygous deficiency of the serine protease inhibitor alpha 1-antichymotrypsin. Am Rev Respir Dis. 1990;141:884–8.
3. Laurell CB, Eriksson S. The electrophoretic alpha 1-globulin pattern of serum in alpha 1-antitrypsin deficiency. Scand J Clin Lab Invest. 1963;15:132–40.
4. Brantly M, Nukiwa T, Crystal RG. Molecular basis of alpha 1-antitrypsin deficiency. Am J Med. 1988;84(Suppl. 6A):13–31.
5. Lomas DA, Evans DL, Finch JT, Carrel RW. The mechanism of Z α_1-antitrypsin accumulation in the liver. Nature. 1992;357:605–7.
6. Teckman JH, Qu D, Perlmutter DH. Molecular pathogenesis of liver disease in α_1-antitrypsin deficiency. Hepatology. 1996;24:1504–16.
7. Stoller JK. Clinical features and natural history of severe α_1-antitrypsin deficiency. Roger S. Mitchell Lecture. Chest. 1997;111(Suppl. 6):123–8S.

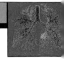

8. Stoller JK, Smith P, Yang P, Spray J. Physical and social impact of alpha 1-antitrypsin deficiency: results of a mail survey of the readership of a national newsletter. Cleve Clin J Med. 1994;61:461–7.

9. Piitulainen E, Tornling G, Eriksson S. Effect of age and occupational exposure to airway irritants on lung function in non-smoking individuals with alpha 1-antitrypsin deficiency (PiZZ). Thorax. 1997;52:244–8.

10. Beighton P. The dominant and recessive forms of cutis laxa. J Med Genet. 1972;9:216–21.

11. Byers PH, Siegel RC, Holbrook KA, Narayama AS, Bornstein P, Hall JG. X-linked cutis laxa: defective cross-link formation in collagen due to decreased lysyl oxidase activity. N Engl J Med. 1980;303:61–5.

12. Reed WB, Horowitz RE, Beighton P. Acquired cutis laxa. Arch Dermatol. 1971;103:661–9.

13. Cupo LN, Pyeritz RE, Olson JL, McPhee SJ, Hutchins GM, McKusick VA. Ehlers–Danlos syndrome with abnormal collagen fibrils, sinus of Valsalva aneurysms, myocardial infarction, panacinar emphysema and cerebral heterotopias. Am J Med. 1981;71:1051–8.

14. Paré JP, Cote G, Fraser RS. Long-term follow-up of drug abusers with intravenous talcosis. Am Rev Respir Dis. 1989;139:231–41.

15. Stern EJ, Frank MS, Schmutz JF, Glenny RW, Schmidt RA, Godwin JD. Panlobular pulmonary emphysema caused by IV injection of methylphenidate (Ritalin): findings on chest radiographs and CT scans. AJR Am J Roentgenol. 1994;162:555–60.

16. Gurney JW, Bates FT. Pulmonary cystic disease: comparison of Pneumocystis carinii pneumatocoeles and bullous emphysema due to intravenous drug abuse. Radiology. 1989;173:27–31.

17. Diaz PT, Clanton TL, Pacht ER. Emphysema-like pulmonary disease associated with human immunodeficiency virus infection. Ann Intern Med. 1992;116:124–8.

18. Wisnieski JJ, Baer AN, Christensen J, et al. Hypocomplementemic urticarial vasculitis syndrome: clinical and serologic findings in 18 patients. Medicine. 1995;74:24–41.

19. Sahebjami H. Emphysema-like changes in HIV (letter). Ann Intern Med. 1992;116:876.

20. Pääkkö P, Ryhänen L, Rantala H, Autio-Harmainen H. Pulmonary emphysema in nonsmoking patients with Salla disease. Am Rev Respir Dis. 1987;135:979–82.

21. Gonzales OR, Gomez IG, Recalde AL, Landing BH. Postnatal development of the cystic lesion of Down syndrome: suggestion that the cause is reduced formation of peripheral air spaces. Pediatr Pathol. 1991;11:623–33.

22. Sveger T. Liver disease in alpha 1-antitrypsin deficiency detected by screening of 200,000 infants. N Engl J Med. 1976;294:1316–21.

23. Brantly ML, Paul LD, Miller BH, Falk BH, Wu M, Crystal RG. Clinical features and history of the destructive lung disease associated with alpha 1-antitrypsin deficiency of adults with pulmonary symptoms. Am Rev Respir Dis. 1988;138:327–36.

24. Fallat RL. Reactive airways disease and alpha 1-antitrypsin deficiency. In: Crystal RG, ed. Alpha 1-antitrypsin deficiency: biology, pathogenesis, clinical manifestations, therapy. New York: Marcel Dekker, Inc.; 1996:259–79.

25. Silverman EK, Pierce JA, Province MA, Rao DC, Campbell EJ. Variability of pulmonary function in alpha 1-antitrypsin deficiency: Clinical correlates. Ann Intern Med. 1989;11:982–91.

26. Foster ME, Foster DR. Bronchiectasis and Marfan's syndrome. Postgrad Med J. 1980;56:718–19.

27. Hubbard RC, Sellers S, Czerski D, Stephens L, Crystal RG. Biochemical efficacy and safety of monthly augmentation therapy for alpha-1 antitrypsin deficiency. JAMA. 1988;260:1259–64.

28. Stone PJ, Morris TA III, Franzblau C, Snider GL. Preliminary evidence that augmentation therapy diminishes degradation of cross-linked elastin in alpha-1-antitrypsin deficient humans. Respiration. 1995;62:76–9.

29. Schwartz Hr, McDuffies FC, Black LF, Schroeter AL, Conn DL. Hypocomplementemic urticarial vasculitis: association with chronic obstructive pulmonary disease. Mayo Clin Proc. 1982;57:231–8.

30. Seersholm N, Kok-Jensen A, Dirksen A. Decline in FEV_1 among patients with severe hereditary α_1-antitrypsin deficiency type PiZ. Am J Respir Crit Care Med. 1995;152:1922–5.

31. Seersholm N, Kok-Jensen A, Dirksen A. Survival of patients with severe alpha 1-antitrypsin deficiency with special reference to non-index cases. Thorax. 1994;49:695–8.

Allergies in Childhood (ISAAC). The study investigated 463,801 children aged 13–14 years in 56 countries. The results showed considerable variability between countries in the prevalence of childhood self-reported asthma (Fig. 40.2). The highest prevalence was about 20 times higher than the lowest. For instance, the highest 12-month prevalences of asthma were from centers in the UK, Australia, New Zealand, and Republic of Ireland (the highest being 36.8%), followed by centers in North, Central, and South America. The lowest prevalences were from participating centers in several Eastern European countries, Indonesia, China, Taiwan, Uzbekistan, India, and Ethiopia (the lowest in these countries being 1.6%). Although the prevalences varied generally in centers in any one country, differences were larger between different countries. Analysis of this difference might ultimately result in the discovery of different risk factors, as has been the case for the development of cancer in epidemiologic studies.

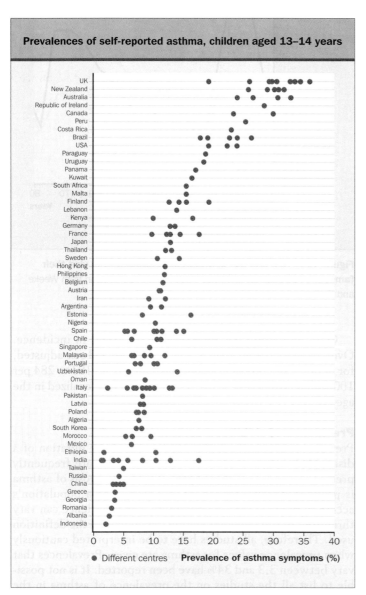

Figure 40.2 12-Month prevalences of self-reported asthma with a written questionnaire, for children aged 13–14 years. (Adapted with permission from The International Study of Asthma and Allergies in Childhood Asthma Steering Committee[1].)

The prevalence of wheezing in childhood has increased over the past decade. However, differences in methodology, definitions, and use of the label 'asthma' may exaggerate the true increase in prevalence. Awareness of asthma in the population may have increased because of widespread publicity. Therefore, the authors of this chapter carefully examined the data to prevent bias, and some studies still showed an increase in prevalence. Analyses of the available data suggest an increase in asthma prevalence from 1970 onward[2].

In Australia in 1969, 19.2% of 7-year-old children had experienced recurrent episodes of wheezing; in New Zealand in 1973, 23% of 9-year-old children had a history of one or more attacks of wheezing. These were cross-sectional studies, and so they do not simply reflect an increase in prevalence. In a UK population study in which 36 regions were investigated in 1982 and again in 1992 using the same methodology[4], a three-fold increase in asthma attacks in children aged 5–11 years occurred, with a 30–60% increase in occasional wheeze and a 30–40% increase in persistent wheeze, which suggests a real increase in asthma prevalence. In the USA, reported prevalence of wheeze among children aged 6–11 years increased significantly from 4.8% between 1971 and 1974 to 7.6% between 1976–1980. In addition, childhood asthma was rare in Africa up to the late 1970s, yet recent studies suggest that the prevalence is in the highest range[2].

Prevalence of adult asthma

Fewer data are available on adults and it is unclear whether the prevalence of asthma is increasing in adults as well. The same considerations in interpreting the results of different studies as noted for childhood asthma apply for adult asthma. The European Community Respiratory Health Study showed considerable variation between countries for adult asthma. Wheezing during the past 12 months was present in 20–27% of the different populations, with more variability for nocturnal dyspnea and attacks of asthma. When airway hyperresponsiveness was taken as a measure of asthma, it was high in New Zealand, Australia, USA, Britain, France, Denmark, and Germany, whereas it was low in Sweden, Italy, and Spain.

Early data from inhabitants of Tristan da Cunha suggest that current asthma has increased from 11% in 1974 to over 20% in 1995. In Sweden, the prevalence of asthma in 18-year-old military conscripts increased by 47% (from 1.8 to 2.8%) between 1971 and 1981. In Finland, investigations in 19-year-old conscripts showed an increase in adult asthma that rose from 0.08% in 1961 to 1.29% in 1966 and then 20-fold up to 1.79% in 1989. It seems unlikely that a rise of this kind relates only to diagnosis, as this would imply that 95% of the cases were undiagnosed in 1966.

A recent study in Greenwich showed that the prevalence of asthma among adults (16–50 years old) has increased since a similar survey in 1986, although with a lower increase[4].

Most studies report that asthma prevalence diminishes with age. Curiously, in some developing countries the prevalence of asthma in adults is higher than that in children. For instance, in Papua New Guinea, the point prevalence of asthma in children in the 1970s was nil and the adult prevalence was only 0.28%. A decade later, the prevalence was 0.6% in children and 7.3% in adults. Severe asthma now also occurs in these adults, especially when exposed to high levels of house dust mite. The striking rise in asthma was not observed in a similar village, in which a four-fold lower mite density in blanket dust occurred. No good explanation exists for this difference in childhood to adulthood asthma ratio, found in almost all other countries.

Prevalence of asthma mortality

Asthma rarely leads to death, as reflected in the mortality rates, which are measured in deaths per 100,000 subjects. For many countries, asthma deaths are less than a few hundred per annum. However, decreasing accuracy occurs in the diagnosis of asthma in decedents older than 35 years of age and only a low percentage of asthma deaths are validated by autopsy. In spite of these and other limitations, much has been learned about mortality rate changes. A large variability in asthma mortality occurs between countries, similar to the large variation of its prevalence. Mortality rates vary from 9/100,000 in former West Germany to 1.5/100,000 in Hong Kong for persons of all ages (Fig. 40.3). A recent Dutch study showed that asthma mortality in the age group 5–34 years decreased between 1980 and 1994, from 3.1 to 1.1 deaths per million people, one of the lowest reported in the literature. A history of severe disease, lack of access to medical care, suboptimal pharmacotherapy, emotional depression, and family disturbance have all been suggested as risk factors for asthma mortality.

On two occasions in the past three decades a substantial increase in mortality in England, Wales, Australia, and New Zealand occurred. This was attributed to a direct toxic effect of high-dose sympathomimetic bronchodilator use, delay in obtaining medical care, and increased exposure to aeroallergens. Whether inhaled β-agonists are associated with or alternatively cause subsequent mortality remains unclear.

In a Danish follow-up study in adults it appeared that cigarette smoking, age, presence of blood eosinophilia, degree of impairment of lung function, and degree of reversibility to β-agonists contributed to asthma mortality. Greater reversibility was a risk factor, in contrast to expectations. It might be that this signifies that asthma was undertreated in these individuals, which supports other data that the outcome of asthma is improved when inhaled corticosteroids are instituted as early as possible.

Risk factors for development of asthma

Since asthma prevalence and mortality are increasing, it seems important to determine which risk factors cause this increase. Many studies have tried to assess risk factors and found evidence that, for example, atopy, hyperresponsiveness, (passive) smoking, and diet could be considered as single risk factors for the presence of asthma. Until recently, only a few studies had assessed the risk for development of asthma using logistic regression analyses in terms of odds ratios. Only in this way can one interpret the relative risks of different factors that all ultimately contribute to the development of disease. These studies are addressed below.

A distinction can be made between inherent factors (atopy, genetic predisposition, gender), causal factors (smoking), and contributing factors (e.g. the load of allergen exposure) as risk factors in the development of asthma (Fig. 40.4).

Atopy

Atopy is characterized by elevated levels of total serum IgE[7], detection of specific IgE against common aeroallergens, and/or positive skin tests to common aeroallergens. In many countries, atopy is the greatest risk factor for asthma in childhood and adulthood (Fig. 40.5). Asthmatics tend to be more atopic than nonasthmatics. In children, the odds ratios for the association between

Factors that contribute to asthma		
Inherent factors	**Causal factors**	**Contributing factors**
Atopy	Smoking	Indoor allergens (domestic mites, animal allergens, cockroach allergens, fungi)
Gender	Respiratory infections	
Hyperresponsiveness	Small birth weight	Outdoor allergens (pollens, fungi)
Genetic abnormalities	Diet	Occupational sensitizers
	Air pollution	
	Level of lung function	

Figure 40.4 Factors that contribute to asthma.

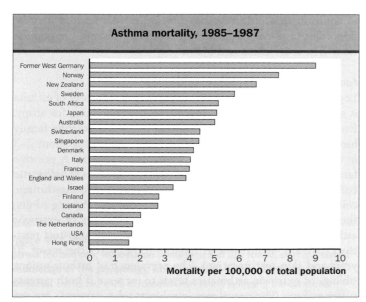

Figure 40.3 Asthma mortality (total population) rate per 100,000, measured in 1985–1987. (Adapted with permission from Seas[6].)

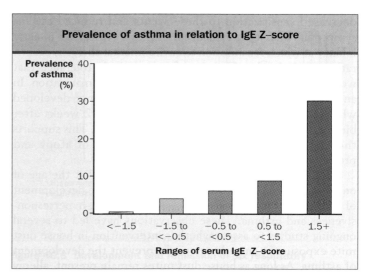

Figure 40.5 Prevalences of asthma in relation to IgE Z-scores (standardized for age and sex) in 1662 Tucson persons who had completely negative skin tests to house dust. (Adapted with permission from Burrows et al.[7])

the sole reason, as it also occurs in those affected by persistent hyperresponsiveness. Another factor might be that atopy interferes with the expression of hyperresponsiveness. In children in Southampton, airway hyperresponsiveness decreased with age from 29.1% at 7 years to 16.5% at 11 years, while the prevalence of atopy increased from 26 to 31.6% over the same period. Thus, although atopy is associated with hyperresponsiveness, and the presence of atopy is a risk factor for its development, it does not fully explain its presence. Finally, the importance of persistent airway hyperresponsiveness in predicting ongoing respiratory symptoms has been demonstrated in two long-term epidemiologic studies[11].

Smoking

Smoking is an acknowledged respiratory irritant[14]. The weight of evidence suggests that home exposure to tobacco smoke is second only to atopy as a major risk factor for childhood asthma. Mechanisms suggested include increased susceptibility to lower respiratory tract infections and increased risk for development of atopy. Thus, parental smoking affects the development of atopy and asthma, and in-utero cigarette smoke exposure and exposure in the first few months of life especially appear to be risk factors for the development of atopy and asthma[14]. Children whose parents smoke have been reported to have many more problems with wheezing, lower respiratory infections, and asthma than children of parents who do not smoke, especially during the first year of life. This effect remains even after controlling for the predictors of childhood wheezing such as day care, season of birth, sharing a bedroom, or parental history of childhood respiratory trouble. In Tucson, Arizona, smoking of more than 10 cigarettes a day was associated with a 2.5 times increased risk of development of asthma before the age of 12 years, as was a lower maximal midexpiratory flow among children of women with 12 years or less of education; this association was not present in women with higher education.

The observation that active smoking during adolescence is associated with shortening of the plateau phase of FEV_1 that generally occurs between 20 and 35 years does, however, suggest an overall negative effect of smoking in adolescence, which may also be present in asthmatics. Further observations show that smoking cessation during adolescence has a positive impact on lung growth.

Early respiratory tract infections

The relationship between respiratory tract infections and the development of asthma is complex. A number of mechanisms have been proposed to explain how viral infections may induce asthma symptoms. Viral infections damage airway epithelium, cause reflex bronchoconstriction from upper airway inflammation, cause local airway generation of proinflammatory cytokines, and enhanced recruitment of inflammatory cells to the airways accompanied by enhanced mediator release, and virus-specific IgE antibody generation may follow. Asthmatic individuals have been reported to have viral infections more frequently. However, atopic infants (eczema and or positive skin test) have not been reported to have more respiratory infections than nonatopic infants during the first year of life. In a prospective study to investigate risk factors for the development of asthma in childhood, respiratory infections appeared

to be important. They had a lasting effect on respiratory symptoms as well as lung function in childhood. Those children whose bronchiolitis was caused by respiratory syncytial virus (RSV) had greater exercise lability than control children who had the same degree of atopy. Wheeze and airway hyperresponsiveness were also increased in children after RSV bronchiolitis, although the prevalences of recognized and treated asthma, and of atopy, were similar in a control group. In addition, viral respiratory tract infection causes exacerbations in asthmatics. Sensitization to the viral agent has been reported to play a role, as production of virus-specific IgE is associated with wheeze for RSV and parainfluenza virus.

In contrast, some circumstantial evidence also indicates that early respiratory tract infections may be a protective factor. Those who have fewer infections early in life may be prone to increased prevalence of atopic disease, a risk factor for the development of asthma in itself. An inverse relationship between the prevalence of atopy and the number of siblings has been reported. This could be related to increased infections in those who have a large number of older siblings, which thus reduces the tendency to develop atopy – further investigation is required[12].

Environmental exposure

It is now well established that episodes of air pollution increase morbidity from asthma. Prevalence of asthma is increased in polluted areas compared with unpolluted areas in Israel. Among several key studies on air pollution and the development of asthma, one compared respiratory illness in the former East and West Germanys. Children in the less-polluted city of Munich had higher rates of wheezing (20 versus 17%), diagnosed asthma (9.3 versus 7.3%), and hayfever (8.6 versus 2.4%) than did children in Leipzig. The latter children had more bronchitis, 30.9 versus 15.9% in Munich. These results may be interpreted as air pollution being a risk factor for atopy and asthma, although other explanations for these data have been given (see paragraph on atopy as a risk factor). However, the study is a cross-sectional one. It may well be that environmental air pollution does not increase the prevalence of atopic status, but enhances the development and duration of clinical symptoms among already sensitized subjects. Another risk factor that might interact with exposure to air pollution is hyperresponsiveness. Both factors were found to be of importance in a recent study in The Netherlands, in which children who had both airway hyperresponsiveness and above median levels of serum total IgE were especially susceptible to air pollution. The effects of air pollution are, however, thought to be smaller than those of indoor environment, since the ISAAC study found no consistent evidence for an effect of industrial air pollution in an area of New Zealand exposed to emissions from paper mills and sulfur fumes.

Level of pulmonary function

Reduced lung function appeared to be a predisposing factor for a first wheezing illness in infants. Martinez et al.[15] prospectively studied 124 newborn infants and found that the risk of a wheezing illness was 3.7 times higher among infants whose airway conductance was in the lowest third compared with those in the highest two thirds. Children who had transient wheezing that resolved by the age of 6 years were more likely to have had initially reduced lung function, whereas children in whom asthma persisted were more likely to be atopic and reduced lung function was not a significant factor. Thus, respiratory tract infection may be a risk factor for wheeze, but not for the development of asthma. Both in children and in adults, low levels of FEV_1 appear to be predictive for continuation of wheezing into adulthood and reduced level of lung function in adulthood, as well as for more rapid decline of FEV_1.

Birth weight

With the increasing survival of premature infants and the associated pulmonary problems, the role of prematurity in asthma has come under increasing scrutiny. Prematurity has been reported to be a risk factor for the development of respiratory symptoms. Mothers of premature infants have a higher prevalence of hyperresponsiveness than mothers of full-term infants. Thus, a genetic or familial factor may have induced respiratory symptoms in premature infants, but prematurity itself was not the cause. A family history of asthma, but not of other allergies, was identified as a predictor for children who have respiratory distress syndrome developing bronchopulmonary dysplasia in one study, but not in another. Other investigators reported that low birth weight and prematurity, regardless of neonatal respiratory disease, are associated with decreased flow rates and airway conductance in childhood. A recent study in Austria reported that low birth weight, a low level of maternal education, and a larger family size predicted a decrease in level of most lung function parameters in children aged between 7.5 and 11 years, which confirmed results obtained in the UK in 1993. This effect could result from gestational age itself, but even after adjustment for this, birth weight remained a major risk factor for reduced lung function. Below a birth weight of 2kg (4.4lb), children had more problems with cough but not wheeze than did age-matched schoolmates.

Diet

Eating fish more than once a week had a protective effect on the development of asthma in Australian children. After adjusting for gender, country of birth, ethnicity, atopy, respiratory infection in the first 21 years of life, and a parental history of asthma, children who ate fresh oily fish with >2% fat had a reduced risk for current asthma. Furthermore, an increased prevalence of methacholine responsiveness was reported in children and adults who had a higher salt intake. In children no relationship was found between asthma and exercise responsiveness. Studies on salt intake in adults are less consistent, and the influence of sodium in the development of asthma remains unclear.

In a prospective study in more than 77,000 women, vitamin E appeared to be protective against asthma, but only when increased intake was part of a diet and not when given as a supplement, which suggests that other factors might be responsible for the observed protective effect.

Occupational exposure

Some studies show that toluene diisocyanate exposure may induce asthma, and that the longer the exposure the less likely is the asthma to remit after stopping exposure. Occupational asthma may account for a considerable part of the total burden of asthma in a population – some 15% of all cases of asthma in Japan are attributed to occupational causes. However, in Western countries the numbers are far lower. In some industries more than 30% of the workers develop asthma, in others the numbers are low or even zero. The level of allergen exposure and the presence of atopy appear to be risk factors in animal workers.

CONCLUSIONS

Asthma is a common disease in the general population and epidemiologic studies show that the prevalence increases both in childhood and adulthood. Risk factors for the development of asthma have been found with consistency in many epidemiologic studies; of these, atopy and smoking are the two most important. One of the most significant factors in intervention to lower the incidence and prevalence of asthma is certainly smoking cessation! Furthermore, hyperresponsiveness and gender are important as inherent factors. Allergen exposure, early respiratory infection, low birth weight, diet, and air pollution all contribute to the risk of development of asthma. A genetic predisposition together with early exposure to allergens in the absence of recurrent infections may lead to an inflammatory process and airway responsiveness associated with asthma. Identification of those individuals at risk should lead to further attenuation of asthma, since appropriate intervention is currently possible, as far as knowledge on putative risk factors exists. It is possible that a better understanding of the genetic factors that contribute to atopy, hyperresponsiveness, and asthma will lead to the prevention of most asthma in the future.

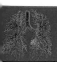
REFERENCES

1. The International Study of Asthma and Allergies in Childhood (ISAAC) Steering Committee. Worldwide variation in prevalence of symptoms of asthma, allergic rhinoconjunctivitis, and atopic eczema: ISAAC. Lancet. 1998;351:1225–32.
2. Woolcock AJ, Peat JK. Evidence for the increase in asthma worldwide. Ciba Found Symp. 1997;206:122–34.
3. Gregg I. Epidemiological aspects. In: Clark TJH, Godfrey S, eds. Asthma. London: Chapman and Hall; 1983:242–84.
4. Burney PGJ, Chinn S, Rona RJ. Has the prevalence of asthma symptoms increased in children? Evidence from the national study of health and growth 1973–86. Br Med J. 1990;300:1306–10.
5. Weeke ER, Pedersen PA. Allergic rhinitis in a Danish general practice. Allergy. 1981;36:375–9.
6. Sears MR Worldwide trend in asthma mortality. Bull Int Lung Dis. 1991;166:79–83.
7. Burrows B, Martinez FD, Halonen M, Barbee RA, Cline MG. Association of asthma with serum IgE levels and skin test reactivity to allergens. N Engl J Med. 1989;320:271–7.
8. Sears MD, Herbison GP, Holdaway MD, et al. The relative risks of sensitization to grass pollen, house dust mite and cat dander in the development of childhood asthma. Clin Exp Allergy. 1989;19:419–24.
9. Landau LI. Risks of developing asthma. Pediatr Pulmonol. 1996;22:314–18.
10. Peat JK. The rising trend in allergic illness: which environmental factors are important? Clin Exp Allergy. 1994;24:797–800.
11. Meijer B, Bleecker ER, Postma DS. Genetics. In: Barnes PJ, Rodger IW, Thomson NC, eds. Asthma. Basic mechanisms and clinical management. San Diego: Academic Press; 1998:35–46.
12. Grol MH, Gerritsen J, Postma DS. Asthma: from childhood to adulthood. Allergy. 1996;51:855–69.
13. Xu X, Rijcken B, Schouten JP, Weiss ST. Airways responsiveness and development and remission of chronic respiratory symptoms in adults. Lancet. 1997;350:1431–4.
14. Strachan DP, Cook DG. Parental smoking and childhood asthma: longitudinal and case–control studies. Thorax. 1998:53:204–12.
15. Martinez FD, Morgan WJ, Wright AL, et al. Dimished lung function as a predisposing factor for wheezing respiratory illness in infants. N Engl J Med. 1988;319:1112–17.

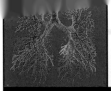

Chapter 41

Asthma: Clinical Features, Diagnosis, and Treatment

Martyn R Partridge

EPIDEMIOLOGY, RISK FACTORS, AND PATHOPHYSIOLOGY

Asthma is a common condition. The clinical features associated with it are not exclusive to it, and objective diagnostic tests are not practical in the very young. Both overdiagnosis and underdiagnosis are common. Effective treatments for the condition exist, but even if correctly prescribed they are often not taken. Like many long-term conditions, asthma represents a challenge to the clinician, but one most likely to be successfully tackled if managed in a partnership with the patient.

The rising prevalence of asthma (Chapter 40) appears to be associated in some way with civilization, Westernization, or modern living. The population's genetic constitution has not changed over the past 20–30 years, and so environmental factors must be activating the inherited predisposition to asthma and other atopic diseases in more people now than ever before. Studies in Zimbabwe and Ghana show increased frequencies of asthma in richer urban areas compared with rural areas, and in the Far East much higher rates of asthma are found in children who live in Hong Kong than among those of similar genetic constitution who live in the neighboring provinces of Southern China.

Maternal smoking is one factor associated with an increased risk of the offspring developing a wheezing illness, but there are other hypothetical causes. Higher rates of asthma occur in populations who take less magnesium and less oily fish in the diet, among those exposed to fewer infections in early life (e.g. the first born in a family), and in those who exhibit less tuberculin skin-test reactivity. Dietary factors and lack of early life exposure to infections may thus render a genetically susceptible individual more prone to asthma, and this enhanced tendency may be activated by other environmental changes. These might include changes in the home environment, for in many countries the more 'closed', less well-ventilated housing allows increased concentrations of allergens or the exhaust gases associated with cooking. Other environmental change may be that associated with poverty (increased exposure to cockroach allergen in poor housing), or to increased traffic pollution.

The major challenge is that of the primary prevention of the condition – that is to identify what activates asthma in increasing numbers of those born with a genetic susceptibility. Once identified, the hope is that suitable environmental avoidance procedures or vaccines can be used to reduce the prevalence. However, the current aim is that of secondary prevention – to ensure that those who have asthma benefit from current knowledge and from the treatments available. This involves well-educated health professionals working in a well-organized,

adequately funded system, and offering treatment in a manner that makes it likely to be taken. An overview of the scope for both primary and secondary prevention and of the basis of the clinical features of asthma is shown in Figure 41.1.

CLINICAL FEATURES

Asthma is defined in physiologic terms as 'a generalized narrowing of the airways, which varies over short periods of time either spontaneously or as a result of treatment'. As an airway disorder its clinical features are common to other airway disorders and

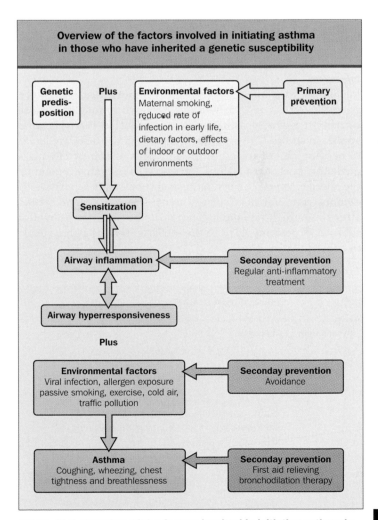

Figure 41.1 Overview of the factors involved in initiating asthma in those who have inherited a genetic susceptibility. The scope is shown for potential primary and secondary interventions.

may include cough, wheezing, tightness in the chest, and breathlessness, but the key feature is the variability of these symptoms and the tendency for them to be worse at night or in the early morning, and to be worse after exercise (Fig. 41.2). The wheeze arises from vibration of the airway walls, the chest tightness and breathlessness reflect reduced airway caliber, and all of these and the cough reflect underlying airway inflammation and airway hyperresponsiveness (AHR). The factors that underlie the development of inflammation and AHR are shown in Figure 41.1. Characteristic pathologic features include the presence in the airway of inflammatory cells, plasma exudation, edema, smooth muscle hypertrophy, mucus plugging, and shedding of epithelium. Such features may be present even in those who have mild asthma, and the characteristic pathologic changes are frequently present even when no symptoms are found. Not only does the presence of these basic changes mean that clinical symptoms can develop at any time, but also increasing indirect evidence shows that the persistence of such untreated inflammatory change may lead to the airway narrowing becoming 'fixed' with time. It is possible that such irreversible change may occur relatively early in the course of the disease.

Exacerbating factors (triggers)

The important risk factors for predisposition to asthma are detailed in Chapter 40. Several of these, and others, can exacerbate or trigger asthma at some stage; a list is given in Figure 41.3.

Infections

In children, viral infections (especially rhinoviruses, respiratory syncytial virus, and influenza virus) are among the most common triggers of asthma and it is probable that the same applies in adults. The adverse effects of such viruses are likely to be through the release from lung cells of similar chemical mediators as occur in asthma and also through enhancement of the allergic response. Even in normal subjects, it is possible to demonstrate enhanced airway irritability for several weeks after viral infections, and it is not difficult to imagine how the addition of postviral AHR to the intrinsic AHR of asthma leads to enhanced symptoms.

Allergic triggers

Once sensitized to an allergen, subsequent re-exposure is likely to worsen an individual's asthma. Common allergens are grass or tree pollen, pets, and house dust and mites. Exposure to only small quantities is sufficient to exacerbate the clinical condition, and avoidance of allergens is extremely difficult. Cat allergen travels widely on other peoples' clothing and is found in circumstances in which cats are not found (e.g. on public transport, in hospital outpatient departments, or in a cinema). Other pet allergens include dogs and small mammals, which may be found not only in the home, but also at school and in the workplace.

Indoor allergens include house dust mites and cockroaches. The former are globally distributed, but it is possible that changes in home design have enhanced exposure in some countries. House dust contains multiple organic and inorganic materials, but the most common domestic mites are the *Dermatophagoides* spp., which feed on human scales. The mites live in soft furnishings and especially thrive in warm, moist surroundings. In other environments, sensitization to cockroach allergen is more common and lifestyle changes (e.g. increased use of central heating) have increased the number of environments in which cockroaches survive and so enhanced the population's potential exposure to them.

Air pollution

Most people spend over 95% of their lives indoors and therefore the adverse effects of pollutants on the clinical features of asthma involve both indoor and outdoor pollution. Indoor pollutants include nitric oxide, nitrogen oxides, carbon monoxide, sulfur dioxide, carbon dioxide, and volatile organic compounds, which may arise from cooking, heating, or the use of insulation materials and paints. Outdoor pollutants may include visible smog or invisible agents that can damage respiratory epithelium, such as nitrogen oxides, ozone, sulfur dioxide, or particulate matter. The magnitude of the role of these agents in triggering attacks of asthma is unclear. While they can certainly make asthma worse, the likelihood is that these triggers have significant effects only in those affected by more severe disease. However, it is possible that pollutants have an adverse synergistic effect, such that exposure to atmospheric pollution may enhance the risk of sensitization to allergens to which an individual is simultaneously exposed.

Clinical features suggestive of asthma	
Investigation	**Outcome**
Medical history	Episodic wheezing, chest tightness, shortness of breath, cough
	Symptoms worsen in presence of aeroallergens, irritants, or exercise
	Symptoms occur or worsen at night, awakening the patient
	Patient has allergic rhinitis or atopic dermatitis
	Close relations have asthma, allergy, sinusitis, or rhinitis
Physical examination	Hyperexpansion of the thorax
	Sounds of wheezing during normal breathing or a prolonged phase of forced exhalation
	Increased nasal secretions, mucosal swelling, sinusitis, rhinitis, or nasal polyps
	Atopic dermatitis/eczema or other signs of allergic skin problem

Figure 41.2 Clinical features suggestive of asthma (Adapted from National Heart, Lung, and Blood Institute[1].)

Factors that may exacerbate asthma	
Factor	**Comment**
Smoking	Active and passive
Infections	Especially rhinoviruses, respiratory syncytial virus, influenza virus
Exercise	Especially on cold dry days
Changes in the weather	Thunderstorms
Pollution	Ozone and sulfur dioxide
Allergens	Pet allergens, house dust and house dust mite, cockroach allergens, pollens
Drugs	Aspirin, nonsteroidal anti-inflammatory agents, β-blockers (oral and ophthalmic)
Occupational factors	Dusty work places, 'cold rooms'

Figure 41.3 Factors that may exacerbate asthma (trigger factors).

Exercise

Exercise is likely to exacerbate or provoke asthma in all ages and in all patients. How prominently exercise is quoted as a trigger depends on the intensity of the exercise and on whether the person with asthma has adjusted his or her lifestyle to avoid this trigger. Exercise-induced asthma is more likely to occur in cold, dry environments (e.g. cross-country running on frosty days) than in a heated indoor swimming pool, and this reflects its likely mechanism – water loss from the airway wall that results in increased osmolarity of surface liquid which induces mediator release. Knowledge that exercise easily induces asthma has led to its frequent use as a diagnostic test (see below).

Occupations

Occupational sensitizing agents may be responsible for the initiation of asthma, but certain occupational environments may also worsen the condition in those who already have it, as discussed in Chapter 62.

Drugs

Some drugs may trigger attacks of asthma. The most severe reactions can be those with β-blocker tablets – topical β-blockers are also used in the treatment of glaucoma and sufficient may be absorbed from this site to have severe effects on airway function.

Up to 3% of those who suffer asthma may be aspirin sensitive, and aspirin (as well as other nonsteroidal anti-inflammatory agents and possibly biphosphonates) may cause severe attacks. The patient may have previously taken aspirin with impunity, but within minutes to hours of a subsequent ingestion, fatal asthma may occur. Such adverse reactions may be more common in women than men and in those who have nasal polyps, but it can affect anyone who has asthma. An additional problem may be cross-reactivity between aspirin sensitivity and use of parenteral hydrocortisone; aspirin-sensitive asthmatics may develop increased airway narrowing if given intravenous hydrocortisone for the treatment of an exacerbation of asthma.

Premenstrual asthma

Worsening of symptoms of asthma may occur in women in the premenstrual and menstrual periods. The peak of worsening symptoms occurs 2–3 days before menstruation begins and correlates with the late luteal phase of ovarian activity, when circulating progesterone and estrogen levels are at their lowest. Such an association may be overlooked by the patient or doctor unless specifically questioned, and in severe cases hospitalization has been shown to have always occurred around this time in an individual's cycle. For most patients, treatment remains of the standard type, if necessary increased in quantity, but progesterone supplementation (orally and by pessary) is necessary in a minority of patients.

Associated clinical conditions

Several important conditions may exacerbate asthma or cause chronic deterioration, or occur in association with it.

Rhinosinusitis

Asthma frequently coexists with rhinosinusitis and the latter may make asthma worse and may impair both the patient's and the health professional's assessment of the asthma. Accurate diagnosis and treatment of rhinosinusitis can lead to significant improvements in accompanying asthma (see Chapter 31).

Churg–Strauss syndrome

Originally described over 40 years ago, this uncommon condition usually has troublesome asthma as a prominent feature, but the other manifestations are rhinitis, peripheral blood eosinophilia, and a systemic vasculitis that may affect the heart, the nervous system, the kidneys, the skin, and joints. Untreated, it can kill or leave permanent disability (see Chapter 48).

Bronchopulmonary aspergillosis

Any patient who has asthma may develop an allergic response to the presence of the fungus *Aspergillus* in the airways. Some patients, however, have severe hypersensitivity reactions to the presence of *A. fumigatus*, which may be carried into the proximal airways where it is trapped in the mucus and incites a profound eosinophilic infiltration in the surrounding airway and lung. Bronchial occlusion frequently occurs, which may give rise to segmental or lobar collapse visible on the chest radiograph. Such episodes are manifest clinically as fever, worsening asthma or chest pain, and episodes can result in significant bronchial wall damage and the development of bronchiectasis of the proximal airways (Fig. 41.4). Diagnosis of bronchopulmonary aspergillosis depends upon detection of positive skin tests to *A. fumigatus*, serum precipitating antibodies, and a peripheral blood eosinophilia in someone who has asthma and chest radiographic abnormalities as described. It is treated with corticosteroid tablets.

Cryptogenic eosinophilic pneumonia

Eosinophilic pneumonia may occur as a complication of bronchopulmonary aspergillosis, as a result of the usage of certain drugs (e.g. nitrofurantoin, sulfasalazine), as a complication of parasitic infections, or represent a cryptogenic eosinophilic pneumonia. While termed 'cryptogenic', this last condition is one that has a characteristic and consistent clinical presentation and has been recognized as a distinctive syndrome for over 30 years. At least 50% of patients who have cryptogenic eosinophilic pneumonia already have asthma and many develop it subsequently to the pneumonia. The characteristic presentation is of fever, breathlessness, weight loss, and profound and drenching night sweats; the chest radiograph shows a classic photographic negative of that seen in pulmonary edema, with peripheral shadowing most marked in the upper zones (see Fig. 41.5; see Chapter 48).

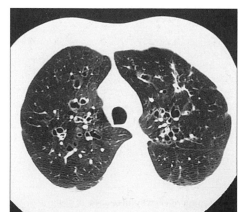

Figure 41.4 Computed tomography scan performed on a patient who has bronchopulmonary aspergillosis. Significant proximal airway bronchiectasis is shown.

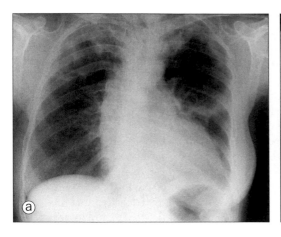

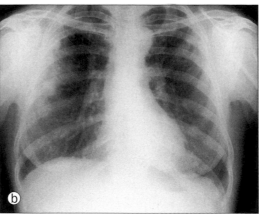

Figure 41.5 Chest radiographs of cryptogenic eosinophilic pneumonia. (a) Predominantly peripheral upper zone shadowing. (b) In this example, it is easier to see how cryptogenic eosinophilic pneumonia may be mistaken for tuberculosis, unless the appropriate tests are performed.

Gastroesophageal reflux

A third of the population have been demonstrated to have gastroesophageal reflux at some stage in some studies. It may be more common in asthma and when present may make asthma worse (see Chapter 15).

DIAGNOSIS, DIFFERENTIAL DIAGNOSIS, AND ASSESSMENT OF SEVERITY

Asthma is only one of very many respiratory diseases, and if considered within the spectrum of all the causes of breathlessness, it must be considered in the context of all cardiorespiratory disorders, as well as anemia, hyperthyroidism, and obesity.

The airway disorders have an important list of differential diagnoses (Fig. 41.6), but it needs to be stressed that features such as cough, wheeze, breathlessness and airway narrowing, and reduced peak flow or obstructive spirometry may occur because of generalized narrowing of the medium and small airways or because of localized obstruction of a larger central airway (Fig. 41.7). Clinically, clues to a localized nature of the airway obstruction may be that the wheezing is asymmetric, monophonic rather than polyphonic, or stridor emanates from the upper airways. Even when the wheezing and airway narrowing appear to be generalized, the list of differential diagnoses must be considered

(see Fig. 41.6). Obliterative bronchiolitis is a rare cause of unexplained, generalized airway narrowing that can occur especially in women who have rheumatoid arthritis, and also occurs as a complication of rejection after lung transplantation (see Chapter 78). In patients who produce large quantities of sputum, the alternate diagnosis of bronchiectasis is considered, and patients who suffer cystic fibrosis occasionally have late presentations and may be misdiagnosed as having asthma. Once all of these diagnoses have been considered, in adults the final differentiation in many cases is that from chronic obstructive pulmonary disease (COPD).

Differentiation of asthma from chronic obstructive pulmonary disease

Some may argue that these conditions are a spectrum in which reversible airways obstruction occurs at one end and fixed narrowing at the other. Furthermore, many patients who have COPD exhibit some reversibility, and many who have asthma develop a fixed component to the airway narrowing. Some of the treatments are also common to the two disorders. However, a more satisfactory approach seems to be to separate the two conditions, as in the Venn diagram shown in Figure 41.8. The reasons for differentiation are that the cause of the two conditions is dissimilar (COPD being essentially due to smoking), the pathologic processes can be quite different (emphysema does not occur in asthma), the natural

Differential diagnosis of airway diseases in the consideration of asthma	
Airway diseases	
Localized	**Generalized**
Vocal cord paresis	Asthma
Laryngeal carcinoma	Chronic obstructive pulmonary disease
Thyroid enlargement	
Relapsing polychondritis	Bronchiectasis
Tracheal carcinoma	Cystic fibrosis
Bronchial carcinoma	Obliterative bronchiolitis
Post-tracheostomy stenosis	
Foreign bodies	
Bronchopulmonary dysplasia	
Obstructive sleep apnea	

Figure 41.6 Differential diagnosis of airway diseases in the consideration of asthma.

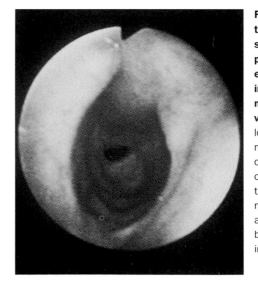

Figure 41.7 Severe tracheal narrowing secondary to prolonged previous endotracheal intubation and mechanical ventilation. The localized nature of this man's airway obstruction was overlooked for some time and he was mistakenly treated for asthma using bronchodilators and inhaled corticosteroids.

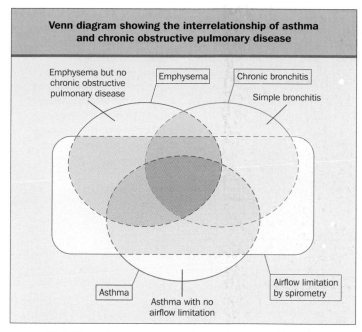

Venn diagram showing the interrelationship of asthma and chronic obstructive pulmonary disease

Emphysema but no chronic obstructive pulmonary disease

Emphysema

Chronic bronchitis

Simple bronchitis

Asthma

Asthma with no airflow limitation

Airflow limitation by spirometry

Figure 41.8 Venn diagram showing the interrelationship of asthma and chronic obstructive pulmonary disease (COPD). An overlap is shown because both are common diseases and both may therefore occasionally occur in the same person. Also, even those people who have COPD show some response to bronchodilators, and in asthma the disease may also consist of a component of irreversible airway narrowing.

history is different (progressive decline in airway caliber is likely in those patients who have COPD who continue to smoke), and the response to treatments is dissimilar in terms of both magnitude and type. Taking a 'prescription-oriented approach' to COPD can often cause both harm (e.g. from side effects of corticosteroid therapies that have only a limited beneficial effect in COPD compared with asthma), and by deflection away from other issues that can help those who suffer COPD (e.g. correct selection of the right type of supplementary oxygen, attention to depression and social factors, and smoking cessation support).

Vocal cord dysfunction

Vocal cord dysfunction is an important condition that can cause serious diagnostic difficulty in both adolescents and adults and, if not recognized, unnecessary overtreatment. Glottic wheezing or vocal cord dysfunction can occur within a spectrum of severity, at one extreme complicating genuinely troublesome asthma and at the other representing a conversion symptom or Munchausen's syndrome. A diagnosis of vocal cord dysfunction is made with considerable care, and in acute cases of wheezing the diagnosis and treatment must always be regarded as that of pure asthma until that diagnosis is disproved[2-4].

Wheezing that arises from the glottis is heard throughout the lung fields when auscultation is performed using a stethoscope, but in cases of vocal cord dysfunction the glottic origin can often be determined by removing the stethoscope from the ears, and standing behind the patient and listening at neck level: the glottic origin of the noise (which often sounds more forced than usual wheezing) becomes apparent. Direct visualization of the glottis by laryngoscopy may reveal the characteristic inspiratory apposition of the cords.

Sometimes those who have asthma make this noise, perhaps because they feel subconsciously the need to impress upon the doctor the severity of their condition. In other patients the noise occurs for psychologic reasons and no evidence of asthma is found. Patients may be of either sex, but are often women in the age range 16–50 years and they may have a paramedical background. Their 'asthma' appears 'resistant' to standard treatments and often they have been admitted to hospital on many occasions and been treated with large doses of corticosteroids and other treatments[5].

Home peak-flow readings may be variable, but show little correlation with attacks or treatment. Spirometry may be similarly variable. Flow–volume curves may show a characteristic 'fluttering' of the inspiratory curve. Measurement of total airway resistance in a body plethysmograph may be diagnostic, for the panting maneuver necessary for such measurement abolishes the vocal cord adduction, and airway resistance can be shown to be normal.

Vocal cord dysfunction is probably much more common than appreciated and if underdiagnosed or mistaken for asthma, overtreatment is likely. Correct diagnosis is essential, and if vocal cord dysfunction is the sole or major part of the wheezing disorder, speech therapy can be helpful.

Investigations used in the diagnosis and assessment of asthma
Peak expiratory flow rate

As asthma is defined in physiologic terms, physiologic tests are required to make the diagnosis. Many of the differential diagnoses listed above have characteristic clinical features, but in other cases asthma is only excluded or confirmed as a diagnosis by establishing whether the patient fulfils the definition of 'generalized airway narrowing that varies over short periods of time either spontaneously or as a result of treatment'. In the great majority of cases, this definition may be fulfilled by measurement of peak expiratory flow rate (PEFR) on more than one occasion in the clinic or surgery, or by the loan of a meter for recording 2–3 times daily at home, or in cases of occupational asthma, at work as well (see Fig. 41.9).

Spirometry

Although less generally available, spirometry is used as the standard measurement of dynamic airflow to detect the presence of airways obstruction and to test for reversibility of flow. Airflow obstruction is established if the forced expiratory volume in 1 second (FEV_1) is <80% predicted, or the ratio of FEV_1 to forced vital capacity is <65% or below the lower limit of normal. If evidence of airway narrowing is detected, response to a bronchodilator must be established, and if positive (>15% response), a diagnosis of asthma is made. In other cases, little spontaneous variation of peak flow may occur over the period of observation, and the response to inhaled bronchodilators may be slight; in these cases, differentiation from COPD, for example, is difficult unless a trial of corticosteroid tablets (see Fig. 41.10) is given. In some cases a prolonged course of high-dose, inhaled corticosteroids (ICSs) can be used as an alternative test of corticosteroid responsiveness.

In some patients, additional tests are needed when asthma is suspected and spirometry normal, when coexisting conditions are suspected, or for other reasons (see Fig. 41.11). If no airway narrowing is apparent at the time of consultation and if the history is unclear, it may help to observe the PEFR at home for 1–2 weeks.

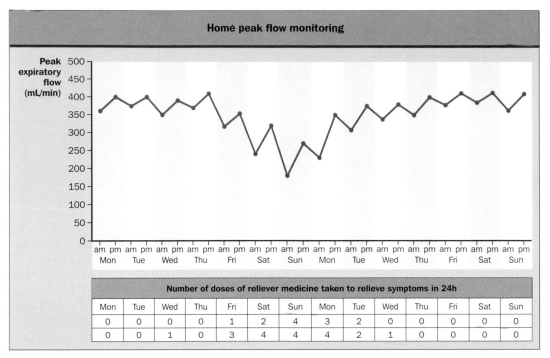

Home peak flow monitoring

Peak expiratory flow (mL/min)

Number of doses of reliever medicine taken to relieve symptoms in 24h

	Mon	Tue	Wed	Thu	Fri	Sat	Sun	Mon	Tue	Wed	Thu	Fri	Sat	Sun
	0	0	0	0	1	2	4	3	2	0	0	0	0	0
	0	0	1	0	3	4	4	4	2	1	0	0	0	0

Figure 41.9 Peak flow readings made twice daily at home by a middle-aged man. The diurnal variation and the day-to-day variation in readings is of such magnitude that there can be no doubt that the patient's airway narrowing fulfilled the diagnostic definition of asthma. (The daily readings are the best of three blows, morning and evening.)

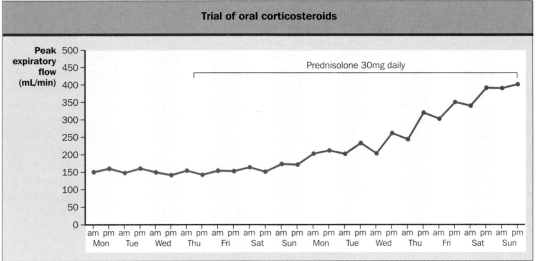

Trial of oral corticosteroids

Peak expiratory flow (mL/min)

Prednisolone 30mg daily

Figure 41.10 Trial of oral corticosteroids. Home peak-flow recordings showed little initial variability. However, after corticosteroids were instituted (within bracket), significant improvement in peak flow occurred, which confirmed a diagnosis of asthma. (The daily readings are the best of three blows, morning and evening.)

Additional tests for suspected asthma

Reason	Test
Patient has symptoms, but spirometry is normal or near normal	Assess diurnal variation of peak flow over 1–2 weeks
	Consider bronchoprovocation with methacholine, histamine, or exercise
Suspect infection, large airway lesions, heart disease, or obstruction by foreign body	Chest radiograph and consider bronchoscopy
Suspect coexisting chronic obstructive pulmonary disease, restrictive defect, or central airway obstruction	Additional pulmonary function tests (e.g. diffusing capacity)
Suspect other factors that contribute to asthma	Allergy tests – skin or *in vitro*
	Nasal examination
	Gastroesophageal reflux assessment

Figure 41.11 Additional tests for asthma if the diagnosis is uncertain. (Adapted from National Heart, Lung, and Blood Institute[1].)

An alternative is to establish whether the airway narrowing can be induced and the diagnostic definition of asthma fulfilled in that way. In some suspected cases of occupational asthma, disease may be induced by careful exposure to small quantities of the probable incriminating agent (i.e. challenge testing).

More commonly airway narrowing and a positive diagnosis of asthma is induced by means of exercise, which can be performed simply, and is applicable to both adults and children old enough to use a peak flow meter. It is best carried out by asking the patient suspected to have asthma to make some baseline peak-flow readings and then to undertake 6 minutes of free running (Fig. 41.12). Any postexercise fall in peak flow is abnormal, but a fall of >15% is regarded as diagnostic of asthma. Peak-flow readings are made at 2 minute intervals for up to 20 minutes after exercise, and if significant asthma is induced bronchodilators are given. False-positive tests do not occur, but a false-negative result can happen so a negative exercise test does not exclude the possibility of asthma at other times.

Results of an asthma exercise test

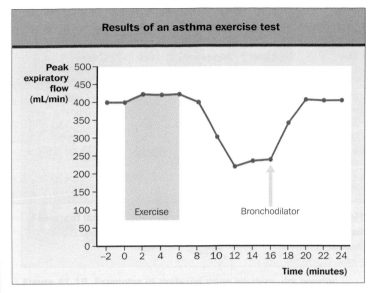

Figure 41.12 Results of an asthma exercise test. Here 6 minutes of free running induced severe asthma in a child who had normal peak flow when first tested.

Flow–volume curves

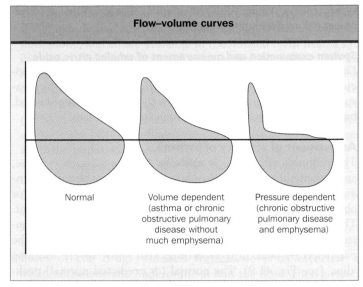

Figure 41.13 Flow–volume curves in some common diseases and their (limited) use in differentiating asthma from some other conditions.

Other lung function tests

Detailed lung function may help in the differentiation of other conditions from asthma. The expiratory flow–volume curve is useful to identify pressure-dependent reduction in expiratory flows – because of loss of elastic recoil forces seen in emphysema (Fig. 41.13). The maneuver is also excellent for identifying upper airway problems (see Chapter 4). However, if the differential diagnosis is from chronic obstructive bronchitis (i.e. pure airway disease, with no emphysema), the expiratory flow–volume curve has a volume-dependent shape (Fig. 41.13) and is similar in both COPD and asthma. In general, measurements of lung volume tend to show an increase in total lung capacity (TLC) with COPD, but both COPD and asthma patients can show increased levels of functional residual capacity and residual volume, the values in asthma increasing with the severity of the disease, but it is unusual for asthmatic patients to show an increase in TLC.

The measurement of the single-breath gas transfer factor (D_{LCO}) is normal in asthma, but can be reduced in COPD, and especially in emphysema.

Lung function tests are rarely diagnostic, but the demonstration of restrictive spirometry and a reduction in lung volumes

excludes asthma and introduces the differential diagnosis of restrictive lung disorders.

Chest radiograph

The chest radiograph in asthma may show larger than normal lungs because of gas trapping, with flattened diaphragms and horizontal ribs – they appear quite distinct from those of restrictive disorders (Fig. 41.14). The chest radiograph can also alert the physician to complications of asthma such as bronchopulmonary aspergillosis, infection, pulmonary eosinophilia, or pneumothorax.

Skin-prick testing

The presence of an allergic condition by skin testing (or by measurement of specific IgE) can help to identifying possible trigger factors for an individual's asthma, but adds little to diagnosis of the underlying condition

Measurement of airway hyperresponsiveness

A cardinal feature of asthma is AHR, but it is not specific to it. Nevertheless, in some centers measurement of AHR is an integral part of asthma management and its establishment in an otherwise

Figure 41.14 Comparative lung sizes on chest radiograph.
(a) Radiograph of a man who has hyperinflation secondary to severe airway narrowing. (b) The small lungs (restrictive disorder) often seen in the very obese.

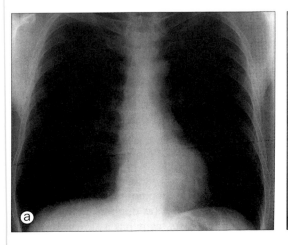

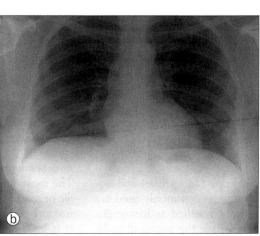

PATHOLOGY

Airways

At autopsy, the typical gross appearance of the lung is one of consolidation. Numerous areas of bronchiectasis filled with mucopurulent material, mucus plugging of the smaller airways, thickening and fibrosis of the airway walls, and the presence of fibrinous pleuritis can be observed in areas where infection has bored through to the pleural surface (Fig. 42.4). Microscopically, obliteration of bronchioles, dilatation of air spaces with destruction of interalveolar septi, diffuse airway occupation by eosinophilic materials, and diffuse interstitial fibrosis are common. In some patients, subpleural blebs and large bronchiectatic cysts may be present. In patients who have experienced prolonged hypoxemia, the vascular changes of pulmonary hypertension also may be evident.

Pancreas

Approximately 95% of CF patients exhibit some degree of exocrine pancreas dysfunction. Enzyme insufficiency leads to maldigestion of protein and fat. Microscopically, a loss of normal anatomy occurs, fibrous fatty tissue diffusely occupies the parenchyma, and small cysts develop from dilated ducts present throughout the organ (hence the term CF of the pancreas; Fig. 42.5).

Hepatobiliary system

In a large number of individuals, the liver appears abnormal microscopically on autopsy. Secretions and bile become inspissated, bile duct proliferation occurs, and inflammatory reaction is present in about 30% of CF patients. Overt nodular cirrhosis is rare and is associated with death in only a small minority (i.e. 1–5%) of CF patients (Fig. 42.6). The gallbladder is commonly hypoplastic (i.e. microbladder), and contains inspissated bile, viscous material, and/or bile stones.

Intestines

Goblet cell hyperplasia and accumulation of the eosinophilic secretions within the crypts in the lumen of the intestine are characteristic in CF. Mucus abnormality may be a factor in the increased tendency of stools to adhere to the walls of the organ.

Reproductive system

Although spermatogenesis can be demonstrated by testicular biopsy, >99% of male CF patients are sterile because of incomplete development of the wolffian ducts. The epididymis and vas deferens are either partially or completely absent; seminal vesicles may be very small or absent as well. Many females are annovulatory secondary to chronic lung disease, although fertility may be as high as 20%. Furthermore, viscous and inspissated cervical mucus may plug the cervical canal and prevent conception.

Upper respiratory tract

Virtually all CF patients experience increased production of secretions and thickening of the mucosal lining of the sinuses. Nasal polyposis occurs in up to 30% of CF patients. Upper respiratory manifestations range from small formations that cause increased posterior nasal drainage to large tumors that completely obstruct the nasal passages. In rare instances, mucoceles

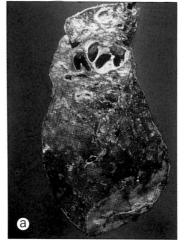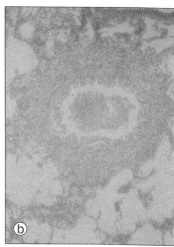

Figure 42.4 Lung pathology. (a) Gross abnormal lung showing bronchiectatic cysts. (b) Microscopic view of a cystic fibrosis lung with small bronchus showing occupation of the lumen. (Courtesy of J Palmer.)

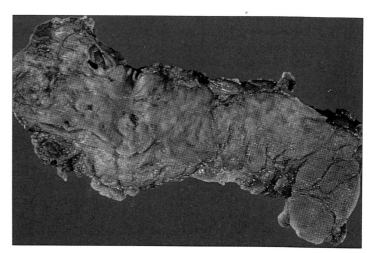

Figure 42.5 Gross cystic fibrosis pancreas pathology.

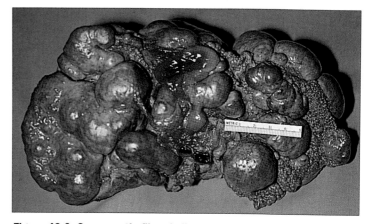

Figure 42.6 Gross cystic fibrosis liver showing nodular cirrhosis. The patient died from hepatic failure.

and ballooning of the sinus cavity may compress the orbit. Infraorbital edema with widening of the nasal bridge should increase clinical suspicion of polyps and more significant sinus disease in CF patients (Fig. 42.7).

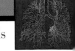

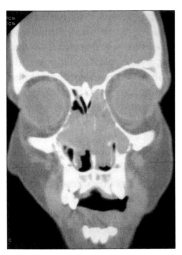

Figure 42.7 Sinus disease in cystic fibrosis. Computed tomography scan showing opacification of the ethymoid sinuses and large nasal polyps in a cystic fibrosis patient.

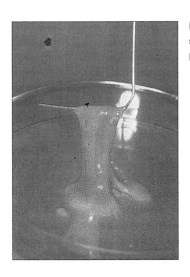

Figure 42.8 Thick tenacious sputum from a cystic fibrosis patient. (Courtesy of J Palmer.)

Lower respiratory tract

Chronic or recurrent bronchiolitis, in the presence of cough, wheezing, tachypnea, and prolonged expiration, is commonly observed in infants who have CF. As growth and aging progress, the contribution of small airways to the overall airway resistance diminishes. Classically, CF is characterized by periodic flare ups of chronic bronchitis. An increase in daily cough, increased lung mucus production, and an increase in sputum become common features in most patients. Sputum ranges from light yellow to deep green and is usually thick and tenacious (Fig. 42.8). Exacerbations are usually triggered by infection with viruses or mycoplasma. During these episodes, cough and expectoration increase, and sputum becomes thicker and more abundant. Patients also may run a low-grade fever, experience increased fatigue (sometimes accompanied by shortness of breath), and exhibit a decrease in or loss of appetite (coupled with weight loss). Wheezing in the presence of crackles in additional lung areas, prolonged expiration, and suprasternal (and occasionally intercostal) retractions also can be present. Chest radiographs may show hyperinflation, increased mucus plugging, and obstruction of the airways.

CLINICAL FEATURES

The abnormal physiology associated with CF affects many body systems; thus, it is not surprising that a variety of complications may be seen in patients who have the disease, although pulmonary abnormalities comprise the major focus of concern. The most common primary clinical manifestations of CF include endobronchial inflammation (i.e. chronic, recurrent airways obstruction and infection), pancreatic insufficiency with intestinal malabsorption, and congenital bilateral absence of the vas deferens in males. Nonpulmonary manifestations also are common and include meconium ileus, malabsorption, fatty infiltration of the liver, focal biliary cirrhosis, glucose intolerance, and a predilection for heat prostration because of severe salt depletion (Fig. 42.9).

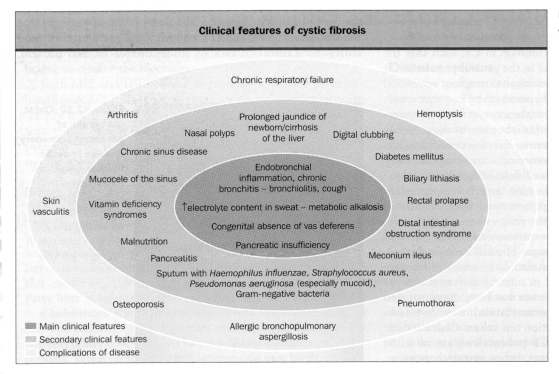

Figure 42.9 Clinical features of cystic fibrosis.

Clinical features of cystic fibrosis

Chronic respiratory failure

Arthritis — Prolonged jaundice of newborn/cirrhosis of the liver — Hemoptysis

Nasal polyps — Digital clubbing

Chronic sinus disease — Diabetes mellitus

Endobronchial inflammation, chronic bronchitis – bronchiolitis, cough

Mucocele of the sinus — Biliary lithiasis

↑electrolyte content in sweat – metabolic alkalosis — Rectal prolapse

Skin vasculitis — Vitamin deficiency syndromes — Congenital absence of vas deferens — Distal intestinal obstruction syndrome

Malnutrition — Pancreatic insufficiency

Pancreatitis — Meconium ileus

Sputum with *Haemophilus influenzae, Straphylococcus aureus, Pseudomonas aeruginosa* (especially mucoid), Gram-negative bacteria

Osteoporosis — Pneumothorax

Allergic bronchopulmonary aspergillosis

Main clinical features
Secondary clinical features
Complications of disease

Pulmonary complications of cystic fibrosis					
Complication	**Cause**	**Management**	**Complication**	**Cause**	**Management**
Pneumothorax	Bursting of sub-pleural blebs	Thoracotomy and chest tube insertion. If no resolution within 48 hours, limited pleural abrasion via thoracoscopy or thoracotomy	Atelectasis	Mucus plugging of proximal bronchus	Antibiotic therapy, energetic chest physical therapy, endoscopy

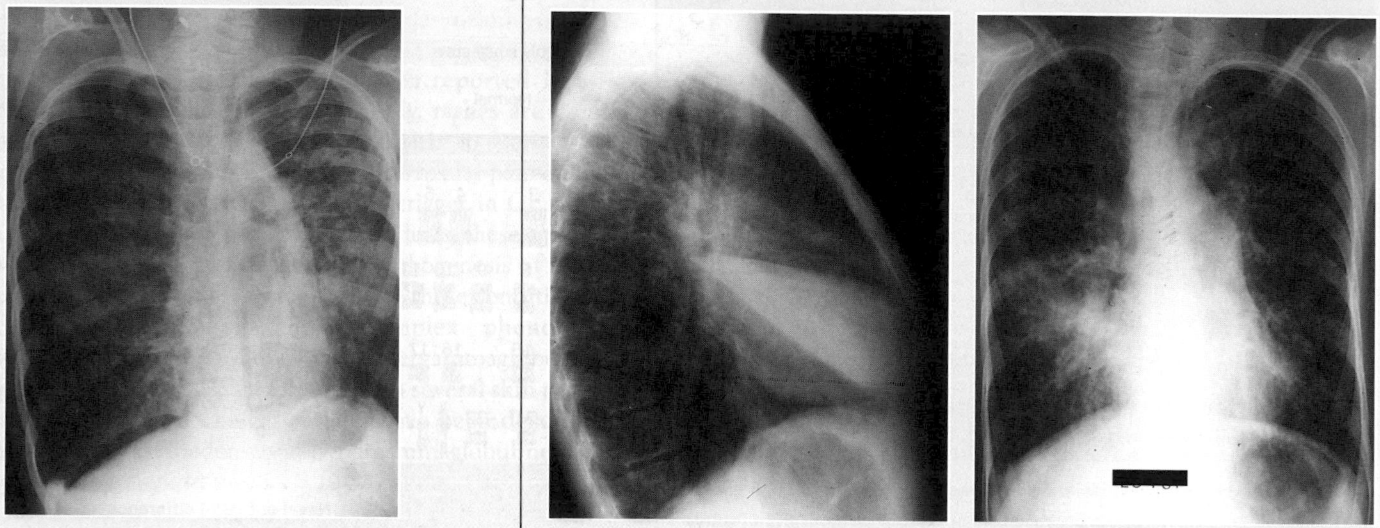

Figure 42.14 Pulmonary complications of cystic fibrosis. This Figure shows two complications of cystic fibrosis. Not shown are hemoptysis and allergic bronchopulmonary aspergillosis.

The goals of general CF care are to prevent or slow the decline of lung function, improve nutritional status, and optimize quality of life. As CF is a disease that affects multiple body systems, a multidisciplinary team can be highly effective in providing continuity of care as patients mature. Cystic fibrosis centers throughout North America and Europe provide a framework of specialized health care sites focused on providing early and aggressive treatment of deterioration and complications, as well as patient education and family support. Additionally, the central gathering of data into national and international registries has expanded our understanding of the epidemiologic characteristics of this condition and facilitated therapeutic advances.

Pulmonary exacerbations

Although no criteria to define a pulmonary exacerbation (PE) are universally accepted, a recent consensus panel developed a list of signs and symptoms that are recognized by clinicians experienced in the management of CF to be commonly associated with PE (Fig. 42.15)[20]. Pulmonary function invariably declines during an exacerbation, and it is the single most important objective marker by which to assess the severity of an exacerbation and the patient's response to treatment. Sputum cultures and bacterial sensitivities are performed routinely at the onset of an exacerbation, and treatment decisions are based on these laboratory results. Oral or inhaled antibiotic therapies are commonly employed when symptoms, signs, and pulmonary function decrements are mild (Fig. 42.16)[21,22]; however, it is important to monitor the patient's progress to ensure clinical improvement. When an exacerbation is severe (or when sputum cultures fail to identify a microbial susceptibility to an oral agent) intravenous antibiotics are administered to the patient (Fig. 42.17)[21,22]. Similarly,

should the clinician determine that home care is suitable, close monitoring of the patient's progress and condition is critical.

In addition to choosing an agent to which the organism is sensitive, CF patients require adequate antibiotic dosages (to achieve bactericidal levels) administered for a sufficient period to achieve a clinical response. While a 2-week course of therapy usually suffices for the patient who has not undergone multiple courses of

Signs and symptoms of pulmonary exacerbation
Increased cough
Increased sputum production and/or a change in appearance of expectorated sputum
Fever [≥100.5°F (≥38°C) for at least 4h in a 24h period] on more than one occasion in the previous week
Weight loss ≥1kg or 5% of body weight associated with anorexia and decreased dietary intake or growth failure in an infant or child
School or work absenteeism (because of illness) in the previous week
Increased respiratory rate and/or work of breathing
New findings on chest examination (e.g. rales, wheezing, crackles)
Decreased exercise tolerance
Decrease in forced expiration volume in 1 second of ≥10% from previous baseline study within past 3 months
Decrease in hemoglobin saturation (as measured by oximetry) of ≥10% from baseline value within past 3 months
New finding(s) on chest radiograph

Figure 42.15 Signs and symptoms of pulmonary exacerbation. (Adapted with permission from Cystic Fibrosis Foundation[20].)

treatment, longer intervals may be necessary for those CF patients who do not achieve a complete response at 14 days or for those patients who have more severe disease. Routinely, CF patients require high-dose antibiotic therapy – which must also be administered in a considerably higher concentration than required for a non-CF patient. This requirement for dosage adjustment results from the metabolic impact of CF on rate of absorption and whole body clearance of antibiotics. Pharmacokinetic studies in CF patients during antibiotic administration have clearly demonstrated that metabolic alterations, unique to the CF population, result in reduced antibiotic concentrations and activity in the sputum when standard doses are administered[23]. To compound

Oral antibiotic treatment in cystic fibrosis			
Antibiotic		**Standard adult dose for cystic fibrosis**	**Organisms targeted**
Penicillins	Amoxicillin–clavulanate	500mg q8h or 875mg q12h	Staphylococcus aureus, Haemophilus influenzae
	Dicloxacillin	500mg q6h	S. aureus
Cephalosporins	Cefaclor	500mg q8h	S. aureus, H. influenzae
	Cephalexin	500mg q6h	S. aureus
	Cefuroxime	500mg q12h	S. aureus, H. influenzae
Others	Azithromycin	500mg on day 1, followed by 250mg/day on days 2–5	S. aureus, H. influenzae
	Chloramphenicol	500mg q6h	Burkholderia cepacia, H. influenzae
	Clarithromycin	500mg q12h	S. aureus
	Doxycycline	100mg q12h	H. influenzae
	Erythromycin	500mg q6h–q8h	S. aureus
	Trimethoprim–sulfamethoxazole	160mg q12h/800mg q12h	S. aureus, H. influenzae, B. cepacia
Quinolones	Ciprofloxacin (not indicated for use in patients <18 years of age)	500–750mg q12h	Pseudomonas aeruginosa, S. aureus, H. influenzae
	Levofloxacin	500mg once daily	S. aureus, H. influenzae, P. aeruginosa
	Ofloxacin	400mg q12h	P. aeruginosa, S. aureus, H. influenza

Figure 42.16 Oral antibiotic treatment in cystic fibrosis. Adapted from Ramsey[21] and Varlotta and Schidlow[22].

Intravenous antibiotic treatment in cystic fibrosis			
Antibiotic		**Standard adult dose for cystic fibrosis**	**Organisms targeted**
Aminoglycosides (dosages given are starting doses; guided by peak and trough serum levels, as indicated			
	Amikacin	20–30mg/kg per day in 2–3 divided doses	Pseudomonas aeruginosa, Haemophilus influenzae
	Gentamicin	6–15mg/kg per day in 2–3 divided doses	P. aeruginosa, H. influenzae
	Tobramycin	6–15mg/kg per day in 2–3 divided doses	P. aeruginosa, H. influenzae
Cephalosporins	Ceftazidime	2g q8h	P. aeruginosa, H. influenzae, Burkholderia cepacia
	Cefuroxime	0.75–1.5g q8h	H. influenzae
Penicillins	Ampicillin–sulbactam	1.5–2.0g q6h	Staphylococcus aureus, H. influenzae
	Nafcillin	1.0–2.0g q6h	S. aureus
	Piperacillin, piperacillin–tazobactam	3.0–4.0g q4h–q6h	P. aeruginosa, H. influenzae
	Ticarcillin, ticarcillin–clavulanate	3.0g q4h–6qh	P. aeruginosa, H. influenzae
	Oxacillin	1.0–2.0g q6h	S. aureus
Other	Aztreonam	1.0–2.0g q6h	P. aeruginosa, H. influenzae
	Chloramphenicol	50mg/kg per day in 4 divided doses	B. cepacia, H. influenzae
	Ciprofloxacin (not indicated for patients <18 years of age)	400mg q12h	P. aeruginosa, H. influenzae, S. aureus
	Clindamycin	600–900mg q8h	S. aureus
	Imipenem–cilastatin	0.5–1.0g q6h	P. aeruginosa, H. influenzae, S. aureus
	Trimethoprim–sulfamethoxazole	12.0–20.0mg/kg per day in 2–4 divided doses	B. cepacia, H. influenzae, S. aureus
	Vancomycin	500mg q6h	S. aureus

Figure 42.17 Intravenous antibiotic treatment in cystic fibrosis. Adapted from Ramsey[21] and Varlotta and Schidlow[22].

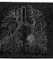

this, the properties of *P. aeruginosa* that relate to coexistent populations of varying drug sensitivities and alginate product (mucoid strains) render the organism more difficult to treat. Furthermore, other agents, such as tobramycin, may be inactivated because binding to free DNA in the infected CF airway secretions[24].

The goal of therapy is to return the patient to baseline, or pre-exacerbation, status. Symptoms, sputum product, and lung function must be evaluated at presentation, midpoint in the treatment course, and when treatment is terminated. Alone, radiographic chest films (which may remain unchanged during an exacerbation) are insufficiently sensitive for the evaluation of therapeutic outcomes[8]. Significant declines in FEV_1 and forced vital capacity can frequently occur, and spirometry is routinely employed to assess the treatment response in a CF patient.

The goal of CF management is to prevent pulmonary deterioration. Despite widespread agreement among CF care givers regarding the importance of aggressive antimicrobial therapy for exacerbations, the use of these agents prophylactically to slow the progression of lung disease and to increase the intervals between exacerbations in patients chronically infected with *P. aeruginosa* has become more widely accepted, albeit controversial. These efforts, in combination with long-term use of mucolytics such as dornase alfa (to decrease the viscosity of airway mucus and reduce the frequency of PEs)[25] and anti-inflammatory agents such as corticosteroids and high-dose ibuprofen[26], have all contributed to better patient outcomes.

For patients who have end-stage disease, bilateral lung transplantation is the only therapeutic alternative[27]. Both organ demand (which far exceeds the number of suitable organs available for transplant and routinely includes a waiting period of 18–24 months) and advance preparation of the patient and family preclude lung transplantation as an emergency procedure. Several other factors, such as portal hypertension, severe malnutrition, and lung colonization with *B. cepacia*, may negate transplant surgery for patients in some centers. Transplant survival data show a 73% survival at 1 year after transplant, 63% at 2 years, and 57% at 3 years, with patients generally enjoying a good quality of life[19].

Nonpulmonary management

As a result of increased metabolic demands created by the work of breathing, battling chronic infection, and imbalances in digestion and nutritional absorption, CF patients may require 120–140% of the recommended daily allowance for caloric intake[28]. Maintaining an unrestricted fat, high-calorie diet, with liberal salt intake and vitamin plus mineral supplementation, is encouraged[29]. Patients affected by exocrine pancreatic deficiency are aided by enzyme replacement therapy; however, the administration of high doses of lipase has been associated with fibrosing colonopathy, and close monitoring is prudent[30]. Children who experience growth failure because of inadequate nutritional intake may benefit from enteral supplemental feedings at nighttime, commonly accomplished via gastrostomy[28].

PROGNOSIS

Despite the research and technologic advances available as we broach the new millennium, CF is still considered a chronic, progressive, lethal disease. Increased understanding of the pathophysiology of this disease, coupled with earlier diagnosis and improved management, have resulted in steady increases in median

survival. Median survival in the USA now exceeds 31 years of age. Canadian and some European countries report median survival rates of upwards of 40 years of age. With the increased detection of patients who show milder disease expression, the development of new therapies to correct the basic ion transport defect, and the advent of lung transplantation, it is reasonable to expect this trend to continue[31].

Currently, survival among males is slightly better than that among females, although the reasons for this remain unclear[32]. These differences in male and female survival rates occur during the age range 1–20 years. No significant predictive difference between males and females has been clearly established for pulmonary function, nutritional status, and airway microbiology, although each of these factors is closely associated with mortality[32]. Factors positively linked to improved longevity include pancreatic sufficiency[33], male sex, absence of colonization with mucoid *P. aeruginosa*, a predominant presentation of gastrointestinal symptoms, appropriate and supportive family functioning and coping, and compliance with treatment regimens. To date, no definitive research has established a link between early diagnosis and improved survival.

Genotype–phenotype relationship

Correlation of genotype and phenotypic expression in CF is confounded by the identification of >600 CF mutations (and the factorial potential for genotypic permutations). Furthermore, individual variability in compensatory homeostatic mechanisms, environmental factors, and other genetic modifiers increase the challenge of identifying these relationships in CF. Several factors, such as age at diagnosis, diversity in presentation, disease severity, and rate of progression appear to be directed by the specific gene mutation.

The high frequency of the $\Delta F508$ mutation has facilitated research to establish genotype–phenotype correlations with this genotype[32]; however, other mutations occur so infrequently that to perform statistically relevant studies is extremely difficult. Knowledge of these >600 CF mutations has, however, facilitated the development of functional classifications on the basis of CFTR protein alterations (see Fig. 42.2).

Pancreatic status has been demonstrated to have the strongest genotype–phenotype correlation yet identified[35]. For example, a strong concordance of pancreatic function status (phenotype) among affected individuals within the same family (genotype) has been documented. The relationship between the phenotypic expression of pulmonary manifestations in CF and genotype is less clear.

Investigational therapeutic approaches

In 1989, a group of US and Canadian scientists cloned and sequenced the CFTR gene. Since that time, an intensive effort has been underway to develop a vector to facilitate correction of the faulty gene. In an attempt to identify a mechanism that can deliver a functional CFTR gene, several vector types are being researched. Presently, these include three types of viral vectors:
- adenoviral vectors (or Ad vectors);
- adeno-associated viral (AAV) vectors;
- retroviral vectors (lentiviruses).

Research is also being carried out on the use of nonviral vectors (liposomes). All of these vectors can be broadly grouped by mechanism of action into two categories. The Ad vectors, liposomes, and molecular conjugates lead to transient expression of the CFTR protein, in which the CFTR gene functions as extrachromosomal (or episomal) DNA in the nucleus. The AAV and retroviral vectors integrate or insert into the host-cell genome. Studies are underway with naturally occurring viruses as well as recombinant vectors, while such issues as efficacy, delivery site, duration of function, immune response, and general safety are being explored.

Gene-assist therapy

Gene-assist therapy focuses on the abnormal gene product, CFTR, and seeks to normalize chloride concentrations in the airway surface fluids (i.e. trafficking), either by repairing the defective protein or by bypassing the cellular defect and opening alternative chloride channels. Early research efforts demonstrated that partial correction of chloride ion transport to the nasal tissues may be possible with the drug 8-cyclopentyl-1,3-dipropylxanthine (CPX), which essentially promotes chloride ion transport and improves CFTR trafficking[36]. Another investigational agent, uridine phosphatidylglycerol (UTP), bypasses the cellular defect and opens alternative chloride channels. The objective of gene-assist therapy is to restore the normal ionic composition of the airway fluid and thereby the activity of endogenous antimicrobial substances that protect against infection.

Protein repair therapy

Recent research has enhanced our understanding of CFTR gene mutations, and protein repair therapy (a relatively new concept) is aimed at manipulating the class mutation defects in CFTR production, folding, trafficking, and/or chloride conduction. For example, class I mutations decrease the production of CFTR protein via stop codons, which prematurely terminate CFTR mRNA. This results in truncated mRNA transcripts that are unstable and usually not translated into proteins[3]. Based on genotype, patients known to carry two class I mutant alleles can be given an agent (aminoglycoside antibiotic) to suppress the 'nonsense' mutations (and thereby prevent the early termination of CFTR mRNA) and permit production of full-length CFTR mRNA protein (see Fig. 42.2)[3,37].

Class II mutations result in accumulation of the mutant CFTR protein in the endoplasmic reticulum, where the protein is degraded[3]. The ΔF508 mutation, a single amino acid deletion of phenylalanine at position 508, is the prototype of this class. It is thought that the premature destruction of ΔF508 results from a block in protein trafficking or from misfolding during translation. The ΔF508 protein is nearly completely degraded (i.e. 99%) by the quality control mechanisms in the endoplasmic reticulum, the role of which is to degrade misfolded or mutant protein. Interestingly, this protein can be recovered by growing cells at subphysiologic temperatures (73.5–80.5°F [23–27°C]), which has led to the development of a number of new therapeutic approaches (see Fig. 42.2). These mutations are severe and associated with pancreatic insufficiency.

Class III mutations are completely defective in regulation and activation of chloride channel activity. Presently, no clinical trials have been announced to specifically address the class III mutations, although compounds that affect the interaction of the nucleotide-binding folds with ATP may prove to be useful in future trials[3]. Furthermore, as several of the class III and IV mutations may prove unresponsive to direct stimulation, it is reasonable to explore the use of gene therapy, rather than protein repair alone, for some of these mutations.

Class IV mutations, associated with milder forms of CF that are characterized by pancreatic sufficiency, comprise CFTR proteins that have reduced conductance for chloride[3]. Although a few agents are currently under investigation, no therapeutic agents for class IV mutations have been announced.

CONCLUSION

Achievements in patient management and traditional therapeutic agents, coupled with advances in our understanding of the pulmonary biology and pathophysiology of CF, have significantly improved the clinical prognosis and quality of life for CF patients. As scientists continue with ongoing molecular and genetics research, the promise of novel therapeutics and strategies via gene therapy and protein repair techniques offers renewed hope in the battle with this most challenging foe.

REFERENCES

1. FitzSimmons SC. The changing epidemiology of cystic fibrosis. J Pediatr. 1993;122:1–9.
2. FitzSimmons SC. Cystic Fibrosis Foundation Patient Registry Annual Data Report 1995. Bethesda: Cystic Fibrosis Foundation; 1996.
3. Zeitlin PL. Therapies directed at the basic defect. Clin Chest Med. 1998;19:6.1–11.
4. Welsh MJ, Ramsey BW. Research on cystic fibrosis: a journey from the Heart House. Am J Respir Crit Care Med. 1998;157:S148–54.
5. Khan TZ, Wagener JS, Bost T, Martinez J, Accurso FJ, Riches DW. Early pulmonary inflammation in infants with cystic fibrosis. Am J Respir Crit Care Med. 1995;151:1075–1082.
6. Govan JRW, Nelson JW. Microbiology of lung infection in cystic fibrosis. Br Med Bull. 1992;48:912–30.
7. Saiman L, Nui WW, Neu HC, et al. Antibiotic strategies to treat multi-resistant Pseudomonas aeruginosa. Pediatr Pulmonol. 1992;8:S286–7.
8. Brasfield D, Hicks G, Soong S, et al. Evaluation of a scoring system of the chest radiographs in cystic fibrosis: a collaborative study. Pediatrics. 1979;63:24–9.
9. Rubinstein S, Moss R, Lewiston N. Constipation and meconium ileus equivalent in patients with cystic fibrosis. Pediatrics. 1986;78:474–9.
10. Kotloff RM. Reproductive issues in patients with cystic fibrosis. Semin Respir Crit Care Med. 1994;15:402–13.
11. Lanng S, Thorsteinnsson B, Nerup J, et al. Diabetes mellitus in cystic fibrosis: effect of insulin therapy on lung function and infections. Acta Paediatr Scand. 1994;83:849–53.

12. Moran A. Diabetes and glucose intolerance in cystic fibrosis. New Insights Into Cystic Fibrosis. 1997;5:1–6.
13. Cystic Fibrosis Foundation. Report of the 1995 Patient Registry. Bethesda: Cystic Fibrosis Foundation; 1996.
14. Cystic Fibrosis Foundation. The diagnosis of cystic fibrosis: consensus statement. In: Clinical practice guidelines for cystic fibrosis. (Consensus Conference Document; Appendix 1, Table 2.) Cystic Fibrosis Foundation; 1996.
15. Cystic Fibrosis Foundation. The diagnosis of cystic fibrosis: consensus statement. In: Clinical practice guidelines for cystic fibrosis. Bethesda: Cystic Fibrosis Foundation; 1997;VII(I):1–5(Appendix 1).
16. Rosenstein BJ, Cutting GR. The diagnosis of cystic fibrosis; a consensus statement. Cystic Foundation Consensus Panel. J Pediatr. 1998;132:589–95.
17. Alton EWFW, Currie D, Logan-Sinclair R, et al. Nasal potential difference: a clinical diagnostic test for cystic fibrosis. Eur Respir J. 1990;3:922–6.
18. Brock DJH. Prenatal screening for cystic fibrosis: 5 years' experience reviewed. Lancet. 1996;347:148–50.
19. Fitzsimmons SC. Cystic Fibrosis Foundation Patient Registry Annual Data Report. 1996. Bethesda: Cystic Fibrosis Foundation; 1997.
20. Cystic Fibrosis Foundation. Microbiology and infectious disease in cystic fibrosis. Clinical Practice Guidelines For Cystic Fibrosis. Bethesda: Cystic Fibrosis Foundation; 1997;V(I):25.
21. Ramsey BW. Management of pulmonary disease in patients with cystic fibrosis. N Engl J Med. 1998;335:179–86.
22. Varlotta L, Schidlow DV. CF lung disease: choosing an antibiotic regimen. J Respir Dis. 1997;18:258–67.
23. Moutin JW, Kerrebijn KF. Antibacterial therapy in cystic fibrosis. Med Clin North Am. 1990;74:837–50.
24. Horrevorts AM, Driessen OM, Michel MF, Kerribijn KF. Pharmacokinetics of antimicrobial drugs in cystic fibrosis: aminoglycoside antibiotics. Chest. 1988;94(Suppl 2):S120–5.
25. Fuchs HJ, Borowitz DS, Christiansen DH, et al. Effect of aerosolized recombinant human DNase on exacerbations of respiratory symptoms and on pulmonary function in patients with cystic fibrosis. N Engl J Med. 1994;331:637–42.
26. Konstan MW, Byard PJ, Hoppel CL, et al. Effect of high-dose ibuprofen in patients with cystic fibrosis. N Engl J Med. 1995;332:848–54.
27. Zuckerman JB, Kotloff RM. Lung transplantation for cystic fibrosis. Clin Chest Med. 1998;19:8.1–20.
28. Ramsey BW, Ranell PM, Pencharz P. Nutritional assessment and management in cystic fibrosis: a consensus report. Am J Clin Nutr. 1992;55:108–16.
29. Peters SA, Rolles CJ. Vitamin therapy in cystic fibrosis – a review and rationale. J Clin Pharmacother. 1993;18:33–8.
30. Borowitz DS, Grand RJ, Durie PR. Use of pancreatic enzyme supplements for patients with cystic fibrosis in the context of fibrosing colonopathy. J Pediatr. 1995;127:681–4.
31. Robinson CB. Is DNA destiny? Clin Chest Med. 1998;19:7.1–8.
32. Rosenstein BJ, Zeitlin PL. Cystic fibrosis. Lancet. 1998;351:277–82.
33. Gaskin KJ, Gurwitz D, Durie PR, et al. Improved respiratory prognosis in patients with cystic fibrosis with normal fat absorption. J Pediatr. 1982;100:857–62.
34. Kerem B, Corey M, Kerem B-S, et al. Relationship between genotype and phenotype in cystic fibrosis – analysis of the most common mutation (ΔF508). N Engl J Med. 1990;23:1517–22.
35. Kristidis P, Bozon D, Corey M, et al. Genetic determination of exocrine pancreatic function in cystic fibrosis. Am J Hum Genet. 1992;50:1178–84.
36. Weatherly MR. Medical topic – CPX: a new 'gene-assist' drug. International Association of Cystic Fibrosis Adults. 1997;51:3–5.
37. Howard M, Frizzell RA, Bedwell DM. Aminoglycoside antibiotics restore CFTR function by overcoming premature stop mutations. Nature Med. 1996;2:467–69.

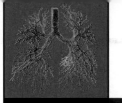

Section 8 Lung Tumors

Chapter 43

Lung Tumors

David E Midthun and James R Jett

INTRODUCTION

Cancer of the lung is the leading cause of cancer death in both women and men in the USA, Canada, and China (Fig. 43.1)[1]. In Australia, France, Germany, Scandinavia, Spain, and the UK, lung cancer is the number one cause of cancer death in men and the second or third cause in women. The prevalence is particularly alarming given that, at the turn of the 20th century, lung cancer was a rare malignancy. As the 5-year survival for lung cancer in the USA and Europe is currently about 13%, the devastation caused by this single cancer type is worth special attention. The frequent presence and lethal nature of lung cancer has thrust it to the forefront of problems in pulmonary medicine.

The term lung cancer is used to describe cancer that arises in the airways or pulmonary parenchyma. Lung cancer is classified into primarily two subgroups: small-cell lung cancer (SCLC) and nonsmall-cell lung cancer (NSCLC). The distinction in subgroups is essential with regard to treatment and prognosis. Approximately 95% of all lung cancers fall into either small-cell or nonsmall-cell categories (Fig. 43.2). Although lung cancer and bronchogenic carcinoma are terms often used synonymously, tumors of other rare cell types comprise the other 5% of cancers that originate in the lung. The majority of this chapter is devoted to a discussion of bronchogenic carcinoma. Carcinoid tumor, lymphoma, mucoepidermoid carcinoma, adenoid cystic carcinoma, hamartoma, and lung metastasis are discussed at the end of the chapter.

EPIDEMIOLOGY, PATHOGENESIS, AND PATHOLOGY

Epidemiology

Cigarette smoke is by far the most significant factor in the causation of lung cancer. The relationship between smoking and lung cancer was initially reported in the 1940s and was further established from epidemiologic research in the 1950s. The first US Surgeon General's *Report on Smoking and Health* was published in 1964 and concluded that cigarette smoking was causally related to lung cancer.

In 1965, 52% of men and 34% of women in the USA over the age of 18 years were cigarette smokers. By 1991, the percentages had declined to 28% for men and 24% for women. Current cigarette use appears to have leveled off at about one quarter of the adult population. Each day in the USA, approximately 3000 teenagers start to smoke. Smoking rates in many countries in Europe and Asia have been and are higher than those in the USA. Approximately 1 out of every 5 deaths in the USA result from smoking, and long-term studies estimate that about half of all regular smokers are eventually killed by their habit.

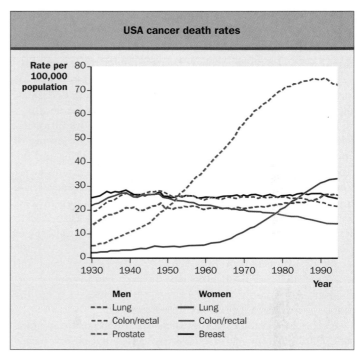

Figure 43.1 USA cancer death rates. (Data from the American Cancer Society[2].)

Figure 43.2 Lung cancer classification.

Lung cancer classification	
Category	Incidence (%)
Small-cell lung cancer	20
Nonsmall-cell lung cancer	75
Adenocarcinoma	35
Squamous cell carcinoma	30
Large-cell carcinoma	10
Others	5
Carcinoid tumors	–
Pulmonary lymphoma	–
Mucoepidermoid carcinoma	–
Adenoid cystic carcinoma	–
Sarcomas	–

Approximately 85% of lung cancer occurs in smokers or former smokers. The Edinburgh Lung Cancer Group reported that of 3070 new patients who had lung cancer, only 74 (2%) were lifelong never smokers. Cigarette smoking is identified as the major cause of each of the histologic types of lung cancer: small cell, squamous cell, large cell, and adenocarcinoma. The risk of developing lung cancer is related to the number of cigarettes smoked, age at which smoking started, and duration of smoking[2]. Cigarette smoke contains more than 4000 chemical constituents, some of which have been identified as carcinogens. Smoking is also associated with the formation of cancers of the larynx, pharynx, mouth, esophagus, pancreas, and bladder. Current smokers have a rate of lung cancer 10–15 times that of someone who has never smoked, and the risk increases to 20–25 times if more than one pack per day of cigarettes is consumed (Fig. 43.3). The British physician study showed the risk of lung cancer remains elevated long after smoking cessation and takes 15 years to approach that of someone who has never smoked[3]. Results of the Multiple Risk Factor Intervention Trial were similar. After 10.5 years of follow-up, 119 men who were smokers or ex-smokers at entry died of lung cancer compared with no lung cancer deaths among men who reported never having smoked. The lag time for a significant reduction in lung cancer death from smoking cessation was many years. Even if cigarette consumption ceased today, the current epidemic of lung cancer would persist for decades.

In passive smoking, side-stream smoke is unintentionally inhaled by someone in the presence of a smoker. A number of epidemiologic studies have evaluated passive smoking and the risk of lung cancer. Studies that involved women who never smoked but who lived with a smoking husband suggest a 1.2–2 times increase in lung cancer risk compared with nonsmoking women in smoke-free homes[4]. Passive smoking is estimated to account for approximately 3000 new cases of lung cancer per year in the USA.

Air pollution from motor vehicles, factory emissions, and wood and coal burning heaters have been shown to contain carcinogens. Air pollution is felt to increase lung cancer risk, but the degree of risk has not been accurately assessed.

A clear association exists between asbestos exposure and lung cancer, although the increased risk is generally not observed until 20 or more years following the initial exposure. A naturally occurring, fibrous silicate ubiquitous in the soil, asbestos was commercially used in the construction industry and for its fire-retardant properties. Certain types of asbestos fibers are more carcinogenic than others. A combination of asbestos exposure and cigarette smoking results in an approximately 50-fold increase in the risk of lung cancer compared with someone who has never smoked and has not been exposed to asbestos.

Radon exposure is perhaps the greatest element of lung cancer risk for nonsmokers who have not been exposed to asbestos. Radon is a decay product of naturally-occurring radium which, in turn, is a breakdown product of uranium. Radon is present in indoor and outdoor air, and the relative risk of lung cancer appears to increase linearly with exposure. The Committee on Biological Effects of Ionizing Radiation has established that radon in the general environment is responsible for 10% of all lung cancers in the USA, placing it as the second most frequent cause of lung cancer. The US Environmental Protection Agency has established acceptable levels for annual exposure to radon and has advised that most houses be tested for radon.

Although no specific, inherited lung-cancer gene has been identified, evidence for familial susceptibility to lung cancer after controlling for cigarette smoking has been found. Squamous cell carcinoma appears to be most associated with familial clustering of lung cancer. Women may be at greater risk than men who have an equivalent smoking history. An increasing number of

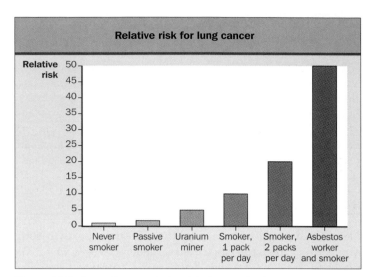

Figure 43.3 Approximate relative risk factors for lung cancer.

genetic abnormalities are recognized in resected lung cancers. Genetic predisposition may result from a difference in carcinogen metabolism, genetic instability of DNA repair processes, or altered oncogene expression. Epidemiologic evidence also demonstrates an increased risk among individuals whose diet is low in β-carotene and vitamin A.

Studies carried out in the 1980s in different institutions showed that chronic obstructive pulmonary disease is a risk factor for lung cancer over and above the risk from cigarette smoking. Presence of airflow obstruction on pulmonary function testing was associated with a 4–6 times greater risk of lung cancer when controlled for cigarette smoking[5]. The association of airflow obstruction and lung cancer was further supported by the Lung Health Study, in which 5800 patients who had mild airway obstruction and a history of smoking were assessed for effectiveness of smoking cessation and anticholinergic therapy. Lung cancer was the leading cause of death during the 5 years of follow-up for this study[6]. Whether airflow obstruction predisposes to lung cancer or whether both arise from a common factor is unclear.

Pathogenesis

The current understanding of the pathogenesis of lung cancer is that of a multistep process of carcinogen-induced genetic damage to cells that proceeds through the three stages of initiation, promotion, and progression. The increased incidence of lung cancer with aging supports a multistep process. Pathologic changes of bronchial epithelium from dysplasia to carcinoma *in situ* in smokers is consistent with a multistep process. The mechanism by which smoking causes lung cancer is not completely understood. Components of cigarette smoke have been shown to initiate and promote the process of carcinogenesis. Genetic changes have also been demonstrated in histologic respiratory epithelial cells of normal appearance obtained from smokers. Deletion of the short arm of chromosome-3 (3p) and -9 (9p) has been identified as early genetic change present in both epithelial cells of normal appearance and lung cancer cells.

Greater recognition of the genetic changes that occur in lung cancer may lead to a better understanding of its pathogenicity. Lung cancers have been shown to contain an average of 30–60 different cellular, genetic abnormalities. Both SCLC and NSCLC have been shown to contain certain consistent chromosomal abnormalities. Although survival with lung cancer correlates best to the stage of disease, large survival discrepancies among patients within a single stage of disease are unexplained and may reflect a specific tumor biology. Research in cancer biology has revealed a number of markers that may be significant in tumor behavior. Predictions of a good or bad outcome have been attempted on the basis of oncogene amplification, level of tumor-associated antigens, specific enzymes and growth factors, rate of cell proliferation, and other biologic factors. Several oncogenes, such as c-*myc*, K-*ras*, and c-*erbB2*, have been identified in association with some lung cancers, but the pathogenic relationship is unclear. Mutations in the tumor suppressor gene p53 are frequently identified in patients who have NSCLC, although conflicting results have occurred as to its association with prognosis. Clarification of these tumor biologic factors may help to focus the estimation of specific patient prognosis.

Pathology

Histopathologic designation of lung cancer is based on the World Health Organization Classification System. A correct histologic diagnosis of lung cancer is imperative to determine treatment and prognosis. Differing cell types are designated by their appearance under light microscopy. An agreement between pathologists in the separation of SCLC and NSCLC occurs in >95% of cases; the latter is composed of squamous cell, adenocarcinoma, and large cell carcinoma. Considerable variation in histologic differentiation in individual cases leads to differences in interpretation. Interobserver variation among pathologists in the recognition of NSCLC subtypes ranges as high as 25–40% of cases.

Adenocarcinoma is currently the most frequent histologic cell type of lung cancer and it comprises 30–35% of lung cancer series. Adenocarcinoma comprises the majority of lung cancers in patients who have never smoked and occurs most commonly in the peripheral aspects of the lung parenchyma as a solitary nodule or mass (Fig. 43.4). The identification of adenocarcinoma requires histologic evidence of neoplastic gland formation or the presence of intracytoplasmic mucin. Bronchoalveolar cell is a subtype of adenocarcinoma and may present as a nodule or mass as well as a pneumonia-like infiltrate (Fig. 43.5). Histologic features of bronchoalveolar cell carcinoma include origin distal to grossly recognizable bronchi, well-differentiated cytologic features, and growth along intact alveolar septa.

Squamous cell carcinoma is the second most common cell type and comprises about 30% of lung cancer. Squamous cell type correlates highly with smoking history and originates most often in the central airways (Fig. 43.6). Patients who have squamous cell carcinoma may have symptoms of airway involvement, show radiographic evidence of airway obstruction, or the tumor may be radiographically occult. Cavitation may be seen in squamous cell as well as in other types of NSCLC (Fig. 43.7) and is not a characteristic of SCLC. The diagnosis of squamous cell carcinoma requires histologic evidence of

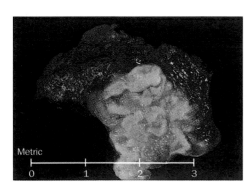

Figure 43.4 Peripheral adenocarcinoma. This wedge resection gross specimen of a peripheral nodule showed grade 2 adenocarcinoma. The patient underwent a lobectomy with formal lymph node dissection.

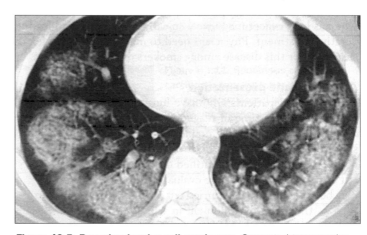

Figure 43.5 Bronchoalveolar cell carcinoma. Computed tomography scan of the chest showing bilateral alveolar infiltrates in a patient who has unresolving pneumonia. Transbronchoscopic biopsy revealed bronchoalveolar cell carcinoma.

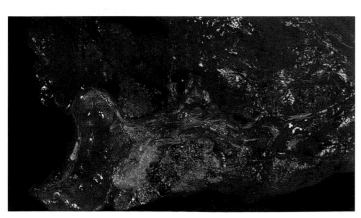

Figure 43.6 Squamous cell lung cancer. Gross specimen of the left lung showing obstruction of the left upper lobe bronchus by tumor and peribronchial extension. Histology showed grade 2 squamous cell carcinoma.

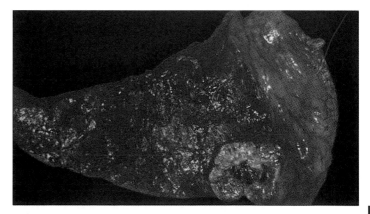

Figure 43.7 Cavitating squamous cell carcinoma. Gross specimen of the right lower lung showing a peripheral, thick-walled cavity with central necrosis. Histology revealed squamous cell carcinoma.

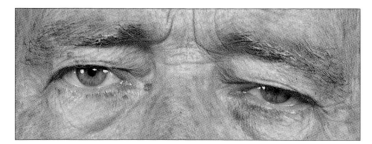

Figure 43.14 Ptosis as part of Pancoast's syndrome. Drooping of this man's left eye is evident as part of Pancoast's syndrome, and meiosis was also present. His computed tomography scan is shown in Figure 43.13.

and fingers. Patients often seek a chiropractor or orthopedist prior to proper diagnosis.

Metastatic effects

Hardly any body tissue is immune from the metastatic presence or effects of lung cancer. Lung cancer may spread by direct extension, through lymphatics, or hematogenously.

Liver

The liver is a frequent site of spread from lung cancer. Autopsy studies have shown evidence of hepatic metastasis in >60% of patients who have small-cell type and about 30% of those who have squamous cell carcinoma of the lung (Fig. 43.15)[9]. The presence of hepatic metastasis at presentation is much less common. Among patients diagnosed to have operable NSCLC in the chest, approximately 5% show computed tomographic evidence of liver metastasis. Involvement of the liver is shown by computed tomography (CT) in about 25% of patients who have SCLC at initial staging. Patients who have liver involvement are often asymptomatic at initial presentation.

Adrenal

Metastasis to the adrenal glands is present at autopsy in 25–40% of patients who have lung cancer (Fig. 43.16)[9]. The usual scenario in adrenal metastasis is a unilateral adrenal mass found during staging CT for lung cancer. Oliver et al. found that of 330 patients who have operable NSCLC, 25 (7.5%) had isolated adrenal masses and eight (2.4%) proved malignant[10]. Even in the setting of initial evaluation for lung cancer, most of the adrenal masses are benign and usually caused by adenomas, nodular hyperplasia, or hemorrhagic cysts. The finding of a unilateral adrenal mass in a patient who has otherwise resectable disease requires a needle biopsy guided by CT to confirm the presence or absence of metastasis.

Bone

Bone metastasis from lung cancer is most common in the small-cell type, but is also frequent in nonsmall-cell types. An osteolytic radiographic appearance is more frequent than an osteoblastic one, and vertebral bodies are the most common bones involved. Approximately 30–40% of patients initially staged for SCLC with a bone scan and bone marrow will have evidence of metastasis[9]. Chest pain, skeletal pain, bone tenderness, and elevated levels of serum calcium or alkaline phosphatase are usually present in patients who have bony metastasis caused by NSCLC. Bone pain and elevated levels of serum calcium or alkaline phosphatase are often absent in patients who have SCLC and bone marrow involvement.

Nervous system

Neurologic manifestations of lung cancer include direct metastatic effects and paraneoplastic syndromes; the latter are discussed in the next section. The presence of central nervous system (CNS) metastasis may be asymptomatic or cause headache, vomiting, seizures, hemiparesis, cranial nerve deficit, or visual field loss. Autopsy series have shown brain metastasis in the range 25–40% for patients who had lung cancer[9]. Squamous cell carcinoma has the least tendency to metastasize to the CNS, and SCLC the greatest. Combined resection may be feasible in selected cases that have operable NSCLC in the chest and a solitary brain metastasis. Various surgical series have shown 2-year survival rates of 25–45%.

Isolated nerve dysfunction may be the result of regional extension of bronchogenic carcinoma. Neoplasm is the most common cause of unilateral vocal cord paralysis, and lung cancer is the most common malignancy. The presence of hoarseness in a smoker raises concern for lung cancer. Extension of lung cancer into the phrenic nerve may result in diaphragm paralysis; patients may report dyspnea or be asymptomatic.

Pleural

Presence of carcinoma cells in the pleural fluid establishes the lung cancer as unresectable. Of patients who have lung cancer, <10% have pleural involvement at presentation. Dyspnea and cough are common symptoms that occur with malignant pleural

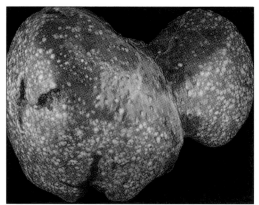

Figure 43.15 Liver metastases from small-cell carcinoma of the lung. The gross autopsy liver specimen from a 50-year-old male smoker shows innumerable metastatic foci of small-cell carcinoma.

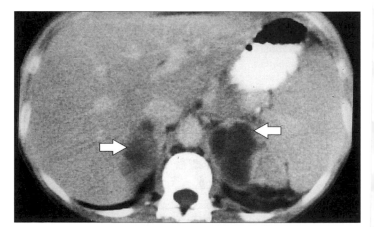

Figure 43.16 Adrenal metastases. Computed tomography scan of the abdomen showing large adrenal metastases (arrows) in a patient who has a lung mass and mediastinal adenopathy. Fine needle aspirate of the adrenal showed adenocarcinoma.

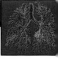

effusions; approximately one fourth of patients who have lung cancer and pleural metastases are asymptomatic (Fig. 43.17). Malignant effusions are typically exudates and may be serous, serosanguineous, or grossly bloody. The simple presence of a pleural effusion in the setting of bronchogenic carcinoma does not establish unresectability. Pleural effusion may result from lymphatic obstruction, postobstructive pneumonitis, or atelectasis. The presence of pleural metastasis needs to be confirmed so that a chance for curative resection is not overlooked (Fig. 43.18). Documented cases of malignancy have shown the yield of pleural fluid cytology to be about 66%[11]. Pleural biopsy adds little to the yield of cytologic examination. In a patient suspected to have malignancy, repeat pleural fluid cytology with or without pleural biopsy is appropriate if the initial study is negative. In the setting of a malignant effusion, a low pleural fluid pH (<7.30) is a poor prognostic sign.

Paraneoplastic syndromes

The remote effects of cancer are those not related to the direct invasion, obstruction, or metastatic effects of tumor, and are generally termed paraneoplastic. Paraneoplastic syndromes related to bronchogenic carcinoma occur in 10–20% of patients (Fig. 43.19).

Musculoskeletal

Clubbing of the digits is a manifestation of lung cancer and other diseases such as congenital heart disease, pulmonary fibrosis, liver disease, hereditary diseases, and others. Clubbing may involve the fingers and toes and consists of selective enlargement of the connective tissue in the terminal phalanges (see Fig. 43.20). Physical findings include loss of the angle between the base of the nail bed and cuticle, rounded nails, and enlarged finger tips. Clubbing is an isolated finding and is usually asymptomatic.

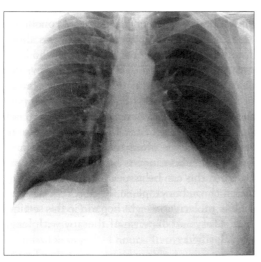

Figure 43.17 Malignant pleural effusion. Chest radiograph showing a left pleural effusion; thoracentesis revealed adenocarcinoma consistent with a lung primary tumor.

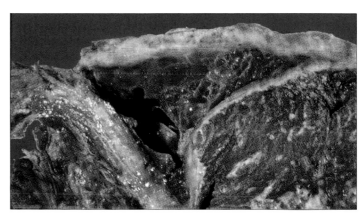

Figure 43.18 Pleural involvement by adenocarcinoma. The gross specimen shows malignant pleural involvement similar to the appearance of mesothelioma (see Fig. 67.4). Histology revealed adenocarcinoma.

Figure 43.19 Paraneoplastic syndromes associated with bronchogenic carcinoma.

Paraneoplastic syndromes associated with bronchogenic carcinoma			
System	**Paraneoplastic syndrome**	**System**	**Paraneoplastic syndrome**
Musculoskeletal	Hypertrophic osteoarthropathy	Neurologic	Lambert–Eaton syndrome
	Polymyositis		Peripheral neuropathy
	Osteomalacia		Encephalopathy
	Myopathy		Myelopathy
Cutaneous	Clubbing		Cerebellar degeneration
	Dermatomyositis		Psychosis
	Acanthosis nigricans		Dementia
	Pruritus	Vascular/hematologic	Thrombophlebitis
	Erythema multiforme		Arterial thrombosis
	Hyperpigmentation		Nonbacterial thrombotic endocarditis
	Urticaria		Thrombocytosis
	Scleroderma		Polycythemia
Endocrinologic	Cushing's syndrome		Hemolytic anemia
	Syndrome of inappropriate antidiuretic hormone secretion		Red cell aplasia
			Dysproteinemia
	Hypercalcemia		Leukemoid reaction
	Carcinoid syndrome		Eosinophilia
	Hyperglycemia/hypoglycemia		Thrombocytopenic purpura
	Gynecomastia		Hypercoagulable state
	Galactorrhea		
	Growth hormone excess	Miscellaneous	Cachexia
	Calcitonin secretion		Hyperuricemia
	Thyroid-stimulating hormone		Nephrotic syndrome

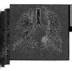
If patients relapse within 6 months of therapy using a platinum-based regimen or if they fail to respond to initial therapy, second-line treatment decisions are more difficult. Response rates to second-line CAV have generally been poor and are ≤ 25%. Early studies reported response rates of 25–35% for single-agent topotecan or paclitaxel in relapse SCLC. The chance of responding to these agents as second-line therapy is increased significantly if the patients responded to initial therapy and if they have been off this prior therapy for 3 months or longer. As no standard second-line therapy is established for SCLC, these patients should, whenever possible, be enrolled in prospective clinical trials to evaluate new therapies.

CLINICAL COURSE AND PREVENTION

Among patients who have lung cancer, the overall 5-year survival is 13%. Taking this into account, the clinical course of most patients who have lung cancer is unpleasantly predictable. The best efforts of the physician, surgeon, and medical and radiation oncologist uncommonly result in a cure or greatly prolonged survival. The two most important prognostic factors are tumor stage and performance scores. Resected stage IA NSCLC has a 5-year survival of approximately 70% compared with 10% for stage I tumors in patients who are not surgical candidates because of medical problems or refusal to undergo surgery[32]. Long-term survival in patients at various stages of lung cancer detected in the absence of symptoms is 35%, versus 10% among those detected in the presence of symptoms. Identification of patients in the preclinical phase of lung cancer is desirable, but a clearly effective screening tool has not been identified. Younger patients and those who have squamous cell type carry a better prognosis among those patients who have operable disease. The prognosis is poor for patients who have NSCLC beyond surgical resectability and in those who suffer SCLC.

Following resection and possible cure for any resectable stage of disease, the risk of developing a second primary lung cancer is 2–3%/year[33]. Accordingly, patients are followed at intervals of 3–4 months for the first 2 years after treatment for the development of recurrent disease. Most lung cancers recur within the first 2 years. After this, patients are followed every 6–12 months for the possible development of late recurrence or a new primary lung cancer. At the present time, no adjuvant therapy has been proven to prolong survival after curative resection, but studies are under way.

Functional status has been shown to be an important predictor of survival. The Karnofsky Performance Status assesses activity and ability for self-care on a scale from 100 to 0. A performance status ≤ 70 (one who is unable to work or pursue normal activities, but who lives at home and carries out self-care) is recognized as an independent predictor of shortened survival. Other performance status scales are in use and have shown the ability to predict survival. These measures help to both focus the estimation of prognosis and determine when treatment is appropriate in advanced stage disease.

Weight loss >10% of body weight and male sex are also independent predictors of shortened survival among patients who have unresectable disease. Poor prognosis is also associated with the presence of distant metastasis to liver, bone, and brain, as is an elevated lactate dehydrogenase. Within a single stage of lung cancer, considerable discrepancies arise in survival between patients, which suggests that other biologic factors are involved

in prognosis. Research into cancer biology has identified a number of markers that may play a role in tumor behavior but, at this point, their roles are unclear.

Recurrence or progression of disease occurs in the vast majority of patients who have lung cancer, which eventually results in death. Patients who suffer squamous cell carcinoma have a higher rate of local failure and a lower rate of distant metastasis when compared with those who have adenocarcinoma or large cell carcinoma. Patients who suffer small-cell carcinoma have a higher rate of distant spread, and approximately 25% die of local tumor complications and the remainder show evidence of carcinomatosis. An investigation of terminally ill patients who had lung cancer gave insight into the role of palliative care[34]. Hyperalimentation was administered in 90% of the patients, oxygen therapy in 78%, and morphine in 40%. The most frequent cause of death in this series was respiratory failure caused by progression of cancer followed by infection, and effusions of the pleura or pericardium. Hospice care can effectively ensure that the patient receives adequate pain control and other palliative measures, while it allows the patient to reside at home. Autopsy series show that approximately one half of patients who have cancer of various cell types have brain metastasis at the time of their demise.

Lung cancer remains a highly preventable disease, since approximately 85% of lung cancer occurs in smokers or former smokers, and so primary prevention remains the avoidance of the cigarette. Efforts at early detection and treatment should not diminish the energy devoted to help patients quit smoking. Smoking rates have fallen in the USA and are showing signs of diminishing elsewhere in the world. Unfortunately, cigarette smoking is highly addictive, and smoking cessation often proves difficult. Physicians may be an important motivator to help patients quit smoking. A 3-minute interview session with a physician can lead to a 5% success rate in smoking cessation when combined with antismoking reading materials and a follow-up visit. Use of supplemental nicotine, group therapy, behavioral training, hypnosis, or acupuncture achieve 1-year abstinence rates of around 20% in controlled trials. A sustained-release form of the antidepressant bupropion showed cessation rates of 44% after 7 weeks of treatment and 23% at 1-year follow-up in a placebo controlled trial[35]. Interestingly, the mean weight gain among patients was 1.5kg compared with 2.9kg in the control group (p =0.02) at the end of 7 weeks of therapy. Clearly, primary prevention by avoidance of smoking or through smoking cessation is the best way to prevent the devastating grip of this disease. Home radon testing may also play a role in reducing an individual's risk for lung cancer.

OTHER LUNG NEOPLASMS AND LUNG METASTASES

Carcinoid tumor

Bronchial carcinoid tumors are low-grade malignant neoplasms comprised of neuroendocrine cells and account for 1–2% of all tumors of the lung. Patients may present with hemoptysis, have evidence of bronchial obstruction, or be asymptomatic (Fig. 43.35). The association of carcinoid syndrome with bronchial carcinoid tumor is rare, as is ectopic production of adrenocorticotropic hormone and Cushing's syndrome. As the tumors are often endobronchial, bronchoscopy commonly obtains tissue effectively, but this is a relatively vascular tumor so caution in

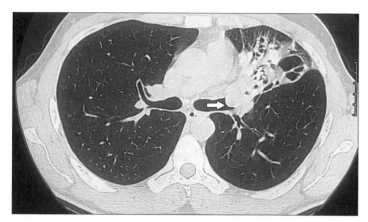

Figure 43.35 Carcinoid tumor. Computed tomography of the chest in a 34-year-old man with a 1-year history of recurrent left upper-lobe pneumonia and hemoptysis. Tumor obstructs the left upper-lobe bronchus (arrow) with associated focal bronchiectasis. Bronchoscopy and subsequent resection revealed carcinoid tumor.

sampling is appropriate. Surgical resection is often curative, and in the absence of nodal metastasis, 5-year survival is 90%[36]. Prognosis is lessened in tumors >3cm or in the presence of nodal metastasis.

When histologic evidence of increased mitotic activity, nuclear pleomorphism, and disorganization is present, lesions are designated as atypical carcinoids, which tend to have a higher rate of metastasis and be larger at the time of diagnosis than typical carcinoid tumors. The 5-year survival with atypical carcinoid tumors is approximately 60–70%, and surgical treatment is desired when feasible.

Pulmonary lymphoma
Primary pulmonary lymphomas account for <1% of all lung cancer and are uniformly non-Hodgkin's lymphomas. In a series of 33 patients from Mayo Clinic, 22 patients had small-cell lymphoma, six had large cell lymphoma, and five had mixed-cell lymphoma[37]. In these patients treated with surgery, surgery plus chemotherapy, or chemotherapy alone, 5-year survival was 77%. Surgical resection of a localized, primary non-Hodgkin's lymphoma may be curative, and chemotherapy appears effective in patients who have bilateral or disseminated disease.

Mucoepidermoid carcinoma
Mucoepidermoid carcinoma is another rare airway neoplasm derived from minor salivary gland tissue in the proximal tracheobronchial tree. As a result of the central airway location, patients usually present with cough, hemoptysis, or obstructive pneumonia. Surgical resection remains the treatment of choice when feasible, and complete resection portends an excellent prognosis[37]. Lesions of low-grade histology are uncommonly associated with nodal metastases.

Adenoid cystic carcinoma
Adenoid cystic carcinoma is the most common salivary gland-like tumor to occur in the lower respiratory tract and accounts for <1% of all primary lung cancers. Adenoid cystic carcinomas usually arise in the lower trachea, main stem, or lobar bronchi, and are rarely peripheral. Presenting symptoms are usually cough, hemoptysis, or evidence of airway obstruction. Surgical resection

is preferred; however, this cell type has a propensity to recur locally and metastasize and is often incompletely resected. Delayed recurrence as long as 15–20 years after initial resection has been reported.

Hamartoma
Hamartoma is the most common benign neoplasm to occur in the lung. Histologically, the lesions consist of a combination of cartilage, connective tissue, smooth muscle, fat, and respiratory epithelium. Most hamartomas are detected when patients are asymptomatic, and the highest incidence is in the sixth or seventh decade. A series of 215 patients from the Mayo Clinic reported that only four patients had symptoms related to the hamartoma[38]. The classic radiographic appearance of popcorn-ball calcification occurs in only about 25% of hamartomas. Approximately 15% show evidence of fat on thin-section CT scanning (Fig. 43.36). Radiographic recognition allows for simple observation in most instances; radiographically indeterminate lesions may be resected for confirmation. Multiple pulmonary hamartomas have been reported rarely.

Lung metastasis
The lung is a frequent site of metastasis from a variety of extrathoracic malignancies. Carcinomas recognized as frequent sources for pulmonary metastases include those of the head and neck, colon, renal, breast, and thyroid, and melanoma. Approximately 10–30% of all malignant nodules resected are metastases. In addition to solitary or multiple nodules, metastatic patterns include lymphangitic, endobronchial, pleural, and embolic. The finding of multiple or innumerable nodules is the most common clinical situation (see Fig. 43.37). Depending on the size and location of the nodules, a diagnosis may be obtained by transthoracic needle aspiration or bronchoscopy. Surgical resection may be appropriate in the setting of a solitary pulmonary metastasis when evidence of other sites of metastatic disease have been excluded. Although randomized studies have not been performed, some evidence suggests improved survival in some patients who have solitary pulmonary metastasis from sarcomas, renal cell carcinoma, breast cancer, and colon cancer.

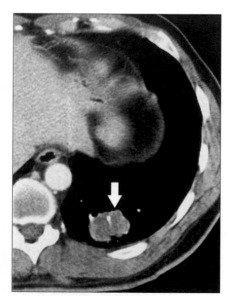

Figure 43.36 Hamartoma. Thin-section computed tomography through this solitary pulmonary nodule reveals evidence of calcification and fat (arrow) consistent with a hamartoma.

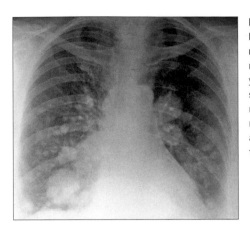

Figure 43.37 Pulmonary metastases. Chest radiograph of a 64-year-old woman showing innumerable nodules from metastatic adenocarcinoma of the thyroid.

PITFALLS AND CONTROVERSIES

Screening for lung cancer

Chest radiography or sputum cytology to screen for lung cancer has not been proven to reduce mortality; however, it is unclear whether the use of such screening has been disproven. In the 1970s, the National Cancer Institute sponsored three large, randomized trials. Participants were men ≥ 45 years of age who had smoked 1 pack of cigarettes per day or more within the year prior to enrollment. The Mayo Lung Project randomized patients to a chest radiograph and 3-day pooled sputum cytology every 4 months in the screened group, and the control group was advised to have an annual chest radiograph and sputum cytology, but had no scheduled follow-up. Johns Hopkins and Memorial Sloan-Kettering were the other two participating centers, and both randomized patients to a dual screen with an annual chest radiograph and 3-day pooled sputum cytology every 4 months versus an annual chest radiograph. None of these trials demonstrated a decreased lung cancer mortality in the screened group, but none of the three centers had an untested control group. In each, the 5-year survival from lung cancer in the screened group was approximately 35%, which is much greater than the historic precedent. Mortality remains the only measure free of bias; however, in the absence of a true control group in the studies, the question remains unanswered. Additional screening trials are currently under way, and new techniques such as monoclonal antibody analysis of sputum, autofluorescent bronchoscopy, and spiral CT scanning are under investigation.

Evaluation of the solitary nodule

The evaluation of a SPN is unclear (see Fig. 43.23). Nodules that are indeterminate following radiographic investigations call for a decision between observation, biopsy, or removal. Newer radiographic techniques will, hopefully, ease the decision making and reduce the incision making. Contrast-enhanced CT as well as contrast-enhanced positron emission tomography and MRI are useful to identify malignancy in the setting of an SPN. The prospective study by Swensen et al. of contrast-enhanced CT reported a sensitivity of 98% and a specificity of 73% in the identification of malignant neoplasms[39]. The test involves the administration of conventional, iodinated contrast material at a specific rate with thin-section CT assessments through the nodule at 1-minute intervals (Fig. 43.38). Malignant neoplasms enhance significantly more (>20 Hounsfield units) than do granulomas and benign neoplasms. The overall accuracy of 93% establishes CT contrast enhancement as a valuable tool in the evaluation of indeterminate SPNs. Positron emission tomography scanning with ^{18}F-fluorodeoxyglucose identifies malignant lesions with a sensitivity of 90–100% and a specificity of 80–89%, but it is currently not widely available and is expensive[40]. Similarly effective in the identification of malignant nodules is MRI with gadolinium–pentetic acid.

Treatment: stage IIIA

One important area that is unclear is the most appropriate treatment for stage IIIA NSCLC. The literature strongly suggests that surgery alone or radiotherapy alone are not optimal treatments. If the patient has a negative mediastinoscopy or CT scan of the chest for adenopathy and is found to have stage IIIA disease at the time of thoracotomy, consideration should be given to postoperative therapy in the setting of a clinical trial. While adjuvant therapy in this setting has not been proven to prolong survival (based on past studies with older chemotherapeutic agents), it is clear that 5-year survival with surgery alone is approximately 25%. In patients who are not operative candidates, the combination of chemotherapy and radiotherapy has been shown to be superior in those of good performance status and minimal weight loss.

Prophylactic cranial irradiation: small-cell lung cancer

Perhaps the most controversial area in therapy for lung cancer is the role of prophylactic cranial irradiation (PCI). Randomized

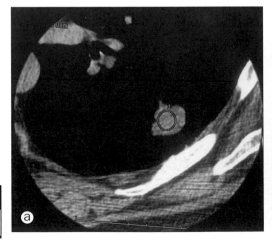
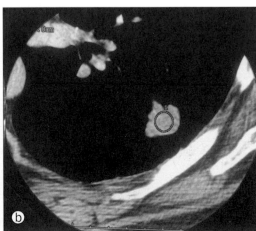

Figure 43.38 Evaluation of a solitary pulmonary nodule with computed tomography (CT) contrast enhancement. (a) Before contrast injection. (b) Following injection of contrast. According to protocol, CT scanning is carried out at 1-minute intervals for 4 minutes and shows an increase in nodule density of 63 Hounsfield units (HU). Enhancement by >20HU is a strong indicator of malignancy. Resection revealed stage IA (T1N0M0) nonsmall-cell lung cancer.

trials have clearly documented that PCI reduces the rate of brain metastasis in patients who have SCLC. However, to date, trials have not clearly shown a survival advantage with PCI. Neurotoxicity adds to the debate. Ataxia, difficulty with concentration, memory problems, and occasional dementia are observed in patients treated with cranial irradiation. Recent trials have employed lower dose and fraction regimens, and preliminary reports have not noted any significant detrimental neurologic sequelae.

At the present time, advocating PCI is inappropriate for a patient who is not in complete clinical remission. Patients who have SCLC and who survive for ≥ 2 years have a 50% likelihood of developing CNS metastasis. If a patient in remission is not given PCI, the patient should be followed carefully for signs and symptoms of CNS metastasis. The highest risk of CNS relapse is within the first 2 years of remission. During the period of observation, some physicians advocate serial CT head scans or MRI of the brain at 3–4 month intervals, although this is an expensive approach.

REFERENCES

1. Landis SH, Murray T, Bolden S, Wingo PA. Cancer statistics 1998. CA, Cancer J Clin. 1998;48:6–29.

2. American Thoracic Society Statement. Cigarette smoking and health. Am J Respir Crit Care Med. 1996;153:861–5.

3. Doll R, Peto R, Wheatley K, Gray R, Sutherland I. Mortality in relation to smoking: 40 years observation on male British doctors. Br Med J. 1994;309:901–11.

4. Janerich DT, Thompson WD, Varela LR, et al. Lung cancer and exposure to tobacco smoke in the household. N Engl J Med. 1990;323:632–6.

5. Tockman MS, Anthonisen NR, Wright EC, Donithan MG. Airways obstruction and the risk for lung cancer. Ann Intern Med. 1987;106:512–18.

6. Anthonisen NR, Connett JE, Kiley JP, et al. Effects of smoking intervention and the use of an inhaled anticholinergic bronchodilator on the rate of decline of FEV1: The Lung Health Study. JAMA. 1994;272:1497–505.

7. Bell DR, Woods RL, Levi JA. Superior vena caval obstruction: a ten-year experience. Med J Aust. 1986;145:566–8.

8. Arcasoy SM, Jett JR. Superior pulmonary sulcus tumors and Pancoast's syndrome. N Engl J Med. 1997;337:1370–6.

9. Hansen HH. Diagnosis in metastatic sites. In: Strauss MJ, ed. Lung cancer: clinical diagnosis and treatment, 2nd edn. Philadelphia PA: Grune and Stratton; 1983:185–200.

10. Oliver TW, Bernardino ME, Miller JI, et al. Isolated adrenal masses in non-small cell bronchogenic carcinoma. Radiology. 1984;153:217–18.

11. Sahn SA. State of the art: the pleura. Am Rev Respir Dis. 1988;138:184–234.

12. Sigurgeirsson B, Lindelof B, Edhag O, Allander E. Risk of cancer in patients with dermatomyositis or polymyositis. N Engl J Med. 1992;326:363–7.

13. Cornuz J, Pearson SD, Creager MA, Cook EF, Goldman L. Importance of findings on the initial evaluation for cancer in patients with symptomatic idiopathic deep venous thrombosis. Ann Intern Med. 1996;125:785–93.

14. Takai E, Yano T, Iguchi H, et al. Tumor induced hypercalcemia and parathyroid hormone related protein in lung carcinoma. Cancer. 1996;78:1384–7.

15. Vinholes J, Guo CY, Purohit OP, Eastell R, Coleman RE. Evaluation of new bone resorption markers in a randomized comparison of pamidronate or clodronate for hypercalcemia of malignancy. J Clin Oncol. 1997;15:131–8.

16. Ayus JC, Krothapalli RK, Arieff AI. Treatment of symptomatic hyponatremia and its relation to brain damage: a prospective study. N Engl J Med. 1987;317:1190–5.

17. Orth DN. Cushing's syndrome. N Engl J Med. 1995;332:791–803.

18. Lucchinetti CF, Kimmel DW, Lennon VA. Paraneoplastic and oncological profiles of patients seropositive for Type 1 anti-neuronal nuclear autoantibodies. Neurology. 1998;50:652–7.

19. American Thoracic Society/European Respiratory Society Statement. Pre-treatment evaluation of non-small cell lung cancer. Am J Respir Crit Care Med. 1997;156:320–32.

20. Mehta AC, Marty JJ, Lee FYW. Sputum cytology. Clin Chest Med. 1993;14:69–85.

21. Mountain CF, Dresler CM. Regional lymph node classification for lung cancer staging. Chest. 1997;111:1718–23.

22. Mountain CF. Revisions in the international system for staging lung cancer. Chest. 1997;111:1710–17.

23. Ginsberg RJ, Rubinstein LV, for Lung Cancer Study Group. Randomized trial of lobectomy versus limited resection for T1 N0 non-small cell lung cancer. Ann Thorac Surg. 1995;60:615–23.

24. Rosell R, Gamez-Codina J, Camps C, et al. A randomized trial comparing preoperative chemotherapy plus surgery with surgery alone in patients with non-small cell lung cancer. N Engl J Med. 1994;330:153–8.

25. Roth JA, Fossella F, Komaki R, et al. A randomized trial comparing perioperative chemotherapy and surgery with surgery alone in resectable stage IIIA non-small cell lung cancer. J Natl Cancer Inst. 1994;86:673–80.

26. Non-Small Cell Lung Cancer Collaborative Group. Chemotherapy in non-small cell lung cancer: a meta-analysis using updated data on individual patients from 52 randomized clinical trials. Br Med J. 1995;311:899–909.

27. Cortese DA, Edell ES. Role of phototherapy, laser therapy, brachytherapy, and prosthetic stents in the management of lung cancer. Clin Chest Med. 1993;14:149–59.

28. Shaw EG, Su JQ, Eagan RT, et al. Prophylactic cranial irradiation in complete responders with small cell lung cancer. J Clin Oncol. 1994;12:2327–32.

29. Lad T, Piantadosi S, Thomas P, et al. A prospective randomized trial to determine the benefit of surgical resection of residual disease following response of small cell lung cancer to combination chemotherapy. Chest. 1994;106(Suppl.):320S–3S.

30. Pignon JP, Arriagada R, Ihde DC, et al. A meta-analysis of thoracic radiotherapy for small cell lung cancer. N Engl J Med. 1992;327:1618–24.

31. Elias AD. Small cell lung cancer: state of the art therapy in 1996. Chest. 1997;112(Suppl.):251S–8S.

32. Flehinger BJ, Kimmel M, Melamed MR. The effect of surgical treatment on survival from early lung cancer: implications for screening. Chest. 1992;101:1013–18.

33. Thomas PA, Rubinstein L for the Lung Cancer Study Group. Malignant disease appearing late after operation for T1N0 non-small cell lung cancer. J Thorac Cardiovasc Surg. 1993;106:1053–8.

34. Homma T, Yoshida S, Yoneda S, et al. The clinical picture of terminally ill patients with lung cancer. Gan No Rhinsho – Jpn J Cancer Clin. 1989;35:891–4.

35. Hurt RD, Sachs DPL, Glover ED, et al. A comparison of sustained-release bupropion and placebo for smoking cessation. N Engl J Med. 1997;337:1195–202.

36. Torre M, Barberis M, Barbieri B, Bonacina E, Belloni P. Typical and atypical bronchial carcinoids. Respir Med. 1989;83:305–8.

37. Miller DL, Allen MS. Rare pulmonary neoplasms. Mayo Clin Proc. 1993;68:492–8.

38. Gjevre JA, Myers JL, Prakash UBS. Pulmonary hamartomas. Mayo Clin Proc. 1996;71:14–20.

39. Swensen SJ, Brown LR, Colby TV, Weaver AL, Midthun DE. Lung nodule enhancement at CT: prospective findings. Radiology. 1996;201:447–55.

40. Dewan NA, Shelhan CJ, Reeb SD, et al. Likelihood of malignancy in a solitary pulmonary nodule: comparison of Bayesian analysis and results of FDG–PET scan. Chest. 1997;112:416–22.

Chapter 44

Approach to Diagnosis

John Britton and Andrew Evans

INTRODUCTION

Diffuse or interstitial lung disease embraces those lung disorders that involve infiltration of alveolar air spaces or thickening of pulmonary interstitial structures. More precise definition of the diffuse lung diseases is difficult, partly because of the disparity of individual disorders involved, and partly because alveolar and interstitial pathology is a recognized component of many lung diseases, for example bacterial pneumonia or primary lung cancer, which are generally and quite appropriately classified elsewhere. The uniting feature of the diffuse lung diseases is that the pathology is relatively widespread and generalized throughout the lungs, and in clinical practice the diffuse lung diseases are usually characterized by and first suspected on the grounds of widely distributed opacification or reticular shadowing on the chest radiograph.

Irrespective of difficulties of definition, the diffuse lung diseases unquestionably cover an immense diversity of lung pathology, which includes disease caused by inhaled materials as in pneumoconiosis or hypersensitivity pneumonitis, by pulmonary involvement in a more generalized multisystem disease, such as the collagen vascular disorders or vasculitides, interstitial infiltration caused by sarcoidosis, amyloid, diffuse malignancy, or tuberculosis, and various other diseases that collectively present a broad range of clinical features and often significant diagnostic difficulty. An appreciable proportion of cases of diffuse lung disease have a characteristic pattern of interstitial inflammation and fibrosis with no recognized cause, and are labeled as idiopathic fibrosing alveolitis [or idiopathic pulmonary fibrosis (IPF), see Chapter 9.45], and also known as cryptogenic fibrosing alveolitis. The majority of diffuse lung diseases run a chronic course, and present with a history of breathlessness or cough dating back over several weeks or months, although more acute presentations do occur.

The diversity of this disease group makes it difficult to provide representative estimates of the size of the disease burden it represents, but a study from Bernalillo County, New Mexico[1], in which interstitial lung diseases were comprehensively ascertained by various methods, found diffuse lung diseases to be prevalent in 81/100,000 adult men and 67/100,000 adult women, and new cases to occur in 32/100,000 and 26/100,000 person-years, respectively. The diffuse lung diseases are therefore less common than the major lung infections, neoplasms, and obstructive airways diseases, but collectively they amount to a significant disease burden for society, and an appreciable workload for the pulmonary physician.

DIFFERENTIAL DIAGNOSIS

The differential diagnosis of diffuse lung disease is extremely extensive, so this discussion can only serve as an approximate guide to the diagnosis of these conditions. In the first place, a standard clinical history and examination usually establishes whether the onset of disease is acute or chronic, and the chest radiograph and other routine clinical investigations all help to establish major alternative diagnoses, such as bacterial pneumonia, tuberculosis, lung cancer, pulmonary edema, or adult respiratory distress syndrome. Many of these diagnoses present relatively acutely and are discussed in detail elsewhere in this book (see Chapters 29, 29, 43, and 69). For the most part, however, the diffuse lung diseases present with a more chronic onset and, although in some cases (such as in the original 'Hamman–Rich' presentation of IPF[2]) the disease can progress rapidly, the clinical history usually points toward a process that began weeks, months, or sometimes years before presentation. For an outline of the major diagnoses that present as diffuse lung disease, see Figure 44.1; although this list is by no means exhaustive, it clearly includes an immense variety of individual and in many cases rare diagnoses.

The occurrence of the individual diffuse lung diseases varies substantially, both in place and time. Occupational lung diseases account for a major proportion of diffuse lung disease, but the prevalence of individual disorders is subject to geographic variation according to local patterns of industrial exposure. Many, such as coal-worker's pneumoconiosis, are becoming less frequent in developed countries as a result of improvements in occupational hygiene and disease screening, while asbestosis among those who work in the production or manufacture of asbestos products has also become much less common in many countries as a result of tight regulation of occupational exposure within the asbestos industry. However, in the UK and the USA exposure to asbestos in building construction, shipyards, maintenance workers, and some other occupational groups remained a significant problem for several years after the introduction of controls in the asbestos industry[3], and may still be common in some countries.

Diffuse lung disease caused by drug exposures is well recognized, particularly in relation to the use of immunosuppressant, cytotoxic, or antimitotic agents, and more recently amiodarone[4]. Pulmonary fibrosis is a common finding in patients who have connective tissue disorders, and diffuse lung disease can sometimes be the presenting feature of these disorders, but usually the clinical features of rheumatoid arthritis or other connective tissue disease are already evident. A substantial proportion of diffuse lung disease is attributable to specific diagnoses, such as sarcoidosis, and a range of individually rare disorders, such as lymphangioleiomyomatosis, eosinophilic granuloma, or alveolar lipoproteinosis; in many cases these diagnoses can only be made with confidence on the grounds of histologic evidence.

With such an extensive and daunting differential diagnosis, it is helpful to return to epidemiologic evidence to place these diagnoses in some perspective. A listing of all of the prevalence

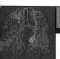

Some recognized causes and differential diagnoses of diffuse lung disease

Cause	Differential diagnosis	
Occupational or other inhalant-related, inorganic	Coal worker's pneumoconiosis	Metal polisher's lung/hard metal fibrosis
	Asbestosis	Berylliosis
	Silicosis	Baritosis (barium)
	Talc pneumoconiosis	Siderosis (iron oxide)
	Aluminum oxide fibrosis	Stannosis
Occupational or other inhalant-related, organic	Bird fancier's lung	Mushroom worker's lung
	Farmer's lung	Maple bark stripper's lung
	Bagassosis (sugar cane)	Malt worker's lung
	Coffee worker's lung	Tea grower's lung
	Tobacco grower's lung	Pituitary snuff-taker's lung
	Fishmeal worker's lung	
Collagen vascular disease related	Systemic lupus erythematosus	Ankylosing spondylitis
	Rheumatoid arthritis	Mixed connective tissue disease
	Scleroderma	Primary Sjögren's syndrome
	Polymyositis	Behçet's syndrome
	Dermatomyositis	Goodpasture's syndrome
Drug related	Amiodarone	Bleomycin
	Propranolol	Busulfan
	Tocainide	Cyclophosphamide
	Nitrofurantoin	Chlorambucil
	Sulfasalazine	Melphalan
	Cephalosporins	Methotrexate
	Gold	Azathioprine
	Penicillamine	Cytosine arabinoside
	Phenytoin	Carmustine
	Mitomycin	Lomustine
	Bromocryptine	
Physical agents/ toxins	Radiation/radiotherapy	Cocaine inhalation
	High concentration oxygen	Intravenous drug abuse
	Paraquat toxicity	
Primary disease diagnoses	Sarcoidosis	Tuberous sclerosis
	Eosinophilic granuloma	Neurofibromatosis
	Amyloidosis	Gaucher's disease
	Lymphangioleiomyomatosis	Niemann–Pick disease
Neoplastic disease	Lymphangitis carcinomatosis	
	Bronchoalveolar cell carcinoma	
Vasculitis related	Wegener's granulomatosis	
	Giant cell arteritis	
	Churg–Strauss syndrome	
Alveolar filling diseases	Alveolar proteinosis	Chronic aspiration
	Lipoid pneumonia	Eosinophilic pneumonia
	Pulmonary lymphoma	Microlithiasis
Disorders of circulation	Pulmonary edema	
	Pulmonary veno-occlusive disease	
Chronic infection	Tuberculosis	Viruses
	Aspergillosis	Parasites
	Histoplasmosis	
Fibrotic disorders of unknown etiology	Acute interstitial pneumonia	Bronchiolitis obliterans organizing pneumonia (BOOP)
	Idiopathic pulmonary fibrosis	
	Lymphocytic interstitial pneumonia	

Figure 44.1 Some recognized causes and differential diagnoses of diffuse lung disease.

Prevalence and incidence of interstitial lung diseases in Bernalillo County, New Mexico

Cause	Interstitial lung disease	Prevalent cases, *n* (%)	Incident cases, *n* (%)
Occupational and environmental	Pneumoconiosis	8 (3.1)	–
	Anthracosis	3 (1.1)	–
	Asbestosis	17 (6.6)	15 (7.4)
	Silicosis	8 (3.1)	6 (3.0)
	Hypersensitivity pneumonitis	–	3 (1.5)
Drug/radiation	Drug-induced interstitial lung disease	5 (1.9)	7 (3.5)
	Radiation fibrosis	1 (0.4)	3 (1.5)
Pulmonary hemorrhage syndromes	Goodpasture's syndrome	–	1 (0.5)
	Vasculitis	–	1 (0.5)
	Hemosiderosis	2 (0.8)	–
	Wegener's granulomatosis	2 (1.2)	6 (3.0)
Connective tissue disease	Mixed connective tissue disease	2 (0.8)	2 (1.0)
	Systemic lupus erythematosus	6 (2.3)	1 (0.5)
	Rheumatoid arthritis	14 (5.4)	10 (5.0)
	Scleroderma	9 (3.5)	3 (1.5)
	Sjögren's syndrome	–	1 (0.5)
	Dermatomyositis/polymyositis	2 (0.8)	1 (0.5)
	Ankylosing spondylitis	–	–
Pulmonary fibrosis	Pulmonary (chronic) Fibrosis/postinflammatory	43 (16.7)	28 (13.9)
	Idiopathic/interstitial fibrosis	58 (22.5)	63 (31.2)
	Interstitial pneumonitis	8 (3.1)	12 (5.9)
Sarcoidosis		30 (11.6)	16 (7.8)
Other	Alveolar proteinosis	1 (0.4)	–
	Amyloidosis	–	–
	Bronchiolitis obliterans	–	1 (0.5)
	Chronic eosinophilic pneumonia	3 (1.2)	1 (0.5)
	Eosinophilic (granuloma) infiltration	2 (0.8)	–
	Infectious/postinfectious interstitial lung disease	3 (1.2)	1 (0.5)
	Lymphocytic infiltrative lung disease	1 (0.4)	–
	Interstitial lung disease, not otherwise specified	29 (11.1)	20 (9.8)
Total		**258**	**202**

Figure 44.2 Numbers of prevalent and incident cases of interstitial lung diseases in Bernalillo county, New Mexico, 10th January 1988 to 9th September 1990. (Adapted with permission from Coultas et al.[1]. Official Journal of American Thoracic Society ©American Lung Association.)

and incidence diagnoses made in the New Mexico study referred to earlier[1] is given in Figure 44.2, which demonstrates that the four most common diagnoses in this population were IPF (22.5%), chronic or postinflammatory fibrosis (16.7%), sarcoidosis (11.6%), and asbestosis (6.6%); together, these accounted for a little over half of all diffuse lung disease diagnoses. A similar pattern is evident in incident (new) cases. Although the identity and relative contributions of specific occupational exposures, such as asbestosis, is likely to be different in other populations, these data are probably representative of the occurrence of diffuse lung disease in most economically developed countries, and demonstrate the rarity of many of the conditions listed in the potential differential diagnosis.

EVALUATION OF A PATIENT

Patients who have diffuse lung disease present to their doctor in several ways, many of which can give important etiologic clues (Fig. 44.3). Most commonly, the presentation is with breathlessness, often with cough, and the possibility of a diagnosis of a diffuse lung disease usually arises in these circumstances because a chest radiograph taken in the process of investigation of the symptoms reveals generalized shadowing. In some cases, however, the diffuse lung disease is identified in the process of investigation for other diseases, such as rheumatoid arthritis or scleroderma, or occurs in an individual in a high-risk occupation that provides a strong indication of a specific pneumoconiosis or other occupational disease. Sometimes, a clear history of exposure to toxins or drugs again points strongly toward the most likely diagnosis.

In many cases, clues from a clinical history and examination, combined with chest radiographic and/or computed tomography (CT) appearances are sufficient to narrow down the list of differential diagnoses considerably. Also, while a confident diagnosis may still require histologic sampling and examination, it is often possible in practice to narrow down the differential diagnosis to the extent that any residual uncertainty does not influence practical decisions on management. At this stage of the diagnostic process some physicians, and some patients, take a pragmatic decision to proceed with therapy, while others opt to strive for greater degrees of diagnostic confidence before commencing therapy. In this respect, practice varies substantially both between and within countries[1,5,6]. With such variation in clinical practice and diversity of the disease under investigation, the following discussion serves only to illustrate the value of different forms of evaluation and investigation in the diffuse lung diseases, rather than to specify what is or is not appropriate or necessary in individual patients.

Clinical history

The most common presenting symptom in diffuse lung disease is breathlessness, but cough is also a feature and can be particularly troublesome in lymphangitis carcinomatosis, extrinsic allergic alveolitis, bronchiolitis obliterans organizing pneumonia (BOOP), and eosinophilic pneumonia. The duration of these symptoms gives some idea of the chronicity of the disease. The standard clinical history also elicits details consistent with current acute infection, risk factors for opportunistic infection, and a past history of tuberculosis or other significant pulmonary disease or infection. It is always worth inquiring about previous chest radiographs and to obtain these if possible, since they often help to identify long-standing disease.

The clinical history should also ascertain as complete an occupational history as possible, exploring details of all lifetime occupations, including temporary and short-term employment, and details of military service. Asbestos exposure is common and has often been extensive in those employed in railway rolling-stock construction, shipyard workers, power station construction and maintenance workers, naval boilermen, and various other specific occupations in which asbestos has played a major role. People previously involved in these occupations usually recall and volunteer their exposure relatively easily. A history of asbestos exposure often has to be sought out more persistently, however, in other groups of workers, such as joiners, carpenters, and other manual workers in the building trade, in whom exposure to asbestos in

the form of roofing and insulation material is not always either appreciated as a significant exposure or recalled as a major component of their work.

Other common occupational causes of pneumoconiosis include coal mining (coal worker's pneumoconiosis), metal polishing (hard metal disease), and 'fettling' or sandblasting of cast iron (silicosis). The occupational history may also identify exposures to organic dusts or allergens linked with extrinsic allergic alveolitis, such as moldy hay (farmer's lung) or mushroom compost (mushroom worker's lung). Extrinsic allergic alveolitis (hypersensitivity pneumonitis) is also commonly caused by exposure to avian proteins, sometimes as a result of specific occupations, but most frequently in people who keep birds as domestic pets or for sport, as in pigeon racing. The clinical history, therefore, needs to explore hobbies and pastimes to complement the occupational history so that potentially relevant exposures can be identified.

Complete drug histories are also necessary to identify or exclude potential drug-related disease. However, although patients may not be able to recall precise details of drugs they have been prescribed, many of the drugs implicated in diffuse lung disease are used in cancer chemotherapy and recall of this generic exposure, if not with precise detail of the specific drugs involved, is not

Important points in the initial evaluation of diffuse lung disease with some specific disease examples		
Evaluation	Aspect	Specific signs
History	All occupations	For example those that involve coal, silica, asbestos, hard metals, organic dusts
	Drugs	For example amiodarone, cytotoxics, gold, nitrofurantoin
	Collagen disease	Rheumatoid arthritis, systemic lupus erythematosus, scleroderma, CREST syndrome, Sjögren's disease
	Physical toxins	Radiotherapy, paraquat, oxygen toxicity
	Geography	Histoplasmosis, parasites, tuberculosis
	Cough	Idiopathic pulmonary fibrosis, asbestosis, lymphangitis, hypersensitivity pneumonitis, infection
	Hemoptysis	Vasculitides
	Breathlessness	Idiopathic pulmonary fibrosis, collagenoses, asbestosis, cancer, pulmonary edema, drugs, infection
	Weight loss	Lymphangitis, advanced disease
Examination	Clubbing	Idiopathic pulmonary fibrosis
	Basal crackles	Idiopathic pulmonary fibrosis, collagenoses, asbestosis, lymphangitis, drugs
	No crackles	Granulomatous diseases, pneumoconiosis, silicosis
	Skin lesions	Erythema nodosum – e.g. sarcoid, tuberculosis
		Telangiectasia – e.g. scleroderma
		Vasculitis – e.g. Wegener's granulomatosis
		Butterfly rash – e.g. systemic lupus erythematosus
	Musculoskeletal	Arthritides, dermatomyositis

Figure 44.3 Important points in the initial evaluation of diffuse lung disease with some specific disease examples.

usually a problem. Since the early 1980s, amiodarone has emerged as one of the more common causes of drug-related diffuse lung disease[4], but the problem is well recognized by clinicians and so the history of exposure is often relatively easy to elicit from medical records if not from the patient. A full past medical history should also elicit details of previous illness in which a patient is likely to have been exposed to high concentrations of oxygen or radiotherapy. Other drugs or pulmonary toxins also need to be considered, including accidental or deliberate paraquat ingestion (which can cause an acute or delayed proliferative bronchiolitis and alveolitis[7]), or inhalation of crack cocaine or heroin (which can cause a number of pulmonary problems including eosinophilic infiltrates, diffuse alveolar hemorrhage, BOOP, and pulmonary edema[8]). Intravenous drug abuse can also result in pulmonary manifestations, which include veno-occlusive disease and talcosis.

Diffuse lung disease frequently occurs in conjunction with, and sometimes in advance of, collagen vascular disease[9]. The clinical history therefore explores details of arthritis and arthralgia, skin disorders, dryness of eyes and mouth, muscular weakness, and other clinical characteristics of rheumatoid arthritis, systemic lupus erythematosus, polymyositis and/or dermatomyositis, Sjögren's syndrome, systemic sclerosis, or other diseases in this category (discussed in more detail in Chapter 11.54). Pulmonary manifestations are also features of Churg–Strauss syndrome, Wegener's granulomatosis, Behçet's disease, and other vasculitides; a history of hemoptysis is common in pulmonary involvement with these disorders, but there may also be an associated history of vasculitic skin rashes, asthma, and nasal discharge and/or bleeding. Evidence of asthma, hemoptysis, skin rashes, and other major features of these vasculitides (see Chapter 10.53) may therefore point toward these diagnoses. Hemoptysis is also a common presenting symptom in Goodpasture's syndrome. Other characteristic features of the history relate to many others of the diagnoses listed in Figure 44.3, including symptoms specific to the primary diagnoses such as sarcoidosis, neurofibromatosis, or lymphangioleiomyomatosis, which are also discussed in Chapters 9.48 and 9.50.

Clinical examination

Findings on clinical examination in diffuse lung disease are, like the differential diagnoses, extremely variable. In some cases, extensive lung shadowing on chest radiographs can occur with virtually no abnormality detectable on clinical examination; sometimes, the converse is the case. Tachypnea and breathlessness on moderate exertion may be observed in any of the diffuse lung diseases, as may the signs of cyanosis or cor pulmonale in advanced disease. Finger clubbing is found in about 50% of those who have IPF or in pulmonary fibrosis associated with collagen vascular disease, but it is rare in sarcoidosis, hypersensitivity pneumonitis, and many other diagnoses. Basal inspiratory crepitations are a more general finding in disease characterized by pulmonary fibrosis, such as IPF or asbestosis, but like finger clubbing they are not generally found in granulomatous diseases such as sarcoidosis, coal worker's pneumoconiosis, or silicosis. Thus, in general the clinical examination can point toward disease that is more fibrotic rather than granulomatous in nature, and may yield specific clues that arise from individual clinical features of some of the diagnoses listed in Figure 44.1. In practice, however, in diagnostic terms and in the context of the initial clinical assessment of the patient who presents with diffuse lung disease,

the clinical examination is usually less helpful than either the clinical history or the chest radiograph.

Chest radiograph

The chest radiograph is probably the single most informative, simple assessment of patients who have diffuse lung disease (Fig. 44.4). In conjunction with a strong clinical history, the chest radiograph is often sufficient to make a confident diagnosis, as for example in coal worker's pneumoconiosis; often, the chest radiograph points strongly toward a particular diagnosis, as in the bilateral hilar lymphadenopathy of sarcoidosis; sometimes, the findings are more diffuse and do not in isolation identify a specific diagnosis, and in a proportion of cases subsequently proved to have diffuse lung disease, the chest radiograph at presentation is normal. Previous radiographs, if available, are extremely helpful in establishing the nature, duration, and progression of disease, particularly (for example) in the postinflammatory fibrosis that can follow tuberculous infection, or in diseases such as sarcoidosis in which characteristic, diagnostic radiologic features may be more evident than in later films of late-stage disease. Examples of chest radiograph appearances in individual diffuse lung diseases appear in the relevant sections of this text. However, a few examples – with different physical signs and symptoms – are shown in Figure 44.5.

The general appearances on the chest radiograph are often categorized according to whether the radiographic pattern suggests

Important investigations for diffuse lung disease with main abnormalities and examples of diseases	
Investigation	**Abnormality and/or disease**
Chest radiograph	Hilar adenopathy
	Size of lungs
	Pleural plaques
	Reticular–nodular shadowing
	Alveolar filling
Blood tests	Erythrocyte sedimentation rate
	Eosinophils
	Autoantibodies
	Anemia
	White cell abnormalities
	Antineutrophil cytoplasmic antibody (ANCA)
	Antiglomerular basement membrane antibodies
	Specific precipitins
Lung function	Pattern – usually restrictive
	Gas transfer
	Hypoxemia, rest and exercise
High-resolution computed tomography scan	Can be virtually diagnostic; also can indicate disease severity
Bronchoalveolar lavage	Infection – tuberculosis, *Pneumocystis carinii*
	Alveolar proteinosis
	Bleeding
	Cell counts (rarely diagnostic)
Transbronchial biopsy	Sarcoidosis, hypersensitivity pneumonitis, cancer, infection (e.g. fungi, tuberculosis)
Open lung biopsy	Definitive

Figure 44.4 Important investigations for diffuse lung disease with main abnormalities and examples of diseases.

alveolar filling or interstitial infiltrates. The appearances of alveolar filling are of a soft, homogeneous shadowing with air bronchograms, sometimes with blurring of mediastinal or diaphragmatic contours; or of a less homogeneous, although still diffuse, pattern of nodular densities because some acini are filled with fluid while others remain air filled. Examples of diseases that produce alveolar shadowing include acute bacterial pneumonia, pulmonary edema, alveolar proteinosis, eosinophilic pneumonia, alveolar cell carcinoma, desquamative interstitial pneumonia (see Chapter 9.45), and pulmonary hemorrhage. Interstitial infiltrates are characterized by more reticular (linear) shadowing, including septal lines, as in IPF, sarcoid, and asbestosis, but may include nodular shadows that are more characteristic of coal worker's pneumoconiosis, silicosis, and miliary tuberculosis. In practice, many diseases display a mixed alveolar and interstitial pattern of shadowing, with nodules of various sizes and density, although the predominant appearance may help to differentiate some of these diagnoses.

Assessment of the size of the lung fields and pattern of distribution of alveolar or interstitial shadowing can also be helpful.

Silicosis, sarcoidosis, and hypersensitivity pneumonitis tend to affect the upper zones of the lung, while IPF, pulmonary fibrosis in conjunction with collagen vascular disease, and asbestosis tend to involve the lower zones. In all of these diagnoses, a general contraction of lung volume can also occur, although this may not be obvious at presentation. Progressive massive fibrosis, Caplan's syndrome, ankylosing spondylitis, post-tuberculous fibrosis, and eosinophilic granuloma also predominantly affect the upper zones of the lung. Enlarged or normal-sized lung fields are seen in lymphangioleiomyomatosis, tuberous sclerosis, neurofibromatosis, eosinophilic granuloma, and IPF in conjunction with chronic obstructive airways disease.

Hilar lymphadenopathy is a characteristic of sarcoidosis, lymphoma, and other malignant disease, while eggshell calcification of hilar nodes is characteristic of silicosis and sarcoidosis. Pleural effusions are seen in collagen vascular disease, infection, pulmonary malignancy, lymphangioleiomyomatosis, and asbestosis, in which pleural thickening, pleural plaques, or mesothelioma may also occur. Pleural disease is notably absent in sarcoid.

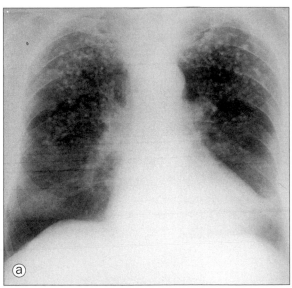

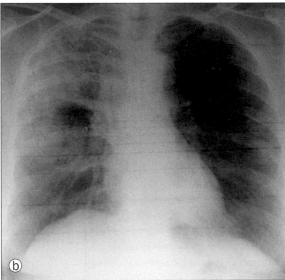

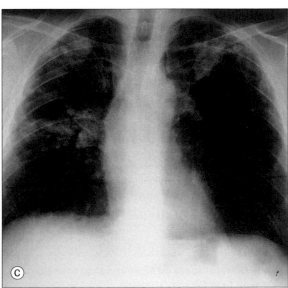

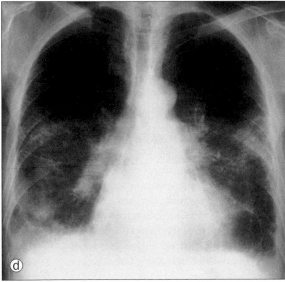

Figure 44.5 Different distributions of radiologic shadowing in diffuse lung diseases. (a) Extensive, predominantly upper lobe, calcified nodules caused by silicosis. The patient had few symptoms and no physical signs.
(b) Middle and upper zone patchy consolidation caused by alveolar cell carcinoma. The patient had a 6-week history of increasing dyspnea and copious watery sputum. Signs of consolidation are present.
(c) Asymptomatic patient who has history of sarcoidosis, but no physical signs. Residual nodular shadowing with cavitation is visible in the right middle and both upper zones.
(d) Extensive, bilateral basal interstitial shadowing with pleural thickening in asbestosis. The patient was dyspneic with a dry cough, which had worsened over 2 years. Bibasal inspiratory crackles were heard on auscultation.

Lung function testing

In most of the diffuse lung diseases, lung function abnormalities tend to be restrictive in pattern with reduced gas transfer and arterial hypoxemia either at rest or on exercise. Some diffuse lung diseases, such as lymphangioleiomyomatosis, can produce an obstructive pattern, while in principle any of the diffuse lung diseases that occur in older patients might be superimposed on pre-existing chronic obstructive airways disease and thus produce a mixed pattern on lung function testing. In alveolar hemorrhage, the gas transfer factor can be markedly increased. In practice, however, aside from providing objective evidence of the presence of abnormal lung physiology, lung function tests do not usually contribute appreciably to the specific diagnosis of individual diffuse lung diseases[10].

Blood tests

Hematology investigations can reveal nonspecific evidence of disease, such as anemia or elevated erythrocyte sedimentation rate or other inflammatory markers, but more specific diagnostic information from blood tests is relatively limited. Eosinophilia is a requirement for the diagnosis of eosinophilic pneumonia, although other causes of eosinophilia with diffuse lung disease occur; the presence of specific allergen precipitins helps to establish a diagnosis of hypersensitivity pneumonitis, but the test is neither sufficiently sensitive nor specific to establish the diagnosis in isolation; autoantibodies or rheumatoid factor are clear markers of collagen vascular disease, but are also often positive in IPF; antineutrophil cytoplasmic antibody helps to confirm a diagnosis of Wegener's granulomatosis, but is also found in other vasculitides. Basement membrane autoantibodies are found in Goodpasture's syndrome.

High-resolution computed tomography

High-resolution computed tomography (HRCT) has revolutionized the diagnosis of diffuse lung disease. By sampling thin, 1–2mm sections of lung, usually at approximately 1cm intervals and using a 'hard', high-resolution algorithm, the HRCT scan provides information representative of the entire lung in a degree of detail often sufficient to make a confident, specific diagnosis. Also, HRCT demonstrates the extent of lung disease, can detect disease that is not yet apparent on the chest radiograph, and, where appropriate, can be a useful guide to percutaneous or transbronchial biopsy of representative lung lesions.

As with the conventional chest radiograph, it is convenient to classify HRCT appearances according to whether they are predominantly nodular or linear, and according to the zones of the lung most affected; in these respects HRCT appearances follow a pattern similar to that outlined above for the chest radiograph. However, with HRCT a much more precise anatomic localization of lesions in relation to lung structures, such as small airways, interlobular septa, the pleura, and other structures, is possible, as is determining whether disease is localized or diffuse throughout the lung, or peripheral or central in distribution. Also, HRCT can define lesions (such as traction bronchiectasis and nodular bronchovascular bundles, subpleural lines, and ground-glass opacification) that were either very difficult or impossible to see on the chest radiograph. In many diffuse lung diseases, such as IPF or hypersensitivity pneumonitis, the overall qualitative appearances on HRCT are relatively distinctive, and the anatomic and histopathologic patterns associated with these appearances are well established[11,12]. Common characteristics of HRCT appearances are presented in Figure 44.6.

Other lung imaging

Gallium scanning, technetium-99m pentetic acid scanning, and other methods of measuring lung permeability are all relatively time consuming and, although abnormal in some diffuse lung diseases, have not been demonstrated to provide specific diagnostic information of more value than the procedures outlined above. Ventilation–perfusion scanning can help in the diagnosis of thromboembolic disease. Real-time nuclear magnetic resonance scanning may also prove to make an important contribution to diagnosis, although this technique is still at a relatively early stage of development.

Bronchoalveolar lavage

Bronchoalveolar lavage (BAL) or sometimes bronchial aspirates obtained via the bronchoscope can be extremely helpful in identifying and isolating infectious causes of diffuse lung disease, such as the various agents that cause bacterial, viral, or fungal pneumonias, mycobacterial disease, or *Pneumocystis carinii* pneumonia; in identifying neoplastic cells in pulmonary malignancy; or in observing bilamellar bodies in alveolar proteinosis. The value of the differential cell count or protein content of BAL

| Common appearances on high-resolution computed tomography in relation to individual diseases ||
Appearance	Disease
Nodules	Sarcoidosis Miliary tuberculosis Bronchiolitis Silicosis Coal worker's pneumoconiosis Eosinophilic granuloma Metastatic disease
Interlobular septal thickening	Idiopathic pulmonary fibrosis Collagen vascular disease Asbestosis Sarcoid Lymphangitis carcinomatosis
Alveolar opacification/ground-glass shadowing	Desquamative interstitial pneumonia Hypersensitivity pneumonitis Alveolar proteinosis Acute bacterial pneumonia Bronchiolitis obliterans organizing pneumonia Eosinophilic pneumonia Alveolar cell carcinoma Drug reactions
Cystic change	Emphysema Lymphangioleiomyomatosis Usual interstitial pneumonia/idiopathic pulmonary fibrosis Collagen vascular disease Asbestosis Eosinophilic granuloma
Pleural involvement	Asbestos disease Amiodarone reaction Collagen vascular disease

Figure 44.6 Common appearances on high-resolution computed tomography in relation to individual diseases.

samples in the diagnosis of other chronic diffuse lung diseases has been extensively explored, however, and found to be less helpful[13]. The total cellular content of BAL fluid in these diseases tends to be increased, with an increased proportion of neutrophils in patients who have IPF or pulmonary fibrosis associated with collagen vascular disease, increased macrophages in silicosis, and relatively normal cell counts in asbestosis (Fig. 44.7). In individual patients, however, these counts are not generally helpful to the diagnostic process and are confounded by the effects of cigarette smoking, which further limits the interpretation of BAL data in these diseases.

Bronchial biopsy

For many of the diffuse lung diseases, a clear diagnosis relies on histologic evidence. Samples of lung tissue for histologic assessment can be obtained by various methods, and with varying degrees of associated morbidity.

Transbronchial biopsy via the flexible bronchoscope, with or without fluoroscopic screening, is probably the simplest and least invasive means of obtaining lung tissue, although the samples are inevitably small and yield only peribronchial tissue. Transbronchial biopsy therefore has a relatively high diagnostic yield in diseases that have a peribronchial distribution, particularly sarcoidosis, and is also often successful in hypersensitivity pneumonitis or lymphangitis carcinomatosis. The main risks associated with this procedure are pneumothorax and hemorrhage, although in practice these are rarely of sufficient severity to cause clinical problems.

Percutaneous needle biopsy is also a relatively simple technique, which can be performed under local anesthetic, often with fluoroscopic, ultrasound, or CT screening, and that allows precise sampling from localized areas of abnormality. Depending on the technique, the samples obtained are again relatively small and are most likely to yield a diagnosis for diseases such as sarcoidosis, malignancy, tuberculosis, vasculitis, BOOP, or other diagnoses in which clear histopathologic evidence can be obtained from small tissue samples. Pneumothorax or hemorrhage are again the major problems of this technique and occur more frequently than with bronchoscopy, particularly when sampling lesions that are relatively deep within the lung or in the presence of coexisting lung disease.

In some cases, either in which the above procedures have failed, more substantial samples of lung tissue are required, or direct inspection of the lung is necessary to identify areas for sampling, open lung biopsy either via thoracotomy or, more recently, by thoracoscopy with video guidance, may be carried out. Mortality and morbidity from biopsy via a thoracotomy is relatively low, but nevertheless occurs, and some patients who have severe diffuse lung disease or other significant concomitant illness may not be suitably fit to proceed with open biopsy by this method. Thoracoscopic techniques are associated with much lower mortality and morbidity, and are rapidly becoming the technique of choice[14-16].

TREATMENT

Treatment of the individual diffuse lung diseases outlined above varies according to disease, and although therapies (such as corticosteroids) are used for several diagnoses, others (such as lung lavage for alveolar proteinosis) are very individual. The specific therapy for individual diffuse lung diseases is therefore discussed elsewhere in the appropriate sections of this book, although a brief summary of typical therapies for the more common diffuse lung diseases is outlined in Figure 44.8.

The approach to therapy in relation to a specific clinical diagnosis also varies considerably between countries for various reasons that relate to accessibility of diagnostic procedures, differences in philosophy and expectation regarding the need for precise diagnosis,

Characteristics of bronchoalveolar lavage fluid				
Characteristic	Idiopathic pulmonary fibrosis	Connective tissue disease	Asbestosis	Silicosis
Cells/mL	↑	↑	–	–
Macrophages/mL	↑	↑	–	↑
Neutrophils/mL	↑	↑	–	–
Lymphocytes/mL	–	–	–	–
Eosinophils present	+	–	–	–
Total protein	↑	↑	–	↑
Immunoglobulin G	↑	↑	↑	↑
Immunoglobulin A	↑	↑	–	↑
Immunoglobulin M	↑	↑	–	–
Albumin	↓	↓	–	–

Figure 44.7 Characteristics of bronchoalveolar lavage fluid in idiopathic pulmonary fibrosis, connective tissue disease, asbestosis, and silicosis. (Adapted with permission from Cherniak et al.[13]. Official Journal of the American Thoracic Society ©American Lung Association.)

Outline guide to the treatment of diffuse lung disease	
Diagnosis	Typical therapy
Pneumoconiosis	Removal from exposure
Hypersensitivity pneumonitis	Removal from exposure Corticosteroids
Collagen vascular disease	Specific therapy to disease
Drug reactions	Removal from exposure Corticosteroids
Sarcoidosis	Corticosteroids
Lymphangioleiomyomatosis	Progesterone
Vasculitic disease	Corticosteroids/immunosuppressants
Alveolar proteinosis	Lung lavage
Pneumonia	Antimicrobial therapy appropriate to infectious agent
Idiopathic pulmonary fibrosis	Corticosteroids/immunosuppressants
Bronchiolitis obliterans organizing pneumonia	Corticosteroids
Eosinophilic pneumonia	Corticosteroids

Figure 44.8 Outline guide to the treatment of diffuse lung disease.

CLINICAL FEATURES

Although Hamman and Rich described a rapidly progressive disease that occurred in relatively young patients (three of the four cases were aged 47 years or under), the typical presentation of IPF in the general population is now in a more elderly age group, and the disease is not always rapid in progression. The presentation and clinical features of IPF in a nationally representative sample of nearly 600 new cases that presented over a 2-year period in the UK have recently been described[9], and show the mean age at presentation to be in the late 60s in both sexes, with a male:female ratio of 1.7:1. The most common presenting symptoms are breathlessness and dry cough of gradual onset, the breathlessness having been present for a median of 9 months before presentation. Finger clubbing is present in approximately 50%, and arthralgia or arthritis, in the absence of more overt clinical evidence of connective tissue disease, in about 20% (Fig. 45.2). In more advanced disease, cyanosis and cor pulmonale may also be present.

The chest radiograph is abnormal at presentation in the great majority of patients who have IPF. Typical chest radiograph appearances are of short, linear (reticular) shadowing, often also with fine nodules, predominantly at the lung bases and usually with associated evidence of reduced lung volume (Fig. 45.3). In more advanced disease the reticular shadowing becomes more prominent, and combines with multiple cystic translucencies to produce the appearance of honeycomb lung. The soft, ground-glass appearance of alveolar shadowing is also sometimes seen, but not usually in isolation from more marked reticulonodular shadowing. In a small proportion of cases subsequently shown to have IPF the chest radiograph is normal.

The characteristic pattern of IPF in terms of lung function should be restrictive, with reduction of vital capacity, forced expiratory volume in 1s (FEV_1), and residual volume. Often at presentation the impairment of FEV_1 and forced vital capacity (FVC) is relatively mild, but measures of gas transfer show a more marked reduction. However, since in practice a high proportion of patients with IPF are or have been active smokers and this has led to some degree of airflow obstruction, in these individuals the lung function tests may reveal a mixed restrictive and obstructive pattern. Arterial blood gas measurements may be normal in early disease, but more commonly demonstrate hypoxemia, and in later stages of disease, hypercapnia.

Up to a third of patients have antinuclear antibodies or rheumatoid factor in their serum at presentation, despite the conventional exclusion of patients who show overt clinical evidence of connective tissue disease from the IPF diagnosis.

DIAGNOSIS

The clinical diagnosis of IPF depends primarily on the identification of symptoms and signs of breathlessness, basal crackles, and often finger clubbing on examination, the characteristic radiographic appearances, and demonstration of restrictive lung function. The clinical history must, however, also explore and exclude other possible causes of interstitial fibrosis, such as the occupational, drug, allergen, and other exposures outlined in Chapter 44. It is thus especially important to establish details of lifetime occupations, as well as a recreational history, to establish whether the patient has been exposed to birds, hay, or

Clinical features at presentation in patients who have idiopathic pulmonary fibrosis				
Features		Males	Females	Total
Age (mean in years)		67	68	67
Symptoms (%)	Breathlessnes	87	92	89
	Cough	73	77	75
	Arthritis/arthralgia	17	24	19
	Asymptomatic	5	4	5
	Finger clubbing	54	40	49
Lung function (% predicted)	Forced expiratory volume in 1s	78	79	78
	Forced vital capacity	78	79	78
	Residual volume	70	74	71
	Diffusing factor for carbon monoxide (DLCO)	48	53	50
	Diffusion coefficient (DLCO/ accessible alveolar volume)	58	65	60
Smoking history	Current	22	13	19
	Ex-smoker	70	36	58
	Never	8	51	24

Figure 45.2 Clinical features at presentation in patients who have idiopathic pulmonary fibrosis. (Information from Johnston et al.[9])

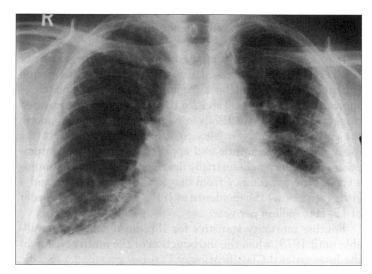

Figure 45.3 Typical chest radiograph appearances in idiopathic pulmonary fibrosis, with reticular and some nodular shadowing at both bases, and some reduction of lung volume. (Radiographs courtesy of Dr Andrew Evans, Nottingham City Hospital.)

other known causes of extrinsic allergic alveolitis, and to obtain a drug history to identify potentially relevant current or previous drug exposures. The history and examination should also seek evidence of skin rashes, arthritis, or arthralgia as markers of connective tissue disease, and general markers of other contributors to breathlessness such as chronic obstructive pulmonary disease, respiratory infections, cardiac disease, primary or metastatic lung cancer, pulmonary embolus or hemorrhage, sarcoid, and other diagnoses (see Fig. 44.1). A full smoking history is also important, since smoking is a risk factor for IPF, and because lung function test data in these patients may show a mixed obstructive and restrictive defect.

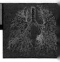

To date no generally agreed or standardized clinical diagnostic criteria have been established for IPF, and to an extent the clinical criteria used in the major descriptive studies of IPF are self-fulfilling, as they have been used to define the cases described. For many years it has been argued that the gold standard for diagnosis of IPF is histopathologic evidence from lung biopsy, which in the majority shows the predominantly interstitial cellular and fibrotic appearance of usual interstitial pneumonia (UIP), but in a minority shows the more cellular air-space involvement of desquamative interstitial pneumonia (DIP; Figs 45.4 & 45.5). Although at present it is not clear whether DIP represents an early stage in the development of UIP, or a completely independent disease process. The relevance of differentiating these pathologic diagnoses is held to be the better prognosis and reported greater likelihood of a response to therapy in DIP[10]. However, in practice it is common to see a mixed appearance of UIP and DIP in different samples from the same individual, or even in the same sample. This, in association with evidence that a clinical response to therapy can be observed in both UIP and DIP, has led many physicians to question the contribution of an open lung biopsy to the diagnosis of IPF and clinical management decisions. Recent improvements in thoracoscopic methods of lung biopsy have reduced the morbidity associated with open lung biopsy procedures, but reservations over the practical consequence of histopathologic findings remain. Transbronchial biopsy does not usually yield a sufficiently substantial sample to make a confident diagnosis of UIP or DIP.

To a large extent, the debate over the role of lung biopsy in the diagnosis of IPF has been overtaken by developments in high-res-

olution computed tomography (HRCT) scanning, which provide a noninvasive means to identify UIPs and DIPs, and to exclude other recognized causes of interstitial lung disease. The HRCT appearances of DIP are of ground-glass attenuation predominantly in the middle or lower zones, sometimes predominantly

Description of usual and desquamative interstitial pneumonias

Usual interstitial pneumonia

Highly variegated structure, often includes the entire spectrum from normal alveolar walls to fibrotic, end-stage lesions in the same tissue sample

Dense pleomorphic interstitial cellular infiltrate including many lymphocytes and monocytes but relatively few eosinophils

Variegated epithelial lining in the small air spaces, ranging from large, rounded cells on less damaged alveolar walls to cuboidal, columnar, ciliated, goblet and squamous cells on more scarred alveolar walls

Few cells, mostly macrophages, in small air spaces

Some proteinaceous exudates, especially in alveoli with early lesions

Desquamative interstitial pneumonia

Relative uniformity of the lesion throughout the tissue sample

Sparse interstitial cellular infiltrate, including an appreciable proportion of plasma cells and eosinophils

Prominent lining of alveoli by large rounded cells

Abundant mononuclear cells filling many small air spaces

Little if any proteinaceous exudate in air spaces or interstitium

Figure 45.4 Description of usual and desquamative interstitial pneumonias. (Information from Carrington et al.[10])

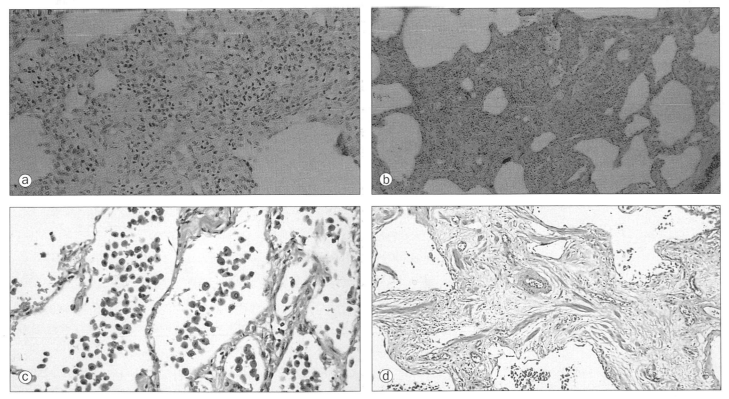

Figure 45.5 Typical histologic appearances of idiopathic pulmonary fibrosis. (a) Pleomorphic cellular interstitial infiltrate in usual interstitial pneumonia (UIP). (b) Interstitial fibrosis in UIP (staining green on Masson trichrome stain). (c) Macrophages in alveolar spaces in desquamative interstitial pneumonia. (d) Advanced interstitial fibrosis in end-stage honeycomb lung. (Courtesy of Dr Colin Clelland, Nottingham City Hospital.)

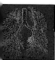

subpleural in distribution. In UIP the HRCT appearances reflect the more predominant fibrosis in this condition, with intralobular interstitial thickening, visible intralobular bronchioles, traction bronchiectasis, and honeycombing, again more marked in the periphery of the lung and in the posterior and lower lung zones (Fig. 45.6)[11]. In practice, HRCT scans of patients who have IPF often show evidence of both DIP and UIP in different areas of the lung. In addition, HRCT sometimes demonstrates slight enlargement of mediastinal lymph nodes.

TREATMENT

The most commonly used interventional therapy for IPF is high-dose corticosteroids, sometimes given in combination with another immunosuppressive agent such as azathioprine. Other immunosuppressants, such as cyclophosphamide, cyclosporin, colchicine, methotrexate, and penicillamine, have also been used.

Despite the widespread use of corticosteroids to treat IPF, no definitive evidence shows that these drugs improve either survival or quality of life in this disease[12]. The available evidence on corticosteroid effects is based entirely on observational studies, none of which has involved a randomized, placebo-controlled, double-blind design. In one of the most widely quoted studies[13], the evidence of benefit was limited to a subgroup of 'good responders' among those who received corticosteroids, but survival among 'poor responders' to corticosteroids was actually worse than that

in untreated patients (Fig. 45.7). The combined survival experience of the corticosteroid-treated group was therefore probably very similar to that of the untreated group. Corticosteroid therapy was associated with significant morbidity, with adverse effects reported in a quarter of those treated.

Despite the lack of randomized, placebo-controlled clinical trial evidence that corticosteroids are beneficial in IPF, these drugs are widely recommended as first-line therapy for this disease, and some investigators argue that placebo-controlled trials of corticosteroids in this disease would now be unethical. Typical corticosteroid doses are 40–60mg/day of prednisolone or equivalent for at least a month, tailing down after stabilization of the disease to around 20mg every other day. Of other proposed therapies for IPF, some have been assessed in randomized controlled trials, usually in comparison with placebo, as an addition to corticosteroids. All are based on small numbers of subjects. Evidence of improved survival relative to placebo therapy has been published with respect to azathioprine, although to a borderline level of statistical significance[14], while a study in a small number of patients found no significant benefit with cyclophosphamide[15]. Evidence of benefit from colchicine, cyclosporin, and methotrexate is limited to case reports of uncontrolled trials. An open, uncontrolled assessment of the antiviral agent ribavirin (tribavirin) concluded no evidence of benefit.

As disease progresses, patients who have IPF can derive some benefit from more general approaches to the management of

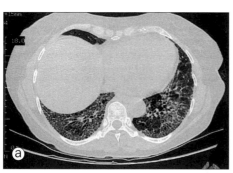
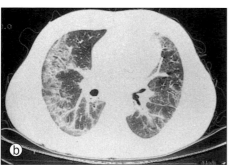
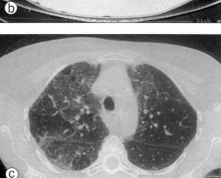

Figure 45.6 High-resolution computed tomography findings in idiopathic pulmonary fibrosis. (a) Interlobular fibrosis and traction bronchiectasis with some honeycombing in usual interstitial pneumonia. (b) More advanced disease with typical peripheral distribution. (c) Soft, ground-glass shadowing in desquamative interstitial pneumonia.

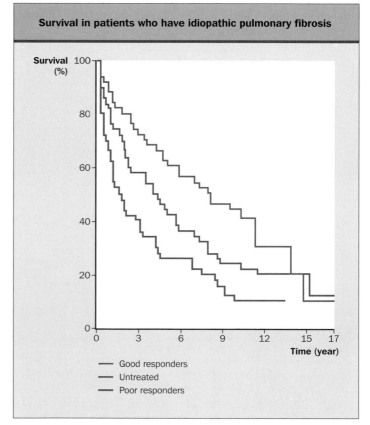

Figure 45.7 Survival in patients who have idiopathic pulmonary fibrosis according to therapy. Patients who receive corticosteroids have been subdivided into 'good responders' and 'poor responders'. Treatment allocation was not randomized. (Adapted with permission from Turner-Warwick et al.[13])

dyspnea and respiratory failure, such as supplemental oxygen, help with mobility outside and inside the home, opiates for respiratory distress, and other general social and nursing support. Radical therapy of IPF by lung transplantation is also an option for some patients, and provides improved quality of life and survival for those who have advanced disease, but is obviously of limited availability.

Potential opportunities for therapeutic intervention in the future include the use of antifibrotic agents such as halofuginone and pirfenidone, and antagonists to cytokines and growth factors thought to be involved in the pathogenesis of pulmonary fibrosis. Antioxidant drugs currently under development, and some existing antioxidants such as N-acetylcysteine, may also have a role. For the present, however, the drug therapy of IPF remains an area of substantial controversy, and some physicians still elect not to intervene with drugs in this disease[9,12,16].

CLINICAL COURSE AND PREVENTION

The clinical course of IPF is variable, but in most cases involves a progressive deterioration to death from respiratory failure. Estimates of life expectancy derived from follow-up of populations of patients who had IPF and attended specialist clinics have usually been about 5 years, but these figures can be substantially biased by the tendency for longer-term survivors to be over-represented in such populations. Typical survival in newly presenting cases of IPF is probably closer to 3 years, which when compared with individuals of similar age and sex represents a loss of normal life expectancy of approximately 7 years[17]. Most of the excess mortality in these patients is directly or indirectly attributable to IPF, but there may also be an increased risk of cardiovascular or lung cancer mortality.

Markers of a poor prognosis include a relatively low FVC, diffusing factor for carbon monoxide, or arterial oxygen level at presentation, male sex, and older age. Evidence of improvement after a trial of corticosteroid therapy is associated with a favorable prognosis and may, in turn, be more likely in those with a relatively cellular histologic pattern on lung biopsy[13], or a predominantly ground-glass pattern of shadowing on HRCT of the lung[18]. Other factors, which include oxygen desaturation on exercise, rapid clearance of inhaled pentetic acid, and low lymphocyte counts in bronchoalveolar lavage fluid samples, may also be related to a poor prognosis, but the additional clinical value of these predictive measures is not clear. It is certainly questionable whether any of these measures, either alone or in combination, determine to any clinically useful degree of confidence whether an individual patient is likely to respond to therapy or not.

Since the etiology of IPF is currently not clearly understood, prevention of this disease is not currently feasible. A number of potentially avoidable risk factors, such as occupational metal or wood dust, or indeed common drugs, have now been identified, but none has yet been established with sufficient confidence to justify attempts at primary prevention. Secondary prevention is also not currently a practical option for IPF, though the implication of viral infections in the pathogenesis of IPF presents potential opportunities for the future.

REFERENCES

1. Hamman L, Rich AR. Acute diffuse interstitial fibrosis of the lungs. Bull Johns Hopkins Hosp. 1944;74:177–204.
2. Scott J, Johnston I, Britton J. What causes cryptogenic fibrosing alveolitis? A case-control study of environmental exposure to dust. Br Med J. 1990;301:1015–21.
3. Coultas DB, Zumwalt RE, Black WC, Sobonya RE. The epidemiology of interstitial lung diseases. Am J Respir Crit Care Med. 1994;150:967–72.
4. Hubbard R, Johnston I, Coultas D, Britton J. Mortality rates from cryptogenic fibrosing alveolitis in seven countries. Thorax. 1996;51:711–16.
5. Coultas, DB, Hughes MP. Accuracy of mortality data for interstitial lung diseases in New Mexico, USA. Thorax. 1996;51:717–20.
6. Iwai K, Mori T, Yamada N, Yamaguchi M, Hosoda Y. Idiopathic pulmonary fibrosis – epidemiologic approaches to occupational exposure. Am J Respir Crit Care Med. 1994;150:670–5.
7. Hubbard R, Lewis S, Richards K, Johnston I, Britton J. Occupational exposure to metal or wood dust and aetiology of cryptogenic fibrosing alveolitis. Lancet. 1996;347:284–9.
8. Hubbard R, Venn A, Smith C, et al. Exposure to commonly prescribed drugs and the etiology of cryptogenic fibrosing alveolitis: a case–control study. Am J Respir Crit Care Med. 1998;157:743–7.

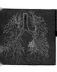
smoking), so that their absence makes the diagnosis of EAA very unlikely. In contrast to type I hypersensitivity to allergens, skin-prick testing has no place in the detection of precipitins[10].

TREATMENT

Acute exacerbations of disease are generally manageable conservatively with bed rest, nonsteroidal anti-inflammatory agents, and supplementary oxygen therapy. In severe cases, mechanical ventilatory support may be required. Spontaneous recovery (over days or weeks, depending on the level of exposure) is the general rule.

The cornerstone of management is to remove the patient from further exposure. While this may be straightforward in some cases, it can be extremely difficult if the patient fears loss of employment or refuses to discontinue a beloved hobby. Furthermore, it is difficult for the physician to insist on complete cessation of exposure since continued exposure does not inevitably result in progressive disease. In an industrial setting it is often possible to reduce exposure significantly by moving the employee to a lower exposure environment, and on farms, simple precautions, such as the thorough drying of hay prior to storage, are often beneficial. Industrial respirators, which filter up to 99% of respirable dust from inhaled air, are helpful but cumbersome to wear for long periods, and are not suitable for heavy manual labor.

Once these measures are in place the patient should be assessed periodically to monitor disease progression or regression. If no evidence of progression is found, the patient may reasonably tolerate existing exposure conditions. However, with evidence of progression, the patient must be advised to cease further exposure. Further management includes investigation of the 'at-risk' environment, with identification of others who have the disease or are at risk.

The role of systemic glucocorticoid therapy at any stage of the disease is unclear. While such therapy accelerates recovery from acute illness following relevant exposure[11], it does not provide any long-term benefit, but it does carry its own added risks. Nevertheless, many patients are given glucocorticoids acutely to hasten improvement. There is also a risk that continual treatment of patients in this fashion makes them complacent about avoiding further exposure.

CLINICAL COURSE AND PREVENTION

If the diagnosis of EAA is made early and further relevant exposure avoided, little risk of permanent lung damage occurs and most changes resolve[12]. It is not always safe to assume, however, that patients will continue to comply with avoidance instructions, so follow up is desirable. Permanent pulmonary dysfunction is relatively uncommon, but occurs in those patients who experience continuous, symptomatic exposure, although even at this stage the majority of such patients do improve if exposure is eliminated and pulmonary fibrosis not advanced. A minority, however, show relentless progression even if exposure is stopped. Unfortunately, many patients do not present with EAA until pulmonary fibrosis is well established and respiratory failure advanced.

PITFALLS AND CONTROVERSIES

The diagnosis of EAA is easy to miss. It is facilitated by maintaining a high index of suspicion and close attention to the patient's occupational and environmental history. In patients who present with an acute, influenza-like illness and impairment of lung function, the differential diagnosis is obviously wide, and the diagnosis of EAA should be considered in patients being investigated for possible viral, bacterial, and fungal pneumonias (especially 'atypical' pneumonias such as psittacosis), tuberculosis, aspiration pneumonia, transient pulmonary infiltrates (such as those associated with collagen vascular diseases, drug reactions, eosinophilic vasculitis, and other vasculitides), and exposure to poisons or other nonorganic industrial dusts. Coexisting asthma, particularly occupational asthma, in such patients may be a source of confusion. Specific differential diagnoses more relevant to the 'at-risk' environment include organic dust toxic syndrome (transient, usually harmless respiratory embarrassment on exposure to very heavy, physically toxic concentrations of microbial spores in contaminated vegetable and cereal produce) and nitrogen dioxide toxicity.

Current controversies in EAA concern the precise pathogenesis of the disease, especially the role of type III, as opposed to type IV, hypersensitivity, the spectrum of the host response in sensitized individuals, and the merits or otherwise of systemic glucocorticoid therapy.

REFERENCES

1. Pepys J, Jenkins PA, Festenstein GN, Lacey ME, Gregory PH, Skinner FA. Farmer's Lung. Thermophilic actinomycetes as a source of 'farmer's lung hay' antigens. Lancet. 1963;ii:607–11.
2. Fink JN. Hypersensitivity pneumonitis. Chest. 1992;13:303–9.
3. Meredith SK, Taylor VM, McDonald JC. Occupational respiratory disease in the United Kingdom 1989: a report to the British Thoracic Society and the Society of Occupational Medicine by the SWORD project group. Br J Indust Med. 1991;48:292–8.
4. Ando M, Arima K, Yoneda R, Tamura M. Japanese summer-type hypersensitivity pneumonitis: geographic distribution, home environment and clinical characteristics of 621 cases. Am Rev Respir Dis. 1991;144:765–9.
5. Suga M, Yamasaki H, Nakagawa K, Kohrogi H, Ando M. Mechanisms accounting for granulomatous responses in hypersensitivity pneumonitis. Sarcoidosis, vasculitis and diffuse lung diseases. 1997;14:131–8.
6. Reynolds HY. Hypersensitivity pneumonitis: correlation of cellular and immunologic changes with clinical phases of disease. Lung. 1991;169(Suppl.):S109–28.
7. Richerson HB, Bernstein IL, Fink JN, et al. Guidelines for the clinical evaluation of hypersensitivity pneumonitis. J Allergy Clin Immunol. 1989;84:839–44.
8. Cormier Y, Lacasse Y. Keys to the diagnosis of hypersensitivity pneumonitis: the role of precipitins, lung biopsy and high-resolution computed tomography. Clin Pulmonary Med. 1996;3:72–7.
9. Hansell DM, Wells AU, Padley SPG, Muller NL. Hypersensitivity pneumonitis: correlation of individual CT patterns with functional abnormalities. Radiology. 1996;199:123–8.
10. Terho EO, Frew AJ. Type III allergy skin testing. Position statement for EAACI subcommittee on skin tests and allergen standardisation. Allergy. 1995;50:392–6.
11. Kokkarinen JI, Tukiainen HO, Terho EO. Effect of corticosteroid treatment on the recovery of pulmonary function in farmer's lung. Am Rev Respir Dis. 1992;145:3–5.
12. Braun SR, doPico GA, Tsiatis A, Horvath E, Dickie HA, Rankin J. Farmer's lung disease: long-term clinical and physiologic outcome. Am Rev Respir Dis. 1979;119:185–91.

Chapter 47

Sarcoidosis

David R Moller

INTRODUCTION

Sarcoidosis is a multisystem disorder of unknown etiology characterized by noncaseating, epithelioid granulomas in affected organs[1]. The disease most commonly affects the lungs and intrathoracic lymph nodes, although granulomatous inflammation may be present in any organ system. Eye and skin involvement is seen in as many as 25% of patients, and symptomatic involvement of other organs occurs less frequently. Clinical, epidemiologic, and family studies support the hypothesis that sarcoidosis is caused by exposure to an environmental, possibly infectious, agent in individuals who have genetic susceptibility to the disease. Although the etiology of sarcoidosis is unknown, the pathogenesis of the granulomatous inflammation involves cytokine-producing CD4+ T-helper-1(TH1) lymphocytes and mononuclear phagocytes. A diagnosis of sarcoidosis is most securely established by a compatible clinical history together with a biopsy that demonstrates noncaseating granulomas in affected organs and the absence of competing diagnoses such as tuberculosis, fungal disease, or malignancy. The clinical course is highly variable, with a disease-related mortality of <1–6%. Corticosteroids remain the mainstay of treatment when sarcoidosis needs to be treated because of organ threatening or chronic progressive disease.

EPIDEMIOLOGY, ETIOLOGY/RISK FACTORS, AND PATHOPHYSIOLOGY

Epidemiology

Sarcoidosis is found worldwide, although striking differences occur in the prevalence of the disease in different geographic areas and racial groups[1–4]. The prevalence of sarcoidosis ranges from 10 to 40/100,000 population in North America, the UK, and southern Europe, but is <10/100,000 in Japan. Higher prevalence rates have been noted in Scandinavian countries and among African–Americans in southeastern USA. In North America, sarcoidosis is 8–10 times more common in African–American populations. In underdeveloped countries where tuberculosis is common, no reliable epidemiologic data are available because of the difficulty in distinguishing these diseases. Worldwide, a slight female predominance is found. Although all ages can be affected, over 80% of patients present between the ages of 20–40 years.

The frequencies of different clinical presentations of sarcoidosis vary among different groups[1–4]. Erythema nodosum, which carries a good prognosis in sarcoidosis, has a particularly high frequency among Scandinavians, Irish female immigrants in the UK, and Puerto Rican women in New York City. In contrast, this presentation is uncommon in patients of African descent and Japanese patients. Lupus pernio, a disfiguring, nodular facial condition associated with chronic sarcoidosis, is more frequent in patients of African descent. Hospital statistics and anecdotal experience suggest that race is an important prognostic indicator, with patients of African descent more likely to have chronic persistent disease and suffer from increased morbidity and mortality than Caucasian patients who have sarcoidosis.

Retrospective studies suggest that sarcoidosis is the direct cause of death in <1–6% of cases. A recent analysis of mortality data from hospitals in the USA from 1979 to 1991 found that 0.02% of the total deaths in the USA were caused by sarcoidosis[5]. Age-adjusted mortality was consistently higher among African–Americans than Caucasians and among women compared with men. In the USA, autopsy studies and hospital data suggest that 40–80% of sarcoidosis deaths are secondary to pulmonary causes such as respiratory insufficiency, cor pulmonale, and massive hemoptysis. In Sweden and Japan, most sarcoidosis deaths are caused by cardiac disease. Uremia from chronic renal failure and hepatic failure are less common causes of death related to sarcoidosis. These statistics are likely to underestimate the problem, given the potential for underdiagnosis of this disease.

Etiology and risk factors

Infection

The cause of sarcoidosis remains unknown[6]. Since sarcoidosis was first described, investigators have postulated an infectious cause of the disease based on the clinical similarities to tuberculosis. However, despite considerable efforts to detect specific infectious agents, no convincing evidence supports an infectious etiology for the disease. Reports of acid-fast organisms, cultivable mycobacterial or cell-wall deficient organisms, and other bacterial, fungal, or viral agents have not been confirmed. High titers of antibodies against many viral and bacterial antigens in sarcoidosis probably reflect generalized B-cell activation and not a causal relationship. Recently, polymerase chain reaction methods have been used to search for traces of genetic elements from microbial organisms; these studies have also been inconclusive, with reports of mycobacterial DNA in a small number of biopsy specimens by some, but not other, investigators[7].

Despite the lack of evidence for a specific infectious cause, seasonal variation, time–space clustering, and occupational associations (e.g. higher incidence in health-care workers) are reported. Such observations support the hypothesis that environmental factors play a role in the etiology of sarcoidosis. A noninfectious, environmental cause of sarcoidosis is suggested by comparison with chronic beryllium disease. This granulomatous lung disease, histologically identical to sarcoidosis, is caused by exposure to beryllium dust in a small proportion of susceptible workers.

Autoimmunity

Other investigators suggest that sarcoidosis is a result of auto-immunity, perhaps from molecular mimicry of autoantigens to proteins from infectious agents. Consistent with this possibility, granulomatous inflammation in sarcoidosis is characterized by dysregulated cytokine production and oligoclonal expansions of T cells at sites of disease. The presence of antinuclear antibodies, rheumatoid factor, hypergammaglobulinemia, and immune complexes in sarcoidosis is cited as evidence that supports an autoimmune origin of sarcoidosis.

Kveim–Siltzbach reaction

In the 1860s, Ansgar Kveim found that the intradermal inoculation of a suspension of sarcoid lymph-node tissue resulted in a nodular skin reaction that contained sarcoid-like granulomas in patients who had suspected sarcoidosis, but not in control individuals. Subsequent investigators found that this reaction (using validated spleen tissue) occurs in 70–80% of patients early in their disease, with a <1% false positive rate[2]. In this reaction, well-formed granulomas take 2–4 weeks to develop. Many attempts have been made to identify the granuloma-inducing factor contained in the Kveim reagent, but precise characterization has yet to be accomplished. Given the concerns of injecting allogeneic material into patients in an era with known retroviral disease, clinical use of this reagent is restricted to a few specialized centers with archived tissue.

Genetic

Substantial evidence exists for a genetic predisposition to sarcoidosis[8]. In a recent USA study, familial clustering of sarcoidosis occurs in 5–16% of patients, with a greater frequency among African–American compared with Caucasian populations. Within the same family, sibling pairs are most commonly affected together, followed by mother–daughter pairs and father–son pairs. Monozygotic twins appear 2–4 times more likely to develop sarcoidosis than dizygotic twins, which strongly suggests a genetic component to the disease. The lack of a clear genetic pattern indicates that susceptibility to sarcoidosis is polygenic and interacts with environmental factors. Inconsistent results have been shown by HLA studies, with associations reported for HLA-DR3 and bilateral hilar adenopathy or erythema nodosum in Swedish patients, HLA-B27 and uveitis, HLA-B13 and chronic disease, HLA-DR5 and Italian patients, and HLA-DRw52 and Japanese patients. More recently, sarcoidosis has been associated with major histocompatibility complex (MHC) haplotypes that contain glutamine at position 69 of the HLA-DPB1 chain, the same association reported to be a risk factor for chronic beryllium disease[9]. Whether detailed MHC haplotype analysis will reveal additional associations with risk or prognosis of sarcoidosis is currently under study.

Pathophysiology

The histologic hallmark of sarcoidosis is the presence of discrete, noncaseating granulomas (Fig. 47.1)[1]. The dominant cell in the central core is the epithelioid cell, thought to be a differentiated form of a mononuclear phagocyte. Mature macrophages and CD4+ lymphocytes are interspersed throughout the epithelioid core, whereas both CD4+ and CD8+ lymphocytes are seen around the periphery of the granuloma. Multinucleated giant cells, which often contain cytoplasmic inclusions such as Schaumann bodies or asteroid bodies, are scattered throughout the inflammatory locus. In the lung, granulomas tend to form along bronchovascular, bronchial submucosal, subpleural, and interlobular septal regions, areas that are rich in lymphatic vessels (see Fig. 47.1b). Hyalinized, relatively acellular ghosts of granulomas are thought to be a later development in granulomatous inflammation.

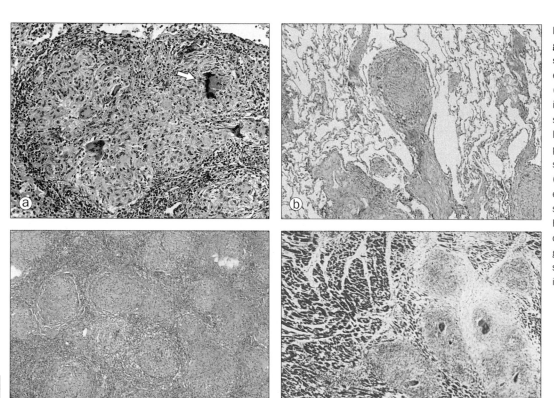

Figure 47.1 Noncaseating granulomatous inflammation in sarcoidosis. (a) Close-up of epithelioid granuloma with giant cells (arrow) and mononuclear cell infiltration. (b) Open-lung biopsy showing granulomas, giant cells, and lymphocytic infiltrates in lung parenchyma and within interlobular septal and subpleural regions. (c) Lymph node biopsy showing extensive replacement with typical sarcoid-type epithelioid granulomas. Fibrinoid necrosis, but not overt caseation, is seen in the center of granulomas. (d) Myocardial biopsy showing patchy granulomatous inflammation with giant cells.

Current concepts of the immunopathogenesis of sarcoidosis have been derived in large part from studies of lung cells and fluid recovered from the alveolar surface by bronchoalveolar lavage (BAL)[10]. Samples of BAL fluid from patients who have sarcoidosis are characterized by an increased proportion of lymphocytes (Fig. 47.2). These lung T cells are predominantly of the CD4+ phenotype, typically with a CD4:CD8 ratio between 3:1 and 10:1, compared with a ratio of 2:1 in healthy individuals. Greater than normal numbers of these lung T cells express the activation markers, very late activation antigen-1 (VLA-1, CD49a) and HLA-DR molecules. Sarcoid lung T cells demonstrate reduced surface density of the CD3:T-cell receptor complex, a hallmark of T cells activated through the T-cell antigen receptor (TCR) pathway. To define disease-specific T cells and potentially identify etiologically relevant antigens, many investigators have analyzed TCR gene expression in sarcoidosis. Results from these studies show that subgroups of patients are characterized by expanded oligoclonal populations of lung, blood, or skin T cells that express specific gene segments from the variable regions of the TCR β-, α-, γ-, or δ-chains[11]. These studies provided the first direct evidence that granulomatous inflammation in sarcoidosis is an antigen-driven response to conventional antigens.

Alveolar macrophages are thought to play a central role in the development of granulomatous inflammation in pulmonary sarcoidosis. Sarcoid alveolar macrophages spontaneously produce tumor necrosis factor-α, interleukin-6 (IL-6), and IL-12, cytokines known to regulate granuloma formation[6,10]. These cells also produce increased amounts of lysozyme, angiotensin-converting enzyme (ACE), and reactive oxygen species. Lung macrophages release increased amounts of fibronectin and insulin-like growth factor-1 (IGF-1) that are important in fibroblast recruitment and replication, as occurs in fibrotic wound healing.

Sarcoidosis as a disorder driven by T-helper-1 cells

A current paradigm in immunology is that the nature of an immune response is determined by the balance of cytokines released by CD4+ (and CD8+) T cells. TH1 cells also produce interferon-γ (IFN-γ) and IL-2, whereas TH2 cells produce IL-4, IL-5, and IL-13 . Human TH1 cytokines are important in cell-mediated immunity and macrophage activation, and TH2 cytokines are important in antibody responses, antihelminthic and allergic responses, and macrophage deactivation. Primarily, macrophages and dendritic cells produce IL-12, which is critical to the initiation of TH1 responses; IL-4 is critical to the development of TH2 responses. Granulomatous immune responses may be driven by either TH1 or TH2 cytokines, largely depending on the nature of the antigenic stimulus (e.g. TH1 in antituberculous and TH2 in antischistosomal immune responses).

Recent evidence supports the concept that sarcoidosis is a dominant TH1 disorder with spontaneous production of IFN-γ and IL-2 by lung T cells and IL-12 by lung macrophages (see Fig. 47.3)[6,10,11]. In contrast, low or undetectable levels of IL-4 and IL-5 occur in most patients who have sarcoidosis. One hypothesis suggests that successful removal of the inciting stimulus by this TH1-dependent response results in resolution of the disease (see Fig. 47.3). In a subgroup of patients, enhanced in-vitro production of transforming growth factor-β (TGF-β) from lung macrophages has been associated with

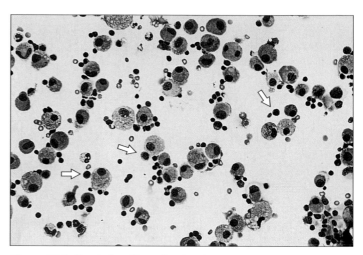

Figure 47.2 Cytospin of bronchoalveolar lavage (BAL) cells from a patient who had sarcoidosis. A larger-than-normal proportion of lung lymphocytes (small, dark-staining cells with unilobular nuclei and scant cytoplasm) is seen (arrows). Larger cells are alveolar macrophages that normally comprise 90% or more of recovered cells from the BAL of healthy individuals.

remission of active disease, suggesting this cytokine may be critical to downregulating the TH1 inflammatory process in sarcoidosis. If the immune response ineffectively removes the stimulating antigens or autoimmunity develops, dysregulated cytokine production driven by a positive feedback loop between IFN-γ and IL-12 results in maintenance of granulomatous inflammation (see Fig. 47.3). A fibrotic outcome may occur in response to unremitting inflammation, with tissue injury from the local release of reactive oxygen species, proteases, and lysosomal products from phagocytic cells in the presence of profibrotic cytokines such as TGF-β and IGF-1 (see Fig. 47.3). Theoretically, fibrosis can be prevented by suppressing the inflammatory response early in the course of the disease. Consistent with this scenario, drugs able to suppress IFN-γ and IL-12 production (e.g. corticosteroids, pentoxifylline, thalidomide) may be beneficial in the treatment of sarcoidosis.

CLINICAL FEATURES

The clinical presentation and natural course of sarcoidosis varies greatly[1-4]. Up to two thirds of patients are asymptomatic, but have sarcoidosis diagnosed after an incidental radiographic finding of bilateral hilar adenopathy or, occasionally, an abnormal liver profile. Symptomatic presentations of sarcoidosis most frequently involve the respiratory system[12-14]. Systemic constitutional symptoms, such as fever, malaise, and weight loss, may be prominent features, particularly in those patients who have Löfgren's syndrome or hepatic sarcoidosis.

Asymptomatic sarcoidosis

Based on population screening with chest radiographs, it is estimated that 30–60% of patients who have sarcoidosis are asymptomatic. Patients in this subgroup are usually noted to have bilateral hilar adenopathy on the chest radiograph. Occasionally, interstitial infiltrates are also seen in association with intrathoracic adenopathy in asymptomatic patients who have sarcoidosis, more commonly in Caucasian individuals.

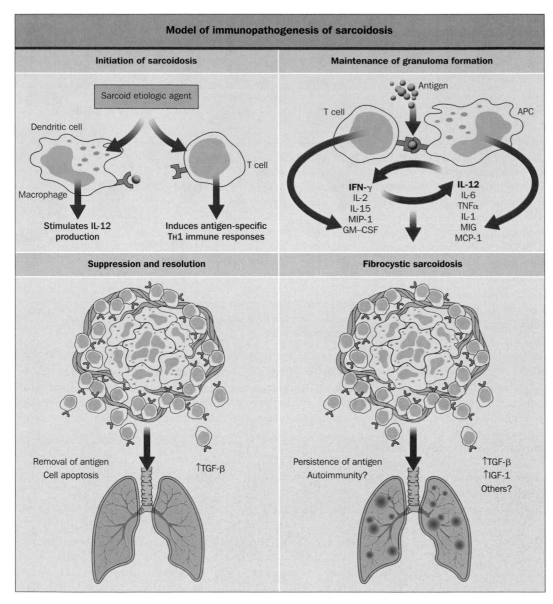

Figure 47.3 Model of the immunopathogenesis of sarcoidosis. Initiation of sarcoidosis involves stimulation of interleukin-12 (IL-12) production from mononuclear phagocytes and dendritic cells and adaptive T-cell immunity to an inciting agent. Maintenance of granuloma formation occurs via a T-helper 1 (TH1) immune response driven by interferon-γ (IFN-γ) and IL-12. Resolution of sarcoidosis occurs after removal of stimulating antigen, suppression of T-cell responses occurs via transforming growth factor-β (TGF-β) and other mediators, and granuloma resorption occurs via cell apoptosis. Fibrotic outcome results from persistent, possibly autoimmune, antigenic stimulation in the presence of TGF-β and other profibrotic mediators. (MIP-1, macrophage inflammatory protein-1; GM–CSF, granulocyte–macrophage-colony-stimulating factor; APC, antigen-presenting cells; MIG, monokine-induced by IFN-γ; MCP-1, monocyte chemotactic protein-1; TNF-α, tumor necrosis factor-α; IGF-1, insulin-like growth factor-1.)

Löfgren's syndrome

Löfgren's syndrome is a well-defined presentation of sarcoidosis that consists of erythema nodosum, polyarthritis, and (in over 90% of cases) bilateral hilar adenopathy. The polyarthritis, which may be severe, commonly involves the ankles, knees, and wrists, sometimes with heel pain and Achilles' tendinitis. Fever and lassitude are often prominent manifestations, and uveitis is found in 50% or more cases. The onset of symptoms is usually abrupt. In most cases, spontaneous remission occurs within several weeks to months. This presentation is common in European and Caucasian populations, but occurs in <5% of patients of African descent who have sarcoidosis.

Pulmonary sarcoidosis

The most common symptoms of pulmonary sarcoidosis are shortness of breath, cough, and chest discomfort (Fig. 47.4). Dyspnea is most marked on exertion and typically progresses in active, untreated disease. Cough is usually nonproductive early in the course of sarcoidosis and can vary greatly in severity. Dyspnea and cough may reflect parenchymal (interstitial) involvement,

endobronchial disease, or both. Chronic sputum production and hemoptysis are more frequent in advanced fibrocystic disease. Chest pain is common, often difficult to describe, and varies in location and severity. Chest tightness and wheezing are frequent in patients who have chronic fibrocystic sarcoidosis or airway hyper-responsiveness. Typically, the physical findings of pulmonary sarcoidosis are few. Lung crackles are heard in <20% of patients, even in those who have advanced disease. Clubbing is rare, but when present it is usually associated with advanced bronchiectasis.

Symptomatic bronchial or tracheal stenosis is rare, but may present with dyspnea, stridor, wheezing, or cough. Lobar atelectasis, usually of the upper or right middle lobes, may be seen. Mechanisms include compression by nearby lymph nodes, fibrotic distortion of major airways, endobronchial disease, or mediastinal fibrosis.

Chronic pulmonary hypertension and cor pulmonale is seen in 1–4% of patients, and usually arise from severe fibrocystic sarcoidosis. Rarely, dyspnea from pulmonary hypertension presents without severe interstitial lung disease. Causes include extrinsic compression of pulmonary vessels by enlarged lymph nodes or fibrosing mediastinitis, or a granulomatous vasculitis of pulmonary

Major clinical features of pulmonary and upper respiratory tract sarcoidosis

Symptoms	Signs	Tests
Dyspnea	Wheezes (occasional)	Lung function
Cough	Crackles (uncommon)	Restrictive impairment
Chest pain	Clubbing (rare)	Obstructive impairment
Sputum production	Stridor	Hypoxemia
	Sinus tenderness	Hypercapnia (late)
Hemoptysis	Cobblestoning, edema, erythema of nasal mucosa, laryngeal structures	Bilateral hilar and mediastinal adenopathy
Hoarseness		Diffuse infiltrates
Nasal congestion	Saddle nose deformity	Upper lobe fibrosis
Sinus pain		Bronchiectasis
		Mycetomas

Figure 47.4 Major clinical features of pulmonary and upper respiratory tract sarcoidosis.

vessels. Superior vena cava syndrome rarely occurs from extensive mediastinal lymphadenopathy and fibrosis as a result of sarcoidosis; more commonly, histoplasmosis or malignancy is the cause.

Chest radiology

Chest radiographs are abnormal in >90% of patients who have sarcoidosis. By international convention, the chest radiograph is divided into the following stages or types (Fig. 47.5)[1–4]:

- stage 0 – normal chest radiograph;
- stage I – bilateral hilar adenopathy;
- stage II – bilateral hilar adenopathy plus interstitial infiltrates;
- stage III – interstitial infiltrates only (non-fibrotic); and
- stage IV – fibrocystic interstitial lung disease.

A normal chest radiograph is found in 5–10% of patients who have sarcoidosis, frequently in those who show extrathoracic manifestations of sarcoidosis. Stage I is seen in 40–50% of cases on initial presentation (Fig. 47.5a). Typically, the hilar adenopathy is discrete, symmetric, and stands away from the right heart border to give the appearance of 'potato nodes'; paratracheal adenopathy, particularly on the right side, is a common accompaniment. A stage II chest radiograph is seen in 20–30% of cases on initial presentation (Fig. 47.5b). Typically, the infiltrates demonstrate fine, linear markings, reticulonodules, or confluent shadows. A mid- or upper-zone predominance is frequently seen and may mimic tuberculosis or histoplasmosis. A stage III chest radiograph has interstitial infiltrates and no discernable hilar adenopathy, and is seen in 10–20% of cases on initial presentation (Fig. 47.5c). Chest radiographs that have extensive fibrocystic changes and scarring are frequently placed under a separate subgroup, stage IV, in recognition of the poor outcome of this group of patients (Fig. 47.5d). Destruction of lung tissue, fibrous traction on airways with upward hilar retraction, and multiple bullous and cystic changes are typically seen.

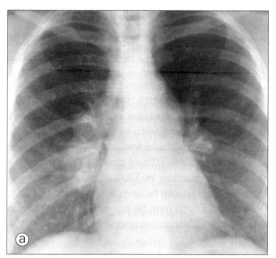

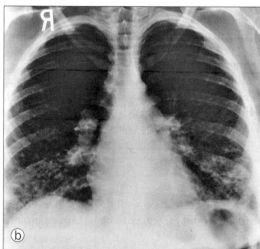

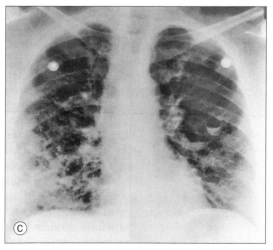

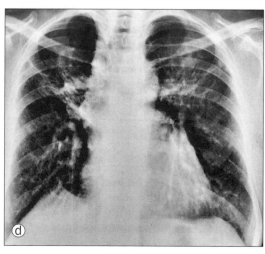

Figure 47.5 Chest radiograph stages of sarcoidosis. (a) Stage I sarcoidosis with bilateral hilar and right paratracheal adenopathy. (b) Stage II sarcoidosis with bilateral hilar adenopathy and reticulonodular infiltrates. (c) Stage III sarcoidosis with bilateral infiltrates without adenopathy. Multiple cystic areas are also seen, which could lead to a classification of stage IV disease. (d) Stage IV fibrocystic sarcoidosis with typical upward hilar retraction and large cystic and bullous changes.

who have chronic sarcoidosis, more frequently in patients of African descent. Other manifestations include posterior uveitis, granulomatous conjunctivitis, or severe chorioretinitis or optic neuritis; these latter conditions may present acutely with blindness.

Cutaneous sarcoidosis

Erythema nodosum is characterized by tender, reddish nodules that are several centimeters in diameter, usually located on the lower extremities. When seen in association with polyarthritis and bilateral hilar lymphadenopathy, Löfgren's syndrome may be diagnosed. Chronic skin sarcoidosis usually manifests as plaques and subcutaneous nodules that have a propensity to involve the skin around the hairline, eyelids, ears, nose, mouth, and extensor surfaces of the arms and legs. Lesions in the scalp are sometimes associated with alopecia. Skin lesions may be either hyperpigmented or hypopigmented and are usually nontender and nonpruritic. Lupus pernio is a particularly disfiguring form of cutaneous sarcoid of the face, with violaceous plaques and nodules that cover the nose, nasal alae, malar areas, and around the eyes. Chronic skin lesions appear more common and severe in patients of African descent.

Cardiac sarcoidosis

Cardiac sarcoidosis appears to be more common in Japan than in other parts of the world; one autopsy series from Japan demonstrated cardiac sarcoidosis in almost 50% of cases, whereas 27% of cases were found to have cardiac involvement in a series from Baltimore[16]. In North America and Europe, cardiac sarcoidosis is clinically apparent in 5% or fewer patients who have sarcoidosis. In one large study, complete heart block was the most common manifestation; ventricular arrhythmias, bundle branch blocks, sudden death, cardiomyopathy, supraventricular arrhythmias, and valvular dysfunction were less common[17]. Rarely, pericardial disease or a process that mimics myocardial infarction was seen. Overall, cardiac sarcoidosis is a major cause of mortality in young adults who have sarcoidosis, primarily from heart block or arrhythmias. Extensive involvement of the myocardium can lead to progressive congestive heart failure and is responsible for most of the other deaths related to cardiac sarcoidosis.

Hepatic sarcoidosis

Noncaseating granulomas are found by percutaneous biopsy in 40–70% of patients, but clinical manifestations are seen in <10% of cases. Symptomatic hepatic sarcoidosis often manifests with fever and tender hepatomegaly. Pruritus can be severe and disabling in a small number of patients. Characteristically, the serum alkaline phosphatase and γ-glutamyl transferase are elevated proportionately higher than aspartate aminotransferase, alanine aminotransferase, and bilirubin, although all patterns can be seen. Hepatic sarcoidosis may mimic primary biliary cirrhosis, except that antimitochondrial antibodies are absent.

Joints and bones

Arthralgias are common in active multisystem sarcoidosis. Acute, often incapacitating, migratory polyarthritis is seen in Löfgren's syndrome. In such instances, joint radiographs are negative, and the arthritis usually regresses within weeks to several months with or without therapy. Persistent joint disease is found in <5% of patients who have chronic sarcoidosis. Pain, swelling, and tenderness of the phalanges of the hands and feet are most common. Joint radiographs may demonstrate 'punched-out' lesions with

cystic changes and marked loss of trabeculae, but with no evidence of erosive chondritis. Cystic lesions of the long bones, pelvis, sternum, skull, and vertebrae rarely occur.

Neurosarcoidosis

Neurosarcoidosis occurs in approximately 5% of patients who have sarcoidosis. The most common manifestation is cranial neuropathy, with bilateral or unilateral 7th nerve (Bell's) palsy seen in 50–70% of cases[18]. The palsy may resolve spontaneously or with corticosteroids, and rarely recurs years later. Optic neuritis, the second most common cranial neuropathy in sarcoidosis, can result in blurred vision, field defects, and blindness. Less commonly, involvement of the glossopharyngeal, auditory, oculomotor, trigeminal, or other cranial nerves occurs. Manifestations of central nervous system (CNS) involvement include mass lesions, aseptic meningitis, obstructive hydrocephalus, and hypothalamic and/or pituitary dysfunction. Seizures, headache, change in mental status, confusion, and diabetes insipidus may be presenting symptoms. Spinal cord compression syndromes are rare, but paraparesis, hemiparesis, and back and leg pain have been described. Peripheral neuropathies account for about 15% of cases of neurosarcoidosis, and often present as mononeuritis multiplex or a primary sensory neuropathy.

Salivary, parotid, and lacrimal gland sarcoidosis

Heerfordt's syndrome, also known as uveoparotid fever, manifests as fever, parotid and lacrimal gland enlargement, uveitis, and bilateral hilar adenopathy. This common presentation of acute sarcoidosis may be associated with cranial neuropathies, usually facial palsy.

Hematologic sarcoidosis

Peripheral lymph node enlargement occurs in 20–30% of patients as an early manifestation of sarcoidosis, but typically undergoes spontaneous remission. Chronic bulky lymphadenopathy occurs <10% of the time. Splenomegaly, occasionally massive, occurs in < 5% of cases. Hypersplenism with anemia and thrombocytopenia are rare and should be investigated for alternative causes. Peripheral leukopenia in sarcoidosis is common, usually as a result of CD4+ lymphopenia from altered trafficking of lymphocytes rather than splenic trapping. Splenomegaly is often associated with hepatomegaly and, less frequently, hypercalcemia, in a characteristic triad that may present without pulmonary involvement. Nonclonal hypergammaglobulinemia is present in 25% or more of patients. Occasionally, common-variable immunodeficiency is found in association with sarcoidosis, and should be suspected in the presence of recurrent pulmonary or sinus infections and splenomegaly. Most patients have cutaneous anergy to recall antigens for mumps, *Candida* spp., *Trichophyton* spp., or tuberculin.

Sarcoid myopathy

Although random muscle biopsies in autopsy series demonstrate muscle granulomas in a majority of patients who have sarcoidosis, symptomatic myopathy with weakness and tenderness is uncommon. Rarely, sarcoidosis can present as a polymyositis with profound weakness and elevated serum creatine kinase and aldolase.

Hypercalcemia, hypercalciuria, and renal disease

Hypercalcemia is present in 2–5% of patients; hypercalciuria is more common. Abnormal calcium regulation is thought to result from an increased conversion of 25-hydroxyvitamin D₃ to the active 1,25-dihydroxyvitamin D₃ by macrophages and epithelioid cells from granulomas. Chronic hypercalcemia or hypercalciuria most commonly manifests as kidney stones. Renal failure from chronic, often asymptomatic, nephrocalcinosis may result if left undetected. Granulomatous involvement of the kidneys is uncommon and usually not a cause of renal failure. Nephrotic syndrome and chronic membranous glomerulonephritis are also associated with sarcoidosis.

DIAGNOSIS

An initial diagnostic evaluation of a patient who has possible sarcoidosis consists of tests to evaluate the presence and extent of pulmonary involvement and to screen for extrathoracic disease (Fig. 47.12)[12,19]. The chest radiograph is an important starting point, since it is abnormal in over 90% of known cases of sarcoidosis and carries prognostic information. Spirometry, diffusing capacity, and lung volume testing are used to detect the presence and extent of parenchymal lung involvement. Flow–volume curves are indicated when laryngeal or upper airway obstruction is possible. Arterial blood gas measurement is not routinely needed unless evidence of moderate or severe pulmonary impairment is found. Oxygen saturation and exercise studies (e.g. 6-minute walk) may help to determine subtle changes in pulmonary involvement in response to treatment or the need for supplemental oxygen, but are not needed for most patients at presentation. An initial slit-lamp examination is recommended in all cases to exclude uveitis, which may be clinically silent. Blood testing is performed to exclude significant hepatic, renal, or hematologic involvement. An electrocardiogram is indicated to detect evidence of arrythmias or heart block from possible cardiac sarcoidosis. A purified protein derivative skin test should be performed to help exclude tuberculosis.

Chest CT is not routinely needed in the evaluation of patients who have suspected pulmonary sarcoidosis[20]. Occasionally, CT is useful to define the pattern of hilar or mediastinal adenopathy to assist the bronchoscopic needle biopsy of mediastinal lymph nodes. Chest CT may also help to define the extent of fibrocystic disease or unusual radiographic features, such as masses, bronchial or tracheal stenosis, atelectasis, or bronchiectasis.

Diagnostic approach
A diagnosis of sarcoidosis is based on a compatible clinical picture, histologic evidence of noncaseating granulomas, and the absence of other known causes of this pathologic response. Tuberculosis, fungal diseases, and lymphoma are usually the most important diseases to be excluded in patients who have chest disease. Chronic beryllium disease, hypersensitivity pneumonitis, and drug reactions must be excluded when the history suggests these possibilities. In the absence of defined multisystem disease, a diagnosis of sarcoidosis is presumed, since local 'sarcoid' reactions may occur in response to infection, tumor, or foreign material.

In general, the easiest accessible biopsy site is used for biopsy confirmation. Biopsy of a skin nodule, superficial lymph node, lacrimal gland, nasal mucosae, conjunctivae, or salivary gland (lip biopsy) can often establish a diagnosis. Biopsy of these sites is generally performed only if the tissue is abnormal, since blind biopsies are usually unhelpful. Biopsy of the liver or bone marrow is nonspecific and are used to support a diagnosis of sarcoidosis only after

Recommended tests for an initial evaluation of sarcoidosis	
Chest radiograph	**Liver function tests**
Pulmonary function tests	Alkaline phosphatase
Spirometry	Aspartate aminotransferase
Diffusing capacity of lung for carbon monoxide	Alanine aminotransferase
Lung volumes	Total and indirect bilirubin
Renal function tests	**Calcium level**
Blood urea nitrogen	**Extrapulmonary organ-specific tests (for symptomatic organ involvement)**
Creatinine	
Urinalysis	Neurosarcoidosis – magnetic resonance imaging with gadolinium enhancement, cerebral spinal fluid examination, nerve conduction studies
Ophthalmologic (slit lamp) examination	
Electrocardiogram	Cardiac sarcoidosis – Holter monitor, 2D-echocardiogram
Purified protein derivative skin test	

Figure 47.12 Recommended tests for an initial evaluation of sarcoidosis.

malignancy and infectious granulomatous diseases or other competing diagnoses have been excluded. When superficial abnormalities are not apparent or it is necessary to exclude infectious or malignant chest disease, bronchoscopic biopsy is usually performed.

Biopsy confirmation of sarcoidosis is usually not necessary in Löfgren's syndrome. An exception to this approach may be found in regions where histoplasmosis is endemic, such as the Mississippi Valley region, where some authorities recommend routine bronchoscopy to exclude infection, particularly before corticosteroid therapy is initiated.

Bronchoscopy
Biopsy by fiberoptic bronchoscopy is now the most frequent procedure used to diagnose pulmonary sarcoidosis because of its relative safety and high yield. The yield of transbronchial biopsy approaches 90% when pulmonary infiltrates are seen radiographically and at least 4–6 transbronchial biopsies are taken (Fig. 47.13)[21]. Studies suggest the yield may approach 50% with stage I chest radiographs, although the absence of infiltrates on chest CT significantly reduces this yield. Recently, several studies emphasized the utility of an endobronchial biopsy, which is safer than a transbronchial biopsy. Endobronchial biopsy directed to abnormal airways (nodularity, mucosal edema, hypervascularity) has a >50% positive yield (see Fig. 47.14). In the absence

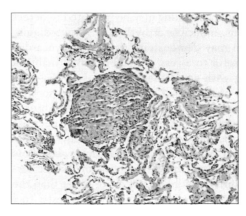

Figure 47.13 Epithelioid granuloma in a transbronchial biopsy from a patient who has sarcoidosis.

been established by rigorous clinical studies. Nonetheless, there is widespread agreement on the basic treatment principles outlined below.

Pulmonary sarcoidosis
Indications for observation are:
- asymptomatic patients who have normal lung function and
- patients who have minimal symptoms and mild functional abnormalities until disease progression.

Indications for treatment are:
- moderate or severe, symptomatic pulmonary disease;
- progressive, symptomatic pulmonary disease; and
- persistent pulmonary infiltrates or abnormal lung function for 1–2 years with mild symptoms (to assess reversibility).

Corticosteroids
Initial treatment of pulmonary sarcoidosis with corticosteroids usually does not require more than prednisone 30–40mg/day[12]. Higher doses are rarely needed. A recommended regimen for treating pulmonary sarcoidosis with corticosteroids is outlined in Figure 47.15. Treatment should ordinarily be continued for a minimum of 8–12 months, since premature tapering is likely to result in relapse of disease. A maintenance dose of 5–15mg/day of prednisone is usually sufficient to suppress persistent pulmonary disease. Alternate-day therapy (e.g. 10–30mg every other day) is suggested by some investigators, although such a regimen may not be effective in a subgroup of patients (who respond to daily dosing) and compliance may be more difficult. Patients who have progressive disease while tapering should be placed on the next highest daily dose that previously resulted in suppression of disease. Intermittent attempts to taper corticosteroids is appropriate in the first several years of treatment, but those patients who have repetitive relapses usually require indefinite suppressive therapy. Patients with advanced fibrocystic disease often have only a modest or no improvement in lung function because of the presence of irreversible fibrosis. However, active granulomatous inflammation is usually seen on open lung biopsy or autopsy when performed in these patients, which strongly argues against the concept of 'burnt-out' fibrocystic disease. A maintenance dose (e.g. 10–20mg/day) is usually indicated in these patients with the goal of preventing or slowing further progression of respiratory insufficiency.

Low-dose corticosteroid therapy is usually well tolerated. The most common complaint is weight gain. Patients are instructed early in the treatment about caloric and salt restriction to minimize this effect. Insomnia and euphoria may also occur; psychosis is rare, but can occur with higher doses. Glaucoma is a potential complication of long-term corticosteroid therapy (or chronic ocular sarcoidosis). Osteoporosis and osteonecrosis are potential complications in patients who have sarcoidosis. Routine use of supplemental calcium and vitamin D supplementation is generally not recommended to avoid the potential for hypercalcemia and hypercalciuria. Potential benefits of newer anti-osteoporosis medications seem likely, although clinical studies are lacking.

Inhaled corticosteroids
Inhaled corticosteroids may help to reduce symptoms of endobronchial sarcoidosis such as cough or airway irritability. A role for inhaled corticosteroids in the treatment of parenchymal pulmonary sarcoidosis is uncertain. Early studies using beclomethasone failed to show benefit, perhaps because of low drug doses. More recently, several studies reported some effectiveness of budesonide, a more potent inhaled corticosteroid, in improving symptoms or lung function in pulmonary sarcoidosis[27]. The effects were modest, dose dependent, and generally involved groups of patients who had mild disease and good prognoses. Other studies failed to demonstrate significant improvement in lung function or chest radiographs, particularly in patients who had more advanced disease. Dysphonia and oral thrush are common with budesonide; systemic side effects have also been documented. Overall, these studies and anecdotal experiences suggest that inhaled corticosteroids cannot be routinely recommended, except possibly for mild disease. Whether potent inhaled corticosteroids will find a place as systemic corticosteroid-sparing agents awaits further study.

Other treatments
Supportive management of patients who have advanced fibrocystic sarcoidosis and cor pulmonale includes supplemental oxygen, diuretics, and bronchodilators for obstructive impairment. Aggressive antibiotic treatment of bronchitis and bronchiectasis is indicated, often employed on a rotating monthly regimen, to reduce the frequency of infectious episodes.

Extrapulmonary sarcoidosis
Indications for treatment are:
- threatened organ failure – severe ocular, cardiac, or CNS disease;
- posterior uveitis or anterior uveitis that does not respond to local corticosteroids;
- persistent hypercalcemia;
- persistent renal or hepatic dysfunction;
- pituitary disease;
- myopathy;
- palpable splenomegaly or evidence of hypersplenism;
- severe fatigue and weight loss;
- painful lymphadenopathy; and
- disfiguring skin disease.

Ocular sarcoidosis
Topical corticosteroids are usually sufficient in anterior uveitis, but oral corticosteroids are necessary in posterior uveitis, chorioretinitis, and optic neuritis. These last two disorders may present as ocular emergencies that require high doses of intravenous corticosteroids initially. Close ophthalmologic follow-up is necessary in all patients who have ocular sarcoidosis.

Cardiac sarcoidosis
Treatment of cardiac sarcoidosis consists of antiarrhythmic therapy, diuretics, and afterload-reducing agents for heart failure, in addition to anti-inflammatory drugs[12,23,26]. Automatic implantable defibrillators can prevent sudden death in individuals who have serious arrhythmias and are indicated in patients at risk for sudden death. A standard approach is to use corticosteroids in moderate doses, based on unpublished and published series that have documented the potential of corticosteroids to reverse heart block, reduce arrhythmias, and improve ejection fraction. Overall improvement in mortality, however, has not been proved by prospective study. Initial therapy might begin with 40–60mg/day followed by a slow taper to a maintenance dose of 15–20mg/day. Methotrexate has also

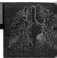

been utilized, although experience remains limited. Extensive fibrosis may result in dilated cardiomyopathy resistant to corticosteroids and cytotoxic drugs. Nonetheless, moderate doses of corticosteroids for maintenance therapy are generally recommended in an attempt to prevent further myocardial granulomatous inflammation and fibrosis.

Neurosarcoidosis
High doses of oral corticosteroids (60–80mg/day) sometimes preceded by several days of high-dose pulse intravenous therapy are often employed for serious CNS involvement[23]. Tapering to more modest doses of corticosteroids is performed over several months, following evidence of suppression by objective criteria (e.g. serial MRI scans or CSF examinations). Neurosarcoidosis tends to be chronic, and requires long-term therapy.

Hepatic sarcoidosis
Persistently elevated liver function tests (e.g. alkaline phosphatase >2–3 times normal) probably should be treated, even in the asymptomatic patient, to prevent progressive hepatic dysfunction and cirrhosis. Low-dose corticosteroids (10–15mg/day) are usually sufficient to suppress hepatic inflammation and prevent progressive organ dysfunction. Hyperglycemia is a frequent complication of corticosteroid therapy in hepatic sarcoidosis and is monitored prospectively.

Hypercalcemia
Persistent hypercalcemia is an indication for treatment because of the risk of nephrocalcinosis or (rarely) acute hypercalcemic crisis. Prednisone in moderate doses is almost always effective; if not, primary hyperparathyroidism should be considered. Case reports also document that chloroquine, hydroxychloroquine (see below), and ketoconazole may effectively treat hypercalcemic sarcoidosis.

Bone and joint sarcoidosis
Corticosteroids usually result in dramatic improvement in symptoms. Over months, new bone formation can occur with a return to a normal radiographic bone appearance. Chloroquine and hydroxychloroquine may also be effective.

Hematologic sarcoidosis
Corticosteroids usually effectively shrink an enlarged spleen, although some splenic enlargement may persist. Hypersplenism also frequently responds, at least in part, to low or moderate doses of corticosteroids.

Special situations
Löfgren's syndrome
Bed rest and nonsteroidal anti-inflammatory drugs are recommended for symptomatic relief of constitutional symptoms and joint pains. Corticosteroids are almost immediately effective, but are recommended only in cases in which symptoms are disabling and unresponsive to nonsteroidal anti-inflammatory drugs. Generally, the corticosteroids can be tapered over a few weeks to months without recrudescence of symptoms.

Mucocutaneous sarcoidosis
The antimalarial drugs, chloroquine and hydroxychloroquine, have been used as first-line drugs for lupus pernio, other disfiguring

sarcoid skin disease, and nasal sarcoidosis[12]. Response rates approximate 50% and are higher with chloroquine than with hydroxychloroquine. Beneficial effects may not be evident for 2–3 months. Chloroquine may be useful in chronic laryngeal sarcoidosis, although corticosteroids are usually used initially to prevent acute airway obstruction. These drugs have not been effective for pulmonary or systemic disease, but may be used in conjunction with low doses of corticosteroids when recalcitrant mucocutaneous disease and pulmonary disease coexist. Ocular toxicity is a major concern with chloroquine, but is rare when low doses are used with periods of drug-free use (see Fig. 47.15). Serial ophthalmologic evaluations are performed every 4–6 months during therapy. Hydroxychloroquine appears to be less efficacious, but its lower toxicity makes it a useful alternative and it may be used without interruption.

Role of cytotoxic and other alternative therapies
Methotrexate
Methotrexate has been used to treat severe sarcoid skin disease with anecdotal success. More recently, methotrexate in low, weekly doses (10–20mg/day) was proposed as an alternative therapy in corticosteroid-resistant pulmonary sarcoidosis[28]. One group found a response rate of 70%, although improvement in some patients was not noted until 6 months of therapy[28]. Randomized clinical trials are not yet reported, and other experiences are not as favorable. Hepatic toxicity, opportunistic infections, and bone marrow suppression have limited enthusiasm for this drug. Given the risk of cirrhosis with long-term therapy, many workers prefer azathioprine when corticosteroid therapy is unsatisfactory.

Azathioprine
Anecdotal experience suggests that azathioprine in a dose of 100–200mg/day may be useful in corticosteroid-resistant sarcoidosis. Low doses of corticosteroids (e.g. 10mg/day prednisone) are usually prescribed concomitantly; beneficial effects usually are apparent by 2–3 months. Bone marrow toxicities, gastrointestinal symptoms, skin rashes, and arthralgias are serious drawbacks, and the drug has a slightly increased risk of malignancy. Nonetheless, since the drug is often well tolerated for prolonged periods of treatment, azathioprine remains the first drug used by many clinicians for severe, corticosteroid-resistant sarcoidosis.

Other cytotoxic and immunosuppressive agents
Chlorambucil and cyclophosphamide have had anecdotal successes in the treatment of progressive sarcoidosis refractory to corticosteroids, although their oncogenic potential suggests their use should be extremely limited. Limited clinical experience with cyclosporin A, a drug known to inhibit T-cell activation, also proved disappointing.

Pentoxifylline
A recent clinical study found that pentoxifylline was beneficial when used alone or with corticosteroids in the initial treatment of sarcoidosis[29]. Anecdotal experience suggests that the drug may be useful in some cases of mild pulmonary or hepatic disease, or as a corticosteroid-sparing agent, although experience remains limited. Gastrointestinal side effects and headache may be troublesome, but given the relative safety of the drug, further studies seem merited.

Diffuse Lung Diseases

cause of LAM is unknown, but its occurrence solely in women and an association with postmenopausal hormonal therapy suggest a pathogenic role for estrogenic hormones and/or abnormal tissue response to these hormones. Also, LAM may occur in association with tuberous sclerosis (TS) in which LAM appears to represent a pulmonary manifestation of TS that is an autosomal-dominant form of congenital hamartomatosis[2]. Those patients with TSC and LAM are also strictly women[2].

Histopathologic examination of lung tissue involved by LAM reveals abnormal proliferation of atypical smooth muscle cells (LAM cells) in the parenchyma as well as around the vessels, airways, and lymphatics (Fig. 49.3). Impingement of smooth muscle proliferation in the latter structures causes hemoptysis, airway obstruction, and chylothorax, respectively. Cystic changes in lung parenchyma may be mediated by airway obstruction and resultant air trapping and/or degradation of elastic fibers in the alveolar walls[3].

The preferred term for primary pulmonary histiocytosis X, pulmonary eosinophilic granuloma, and Langerhans' cell granulomatosis is LCH. Two broad categories of histiocytic disorders exist: disorders of varied biologic behavior and malignant disorders. Each category is further subdivided according to whether the abnormal cells are derived from the dendritic cell or of macrophage lineage – LCH is considered a dendritic-cell-related disorder of varied biologic behavior.

Langerhans' cells are present in the normal lung, almost exclusively intercalated between epithelial cells of the airways, and they have potent antigen-presenting capabilities. Langerhans' cells are differentiated from dendritic cells by their characteristic pentalaminar, plate-like cytoplasmic organelles (Birbeck granule or X-body) seen by electron microscopy, and their strong expression of the CD1a antigen on the cell surface. They also stain with S-100 and CD45 antibodies. The cause of LCH is not known and it results in excessive proliferation of Langerhans' cells. The isolated pulmonary form that occurs in adults is considered a LCH variant and is strongly associated with cigarette smoking. In this chapter the pulmonary form is referred to as LCH, but it should be understood that LCH is not one disease. Most studies have shown >90% of patients who have LCH to be current or previous cigarette smokers who are typically in their third or fourth decades of life[4,5]. Cigarette smoking has been shown to increase the number of Langerhans' cells in the lung parenchyma. Although certain forms of LCH probably represent monoclonal proliferations of Langerhans' cells, it is not known whether this is true for the isolated pulmonary form of LCH. Morphologic studies show proliferating Langerhans' cells involved in a bronchocentric process accompanied by mixed cellular infiltrates (Fig. 49.4). Adjacent blood vessels and lung parenchyma are also involved. As this granulomatous-like reaction evolves, collagen fibrosis and scarring occur, with associated paracicatricial air-space enlargement that accounts for the concomitant cystic changes.

Although LIP was initially described as an unusual form of idiopathic interstitial pneumonia, it appears that this disorder

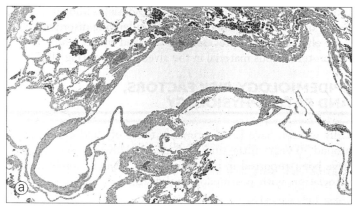

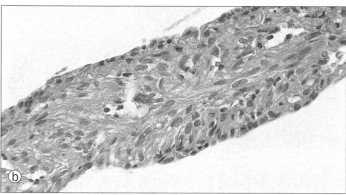

Figure 49.3 Histopathology of lymphangiomyomatosis (LAM).
(a) Low-magnification photomicrograph of LAM showing cystic spaces surrounded by a variably thick wall containing proliferating spindle cells. Hemosiderin pigment is present in adjacent air spaces, which attests to the presence of alveolar hemorrhage. (b) Higher-magnification photomicrograph showing smooth muscle cells within thickened peribronchiolar interstitium in LAM.

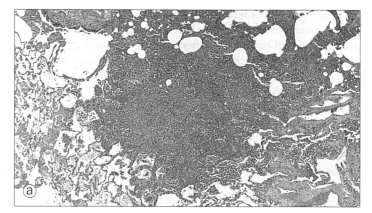

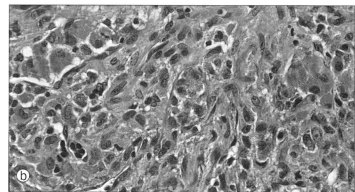

Figure 49.4 Histopathology of Langerhans' cell histiocytosis (LCH).
(a) Low-magnification photomicrograph showing stellate, bronchocentric nodule in LCH. (b) High-magnification photomicrograph showing a polymorphic, interstitial infiltrate in LCH. The cellular infiltrate includes a mixture of mononuclear cells and eosinophils. Langerhans' cells predominate and are differentiated by highly convoluted nuclei with nuclear grooves, which result in nuclear configurations that resemble crumpled paper or coffee beans.

can be associated with a variety of underlying conditions, which include human immunodeficiency virus (HIV) infection, Sjögren's syndrome, Hashimoto's thyroiditis, chronic active thyroiditis, primary biliary cirrhosis, myasthenia gravis, and other disorders[6-8]. It may also occur in an idiopathic form. In some cases, LIP is thought to transform into lymphoma or represent lymphoma *de novo*[7]. Epstein–Barr virus genome has been identified in some patients who have LIP. The majority of HIV-negative patients who have LIP are adults in their fourth to seventh decades[8,9]. Women are more commonly affected than men by 2:1; however, those who have LIP in association with HIV infection tend to be younger with a male predominance.

Alveolar proteinosis is an uncommon disorder that occurs in patients over a wide age range, but mostly between the ages of 20 and 50 years[10]. Few familial cases have been reported, men are affected about twice as often as women, and it has been reported in virtually all industrialized countries. It is restricted to the lungs and is characterized by accumulation of acellular, lipoproteinaceous material in the alveolar spaces. Alveolar proteinosis can be seen in a primary (idiopathic) form. Secondary alveolar proteinosis may occur in association with pulmonary infections, exposure to inhaled chemicals (insecticides) and minerals (silica, aluminum dust, titanium), hematologic disorders (lymphoma, leukemia), and HIV infection[10]. Pathogenesis is thought to be mediated by disrupted clearance and/or excessive secretion of surfactant-like material that involves alveolar macrophages and type II alveolar pneumocytes.

CLINICAL FEATURES

The characteristic presentation of LAM includes progressive breathlessness and recurrent pneumothoraces. Less common symptoms include chest pain, cough, hemoptysis, pleural effusions (usually chylous), chylous ascites, and (rarely) chyloptysis. Physical examination is usually unremarkable unless a pleural effusion is found, or occasional wheezes or basal crackles. Those patients who have LAM associated with TS usually show pathognomonic findings, which include facial angiofibromas, periungual or ungual fibromas, and retinal astrocytomas[2].

The vast majority of patients who have LCH are current or past smokers and commonly present with dyspnea and cough. A history of pneumothorax is obtained in about one fourth of patients[4,5,11]. Other symptoms may include wheezing, fever, fatigue, weight loss, chest pain, and hemoptysis. In the early stages of the disease, up to one fourth of patients may be asymptomatic or have mild, nonspecific symptoms[4]. On examination, crackles, wheeze, and digital clubbing are sometimes present. Bone lesions may be identified in about 10% of patients who have LCH, and diabetes insipidus also in about 10%.

Most patients affected by LIP are symptomatic at presentation, with breathlessness and cough[7,8,12]. Less common symptoms include weight loss, fever, and chest pain. On examination, bibasilar crackles are heard in most patients[7,12], but digital clubbing is unusual, as is pneumothorax. Other physical signs present may be related to an associated disorder. Dysproteinemia, most commonly polyclonal hypogammaglobulinemia, is found in the majority of patients[7,12]. Rheumatoid factor and antinuclear antibody titers may be elevated in those who have Sjögren's syndrome in association with LIP[12].

Clinical presentation of alveolar proteinosis is nonspecific, with dyspnea and a dry cough in most patients. Less common

symptoms include chest pain, hemoptysis, weight loss, chills, and arthralgias[10]. Fever is also unusual and should raise the possibility of a superimposed process, such as an infection. Crackles occur over the involved areas of lung in about 20% of patients. Digital clubbing occurs in about 30% and cyanosis is seen with severe disease. Mildly elevated serum lactate dehydrogenase level is common, and recent studies have found elevated serum levels of lung surfactant A and D (SP-A and SP-D) in patients who have alveolar proteinosis in comparison with healthy volunteers. However, this finding is not specific and can occur in patients who have idiopathic pulmonary fibrosis, interstitial lung disease associated with connective tissue diseases, and other conditions[13]. Patients affected by alveolar proteinosis may have periodic acid–Schiff (PAS)-positive material or elevated SP-A levels in their sputum, but these findings are also nonspecific.

Chest radiographs of patients who have LAM are usually abnormal and show diffuse reticular and nodular densities, without sparing of the costophrenic angles (Fig. 49.5). As the disease progresses, cystic changes may become apparent together with signs of hyperinflation. These infiltrates may be accompanied by pneumothorax and/or pleural effusions. However, in early disease, the chest radiograph may be entirely normal. High-resolution computed tomography (HRCT) of the chest reveals well-defined cystic spaces throughout both lungs, even in those patients who have normal chest radiographs (Fig. 49.6)[14]. Cystic changes are diffuse with no sparing of the costophrenic angles.

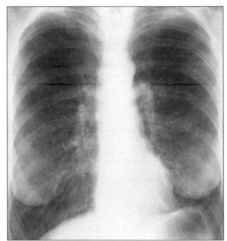

Figure 49.5
Lymphangiomyomatosis (LAM). This posteroanterior chest radiograph of a 37-year-old woman who has LAM shows hyperinflation and diffuse reticular infiltrates.

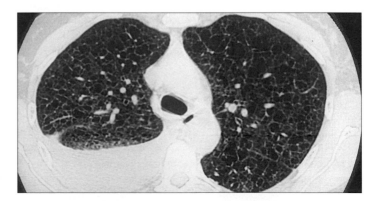

Figure 49.6 Lymphangiomyomatosis. High-resolution computed tomogram of a 42-year-old woman who has tuberous sclerosis complex with lung involvement (lymphangiomyomatosis) showing diffuse cystic changes and a right pleural effusion (chylothorax).

The cysts have uniformly thin walls and measure a few millimeters to several centimeters in diameter. Most are round, but they can coalesce into bizarre shapes as the disease progresses. Pleural effusions, pneumothoraces, and mediastinal adenopathy, which sometimes are not apparent on the chest radiograph, may also be seen. Most of the lung parenchyma between the cystic spaces appears normal. No difference is found in the appearance of the lungs of those patients who have LAM with underlying TS compared with those who do not[2]. When a CT of the chest is performed in a woman suspected of having LAM, it is useful to extend the scanning to include the kidneys as one third or more of patients have renal angiomyolipomas even in the absence of underlying TS. Also, CT of the abdomen may reveal unsuspected retroperitoneal lymphangiomyomas or adenopathy.

In patients who have LCH, typical findings on chest radiography include reticulonodular infiltrates, most prominent in the middle and upper zones (Fig. 49.7)[5]. Often the costophrenic angles are spared and the lung volume appears normal or increased. As the disease advances, cystic changes and bullae appear. Pleural disease (except for pneumothorax) or adenopathy are unusual. Predilection for the middle and upper lung zones is confirmed by HRCT of the chest, which also shows thin-walled cysts and nodules (with or without cavitation), reticular densities, as well as some areas of ground glass opacity (Fig. 49.8). The shape of the cysts are irregular and more complex than those seen in LAM.

In patients who have LIP, chest radiography reveals reticulonodular opacities in the basal zones[7,8,12]. Superimposed, patchy alveolar (Fig. 49.9) or nodular infiltrates are present in about half of the patients[12]. Other patterns, which include nodules and mixed infiltrates, may also be seen, with honeycombing in advanced cases[12]. Mediastinal or hilar adenopathy and pleural effusions are infrequent in HIV-negative patients. However, intrathoracic adenopathy may be seen in up to 29% of HIV-infected patients who have LIP[15].

The chest radiographs of patients who suffer alveolar proteinosis usually display bilateral alveolar infiltrates (Fig. 49.10). Less commonly, an interstitial pattern may be seen. These abnormalities are often more prominent in the perihilar regions in a 'bat-wing' pattern and may be mistaken for pulmonary edema[10]. About one third of patients have asymmetric or unilateral infiltrates. Ground glass and/or consolidative infiltrates in a patchy or diffuse distribution are found on HRCT of the chest[10,16]. Distinct central or peripheral distribution is usually not seen[16], but sharp demarcation of the infiltrates from surrounding normal lung tissue is commonly observed. Reticular opacities or interlobular septal thickening are also associated with alveolar proteinosis.

Pulmonary function testing in patients who have LAM usually reveals changes caused by airways obstruction and a decreased diffusing capacity. Lung volumes are generally increased with evidence of air trapping. Hypoxemia is seen in late stages of the disease. Both obstructive and restrictive changes may occur in patients affected by LCH. The effects of cigarette smoking may be superimposed and difficult to differentiate from the effects of LCH itself. Diffusing capacity is usually abnormal[4,5,11]. Exercise performance is commonly impaired and may reflect pulmonary vascular dysfunction[11].

Pulmonary function testing typically reveals restrictive changes with a reduced diffusion capacity in patients who have LIP and alveolar proteinosis. In addition, gas exchange is commonly reduced in patients who have alveolar proteinosis with a low arterial oxygen tension and elevated shunt fraction.

DIAGNOSIS

The diagnosis of LAM, LCH, LIP, and alveolar proteinosis may be strongly suspected on epidemiologic, clinical, radiographic, and physiologic features. For example, diffuse interstitial infiltrates in

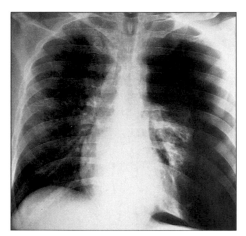

Figure 49.7 Langerhans' cell histiocytosis. Posteroanterior chest radiograph of a 25-year-old male smoker who presented with dyspnea. Massive left pneumothorax and interstitial infiltrates are seen in the right lung.

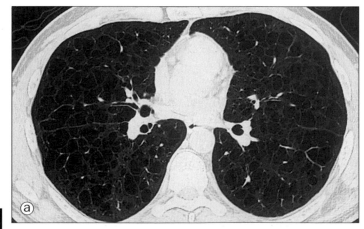

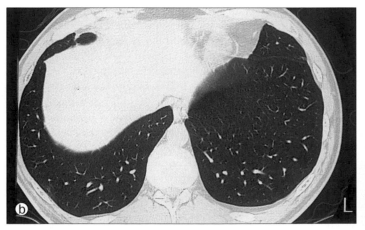

Figure 49.8 Langerhans' cell histiocytosis. High-resolution computed tomograms of the same patient shown in Figure 49.7 taken 6 years after presentation. (a) Diffuse cystic changes are seen with (b) relative sparing of bibasilar regions.

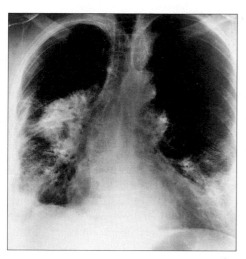

Figure 49.9 Lymphoid intersitital pneumonia (LIP). Posteroanterior chest radiograph of a 73-year-old woman with LIP showing consolidative infiltrates in the right mid-lung and base as well as left lung base.

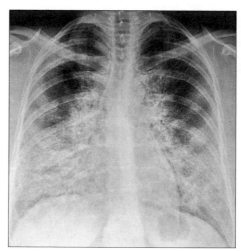

Figure 49.10 Pulmonary alveolar proteinosis. Posteroanterior chest radiograph of a 53-year-old woman who has pulmonary alveolar proteinosis shows diffuse alveolar infiltrates. She presented with progressive exertional dyspnea of 1.5 years' duration.

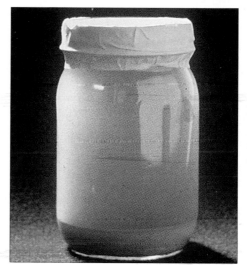

Figure 49.11 Lung lavage fluid in pulmonary alveolar proteinosis. A sample of lung lavage fluid in pulmonary alveolar proteinosis showing the typical cloudy appearance and sediment that forms over 30 minutes.

a nonsmoking woman of childbearing age who has a history of recurrent pneumothoraces strongly suggest LAM. Similarly, diffuse interstitial infiltrates predominantly in the middle and upper lung fields and sparing the costophrenic angles with normal or increased lung volume in a young adult smoker suggests the diagnosis of LCH. A never-smoked history makes the diagnosis of LCH very unlikely. Predominantly bibasilar reticulonodular infiltrates with superimposed patchy alveolar opacities in a middle-aged individual with dysproteinemia suggest LIP. The diagnosis of alveolar proteinosis should be considered in a patient who has chronic perihilar alveolar infiltrates and no evidence of congestive heart failure or infection

The diagnoses of these four disorders generally require histologic confirmation, but the use of HRCT and bronchoalveolar lavage (BAL) provides some exceptions to this rule – the former is very useful in the evaluation of diffuse lung disease. Diffuse cystic changes with no sparing of the costophrenic angles in the lungs of a woman of childbearing age can be nearly pathognomonic, especially if renal angiomyolipomas coexist. Nonetheless, biopsy confirmation of LAM is generally recommended as occasional cases of LCH or metastatic sarcoma may be difficult to differentiate from LAM on HRCT. Transbronchial lung biopsy may suffice for this purpose, especially if the lung biopsy specimen stains positively for the HMB-45 marker, which is highly sensitive and specific for LAM. Similarly, the features seen on the HRCT for LCH, LIP, and alveolar proteinosis may be highly suggestive of these disorders.

Alveolar proteinosis and LCH may be confirmed by BAL. Although Langerhans' cells can be found in other disorders, which include idiopathic pulmonary fibrosis, the presence of 5% CD1a-positive cells in the BAL fluid is highly specific for LCH[7]. If this criterion is not met, histologic confirmation of LCH is pursued by lung biopsy. The histologic hallmark of LCH is the presence of Langerhans' cells. Transbronchial biopsy may provide adequate tissue, but requires a high index of suspicion and an experienced pathologist for proper interpretation. If transbronchial lung biopsy samples or BAL fluid do not confirm the diagnosis, open (or thoracoscopic) lung biopsy or biopsy of bone lesions, if present, may provide diagnostic material.

In an appropriate clinical setting, the diagnosis of alveolar proteinosis may be made by BAL, which typically yields a milky effluent (Fig. 49.11). Under light microscopy, this fluid

shows large amounts of PAS-positive lipoproteinaceous material. Transbronchial biopsy also provides the diagnosis in most cases and demonstrates accumulation of granular, PAS-positive, lipoproteinaceous material within the alveolar spaces with preserved alveolar architecture. Open lung biopsy is now being used less frequently to confirm the diagnosis of alveolar proteinosis. In the absence of a superimposed infection, very few inflammatory cells are seen in the lung tissue. Thickening of the alveolar septa and interstitial fibrosis may be seen in some cases. Although the radiographic features may be suggestive of alveolar proteinosis, other disorders such as sarcoidosis, pulmonary edema, infections, bronchoalveolar cell carcinoma, pneumoconiosis, and other diffuses diseases may have a similar appearance.

The diagnosis of LIP requires a lung biopsy (see Fig. 49.12). Although a transbronchial biopsy may suffice, open (or thoracoscopic) lung biopsy is frequently needed. Infectious processes should be excluded. Immunohistochemical stains are valuable in the differentiation of LIP from other lymphoproliferative disorders, which include malignant lymphoma, pseudolymphoma, chronic lymphocytic leukemia, and multiple myeloma. In patients who have LIP, BAL typically shows lymphocytosis, but this is nonspecific.

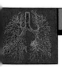

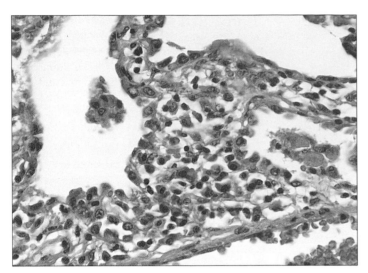

Figure 49.12 Histopathology of lymphoid interstitial pneumonia (LIP). High-magnification photomicrograph showing LIP. The expanded alveolar septum contains an infiltrate of mononuclear cells that, in this example, includes mainly mature plasma cells.

TREATMENT

The treatment of choice for LAM is hormonal manipulation, typically intramuscular medroxyprogesterone injections at a dose of 400mg/month. Those patients who have chylothorax appear to respond best to hormonal therapy. Gonadotropin-releasing hormone analogs, such as leuprolide, has also been used, but tamoxifen and oophorectomy are less frequently employed. Patients who suffer recurrent pneumothoraces or chylothorax may require pleurodesis. Lung transplantation is an option for patients affected by advanced LAM[17]. Few cases of recurrent LAM in the allograft have been reported.

Although corticosteroid therapy has been used in the treatment of patients who have LCH, it is of uncertain benefit. Smoking cessation should be strongly encouraged and may prevent disease progression. Radiation therapy for bone lesions provides symptomatic relief. In those patients who suffer progressive disease, cytotoxic drugs have been used but without much impact.

Most patients affected by LIP are treated with corticosteroids with or without chlorambucil. The response has been variable, but clinical and radiographic improvement may be seen in some individuals on corticosteroid therapy[12]. Chlorambucil and other cytotoxic agents probably provide no significant benefit[12].

Treatment of choice in patients who have alveolar proteinosis is whole lung lavage[10]. This is performed under general anesthetic via a bronchoscope passed down an endotracheal tube and usually lasts 1–2 hours, during which time repeated instillation and drainage of the lung with up to 20–30L of isotonic saline is performed[10]. Only one lung is lavaged at a session, with the other lung treated similarly 2–3 days later if necessary. Chest percussion during the lavage procedure may help. An extracorporeal membrane oxygenator has been used during lavage in those patients who suffer severe alveolar proteinosis. Most patients show clinical, physiologic, and radiographic improvement after lung lavage. Corticosteroid therapy has no beneficial effect.

CLINICAL COURSE AND PREVENTION

The clinical course varies greatly among these four diffuse lung diseases. Most patients affected by LAM have slow progression of their disease. Recent studies report survival rates of 38–78%, 8.5 years after the onset of symptoms. The authors' experience suggests that the rate of progression varies among individuals who have LAM. In addition, postmenopausal women tend to have a more benign course. Exogenous estrogens may exacerbate the disorder and should be avoided.

The rate of decline in forced expiratory volume in 1 second (FEV_1) in a UK series of 45 patients (of whom 35 had data when premenopausal and 10 when postmenopausal) was 118mL/year. The women taking progesterone showed a slower rate of decline of lung function, although this was only significant for the diffusion capacity for carbon monoxide (S Johnson, personal communication). However, the rarity of this disease (1 in 1 million women) makes these studies hard to perform.

In a recent review of 34 patients who have LAM and who underwent lung transplantation, survival rates were 69% and 58% at 1 and 2 years after transplantation, respectively. Mean age at transplantation was 40 years (range, 24–55 years). The average interval between the onset of symptoms and transplantation was 11 years (range, 3–24 years). About half the patients had substantial pleural adhesions that caused intraoperative difficulties. Recurrent pneumothorax in the remaining native lung and chylothorax were the main postoperative problems[17]. Recurrent LAM in the allograft was diagnosed in one patient.

A substantial variation is found in the natural history of LCH. Patients who are relatively young or old, as well as those who have multisystem involvement, have a worse prognosis, and those patients affected by only pulmonary involvement follow a more benign course[11]. Cigarette smoking should be discouraged.

Patients who have LIP also run a variable course. Progressive disease may result in end-stage honeycombing. Some patients diagnosed to have LIP probably have lymphoma from the outset, but cases of LIP transforming to lymphoma have occurred. Death may result from progressive lung involvement with cor pulmonale, malignant lymphoma, or complications of treatment. Those individuals who suffer LIP and HIV infection usually die from complications of the HIV infection.

Spontaneous resolution occurs in about one third of patients who have alveolar proteinosis. In those patients who undergo therapeutic lung lavage, more than half have no recurrence. Death from progressive disease, pulmonary fibrosis, and respiratory failure is rare. Superimposed infection, such as nocardiosis, may occur. Lung transplantation is an option in those individuals affected by progressive disease. A case of recurrent alveolar proteinosis following double lung transplantation has been reported.

PITFALLS AND CONTROVERSIES

Given the similarities between LAM that occurs in patients who have TS and in those who do not, it has been questioned whether LAM may be a marker or 'forme fruste' of TS. Renal angiomyolipomas are seen frequently in patients who suffer TS as well as in those who have LAM and no stigmata of TS. Molecular genetic studies are in progress to answer this question. Although the 'LAM cell' has previously been thought to be of smooth muscle origin, it may be a distinctive cell type, called perivascular epithelioid cell.

It remains unclear whether the isolated pulmonary form of LCH is a neoplastic disorder or not.

The diagnosis of LIP should not be made without immunohistochemical staining to exclude lymphoma.

OTHER RARE DIFFUSE LUNG DISEASES

Neurofibromatosis

Neurofibromatosis is a variably expressed autosomal dominant disorder characterized by café-au-lait spots, subcutaneous neurofibromas, axillary freckling, and iris hamartomas (Lisch nodules)[18]. Thoracic involvement is estimated to occur in 10–15% of patients who show manifestations, which include a predominantly bibasilar interstitial fibrosis in middle-aged patients, apical bullous disease alone or in conjunction with interstitial fibrosis, kyphoscoliosis, and meningoceles. Intrathoracic neurofibromas may occur in the pulmonary parenchyma, either as primary or as metastatic lesions, in the posterior mediastinum, and on the chest wall.

The remaining disorders described in this section are a diverse group of diseases, the pulmonary manifestations of which stem from excessive accumulation of various types of material in the respiratory system.

Pulmonary alveolar microlithiasis

Pulmonary alveolar microlithiasis results from the unexplained and extensive intra-alveolar deposition of concentrically lamellated calcium phosphate spheres, which produces a distinctive calcific, micronodular infiltrate on the chest radiograph. Most patients are asymptomatic, yet dyspnea, cough, and right-sided cardiac failure may occur in later stages with interstitial fibrosis. Microlith expectoration is uncommon[19]. A familial incidence occurs in approximately 50% of cases[19], and diagnosis is usually made on the unique chest radiographic appearance (Fig. 49.13). Supporting evidence can be obtained by transbronchial lung biopsy or by the demonstration of extensive pulmonary uptake during technetium-99m diphosphonate scanning. No therapy is known, although lung transplant has been attempted.

Amyloid

Amyloid, a fibrillar, homogeneous, proteinaceous material, usually derived from immunoglobulin light chains, can deposit in the tracheobronchial tree or pulmonary parenchyma in either localized or diffuse patterns. This accumulation can be part of a systemic process (primary systemic amyloidosis, secondary amyloidosis, familial amyloidosis) or be isolated to the lung (localized pulmonary amyloidosis)[20]. The incidence of pulmonary amyloid deposition with secondary and familial amyloidosis is low, while pulmonary involvement by primary systemic amyloidosis is common and usually takes the form of diffuse, alveolar, septal amyloid accumulation that manifests radiographically as reticular or reticulonodular infiltrates[20]. Pleural effusions may also occur because of simultaneous pleural involvement or from heart failure caused by cardiac amyloid deposition. Prognosis is poor for those primary systemic amyloidosis patients who have pulmonary involvement[20].

A diffuse interstitial pattern is rare with localized pulmonary amyloidosis. Instead, pulmonary parenchymal involvement manifests as single or multiple nodules, which are often detected incidentally on the chest radiograph[20]. These nodules may grow slowly, cavitate, or calcify. Localized amyloid masses or multifocal, submucosal plaques characterize the tracheobronchial forms of localized pulmonary amyloidosis[20]. Diffuse endobronchial involvement is recognized bronchoscopically by shiny, pale plaques with scattered focal stenoses. Symptoms depend upon the extent of luminal compromise, and include dyspnea, cough, hemoptysis, wheeze, atelectasis, and recurrent pneumonia. Severe localized stenosis can be treated with repeated bronchoscopic resection, perhaps incorporating laser ablation, or surgery[20]. Other pulmonary manifestations of amyloid deposition, whether caused by a systemic or localized process, are mediastinal and/or hilar adenopathy, mediastinal masses, and macroglossia that results in obstructive sleep apnea.

Tracheobronchial and diffuse parenchymal forms of pulmonary amyloidosis can be safely diagnosed at bronchoscopy, although the endoscopist must be prepared for potential bleeding[20]. Lung nodules are diagnosed by needle aspiration or resection. Biopsy material reveals the characteristic apple–green birefringence with polarized microscopy after staining with Congo red.

Hermansky–Pudlak syndrome

The Hermansky–Pudlak syndrome is a triad of oculocutaneous albinism, platelet aggregation dysfunction, and visceral ceroid deposition. It is an autosomal recessive disorder with a high frequency among Puerto Ricans. Progressive interstitial fibrosis may develop during the second and fourth decades, for which there is no reliable treatment[21]. The interstitial lung disease is felt to be related to the interaction of alveolar macrophages with ceroid, a material derived from incompletely processed lysosomal membranes. Such ceroid-laden macrophages have been demonstrated by Fontana–Masson staining of BAL fluid.

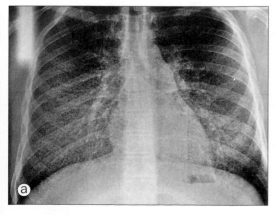

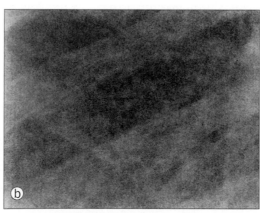

Figure 49.13 Pulmonary alveolar microlithiasis. (a) Posteroanterior chest radiograph of an 18-year-old asymptomatic man who has pulmonary alveolar microlithiasis showing numerous tiny opacities present throughout both lungs. (b) Magnified view of the right lower lung showing numerous opacities that measure <1mm.

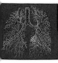

Lipoid storage disorders

Several autosomal-recessive, inborn errors of sphingolipid metabolism may have pulmonary manifestations that result from the intracellular accumulation of metabolic products induced by enzymatic defects. Gaucher's disease is caused by a deficiency of β-glucosidase, which leads to the formation of the characteristic Gaucher cell, a reticuloendothelial cell packed with glucose-1-ceramide. With Niemann–Pick disease, deficiencies in sphingomyelinase or cholesterol esterification lead to the development of foamy appearing cells. Reticular or reticulonodular infiltrates can occur in Gaucher's and Niemann–Pick disease, as alveolar macrophages filled with material accumulate in the interstitium and alveolar spaces[22,23]. Patients who have Fabry's disease, an X-linked sphingolipidosis caused by the absence of α-galactosidase A, may exhibit airflow obstruction and reduced diffusing capacities[24]. In general, the pulmonary manifestations in these metabolic disorders are incompletely described, have a variable course, may occur in childhood, and are often overshadowed by the extrapulmonary manifestations.

REFERENCES

1. Liebow A, Carrington C. Diffuse pulmonary lymphoreticular infiltrations associated with dysproteinemia. Med Clin North Am. 1973;57:809–43.

2. Castro M, Shepherd CW, Gomez MR, Lie JT, Ryu JH. Pulmonary tuberous sclerosis. Chest. 1995;107:189–95.

3. Kalassian KG, Doyle R, Kao P, Ruoss S, Raffin TA. Lymphangioleiomyomatosis: new insights. Am J Respir Crit Care Med. 1997;155:1183–6.

4. Friedman PJ, Liebow AA, Sokoloff J. Eosinophilic granuloma of lung: clinical aspects of primary pulmonary histiocytosis in the adult. Medicine. 1981;60:385–96.

5. Travis WD, Borok Z, Roum JH, et al. Pulmonary Langerhans' cell granulomatosis (histiocytosis X): a clinicopathologic study of 48 cases. Am J Surg Pathol. 1993;10:104–7.

6. Koss MN. Pulmonary lymphoid disorders. Semin Surg Pathol. 1995;12:158–71.

7. Nicholson AG, Wotherspoon AC, Diss TC, et al. Reactive pulmonary lymphoid disorders. Histopathology. 1995;26:405–12.

8. Koss MN, Hochholzer L, Langloss JM, Wehunt WD, Lazarus AA. Lymphoid interstitial pneumonia: clinicopathological and immunopathological findings in 18 cases. Pathology. 1987;19:178–85.

9. Thompson GP, Utz JP, Rosenow EC III, Myers JL, Swensen SJ. Pulmonary lymphoproliferative disorders. Mayo Clin Proc. 1993;68:804–17.

10. Wang BM, Stern, Schmidt RA, Pierson DJ. Diagnosing pulmonary alveolar proteinosis: a review and an update. Chest. 1997;111:460–6.

11. Crausman RS, Jennings CA, Tuder RM, Ackerson LM, Irvin CG, King TE Jr. Pulmonary histiocytosis X: pulmonary function and exercise physiology. Am J Respir Crit Care Med. 1996;153:426–35.

12. Strimlan CV, Rosenow EC 3rd, Weiland LH, Brown LR. Lymphocytic interstitial pneumonitis: review of 13 cases. Ann Intern Med. 1978;88:616–21.

13. Honda Y, Kuroki Y, Matsura E, et al. Pulmonary surfactant protein D in sera and bronchoalveolar lavage fluids. Am J Respir Crit Care Med. 1995;152:1860–6.

14. Muller NL, Chiles C, Kullnig P. Pulmonary lymphangiomyomatosis: correlation of CT with radiographic and functional findings. Radiology. 1990;175:335–9.

15. Carignan S, Staples CA, Muller NL. Intrathoracic lymphoproliferative disorders in the immunocompromised patient: CT findings. Radiology. 1995;197:53–8.

16. Lee KN, Levin DL, Webb WR, Chen D, Storto ML, Golden JA. Pulmonary alveolar proteinosis: high-resolution CT, chest roentgenographic, and functional correlations. Chest. 1997;111:989–95.

17. Boehler A, Speich R, Russi EW, Weder W. Lung transplantation for lymphangioleiomyomatosis. N Engl J Med. 1996;335:1275–80.

18. Riccardi VM. von Recklinghausen's neurofibromatosis. N Engl J Med. 1981;305:1616–27.

19. Prakash UBS, Barham SS, Rosenow EC III, Brown NL, Payne WS. Pulmonary alveolar microlithiasis: a review including ultrastructural and pulmonary function studies. Mayo Clin Proc. 1983;58:290–6.

20. Utz JP, Swenson SJ, Gertz MA. Pulmonary amyloidosis: the Mayo Clinic experience from 1980 to 1993. Ann Intern Med. 1996;124:407–13.

21. Gahl WA, Brantly M, Kaiser-Kupfer MI, et al. Genetic defects and clinical characteristics of patients with a form of ocular cutaneous albinism (Hermanski–Pudlak syndrome). N Engl J Med 1998;338:1258–64.

22. Santamaria F, Parenti G, Guidi G, et al. Pulmonary manifestations of Gaucher disease: an increased risk for L444P homozygotes? Am J Respir Crit Care Med 1998;157:985–9.

23. Long RG, Lake BD, Pettit JE, Scheuer PT, Sherlock S. Adult Niemann–Pick disease. Am J Med. 1977;62:627–35.

24. Rosenberg DM, Ferrans VJ, Fulmer JD, et al. Chronic airflow obstruction in Fabry's disease. Am J Med. 1980;68:898–904.

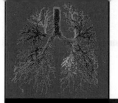

Section 10 Pulmonary Vascular Disorders, Vasculitides, and Hemorrhage

Chapter 50 Pulmonary Embolism

Christian J Herold, Alexander A Bankier, Otto C Burghuber, Erich Minar, and Herbert H Watzke

INTRODUCTION

Pulmonary embolism (PE) is caused by the obstruction of the pulmonary artery(s) by clots from the veins of the systemic circulation that embolize to the lungs. Although obstructive material other than blood can cause PE in certain situations (e.g. fat embolism following severe trauma, postpartum amniotic fluid), venous thromboembolism (VTE) is by far the most common cause. However, the differential diagnosis of PE is broad and can present significant difficulties in accurate diagnosis (Fig. 50.1)[1]. In addition, accurate diagnosis is complicated by the fact that a PE can present in a variety of ways, depending on the size, location, number of emboli, and the underlying condition of the patient (Fig. 50.2)[2]. For clinical purposes, PE and deep venous thrombosis (DVT) represent variations of the common clinical entity VTE. Significant morbidity and mortality can result from PE, particularly when it is unrecognized or undertreated. Research has focused on the prevention, diagnosis, and treatment of this condition and has led to a reduction in mortality from PE.

EPIDEMIOLOGY, RISK FACTORS, PRIMARY PREVENTION, AND PATHOPHYSIOLOGY

Epidemiology
In the USA, PE is common – causing 50,000 deaths annually, and 300,000–600,000 hospitalizations each year are associated with PE and/or DVT. Similar statistical data are available from several European countries. Age-adjusted hospital diagnosis rates and mortality rates from PE are higher in men than in women and are higher in African–Americans than in Caucasians. The incidence rate of PE is also age-dependent, with rates of 130/100,000 in those aged 65–69 years, and 280/100,000 in those aged 85–89 years[3]. Mortality rates from PE have changed in the past few decades – they doubled from 1962 to 1974 and then declined by 25% between 1974 and 1979[4], with a further small decline thereafter. This pattern is paralleled by the decline in incidence rates of PE, which were 92/100,000 population in 1975 and 51/100,000 in 1995, which suggests that the decline in incidence is the primary reason for the decline in death rates from PE. This is further supported by primary prevention trials of postoperative VTE, which show consistent rates of mortality for patients who have suffered PE in the past two decades. Consequently, the identification and avoidance of clinical situations that carry a high risk for PE and/or the development of strategies to prevent high-risk states may be the best strategies to combat mortality.

Risk factors
The clinical significance of a risk factor is determined by its prevalence in the population and by the relative risk it confers to the carrier. These two key features are important for both genetic and acquired risk factors.

Genetic risk factors
A family history of VTE is a strong positive predictor for PE because of the inherited defects in proteins, many of which are

Differential diagnosis of acute pulmonary embolism
Myocardial infarction
Pneumonia
Congestive heart failure
Asthma and chronic obstructive pulmonary disease
Intrathoracic cancer
Pleuritis/pericarditis
Rib fracture
Pneumothorax
Musculoskeletal pain

Figure 50.1 Differential diagnosis of acute pulmonary embolism.

Incidence of symptoms and signs in angiographically proved pulmonary embolism		
	Symptom/sign	Percentage
Symptoms	Chest pain	88
	Pleuritic chest pain	74
	Dyspnea	84
	Cough	53
	Hemoptysis	30
	Syncope	13
Signs	Tachypnea	92
	Crackles	58
	Rales	48
	Tachycardia (>100/min)	44
	Fever (>37.8°C)	43
	Gallop	34
	Phlebitis	32
	Edema	24

Figure 50.2 Incidence of symptoms and signs in angiographically proved pulmonary embolism. (Data from Bell et al.[2])

involved in the regulation of the coagulation cascade (Fig. 50.3)[5]. However, such defects do not explain all cases of familial thrombosis, and other genetic defects must exist. Testing for genetic risk factors is considered in patients who have established PE and one or more of the following typical features of hereditary thrombophilia: VTE at a young age; family history of VTE; no evidence for acquired risk factors for VTE; and PE that originates from a spontaneous venous thrombosis other than leg vein thrombosis.

Antithrombin III

Antithrombin III (ATIII) is an important coagulation inhibitor. Its deficiency is inherited in an autosomal-dominant manner with incomplete penetrance. It increases the risk of VTE fivefold and is found in 1.1% of unselected patients who have VTE. Thus, although rare, ATIII deficiency is associated with an increased risk for VTE.

Protein C and Protein S

The antithrombotic properties of protein C (PC) and protein S (PS) are related to inactivation of the activated factors V and VIII by the serin protease-activated PC (APC); PS is the cofactor in this reaction. Both PC and PS deficiencies are inherited in an autosomal-dominant manner. A sixfold risk of VTE is conferred by PC deficiency. The prevalence of PS deficiency is unknown, and it is associated with only a slightly increased risk of DVT. The cumulative incidence of VTE at age 40 years is 10%.

Activated protein C resistance

Resistance of activated factor V toward its proteolytic degradation by activated PC is an inherited risk factor for VTE. A single point mutation in the factor V gene results in the substitution of arginine at position 506 by glutamine (so called factor V Leiden). This amino acid change takes place at the site where the activated factor V protein is proteolytically cleaved by APC, and thus inhibits the proper degradation of this abnormal molecule. This mutation is found among Caucasians with a prevalence of 2400–7000/100,000 population, and occurs in 21% of patients who present with VTE.

Prothrombin G20210A

A single nucleotide change in the 3'-untranslated region of prothrombin (guanosine to adenosine at nucleotide 20210 of the prothrombin gene) results in elevated prothrombin levels and is associated with a fivefold increase in risk for DVT. The prevalence of this defect is 2300/100,000 population.

Hyperhomocystinemia

Hyperhomocystinemia is a risk factor for VTE, with a high prevalence and a two-fold elevated relative risk. It can be acquired through diminished intakes of folic acid or vitamins B_{12} and B_6, or it can be genetic through defects in enzymes that affect homocysteine disposal. Among the genetic defects, cystathionine β-synthetase deficiency is the most common entity. In the homozygous state, hyperhomocystinemia is associated with the early onset of VTE and a high relative risk of arterial thrombosis. However, its frequency is extremely low. Heterozygotes are much more prevalent and have a mild hyperhomocystinemia, which increases the relative risk of VTE.

Factor VIII

An increased level of factor VIII is an independent risk factor for VTE, with a relative risk of 4.8.

Blood group

Carriers of blood groups other than group O have a twofold increased risk of DVT compared with those who have blood group O.

Combination of genetic risk factors

The high prevalence of some of the hereditary risk factors for VTE increases the chances of a combination of two or more genetic defects. For example, a heterozygous state for factor V Leiden was detected in 10–15% of patients who carry heterozygous PC deficiency and in 22% of patients who had PS deficiency. Patients who carry combined defects present with thrombosis at a younger age and have a higher frequency of thrombotic events than do patients who have single defects. The same findings have been reported for a combination of heterozygous ATIII deficiency and cosegregating factor V Leiden.

Acquired risk factors

Acquired risk factors in hospitalized patients are given in Figure 50.4.

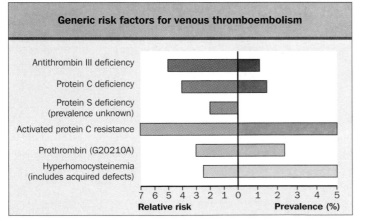

Generic risk factors for venous thromboembolism

Figure 50.3 **Genetic risk factors for venous thromboembolism.** (Data from the Leiden thrombophilia study for heterozygous defects[6].)

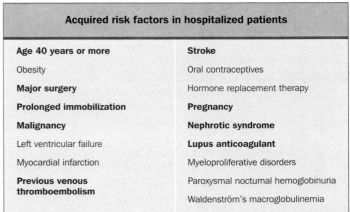

Acquired risk factors in hospitalized patients	
Age 40 years or more	**Stroke**
Obesity	Oral contraceptives
Major surgery	Hormone replacement therapy
Prolonged immobilization	**Pregnancy**
Malignancy	**Nephrotic syndrome**
Left ventricular failure	**Lupus anticoagulant**
Myocardial infarction	Myeloproliferative disorders
Previous venous thromboembolism	Paroxysmal nocturnal hemoglobinuria
	Waldenström's macroglobulinemia

Figure 50.4 **Acquired risk factors in hospitalized patients.** Conditions that carry a particularly high relative risk are highlighted in bold. (Adapted from Anderson et al.[7])

Surgery and trauma

Surgery, whether elective or post-traumatic, is the most significant acquired risk factor for VTE. Surgery is performed on an ever-increasing number of patients (high prevalence) and, at the same time, confers a substantial risk of VTE (high relative risk); several thrombogenic factors account for this:

- blood stasis in the lower extremities is caused by preoperative, intraoperative, and postoperative immobilization, or by cast immobilization following trauma;
- general anesthetic itself disturbs the delicate balance between the level of coagulation factors and their inhibitors, and thereby generates a prothrombotic state;
- local tissue trauma and vessel damage releases tissue factors that cause a hypercoagulable state.

Thus, the risk of PE after surgery or trauma is related, on the one hand, to specific surgical factors such as the site and extent of the trauma, the actual surgical procedure, and the time of perioperative immobilization. On the other hand, it is also related to patient-specific factors such as age, underlying disease, and other medical conditions. The interplay of these factors determines the actual risk of VTE for an individual surgical patient[8].

Medical conditions

Autopsy studies show that the vast majority of patients who die from PE in hospital had underlying medical illnesses as opposed to surgical conditions. The most frequent medical conditions associated with an increased risk for DVT can occur singly or in combination (e.g. left ventricular failure and immobilization). In addition, increasing age contributes to the risk of VTE and must be accounted for when thrombotic risk is estimated in a given individual.

Gynecology

During pregnancy and in the month after delivery, PE is a major risk factor and is still the most prevalent cause of maternal mortality.

Oral contraceptives

The estrogen content of oral contraceptives increases the risk of VTE sevenfold, which is particularly important in women who undergo elective surgery. The risk is further increased if the patient is also heterozygous for factor V Leiden – 30-fold compared with women who do not take the contraceptive pill and have a normal factor V genotype.

Primary prevention

The need for primary prevention is determined by the thrombotic risk of the clinical situation (surgery, stroke, delivery, etc.) in conjunction with the patient's profile of thromboembolic risk factors (genetic and/or acquired). Areas that carry a high risk for VTE, such as orthopedic surgery, demand maximum prophylactic measures for patients who have no predisposing thromboembolic risk factors. Conditions that carry a low risk for VTE, such as pneumonia, need prophylactic measures only when additional acquired risk factors (immobilization, left ventricular failure, advanced age, etc.) and/or genetic risk factors (ATIII deficiency, etc.) are present.

Post-traumatic and elective orthopedic surgery carry the highest risk for postoperative PE. Since orthopedic procedures are standardized, the efficacy of various prophylactic measures for PE have been extensively tested in this setting (Fig. 50.5)[9]. It is evident that medical prophylaxis with heparin is the treatment of choice for the primary prevention of VTE; aspirin is of no value in such cases.

For patients who undergo orthopedic surgery, low-molecular-weight heparins (LMWHs) are superior to unfractionated heparins (UFHs). The incidence of postoperative PE was reduced from 4.1% in patients who received UFH to 1.7% in patients who received LMWH (relative risk, 0.43)[6,7,10], with a concomitant reduction in fatal PEs and no increased risk of perioperative bleeding (Fig. 50.6). The same is true for patients who have severe trauma and those who suffer spinal cord injuries. Hirudin may be superior to LMWHs in the primary prophylaxis of VTE in orthopedic patients.

To prevent postoperative VTE, LMWHs are not superior to UFHs in general surgery, obstetrics, or gynecology. However, several other advantages of LMWHs make them the drug of choice in such cases. Their excellent bioavailability leads to a highly predictive anticoagulant response and makes laboratory tests unnecessary. Their long half-life provides protection from VTE for 24 hours after a single subcutaneous dose. In addition, the risks of osteoporosis and heparin-associated thrombocytopenia are much less than with UFHs.

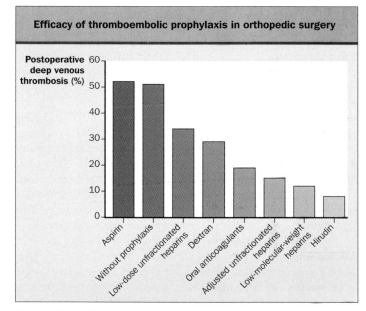

Figure 50.5 Efficacy of thromboembolic prophylaxis in orthopedic surgery.

	Perioperative frequency of pulmonary embolism and fatal pulmonary embolism without prophylaxis			
	Without prophylaxis		**Prophylaxis with low-molecular-weight heparin**	
Type of surgery	Incidence of pulmonary embolism (%)	Incidence of fatal pulmonary embolism (%)	Incidence of pulmonary embolism (%)	Incidence of fatal pulmonary embolism (%)
Post-traumatic orthopedic	6.9	4	–	–
Elective orthopedic	4	1.65	1.7	<1
General	1.6	0.87	0.23	<0.1

Figure 50.6 The perioperative frequency of pulmonary embolism and fatal pulmonary embolism without and with low molecular weight heparin prophylaxis.

Also, LMWHs can be administered safely preoperatively. Preliminary data suggest even greater protection from VTE without increased perioperative bleeding when LMWHs are given prior to surgery. The optimum duration of prophylaxis following surgery has been addressed in many studies. Discontinuation of prophylactic treatments after discharge from the hospital leads to a peak of occasionally fatal thromboembolic complications within 2 weeks. These events can be significantly reduced by prolonging prophylactic treatment with LMWHs for 4 weeks postoperatively. Nonmedical prophylaxis, such as graduated compression stockings, intermittent pneumatic compression, or foot impulse pumps, are valuable in various postoperative risk categories, particularly for patients who have contraindications to anticoagulants.

CLINICAL FEATURES AND DIAGNOSIS

Diagnosis of acute pulmonary embolism

Clinical suspicion is of crucial importance to guide diagnostic testing. In autopsy studies, rates of 62 and 84% were reported for over- and underdiagnosis, respectively. Furthermore, the Prospective Investigation of Pulmonary Embolism Diagnosis (PIOPED)[11] study showed that the combination of clinical probability with lung scan probability establishes the likelihood of PE more accurately. Therefore, to suspect PE in the initial examination is essential for an early diagnosis, with confirmation given by subsequent examinations [e.g. lung scan, pulmonary angiography (PA), computed tomography, etc.]. The interpretation criteria for ventilation–perfusion scans in the PIOPED study are tabulated in Chapter 3 (Fig. 3.6).

The preliminary procedures employed in suspected PE include a good medical history (to identify patients at risk), recognition of common symptoms, physical findings, standard laboratory tests, chest radiography, electrocardiography (ECG), arterial blood gas analysis, echocardiography, and examination of the lower extremities (compression ultrasound and venography).

Medical history

The congenital, prothrombotic coagulopathies (see above) need to be suspected if a family history is apparent, particularly in a young person who carries no acquired risk factor.

Acquired major risk factors for VTE include pelvic and lower extremity fracture or surgery (especially hip and knee replacement), surgical procedures that required more than 30 minutes of general anesthetic, and any cause of prolonged immobility or venous stasis. More modest risk is imposed during the third trimester of pregnancy, the postpartum period, and by cancer, obesity, and the use of estrogen-containing medications.

Symptomatology

The most common symptoms (see Fig. 50.2) are unexplained acute dyspnea, tachypnea (>20 breaths/minute), or substernal chest discomfort – 97% of symptomatic patients who have PE show one or more of these[12]. Shock or syncope is rare and is associated with massive PE. Hemoptysis, often found with an infiltrate localized in the periphery of the lung, is associated with smaller emboli that involve segmental or subsegmental vessels. In fact, pleurisy and hemoptysis are uncommon manifestations of pulmonary infarction, which occurs in a minority of patients who have embolism. In addition, a significant proportion of patients affected by PE may be asymptomatic.

Findings at physical examination

The physical findings in PE are also nonspecific. They may include tachycardia, a pleural rub and rales, a right-sided gallop, and an increased pulmonary component of the second heart sound, with perhaps a right ventricular 'tap' palpable on the right sternal border in massive PE associated with pulmonary hypertension. With right ventricular failure, fixed splitting of the second sound, a right ventricular S3, an elevated jugular venous pulse, and a tender liver may occur. Fever is uncommon if no complicating infection or infarction is present.

Standard laboratory tests

Standard laboratory tests contribute little specific. Leukocytosis and elevation of the sedimentation rate are rarely present without infarction. Plasma D-dimer measurement (a degradation product of cross-linked fibrin) has been used in suspected PE[13], as its level is highly sensitive for acute VTE. Hence, a normal D-dimer level (<500ng/L) probably excludes VTE. In contrast, a high D-dimer level is not helpful because so many other diseases exhibit high levels.

Electrocardiography

Abnormalities of ECG are also nonspecific. The classic electrocardiographic findings of acute right ventricular strain are observed in some patients who have massive PE. However, ECG is useful to exclude competing diagnoses – myocardial infarction or a rapid atrial arrhythmia, with the caveat that T-wave inversion may suggest an early myocardial infarct, and embolism may induce atrial flutter or fibrillation. Characteristic electrocardiographic findings in acute PE (Fig. 50.7) include right ventricular strain pattern with a negative T wave and/or ST segment depression in leads V1–V3, or incomplete or complete right bundle branch block[14,15]. In the limb leads, P pulmonale, and/or rotation of the QRS axis to the right with a deep S wave in lead I, and/or the development of the so called SI–QIII–TIII pattern are found. This pattern comprises a deep S wave in lead I, a deep Q wave in lead III, and an inverted T wave in lead III, and can be very similar to that in posterior myocardial infarction. Ultimately, PE often is accompanied by sinus tachycardia, and sometimes by paroxysms of atrial flutter or fibrillation.

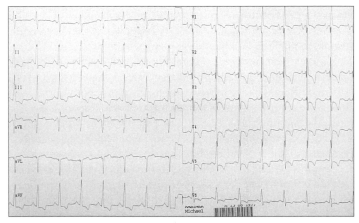

Figure 50.7 Characteristic electrocardiographic findings in acute pulmonary embolism. Right ventricular strain is seen in the precordial leads, P pulmonale in limb leads II and III, and right axis deviation.

Chest radiography

Chest radiography may demonstrate signs compatible with PE (and raise the level of clinical suspicion), may demonstrate or exclude other diseases potentially responsible for a patient's symptoms, and is needed to evaluate a V/Q scan adequately.

A chest radiograph from a patient who is suspected to have PE is neither sensitive nor specific. Notably, a negative chest radiograph is a common presentation of PE, because changes only occur when a fairly large segmental or even more proximal vessel is occluded, or when obstruction of many small vessels impairs pulmonary hemodynamics. However, up to 80% of patients who have confirmed PE have an abnormal chest radiograph[15]. Findings may include loss of lung volume with plate-like atelectasis and/or diaphragmatic elevation, and pleural effusion. Less often, a prominent pulmonary hilus (which represents a large central pulmonary artery) with little tapering of vessels ('Fleischner's sign') can be seen and may or may not be associated with peripheral regional oligemia ('Westermark's sign'). Infarcts are rare and, if present, appear as peripheral, wedge-shaped densities ('Hampton's hump'). Most commonly, radiographic abnormalities in PE are located in the lower portion of the chest, since approximately 90% of all emboli are lodged in lower lobe vessels.

Unfortunately, none of the above signs have a high-enough specificity to allow a straightforward diagnosis of PE. Radiographic abnormalities, including pleural effusion or plate-like atelectasis, may also be found in other thoracic or even abdominal disorders. Nevertheless, the chest radiograph fulfills a very distinct role in the evaluation of patients suspected to have PE, and provides potentially important information on a patient's pulmonary and cardiovascular state (Fig. 50.8).

Arterial blood gas analysis

In the vast majority of patients who have acute PE, the partial pressures of arterial blood gases demonstrate hypocapnia and respiratory alkalosis. The PaO_2 when breathing room air drops with massive PE, but in submassive embolism it may be normal or near normal if no underlying pulmonary disease is present[16]. Hypoxemia is very common in cardiopulmonary disease, but it is not specific and should be interpreted with caution in the assessment of PE.

Doppler echocardiography

Echocardiography, both transthoracic and, in particular, transesophageal, may identify thrombi in the central pulmonary arteries; it does not reliably identify emboli in the lobar and segmental arteries. Echocardiography may prove useful in massive PE associated with pulmonary hypertension. It can be performed rapidly at the bedside and may reveal significant disease. Doppler echocardiographic features that suggest acute massive PE include:
- a dilated, hypokinetic right ventricle;
- absence of right ventricular hypertrophy;
- distortion of the interventricular septum toward the left ventricle (mainly in diastole);
- presence of tricuspid regurgitation with increased flow velocity (3–3.5m/s) compatible with mild-to-moderate elevation of pulmonary artery systolic pressure; and
- absence of significant pathologic left ventricular conditions.

Diagnosis of deep venous thrombosis

More than 90% of all emboli arise from DVT, which is a progressive process that usually begins in the deep veins of the calf and propagates through the popliteal and into the iliofemoral system. Thrombosis of the popliteal or more proximal veins is more likely to cause PE. Consequently, the approach to the diagnosis of PE must also include a search for DVT of the lower extremities.

Although DVT can be silent, symptoms include leg pain, tenderness, and swelling, while the major signs are edema, discomfort in the calf upon forced dorsoflexion of the foot (Homan's sign), venous distension of subcutaneous vessels, discoloration, and a palpable cord (Fig. 50.9). Imaging evaluation is by B-mode compression ultrasonography (CUS), which not only establishes the diagnosis, but also (when it is repeatedly negative), identifies a low-risk group for subsequent PE or proximal DVT. Consequently, the test can be used to stratify the risk of individuals suspected to have PE for subsequent morbid events over a 3-month period. B-mode CUS is so reliable, inexpensive, and safe that it has rapidly supplanted leg phlebography as the gold standard. Phlebography, therefore, is reserved for those situations in which the ultrasound examination is normal despite high clinical suspicion for DVT.

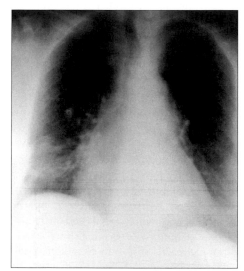

Figure 50.8 Multiple atelectatic lines in the right lower zone of the chest radiograph of a patient who has acute pulmonary embolism.

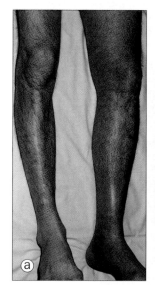
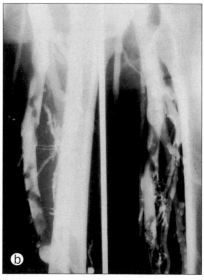

Figure 50.9 Deep venous thrombosis. (a) Leg edema, venous distension of subcutaneous vessels, and skin discoloration are seen. (b) Phlebography of the same patient. Multiple filling defects are seen in the femoral vein. These defects correspond to thrombi.

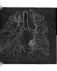
Pulmonary Vascular Disorders, Vasculitides, and Hemorrhage

Common clinical syndromes of acute pulmonary embolism

The clinical features of acute PE can be divided into several syndromes, but they have considerable overlap (Fig. 50.10).

Massive pulmonary embolism

When encountered in its classic form in a predisposed patient, acute massive PE that obstructs >60–70% of the pulmonary circulation is rarely a diagnostic problem. The common features are profound dyspnea, tachypnea, tachycardia, and, occasionally, hypotension. Syncope, cardiogenic shock, and cardiac arrest (particularly with electromechanical dissociation) are life-threatening events that lead to death in most cases. Signs of acute right ventricular failure are usually present. The differential diagnosis includes acute myocardial infarction, superior vena caval syndrome, pericardial tamponade, hypovolemia, and sepsis. The classic electrocardiographic finding in patients who have massive PE may be present (see above). The chest radiograph is not often helpful, whereas the diagnosis may be established by two-dimensional echocardiography, which shows a thrombus in the central part of a pulmonary artery. Indirect echocardiographic features include a dilated, hypokinetic right ventricle, absence of right ventricular hypertrophy, distortion of the interventricular septum toward the left ventricle, and the presence of tricuspid regurgitation.

Submassive pulmonary embolism

Acute, transient unexplained dyspnea and tachycardia

The most difficult diagnostic challenge is posed by transient, mild, or moderate pulmonary hypertension caused by submassive PE. If PE obstructs <60% of the pulmonary circulation, acute right ventricular failure does not occur, which makes the diagnosis of submassive PE difficult. No clinical signs of right ventricular failure are found, and ECG remains normal. If pulmonary infarction has not occurred, pleuritic chest pain is absent and no abnormalities are found on chest radiography or ECG. In such cases, the clinician must rely on the clinical symptoms of sudden onset of dyspnea, tachypnea, and possibly tachycardia and anxiety. The differential diagnosis includes left ventricular failure, pneumonia, and the hyperventilation syndrome. Patients who present with dyspnea caused by acute PE may also be hypoxic.

Pulmonary hemorrhage or infarction

Pulmonary infarction occurs with pleuritic chest pain, with or without dyspnea, and occasionally hemoptysis. The clinical diagnosis of infarction caused by PE cannot be confirmed unless an infiltrate is present on the chest radiograph. Signs of right ventricular failure are absent. Examination of the lungs may reveal rales, wheezes, or evidence of pleural effusion or a friction rub. The most useful laboratory tests include arterial blood gas tensions, differential white blood cell count (WBC), and chest radiography. The arterial blood gas partial pressures usually demonstrate hypocapnia and respiratory alkalosis, whereas PaO_2 may be normal. The WBC and differential count help to diagnose bacterial pneumonia, although a high WBC does not rule out PE.

No symptoms (silent pulmonary embolism)

It has been argued that approximately 10% of patients who have submassive PE may show no symptoms at all; thus, it is crucial to reevaluate these patients periodically.

Chronic thromboembolic pulmonary hypertension

Recurrent PE causes chronic pulmonary hypertension associated with a clinical syndrome of progressive right ventricular failure and cor pulmonale. This develops insidiously and diagnosis is often made only when the disease is far advanced.

Definition of clinical probability

Although no algorithms to estimate the clinical probability of PE are validated, it has been suggested[17] that a high-probability patient (80–100%) shows a plausible risk factor, one or more of the common screening findings, and a radiographic or gas-exchange abnormality. A low-probability patient (1–19%) shows no risk factor, clinical symptoms or findings that are explainable by another disease, or radiographic or gas-exchange abnormalities that are also explainable by another condition. Intermediate category patients (20–79% probability) are those who do not meet the criteria for either of the above categories (Fig. 50.11). Consequently, the integrated approach to the diagnosis of VTE relies both on the clinical estimation of probability and on the use of the two major screening tests – that is, perfusion lung scans and B-mode CUS of the lower extremities.

Common clinical syndromes of acute pulmonary embolism				
	Massive pulmonary embolism		Submassive pulmonary embolism	
	With/without hypotension and shock	With transient dyspnea and tachycardia	With pulmonary hemorrhage or infarction	Without any symptoms
Symptoms	Dyspnea, tachypnea, syncope, +/- shock, cardiac arrest	Dyspnea, anxiety, tachypnea	Pleuritic chest pain, hemoptysis	None
Clinical signs	Tachycardia, splitting 2nd heart sound, right ventricular–S3, elevates jugular venous pulse, tender liver	Tachycardia	Rales, wheezes, pleural friction rub	None
Differential diagnosis	Myocardial infarction, pericardial tamponade, hypovolemia, superior vena caval syndrome	Left ventricular failure, pneumonia, hyperventilation syndrome	Pneumonia	None
Electrocardiogram	Negative T wave in V1–V3, S1–Q3 type, P-pulmonale, incomplete or complete right bundle branch block	Normal	Normal	Normal
Chest radiograph	May be 'knuckle' or Westermark sign	Normal	Pulmonary infiltrate	Normal
Arterial blood gas tension	Often hypoxemia despite hypocapnia, Aa-oxygen gradient↑	Hypoxemia, often Aa-oxygen gradient↑	Hypocapnia, respiratory alkalosis	Normal
Echo	Dilated, hypokinetic right ventricule, no right ventricular hypertrophy, distortion of interventricular septum, TI	Normal	Normal	Normal

Figure 50.10 Common clinical syndromes of acute pulmonary embolism.

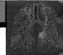

Estimation of clinical probability in acute pulmonary embolism	
Category	**Finding**
High probability (80–100%)	Risk factor present
	Otherwise unexplained dyspnea, tachypnea, or pleuritic chest pain
	Otherwise unexplained radiographic or blood-gas abnormality
Intermediate probability (20–79%)	Neither high nor low clinical probability
Low probability (1–19%)	Risk factor not present
	Dyspnea, tachypnea, or pleuritic chest pain may be present, but explainable by another condition
	Radiograph or blood-gas abnormality may be present, but explainable by another condition

Figure 50.11 Estimation of clinical probability in acute pulmonary embolism. (Data from Hyers[17].)

Imaging in venous thromboembolism
General principles

In patients who have suspected VTE, it is of paramount importance to identify those patients in whom PE and/or DVT is present and who therefore receive anticoagulant treatment. In principle, the diagnosis of either PE or DVT alone suffices to institute therapy. Nevertheless, an examination of the complementary portion of the vascular bed (i.e. the lower extremity veins in PE, or the pulmonary arteries in DVT) may provide important information for the treatment plan, duration of anticoagulation therapy, and use of alternative treatment options in cases of treatment failure. For example, in patients who have PE, it may be important to know whether a thrombus load occurs in the lower extremity veins with the potential to cause recurrent (and potentially fatal) PE. Likewise, the diagnosis of PE in a patient who has DVT may have significant therapeutic implications in the case of a recurrent event, which represents treatment failure (and is an indication for a vena cava filter).

Of equal importance is the selection of cases in which the exclusion of PE and DVT obviates the need for treatment, since long-term anticoagulation carries significant risks, such as hemorrhage. Thus, for management, a multimodality approach is required in many cases to achieve a coherent diagnosis based on the findings in the pulmonary arterial bed and the lower extremity veins.

Since few clinical signs that suggest PE or DVT are reliable enough to confirm or exclude the disease, imaging modalities play a major role in patients suspected to have these disorders. Requirements of the 'ideal' imaging modality are multiple – availability; high sensitivity and specificity; good positive and negative predictive values; cost effectiveness; low invasiveness; and patient acceptance. In addition, the imaging modality should help to depict other diseases that may be the cause of the patient's complaints. Unfortunately, none of the imaging modalities available to date fulfill all these criteria.

Imaging for pulmonary embolism
Chest radiograph
For a discussion of the use of chest radiography in PE, see the section on clinical diagnosis.

Scintigraphy
In patients who have suspected PE, the first-line imaging evaluation usually includes a chest radiograph and V̇/Q̇ scintigraphy.

The latter couples the scintigraphic assessment of lung perfusion (in which the diagnosis of PE is not based on the direct visualization of the embolus, but rather on the detection of perfusion abnormalities subsequent to the embolic event) with the pattern of lung ventilation. The two studies are analyzed together and, in cases of PE, classically display a mismatch between perfusion and ventilation, that is a lung segment distal to an obstructing embolus is not perfused, but is still ventilated (Fig. 50.12).

Although V̇/Q̇ scans do not confirm or exclude PE, they give an estimate of its likelihood. In most classifications, the results of V̇/Q̇ scanning are reported to show high (>90%), intermediate, or low (<10%) probability, or to be normal. In clinical practice, the results of V̇/Q̇ scintigraphy are most usefully interpreted together with the clinical estimate of the likelihood of acute PE (pretest probability). It has been shown that a normal perfusion scan virtually excludes clinically relevant PE[18]. Also, PE may be confidently excluded in patients whose scan shows a low probability and who have a low clinical suspicion of acute PE[11]. Conversely, a high-probability scan (together with a high clinical suspicion of acute PE) is sufficiently reliable to initiate anticoagulant treatment[11].

The clinical relevance of V̇/Q̇ scintigraphy is limited because only 25–40% of patients referred with acute PE fall into the above categories. The remaining cases (the majority) either show intermediate probability results or a clinical assessment that suggests a probability of PE discordant with the probability indicated by the V̇/Q̇ scan. In these patients, the average risk for PE is high (approximately 34%) and a diagnosis must be made using another

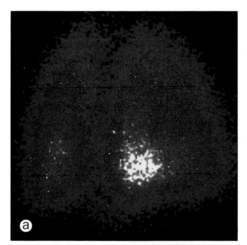

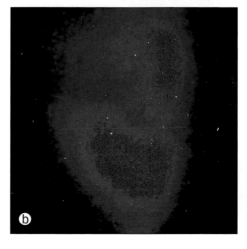

Figure 50.12 Ventilation and perfusion scans in a patient who has multiple pulmonary emboli. (a) Ventilation scan is normal. (b) Perfusion scan shows large segmental defect caused by an embolus in a segmental pulmonary artery.

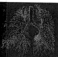
8   International Consensus Statement. Prevention of venous thromboembolism. Int Angiol. 1997;16:3–38.

9   Hirsh J. Prevention of venous thrombosis in patients undergoing major orthopaedic surgical procedures. Acta Chir Scand. 1990;556 (Suppl.1):30–5.

10 Nurmohamed M, Rosendaal F, Büller H, et al. The efficacy and safety of low molecular weight heparin versus standard heparin in general and orthopaedic surgery. Lancet. 1992;340;152–6.

11 PIOPED Investigators. Value of ventilation/perfusion scan in acute pulmonary embolism: results of the prospective investigation of pulmonary embolism diagnosis. JAMA. 1990;263:2753–9.

12 Stein PD, Henry JW, Gottschalk A. The addition of clinical assessment to stratification according to prior cardiopulmonary disease further optimizes the interpretation of ventilation/perfusion lung scans in pulmonary embolism. Chest. 1993;104:1472–6.

13 Perrier A, Bounameaux H, Morabia A, et al. Diagnosis of pulmonary embolism by a decision analysis-based strategy including clinical probability, D-dimer levels, and ultrasonography: a management study. Arch Intern Med. 1996;156:531–6.

14 Ferrari E, Imbert A, Chevalier Th, Mhoubi A, Morand Ph, Baudouy M. The ECG in pulmonary embolism – predictive value of negative T waves in precordial leads – 80 case reports. Chest. 1997;111:537–43.

15 Greenspan RH, Ravin CE, Polansky SM, et al. Acuracy of chest radiography in the diagnosis of pulmonary embolism. Invest Radiol. 1982;17:539–43.

16 Urokinase pulmonary embolism trial. Circulation. 1973;47(Suppl. 2):86.

17 Hyers Th. Diagnosis of pulmonary embolism. Thorax. 1995;50:930–2.

18 Hull RD, Raschok GE, Caotes G, Pajy AA. Clinical validity of normal perfusion lung scan in patients with suspected pulmonary embolism. Chest. 1990;97:23–6.

19 Novelline RA, Baltarowich OA, Althanasoulis CA, Waltman AC, Greenfield AJ, McKusick KA. The clinical course of patients with suspected pulmonary embolism and a negative pulmonary arteriogram. Radiology. 1978;126:561–7.

20 Hudson ER, Smith TP, McDermott VG, et al. Pulmonary angiography performed with iopamidol: complications in 1434 patients. Radiology. 1996;198:61–5.

21 Sostman HD, Ravin CE, Sullivan DC, et al. Use of pulmonary angiography for suspected pulmonary embolism: influence of scintigraphic diagnosis. AJR Am J Roentgenol. 1982;139:673–7.

22 Henschke CI, Mateescu I, Yankelevitz DF. Changing practice patterns in the workup of pulmonary embolism. Chest. 1995;107:940–5.

23 Schluger N, Henschke C, King T, et al. Diagnosis of pulmonary embolism in a large teaching hospital. J Thorac Imaging. 1994;9:180–4.

24 Rémy-Jardin M, Rémy J, Wattinne L, Giraud F. Central pulmonary thromboembolism: diagnosis with spiral volumetric CT with the single-breath-hold technique – comparison with pulmonary angiography. Radiology. 1992;185:381–7.

25 Steiner P, Phillips F, Wesner D,et al. Primary diagnosis and follow-up in acute pulmonary embolism: comparison of digital subtraction angiography and spiral CT. Rofo Fortschr Geb Rontgenstr Neuen Bildgeb Verfahr 1994;161:285–91.

26 Van Rossum AB, Pattynama PM, Ton ER, et al. Pulmonary embolism: validation of spiral CT angiography in 149 patients. Radiology. 1996,201.467–70.

27 Goodman LR, Curtin JR, Mewissen MW, et al. Detection of pulmonary embolism in patients with unresolved clinical and scintigraphic diagnosis: helical CT versus angiography. AJR Am J Roentgenol. 1995;164:1369–74

28 Rémy-Jardin M, Rémy J, Deschildre F, et al. Diagnosis of pulmonary embolism with spiral CT: comparison with pulmonary angiography and scintigraphy. Radiology. 1996;200(3):699–706.

29 Drucker EA, Rivitz SM, Shepard JO, et al. Acute pulmonary embolism: assessment of helical CT for diagnosis. Radiology. 1998;209:235–41.

30 Mayo JR, Rémy-Jardin M, Muller NL, et al. Pulmonary embolism: prospective comparison of spiral CT with ventilation–perfusion scintigraphy. Radiology. 1997; 205:447–52.

31 Bankier AA, Janata K, Fleischmann D, et al. Severity assessment of acute pulmonary embolism with spiral CT: evaluation of two modified angiographic scores and comparison with clinical data. J Thorac Imaging. 1997;12:150–8.

32 Oser RF, Zuckerman DA, Gutierrez FR, Brink JA. Anatomic distribution of pulmonary emboli at pulmonary angiography: implications of cross-sectional imaging. Radiology. 1996;199:31–5.

33 Van Erkel AR, Van Rossum AB, Bloem JL, et al. Spiral CT angiography for suspected acute pulmonary embolism: a cost-effectiveness analysis. Radiology. 1996;201:29–36.

34 Erdman WA, Peshok RM, Redman HL, Bonte F, Meyerson M, Jayson HT. Pulmonary embolism: comparison of MR images with radionuclide and angiographic studies. Radiology. 1994;190:499–508.

35 Dauzat M, Laroche JP, Deklunder G, et al. Diagnosis of acute lower limb thrombosis with ultrasound: trends and controversies. J Clin Ultrasound. 1997;25:343–58.

36 Agnelli G. Anticoagulation in the prevention and treatment of pulmonary embolism. Chest. 1995;107(Suppl.):39–44.

37 Barritt DW, Jordan SC. Anticoagulant drugs in the treatment of pulmonary embolism. A controlled trial. Lancet. 1960;i:1309–12.

38 The Columbus Investigators. Low-molecular-weight heparin in the treatment of patients with venous thromboembolism. N Engl J Med. 1997;337:657–62.

39 Simonneau G, Sors H, Charbonnier B, et al. A comparison of low-molecular-weight heparin with unfractionated heparin for acute pulmonary embolism. N Engl J Med. 1997;337:663–9.

40 Goldhaber SZ. Contemporary pulmonary embolism thrombolysis. Chest. 1995;107(Suppl. 1):S45–51.

41 Konstantinides St, Geibel A, Olschewski M, et al. Association between thrombolytic treatment and the prognosis of hemodynamically stable patients with major pulmonary embolism. Results of a Multicenter Registry. Circulation. 1997;96:882–8.

42 Tow DE, Wagner NH Jr. Recovery of pulmonary arterial blood flow in patients with pulmonary embolism. N Engl J Med. 1967;276:1053–9.

43 Carson JL, Kelley MA, Duff A, et al. The clinical course of pulmonary embolism. N Engl J Med. 1992;326:1240–5.

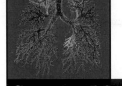
Chapter 51 Pulmonary Hypertension

Andrew Jones and Timothy Evans

Pulmonary hypertension is defined as a mean pulmonary artery pressure >3.3kPa (>25mmHg) at rest, or >4.0kPa (>30mmHg) on exercise. It can occur secondary to many disease processes (i.e. secondary pulmonary hypertension), or in the absence of such conditions [i.e. primary pulmonary hypertension (PPH); Fig. 51.1]. Although this classification is widely accepted, it groups together numerous conditions that are pathologically and physiologically distinct solely because their etiologies are unknown, and it classifies many conditions that have similar pathophysiologic features into different groups. Confusion also arises because some authors restrict the term 'primary' to true idiopathic disease, but others use it to infer that the disease process originates in the pulmonary vessels, even though a cause (e.g. a toxin or collagen vascular disease) may be identified. In this chapter, following the World Health Organization (WHO) report of 1973, the term 'primary' is restricted to those cases of pulmonary hypertension in which the cause remains unknown[1]. Thus, PPH becomes a diagnosis of exclusion.

Classification of pulmonary hypertension

Primary pulmonary hypertension

Secondary pulmonary hypertension

Lung disease
  Parenchymal lung disease
  Disorders of ventilation
  Congenital abnormalities
  Hypoxia-induced (i.e. altitude)

Heart disorders
  Disorders of left-heart filling
  Congenital systemic-to-pulmonary shunts

Thromboembolic disease or obstruction of pulmonary vessels
  Pulmonary thromboembolism
  Mediastinal fibrosis
  Congenital stenosis
  Foreign bodies
  Tumor
  Hemoglobinopathies
  Schistosome eggs

Collagen vascular disease and pulmonary vasculitides

Exogenous substances
  Anorexic agents
  Toxic rapeseed oil
  L-Tryptophan
  Crack cocaine

Human immunodeficiency virus infection

Portal hypertension

Figure 51.1 Classification of pulmonary hypertension.

EPIDEMIOLOGY, RISK FACTORS, AND PATHOPHYSIOLOGY

Epidemiology

PPH is rare (i.e. 1–2/million people). It can present at any age, but the peak incidence is in the third and fourth decades. Note, however, that 9% of the patients included in the US National Institutes of Health (NIH) PPH registry were ≥ 60 years when first diagnosed. In childhood, the sex distribution is almost equal, but in adults the female-to-male ratio is approximately 2:1.

Risk factors

Although most cases of PPH are sporadic, familial disease, inherited in an autosomal dominant pattern, accounted for 6% of the 187 cases in the NIH registry[2]. The phenomenon of 'genetic anticipation' was seen in these families, that is, subsequent generations were more severely affected and often had an earlier onset of disease. No definite racial or geographic differences have been confirmed, although several studies suggest a greater incidence in Afro-Caribbean females, perhaps because they are more prone to autoimmune disease than Caucasians.

Pathology

In 1973 the WHO classified PPH into three pathologic subsets[1] – plexogenic pulmonary arteriopathy, pulmonary veno-occlusive disease (PVOD), and pulmonary capillary hemangiomatosis.

Although plexogenic pulmonary arteriopathy was once thought to be the hallmark of PPH, and a *sine qua non* for diagnosis, it is now recognized as being only one of many histologic manifestations of the condition. Plexogenic arteriopathy is not specific to PPH, as it is also found in secondary forms of pulmonary hypertension and, accordingly, it may reflect a nonspecific response of the pulmonary vasculature to hemodynamic injury. Thrombosis, both intraluminal and organized, is a common finding in PPH, which may result in diagnostic confusion.

In a small proportion of cases, the predominant histopathologic changes are occlusive intimal lesions that occur in the pulmonary veins with arterialization of these vessels. Such patients are given the diagnosis of PVOD. Venous obstruction results in capillary congestion, alveolar hemorrhage, and interstitial and alveolar edema, and accounts for the distinctive clinical presentation of these patients (see below). Predominantly affecting children or young adults, PVOD is rare and may be familial. The underlying cause remains unknown, but there are associations with chemotherapeutic agents, oral contraceptives, bone marrow transplantation, human immunodeficiency virus (HIV) infection, and as a sequel to respiratory viral infection. The coexistence of plexogenic arteriopathy with PVOD in cases of PPH associated

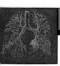
with HIV infection, or following ingestion of contaminated rape seed oil, has led some investigators to suggest that the arterial lesions are not secondary, but are part of a wider injury to the entire pulmonary endothelium, and that the condition would be better termed pulmonary occlusive angiopathy.

Pulmonary capillary hemangiomatosis is an extremely rare condition characterized by the proliferation of thin-walled microvessels that infiltrate the peribronchial–perivascular interstitium, lung parenchyma, and pleura. These microvessels infiltrate the walls of pulmonary veins, which results in medial expansion, destruction of medial elastic fibers, and fibrous luminal obstruction. In addition, medial and intimal thickening of muscular arteries and muscularization of arterioles occur. The proliferating microvessels are prone to bleeding, which results in hemoptysis and accumulation of hemosiderin-laden macrophages in alveolar spaces. This condition may occur spontaneously, or in families, with an autosomal recessive pattern of inheritance.

Pathogenesis

The pathogenesis of PPH remains speculative (Fig. 51.2). Three elements combine to produce the increased vascular resistance – vasoconstriction, vascular remodeling, and *in situ* thrombosis. In recent years much attention has been turned to the endothelium, which is now known to have important reg-

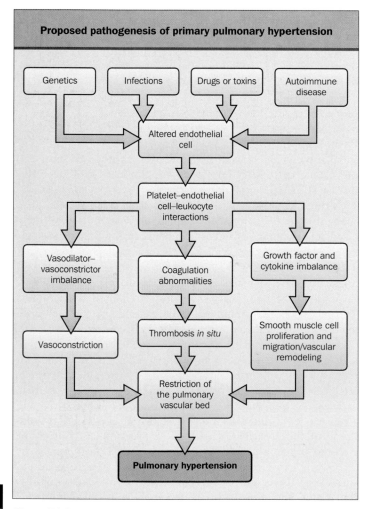

Figure 51.2 Proposed pathogenesis of primary pulmonary hypertension.

ulatory functions, including control of vessel tone and platelet function, and possibly modulation of vascular remodeling[3]. The endothelium is known to elaborate a number of vasoactive mediators, so endothelial dysfunction could result in an imbalance between the production of vasoconstrictor and vasodilator substances, thereby causing vasoconstriction. A reversal of the normal ratio of metabolites of thromboxane (vasoconstrictor) to prostacyclin (vasodilator)[4], impaired endothelial production of the endogenous vasodilator nitric oxide[5], and decreased endothelial clearance of the pressor substance endothelin-1[6], have all been associated with pulmonary hypertension of varying types.

The endothelium is intimately involved in the control of platelet function and coagulation, and endothelial damage may result in a prothrombotic state within the pulmonary vasculature, and *in-situ* thrombosis. Endothelial cell products may modulate vascular remodeling. Thus, endothelin-1 is known to promote smooth muscle cell growth, and nitric oxide and epoprostenol may have opposing effects[3].

Other factors are also likely to be involved, including inflammatory cells that produce chemokines, such as interleukin-1, and growth factors (transforming growth factor-β and fibroblast growth factor)[3].

The exact trigger for the development of PPH remains undefined. Indeed, given the right predisposing conditions, several factors may initiate the condition. Thus, pulmonary hypertension identical to PPH occurs in conjunction with connective tissue diseases, following the ingestion or inhalation of certain drugs or toxins, and as a result of certain infections, including HIV. Individual susceptibility as a prerequisite is suggested by associations with sex, familial PPH, autoimmune disease, and by the fact that not all those exposed to such trigger factors go on to develop the condition.

Pathophysiology

The normal pulmonary circulation is a high-flow, low-resistance system. Pulmonary blood flow can increase three-to-five fold, with minimal changes in pulmonary artery pressures, because of recruitment and distention of the pulmonary vasculature. Normally, the right ventricle does not have to generate significant systolic pressures and is therefore a thin-walled cavity that can accommodate large changes in venous return with little change in filling pressures. Prolonged pulmonary hypertension reduces the cross-sectional area and the distensibility of the pulmonary vasculature. Initially, cardiac output may remain normal at rest, via a compensatory tachycardia and right ventricular hypertrophy, but it fails to increase appropriately with exercise, despite a rise in right ventricular filling pressures. Increased heart rate and systolic pressures may compromise right ventricular myocardial blood flow, which results in right ventricular ischemia. Eventually, cardiac output becomes depressed, even at rest, as right ventricular afterload increases. Increased right ventricular pressures can, by causing septal shift, impair left ventricular filling and performance, and produce a small rise in left ventricular filling pressures. Fluid retention occurs secondary to the low output state, which results in peripheral edema, hepatic congestion, and ascites. Most patients succumb to right ventricular failure, but sudden death is seen in approximately 7%. Common precipitating events are believed to be arrhythmias and pulmonary emboli.

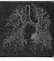

CLINICAL FEATURES

History

Early diagnosis is difficult because of the nonspecific nature of the symptoms, and the subtle findings on physical examination. In the NIH registry the mean length of time from onset of first symptoms to diagnosis was >2 years. In 10% of cases symptoms preceded diagnosis by >3 years[2]. Dyspnea is the presenting complaint in 60% of patients, and is eventually reported by virtually all as the disease progresses. It may be graded I–IV according to the New York Heart Association (NYHA) criteria, and reflects both the severity of the pulmonary hypertension and the prognosis. Fatigue is common. Angina occurs in 47% of patients, and is usually caused by right ventricular ischemia. Coronary angiography is generally normal. Syncope or presyncope, especially on exertion, is an ominous complaint, and indicates severe limitation of cardiac output. Although initial reports suggested otherwise, Raynaud's phenomenon occurs with no greater frequency than in the general population.

Physical examination

Physical findings may be few and subtle in the earliest stages of the condition. With progression, tachycardia occurs, with a low-volume pulse. Low cardiac output results in poor peripheral perfusion, with cold extremities and peripheral cyanosis. Central cyanosis is common, but finger clubbing is not a feature, and its presence should alert the examiner to consider conditions that result in secondary pulmonary hypertension. The jugular venous pressure is often raised. A parasternal heave may be found on palpation, along with a palpable pulmonary component of the second heart sound (P2). Auscultation reveals a loud P2, and right ventricular gallops (i.e. S3 or S4) are present in more severe cases. Tricuspid regurgitation is very common, and evidence may also be found for pulmonary valvular insufficiency (i.e. Graham Steell's murmur, which arises from dilatation of the pulmonary valve ring). Peripheral edema and ascites may be present in severe disease. Careful examination also aims to exclude other secondary causes of pulmonary hypertension, in particular those associated with the connective tissue diseases.

DIAGNOSIS

Subsequent investigation has two specific aims – to confirm and document the severity of the pulmonary hypertension, and to identify or exclude all secondary causes of the condition, thus allowing the diagnosis of PPH to be made. An appropriate approach is presented in Fig. 51.3.

Electrocardiogram

The electrocardiogram typically shows right-axis deviation with evidence of right ventricular hypertrophy and strain, although the degree of these changes does not always reflect the severity of the pulmonary hypertension.

Chest radiography

Chest radiography is abnormal in over 90% of cases. Prominence of the main pulmonary arteries (90%), enlargement of the hilar vessels (80%), and peripheral pruning (51%) are the most common abnormalities (see Fig. 51.4). Of patients enrolled in the NIH registry, only 6% had a normal chest radiograph.

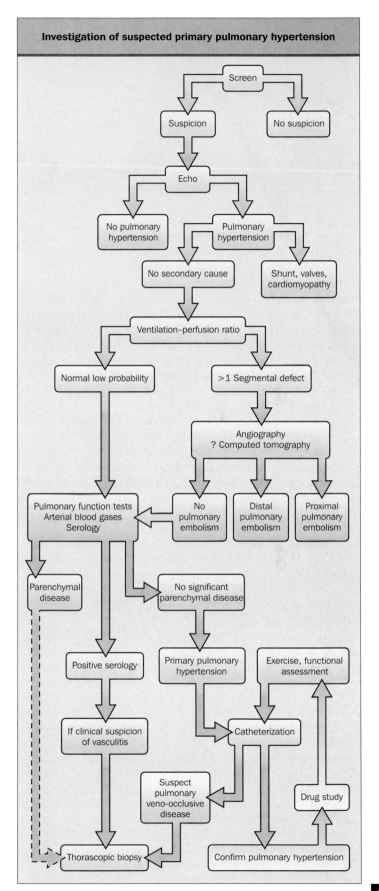

Figure 51.3 Approach to investigate suspected primary pulmonary hypertension. Adapted with permission from Rubin LJ. Primary pulmonary hypertension. Chest 1993;104:236–50.

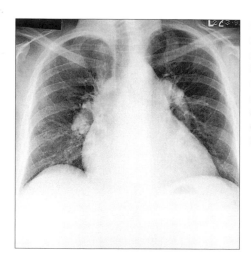

Figure 51.4 Chest radiograph in primary pulmonary hypertension. Enlargement of the proximal pulmonary arteries (spurious cardiomegaly caused by poor inspiration).

Pulmonary function tests

Although mild restrictive defects and evidence of minor small airways dysfunction can be seen in PPH, more significant abnormalities suggest an alternative diagnosis. Significant impairment of gas exchange may occur, with reduced transfer capacity of the lung for carbon monoxide, hypoxemia, hypocapnia secondary to alveolar hyperventilation, and an increased alveolar–arterial oxygen (P_{AO_2}–P_{O_2}) gradient. Severe hypoxemia in PPH may result from intracardiac shunting caused by a patent foramen ovale, or may be a consequence of severely depressed cardiac output with resultant mixed venous hypoxemia[2].

Cardiopulmonary exercise test

If a cardiopulmonary exercise study is performed, it reveals reduced maximal oxygen consumption, high minute ventilation, low anaerobic threshold, and increased P_{AO_2}–P_{O_2} gradient, which widens further on exercise. However, the specificity and sensitivity of such studies to pulmonary hypertension remain to be determined. By contrast, the 6 minute walk test shows a correlation between the distance achieved and disease severity, and can be used to monitor disease progression or response to therapy.

Echocardiography

Transthoracic echocardiography is important to rule out cardiac causes of pulmonary hypertension, as well as to provide a noninvasive estimation of right ventricular function and pulmonary artery pressure. Typically, right ventricular and right atrial enlargement are apparent, with a normal left ventricular cavity size. In severe cases, intraventricular septal curvature may be reversed, and the left ventricular cavity compromised. Pulmonary and tricuspid regurgitation can be identified and quantified using Doppler techniques, which permit the noninvasive estimation of pulmonary artery pressures from assessments of the degree of tricuspid regurgitation[7]. Such studies also provide an index of disease progression, so removing the need for repeated, invasive catheter studies. Although more invasive and more expensive, transesophageal echocardiography provides a superior assessment of structural cardiac defects, and is used to exclude proximal (large) pulmonary thromboembolism.

Lung scanning

Ventilation–perfusion scintigraphy is essential to exclude chronic thromboembolic disease. In PPH, the scan is typically normal, or displays only minor, patchy perfusion defects[2]. In patients who have pulmonary hypertension because of thromboembolic disease, at least one, but often more, major segmental or subsegmental mismatches in ventilation–perfusion relationships is seen (Figs 51.5 & 51.6). A normal or low probability scan effectively excludes thromboembolic disease. In uncertain cases, pulmonary angiography or, increasingly, contrast-enhanced spiral computed tomography (CT), are employed.

If the lung scan shows one or more segmental ventilation–perfusion mismatches, pulmonary angiography is performed to rule out chronic thromboembolic disease (Fig. 51.7). In experienced hands the procedure is quite safe, even in patients who have high pulmonary pressures and low cardiac outputs.

Computed tomography

Recent experience indicates that contrast-enhanced, continuous volume (i.e. spiral) CT scanning provides a less invasive alternative to pulmonary angiography in the investigation of suspected pulmonary thromboembolic disease, as thrombi in the proximal pulmonary arteries can be readily identified by CT. Interpretation of the spiral CT images is highly observer dependent and, at best, only sixth- or seventh-generation pulmonary arteries can be visualized confidently (Fig. 51.8).

Heart catheterization

Pulmonary arterial catheterization is an essential procedure, not only to confirm the presence and degree of pulmonary hypertension, but also to guide therapy and estimate prognosis. Pulmonary arterial pressures are often increased to three times normal, right atrial pressure is elevated, and cardiac output is reduced[2]. Left-sided pressures are usually normal, but severe dilatation of the right ventricle can compress the left-sided chambers, resulting in a slight increase in diastolic filling pressure. Pulmonary capillary occlusion pressure is usually normal in PPH, and may not be elevated even in PVOD because of the patchy nature of this condition.

Serology

Antinuclear antibody testing is frequently positive in patients who have PPH (29% in the NIH registry), despite the absence of connective tissue disease. These are usually of a nonspecific pattern, and are present in low titers.

TREATMENT

General

The rarity and life-threatening nature of PPH mandates that patients be managed in a regional center that has experience with the condition. Education is a critical aspect of care, as patients must live as active a life as possible, but at the same time must avoid excess physical exertion, which can result in a marked increase in pulmonary artery pressure and precipitate arrhythmias. Altitude, with its associated hypoxia, must be avoided. Commercial air travel is generally safe for those affected by only mild or moderate disease, although supplementary oxygen should be available, and a fitness-to-fly test prior to the trip should be considered. Pregnancy, in particular the postpartum period, is poorly tolerated and effective birth control is therefore essential, but oral contraceptives should be avoided since they can produce prothrombotic changes that could potentially aggravate the condition. When ventricular failure develops, with the resultant

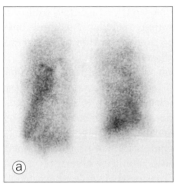
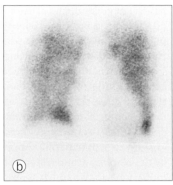
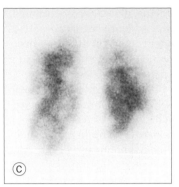
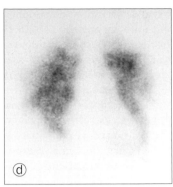

Figure 51.5 Typical ventilation–perfusion scans in primary pulmonary hypertension. (a, b) Normal ventilation scans; (c, d) patchy subsegmental defects on corresponding perfusion scans.

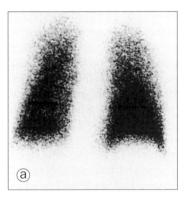
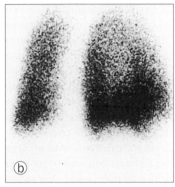
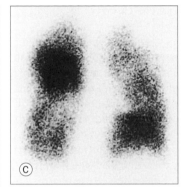
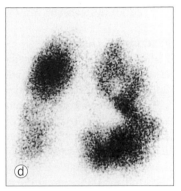

Figure 51.6 Chronic thromboembolic pulmonary hypertension. (a, b) Normal ventilation scans; (c, d) multiple segmental (or larger) defects on corresponding perfusion scans.

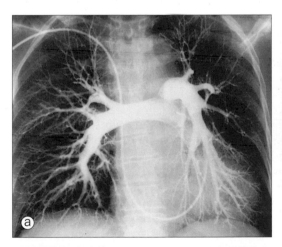
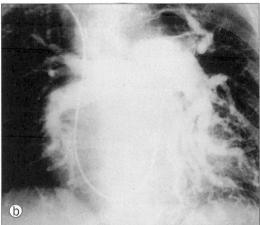

Figure 51.7 Pulmonary angiograms. (a) Normal and (b) in primary pulmonary hypertension, with marked peripheral pruning of pulmonary vasculature.

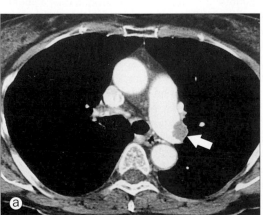
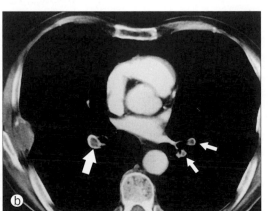

Figure 51.8 Spiral computed tomography with contrast. (a) Massive filling defect in the main pulmonary artery (arrow). (b) Filling defects in lobar (large arrow) and segmental (small arrows) pulmonary arteries.

hepatic congestion and peripheral edema, diuretics are warranted, but must be prescribed with caution as right ventricular performance may become highly dependent upon preload, and over-aggressive diuresis may markedly reduce cardiac output. Pressure stockings may be helpful in some patients.

The use of cardiac glycosides in PPH is controversial, although some investigators recommend their use to counteract the negative inotropic effects of calcium-channel blocking agents when these are used as pulmonary vasodilators[8]. The risk of digitalis toxicity may be aggravated by the concomitant use of diuretics in this group of patients.

There is no rationale for long-term oxygen administration because patients who have PPH are rarely hypoxemic at rest, except when the condition becomes advanced. Most patients desaturate on exercise, however, and for some of these, supplemental oxygen may reduce dyspnea and improve exercise capacity.

Vasodilator therapy

The rationale for using vasodilators is based on the premise that vasoconstriction is an important contributor to the pathophysiology of the condition. Unfortunately, there is no way to predict who might respond to treatment, and the agents employed are all associated with considerable risk for morbidity and mortality. The standard approach to identifying those patients who are likely to benefit from long-term vasodilator therapy is to use a potent, short-acting, titratable vasodilator, the effects of which are confined to the pulmonary circulation. Since these acute pharmacologic tests are not without risk, they should be performed by experienced clinicians using invasive hemodynamic monitoring in an appropriate setting. Repeated measurements of pulmonary artery and right atrial pressures, systemic blood pressure, arterial oxygenation, and cardiac output are made in response to increasing doses of the test drug. In practice, the short half-lives and relative pulmonary selectivity of the agents employed enables any adverse effects to be reversed quickly by discontinuing the drug. Several vasodilators have been employed, including inhaled nitric oxide, intravenous epoprostenol, and intravenous adenosine (Fig.

51.9)[9]. In general, the acute response to these agents is useful in predicting the response to longer-acting, orally-administered compounds[10]. Empiric oral vasodilator therapy, without prior acute vasoreactivity testing, is strongly discouraged.

At present, no criteria to define a beneficial response to an acute vasodilator challenge are uniformly accepted. Most investigators agree that the goal of such therapy is to decrease pulmonary arterial pressures and to increase cardiac output, without decreasing systemic pressures. This is achievable in only approximately 25% of patients[8]. Approximately 25% of patients respond by developing either systemic hypotension with no effect on pulmonary hemodynamics, or by increasing their pulmonary arterial pressures because of an increased cardiac output. These patients are thought to have 'fixed' pulmonary vascular disease, and vasodilator therapy is not thought to be beneficial, and may actually be harmful. The remaining 50% of cases respond to vasodilators by increasing their cardiac output without changing their pulmonary vascular pressures. Although exercise tolerance and right ventricular function may improve in such patients, the long-term benefits of such changes remain unclear[10].

The most commonly used agents for long-term vasodilator therapy are the calcium-channel antagonists nifedipine and diltiazem[1]. The dose required to produce a beneficial response tends to greater than that generally used to treat systemic hypertension or coronary artery disease (Fig. 51.9), although a wide variation exists in requirement and tolerance between individual patients. Verapamil has marked negative inotropic effects and should be avoided in these patients, and angiotensin-converting enzyme inhibitors have little effect in PPH, at least acutely. Oral vasodilator therapy is generally titrated to patient tolerance, in particular systemic hypotension. Other side effects include edema formation and worsening hypoxemia. Hypoxemia may develop as a result of a decrease in cardiac output (with a concomitant decrease in mixed venous oxygen content), worsening ventilation–perfusion matching due to generalized pulmonary vasodilation, or possibly by increased shunting through a patent foramen ovale, if the systemic vasodilating effects reduce left atrial pressures.

Recently, continuous intravenous epoprostenol has been used as a long-term therapy. In a 3-month, randomized, open-label trial, patients with NYHA grade III or IV dyspnea treated with a continuous infusion of epoprostenol (in addition to standard therapy, which included oral vasodilators) had improved hemodynamic parameters and better exercise tolerance, quality of life, and survival, compared with a similar group treated with conventional therapy alone[11]. Longer-term hemodynamic benefits have also been reported, although the dosage may need to be increased for these to be maintained[12].

Improvements in long-term hemodynamics may occur in patients who receive epoprostenol despite finding little or no response to acute infusion. Possible mechanisms include the inhibitory effect of epoprostenol on platelet aggregation, or possible beneficial effects on vascular remodeling. Unlike calcium-channel blocker therapy, which is only instituted after observing a beneficial acute response, treatment with continuous epoprostenol can be considered even in the absence of acute effects. The exceptions to this statement are the small subgroup of patients who have PVOD, in whom epoprostenol may cause acute pulmonary edema, presumably by increasing pulmonary blood flow in the presence of a fixed downstream obstruction.

Vasodilators frequently used in the investigation and management of primary pulmonary hypertension			
Drug	**Route**	**Dose range**	**Half-life**
Epoprostenol[a]	Intravenous	2–20ng/kg of body weight/minute	3–5 minutes
Adenosine	Intravenous	50–200µg/kg of body weight/minute	5–10 seconds
Nitric oxide	Inhaled	5–80 parts per million	15–30 seconds
Nifedipine[b]	Oral	30–240mg/day	2–5 hours
Diltiazem[b]	Oral	120–900mg/day	2–4.5 hours

[a]The dose range shown is for a short-term infusion; the dose range for long-term infusions often exceeds 100–150ng/kg per minute.
[b]The half-life shown refers to conventional preparations; sustained-release preparations may be administered once daily.

Figure 51.9 Vasodilators frequently used in the investigation and management of primary pulmonary hypertension. Dose ranges, routes of administration, and half lives. (Reproduced with permission from Rubin[9]. ©1997 Massachusetts Medical Society. All rights reserved.)

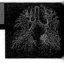

Epoprostenol must be administered by continuous infusion, since it has a short half-life (3–5 minutes) and is inactivated by the low pH of the stomach. This requires the placement and maintenance of a central venous catheter connected to a portable infusion pump. Minor adverse effects are relatively common, including flushing, skin rashes, joint and jaw pain, and diarrhea. More serious adverse effects include catheter-related infections, venous thrombosis, and pump malfunction, which results in under- or overdosing. Interruption of the infusion, because of either pump failure or line occlusion, may lead to rebound pulmonary hypertension, which can be fatal[11–13]. As a result of these and other difficulties, only those patients who remain in NYHA classes III or IV, despite maximal 'conventional' therapy (i.e. anticoagulants, diuretics, oral vasodilators, cardiac glycosides, and supplemental oxygen) are presently potential candidates for long-term epoprostenol therapy (Fig. 51.10).

Anticoagulation

Extensive thrombosis is a common histopathologic finding in patients who suffer PPH. In addition, patients who have PPH are at increased risk of thromboembolic events because of diminished venous return, high right-sided filling pressures, a dilated and poorly contracting ventricle, sluggish pulmonary blood flow, and relative degree of inactivity. Even a small embolic event may have serious consequences because of the lack of pulmonary vascular reserve. A large retrospective study[14], as well as a recent small, nonrandomized, prospective study[8], found that patients treated with oral anticoagulants had an improved survival compared with those who were not. Warfarin is the anticoagulant of choice, with doses adjusted to achieve an international normal-ized ratio of 2–3 (Fig. 51.10). In patients who suffer adverse effects from warfarin, or in whom the risk of bleeding is deemed to be increased, twice-daily subcutaneous heparin may be an alternative. Initial studies suggest that low-molecular-mass heparins cause fewer long-term side effects (e.g. osteoporosis, thrombocytopenia).

Transplantation

Both lung and combined heart–lung transplantation are performed in patients who have PPH, with comparable survival rates[15]. Even markedly impaired right-ventricular function may improve following single or double lung transplant. Mortality is higher for patients who have PPH than for those who receive transplants for other conditions, the main complication being obliterative bronchiolitis. To date, no recurrence of PPH following transplantation has been reported. The decision of when to perform transplantation is difficult, especially in the light of the improved survival seen with recently introduced medical therapies. In general, transplantation is only considered when all medical therapies have failed[16] (Fig. 51.10).

CLINICAL COURSE AND PREVENTION

Historically, the course of PPH has been one of an unrelenting, progressive deterioration with a median survival of 2.5 years[2]. Following the introduction of newer therapies, however, survival has improved. Long-term anticoagulation seems to double the predicted 3-year survival[14], and patients who respond to calcium-channel blockers have a 5-year survival approaching 95%[8]. Continuous intravenous infusion of epoprostenol in NYHA class

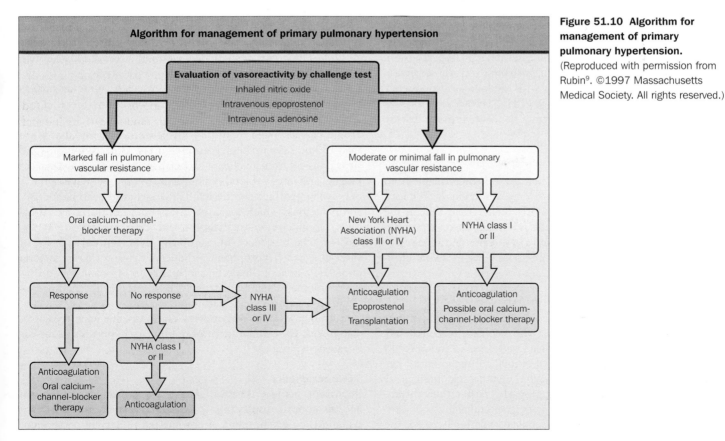

Figure 51.10 Algorithm for management of primary pulmonary hypertension.

III and IV patients doubled their 5-year survival, compared with historical controls (54 versus 27%)[13]. Patients who undergo heart–lung transplantation have 1- and 5-year survival rates of 68–77 and 22–38%, respectively.

Several factors identifiable at presentation predict shorter survival, including:

- higher pulmonary vascular resistance and pressures;
- absence of a favorable response to vasodilator therapy;
- worse NYHA classification;
- elevated right atrial pressure;
- decreased cardiac output (<2.0L/min per m^2);
- pulmonary arterial oxygen saturation $<63\%$;
- distance walked in the 6 minute walking test[2].

PITFALLS AND CONTROVERSIES

Classification

Misclassification of pulmonary hypertension remains the greatest pitfall. It is essential that all secondary causes are vigorously sought and excluded, as the distinction between primary and secondary pulmonary hypertension has important implications regarding management and prognosis. A few specific examples of secondary pulmonary hypertension are worth further discussion.

Autoimmune disorders

Pulmonary hypertension has been reported in association with many connective tissue disorders, which include scleroderma (particularly the CREST variant of Calcinosis cutis, Raynaud's disease, Esophageal dysmotility, Sclerodactyly, and Telangiectasis), systemic lupus erythematosus, mixed connective tissue disease, and, to a lesser extent, with rheumatoid arthritis, polymyositis, and dermatomyositis. The pulmonary hypertension can occur in the absence of any associated pulmonary fibrosis.

The strongest association seems to be with the disorders linked with Raynaud's disease, occuring exclusively in females and often predating the development of pulmonary hypertension. Histologic findings may be indistinguishable from those seen in PPH. These associations, together with the increased frequency of positive antinuclear antibodies in PPH, has lead some authors to suggest that PPH may be a form of connective tissue disease confined to the lung.

Human immunodeficiency virus

Severe pulmonary hypertension, clinically indistinguishable from PPH, is well documented in HIV-infected individuals. The estimated incidence is 0.5%, significantly higher than that in the general population[17]. The pathogenesis remains obscure. Studies have failed to find evidence of direct HIV infection of vascular structures. The association raises the possibility of a viral etiology for PPH.

Portal hypertension

Pulmonary hypertension has been reported in 2–10% of patients admitted with hepatic cirrhosis[17,18]. The mechanism is unknown, although cirrhosis is commonly diagnosed prior to the onset of pulmonary hypertension. Repeated emboli from the portal circulation has been suggested, although the pathologic findings are typically those of plexogenic arteriopathy rather than thromboembolism. Another possibility is that an endogenous or exogenous vasoconstrictor in the splanchnic circulation bypasses the liver and subsequently effects the pulmonary vasculature. However, attempts to produce pulmonary hypertension by surgically creating portal hypertension in animal models have failed.

Drug- or toxin-induced pulmonary hypertension

In the late 1960s, a 20-fold increase in the incidence of unexplained pulmonary hypertension was seen following the introduction of the appetite suppressant aminorex fumarate (2-amino-5-phenyl-2-oxazoline) in Switzerland, Austria, and West Germany. The histology was indistinguishable from the plexogenic arteriopathy of PPH. Aminorex resembles ephedrine and amphetamine in structure, and the release of catecholamines from endogenous stores was suggested as a cause, but attempts to reproduce chronic pulmonary hypertension with prolonged administration of aminorex to animals failed. This, and that only 2% of patients who take aminorex develop pulmonary hypertension, suggests that affected individuals are predisposed to vasoconstriction or to proliferation of the pulmonary vasculature in response to an offending agent.

Pulmonary hypertension has also been linked with use of the anorexic agents fenfluramine and dexfenfluramine[19], which were recently taken off the market in the USA.

A multisystem disorder occurred in Spain in 1981, related to the ingestion of illegally marketed rapeseed oil. The syndrome presented initially as pneumonia, with respiratory distress and pulmonary infiltrates, but individuals failed to respond to conventional therapy. A second stage of fever, myalgia, and neurologic deficits followed, and the syndrome was often associated with pulmonary hypertension. A later stage resembled scleroderma[20]. A total of 20,068 cases were registered, of whom 835 died. Pulmonary hypertension was seen in 20% within the first 3–4 months. Follow-up studies on a subset of 322 patients found that 8% developed pulmonary hypertension, although in most cases it regressed with time and only 2% developed a malignant form. Pathologically, the condition most closely resembled PVOD. The toxin responsible was not identified, although oleoanilides or their metabolites were implicated.

L-Tryptophan is a food supplement used for ailments such as premenstrual syndrome, insomnia, and depression. Since an epidemic in New Mexico in 1989, it has been linked with a syndrome characterized by diffuse myalgia and eosinophilia. More than 1500 cases have been registered in the USA. Symptoms and signs progress from an abrupt onset of incapacitating myalgia and fatigue, and intense blood eosinophilia, to the later development of polyneuropathy, scleroderma-like skin changes, and pulmonary complications, which include eosinophilic infiltrates and effusions, vasculitis, interstitial disease, and chronic pulmonary hypertension. The frequency of pulmonary hypertension is 5–7% of those affected. Tryptophan is produced by the action of bacteria on several nutrients, including anthranilic acid, a compound similar to aniline, which was strongly implicated in the pathogenesis of the syndrome seen with rapeseed oil.

Solvent abuse and inhalation of 'crack' cocaine have been associated with the development of pulmonary hypertension, as has intravenous drug use[21].

Sickle cell disease

Recurrent sickle crises complicated by pulmonary embolism and thrombosis results in microvascular destruction and fibrosis, and the development of chronic pulmonary hypertension.

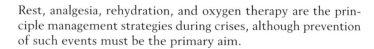

Rest, analgesia, rehydration, and oxygen therapy are the principle management strategies during crises, although prevention of such events must be the primary aim.

Tropical disease and pulmonary hypertension

Several tropical, parasitic infections, which include schistosomiasis, filariasis, and other helminthic infections, can produce a marked granulomatous inflammatory response in the lung. If left untreated, pulmonary hypertension may result, often many years after the acute response. A careful history should suggest or exclude the likelihood of tropical disease, especially if combined with an eosinophil count. Treatment depends on eradication of the underlying organism.

Angiography

Misinterpretation of pulmonary angiograms is another important pitfall, because of the possibility that central thrombi can be seen in PPH caused by the low cardiac output state. Accordingly, angiography should only be performed and interpreted by physicians experienced in the study of patients who have PPH.

Anticoagulation

A final pitfall is that, with progressive disease, right-sided heart failure may lead to hepatic congestion, which can impair hepatic function and alter the extent of anticoagulation observed with warfarin therapy. Accordingly, more frequent monitoring of prothrombin times is warranted.

REFERENCES

1.   Hatano S, Strasser T. Primary pulmonary hypertension: WHO committee report. Geneva: World Health Organization; 1975.
2.   Rich SA, Dantzker DR, Ayres SM, et al. Primary pulmonary hypertension: a National Prospective Study. Ann Intern Med. 1987;107:216–23.
3.   Voekel NF, Tuder RM. Cellular and molecular mechanisms in the pathogenesis of severe pulmonary hypertension. Eur Respir J. 1995;8:2129–38.
4.   Christman BW, McPherson CD, Newman JH, et al. An imbalance between the excretion of thromboxane and prostacyclin metabolites in pulmonary hypertension. N Engl J Med. 1992;327:70–5.
5.   Giaid A, Salch D. Reduced expression of endothelial nitric oxide synthase in the lungs of patients with pulmonary hypertension. N Engl J Med. 1995;333:214–21.
6.   Giaid A, Yanagisawa M, Langleben D, et al. Expression of endothelin-1 in the lungs of patients with pulmonary hypertension. N Engl J Med. 1993;328:1732–9.
7.   Berger M, Haimowitz A, Van Tosh A, Berdoff RL, Goldberg E. Quantitative assessment of pulmonary hypertension in patients with tricuspid regurgitation using continuous wave Doppler. J Am Coll Cardiol. 1984;6:359–65.
8.   Rich SA, Kaufmann E, Levy PS. The effect of high doses of calcium channel blockers on survival in primary pulmonary hypertension. N Engl J Med. 1992;327:76–81.
9.   Rubin LJ. Primary pulmonary hypertension. N Engl J Med. 1997;336:111–17.
10.   Barst RJ. Pharmacologically induced pulmonary vasodilatation in children and young adults with primary pulmonary hypertension. Chest. 1986;89:497–503.
11.   Barst RJ, Rubin IJ, Long WA, et al. A comparison of continuous epoprostenol (prostacyclin) with conventional therapy for primary pulmonary hypertension. N Engl J Med. 1996;334:296–301.
12.   Barst RJ, Rubin LJ, McGoon MD, Caldwell EJ, Long WA, Levy PS. Survival in primary pulmonary hypertension with long term continuous intravenous prostacyclin. Ann Intern Med. 1994;121:409–15.
13.   Rubin LJ, Mendoza J, Hood M, et al. Treatment of primary pulmonary hypertension with continuous intravenous prostacyclin (epoprostenol): results of a randomized trial. Ann Intern Med. 1990;112:485–91.
14.   Fuster V, Steele PM, Edwards WD, Gersh BJ, McGoon MD, Frye RI. Primary pulmonary hypertension: natural history and the importance of thrombosis. Circulation. 1984;70:580–7.

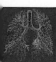

15. Hosenpud JD, Novick RJ, Bennet LE, Keck BM, Fiol B, Daily OP. The registry of the International Society for Heart and Lung Transplantation: thirteenth official report – 1996. J Heart Lung Transplant. 1996;15:655–74.

16. Speich MD, Jenni R, Opravil M, Pfab M, Russi EW. Primary pulmonary hypertension in HIV infection. Chest. 1991;100:1268–71.

17. Naeije RL, Melot C, Hallemans R, Mols P, Lejeune P. Pulmonary haemodynamics in liver cirrhosis. Semin Respir Med. 1985;7:164–70.

18. Hadengue A, Benhayoun MK, Lebrec D, Benhamou JP. Pulmonary hypertension complicating portal hypertension. Gastroenterology. 1991;100:520–8.

19. Abenhaim L, Moride Y, Brenot F. Appetite suppressant drugs and the risk of primary pulmonary hypertension. N Engl J Med. 1996;335:609–16.

20. Gomez-Sanchez MA, Saene de la Calzada C, Gomez-Panjualo C, Martinez-Tello FJ, Mestre de Juan MJ, James TN. Clinical and pathologic manifestations of pulmonary vascular disease in the toxic oil syndrome. J Am Coll Cardiol. 1991;18:1539–45.

21. Schaiberger PH, Kennedy TH, Miller FC, Gal J, Petty TL. Pulmonary hypertension associated with long-term inhalation of crack cocaine. Chest. 1993;104:614–16.

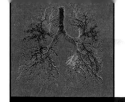

Chapter 52

Pulmonary Vasculitis and Hemorrhage

Marvin I Schwarz

PULMONARY VASCULITIDES

Epidemiology, risk factors, and pathophysiology

The pulmonary vasculitides are one component of a group of systemic disorders (Fig. 52.1) characterized by vascular inflammation, which leads to tissue necrosis and eventual end-organ dysfunction[1,2]. Although pulmonary vasculitis can complicate an established autoimmune disorder (the connective tissue diseases), the others etiologies listed in Figure 52.1 occur with no definable, underlying cause. Although this category of diseases has been recognized for over 60 years, specific etiologies, or even identifiable risk factors, have not been found. In general, the vasculitides are uncommon and involve the lung with a variable frequency (see Fig. 52.1)[3,4]. It does appear, however, that the incidence of systemic vasculitis is increasing, but this most likely relates to the widespread use of testing for antineutrophil cytoplasmic antibody (ANCA), antibodies found in the serum of four of these disorders (Wegener's granulomatosis, microscopic polyangiitis, polyarteritis nodosa, and Churg–Strauss syndrome). The projected annual incidence for most of the disorders ranges from two to 13 cases per million population.

Vasculitis implies inflammation and then eventual necrosis of the vascular walls. If medium- or large-diameter vessels are involved, infarction, necrosis, and end-organ dysfunction result. When vessels of smaller diameter are affected (i.e. capillaries, arterioles, and venules), loss of vascular integrity and leakage of blood into the tissue result. Such vasculitis in small-diameter vessels in the lung is referred to as pulmonary or alveolar capillaritis, producing the clinical syndrome of diffuse alveolar hemorrhage (DAH). When vasculitis occurs in small-diameter vessels of the skin, it is referred to as leukocytoclastic vasculitis and manifests as visible, raised, palpable purpura, and sometimes as petechiae. In the kidney, small-vessel involvement results in a focal, segmental, necrotizing glomerulonephritis, which can be either subclinical (manifesting only as hematuria, red blood cell casts, and protein in the urine) or present as renal insufficiency, which sometimes requires dialysis. Any organ system may be affected by the vasculitic process.

A granulomatous vasculitis that involves blood vessels of small and medium diameter is the characteristic histologic feature of Wegener's granulomatosis. Here, in addition to vascular inflammation and tissue necrosis, a necrotizing granulomatous process occurs in the tissue adjacent to, and within the wall of, the affected blood vessel. An area of central necrosis, surrounded by mixed acute and chronic inflammatory cells, palisading histiocytes, and giant cells (see Fig. 52.2) is characteristic of Wegener's granulomatosis, and is most readily apparent in tissue obtained from the lung, which is involved

The systemic vasculitides and relative frequencies of lung involvement				
Entity	Serum antineutrophil cytoplasmic antibody	Vessels involved	Cases/million per year	Lung involvement
Takayasu's arteritis	No	L and M	?	Common
Giant cell arteritis	No	L and M	13	Rare
Behçet's syndrome	No	L, M, and S	?	Uncommon
Wegener's granulomatosis	Yes	M and S	3–9	Common
Churg–Strauss syndrome	Yes	M and S	2–3	Common
Polyarteritis nodosa	Yes	M and S	3–4	Rare
Collagen vascular disease	No	M and S	12	Common
Kawasaki's disease	No	M	?	Rare
Necrotizing sarcoid granulomatosis	No	M	?	Common
Microscopic polyangiitis	Yes	S	3	Common
Isolated pauci-immune pulmonary capillaritis	Yes/no	S	?	Common
Henoch–Schönlein purpura	No	S	?	Uncommon
Cryoglobulinemia	No	S	2–3	Rare
Goodpasture's syndrome	Yes/no	S	?	Common

Figure 52.1 The systemic vasculitides and relative frequency of lung involvement. L, large-diameter pulmonary arteries (major branches); M, medium-diameter muscular pulmonary arteries; S, small-diameter pulmonary vessels (arterioles, venules, and capillaries).

in 75–90% of cases[5,6]. Renal tissue may only show a vasculitis of small-diameter vessels (capillaritis) that appears as focal, segmental necrotizing glomerulonephritis, often with crescent formation (see Fig. 52.3). Such renal findings are nonspecific and common to many of the systemic vasculitides. Another form of systemic vasculitis, which often affects the lung and also causes granulomatous inflammation, is the Churg–Strauss syndrome. Here, inflammation of medium- and small-diameter vessels includes numerous eosinophils and is associated with eosinophilic pneumonia. Giant cell arteritis, the most common type of vasculitis, is also granulomatous in character; however, it rarely involves the lungs. Necrotizing sarcoid granulomatosis is another example of a granulomatous vasculitis that involves

Diagnosis

To establish a diagnosis of DAH is not difficult in patients who present with hemoptysis, radiographic diffuse pulmonary infiltrates, falling hematocrit, and sequential hemorrhagic BAL. In those without hemoptysis, however, the BAL differentiates DAH from other acute infectious and noninfectious pulmonary processes. Figure 52.13 outlines the expected findings for the more common causes of DAH.

Treatment

Treatment for the systemic vasculitides and the DAH associated with collagen vascular disease is identical to that already described for vasculitis in the previous section of this chapter. One major addition is the use of plasmapheresis in patients who have Goodpasture's syndrome. In patients who have collagen vascular disease and DAH induced by Wegener's granulomatosis, plasmapheresis is ineffective. To treat diffuse DAH induced by alveolar damage, high-dose intravenous methylprednisilone is recommended (see previous section). Mitral stenosis that causes DAH requires surgical intervention. Patient's who have Goodpasture's syndrome must stop smoking.

Clinical course and prevention

The outcome of a systemic vasculitis or collagen vascular disease is adversely affected if DAH occurs. Over half of these patients require mechanical ventilation and death frequently results from respiratory and renal failure, or from a superimposed infection that occurs because of the immunosuppressive therapies. Only 50% of patients who have SLE survive the initial episode of DAH. In Wegener's granulomatosis and microscopic polyangiitis, the initial mortality is 25–30%. Furthermore, 5-year survival is also reduced (65%). The mortality and survival data are more encouraging for isolated pauci-immune pulmonary capillaritis.

In Goodpasture's syndrome, 2-year survival is 50%. Lower survivals in Goodpasture's syndrome are expected in patients who have severe renal failure and persistent DAH. An early mortality (25%) is expected in IPH, but 50% survive 5 years.

The only known preventive approach that can be suggested for patients who have this group of disorders is smoking cessation for patients who suffer Goodpasture's syndrome.

Pitfalls and controversies

In adults who have isolated DAH but who do not show evidence of drug exposure, mitral stenosis, or coagulopathy, a lung biopsy to differentiate between IPH, isolated pauci-immune pulmonary capillaritis, and Goodpasture's syndrome that has no renal involvement is performed. For those patients who present with isolated DAH, open or thoracoscopic lung biopsy is performed after the exclusion of mitral valve disease, coagulopathy, potential drug exposure, or conditions that can lead to diffuse alveolar damage. The clinical and radiographic features of pulmonary veno-occlusive disease can be confused with mitral stenosis.

Two potential pulmonary complications are related to recurrent DAH. One is pulmonary fibrosis that causes a progressive restrictive lung disease, and the other is a progressive obstructive lung disease in patients who have recurrent DAH because of pulmonary capillaritis. It is unclear why recurrent bleeding in the lung causes interstitial fibrosis. In iron-overload states, such as transfusion hemosiderosis or primary hemochromatosis, pulmonary fibrosis does not occur. Obstructive lung disease is thought to arise from the development of emphysema in patients who have pulmonary capillaritis caused by the release of neutral proteases from destroyed neutrophils and ANCA inhibition of antiproteases[25].

The use of plasmapheresis in patients who have microscopic polyangiitis is unclear.

Diagnosis of diffuse alveolar hemorrhage											
Disease	**Glomerulo-nephritis**	**Arthritis**	**Dermat-ologic vasculitis**	**Anti-nuclear antibody**	**Rheuma-atoid factor**	**Serum complement**	**Antibasement antibody syndrome**	**Cytoplasmic antineutrophil cytoplasmic antibody**	**Perinuclear antineutrophil cytoplasmic antibody**	**Antideoxy-ribonucleic acid antibody**	**Tissue immuno-complex antibody**
Wegener's granulomatosis	+	+	+	±	±	Within normal limits	–	+	±	–	–
Microscopic polyangiitis	+	+	+	±	±	Within normal limits	–	–	+	–	–
Systemic lupus erythematosus	+	+	±	+	±	Low	–	–	±	+	+ (granular)
Goodpasture's syndrome	+	–	–	–	–	Within normal limits	+	±	±	–	+ (linear)
Henoch–Schönlein purpura	+	±	+	–	–	Within normal limits	–	–	–	–	+ (IgA)
Idiopathic pauci-immune pulmonary capillaritis	–	–	–	–	–	Within normal limits	–	–	–	–	–
Idiopathic pulmonary hemosiderosis	–	–	–	–	–	Within normal limits	–	–	–	–	–
Pulmonary veno-occlusive disease	–	–	–	±	±	Within normal limits	–	–	–	–	Occasional

Figure 52.13 Diagnosis of diffuse alveolar hemorrhage. (Information from Schwarz et al.[24])

REFERENCES

1. Specks V. Pulmonary vasculitis. In: Schwarz MI, King TE, eds. Interstitial lung disease, 3rd edn. London: BC Decker; 1998:507–34.

2. Hunder G, Arend WP, Bloch DA, et al. The American College of Rheumatology 1990 criteria for the classification of vasculitis. Arthritis Rheumatol. 1990;33:1088–107.

3. Jennette JC, Falk RJ, Andrassy K, et al. Nomenclature of systemic vasculitides: a proposal of an international consensus conference. Arthritis Rheum. 1994;37:187–92.

4. Watts RA, Carruthers DM, Scott DGI. Epidemiology of systemic vasculitis: changing incidence or definition? Semin Arthritis Rheum. 1995;25:28–34.

5. Mark EJ, Matsubara O, Tan-Liu NS, Fienberg R. The pulmonary biopsy in the early diagnosis of Wegener's (pathergic) granulomatosis: a study base in 35 open lung biopsies. Hum Pathol. 1988;19:1065–71.

6. Travis WD, Hoffman GS, Leavitt RY, et al. Surgical pathology of the lung in Wegener's granulomatosis. Am J Surg Pathol. 1991;15:315–33.

7. Gaudin PG, Askin FB, Falk RJ, et al. The pathologic spectrum of pulmonary lesions in patients with anti-neutrophil cytoplasmic autoantibodies specific for anti-proteinase 3 and antimyeloperoxidase. Am J Clin Pathol. 1995;104:7–16.

8. Hauschild S, Schmitt WH, Csernok E, et al. ANCA in systemic vasculitidies, collagen vascular diseases, rheumatic disorders and inflammatory bowel diseases. Adv Exp Med Biol. 1993;336:245–51.

9. Falk RJ, Hagan S, Carey TS, et al. Clinical course of anti-neutrophil cytoplasmic antibody associated glomerulonephritis and systemic vasculitis. Ann Intern Med. 1990;113:656–63.

10. Hoffman GS, Kerr GS, Leavett. Wegener's granulomatosis: an analysis of 158 patients. Ann Intern Med. 1992;116:488–98.

11. Daum DE, Specks, Colby TV, et al. Tracheobronchial involvement in Wegener's granulomatosis. Am J Respir Crit Care Med. 1995;151:522–6.

12. Cordier JR, Valeyre D, Guillevin L, et al. Pulmonary Wegener's granulomatosis. A clinical and imaging study of 77 cases. Chest. 1990;97:906–12.

13. Nishino H, Rubino FA, DeRemee RA, et al. Neurologic involvement in Wegener's granulomatosis: an analysis of 324 patients seen at the Mayo Clinic. Ann Neurol. 1993;33:4–9.

14. Lanham JG, Elkin KB, Pusey CD, Hughes GR. Systemic vasculitis with asthma and eosinophilia: a clinical approach to the Churg–Strauss syndrome. Medicine. 1984;63:65–81.

15. Fauci AS, Haynes BF, Katz P, Wolff SM. Wegener's granulomatosis: prospective clinical and therapeutic experience with 85 patients for 21 years. Ann Intern Med. 1983;98:76–85.

16. Stegeman CA, Cohen-Tervant JW, DeJing PE, et al. Trimethoprim–sulfamethoxazole (co-trimethoxazole) for the prevention of relapses in Wegener's granulomatosis. N Engl J Med. 1996;335:16–20.

17. Schwarz MI. Diffuse alveolar hemorrhage. In: Schwarz MI, King TE, eds. Interstitial lung disease, 3rd edn. Hamilton: BC Decker; 1998:535–8.

18. Travis WD, Colby TV, Lombard C, Carpenter HA. A clinicopathologic study of 34 cases of diffuse pulmonary hemorrhage with lung biopsy information. Am J Surg Pathol. 1990;14:1112–5.

19. Savage COS, Winearls CG, Evans DV, et al. Microscopic polyarteritis: presentation, pathology and prognosis. Q J Med. 1985;56:467–83.

20. Zamora MR, Warner ML, Tuder R, Schwarz MI. Diffuse alveolar hemorrhage and systemic lupus erythematosus: clinical presentation, histology, survival and outcome. Medicine. 1997;76:192–201.

21. Kelly PT, Haponik EF. Goodpasture's syndrome: molecular and clinical advances. Medicine. 1994;73:171–85.

22. Jennings CA, King TE, Tuder R, Cherniack RM, Schwarz MI. Diffuse alveolar hemorrhage with underlying isolated, pauciimmune pulmonary capillaritis. Am J Respir Crit Care Med. 1997;155:1101–9.

23. Thadani V, Borrow C, Whitaker W, et al. Pulmonary venoocclusive disease. Q J Med. 1975;44:133–59.

24 Schwarz MI, Cherniack RM, King TE. Diffuse alveolar hemorrhage and other rare pulmonary infiltrative disorders. In: Murray J, Nadel J, eds. Textbook of respiratory medicine, 2nd edn.Philadelphia:WB Saunders; 1993:1889–912.

25. Schwarz MI, Mortenson RL, Colby TV, et al. Pulmonary capillaritis: the association with progressive airflow limitation and hyperinflation. Am Rev Respir Dis. 1993:548:507–11.

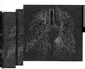
Immunosuppressive therapy for the major pulmonary complications of connective tissue diseases				
Drug	**Dose**	**Duration**	**Comments**	**Monitoring**
Azathioprine	2.5mg/kg per day; max 200mg/day	Continuous	Maximal effect may not be evident for 6–9 months, but has better adverse-effect profile than cyclophosphamide; may be used long term; starting dose 50mg daily with monitoring full blood count in case of thiopurine methyltransferase deficiency, maintenance dose from 1 month	Full blood count Liver function tests
Cyclophosphamide, p.o.	2mg/kg per day	Variable	Oral cyclophosphamide may be used continuously or substituted at 3 months for azathioprine because of more favorable adverse-effect profile in diffuse interstitial lung disease	Full blood count
Cyclophosphamide, i.v.	15mg/kg monthly for 1–6 months	Variable	Intravenous therapy for rapid induction of remission at 2–4mg/kg per day for 3–4 days, especially for vasculitis; pulsed i.v. cyclophosphamide may be given at 1–3 monthly intervals, with better adverse-effect profile and lower long-term cumulative dose, particularly in nonvasculitic disease	Liver function tests Urinalysis for blood
Cyclosporin A	5mg/kg per day	Continuous	Bioavailability variable, thus blood monitoring necessary; may be used in combination with prednisolone	Blood pressure Urea and creatinine Cyclosporin level
Methotrexate	7.5–25mg/week	Continuous	Little information to support use except as second-line therapy after first-line treatment; pulmonary toxicity may be limiting	Full blood count Liver function tests
Prednisolone	1mg/kg per day or 20mg alternate days	Continuous	Prednisolone used alone in high dose for cellular diffuse interstitial lung disease and then titrated to control; in conjunction with immunosuppressants, the low-dose regimen is used	Blood pressure Blood glucose Weight
Methylprednisolone, i.v.	500–1000mg daily	3–5 days	Used for aggressive induction of remission, particularly for vasculitis or acute pneumonitis, then followed by maintenance therapy of prednisolone or prednisolone plus immunosuppressive agent	

Figure 53.17 Immunosuppressive therapy. Common drugs used in the treatment of the major pulmonary complications of connective tissue diseases.

should not be expected to do more than stabilize obliterative bronchiolitis at best.

High-dose corticosteroids given intravenously at the inception of treatment is the mainstay of treatment for organizing pneumonia. Response is usually rapid and complete (see Fig. 53.18), but the condition may have a relapsing, remitting course once corticosteroids are tapered. Occasionally, immunosuppression is required as a corticosteroid-sparing strategy.

Vessel disease

Vasculitis must be treated aggressively – the most accepted regimen is high-dose corticosteroids, together with oral or pulsed cyclophosphamide. Other medications and approaches include azathioprine (often after 3 months of cyclophosphamide), methotrexate, plasmapheresis, and intravenous immunoglobulin.

Vessel disease in PSS is treated differently because it is not a vasculitis. Vasodilators such as captopril and nifedipine are effective in acute studies, and more modestly so in longer term trials, but the high doses required for meaningful improvements in pulmonary vascular resistance often produce unacceptable side effects, such as systemic hypotension and peripheral edema. Clinically significant benefit has not yet been demonstrated, although studies with continuous infusion of prostacyclin are in progress. Calcitonin gene-related peptide has also been tried. At present, pulmonary hypertension continues to be a major cause of mortality in PSS.

Anticoagulation is indicated when pulmonary hypertension is documented.

Pleural disease

Large, persistent, or symptomatic effusions may rarely require treatment with systemic corticosteroids or other immunosuppressive agents. Occasionally, intercostal catheter drainage and pleurodesis have been used.

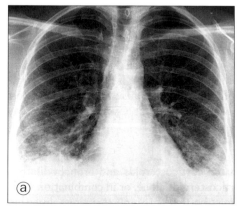
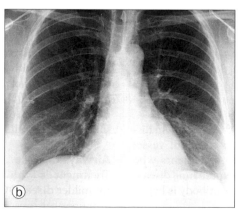

Figure 53.18 Organizing pneumonia.
(a) Radiographically, organizing pneumonia is characterized by diffuse patchy bilateral consolidation. Lung biopsy is required to confirm the diagnosis as there are multiple causes of bilateral consolidation. (b) The radiograph (see biopsy clip, right mid zone) reveals marked radiologic clearance after treatment with corticosteroids.

CLINICAL COURSE AND PREVENTION

The treatment of lung disease in CTD can give rise to two pulmonary complications – opportunistic infection and idiosyncratic, drug-induced lung disease (Fig. 53.19)[23]. Infection is relatively easy to exclude. Differentiation of drug-induced from disease-induced lung problems is more difficult because of the wide range of drug effects that can also affect all compartments. Symptoms are usually subacute. Clinical signs and the results of lung function tests are dependent on the specific compartment(s) involved. Peripheral blood eosinophilia may be seen with methotrexate, but blood tests are not helpful in general. Characteristically, BAL returns an excess of lymphocytes that are predominantly CD8-positive, and eosinophilic parenchymal infiltration is reflected in BAL. Occasionally, biopsy is needed to confirm the pattern of disease. As a general rule, if a patient is receiving any therapy at, or prior to, the time of presentation with pulmonary complaints or findings, drug-induced disease must always be considered. Treatment is drug withdrawal, but occasionally, in severe cases, corticosteroid treatment is required.

Supportive therapy should include assistance with cessation of smoking and the early treatment of infection and heart failure. Influenza and pneumococcal vaccinations are recommended. Long-term oxygen therapy is considered if hypoxia is chronic, as this provides general systemic support, especially of renal function.

Transplantation, either single lung or heart–lung, is considered if the systemic aspects of the CTD disease are not severe and are under satisfactory control. Adequate renal function is essential.

Smoking cessation is critical in patients who have RA, since lung involvement in this condition seems to be more common in smokers. Patients who have PSS, DM/PM, or mixed CTD should have maximal prophylaxis against esophageal reflux and aspiration.

PITFALLS AND CONTROVERSIES

The major pitfall associated with caring for patients who have CTD-associated lung disease is that the lung problem is frequently diagnosed at a far-advanced stage, which limits the possibility of meaningful therapeutic intervention. Patients who have CTD should be frequently screened for pulmonary involvement, even in absence of symptoms.

Another problem is the difficulty in differentiating CTD-associated lung disease from disease caused by a medication used to treat the CTD. Although it seems prudent to monitor patients who receive such agents on a regular basis, the utility of such an approach has not yet been documented.

Advances in diagnosis, treatment, or possible prevention of CTD-associated lung diseases are limited by lack of knowledge. For progress to be made, more epidemiologic data are needed to define the true prevalence and incidence rates of the various types of lung involvement. Accordingly, all patients who have CTD should be screened for lung diseases with at least a chest radiograph and exercise oximetry, and any evidence of lung problems should be followed up with a full evaluation. It may be necessary to utilize lung biopsy more frequently than is the general rule, so that specific lung conditions may be identified. Finally, prospective, randomized clinical trials are needed to evaluate the therapies summarized above. The paucity of patients who have CTD-associated lung disease requires that such trials will, of necessity, be multicenter.

Toxicity of drugs commonly used to treat connective tissue diseases and patterns of lung disease					
Pulmonary effect	Drug				
	Penicill-amine	Metho-trexate	Gold	Cyclophos-phamide	Sulfa-salazine
Hypersensitivity pneumonitis		+	+		
Pulmonary infiltrate with eosinophilia	++	++	+	+	+
Fibrosing alveolitis	++	++	+	+	+
Obliterative bronchiolitis	+		+		
Organizing pneumonia	+		+		+
Pleural effusion/thickening	+	+		+	+
Alveolar hemorrhage/vasculitis	++				+
Anaphylaxis/bronchospasm	+	+		+	
Acute pulmonary edema		+		+	+

Figure 53.19 Drug toxicity. Patterns of lung disease that have been reported as adverse effects of drugs commonly used to treat connective tissue diseases. Bold entries indicate the most common pulmonary complication of treatment with these drugs.

REFERENCES

1. Corrin B. Pathology of interstitial lung disease. Semin Respir Crit Care Med. 1994;15:61–76.
2. Remy-Jardin M, Remy J, Cortet B, et al. Lung changes in rheumatoid arthritis: CT findings. Radiology. 1994;193:375–82.
3. Green RJ, Ruoss SJ, Kraft SA, et al. Pulmonary capillaritis and alveolar haemorrhage. Update on diagnosis and management. Chest. 1996;110:1305–16.
4. Lynch PJ, DeRemee RA, eds. Immunologically mediated pulmonary diseases. Philadelphia: JB Lippincott; 1991.
5. Cannon GW, Zimmerman GA, eds. The lung in rheumatic diseases. New York, Basel: Marcel Dekker; 1990.
6. Klippel JH, Dieppe PA, eds. Rheumatology. London: Mosby; 1994.
7. Wells AU, Hansell DM, du Bois RM. Interstitial lung disease in the collagen vascular diseases. Semin Respir Crit Care Med. 1993;14:333–43.
8. Anaya JM, Diethelm L, Ortiz LA, et al. Pulmonary involvement in rheumatoid arthritis. Semin Arthritis Rheum. 1995;24:242–54.
9. Wells AU, Hansell DM, Rubens MB, et al. Fibrosing alveolitis in systemic sclerosis: indices of lung function in relation to extent of disease on computed tomography. Arthritis Rheum. 1997;40:1229–36.
10. Kane GC, Varga J, Conant EF, et al. Lung involvement in systemic sclerosis (scleroderma): relation to classification based on extent of skin involvement or autoantibody status. Respir Med. 1996;90:223–30.

11. Clements PJ, Furst DE, eds. Systemic sclerosis. Baltimore: Williams and Wilkins; 1996.

12. Derderian SS, Tellis CJ, Abbrecht PH, et al. Pulmonary involvement in mixed connective tissue disease. Chest. 1985;88:45–8.

13. Marguerie C, Bunn CC, Beynon HLC, et al. Polymyositis pulmonary fibrosis and autoantibodies to aminoacyl tRNA synthetase enzymes. Q J Med. 1990;77:1019–38.

14. Tanoue LT. Pulmonary involvement in collagen vascular disease: a review of the pulmonary manifestations of the Marfan syndrome, ankylosing spondylitis, Sjögrens syndrome and relapsing polychondritis. J Thorac Imaging. 1992;7:62–77.

15. Wells AU, Hansell DM, Harrison NK, et al. Clearance of DTPA predicts the clinical course of fibrosing alveolitis. Eur Respir J. 1993;6:797–802.

16. Vitalli C, Viegei G, Tassoni S, et al. Lung function in different connective tissue diseases. Clin Rheumatol. 1986;5:181–8.

17. Roca J, Whipp BJ, ERS Task Force. Clinical exercise testing with reference to lung diseases: indications standardisation and interpretation strategies. Eur Respir J. 1997;10:2662–89.

18. Wallaert B, Hatron P-Y, Grosbois J-M, et al. Subclinical pulmonary involvement in collagen vascular diseases assessed by bronchoalveolar lavage. Am Rev Respir Dis. 1986;133:574–80.

19. Yousem SA, Colby TV, Carrington CB. Lung biopsy in rheumatoid arthritis. Am Rev Respir Dis. 1985;131:770–7.

20. du Bois RM. Diffuse lung disease: an approach to management. Br Med J. 1994;309:175–9.

21. Lynch JP II,I McCune WJ. Immunosuppressive and cytotoxic pharmacotherapy for pulmonary disorders. Am J Respir Crit Care Med. 1997;155:395–420.

22. Walters EH, du Bois RM. Immunology and management of interstitial lung diseases. London: Chapman and Hall; 1995.

23. Foucher P, Biour M, Blayac JP, et al. Drugs that may injure the respiratory system. Eur Respir J. 1997;10:265–79.

Chapter 54

Pregnancy

Stephen Lapinsky and Arthur Slutsky

The pregnant patient who has pulmonary disease presents a unique challenge to the physician, with regard to altered maternal physiology, the occurrence of diseases specific to pregnancy, and the need to consider two patients in all therapeutic decisions. In this chapter the focus is on the changes in pulmonary physiology associated with pregnancy, certain pregnancy-specific disorders, and other pulmonary diseases encountered in the pregnant patient.

PULMONARY PHYSIOLOGY

Physiologic changes in pregnancy

Hormonal changes in pregnancy affect the upper respiratory tract, and cause airway hyperemia, edema, and increased friability. Estrogens are likely responsible for many of these effects, by producing capillary congestion and hyperplasia of mucus glands. Changes to the thoracic cage result both from the enlarging uterus and from hormonal effects that produce ligamentous laxity. The diaphragm is displaced cephalad by up to 4cm, but the potential loss of lung capacity is partially offset by an increase in the anteroposterior and transverse diameters, and by widening of the subcostal angle (Fig. 54.1)[1]. Despite these anatomic changes, diaphragmatic function remains normal and diaphragmatic excursion is not reduced[2]. The maximum transdiaphragmatic inspiratory pressures that can be generated near term are similar to values generated by patients who are not pregnant. The changes in the chest wall return to normal within 6 months of delivery, although the costal angle may remain widened.

The above changes in the thorax produce a progressive decrease in functional residual capacity (FRC), which is reduced by 10–25% by term (see Fig. 54.2)[1]. Residual volume decreases slightly, but the major change is in expiratory reserve volume. These alterations are measurable at 16–24 weeks gestation, and progress to term. The increased diameter of the thoracic cage and the preserved respiratory muscle function allow the vital capacity to remain unchanged, and total lung capacity decreases only minimally. Measurements of airflow and lung compliance are not affected, but chest wall and total respiratory compliance are reduced in the third trimester because of the chest wall changes and increased abdominal pressure[3]. Inconsistencies in results reported in studies of diffusing capacity during pregnancy are likely to arise from the effects of anemia, variable changes in intravascular volume, and the increase in cardiac output. A small increase may be noted in early pregnancy with a subsequent decrease to normal values by term.

Minute ventilation increases markedly in pregnancy, beginning in the first trimester and reaching 20–40% above baseline at term (see Fig. 54.2). The change is associated with an increase in tidal volume of about 30–35%[4]. These changes are mediated by

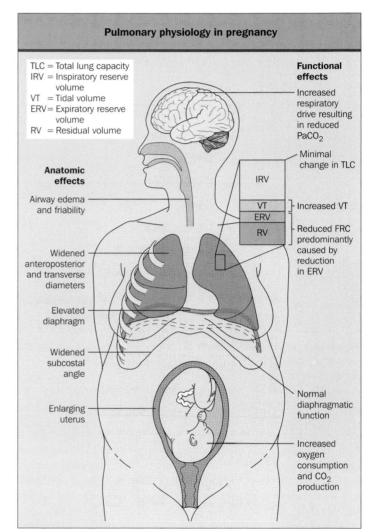

Pulmonary physiology in pregnancy

TLC = Total lung capacity
IRV = Inspiratory reserve volume
VT = Tidal volume
ERV = Expiratory reserve volume
RV = Residual volume

Anatomic effects

Airway edema and friability

Widened anteroposterior and transverse diameters

Elevated diaphragm

Widened subcostal angle

Enlarging uterus

Functional effects

Increased respiratory drive resulting in reduced $PaCO_2$

Minimal change in TLC

IRV

VT — Increased VT
ERV

RV — Reduced FRC predominantly caused by reduction in ERV

Normal diaphragmatic function

Increased oxygen consumption and CO_2 production

Figure 54.1 Pulmonary physiology in pregnancy. Anatomic and functional effects of pregnancy that influence pulmonary physiology.

the increase in respiratory drive that results from elevated serum progesterone levels. A respiratory alkalosis with compensatory renal excretion of bicarbonate results, with partial pressure of carbon dioxide ($PaCO_2$) falling to 3.7–4.3kPa (28–32mmHg) and plasma bicarbonate falling to 18–21mmol/L[4]. Alveolar-to-arterial oxygen tension differences (PAO_2–PaO_2) are similar to nonpregnant values, and mean PaO_2 generally exceeds 13.3kPa (100mmHg) at sea-level throughout pregnancy. Mild hypoxemia and an increased PAO_2–PaO_2 may develop in the supine position because of airway closure as FRC diminishes near term. A recent study, carried out at moderate altitude, suggests that shunt is

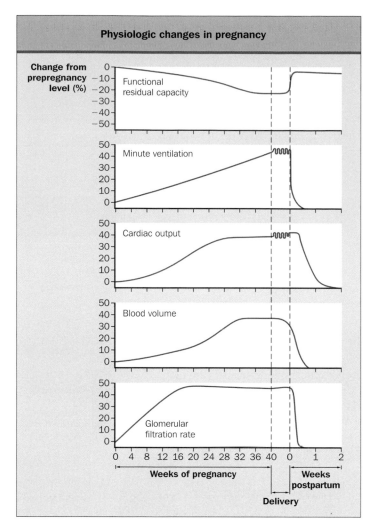

Physiologic changes in pregnancy

Figure 54.2 Physiologic changes in pregnancy. Shown are some of the physiologic changes that occur during pregnancy and the postpartum period. (Reproduced with permission from Lapinsky SE, Kruczynski K, and Slutsky AS. Critical care in the pregnant patient. Am J Respir Crit Care Med. 1995;152:427–55.)

normally increased in the third trimester to about 15%, and is not changed significantly by posture[5]. Oxygen consumption increases, beginning in the first trimester, and reaches 20–33% above baseline by the third trimester, because of fetal demands and maternal metabolic processes. The combination of a reduced FRC and increased oxygen consumption lowers oxygen reserve, which renders the pregnant patient susceptible to the rapid development of hypoxia in response to hypoventilation or apnea[1].

During labor, hyperventilation increases and tachypnea (caused by pain or anxiety) may result in marked respiratory alkalosis. Superimposed metabolic alkalosis can be produced by volume depletion and vomiting. Alkalosis adversely affects fetal oxygenation by reducing uterine blood flow. In some patients, severe pain and anxiety may lead to rapid, shallow breathing with alveolar hypoventilation, atelectasis, and mild hypoxemia. Achieving adequate pain relief with narcotics or epidural analgesia blunts the ventilatory response, and can correct the gas exchange abnormalities associated with active labor. The pregnancy-associated changes in lung function reverse significantly in the first 72 hours postpartum, and return to baseline within a few weeks.

Dyspnea in pregnancy

Dyspnea is a common complaint in women who have otherwise normal pregnancies, and often is an isolated symptom that results from the normal physiologic changes in the respiratory system. Although a number of mechanisms have been proposed, the symptom most likely arises from a normal perception of the increased minute ventilation that accompanies pregnancy[6].

PREGNANCY-SPECIFIC DISORDERS

Amniotic fluid embolism

Epidemiology and pathophysiology

Amniotic fluid embolism is a rare (between 1/8,000 and 1/80,000 live births), but potentially catastrophic obstetric complication (mortality 10–86%)[7] that may account for 10% of maternal deaths. Amniotic fluid embolism is usually associated with labor and delivery, but it may also occur with uterine manipulations, uterine trauma, or in the early postpartum period[8]. The mechanism appears to involve amniotic fluid that enters the vascular circulation through endocervical veins or uterine tears. Particulate cellular contents or humoral factors in the amniotic fluid produce acute, pulmonary hypertension, both by obstructing the pulmonary vessels and by causing vascular spasm (Fig. 54.3). Acute, left-ventricular dysfunction may also occur[9], either secondary to the initial pulmonary embolic event or in response to humoral events mediated by cytokines. It was recently suggested that the cardiovascular changes of amniotic fluid embolism closely resemble those of anaphylaxis, and sensitivity to amniotic fluid contents may be responsible[7].

Clinical features

The clinical presentation usually involves the sudden onset of severe dyspnea, hypoxemia, and cardiovascular collapse, often accompanied by seizures. Less common presentations are with hemorrhage caused by disseminated intravascular coagulation, or with fetal distress[8]. Up to half of the patients may die within the first hour, and cardiac arrest during this period is common.

Diagnosis

The diagnosis of amniotic fluid embolism is usually based on observing the typical clinical picture. Fetal squames in a wedged pulmonary capillary aspirate have been used to confirm the diagnosis, but this does not appear to be a specific finding. Newer, less invasive diagnostic tests may soon be available (e.g. monoclonal antibodies to fetal mucin, measurement of maternal serum zinc coproporphyrin).

The differential diagnosis includes septic shock, pulmonary thromboembolism, abruptio placentae, tension pneumothorax, or a myocardial ischemic event.

Treatment

Treatment involves routine resuscitative and supportive measures, with prompt attention to adequate oxygenation, mechanical ventilation, and inotropic support. No specific therapy has been shown to be effective, but some suggest a role for corticosteroids[7]. In view of the inconsistent hemodynamic findings, invasive monitoring may be of value.

Clinical course and prevention

Survivors of the initial resuscitation are likely to develop the complications of disseminated intravascular coagulation and/or

Pathophysiology of amniotic fluid embolism

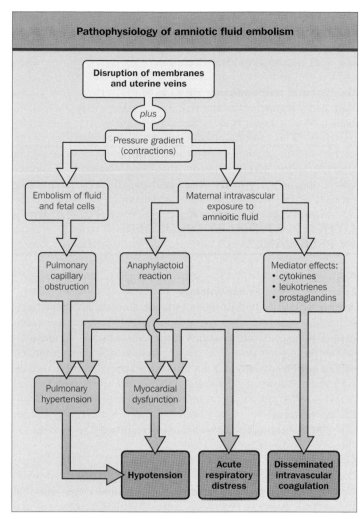

Figure 54.3 Pathophysiology of amniotic fluid embolism. Proposed pathophysiologic mechanisms for the development of circulatory shock caused by amniotic fluid embolism.

Acute respiratory distress in pregnancy

Disorder	Distinguishing features
Amniotic fluid embolism	Cardiorespiratory collapse, seizures, disseminated intravascular coagulopathy
Pulmonary edema secondary to pre-eclampsia	Hypertension, proteinuria
Tocolytic pulmonary edema	Tocolytic administration, rapid improvement
Aspiration pneumonitis	Vomiting, aspiration
Peripartum cardiomyopathy	Gradual onset, cardiac gallop
Venous thromboembolism	Evidence of deep venous thrombosis; positive ventilation–perfusion scan, venous Doppler's, angiogram
Pneumomediastinum	Occurs during delivery, subcutaneous emphysema
Air embolism	Sudden hypotension, cardiac murmur

Figure 54.4 Causes of acute respiratory distress related to pregnancy and labor.

often in response to maternal tachycardia and/or hypotension induced by β-stimulation and reduced oncotic pressure. Gluco-corticoids are often administered in preterm labor to enhance fetal lung maturity and may compound fluid retention[10].

Clinical features
The clinical presentation is of acute respiratory distress with features of pulmonary edema. No specific features characterize this condition.

Diagnosis
The diagnosis is a clinical one, made in the presence of acute pulmonary edema occurring in the appropriate clinical situation. The differential diagnosis includes cardiogenic pulmonary edema, amniotic fluid embolism, and other conditions (Fig. 54.4). Failure of the pulmonary edema to resolve in 12–24 hours prompts a search for alternative causes.

Treatment and clinical course
The β-agonist must be discontinued, whereupon pulmonary edema should resolve rapidly; additional treatment is supportive and includes diuresis. Early recognition and management should reduce the need for invasive, hemodynamic monitoring and mechanical ventilation.

Pitfalls and controversies
Recent studies suggest that tocolytics do not improve the outcome in preterm labor[11]. Accordingly, prolonged use of these agents may become less common. The condition remains of physiologic interest as the pathophysiology has not yet been clarified.

Pre-eclampsia and pulmonary edema
Epidemiology and pathophysiology
Pulmonary edema may rarely occur in association with pre-eclampsia (i.e. perhaps 3% of pre-eclamptic patients)[12]. The pre-eclamptic patient is usually volume depleted, and pulmonary edema most commonly occurs in the early postpartum period, and is often associated with aggressive, intrapartum fluid replacement. Other factors that may contribute to the pathogenesis include reduced serum albumin, elevated left ventricular afterload, and systolic

acute respiratory distress syndrome (ARDS). Neurologic damage caused by hypotension and hypoxemia is common.

Pitfalls and controversies
Predisposing factors, pathophysiology, and therapy of this condition are poorly understood. Accordingly, given that only supportive therapy can be undertaken, little can be done to prevent the condition or to reduce its morbidity or mortality. Concerns regarding use of Swan–Ganz catheters, oxygen toxicity, and/or ventilator-induced acute lung injury apply to the resuscitative measures used in this setting.

Tocolytic pulmonary edema
Epidemiology and pathophysiology
β-Adrenergic agonists, particularly ritodrine and terbutaline, are used to inhibit uterine contractions in preterm labor. A complication of β-agonists that is unique to pregnancy is the development of pulmonary edema[9]. The frequency of tocolytic-induced pulmonary edema varies in published series, from 0.3 to 9%[9,10]. Postulated mechanisms include prolonged exposure to catecholamines, which causes myocardial dysfunction, increased capillary permeability, large volumes of intravenous fluid administration,

and diastolic myocardial dysfunction (Fig. 54.5). Increased capillary permeability may also occur, aggravated by concomitant conditions such as sepsis, abruptio placentae, or massive hemorrhage.

Pulmonary edema has been described in chronically hypertensive, obese, pregnant patients who develop pre-eclampsia. Diastolic left ventricular dysfunction results from both the hypertension and the obesity, and pulmonary edema is precipitated by volume overload of pregnancy and hemodynamic stresses of pre-eclampsia[13].

Clinical features
The presentation is of acute respiratory distress in the pre-eclamptic patient, often in the early postpartum period.

Diagnosis
Pre-eclampsia is characterized by hypertension, proteinuria, and peripheral edema, usually in the third trimester.

Treatment and clinical course
The standard approach is to restrict fluid, and to administer supplemental oxygen and diuresis. Invasive monitoring may be useful if inotropic or vasodilator therapy becomes necessary, particularly in the presence of renal dysfunction. Aggressive diuresis must be avoided, as filling pressures cannot be reduced to the point of compromising cardiac output and reducing placental perfusion. The ultimate treatment of pre-eclampsia is delivery of the fetus.

Pitfalls and controversies
The 'best' approach to fluid therapy is controversial. Volume replacement may be necessary as these patients may be markedly volume depleted, particularly if vasodilators are used. Excessive fluid replacement may precipitate pulmonary or cerebral edema, however. Accordingly, many recommend invasive hemodynamic monitoring.

Peripartum cardiomyopathy
Cardiac failure may occur in the absence of pre-existing heart disease as a result of the hypertension of pregnancy, and/or from peripartum cardiomyopathy. This idiopathic condition presents in the last month of pregnancy or in the postpartum period, and is associated with increased mortality. During labor and the early postpartum period, tachycardia and increased cardiac output may precipitate pulmonary edema.

Gestational trophoblastic disease
Pulmonary hypertension and pulmonary edema may complicate benign hydatidiform mole, caused by trophoblastic pulmonary embolism. This most commonly occurs during evacuation of the uterus, and the incidence of pulmonary complications is higher in later gestations. Molar pregnancy may be associated with choriocarcinoma, which can produce multiple, discrete pulmonary metastases, and occasionally pleural effusions.

OTHER PULMONARY DISORDERS IN PREGNANCY

Asthma
Epidemiology and pathophysiology
Asthma affects 5–10% of the population and can, accordingly, be expected to affect a similar proportion of pregnant women; during pregnancy, asthma may improve, worsen, or remain[14]. While pregnancy does not affect airflow in normal subjects, airway hyperreactivity can be altered. Asthma severity usually returns to pre-pregnancy levels within 3 months postpartum.

Clinical features
The clinical features of asthma during pregnancy are the same as those in patients who are not pregnant.

Diagnosis
Objective assessment using pulmonary function tests is essential to assess the presence of airflow obstruction. The incidence of gastroesophageal reflux is increased in both frequency and severity during pregnancy, so the appropriate symptoms should be sought.

Treatment
Management is similar to that in patients who are not pregnant (Fig. 54.6)[15,16], and includes adequate monitoring, avoidance of precipitating factors, and adequate education. While physicians may be reluctant to prescribe medications during pregnancy, poorly controlled asthma is potentially more dangerous for the fetus[15]. Inhaled corticosteroids remain the mainstay of therapy. Beclomethasone has been used in pregnant patients for many years without significant adverse effects. The use of a spacer device is encouraged, to reduce local side effects and systemic absorption. While animal data suggest a small risk of cleft palate with systemic corticosteroid use, this has not been demonstrated in humans. Short courses of prednisone should be used to manage poorly controlled asthma where clinically indicated. Inhaled β-agonists appear safe and should be used as required for symptomatic relief. Acute attacks are treated by ensuring adequate oxygenation, closely monitoring the fetus, and administering appropriate medications. Antireflux measures may markedly reduce asthmatic symptoms.

Clinical course and prevention
An increased incidence of preterm births, low birth weight, and increased perinatal mortality have been reported, largely related to poor asthma control. Acute exacerbations may be associated with hypoxemia which may, in turn, compromise the fetus.

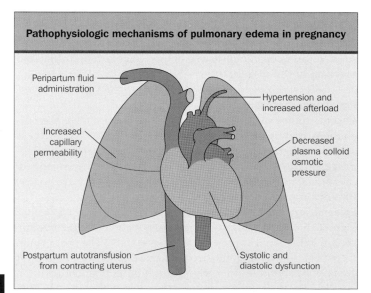

Pathophysiologic mechanisms of pulmonary edema in pregnancy

Peripartum fluid administration

Hypertension and increased afterload

Increased capillary permeability

Decreased plasma colloid osmotic pressure

Postpartum autotransfusion from contracting uterus

Systolic and diastolic dysfunction

Figure 54.5 Pathophysiologic mechanisms responsible for the development of pulmonary edema in pre-eclampsia.

Asthma therapy in pregnancy		
Drug	**Clinical use**	**US Food and Drug Administration Classification**
Inhaled bronchodilators		
Albuterol (salbutamol)	Common	C
Terbutaline	Common	B
Ipratropium	Occasional	C
Inhaled corticosteroids		
Beclomethasone	Common	C
Budesonide	Less experience and data	C
Fluticasone	Limited experience and data	C
Theophylline	Uncommon	C
Cromolyn (cromoglycate)	Occasional	B
Systemic corticosteroids	If necessary	B

Figure 54.6 Asthma therapy in pregnancy. Clinically used drugs and US Food and Drug Administration classification of drug safety in pregnancy. (Category A, human studies fail to demonstrate fetal harm; B, animal studies fail to demonstrate harm, but no human studies or animal studies demonstrate risk not shown in human studies; C, animal studies demonstrate risk or insufficient data available – drugs may be used if benefit outweighs risk; D, human studies demonstrate risk – drugs may be used if benefits justify the risks; X, contraindicated in pregnancy.)

Pitfalls and controversies

Concerns for fetal effects of drugs should not cause physicians and patients to avoid inappropriately the use of effective pharmacologic therapy. Gastroesophageal reflux, a potentially preventable cause of asthma, is frequently overlooked.

Pulmonary thromboembolic disease

Epidemiology and pathophysiology

Pulmonary thromboembolism occurs in up to 1.3% of pregnancies, both during pregnancy and in the postpartum period; it is an important cause of maternal mortality[17]. The increased incidence results from a hypercoagulable state that occurs with pregnancy, from hormonally mediated venous stasis, and from local pressure effects of the uterus on the inferior vena cava. Pulmonary embolism occurs more frequently in the early postpartum period than during pregnancy, particularly after cesarean section[18]. Deep venous thrombosis occurs with almost equal frequency in all trimesters.

Clinical features

The presentation is similar to that in the patient who is not pregnant. However, the clinical diagnosis of deep venous thrombosis and pulmonary embolism is notoriously inaccurate. The overwhelming predilection for left-leg deep venous thrombosis in pregnancy is likely to be the result of anatomic factors[17].

Diagnosis

Investigation of suspected pulmonary embolism follows a similar approach to that in the patient who is not pregnant, and the diagnosis must be pursued aggressively. Duplex ultrasound is useful for the diagnosis of deep venous thrombosis, although venous Doppler can give false-positive results because of venous obstruction by the gravid uterus[17]. Ventilation–perfusion scanning can be performed with <0.5mGy (<50mrad) exposure to the fetus and, if necessary, a pulmonary angiogram via the brachial route may be carried

Management of thromboembolic disease in pregnancy – fetal risk of diagnostic procedures		
Investigation	**Fetal radiation exposure (mGy)**	**Comments**
Duplex ultrasound	Nil	Initial procedure of choice, false positives from ultrasound alone
Chest radiograph (abdomen shielded)	0.01–0.08	Minimal risk
Ventilation–perfusion scan		
Perfusion	0.06–0.12	Low risk, begin with perfusion scan
Ventilation	0.04–0.35	
Pulmonary angiogram		
Brachial route	c. 0.5	Perform if indicated
Femoral route	2.2–4.0	

Figure 54.7 Management of thromboembolic disease in pregnancy. Fetal risk of diagnostic procedures.

Management of thromboembolic disease in pregnancy – treatment of pulmonary thromboembolism		
Therapy	**US Food and Drug Administration classification**	**Comments**
Heparin	C	Treatment of choice
Low-molecular-mass heparin	B/C	Increasing evidence of safety
Warfarin	X	Embryopathy and central nervous system abnormalities
Thrombolytics	C	Consider in acute, life-threatening situations

Figure 54.8 Management of thromboembolic disease in pregnancy. Treatment of pulmonary thromboembolism. (Category A, human studies fail to demonstrate fetal harm; B, animal studies fail to demonstrate harm, but no human studies or animal studies demonstrate risk not shown in human studies; C, animal studies demonstrate risk or insufficient data available – drugs may be used if benefit outweighs risk; D, human studies demonstrate risk – drugs may be used if benefits justify the risks; X, contraindicated in pregnancy.

out with similarly low fetal exposure (Fig. 54.7)[19]. Such levels of exposure are not associated with teratogenicity, although an increased incidence of childhood leukemia has been documented with fetal exposure of <50mGy (<5000mrad)[19].

Treatment

Warfarin therapy during the first trimester has been associated with development of an embryopathy, and central nervous system abnormalities have been described with second and third trimester exposure. Accordingly, warfarin should be avoided (Fig. 54.8). The anticoagulant of choice is heparin, which does not cross the placenta, is not associated with adverse fetal outcome, and can be readily reversed[20]. Low molecular weight heparins do not appear to cross the placenta, and increasing clinical evidence suggests that they are both safe and effective in pregnancy[21].

When administered with adequate precautions, streptokinase, urokinase, and tissue plasminogen activator have been used successfully without major hemorrhagic complications or significant

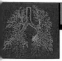

adverse effects on the fetus or placenta[22]. Use of these agents should nevertheless be limited to life-threatening situations. Where clinically indicated, transvenous placement of an inferior vena cava filter can be performed, although there is some risk of dislodgment because of the dilated venous system and pressure effects during labor.

Clinical course and prevention

Women who have a known hypercoagulable state and those who had a previous thromboembolism are at increased risk and should receive prophylaxis with anticoagulation throughout pregnancy.

Pitfalls and controversies

The use of radiologic investigations during pregnancy remains a concern, for both physician and mother. It is nevertheless important to establish a diagnosis of pulmonary embolism because of the major implications if such a diagnosis is missed, and the effects of unnecessary therapy on the health of mother and fetus.

Lower respiratory tract infections
Epidemiology and pathophysiology

Lower respiratory tract infections are an infrequent occurrence, but an important cause of indirect obstetric death. The pregnant patient is susceptible to the usual bacterial pathogens such as *Streptococcus pneumoniae*, *Haemophilus influenzae*, and *Mycoplasma pneumoniae*; less common diseases include varicella pneumonia (Fig. 54.9) and coccidioidomycosis (with dissemination). *Pneumocystic carinii* pneumonia is seen in HIV-positive patients. Pregnancy does not appear to affect the course or incidence of reactivation of tuberculosis.

Clinical features

The clinical features are similar to those in patients who are not pregnant. Although dyspnea is common in pregnancy, the respiratory rate is not elevated by the pregnant state.

Diagnosis

A chest radiograph is essential for the diagnosis of lower respiratory tract infections, and must be considered in any pregnant woman who has a clinical presentation suggestive of pneumonia. Further diagnostic investigations include the usual microbiologic cultures, sputum microscopy, and serologic tests.

Treatment

Tetracyclines should be avoided in pregnancy. Treatment of varicella pneumonitis is with acyclovir, which decreases mortality and has not been associated with fetal anomalies[23]. Coccidioidomycosis is associated with an extremely high mortality and disseminated disease should be treated with antifungal agents. *Pneumocystis carinii* pneumonia requires treatment with trimethoprim–sulfamethoxazole with folate supplementation, as well as with corticosteroids if indicated clinically. While folic acid antagonists and sulfas carry risks for the fetus, pentamidine is associated with higher risks for mother and fetus. Tuberculosis treatment is with isoniazid and rifampin (rifampicin), which have a low risk of adverse fetal effects, as well as ethambutol initially, until sensitivities are available[24].

Clinical course and prevention

While pneumonia is associated with an increased risk of mortality, this is probably attributable to underlying diseases rather

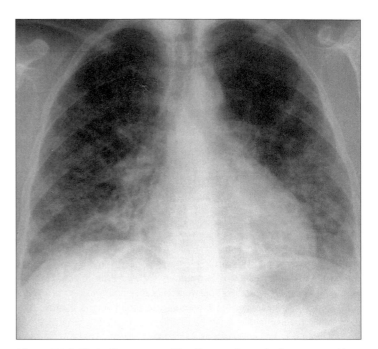

Figure 54.9 Varicella pneumonitis. Chest radiograph of a woman with varicella pneumonitis which developed at 29 weeks gestation. Note the diffuse, bilateral, fluffy nodular infiltrate. (Courtesy of Dr M. Steinhardt, Mount Sinai Hospital, Toronto.)

than to the pneumonia *per se*. Fetal complications may occur, as may preterm labor. Transplacental transmission of varicella-zoster occurs uncommonly (<5%), but can produce limb deformities and neurologic involvement. The nonimmune pregnant woman exposed to varicella-zoster should receive prophylaxis with varicella-zoster immunoglobulin within 96 hours of exposure, and acyclovir if she develops clinical disease. Unlike the treatment of active disease, tuberculosis prophylaxis can usually be deferred until after pregnancy, except in the case of recent exposure or skin-test conversion.

Pitfalls and controversies

When investigating and managing lower respiratory tract infections it is important to consider effects on the fetus (i.e. radiation exposure, drug toxicities), but necessary evaluations and interventions should not be avoided inappropriately.

Acute respiratory distress syndrome in pregnancy
Epidemiology and pathophysiology

The pregnant patient is at risk of developing ARDS from a number of pregnancy-associated problems (Fig. 54.10)[25]. Iatrogenic factors such as excessive fluid administration and tocolytic therapy may contribute, as may a reduced albumin level.

Clinical features

The clinical features are similar to those in the patient who is not pregnant.

Diagnosis

The diagnosis is by the usual criteria of hypoxemia in the presence of diffuse pulmonary infiltrates and in absence of an increased wedge pressure. A detailed history is critical to identification of the underlying problem.

Acute lung injury in pregnancy	
Relationship to pregnancy	Injury
Pregnancy specific	Preeclampsia
	Amniotic fluid embolism
	Chorioamnionitis
	Trophoblastic embolism
Risk increased by pregnancy	Gastric acid aspiration
	Pyelonephritis
	Sepsis
	Air embolism
	Massive hemorrhage
Nonspecific	Trauma
	Drugs/toxins
	Pancreatitis

Figure 54.10 Causes of acute lung injury in pregnancy. Listed are pregnancy-specific diseases, conditions that are more common in pregnancy, and conditions not related to pregnancy.

Treatment

There are no major differences between the management of pregnant patients who have ARDS and that in those who are not pregnant, other than the need for continuous assessment of the fetus. When administering pharmacologic therapy, it is critical to assess the effects on both the fetus and the mother. Ventilatory management includes consideration of the normal physiologic changes of pregnancy. Adequate maternal oxygen saturation is essential for fetal well-being. Alkalosis has an adverse effect on placental perfusion and should be limited. Acidosis appears to be reasonably well tolerated by the fetus. Fetal delivery may benefit both the mother and the fetus. Epidural anesthetic may reduce the increased oxygen demand produced by uterine contractions.

Clinical course and prevention

Survival appears to be similar or better than that in the general population, possibly because of the young age of the patients and the reversibility of many of the predisposing conditions.

Pitfalls and controversies

Specific causes of ARDS that pertain to pregnancy should be sought when assessing patients who have this syndrome. When women of childbearing age present with ARDS, they should be checked for pregnancy.

Pleural disease

While pleural effusions may accompany obstetric complications, such as pre-eclampsia and choriocarcinoma, a significant proportion of women develop small, asymptomatic pleural effusions in the postpartum period. These result from the increased blood volume and reduced colloid osmotic pressure that occur in pregnancy, as well as from impaired lymphatic drainage caused by Valsalva's maneuvers during labor[26]. Moderate size effusions, or the presence of symptoms should prompt a full clinical evaluation. The repeated Valsalva's maneuvers of labor may also cause spontaneous pneumothorax and pneumomediastinum, particularly in patients affected by predisposing conditions such as asthma. This diagnosis should be considered in the patient who develops chest discomfort and dyspnea during, or immediately following, delivery.

Interstitial lung disease

Interstitial lung disease generally occurs in women who are older than their childbearing years. When it exists in pregnant women, however, certain physiologic aspects must be considered. A reduced diffusing capacity may cause difficulty meeting the increased oxygen-consumption requirements of pregnancy. Any pulmonary hypertension carries increased risks as cardiac output must increase during pregnancy. Little data exist on the management and outcome in these patients, but restrictive lung disease appears reasonably well tolerated in pregnancy[27]. Patients who have a vital capacity <1L and those who have pulmonary hypertension should consider avoiding pregnancy[28]. Lymphangioleiomyomatosis and systemic lupus erythematosus may worsen as a result of pregnancy.

Management involves careful assessment and monitoring of respiratory and cardiovascular status. Exercise intolerance is common, and patients may require supplemental oxygen therapy early in pregnancy to avoid hypoxemic episodes, which may be dangerous for the fetus. During labor, maternal effort should be limited, and oxygen saturation must be monitored. Invasive hemodynamic monitoring may be indicated in the presence of pulmonary hypertension.

Obstructive sleep apnea

Pregnancy may be complicated by obstructive sleep apnea (OSA), with potential adverse effects for both the mother and fetus[29]. In general, apnea and hypopnea are uncommon in pregnancy, because of the respiratory stimulatory effect of progesterone. Usually, OSA is confined to obese patients, perhaps being precipitated by the pregnancy-associated airway mucosal edema and vascular congestion. An association occurs between OSA and pre-eclampsia, probably because of the generalized edema that occurs. Nocturnal hypoxemia may adversely affect the fetus, and poor fetal growth has been documented in these patients. Treatment with nasal continuous positive airway pressure (continuous positive airway pressure) is safe and effective. Snoring is not associated with fetal risk and is not a good marker for OSA in pregnant women[29].

Cystic fibrosis

Advances in the management of patients who have cystic fibrosis have extended life expectancy into the childbearing age. Although fertility is impaired, contraception and planned pregnancy should be considered in the management of these patients. Available data indicate that pregnancy does not increase mortality in patients who have stable disease, but poor outcomes can occur in those affected by advanced disease[30,31]. Those who have a forced vital capacity <50% of predicted and pulmonary hypertension prior to pregnancy are at greatest risk[30]. Perinatal mortality is increased, related largely to preterm delivery that occurs spontaneously, or to maternal complications of cystic fibrosis. Management requires a multidisciplinary approach, with careful attention to nutrition, glucose monitoring, and genetic counseling. Respiratory exacerbations require early aggressive therapy, with due consideration of the potential fetal toxicity of antibiotics such as aminoglycosides and quinolones, and the altered maternal pharmacokinetics[32].

Gastric aspiration

Gastric acid aspiration may occur during labor due to delayed gastric emptying, reduced lower esophageal sphincter tone and the effects of increased intra-abdominal pressure. The presentation is

Routine laboratory evaluation of bronchoalveolar lavage specimens after hematopoietic stem cell transplantation	
Pathology	Stains
	Wright–Giemsa stain
	Papanicolaou stain
	Silver stain
	Modified Jimenez stain (or other stain suitable for detecting Legionella spp.)
	Monoclonal fluorescent antibody stain for Pneumocystis carinii (consider in exceptional setting)
Microbiology	Stains
	Gram stain
	Wet mount potassium hydroxide stain or calcofluor white stain
	Modified acid-fast stain
	Fluorescent antibody stain for Legionella spp.
	Culture
	Bacterial (aerobic), semiquantitative method
	Fungal
	Legionella spp. (chocolate yeast extract)
	Acid-fast
Virology	Fluorescent antibody stains
	Cytomegalovirus
	Herpes simplex virus
	Respiratory syncytial virus, parainfluenza and influenza viruses pooled antibodies
	Culture (rapid centrifugation technique preferred)
	Cytomegalovirus
	Herpes simplex virus
	Adenovirus
	Respiratory syncytial virus, parainfluenza, and influenza viruses (in appropriate clinical setting)

Figure 55.11 Routine laboratory evaluation of bronchoalveolar lavage specimens after hematopoietic stem cell transplantation. Fluorescent antibody stains may be supplemented or replaced by enzyme immunoassays as available for detecting respiratory syncytial virus, parainfluenza virus, and influenza virus. Culture for viruses may be replaced with fluorescent antibody stains or enzyme immunoassay alone if culture facilities are unavailable.

Pulmonary infection is confirmed with cytology, histology, or culture. In addition to bacterial, fungal, and cytologic stains, a quantitative bacterial culture should be performed (Fig. 55.11). These specimens should also be processed with rapid detection techniques for viral pathogens. Direct fluorescent monoclonal antibody stains and centrifugation culture (shell vial) are indicated if the patient or donor are seropositive for CMV. Outbreaks of viral pneumonias due to respiratory syncytial virus and parainfluenza virus have recently been recognized in HSCT units. Bronchoalveolar lavage, as well as nasopharyngeal and throat swabs for virologic studies, should be performed to exclude treatable pulmonary infection, especially during autumn and winter.

Focal infiltrates

Focal, multifocal, or patchy infiltrates after HSCT frequently represent bacterial or fungal infection[20]. Bacteria are an unusual cause of diffuse infiltrates. The proportion of focal infiltrates that resolve spontaneously or with empiric antibacterial therapy is unknown. Focal radiographic lesions with a mass-like appearance that develop or persist despite antibiotics at any time after HSCT are, in the

Invasive pulmonary aspergillosis after hematopoietic stem cell transplantation: the bronchogenic carcinoma equivalent
Presentation most often focal
Patients have identified risk factors
Chemotherapy alone of limited value
Cause of death
Spread to brain or heart
Erosion into vessels (causing hemoptysis)
Consider surgical resection
Potentially curative
'Debulking' of devascularized tissue

Figure 55.12 Invasive pulmonary aspergillosis after hematopoietic stem cell transplantation: the bronchogenic carcinoma equivalent.

majority of cases, due to pulmonary fungal infection. The incidence of invasive fungal infections after HSCT has increased to more than than 11%[21]. Occasionally, Legionella, Pseudomonas and (rarely) Nocardia spp. are identified within localized lesions.

Noninfectious causes of focal lung lesions after HSCT include resolving (sterile) abscess, lymphoma or Hodgkin's disease, and organizing pneumonia with bronchiolitis obliterans. A clinical history of recent bacteremia, previous solid tumor, and clinical acute pneumonia that is resolving are important clues to the differential diagnosis. Unfortunately, the absence of fever and clinical symptoms does not exclude the diagnosis of filamentous fungal infection.

Hematopoietic stem cell transplantation recipients with focal pulmonary lesions should be evaluated aggressively because there is a high probability of infection. Computed tomogram scanning of the chest should usually be included in the diagnostic evaluation. A fungal infection often has a mass-like appearance with a zone of attenuation that is highly suggestive of tissue invasion. Additional lesions that are not appreciated on plain chest radiography may also be seen.

The diagnostic approach to localized lesions is dictated by the radiographic appearance and their locations. Areas of apparent bronchopneumonia are approached with fiberoptic bronchoscopy and BAL, whereas peripheral, consolidated lesions are amenable to percutaneous needle aspiration for diagnosis (see Fig. 55.10). A nondiagnostic result by any technique warrants repeated attempts or alternative measures for diagnosis should be tried. If bronchoscopy or needle aspirations are not diagnostic, the most definitive study is biopsy at thoracotomy. Surgical resection should be considered when the pulmonary lesions could be removed completely because this may be both diagnostic and curative in patients with a localized fungal infection (Fig. 55.12).

The presentation of basilar infiltrates without mass-like consolidation that occur within the first several weeks after marrow infusion in the setting of oral mucositis should prompt evaluation for recurrent aspiration. A history of recurrent cough induced by attempts at swallowing or nocturnal paroxysms of cough in the setting of severe mucositis is common. The appropriate approach to such patients is conservative – moderating the administration of sedatives, encouraging pulmonary toilet, and avoiding mucosal bleeding by adequate platelet support. Most patients receive broad-spectrum antibiotics. Rarely, tracheal intubation is required to avoid massive aspiration in a profoundly obtunded patient or acute airway obstruction in the presence of severe upper airway bleeding.

RESPIRATORY FAILURE WITHOUT INFILTRATES

Air-flow limitation and bronchiolitis

Several centers report that 6–10% of allogeneic marrow recipients develop chronic air-flow limitation Most of these cases are among long-term survivors with chronic GVHD. In 70% of the reported cases, the histology of the lungs was obliterative bronchiolitis. The obliterative bronchiolitis lesions in the lungs of marrow transplantation recipients are occasionally, but not always, accompanied by interstitial infiltrates of mononuclear cells. However, interstitial fibrosis and bronchitis without obliteration has also been noted among patients with air-flow limitation. Air-flow limitation with obliterative bronchiolitis has been reported after autologous marrow transplantation[22]. Based on these findings, new-onset air-flow limitation, not the presence of obliterative bronchiolitic lesions, is the hallmark of this problem.

The etiology of obliterative bronchiolitis after marrow transplantation is unknown. Those causes recognized in otherwise normal hosts (e.g. recurrent aspiration, viral infection with influenza, adenovirus or measles, and bacterial or mycoplasma infection) have not been found consistently in marrow recipients with obliterative bronchiolitis. Immunologic mechanisms inducing bronchial epithelial injury are suggested by the strong association between chronic GVHD and the development of obliterative bronchiolitis. Factors associated with the increased risk of GVHD, such as increasing age and HLA-nonidentical marrow grafts, are not independent risk factors for the development of obliterative bronchiolitis. The lung epithelium may be the target of immune-mediated-injury in chronic GVHD through the expression of Ia antigens and subsequent activation of donor cytotoxic T lymphocytes. The reported association with the administration of methotrexate also raises the possibility of direct drug-related injury to the pulmonary bronchial epithelium. Furthermore, there is a higher incidence of decreased levels of IgG among patients with obliterative bronchiolitis than that seen in other marrow recipients. This hypogammaglobulinemia may be a manifestation of the immunologic lesion responsible for the airway disease or it may merely be related to the presence of chronic GVHD.

Air-flow limitation is occasionally seen within 100 days of transplant. Histology is available for fewer of these cases, and the defect is possibly related to airway infection. This early presentation is often associated with acute GVHD.

Clinical presentation and course

Typical manifestations of air-flow limitation due to obliterative bronchiolitis after marrow transplantation are[11]:
- insidious progression of tachypnea;
- dyspnea on exertion; and
- dry, nonproductive cough.

Fever is not common. Physical findings may be minimal. Scattered expiratory wheezing and occasionally diffuse inspiratory crackles may be heard, but chest auscultation is sometimes normal. The chest radiograph is commonly interpreted as normal; however, recent studies reveal almost all affected children have typical abnormalities noted on high-resolution chest CT scans[23].

The diagnosis of air-flow limitation is made among marrow transplantation recipients by routine pulmonary function testing. When the presentation is more than 150 days after marrow trans-

plantation, evidence of chronic GVHD is usually present, although the condition may occur at any time after transplantation.

The syndrome is often progressive and results in death from respiratory failure. A more rapid onset and faster rate of progression is associated with worse outcome[24]. Control of chronic GVHD with increased immunosuppression may achieve stabilization of the airway disease. Patients with gradual declines in air flow tend to have courses that are more benign. Marrow recipients with the onset of air-flow limitation beyond 150 days after transplantation tend to have a more gradual decline in lung function. Air flow may stabilize in 50% of these patients. Reversal of the abnormality is reported in only 8% of cases.

Treatment

There are no prospective studies of the treatment of new-onset air-flow limitation after marrow transplantation. Reduced air flow in the presence of chronic GVHD is managed primarily by controlling the GVHD with increased immunosuppression (Fig. 55.13). Air-flow limitation has improved in some patients with increased immunosuppression. Experience with obliterative bronchiolitis among the recipients of heart–lung transplant suggests the addition of azathioprine (1.0–1.5mg/kg per day) to cyclosporine may be effective in arresting the decline in air flow in these patients. In addition, aerosolized bronchodilator treatment for symptomatic patients is appropriate. Early and aggressive antibiotic treatment for any potential lower respiratory infection should be initiated. Prophylactic trimethoprim–sulfamethoxazole (cotrimoxazole; or another form of prevention of *P. carinii* infection) should be continued for the duration of immune suppression. Routine intravenous replacement of immunoglobulin for those with low class or subclass levels is usual.

Similar immunosuppressive management is recommended for the air-flow limitation that develops early in the transplant course in the absence of chronic GvHD. Evaluation for possible airway infection by respiratory viruses or fungus should be undertaken in rapidly developing obstruction, especially in the presence of acute GvHD.

Early recognition and treatment may improve outcome. Therefore, routine spirometry after marrow transplantation

Approach to treatment of airflow limitation after hematopoietic stem cell transplantation	
1.	Control associated chronic graft-versus-host disease (cyclosporin-A, FK-506)
2.	Prophylaxis for *Pneumocystis carinii* pneumonia
3.	Treat any intercurrent respiratory infection
4.	Augment low serum immunoglobulin levels
5.	Administer aerosolized adrenergic agonists to symptomatic patients
6.	Prednisone (or its equivalent) 1–1.5mg/kg per day (up to 100mg per day) for 4–6 weeks
7.	Repeat pulmonary function testing monthly
8.	If there is no improvement or if there is deterioration after 1month of corticosteroid therapy, begin azathioprine (up to 3mg/kg per day, 200mg/day maximum)
9.	If there is no response, add mycophenolate mofetil or thalidomide

Figure 55.13 Approach to treatment of air-flow obstruction after hematopoietic stem cell transplantation.

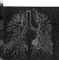

3. Meyers JD. Infection in bone marrow transplant recipients. Am J Med. 1986;81(Suppl. 1A):27–38.

4. Crawford SW, Hackman RC, Clark JG. Open lung biopsy diagnosis of diffuse pulmonary infiltrates after marrow transplantation. Chest. 1988;94:949–53.

5. Winston D, Ho W, Bartoni K, et al. Ganciclovir prophylaxis of cytomegalovirus infection and disease in allogeneic bone marrow transplant recipients. Ann Intern Med. 1993;118:179–84.

6. McWhinney PH, Kibbler CC, Hamon MD, et al. Progress in the diagnosis and management of aspergillosis in bone marrow transplantation: 13 years' experience. Clin Infect Dis. 1993;17:397–404.

7. Kantrow SP, Hackman RC, Boeckh M, Myerson D, Crawford SW. Idiopathic pneumonia syndrome: the changing spectrum of lung injury after marrow transplantation. Transplantation. 1997;63:1079–86.

8. Crawford SW, Pepe M, Lin D, Benedetti F, Deeg HJ. Abnormalities of pulmonary function tests after marrow transplantation predict non-relapse mortality. Am J Respir Crit Care Med. 1995;152:690–5.

9. Przepiorka D, Anderlini P, Ippoliti C, et al. Allogeneic blood stem cell transplantation in advanced hematologic cancers. Bone Marrow Transplant. 1997;19:455–60.

10. Crawford SW, Fisher L. Predictive value of pulmonary function tests before marrow transplantation. Chest. 1992;101:1257–64.

11. Clark JG, Crawford SW, Madtes DK, Sullivan KM. Obstructive lung disease after allogeneic marrow transplantation: clinical presentation and course. Ann Intern Med. 1989;111:368–76.

12. Badier M, Guillot C, Delpierre S, et al. Pulmonary function changes 100 days and one year after bone marrow transplantation. Bone Marrow Transplant. 1993;12:457–61.

13. Crawford SW, Schwartz DA, Petersen FB, Clark JG. Mechanical ventilation after marrow transplantation: risk factors and clinical outcome. Am Rev Respir Dis. 1988;137:682–7.

14. Lee CK, Gingrich RD, Hohl RJ, Ajram KA. Engraftment synrome in autologous bone marrow and peripheral stem cell transplantation. Bone Marrow Transplant. 1995;16:175–82.

15. Robbins RA, Linder J, Stahl MG, et al. Diffuse alveolar hemorrhage in autologous bone marrow transplant recipients. Am J Med. 1989;87:511–18.

16. Jules-Elysee K, Stover DE, Yahalom J, White DA, Gulati SC. Pulmonary complications in lymphoma patients treated with high-dose therapy and autologous bone marrow transplantation. Am Rev Respir Dis. 1992;146:485–91.

17. DeLassence A, Fleury-Feith J, Escudier E, et al. Alveolar hemorrhage: diagnostic criteria and results in 194 immunocompromised hosts. Am J Respir Crit Care Med. 1995;151:151–63.

18. Agusti C, Ramirez J, Picado C, et al. Diffuse alveolar hemorrhage in allogeneic bone marrow transplantation: a post-mortem study. Am J Respir Crit Care Med. 1995;151:1006–10.

19. Metcalf JP, Rennard SI, Reed EC, et al. Corticosteroids as adjunctive therapy for diffuse alveolar hemorrhage associated with bone marrow transplantation. Am J Med. 1994;96:327–34.

20. Crawford SW, Hackman RC, Clark JG. Biopsy diagnosis and clinical outcome of focal pulmonary lesions after marrow transplantation. Transplantation. 1989;48:266–71.

21. Wald A, Leisenring W, van Burick J, Bowden RA. Epidemiology of *Aspergillus* infections in a large cohort of patients undergoing bone marrow transplantation. J Infect Dis. 1997;175:1459–66.

22. Paz HL, Crilley P, Patchefsky A, Schiffman RL, Brodsky I. Bronchiolitis obliterans after autologous bone marrow transplantation. Chest. 1992;101:775–8.

23. Sargent MA, Cairns RA, Murdoch MJ, et al. Obstructive lung disease in children after allogeneic bone marrow transplantation: evaluation with high-resolution CT. Am J Roentgenol. 1995;164:693–6.

24. Hackman RC, Madtes DK, Petersen FB, Clark JG. Pulmonary veno-occlusive disease following bone marrow transplantation. Transplantation. 1989;47:989–92.

25. Seber A, Khan SP, Kersey JH. Unexplained effusions: association with allogeneic bone marrow transplantation and acute or chronic graft-versus-host disease. Bone Marrow Transplant. 1996;18:826.

26. Weiss SW, Hert RC, Gianola FG, Clark JC, Crawford SW. Complications of fiberoptic bronchoscopy in thrombocytopenic patients. Chest 1993;104:1025–8.

27. Faber-Langendoen K, Caplan AL, McGlave PB. Survival of adult bone marrow transplant patients receiving mechanical ventilation: a case for restricted use. Bone Marrow Transplant. 1993;12:501–7.

28. Crawford SW, Schwartz DA, Petersen FB, Clark JG. Mechanical ventilation after marrow transplantation: risk factors and clinical outcome. Am Rev Respir Dis. 1988,137:682–7.

29. Rubenfeld GD, Crawford SW. Withdrawing life-support for mechanically ventilated bone marrow transplant patients: a case for evidence-based guidelines. Ann Intern Med. 1996;125:625–33.

Chapter 56

Pulmonary Complications of Hematologic Problems

Thomas K Aldrich

The hematologic system includes all of the cellular components of the blood – erythrocytes, leukocytes, and platelets, and factors related to the thrombotic–thrombinolytic system. Each has its characteristic pulmonary manifestations and complications.

RED CELL DISORDERS

Anemia

Anemia of any cause reduces the oxygen-carrying capacity of blood. Once the patient reaches the limits of his or her ability to compensate by increasing cardiac output and oxygen extraction, delivery of oxygen to metabolizing tissues can become limited. The consequences include reduced exercise tolerance and increased risk of myocardial and other tissue ischemia. The major pulmonary consequence of anemia is increased severity of arterial hypoxemia in the setting of conditions that cause shunt or low ventilation/perfusion ratios (V/Q). This occurs because the reduced oxygen carrying capacity of the blood requires increased extraction of oxygen at the tissue level, which thus lowers the venous oxygen content. Blood with a low mixed venous saturation that subsequently perfuses areas of shunt or regions of low V/Q continues to have a low oxygen content, and thereby reduces the oxygen content in the pulmonary venous blood by further diluting the oxygen content in blood that comes from areas with more normal gas exchange. In addition, the high cardiac output associated with anemia may, in the setting of an abnormal diffusing capacity, shorten the pulmonary capillary transit time to the extent that full equilibration of alveolar oxygen with pulmonary capillary blood may not occur. Accordingly, although anemia does not cause hypoxemia in and of itself, it accentuates the degree of pre-existing hypoxemia produced by shunt, low V/Q, and abnormal diffusion.

Erythrocythemia

Just as anemia potentially impairs delivery of oxygen to metabolizing tissues, erythrocythemia has the potential to improve oxygen delivery and does so in subjects who have impaired oxygen delivery to the site in the kidney in which erythropoietin production occurs. Erythrocythemia can therefore occur in response to the reduced barometric pressure inherent in living at high altitude, any pulmonary condition or ventilatory drive problem that reduces arterial oxygen content, any cardiac disease that reduces oxygen delivery, renal artery stenosis, smoking-induced carboxyhemoglobinemia, and (occasionally) mutant hemoglobins. It also occurs in a number of erythropoietin-secreting tumors (e.g. hepatic and renal cell carcinoma), as well as in polycythemia vera.

Since cyanosis depends upon the concentration, rather than the percentage, of reduced hemoglobin, and as reduced hemoglobin concentrations may be extremely high despite only slight reductions in saturation, patients who have erythrocythemia are often severely cyanotic. By increasing blood viscosity, erythrocythemia may worsen pulmonary hypertension, impair cardiac output, and probably impair microvascular perfusion, especially in the brain. Thus, when excessive, erythrocythemia may actually worsen rather than improve oxygen transport. It is still unclear how high the hemoglobin concentration must be to have deleterious effects on oxygen transport, but most investigators recommend phlebotomy when the hematocrit exceeds 60%.

Abnormal hemoglobins, including sickle cell disease

A number of genetic hemoglobinopathies have been described, including mutant hemoglobins with abnormally high or low oxygen affinity, thalassemias (abnormal globin-chain synthesis), with their characteristic hemolysis and anemia, and (most importantly for pulmonologists) sickle cell disease[1].

Sickle cell disease is caused by the substitution of valine for glutamic acid as the sixth amino acid in the β-globin chain. It is common in Subsaharan Africa, but is also seen in Saudi Arabia, Israel, India, Greece, and Sicily. About 12% of African–Americans are heterozygous, and about 0.25% are homozygous.

Hemoglobin S itself does not have abnormal oxygen affinity, but red cells with high concentrations of hemoglobin S show strong right shifts of their oxyhemoglobin dissociation curves, in part because of elevated 2,3-diphosphoglycerate levels, and in part because of an accentuated Bohr effect. Moreover, under hypoxic conditions, hemoglobin S forms insoluble polymers that have severely impaired oxygen affinity. The result may be a potentially beneficial enhancement of oxygen unloading at the tissue level, but high concentrations of the hemoglobin S polymer within erythrocytes impairs cell deformability, and can cause the red cells to assume bizarre shapes (see Fig. 56.1). Under hypoxic conditions, patients who have sickle cell disease are at risk for microvascular occlusion in a number of organs, which include the lung, as a result of the hypoxia-induced impairment in deformability of sickle cells and their excessive endothelial adhesiveness. Heterozygotes (persons who have sickle trait) produce more than 60% normal hemoglobin A and are generally asymptomatic, but may be at increased risk of pulmonary embolism, especially if exposed to hypoxia.

About 50% of SS homozygotes and compound heterozygotes (hemoglobin SC disease or sickle-β-thalassemia) suffer at least one episode of the acute chest syndrome, characterized by severe, pleuritic chest pain, fever, leukocytosis, pulmonary infiltrates, and hypoxemia (see Fig. 56.2). In many cases, the syndrome

Pulmonary Manifestations of Systemic Conditions

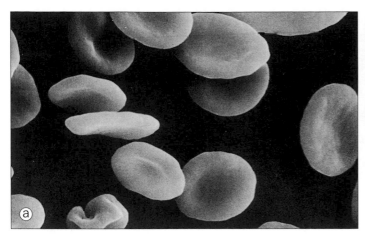

Figure 56.1 Sickle cell anemia. Scanning electron microscopy of a sample of red cells from a patient who has sickle cell disease under (a) oxygenated and (b) deoxygenated conditions. Although most cells assume a normal discoid shape when well oxygenated, some 'irreversibly sickled cells' remain in the oxygenated sample. Under hypoxic conditions, all cells show spicules, sickle shapes, or other bizarre conformations. (Courtesy of Dr Mary Fabry.)

appears to be triggered by vaso-occlusive crisis or by pulmonary infection, often caused by atypical organisms. The pathophysiology is obscure, but probably involves nonembolic pulmonary microvascular occlusion, brought about either by abnormal adhesiveness of sickle cells, perhaps enhanced by cytokines liberated during infection, or by mechanical entrapment of abnormally nondeformable sickle cells in regions of alveolar hypoxia, perhaps elicited by pneumonia, or by atelectasis or regional hypoventilation associated with splinting or narcotics.

Severe cases of acute chest syndrome are often associated with evidence of bone marrow embolization, which originates from infarcts in the spine, rib, or other bones. Preliminary evidence suggests that bone marrow embolization may promote extraordinarily high plasma activity of the enzyme phospholipase A_2, which has been implicated as a possible contributing cause of sepsis-associated pulmonary edema in nonsickle cell patients; perhaps phospholipase A_2 plays a crucial pathogenic role in at least some cases of acute chest syndrome.

Treatment consists of oxygen supplementation, analgesia administration, and hydration. Antibiotics are usually recommended, even if no sputam is produced. Exchange transfusion is used to reduce the amount of hemoglobin S to <30%. Recently, in moderate to severe cases, hydroxyurea, which increases production of fetal hemoglobin, and thereby interferes with sickling, has been found to reduce the incidence and severity of sickle cell crises and may also reduce the risk of acute chest syndrome. Additional clinical manifestations of SS disease include left ventricular enlargement and diastolic dysfunction, attributed to possible microvascular occlusion in the coronary circulation. Pulmonary hypertension and pulmonary fibrosis, possibly as sequelae to recurrent episodes of acute chest syndrome, are also common.

LEUKOCYTE DISORDERS

Leukocytes, especially nonlymphocytic leukocytes, can contribute to lung disease when they are present in excessive number or when they are abnormally activated. Also, by allowing unchecked pulmonary and systemic infection, deficiency of leukocytes is often associated with pneumonia or septicemia-related pulmonary infiltrates.

Acute chest syndrome of sickle cell disease			
Manifestations	**Precipitating factors**	**Pathogenetic factors**	**Treatment**
Chest pain	Vaso-occlusive crisis	Pulmonary microvascular occlusion	Antibiotics
Dyspnea	Infection		Fluids
Fever	Bone marrow embolization	Ischemia	Analgesics
Pulmonary infiltrates	Regional alveolar hypoxia	Thrombosis	Bronchodilators
Hypoxemia		Cytokines	Incentive spirometry
Fall in hemoglobin		Neutrophils	Oxygen
		Platelets	Ventilatory support
		Phospholipase A_2?	Transfusion

Figure 56.2 Acute chest syndrome of sickle cell disease.

Hematologic malignancies

In nonlymphocytic leukemias, when the white blood cell (WBC) count exceeds 50,000/mm^3, patients are at risk for leukostasis, a syndrome of fever, pulmonary infiltrates, and hypoxemia, which results at least in part from pulmonary vaso-occlusion by leukocytes. When WBC count exceeds 200,000/mm^3, leukostasis is virtually always present. Often, associated abnormalities of fibrinolysis are found, which may trigger the syndrome, and that may play a pathogenetic role by promoting leukocyte–endothelial adherence. In addition to chemotherapy, treatment requires urgent leukopheresis, as the response to medications alone is too slow.

Assessment of the degree of hypoxemia is complicated in patients who have leukocytosis (particularly when WBC count exceeds 100,00/mm^3), because of the potential for ongoing WBC metabolism to reduce the PaO_2 measured in blood samples, even when these are kept on ice. Whenever severe leukocytosis is present, or at least when hypoxemia is documented in patients who have severe leukocytosis, the arterial blood sample should be treated with potassium cyanide, which stops the metabolism and eliminates the possibility of this artifact.

Just as in other malignancies, patients who have hematologic malignancies often suffer respiratory complications, which may be the result of spreading of the primary disease to the lungs or mediastinal nodes, of infection as a consequence of immuno-compromise, or of toxic effects of radiotherapy or antineoplastic chemotherapy[2] (Fig. 56.3). These complications are discussed at greater length in Chapter 77. The pulmonary toxicity of treatment of M5 leukemia requires specific comment, as up to 25% of patients who receive all-*trans*-retinoic acid (tretinoin) therapy develop dyspnea, fever, pulmonary infiltrates, and hypoxemia.

Transfusion reactions

Acute hemolytic transfusion reactions generally occur when the ABO antigens on the transfused red blood cells are incompatible with circulating antibodies in the recipient. Such reactions are manifested by chills, dyspnea, chest or back pain, and hypotension, and are generally accompanied by fever and tachycardia. Laboratory studies indicate disseminated intravascular coagulation (DIC), which includes hemoglobinemia, hemoglobinuria, hyperbilirubinemia, and a positive direct Coomb's test. Delayed hemolytic reactions (i.e. from 2 days up to 2 weeks following the transfusion) can occur when antigens on newly transfused red blood cells produce an anamnestic response in patients who have previously been alloimmunized. These reactions are milder, and present with fever, a positive direct Coomb's test, and elevations of lactic dehydrogenase and bilirubin.

With the exception of hemolytic reactions caused by incompatible red cells, most transfusion reactions result from leukoagglutinins (i.e. immunoglobulins that are directed against neutrophils). Most commonly, the leukoagglutinin is transferred with donor plasma and reacts with recipient neutrophils, but, in a small percentage of cases, the reverse may occur. Nonhemolytic reactions occur in approximately 1% of transfusions, but are more common in previously alloimmunized patients (e.g. recipients of previous transfusions, women who have been pregnant), and in patients who have neoplasms or other diseases that may be associated with autoantibody production. In most instances the major manifestation is fever. On occasion, however, anaphylaxis and/or transfusion-related acute lung injury can occur.

Experimentally, it is clear that complement fragments and other cytokines can activate neutrophils to cause alveolar damage and consequent pulmonary edema in isolated, ventilated, and perfused lungs, as well as in intact animals (Fig. 56.4) In clinical medicine, it is suspected that neutrophils play a major role in the pathogenesis of noncardiogenic pulmonary edema after a variety of toxic exposures, during sepsis, after fat embolism, and in the postperfusion syndrome[4]. Although the occurrence of pulmonary edema in patients and experimental preparations with few or no neutrophils demonstrates that neutrophils are not absolutely required for lung injury, there is little doubt that neutrophils accelerate and often initiate alveolar damage under many clinical conditions. Patients in need of repeated transfusion and who have a history of severe, nonhemolytic reactions, may do better if they receive leukocyte-depleted transfusions.

Non-neutrophil leukocytes can also contribute to respiratory disease. In a number of hypereosinophilic conditions eosinophils are thought to produce acute or subacute alveolar damage in much the same way as neutrophils. Alveolar macrophages, derived from blood monocytes, are thought to play important roles in more chronic conditions, such as sarcoidosis and hypersensitivity pneumonitis. Although lymphocytes *per se* appear to be relatively less toxic to the lungs than are neutrophils, at least when present in large numbers in leukemia, they play crucial roles in the pathogenesis of a number of immunologically mediated diseases, notably asthma.

PLATELET DISORDERS

As with leukocytes, platelets or the lack of platelets can contribute to lung disease. Platelets produce a host of vasoactive and other mediators, which (often through interaction with mediators produced by leukocytes) can result in lung injury either directly or by promotion and facilitation of inflammatory reactions.

Common pulmonary complications of hematologic malignancies				
Condition	Leukostasis	Spread of primary tumor to chest	Radiation or chemotherapy-induced lung injury	Common pneumonias
Lymphocytic leukemia	No	Occasionally in chronic lymphocytic leukemia	Uncommon	Encapsulated bacteria
Nonlymphocytic leukemia	Yes	Uncommon	Frequent	Gram-negative bacteria *Aspergillus* spp.
Hodgkin's lymphoma	No	Frequently to nodes, occasionally to lung	Frequent	Variable
Non-Hodgkin's lymphoma	No	Frequently to nodes, occasionally to lung	Uncommon	Encapsulated bacteria, fungi, cytomegalovirus
Mutiple myeloma	No	Occasionally to rib	Uncommon	Encapsulated bacteria, *Pneumocystis carinii* pneumonia

Figure 56.3 Common pulmonary complications of hematologic malignancies.

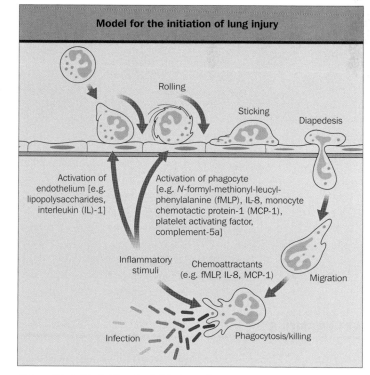

Figure 56.4 Model for the initiation of lung injury. Cytokine activation of neutrophils leads to their evascularization and degranulation. The granule contents amplify the inflammatory reaction. (Adapted with permission from Canonico and Brigham[3].)

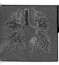

Furthermore, platelet aggregates, formed as a result of abnormal platelet activation, have the potential to serve as microemboli, which contributes to the pulmonary hypertension of noncardiogenic pulmonary edema.

Patients with severe thrombocytopenia have a risk of hemoptysis, particularly after transbronchial lung biopsy. However, spontaneous life-threatening pulmonary hemorrhage is quite unusual in the absence of other structural lung or bronchial disease.

COAGULOPATHIES

Both deficiency and excesses of various clotting factors can affect the respiratory system. Bleeding is the major risk for patients who have inherited or acquired clotting factor deficiency, but, as in thrombocytopenia, serious pulmonary hemorrhage is not common in the absence of an identifiable structural lesion.

The major risk of the various hypercoaguable states is deep venous thrombosis and pulmonary embolism, discussed in Chapter 50. Abnormal balance of clotting factors and abnormal activation of factors is a feature of sepsis-associated DIC, and may well participate in the pathogenesis of sepsis-associated noncardiogenic pulmonary edema.

CONCLUSION

The lung, the only organ that receives and filters the entire cardiac output, is uniquely at risk for complications related to abnormalities of blood components. All types of hematologic disease have potential pulmonary manifestations, most notably sickle cell disease, hematologic malignancies, transfusions, and sepsis-associated abnormalities in leukocytes, platelets, and clotting factors.

REFERENCES

1. Aldrich TK, Nagel RL. Pulmonary complications of sickle cell disease. In: Bone RC, Dantzker DR, Matthay RA, George RB, Reynolds HY, eds. Pulmonary and critical care medicine. St Louis: Mosby; 1998, Section L, Chapter 5:1–10.
2. Wickremasinghe M. Respiratory complications associated with haematological malignancies. Thorax. 1997;52:390–1.
3. Canonico AE, Brigham KL. Biology of acute lung injury. In: Crystal RG, West JB, Barnes PJ, Weibel ER, eds. The lung: scientific foundations, 2nd edn. Philadelphia: Lippincott–Raven; 1997:2475–98.
4. Kollef MH, Schuster DP. The acute respiratory distress syndrome. N Engl J Med. 1995;332:27–37.

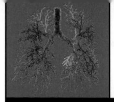

Chapter 57

Hepatic and Biliary Disease

Roberto Rodriguez-Roisin

EPIDEMIOLOGY, RISK FACTORS, AND PATHOPHYSIOLOGY

Epidemiology

A variety of pulmonary problems occur in conjunction with a number of chronic liver or biliary diseases (Fig. 57.1). The prevalence of gas exchange abnormalities in patients who have advanced liver disease is approximately 70%, and as many as 50% complain of dyspnea either at rest or with exercise[1]. Although mild hypoxemia is relatively common, arterial partial pressures of oxygen (PaO_2) <7.8kPa (<60mmHg) are found in only 10–30% of patients[2], unless an underlying cardiopulmonary problem is present. Diffusion abnormalities are also common. The prevalence of the hepatopulmonary syndrome may be as high as 45% when transesophageal echocardiography is used to establish the diagnosis[2]. Transudative pleural effusions occur in approximately 6% of patients who have cirrhosis and ascites[3]. Pulmonary hypertension has been found in up to 4% of patients who suffer portal hypertension. The prevalence of pulmonary manifestations of the other hepatic and biliary diseases outlined in Figure 57.1 is not well characterized, but is seemingly quite low.

Risk factors

Pulmonary disease in conjunction with primary biliary cirrhosis is rare in the absence of co-existent Sjögren's syndrome, in which case as many as 50% have airflow limitation[4]. No other risk factors for the pulmonary manifestations of hepatic or intestinal disease have been identified.

Pathophysiology

The pathophysiology of the pulmonary manifestations of hepatic and biliary diseases is unknown (with the exception of the recognized transdiaphragmatic pathways by which ascitic fluid,

Pulmonary complications of gastrointestinal disease	
Gastrointestinal disease	**Pulmonary complications**
Cirrhosis	Hepatopulmonary syndrome Portopulmonary hypertension Pleural effusion
Primary biliary cirrhosis	Bronchitis Interstitial pneumonitis and fibrosis Chest wall deformities
Viral hepatitis	Pleuritis Interstitial pneumonitis and fibrosis (rare)
Sclerosing cholangitis	Bronchitis and bronchiectasis
α_1-Antitrypsin deficiency	(see Chapter 39)

Figure 57.1 The pulmonary complications of gastrointestinal disease.

formed as a result of portal hypertension in conjunction with low osmotic pressure, moves into the pleural space, which explains cirrhosis-related effusions)[3]. Hypotheses to explain the hepatopulmonary syndrome are that the progressively diseased liver either fails to metabolize a pulmonary vasodilator or a pulmonary vascular growth factor present in the portal venous blood, or that the diseased liver actually produces such substances. Locally produced (i.e. pulmonary) mediators may also contribute as concentrations of exhaled nitric oxide are greater in patients who have end-stage liver disease as well as the hepatopulmonary syndrome than in those who do not, and the concentration of exhaled NO is negatively correlated with pulmonary vascular resistance[5].

Portopulmonary hypertension might result from the entry of a pulmonary vasoconstrictor into the pulmonary arterial blood because the diseased liver fails to metabolize the substance, and/or because collaterals develop as a result of portal hypertension, which allow portal venous blood to bypass the liver.

CLINICAL FEATURES

Hepatopulmonary syndrome

The hepatopulmonary syndrome is defined as the clinical triad of liver disease, arterial hypoxemia, and generalized intrapulmonary vascular dilatations (both precapillary and capillary vessels, with surrounding normal pulmonary parenchyma), in the absence of intrinsic cardiopulmonary disease (see Fig. 57.2)[6]. The syndrome may be found in association with any type of chronic liver disease, but is most commonly encountered in patients who have cirrhosis. The majority of patients have cutaneous cyanosis, finger clubbing, and a hyperkinetic circulatory status, in addition to the typical stigmata of severe liver dysfunction, abnormal liver function tests, and portal hypertension[2]. They may complain of shortness of breath and platypnea. Cutaneous spider angiomata are considered to be a clinical marker of the pulmonary hemodynamics and gas exchange abnormalities found in these patients[7]. The more severe the hepatic failure the greater the severity of the hepatopulmonary syndrome.

Portopulmonary hypertension

Portopulmonary hypertension is defined as pulmonary hypertension [pulmonary arterial mean pressure >3.33kPa (25mmHg) at rest] that occurs in the setting of portal hypertension from any cause. It is an uncommon complication of portal hypertension (between 1 and 4%), but the prevalence in the cirrhotic population is clearly greater than that in normal individuals. The principal lesion is a nonspecific plexiform arteriopathy[8,9].

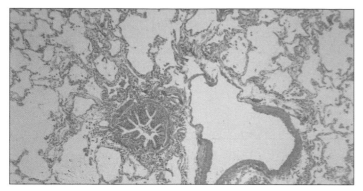

Figure 57.2. Lung biopsy from a patient who has hepatopulmonary syndrome. Note the presence of a markedly dilated pulmonary artery, under normal conditions always smaller than the neighboring airway, close to a normally structured bronchiole, both immersed in an intact pulmonary architecture (hematoxylin—eosin).

Pleural effusion (hepatic hydrothorax)

Effusions in the setting of chronic liver disease are virtually always associated with ascites. Although they occur predominantly on the right side, they may be bilateral on occasion, and may rarely occur on the left. Hepatic hydrothoraces may occasionally be massive in volume, but are more commonly small or modest in size, and generally have no substantive effect on gas exchange.

Chronic hepatitis

Bronchoalveolar lavage of patients who have chronic hepatitis (generally from hepatitis C virus) shows an increase in lymphocytes and eosinophils, and both lymphocytic pneumonitis and fibrosing alveolitis have been observed pathologically[10], along with an autoimmune pleuritis[11].

Primary biliary cirrhosis

Patients who have primary biliary cirrhosis may have a lymphocytic alveolitis documented by bronchoalveolar lavage (similar in nature to that seen in sarcoidosis), and reduced diffusion, in the absence of clinical symptoms or chest radiographic abnormalities[12]. Those who have concomitant Sjögren's syndrome may present with fever, cough, sputum production, and dyspnea. Lymphocytic interstitial pneumonitis, fibrosing alveolitis, organizing pneumonitis, and granulomatous inflammation have been seen on biopsy. On occasion, the pulmonary manifestations may appear prior to the hepatic disease[13]. Abnormal calcium metabolism that results from the biliary disorder may cause osteopenia, which in turn deforms the thoracic cage and causes a restrictive pulmonary disorder.

Sclerosing cholangitis

Patients who have sclerosing cholangitis may develop cough, with or without sputum production, and may rarely complain of dyspnea. Since sclerosing cholangitis is commonly associated with ulcerative colitis, and airflow limitation and bronchiectasis have been reported with both conditions, it is not possible to determine whether the pulmonary manifestations result from the cholangitis or from the colitis[14].

DIAGNOSIS

Steps in the evaluation of patients with liver disease who have gas-exchange abnormalities are given in Figure 57.3. Patients who have end-stage liver disease commonly have reduced diffusion[15]. Spirometry can show obstructive and, in the setting of ascites, restrictive abnormalities[16].

Hepatopulmonary syndrome

Finding severe hypoxemia in a patient who has any type of liver disorder is highly suggestive of the hepatopulmonary syndrome.

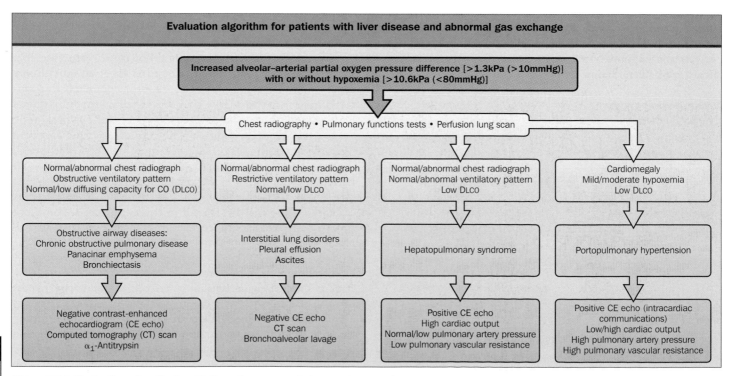

Evaluation algorithm for patients with liver disease and abnormal gas exchange

Increased alveolar–arterial partial oxygen pressure difference [>1.3kPa (>10mmHg)] with or without hypoxemia [>10.6kPa (<80mmHg)]

Chest radiography • Pulmonary functions tests • Perfusion lung scan

Normal/abnormal chest radiograph Obstructive ventilatory pattern Normal/low diffusing capacity for CO (DLCO)	Normal/abnormal chest radiograph Restrictive ventilatory pattern Normal/low DLCO	Normal/abnormal chest radiograph Normal/abnormal ventilatory pattern Low DLCO	Cardiomegaly Mild/moderate hypoxemia Low DLCO
Obstructive airway diseases: Chronic obstructive pulmonary disease Panacinar emphysema Bronchiectasis	Interstitial lung disorders Pleural effusion Ascites	Hepatopulmonary syndrome	Portopulmonary hypertension
Negative contrast-enhanced echocardiogram (CE echo) Computed tomography (CT) scan α_1-Antitrypsin	Negative CE echo CT scan Bronchoalveolar lavage	Positive CE echo High cardiac output Normal/low pulmonary artery pressure Low pulmonary vascular resistance	Positive CE echo (intracardiac communications) Low/high cardiac output High pulmonary artery pressure High pulmonary vascular resistance

Figure 57.3 Evaluation of patients with liver diseases and abnormal gas exchange.

The criteria proposed for the diagnosis include[6]:
- presence of a chronic liver disease;
- no intrinsic cardiopulmonary disease;
- chest radiograph that is normal or shows mild interstitial opacities;
- elevated alveolar-to-arterial difference in oxygen partial pressures with or without arterial hypoxemia; and
- positive contrast-enhanced echocardiogram or evidence of intravenous radiolabeled microspheres in extrapulmonary sites.

Supplementary features that support the diagnosis include an abnormal diffusing capacity, a high cardiac output and low systemic arterial pressure, normal or low pulmonary arterial pressures, and a poor hypoxic pulmonary vascular response. These patients also have a low $PaCO_2$, and spirometry and lung volumes are normal or near normal. When the condition is mild, the predominant physiologic mechanism that accounts for the hypoxemia is ventilation–perfusion heterogeneity (with overperfusion of alveoli relative to their ventilation). Such patients increase their PaO_2 when breathing 100% oxygen. When the hypoxemia is more severe, the pathophysiology is that of shunt, along with diffusion limitation (which can be explained by the increased diffusing distance inherent in dilated vessels, together with reduction in time for oxygen equilibration that is caused by the increased cardiac output)[15]. Breathing 100% oxygen has no substantive effect on the PaO_2 if the predominant mechanism is shunt, but increases it if the problem is diffusion limitation, since oxygen administration increases the alveolar-to-capillary driving pressure.

Many patients who have the hepatopulmonary syndrome have bilateral, basilar nodular, or reticulonodular opacities on their chest radiographs that can be shown by other techniques to represent the abnormal vessels[17]. The pulmonary vessels in the apices and bases of these patients may be equally engorged, as can the central pulmonary arteries on occasion. Conventional computed tomograms of the chest can be extremely helpful as they can confirm the presence of distal vascular dilatations, with an abnormally large number of visible terminal branches that extend to the pleural surface, and exclude a number of other intrinsic pulmonary disorders that can show similar radiographic and clinical manifestations. The most sensitive semi-invasive diagnostic test is transesophageal echocardiography. Positive studies demonstrate echoes that result from air microbubbles or indocyanine green that appear in the left atrium within 3–6 beats of their visualization in the right cardiac cavities (Fig. 57.4). Normally, echos are not found in the left heart chambers, since the microbubbles are trapped in the pulmonary capillary. The transesophageal echos can also clearly differentiate between the intrapulmonary vascular deformities seen in patients who have chronic liver disease from intracardiac malformations (a distinction not possible using radionuclide scanning).

Portopulmonary hypertension

Most patients who have portopulmonary hypertension have cardiomegaly, large main pulmonary arteries, and minimal hypoxemia[18]. Electrocardiograms may show evidence of increased right ventricular afterload (e.g. right atrial enlargement, right axis deviation, right ventricular hypertrophy). On occasion, the pulmonary hypertension is only detectable by echocardiography. Routine echocardiographic screening is not warranted in patients who have cirrhosis, but should be strongly considered in those being evaluated for transplantation, as the presence of pulmonary hypertension may increase the morbidity and mortality of the operation.

TREATMENT

Hepatopulmonary syndrome

Anecdotal reports of a variety of vasoconstricting medications, including almitrine, prostaglandins, indomethacin, somatostatin, cyclophosphamide, propranolol, garlic preparations, and methylene blue, have shown no substantial improvement[2]. Lack of success has also been reported after embolization of arteriovenous fistulae or plasma exchange[2]. Improvement in some, but not all, patients has been reported following liver transplantation[19].

Portopulmonary hypertension

No pharmacologic management of this condition has yet been found, and the outcome following liver transplantation is poor (see below).

Pleural effusion

For most patients who have hepatic hydrothorax, therapy is to minimize the accumulation of ascites (i.e. salt restriction,

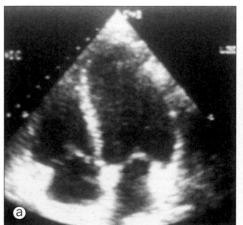
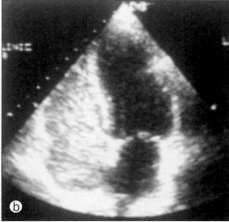
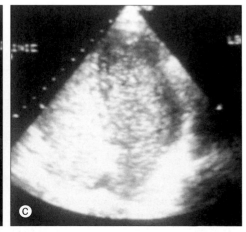

Figure 57.4 Patient who has hepatopulmonary syndrome (HPS). (a) Contrast-enhanced echocardiography using agitated saline injected through a peripheral vein in a patient who has HPS showing normal four-chamber views; also note (b) opacification of right heart cavities and (c) delayed opacification of the left ones. The echogenic presence of air microbubbles in the left heart chambers is strongly suggestive of intrapulmonary vascular dilatations with or without the presence of anatomic arteriovenous malformations, and excludes intracardiac communications.

diuretics, aldosterone antagonists). On occasion, large-volume effusions (and/or ascites) may require drainage solely to improve pulmonary function. Recurrent, severe pleural fluid accumulations have recently been approached by obliterating the diaphragmatic deformities via videothoracoscopic techniques, and transthoracic intrahepatic portosystemic shunting[20].

CLINICAL COURSE AND PREVENTION

In most instances the patient's clinical course is more closely related to their primary hepatic or biliary disorder than to the pulmonary manifestations of the specific condition. The major exception to this rule is the pulmonary hypertension associated with cirrhosis, which carries a poor prognosis. Anecdotal reports of patients who spontaneously recover from the hepatopulmonary syndrome occur, although in other patients the condition is progressive and causes life-threatening hypoxemia.

No preventive measures are know for any of the conditions outlined in Figure 57.1.

PITFALLS AND CONTROVERSIES

Up to 14% of patients who receive methotrexate for primary biliary cirrhosis or sclerosing cholangitis may develop drug-induced pulmonary disease[22].

Liver transplantation in patients who have portopulmonary hypertension has been associated with an extremely poor prognosis, with death from right ventricular failure which, in turn, results from the increased venous return to the right heart in face of function-limiting afterload. Many transplant centers routinely obtain transthoracic echocardiography on all liver transplant candidates and exclude those who have pulmonary hypertension.

REFERENCES

1. Hourani JM, Bellamy, PE, Tashkin DP, Batra P, Simmons MS. Pulmonary dysfunction in advanced liver disease: frequent occurrence of an abnormal diffusing capacity. Am J Med. 1991;90:693–700.
2. Castro M, Krowka MJ. Hepatopulmonary syndrome: a pulmonary vascular complication of liver disease. Clin Chest Med. 1996;17:35–48.
3. Johnston RF, Loo RV. Hepatic hydrothorax. Studies to determine the source of the fluid and report of thirteen cases. Ann Intern Med. 1964;61:385–401.
4. Rodriguez-Roisin R, Parés A, Bruguera M, et al. Pulmonary involvement in primary biliary cirrhosis. Thorax. 1981;36:208–212.
5. Rodriguez-Roisin R, Barberà JA. Hepatopulmonary syndrome: is NO the right answer? Gastroenterology. 1997;113:682–4.
6. Rodriguez-Roisin R, Agustí AGN, Roca J. The hepatopulmonary syndrome: new name, old complexities. Thorax. 1992;47:897–902.
7. Rodriguez-Roisin R, Roca J, Agustí AGN, Mastai R, Wagner PD, Bosch J. Gas exchange and pulmonary vascular reactivity in patients with liver cirrhosis. Am Rev Respir Dis. 1987;135:1085–92.
8. Castro M, Krowka MJ, Schroeder DR, et al. Frequency and complications of increased pulmonary artery pressures in liver transplant patients. Mayo Clin Proc. 1996;71:543–51.
9. Kuo P. Pulmonary hypertension: considerations in the liver transplant candidate. Transplant Int. 1996;9:141–50.
10. Kubo, K, Yamaguchi S, Fujimoto K, et al. Bronchoalveolar lavage fluid findings in patients with chronic hepatitis C virus infection. Thorax. 1996;51:312–14.
11. Turner-Warwick M. Fibrosing alveolitis and chronic liver disease. Q J Med. 1968;37:133–49.
12. Wallaert B, Bonniere WB, Cortot PL, Tonnel AB, Voisin C. Primary biliary cirrhosis. Subclinical inflammatory alveolitis in patients with normal chest roentgenograms. Chest. 1986;90:842–8.
13. Izdebska-Makosa Z, Zielinski U. Primary biliary cirrhosis in a patient with interstitial lung fibrosis. Chest. 1987;92:766–7.
14. Wiesner RH, LaRusso NF. Clinicopathologic features of the syndrome of primary sclerosing cholangitis. Gastroenterology. 1980;79:200–6.
15. Agustí AGN, Roca J, Rodriguez-Roisin R. Mechanisms of gas exchange impairment in patients with liver cirrhosis. Clin Chest Med. 1996;17:49–66.
16. Agustí AGN, Roca J, Bosch J, Rodriguez-Roisin R. The lung in patients with cirrhosis. J Hepatol. 1990;10:251–7.
17. McAdams P, Erasmus J, Crokett R, Mitchell J, Godwin JD, McDermott VG. The hepatopulmonary syndrome: radiologic findings in 10 patients. AJR Am J Roentgenol. 1996;166:1379–85.
18. Krowka MJ. Hepatopulmonary syndrome versus portopulmonary hypertension: distinctions and dilemmas. Hepatology. 1997;25:1282–4.
19. Rodriguez-Roisin R, Krowka MJ. Is arterial hypoxaemia due to hepatic disease an indication for liver transplantation? A new therapeutic approach. Eur Respir J. 1994;7:839–42.
20. Krowka MJ. Recent pulmonary observations in α_1-antitrypsin deficiency, primary biliary cirrhosis, chronic hepatitis C, and other hepatic problems. Clin Chest Med. 1996;17:67–82.
21. Sharma A, Provenzale D, Mukusick A, Kaplan MM. Interstitial pneumonitis after low dose methotrexate therapy in primary biliary cirrhosis. Gastroenterology. 1994;107:266–70.

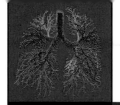

Inflammatory Bowel Diseases

Philippe Camus and Thomas V Colby

INTRODUCTION

Respiratory manifestations in inflammatory bowel diseases (IBDs) include:

- 'specific' inflammatory reactions, which probably reflect the systemic nature of IBDs; and
- lung disease induced by one or more of the medications used to treat the IBD [e.g. sulfasalazine (salycilazosulfapyridine) may induce eosinophilic pneumonia, and mesalazine can induce bronchiolitis obliterans and organizing pneumonia and/or chest pain][1].

EPIDEMIOLOGY

Ulcerative colitis (UC) is the IBD most often associated with lung problems[1]. Although there is some similarity between UC and Crohn's disease[2-5], pulmonary involvement is less common and more often granulomatous in nature in patients who have Crohn's disease[6].

Chronologically, respiratory involvement can develop at any time during the course of the IBD. In about 80% of cases, however, the onset of pulmonary symptoms follows the diagnosis of IBD by months to years. In some instances, concomitant and brisk onset of lung and bowel symptoms occurs. Importantly, patients who have prior colectomy are not immune to the development of IBD-associated lung involvement, and lung symptoms can develop as early as a few days and up to many years after colectomy[1]. Sometimes, the link between the bowel and lung diseases may be difficult to appreciate, especially in a patient who has a very remote history of colectomy. Collectively, patients who have prior colectomy tend to develop airways disease, and noncolectomy patients tend to develop parenchymal disease. Acute flares of the IBD may be associated with transient serositis. The similarity between the colonic and respiratory lesions, and that pulmonary involvement can develop even after colectomy point to the systemic nature of IBDs.

CLINICAL FEATURES

Respiratory involvement in IBD is mostly inflammatory in nature, and can involve the airways, lung parenchyma, or serosal surfaces. Involvement of the bronchial tree ranges from subglottic inflammation and stenosis to large airway inflammation with chronic productive cough, or small airways disease with attending severe chronic obstruction to airflow. Involvement at several levels of the bronchial tree is common. Typical symptoms consistent with the airway inflammation include a hacking cough, productive of variable amounts of mucopurulent sputum, diffuse wheezes, and rhonchi. The amount of sputum is sometimes large enough to interfere with normal social activities. Upper airway stenosis typically results in cough, hoarseness, and stridor. Rapidly progressive stenosis can present with asphyxia. The rare patient who has small airways disease usually presents with variable sputum production. These airway problems are encountered more commonly in patients who have UC than in those who have Crohn's disease.

Interstitial lung disease [including bronchiolitis obliterans organizing pneumonia (BOOP)] is characterized by diffuse or predominantly upper lobe infiltrates or masses, which can present with acute respiratory failure in some instances. Typically, the interstitial lung disease of Crohn's disease is granulomatous, and may mimic parenchymal sarcoidosis. Necrobiotic nodules are peculiar UC-associated lesions that present as acute sterile neutrophilic aggregates in the lung parenchyma, and resemble pyoderma gangrenosum of the skin[1]. Significant serositis is usually characterized by acute chest pain and fever. If myocarditis is present, arrhythmia and/or heart failure may be seen.

DIAGNOSIS

Endoscopy is the key to diagnosis in most if not all cases that have large airways involvement. Regardless of the anatomic level, the degree of macroscopic inflammation ranges from simple redness of the bronchial mucosa to exuberant pseudotumoral granulation tissue with a marked tendency to bleed. The airway narrowing may be so severe as to prevent the insertion of a fiberoptic bronchoscope beyond the area of inflammation. In patients who have pure small airways disease, endoscopy is usually entirely normal. Typically, bronchoalveolar lavage yields huge numbers of neutrophils in most cases.

The chest radiograph is often normal in patients who have upper airway obstruction, but radiographs and computed tomography (CT) scans of the trachea demonstrate the stenotic area. In large airway involvement, the chest radiograph ranges from normal to a pattern of increased bronchial markings or bibasilar bronchiectasis. Bronchoceles with dichotomous branched shadows are commonly seen (see Figs 58.1 & 58.2).

Pulmonary function tests show a predominantly obstructive pattern that is little influenced by bronchodilators and roughly correlates with the extent of involvement seen at endoscopy.

Biopsy of the bronchial mucosa shows an extensive submucosal inflammation by mononuclear cells and neutrophils, which is responsible for the reduced patency of the airways. In patients with early small airways disease, the lung biopsy usually demonstrates diffuse panbronchiolitis, a lesion characterized by inflammatory cuffing of the small airway, associated with an interstitial infiltrate of foamy macrophages. After some time, bronchioles are obliterated and demonstrate a pattern of bronchiolitis obliterans.

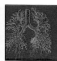

REFERENCES

1. Camus P, Piard F, Ashcroft T, Gal AA, Colby TV. The lung in inflammatory bowel disease. Medicine (Baltimore). 1993;72:151–83.

2. de Wazières B, Fest T, Morin G, Vuitton DA, Dupond JL. Crohn's disease with initial upper airway, tracheal and cutaneous localizations mimicking Wegener's granulomatosis. Eur J Intern Med. 1993;4:59–62.

3. Lamblin C, Copin M-C, Billaut C, et al. Acute respiratory failure due to tracheobronchial involvement in Crohn's disease. Eur Respir J. 1996;9:2176–8.

4. Hotermans G, Benard A, Guenanen H, Demarcq-Delerue G, Malart T, Wallaert B. Nongranulomatous interstitial lung disease in Crohn's disease. Eur Respir J. 1996;9:380–2.

5. Eaton TE, Lambie N, Wells AU. Bronchiectasis following colectomy for Crohn's disease. Thorax. 1998;53:529–31.

6. Calder CJ, Lacy D, Raafat F, Weller PH, Booth IW. Crohn's disease with pulmonary involvement in a 3-year-old boy. Gut. 1993;34:1636–8.

7. Rickli H, Fretz C, Hoffman M, Walser A, Knoblauch A. Severe inflammatory upper airway stenosis in ulcerative colitis. Eur Respir J. 1994;7:1899–902.

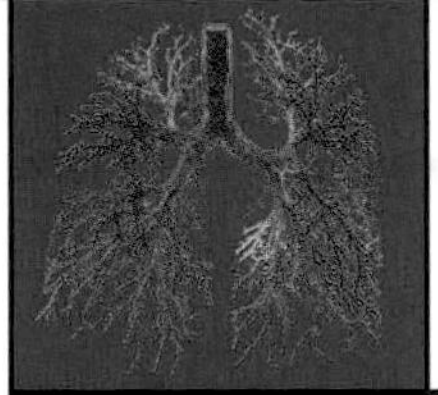

Chapter 59

Disability Evaluation

Robin Rudd

In patients who have occupational respiratory disease it is often necessary to assess disability so that compensation and fitness for work can be determined. In considering respiratory disability, it is important to differentiate between the impairment of respiratory function that exists and the disability that results from the impairment. Respiratory disability is defined by the World Health Organization as a reduction in exercise capacity secondary to impaired lung function, and the resultant social and occupational disadvantage is designated as a handicap[1]. The assessment of respiratory disability requires information about impairment of respiratory function and its effect on exercise performance. The former is easily obtained by standard tests of static lung function. The latter is obtained by interviews with the subject, but much effort has been expended on trying to devise more objective methods.

ASSESSMENT OF LUNG FUNCTION IMPAIRMENT

Impairment of respiratory function is assessed by a range of lung function tests, the results of which are commonly interpreted by comparison with reference values. These are values determined in subjects who have no known respiratory disease or respiratory symptoms. In some, but not all, series used to determine reference values smokers have been excluded. It is important to appreciate that reference values represent only the mean of a population of similar age, sex, and height so that, by definition, some healthy individuals have values well above or below the reference value.

Rating scales for impairment of respiratory function have been formulated by working groups of the American Thoracic Society[2] (ATS) and European Society for Clinical Respiratory Physiology[3] (SEPCR). The proposals differed in their definitions of the lower limit of normal, being 20% and 1.64 standard deviations (SD), respectively, below the reference value. The latter has more statistical validity since it defines the lowest 5% of the population at any age, whereas a criterion based upon percentage predicted defines more patients as abnormal with increasing patient age. The categories of impairment defined by the two scales are shown in Figure 59.1. As well as being statistically questionable, these grades are arbitrary and their descriptions were not accompanied by evidence that validated their selection to reflect loss of exercise capacity. Only a weak correlation is found between loss of lung function and the resultant loss of exercise capacity[4]. These guidelines relate to persons who have chronic stable respiratory disease and are inappropriate for patients who have asthma, whose impairment by definition is variable. The ATS has proposed a scoring system for the evaluation of disability in patients who have asthma[5].

Impairment of lung function as defined by the American Thoracic Society and European Society for Clinical Respiratory Physiology

Impairment	American Thoracic Society	European Society for Clinical Respiratory Physiology
None	FEV_1, FVC, and $DLCO$ >80%; FEV_1% >75%	> Reference value – 1.64 standard deviations
Mild	FEV_1, FVC, or $DLCO$ 60–79%; FEV_1% 60–74%	Not normal, but >60% reference value
Moderate	FEV_1, FEV_1%, or $DLCO$ 41–59%; or FVC 51–59%	40–59% reference value
Severe	FEV_1, FEV_1%, or $DLCO$ <40%; or FVC <50%	<40% reference value or FVC <50%

FEV_1, forced expiratory volume in 1s; FVC, forced vital capacity; $DLCO$, diffusing capacity of lung for carbon monoxide; FEV_1%, FEV_1/FVC%.

Figure 59.1 Impairment of lung function as defined by the American Thoracic Society and European Society for Clinical Respiratory Physiology. The rating is based upon the index that deviates most from normality.

ASSESSMENT OF EXERCISE ABILITY

Questionnaires

Assessment of disability includes an assessment of the extent to which exercise capacity is impaired. The simplest, structured method to assess limitation of exercise capacity is to use a validated questionnaire. One of the earliest and most widely used is that devised by the Medical Research Council in the UK[6], of which the questions about breathlessness are given in Figure 59.2. A more detailed questionnaire that assesses grades of breathlessness was devised by McGavin et al. (see Fig. 59.3)[7].

Medical Research Council questionnaire on respiratory symptoms – breathlessness

Question

Are you troubled by shortness of breath when hurrying on level ground or walking up a slight hill?

If yes

Do you become short of breath walking with other people of your own age on level ground?

If yes

Do you have to stop for breath when walking at your own pace on level ground?

Figure 59.2 The Medical Research Council questionnaire on respiratory symptoms – breathlessness.

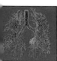
6. Medical Research Council. Questionnaire on respiratory symptoms. London: Medical Research Council; 1986.

7. McGavin CR, Artvinli M, Naoe H, McHardy GJR. Dyspnoea, disability, and distance walked: comparison of estimates of exercise performance in respiratory disease. Br Med J. 1978;2:241–3.

8. Cotes JE. The ventilatory cost of activity. Br J Ind Med. 1975;32:220–3.

9. Butland RJ, Pang J, Gross ER, Woodcock AA, Geddes DM. Two-, six, and 12-minute walking tests in respiratory disease. Br Med J. 1982;284:1607–8.

10. Cotes JE. Rating respiratory disability: a report on behalf of a working group of the European Society for Clinical Respiratory Physiology. Eur Respir J. 1990;3:1074–7.

11. Jones NL, Makrides L, Hitchcock C, Chypchar T, McCartney N. Normal standards for an incremental progressive cycle ergometer test. Am Rev Respir Dis. 1985;131:700–8.

12. Weller JJ, el-Gamal FM, Parker L, Reed JW, Cotes JE. Indirect estimation of maximal oxygen uptake for study of working populations. Br J Ind Med. 1988;45:532–7.

13. Cotes JE, Chinn DJ, Reed JW, Hutchinson JEM. Experience of a standardised method for assessing respiratory disability. Eur Respir J. 1994;7:875–80.

14. King B, Cotes JE. Relation of lung function and exercise capacity to mood and attitudes to health. Thorax. 1989;44:402–9.

15. Cotes JE. Assessment of disablement due to impaired respiratory function. Bull Eur Physiopathol Respir. 1975;11:210–17P.

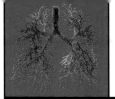
Chapter 60

Silicosis and Coal Workers' Pneumoconiosis

Daniel E Banks and William WL Chang

INTRODUCTION

Silicosis and coal workers' pneumoconiosis (CWP) result from the inhalation of mineral dusts, but despite their similar radiographic and clinical presentations, the pathologic features and natural histories may be quite different. Requirements for the diagnosis of both diseases are the same and include:

- a history of significant exposure, usually for 10 years or more, to either coal (typically in underground coal mining) or crystalline silica dust (often in mining, but in any occupation where exposure to silica particles occurs);
- radiographic features consistent with these illnesses (the parenchymal radiographic features of silicosis and CWP are identical); and
- the absence of illnesses that may mimic these diseases (primarily infections with a predominantly miliary radiographic pattern, such as tuberculosis, fungal infections, or sarcoidosis).

Symptoms such as cough, dyspnea, sputum, or respiratory impairment are of no discriminating value, but crackles and clubbing are not part of CWP or silicosis and should alert the clinician to the presence of other pulmonary diseases[1].

PATHOPHYSIOLOGY

Coal is formed by the accumulation of vegetable matter covered by sedimentary rock (creating an anaerobic environment) and subjected to pressure and temperature over time. The matter dries, becomes warmer, and loses oxygen and water content, all the while increasing the relative carbon content. This process of 'coalification' follows a transformation of vegetable matter (primarily wood) into peat, then lignite, bituminous coal, and finally anthracite coal. In the most simple terms, coal comprises moisture (which lessens with time), carbon, and mineral contaminants, with the overall composition varying with the coal seam. Dusts of high rank, such as anthracite, typically contain more silica than dusts of lesser rank, such as bituminous, and the anthracite seams often have roofs and floors of quartz, which contaminate the coal during mining.

The histopathologic hallmark of CWP is the coal macule. The coal macule is a focal collection of coal dust-laden macrophages at the division of respiratory bronchioles that may exist within alveoli and extend into the peribronchiolar interstitium with associated reticulin deposits and focal emphysema. Focal emphysema is the term used for the airspace enlargement that occurs adjacent to the coal macule[2] (Fig. 60.1).

Particles of silica and coal dust cause lung damage through:

- the direct cytotoxicity of the dust;
- cell death, with the ensuing release of oxidants, enzymes, and cell membrane constituents; and
- stimulation of cytokine release from alveolar macrophages to recruit effector cells (other macrophages or neutrophils) and stimulate fibroblast proliferation and collagen synthesis in the area of dust deposition.

When either coal or silica dust is cleared, free radicals are generated and present on the surface of the fractured particle. Excessive release of these reactive species may overwhelm the naturally protective antioxidant system within the lung and begin the process of inflammation and fibrosis. The coal particle is less fibrogenic than the silica particle, yet excessive exposures over a period of time overwhelm effective clearance mechanisms. Importantly, the free radicals generated by crushing anthracite coal are more numerous than those generated by crushing bituminous coal, leading to the suggestion that exposure to anthracite coal has a greater potential for causing fibrosis[3].

Silica is formed from the reaction of silicon with oxygen. It is an abundant mineral found in high concentrations of the free crystalline form in quartz, flint, chert, opal, chalcedony, and diatomite. Combined forms of silica are called silicates and include asbestos, talc, and kaolin. Inhalation of silicates may cause pneumoconiosis but with radiographic presentations that may be distinct from those in silicosis.

The histologic hallmark of silicosis is the silicotic nodule (see Fig. 60.2). This lesion has the whorled appearance that has been

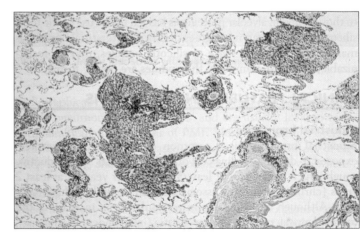

Figure 60.1 Macular lesion of coal workers' pneumoconiosis. The macular lesion seen near the center consists of collections of macrophages that are laded with coal dust and that completely fill alveolar spaces and extend into the connective tissue surrounding the respiratory bronchioles. The deposition of a small amount of collagen is also present. In the nearby areas, focal emphysema is noted. A bronchiole and an accompanying artery are seen at the right upper portion. Collections of macrophages laden with coal dust are also evident in the perivascular areas.

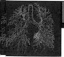
Major asbestos uses and sources of exposure		
Environment	**Type of exposure**	**Source of exposure**
Occupational	Asbestos–cement products	Construction industry (sheeting used in roofing and cladding of structural materials, molded into roof tiles, pipes, gutters; filler for wall cracks, cement, joint compound, adhesive, caulking putty)
	Floor tiling	Filler and reinforcing agent in asphalt flooring, vinyl tile, adhesive
	Insulation, fireproofing	Insulators, pipefitters
		Construction industry (pipes, boiler covers, ship bulkheads, sprayed on walls and ceilings as fireproofing, sound-proofing)
	Textiles	Fireproof textiles used in clothing, blankets
	Paper products	Roofing felt, wall coverings, mill board, insulating paper
	Friction materials	Brake linings
	Rubber, plastic manufacture	Filler in rubber and plastics
	Building trades, secondhand exposure	Building maintenance activities, pipefitting, electrical repair, boiler tending and repair, power station maintenance
		Carpenters, plumbers, welders
Domestic	'Fouling the nest'	Carry home asbestos in hair and clothes of exposed workers results in exposure to family members
	Secondhand exposure	Residential remodeling, removal, handling of frayed, friable asbestos in homes can cause environmental exposure
General	Contaminated buildings	Found in low levels in buildings under normal use
		Elevated exposures from remodeling, renovation, asbestos removal, disturbance of contaminated materials such as acoustic ceiling tiles, vinyl floor tiles, paints, plaster, pipes, boilers, steel beams
	Geologic exposure	Living near asbestos mines or cement factories, or in geographic areas in which naturally occurring asbestos is found in ambient air
	Urban environment	Ambient air levels slightly higher in cities, perhaps because of automotive brakes, and high concentration of industry and construction

Figure 61.2 The major environmental and occupational sources of asbestos exposure. Categorization is based on exposures in the workplace, home, or general environment.

fibers (Fig. 61.3). Gray streaks of fibrosis can be seen in the parenchyma, along interlobar and interlobular septa. Later, the pleural surface becomes more nodular in appearance and the parenchyma loses volume and elasticity, and forms more fibrotic scars and honeycombing. The gross pathologic appearance is most obvious in the lower lung zones bilaterally, with the worst disease nearest to the pleura. The pathology definition remains unclear[3,4]. The College of American Pathologists has defined four grades of severity describing interstitial and airway changes.

Although histologic evidence of pulmonary fibrosis may occasionally be obtained in the course of clinical evaluation, routine lung biopsy and lavage are not recommended, and microscopic evidence is rarely required to diagnose asbestosis[3,5].

Occasionally, the determination of asbestos fibers in lung tissue, bronchoalveolar lavage, or sputum may be used to document past exposure, although these measurements are not usually relied upon or required for the clinical diagnosis of asbestosis. Under light microscopy or using transmission electron microscopy, uncoated fibers or fibers coated with ferritin protein may be detected. These latter so-called asbestos bodies or ferruginous bodies are nonspecific, as they can be found in occupationally unexposed individuals, in occupationally exposed individuals who have no asbestos-related lung disease, and in workers who suffer asbestosis. Generally, the most exposed and most severely affected individuals have higher asbestos fiber counts, but a significant inter-laboratory variability is found in these measures.

Pathogenesis

Some of the major events thought to be involved in the pathogenesis of asbestosis are summarized in Figure 61.4. Within minutes after asbestos fibers have been inhaled, a local tissue response is initiated at the bifurcations of terminal bronchioles and alveolar ducts. The first changes occur in epithelial cells and then in alveolar macrophages as they attempt to engulf and are pierced by the fibers. In addition to cell death, which leads to the release of macrophage contents, asbestos-activated macrophages release reactive oxygen species that directly damage the tissue through peroxidation and direct cytotoxicity[1,6]. Asbestos can also induce toxicity by mechanisms independent of its ability to promote reactive oxygen species.

Increasing numbers of alveolar macrophages accumulate within 48 hours of first exposure. With chronic inhalation, a

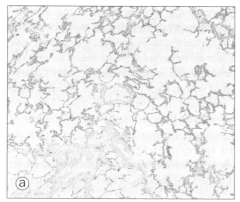

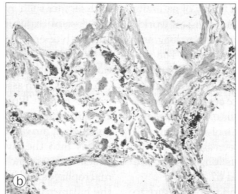

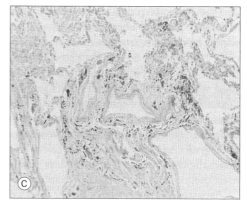

Figure 61.3 Histology of asbestosis. (a) In this grade 1 lesion, fibrosis is limited to the peribronchiolar tissue and the walls of the respiratory bronchioles (hematoxylin and eosin). (b) Enlargement of a grade 1 lesion illustrates presence of asbestos bodies (hematoxylin and eosin). (c) In this grade 3 lesion, fibrosis extends into the interstitial space between the respiratory units and into the alveolar ducts (hematoxylin and eosin). (Courtesy of Dr Val Vallythan, National Institute for Occupational Safety and Health, Morgantown, West Virginia.)

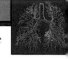

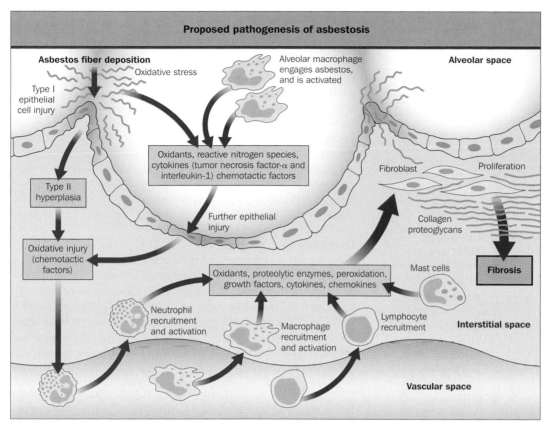

Figure 61.4 **Proposed pathogenesis of asbestosis.**
Asbestos fibers deposit at branch points in the distal airways and alveolar ducts, which prompts an inflammatory cascade characterized by cellular activation, recruitment, and injury. The result is fibroblast proliferation and extracellular matrix deposition in the interstitial space.

localized fibrosing alveolitis in the peribronchiolar region develops, followed by diffuse fibrotic scarring. Increasing the dose of asbestos increases the cellular response. A cascade of events ensues, in which the macrophages and neutrophils release various cytokines (such as interleukin-8 and interferon-γ), chemokines, oxidants, and growth factors (such as fibronectin, platelet-derived growth factor, insulin-like growth factor, transforming growth factor-β, tumor necrosis factor-α, and fibroblast growth factor). These attract and alter the function of other inflammatory cells and resident cells, and thus promote inflammation and fibrosis. The response of fibroblasts to these signals is to proliferate and produce the constituents of extracellular matrix (e.g. collagen, proteogylcans) in the pulmonary interstitium. Resident cells themselves are both targets and perpetrators of the fibrotic response. The pathogenesis of the chronic fibrotic response remains sketchy. However, it is clear that this chronic response is progressive and that, apart from macrophages, neutrophils, and epithelial cells, a number of other cell types, such as lymphocytes and mast cells, contribute to the cycle of lung remodeling and fibrosis. Multiple, functionally overlapping, redundant inflammatory events occur in the lung simultaneously during the period of fibrogenesis. The consequence is an irreversible alteration in the structure and function of the lung.

Clinical features

Asbestosis is the pulmonary fibrotic disease that results from asbestos exposure. It affects the lungs symmetrically and is typically diagnosed on the basis of a consistent occupational or environmental history of asbestos exposure plus evidence of pulmonary fibrosis, usually by chest radiography[5,7]. The latency period from first exposure to clinical disease is 10–20 years, but can be up to 40 years or more, with shorter latency and more severe disease seen in those workers who have the highest inhalational exposures. In some situations the exposure history may be difficult to document. If needed, further evidence of occupational exposure can be verified by identifying high numbers of asbestos bodies in bronchoalveolar lavage fluid, sputum, or lung tissue, as discussed above. Evidence of bilateral pleural plaques is pathognomonic for previous asbestos exposure. The radiographic finding of bilateral interstitial markings in the lower lung zone is sufficient radiographic evidence of asbestosis, although (as discussed below) other tools such as computed tomography (CT) and measures of lung physiology also aid diagnosis.

The most common symptoms of asbestosis are the insidious onset of dyspnea on exertion (and eventually at rest), dry cough which can be paroxysmal, and fatigue. Hemoptysis, chest pain, and weight loss are not common and should raise suspicion of asbestos-related malignancy. Although physical abnormalities are uncommon at the early stages of asbestosis, over time these patients may develop dry, bilateral basilar rales at end inspiration, digital clubbing in approximately one half of cases, cyanosis, and signs of cor pulmonale.

Radiologic findings

Radiographically, asbestosis typically presents in the lower lobes with irregular 'reticular' markings toward the lung periphery and costophrenic angles (see Fig. 61.5). Linear opacities that resemble extensions of vascular markings may assume a net-like appearance. In early or less severe disease, the mid and upper lung zones may appear relatively spared. With progression, the linear and irregular opacities thicken and spread to the mid lung zones, but rarely to the apex. The International Labor Organization (ILO) International Classification of Radiographs[8] characterizes each type of irregular opacity based on increasing size and thickness as

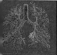

Occupational and Environmental Lung Diseases

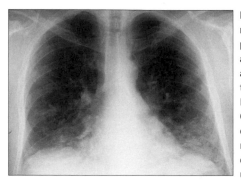

Figure 61.5 Chest radiograph illustrating parenchymal abnormalities in asbestosis. Descriptive terms from the International Labor Organization's classification for the radiographic appearance of pneumoconioses are used here (see Chapter 60, Fig. 60.3). Coarse 'u' and 't' reticular opacities can be seen in the lower lung zones. In this advanced case, the profusion of small opacities is 3/3.

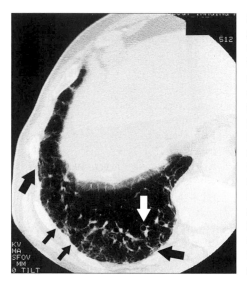

Figure 61.6 Asbestosis. High-resolution computed tomography (CT) of an asbestos-exposed worker who has asbestosis and mild pleural thickening. Patchy subpleural accentuation of interstitial markings (thick arrows) with honeycombing (thin arrows) and traction bronchiectasis (white arrow) are classic for the CT appearance of advanced asbestosis.

's', 't', or 'u,' and on a scale of profusion (number) of opacities from normal profusion (0/–, 0/0, 0/1) to severe (3/2, 3/3, 3/+; see Chapter 60, Fig. 60.3 for classification details). When irregular opacities are seen on the chest radiograph in conjunction with pleural thickening, the radiograph can be considered virtually pathognomonic for asbestosis. However, the chest radiograph lacks sensitivity, since 15–20% of symptomatic, biopsy-proved cases have normal chest radiographs. Focal masses are uncommon except those caused by rounded atelectasis.

Computed tomography

High-resolution computed tomography (HRCT), obtaining 1–3 mm slices, has superior sensitivity to the plain chest radiograph in detection of the fine reticular opacities in this disease. Of asbestos-exposed workers who have normal chest radiographs, 10–30% have HRCT scans that suggest underlying interstitial disease[9,10]. Thus, the HRCT can prove useful when the clinical index of suspicion for asbestosis is high, but the chest radiograph appears normal. The most common HRCT findings in asbestosis are short, peripheral septal lines, subpleural curvilinear lines, peripheral cystic lesions (honeycombing), parenchymal bands adjacent to areas of pleural thickening, and bronchiolar thickening (Fig. 61.6). The density of interstitial abnormalities found on HRCT has been shown to correlate with the symptoms, and with physiologic and inflammatory indicators of asbestosis[11,12], although in general both the chest radiograph and the HRCT show only a limited correlation with disease severity measured physiologically.

Pulmonary physiology

The earliest physiologic changes include small airways dysfunction [e.g. decreased forced expiratory flow ($FEF_{25-75\%}$)]. As the disease progresses, restriction (diminished total lung capacity and forced vital capacity) is observed, as is worsening gas exchange as measured by diffusing capacity, and by exercise- and rest-associated arterial blood gas partial pressures. These parameters do not necessarily show the same degree of abnormality. Measures of gas exchange are generally more sensitive than are measures of lung volumes in this disorder. Isolated, severe, obstructive airway disease is usually not attributable to asbestosis alone, although airflow obstruction can be observed with or without restriction, and occurs even in asbestos-exposed workers who were nonsmokers. The degree of airflow obstruction is related to the dose of exposure.

Diagnosis

The long latency between asbestos exposure and development of asbestosis and the gradually progressive nature of the symptoms mean that this disease has a tendency to remain undetected until fairly late in its course. Efforts to conduct workplace surveillance using the chest radiograph and ILO readings of these films has improved disease detection. The diagnosis is based on a consistent history of exposure to asbestos, with sufficient latency, and evidence of interstitial fibrosis. A careful work and environmental history holds the key to determining whether past exposure has occurred. As discussed above, the presence of bilateral pleural plaques or demonstration of asbestos bodies in lavage or on biopsy can also aid in the assessment of exposure. While most algorithms for diagnosis of asbestosis suggest that the combination of histologic material plus mineralogic assessment is the most sensitive and specific method of diagnosis, frequently such biopsy material is unavailable and unnecessary in making a probable determination of disease. Even the lung pathology should be considered in context with clinical data. The main considerations in the histologic differential diagnosis include the other pneumoconioses and other causes of pulmonary fibrosis such as pharmaceutical drugs, oxygen, metal dusts, infectious agents, autoimmune disorders, and idiopathic pulmonary fibrosis.

In the absence of lung histology and mineralogic analysis, the clinical diagnosis of asbestosis can be made with reasonable confidence based on:

- history of significant asbestos exposure;
- appropriate time interval between exposure and disease detection (latency); and
- radiographic evidence of bilateral lung fibrosis by chest radiograph or HRCT (especially with coexisting pleural plaques).

Helpful, but less essential, criteria include evidence of restrictive lung function, abnormalities of gas exchange, bilateral inspiratory crackles (rales), and digital clubbing.

Treatment

Presently, no cure exists for asbestosis and no benefit from the use of corticosteroids or other immunosuppressive therapy has been documented. Once exposure and early disease have occurred, no prophylatic measures are available.

Medical management in cases of asbestosis focuses on:

- supplemental oxygen therapy in the face of hypoxemia and/or pulmonary hypertension;
- treatment of intercurrent infections;
- treatment of right ventricular failure in advanced disease;

- immunization for influenza and pneumococcal infections;
- appropriate medical documentation of the degree of physical impairment and appropriate advice to the patient to apply for workers' compensation benefits if exposure was occupational;
- education on the signs and symptoms of lung cancer and mesothelioma;
- assistance in smoking cessation among current smokers who have asbestosis, to help reduce the risk of lung cancer; and
- cessation of ongoing asbestos exposure is advisable, since it may slow disease progression, based on experimental evidence[13].

Clinical course

The prognosis for patients with asbestosis varies widely. It is dependent, in part, on the magnitude of exposure. In 1906, the disease was almost uniformly fatal by the third decade of life. However, with fewer exposures and lower exposure times, and with superior detection and supportive care, few patients demonstrate such severe progression of their disease. After removal from exposure, progression is usually slow, and occurs in 5–40% of patients over approximately a decade of follow up. Thus, if clinical deterioration occurs over a period of days or weeks, the clinician must look first for other explanations, such as infection or malignancy. Many patients may remain mildly symptomatic for many years, and show little or no objective signs of disease progression, while others show steady, inexorable decline in lung function, gas exchange, worsening symptoms, development of end-stage respiratory insufficiency, and cor pulmonale with right ventricular failure.

Patients who suffer asbestosis are at increased risk of intercurrent lung infections and lung cancer. The best prognosis is found in those workers who have the lowest ILO profusion scores (i.e. chest radiographs that show the fewest irregular opacities) at time of termination of exposure. Tobacco smoking contributes to radiographic evidence of disease severity. Greater age at time of diagnosis is a strong predictor of progression; both smoking and exposure contribute relatively smaller, yet significant, effects also[14]. Multiple studies demonstrate that those with the greatest average and cumulative dust exposures tend to have the higher initial profusions of small opacities on chest radiographs and more rapid disease progression.

Based on National Center for Health Statistics data through 1992, for US residents the age-adjusted mortality rate attributable to asbestosis began to plateau in the 1990s, but only after having risen from an age-adjusted mortality rate of 0.44/1,000,000 population in 1968 to 3.01/1,000,000 in 1990. Mortality rates are much higher among men than among women, and the age at which people die of asbestosis has risen from a median of 60 years in 1968 to approximately 74 years in 1992. In 1992, asbestosis resulted in nearly 12,000 years of potential life lost to life expectancy[15]. Lung cancer is a significant contributing cause of increased mortality in asbestosis patients.

ASBESTOS-RELATED, NONMALIGNANT PLEURAL DISORDERS

The most common pleural changes caused by asbestos are pleural plaques, with or without pleural calcification and diffuse pleural thickening[16]. Once thought of as markers of exposure, these pleural changes are now known to contribute to the lung function abnormalities seen in asbestos-exposed workers. Both types of pleural alteration contribute independently to restrictive lung physiology (reduced vital capacity), reduced lung compliance, and diminished diffusing capacity[17,18]. Of asbestos-exposed construction workers, 20–60% demonstrate chest radiographic evidence of pleural disease, which is remarkable in light of the insensitivity of the radiograph.

Circumscribed pleural plaques that involve the parietal pleura are usually symmetric and bilateral, most commonly between the fifth and eighth ribs toward the posterolateral aspects of the thorax (Fig. 61.7); they also frequently involve the diaphragmatic pleura (Fig. 61.8). These lesions remain discrete. Thus, if radiographic evidence of more diffuse thickening is found, either mesothelioma or diffuse pleural thickening must be considered. Histologically, pleural plaques are hyalinized, acellular, avascular masses, and rarely contain asbestos bodies. They have a tendency to calcify, which can be mistaken for nodular infiltrates on the chest radiograph. Although the ILO classification system has an elaborate section devoted to characterization of pleural abnormalities on the chest radiograph, inter-reader agreement is relatively low. Since HRCT is more sensitive than chest radiography in the detection of pleural plaques, it helps to determine past asbestos inhalation, since these plaques are pathognomonic for that exposure. Also, HRCT helps to differentiate plaques from extrapleural fat pads. Asbestosis can occur in the absence of pleural disease and, inversely, pleural disease can occur without underlying pulmonary fibrosis, although

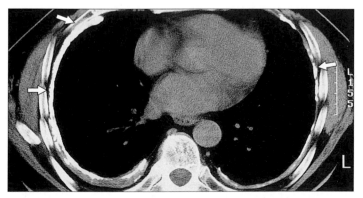

Figure 61.7 Pleural plaque. A conventional computed tomography scan of an asbestos worker shows extensive bilateral pleural calcifications (arrows).

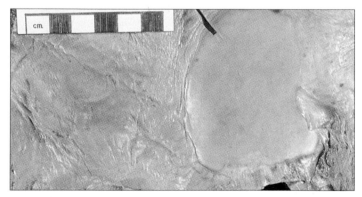

Figure 61.8 The gross pathologic appearance of a pleural plaque adjacent to the diaphragm of a construction worker. The benign pleural plaques that form as a consequence of asbestos inhalation have a smooth, shiny appearance and are usually well circumscribed.

autopsy studies suggest that when pleural changes are seen there is often histologic evidence of asbestosis even if the radiograph is normal. Pleural plaques rarely, if ever, undergo malignant transformation.

Diffuse pleural thickening involves both parietal and visceral pleura and is strongly associated with prior, benign asbestos pleural effusions. It may also develop when subpleural parenchymal fibrosis extends to the visceral pleura. Diffuse pleural thickening is most commonly located in the lower thorax, can blunt the costophrenic angles, and may be either unilateral or bilateral. As it is so diffuse, this form of pleural thickening can produce dyspnea on exertion and dry cough, as well as loss of lung function. Other conditions that can induce similar diffuse thickening include past tuberculosis, thoracic surgery, chest trauma with hemorrhage, adverse drug reactions, and infection.

Following direct contact of asbestos fibers and the pleural space, an inflammatory, exudative, and often hemorrhagic effusion can develop. It is asymptomatic in two thirds of cases, but can be associated with acute chest pain with or without fever. It can occur in the presence or absence of asbestosis. Its incidence in asbestos-exposed workers has been estimated to be <5%. While it can be the first manifestation of asbestos-related disease, the mean latency for benign, asbestos-related pleural effusions is 30 years[19]. These effusions often resolve spontaneously, but recur in approximately one third of cases. The regression may be associated with pain. The consequences include not only diffuse pleural thickening, but also the formation of adhesive fibrothorax. Benign pleural effusion is considered a diagnosis of exclusion.

Rounded atelectasis, while uncommon, is important to recognize because of its tendency to mimic lung tumors[20]. It is thought to occur when visceral pleural thickening invaginates and folds upon the lung parenchyma, resulting in atelectasis – CT is the preferred method of detecting its typical cicatricial pattern. Malignancy has only rarely been described in areas of rounded atelectasis.

PREVENTION

The threshold of asbestos exposure below which asbestosis will not occur is unclear, and so any asbestos exposure carries some potential risk of asbestos-related disease. Prevention is superior to treatment of disease, as there is no cure. The best preventive measure is to eliminate inhalational exposure by:

- not working with asbestos;
- not disturbing asbestos in buildings or other locations where it has been used in the past;
- encapsulating exposed areas of friable asbestos; and
- having asbestos removed by those experienced in asbestos abatement technologies.

Substitute materials that have less toxicity must be considered in industrial applications. When asbestos substitutes are not available, appropriately designed and maintained engineering controls must be used, such as local exhaust ventilation systems. Personal respiratory protection is appropriate for short periods of exposure or when other controls are not feasible. Such respirators must be appropriately fitted to the individual and tested for the degree of protection they afford the worker, by quantitative fit-testing. Showering and changing of work clothes at the end of work shifts help to eliminate take-home exposures. Workers must be educated about the combined risks of asbestos exposure and smoking, and must be counseled to avoid future asbestos exposure. Companies that use asbestos must strictly comply with government regulations as to the permissible exposure limits and appropriate medical surveillance of workers.

REFERENCES

1. Schwartz DA, Peterson MW. Asbestosis and asbestos-induced pleural fibrosis. In: Schwarz MI, King TE Jr, eds. Interstitial lung disease, 3rd edn. Hamilton: BC Decker; 1998:351–66.
2. Veblen DR, Wylie AG. Mineralogy of amphiboles and 1:1 layer silicates. In: Guthrie GD Jr, Mossman BT, eds. Health effects of mineral dusts. Reviews in Mineralogy, Vol. 28. Washington, DC: Mineralogical Society of America; 1993:275–308.
3. Craighead JE, Abraham JL, Churg A, et al. The pathology of asbestos-associated disease of the lung and pleural cavities: diagnostic criteria and proposed grading scheme. Arch Pathol Lab Invest. 1982;106:544–95.
4. Hammar SP. Controversies and uncertainties concerning the pathologic features and pathologic diagnosis of asbestosis. Semin Diagn Pathol. 1992;9:102–9.
5. Murphy RL, Becklake MR, Brooks SM, et al. The diagnosis of nonmalignant diseases related to asbestos. Am Rev Respir Dis. 1986;134:363–8.
6. Mossman BT, Churg A. Mechanisms in the pathogenesis of asbestosis and silicosis. Am J Respir Crit Care Med. 1998;157:1666–80.
7. Affairs COS. A physician's guide to asbestos-related diseases. JAMA. 1984;252:2593–7.
8. International Labor Office (ILO)/University of Cincinnati: International classification of radiographs of pneumoconiosis 1980, No.22 revised, Occupational safety and health series. Geneva: International Labor Office; 1980.
9. Staples CA, Gamsu F, Ray CS, Webb WR. High resolution computed tomography and lung function in asbestos-exposed workers with normal chest radiographs. Am Rev Respir Dis. 1989;139:1502–8.
10. Bégin R, Ostiguy G, Filion R, Colman N, Bertrand P. CT scan in early asbestosis. Br J Indust Med. 1993;50:689–98.
11. McCloud TC. Asbestos-related pleura and parenchymal fibrosis: detection with high-resolution CT. Invest Radiol. 1989;24:636–7.
12. Hartley PG, Galvin JR, Hunninghake GW, et al. High-resolution CT-derived measures of lung density are valid indexes of interstitial lung disease. J Appl Physiol. 1994;76:271–7.
13. Bégin R, Cantin A, Massé S. Influence of continued asbestos exposure on the outcome of asbestosis in sheep. Exp Lung Res. 1991;17:971–84.
14. Sluis-Cremer GK, Hnizdo E. Progression of irregular small opacities in asbestos miners. Br J Indust Med. 1989;46:846–52.
15. Division of Respiratory Disease Studies, National Institute for Occupational Safety and Health (NIOSH). Work-related lung disease surveillance report 1996. Washington, DC: U.S. Government Printing Office, DHHS (NIOSH) Publication No. 96–134; 1996:11–31.
16. Schwartz DA. New developments in asbestos-induced pleural disease. Chest. 1991;99:191–8.
17. Rosenstock L, Barnhart S, Heyer NJ, et al. The relation among pulmonary function, chest roentgenographic abnormalities, and smoking status in an asbestos-exposed cohort. Am Rev Respir Dis. 1988;138:272–7.
18. Schwartz DA, Fuortes LJ, Galvin JR, et al. Asbestos-induced pleural fibrosis and impaired lung function. Am Rev Respir Dis. 1990;141:321–6.
19. Hillerdal G. Non-malignant asbestos pleural disease. Thorax. 1981;36:669–75.
20. Mintzer RA, Cugell DW. The association of asbestos-induced pleural disease and rounded atelectasis. Chest. 1982;81:457–60.

Section 12 Occupational and Environmental Lung Diseases

Chapter 62 Occupational Asthma

Moira Chan-Yeung and Jean-Luc Malo

INTRODUCTION

Interest in occupational asthma (OA) has grown recently for several reasons. The prevalence of asthma has increased progressively during the past two decades and occupational exposure may be a contributing factor. The list of agents that can cause OA is steadily lengthening, and OA has become the most prevalent occupational lung disease in many developed countries, resulting in an increased burden to society. Moreover, OA is an excellent model to study the epidemiology, pathophysiology, genetics, and other aspects of asthma in humans.

The definition of OA is a disease characterized by variable airflow limitation and/or bronchial hyperresponsiveness caused by agents and conditions attributable to a particular working environment and not to stimuli encountered outside the workplace[1]. Individuals who have pre-existing or concurrent asthma are excluded by this definition.

The pathogenic mechanisms of OA provide a categorization – immunologically or nonimmunologically mediated. Immunologically-mediated OA is characterized by a latency period, while nonimmunologically mediated OA has no latency period.

EPIDEMIOLOGY, RISK FACTORS, AND PATHOPHYSIOLOGY

The most common form of occupational lung disease in developed countries is OA. It has been estimated that 5–15% of adult-onset asthma is caused by occupational exposure[2,3]. Several types of studies have been used to estimate the frequency of immunologic OA – population based-surveys, cross-sectional surveys in high-risk workplaces, registry based on physician reporting, and medicolegal statistics. Some results of these approaches are summarized in Figure 62.1[2]. In general, the prevalence of OA caused by agents of high molecular weight is <5% and that by those of low molecular weight is 5–10%. Reactive airways dysfunction syndrome (RADS) or irritant-induced asthma accounted for 17% of 154 consecutive cases of OA in one series[4]; this is the most common form of nonimmunologically induced asthma.

The degree of exposure is the most important determinant of OA. It is now possible to measure levels of exposure by personal sampling using a direct chemical-analytic method or, in the case of protein-derived allergens, by immunologic methods. Some agents appear to be more potent in inducing sensitization than others.

Pathophysiology

A latency period characterizes OA induced by immunologic mechanisms. Only a small proportion of the exposed subjects are affected and exposure to a minute quantity of the offending agent can result in a severe asthmatic reaction. While some agents induce asthma through the production of specific immunoglobulin E (IgE) antibodies, in others the immunologic mechanisms responsible have not yet been identified.

Immunologic, IgE mediated

Occupational agents of high molecular weight act as complete antigens and induce production of specific IgE antibodies. The best examples are laboratory animals and flour. Some occupational agents of low molecular weight, which include platinum salts, trimellitic anhydride, and other acid anhydrides also induce specific IgE antibodies. They probably act as haptens and bind with proteins to form complete antigens.

Reactions between specific IgE antibodies and antigens lead to a cascade of events that result in the release of inflammatory

Frequency of occupational asthma				
Survey type	Population	Number of subjects	Participation (%)	Prevalence
Population-based	Spain	2646	61	5.0–7.7%
	New Zealand	1609	64	1.9–3.1%
Registry based on voluntary reporting	United Kingdom	554	Not relevant	22/million per year
	Quebec	287	Not relevant	60/million per year
	British Columbia	124	Not relevant	92/million per year
	Sweden	1010	Not relevant	80/million per year
Survey in high-risk workplaces[4]	Agents of high molecular weight			
	Snow-crab processors	303	97	15%
	Clam/shrimp	57	93	4%
	Psyllium (pharmacists)	130	93	4%
	Psyllium (nurses)	194	91	4%
	Guar gum	151	96	3%
	Agents of low molecular weight			
	Isocyanates	51	100	12%
	Spiramycin	51	100	8%
	White cedar	31	94	10%
Medicolegal	Quebec	c. 60/year	Not relevant	c. 20/million per year
	Finland	352	Not relevant	c. 156/million per year

Figure 62.1 Frequency of occupational asthma.

mediators and influx of cells in the airway; this produces airway inflammation and development of airway hyperresponsiveness, as in asthma caused by common allergens. No differences are apparent in the pathogenetic mechanisms between OA induced by high-molecular-weight occupational agents and those of allergic nonoccupational asthma (see Chapter 40).

Immunologic, nonIgE mediated

Many low-molecular-weight agents, such as isocyanates and plicatic acid (responsible for Western red cedar asthma), have been shown to cause OA, and yet specific IgE antibodies cannot be found or are found in only a small percentage of the affected subjects. The significance of these antibodies in the pathogenesis of asthma is not clear.

Bronchial biopsies of subjects who suffer OA have shown activation of T lymphocytes, which suggests that T lymphocytes may play a direct role mediating airways inflammation[5]. This hypothesis has been substantiated by the finding of proliferation of peripheral blood lymphocytes when stimulated with the appropriate antigen in a proportion of affected subjects who have nickel-induced asthma and Western red cedar asthma. In isocyanate-induced asthma, increases of CD8-positive cells and eosinophils were found in the peripheral blood of the subjects during a late asthmatic reaction induced by exposure testing[5]. Cloning of T lymphocytes from the bronchial biopsies of these subjects showed that the majority of the clones exhibited the CD8 phenotype, which produced interferon-γ (IFN-γ) and interleukin-5 (IL-5), with very few clones that produced IL-4[5]. This provides supportive evidence that CD8 lymphocytes may play a direct role in OA, without the need to produce IgE antibodies.

Some low-molecular-weight agents have pharmacologic properties that cause bronchoconstriction. For example, isocyanates may block the β_2-adrenergic receptor. Isocyanates and other occupational agents may also stimulate sensory nerves to release substance P and other peptides, which have been shown to inhibit the neutral endopeptidases necessary for the inactivation of neuropeptides. Neuropeptides affect many cells in the airways and cause cough, smooth muscle contraction, and mucus production in subjects who have asthma. Thus, some occupational agents such as the isocyanates may induce asthma through more than one mechanism.

An autopsy study of the lung of one subject who had isocyanate-induced asthma and died after re-exposure showed denudation of airways epithelium, subepithelial fibrosis, and infiltration of the lamina propria by leukocytes (mainly eosinophils and diffuse mucous plugging of the bronchioles), similar to the lungs of patients who die from nonoccupational asthma[6]. Bronchial biopsies of 18 subjects who had proven OA also showed extensive epithelial desquamation, ciliary abnormalities of the epithelial cells, smooth muscle hyperplasia, and subepithelial fibrosis (Fig. 62.2)[7]. The total cell count, and number of eosinophils and lymphocytes were increased compared with those of healthy controls.

Nonimmunologic

Absence of latency characterizes OA caused by nonimmunologic mechanisms. The underlying mechanism of RADS is not known. It has been postulated that extensive denudation of the epithelium in these conditions leads to airways inflammation and airways hyperresponsiveness for several reasons, which include loss of the epithelial-derived relaxing factors, exposure of the nerve endings

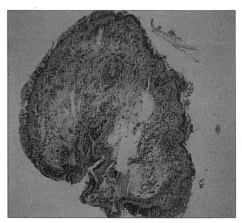

Figure 62.2 Bronchial biopsy of patient who had occupational asthma caused by toluene di-isocyanates. After removal from exposure, partial desquamation of the epithelium, thickened basement membrane, and some cellular infiltration were found.

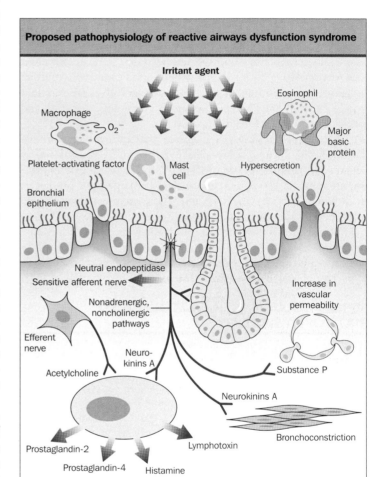

Figure 62.3 Proposal for the pathophysiology of reactive airways dysfunction syndrome.

(leading to neurogenic inflammation), and nonspecific activation of mast cells with release of mediators and cytokines (Fig. 62.3).

Sequential changes in the airways of subjects who have RADS or irritant-induced asthma have been described[8]. In the acute phase of RADS, rapid denudation of the mucosa with fibrinohemorrhagic exudate in the submucosa is followed by regeneration of the epithelium with proliferation of basal and parabasal cells and subepithelial edema (Fig. 62.4). In the chronic phase of RADS, the airways wall thickens markedly (Fig. 62.5)[8]. In a study of irritant-induced asthma caused by multiple exposure to an irritant, inflammatory

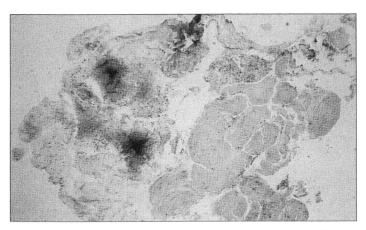

Figure 62.4 Bronchial biopsy taken 3 days after an acute accidental inhalation of a high concentration of chlorine. This shows almost complete desquamation of bronchial mucosa with fibrinohemorrhagic deposit (Weigert–Masson stain).

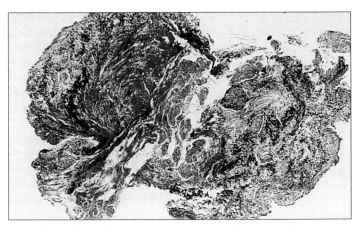

Figure 62.5 Bronchial biopsy taken 2 years after an acute accidental inhalation of chlorine showing severe desquamation of epithelial cells. Smooth muscle cells are surrounded by reticulocollagenic fibrous tissue (Weigert–Masson stain).

infiltrate with eosinophils and lymphocytes, as well as diffuse deposition with collagen fibers, were found[9].

CLINICAL FEATURES

Many agents can cause OA, and those that cause immunologically mediated OA include a broad spectrum of protein-derived as well as natural and synthetic chemicals used in various workplaces. Extensive lists of causative agents and workplaces have been published and a database on computer diskette has been made available by professional agencies[10]. The most common workplaces and agents to cause immunologically mediated OA are listed in Figure 62.6. Such agents can be classified according to their molecular weight – high (>5000Da) and low (<5000Da).

Figure 62.7 shows some of the agents reported to have given rise to RADS[12]. All agents in exceedingly high concentrations can theoretically cause OA through nonimmunologic mechanisms, especially those agents that occur in vapor or gaseous forms, such as chlorine and ammonia.

The clinical signs and symptoms of OA are similar to those of other types of asthma. However, it is not uncommon for rhinitis to occur several months before the onset of asthma. At the onset of the illness, many patients present with cough, wheeze, and shortness of breath after working hours, with improvement during the evening. Their symptoms improve whenever they are away from work and recur when they return to work. As they continue to be exposed, symptoms tend to occur earlier during the shift. In some individuals, symptoms may develop immediately upon exposure to the causative agent. At this stage, no remission of symptoms occurs during weekends – a much longer period is necessary for improvement to take place.

Common agents that cause immunologically mediated occupational asthma and at-risk occupations	
Agent	**Workers at risk**
High molecular weight	
Cereals	Bakers, millers
Animal-derived allergens	Animal handlers
Enzymes	Detergent users, pharmaceutical workers, bakers
Gums	Carpet makers, pharmaceutical workers
Latex	Health professionals
Seafoods	Seafood processors
Low molecular weight	
Isocyanates	Spray painters, insulation installers, manufactures of plastics, rubbers, foam
Wood dusts	Forest workers, carpenters, cabinetmakers
Anhydrides	Users of plastics, epoxy resins
Amines	Shellac and lacquer handlers, solderers
Fluxes	Electronic workers
Chloramine-T	Janitors, cleaners
Dyes	Textile workers
Persulfate	Hairdressers
Formaldehyde, glutaraldehyde	Hospital staff
Acrylate	Adhesive handlers
Drugs	Pharmaceutical workers, health professionals
Metals	Solderers, refiners

Figure 62.6 Common agents that cause immunologically mediated occupational asthma and at-risk occupations. (Reproduced with permission from Chan-Yeung and Malo[11]. ©1995 Massachusetts Medical Society. All rights reserved.)

Agents responsible for reactive airways dysfunction syndrome		
Acetic acid	Diesel exhaust	Spray paint
Sulfuric acid	Diethylaminoethanol	Sulfur dioxide
Chloridric acid	Epichlorohydrin	Gas (chlorine, mustard, phosgene, etc.)
Heated acid	Ethylene oxide	Fire/smoke
Ammonia	Isocyanates	Floor sealant
Bleaching agent	Metal remover	Formol–Zenker
Chlorine	Oxide (calcium)	Cleaning mist
Chloropicrin	Paints (heated)	Hydrazine
Cleaning agents	Phthalic anhydride	

Figure 62.7 Agents responsible for reactive airways dysfunction syndrome. (Information from Lemiere et al.[12])

The clinical presentations of subjects whose OA results from IgE-mediated and from non-IgE-mediated causes are different. The latency period is longer for agents of high molecular weight than for those of low molecular weight. The temporal pattern of bronchial reactions on specific inhalation challenges in the laboratory is different. Immediate or dual reactions occur more frequently for high-molecular-weight agents, while isolated late or atypical reactions develop for low-molecular-weight agents.

The presence of sensitization to occupational agents can be detected either by skin tests or by radioallergoabsorbent (RAST) or enzyme-linked immunosorbent assay tests. In subjects who have compatible clinical histories of OA and bronchial hyper-responsiveness, a positive skin or RAST test probably has a diagnostic accuracy close to 80%. Unfortunately, very few standardized materials for skin tests or for RAST tests in OA are commercially available.

Atopic subjects are much more prone to develop sensitization to agents of high molecular weight[13]. Smoking predisposes workers to sensitization to some agents, which include platinum salts[13]. However, nonatopic subjects and nonsmokers are more often affected in OA caused by agents that induce asthma through non-IgE-mediated mechanisms[13]. Certain HLA class II antigens have been reported to confer susceptibility to, while others provide protection from OA caused by low-molecular-weight compounds[5].

The cause of RADS is acute airways injury from accidental exposure to a high dose of irritants[14]. The typical clinical presentation is the development of symptoms of asthma within a few hours of acute exposure in a subject who has no history of any respiratory symptoms. The symptoms of asthma usually last for more than 3 months, associated with nonallergic bronchial hyper-responsiveness.

DIAGNOSIS

It is necessary to confirm the diagnosis of OA using objective means for several reasons. The diagnosis of OA has considerable socioeconomic implications to the worker and family; it usually means a change of job in most instances, with its financial consequences. In Quebec, each accepted claim of OA costs the compensation board US$35,000 equivalent; thus, it is costly to the society. Asthma is a common disease that affects 6–8% of the adult population in Canada and higher proportions in other parts of the world. The combination of asthma and working in an environment with an agent known to give rise to OA does not make the diagnosis of OA.

An occupational cause should be suspected for all new cases of adult-onset asthma. A detailed occupational history on past and current exposure to possible causal agents in the workplace, work processes, and specific job duties must be obtained. In addition, the intensity, frequency, and peak concentrations of exposure in the workplace are assessed qualitatively. Information can be requested from the work site, including material safety data sheets, although (in some instances) the information is incomplete on all constituents of the product. Computerized databases and published lists of agents and workplaces are very useful. Walk-through visits of the workplace may be necessary. Industrial hygiene data and employee health records can be obtained.

Open medical questionnaires are fairly sensitive but not specific tools for diagnostic purposes. Temporal associations are not suffi-

cient to diagnose work-related asthma. Ocular and nasal symptoms often accompany respiratory symptoms, are more frequent in OA caused by high molecular weight than by low molecular weight agents, and usually precede the onset of asthma symptoms.

An individual suspected to have OA may be best assessed by a specialist in this area, the role of whom is to confirm the diagnosis of OA by objective means if possible and to assess impairment and/or disability. A delay in referral may jeopardize the chance to confirm the diagnosis using objective measurements, as the subject may have left the workplace and have recovered or the working conditions may have changed.

An algorithm for the clinical investigation of OA is given in Figure 62.8. The advantages and pitfalls of the various tools used to confirm the diagnosis of OA are listed in Figure 62.9. For high-molecular-weight agents, skin tests to detect immediate reactivity and/or measurements of specific IgE antibodies are important tools. Although having immediate skin reactivity to an inhalant only reflects immunologic 'sensitization' and not necessarily the disease, it has been shown that having both immediate skin reac-

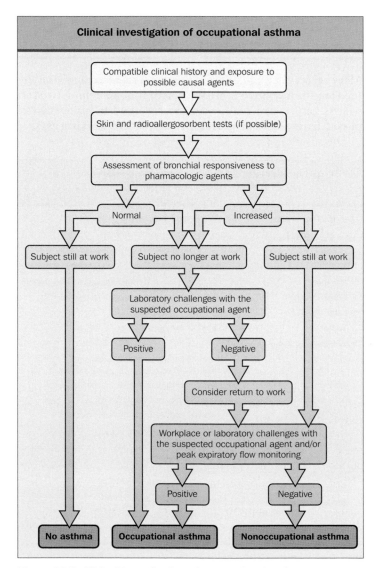

Figure 62.8 Clinical investigation of occupational asthma.

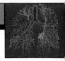

Advantages and disadvantages of diagnostic methods in occupational asthma		
Method	**Advantages**	**Disadvantages**
Questionnaire	Simple, sensitive	Low specificity
Immunologic testing	Simple, sensitive	Only for agents of high molecular weight and for some of low molecular weight; identifies sensitization, not disease; no 'standardized' and commercially available agents
Bronchial responsiveness to methacholine/histamine	Simple, sensitive	Not specific for asthma or occupational asthma; occupational asthma not ruled out by a negative test if workers are no longer exposed
Measurement of forced expiratory volume in 1s (FEV_1) before and after a work shift	Simple, inexpensive	Low sensitivity and specificity
Peak expiratory flow monitoring	Relatively simple, inexpensive	Requires patient's cooperation and honesty; not as sensitive as FEV_1 or a computerized method to assess airway caliber to interpret changes
Specific inhalation challenges in a hospital laboratory	If positive, confirmatory	Diagnosis not ruled out by a negative confirmatory test; (e.g. if wrong agent or subject no longer at work); expensive; few referral centers
Serial FEV_1 measurement at work under supervision	If negative, rules out diagnosis when patient tested under usual work	A positive test may be result from conditions irritation; requires collaboration of employer

Figure 62.9 Advantages and disadvantages of diagnostic methods in occupational asthma. (Reproduced with permission from Chan-Yeung and Malo[11]. ©1995

tivity and increased bronchial hyperresponsiveness results in an 80% likelihood of developing an asthmatic attack on laboratory exposure to this agent[15]. Unfortunately, reagents used for skin and *in-vitro* testings are not standardized and are generally prepared from occupational agents in individual laboratories.

The absence of nonallergic bronchial hyperresponsiveness in a subject at the end of 2 weeks of working under the usual conditions virtually excludes the diagnosis of asthma and OA. If there is nonallergic bronchial hyperresponsiveness, further testing is required. Measuring spirometry before and after a work shift has not been found to be sensitive or specific. Two options can be considered for objective confirmation, depending on availability (see Fig. 62.8). Exposure to the suspected agent under control conditions in a hospital laboratory can be carried out, as originally described by Pepys and Hutchcroft[16]. Attempts have been made to improve specific challenge tests by exposing subjects in the laboratory to low and stable levels of dry or wet aerosols and vapors to avoid nonspecific reactions. However, these tests can be falsely negative if a wrong agent is used for the test or if the subject has been away from work for too long, although such occurrences are rare. If this is the case, the subject is instructed to return to the workplace if feasible, and specific laboratory or work site challenges repeated at a later time.

Burge[17] and coworkers were the first to propose the use of serial measurements of peak expiratory flow (PEF) using portable devices for the diagnosis of OA. An example of serial PEF recording is shown in Figure 62.10. Although relatively good correlation is found between results of serial PEF monitoring and OA as confirmed by specific inhalation challenges in the laboratory, several limitations and pitfalls occur in PEF monitoring (see Fig. 62.9). When PEF monitoring is suggestive of OA and specific inhalation challenges in the laboratory are not possible or negative, it is advisable to confirm OA by sending a technician to the workplace and record spirometry serially throughout a work shift. The use of computerized peak flow

meters helps to overcome some of the problems of PEF monitoring. Combination of PEF monitoring with serial assessments of nonallergic bronchial responsiveness can provide further objective evidence, although this does not add to the sensitivity and specificity of PEF monitoring alone.

TREATMENT

The ideal treatment for patients who have OA is removal from the causal exposure permanently, with retraining for alternative employment if necessary. Larger companies may be able to relocate the patient to another job in the same plant or another plant that has no exposure; they may also be able to improve ventilation, or change work practices to eliminate or reduce exposure, but usually this is not possible for smaller companies. Any patient who has OA and remains in the same job must have respiratory protection and close medical follow-up. Worsening of asthma should lead to immediate removal from exposure. Pharmacologic treatment of patients who have OA is similar to that for other types of asthma. Although removal from exposure generally results in improvement, patients may continue to require medication and have airflow limitation or nonallergic bronchial hyperresponsiveness.

Once the diagnosis is made, physicians should counsel patients concerning compensation; the specifics vary from country to country. The appropriate public health authority should be notified, and such agencies need to initiate surveillance programs once sentinel cases have been identified. Patients should also be referred to compensation boards or similar agencies where appropriate. Patients are evaluated for temporary impairment when their asthma is under control, and evaluation for permanent impairment and disability takes place when improvement is maximal, which may take 1–2 years. The guidelines for assessment of impairment and disability for patients who have chronic irreversible lung diseases are inappropriate for those who have asthma. The American Thoracic Society guidelines attempt to take into account all the special

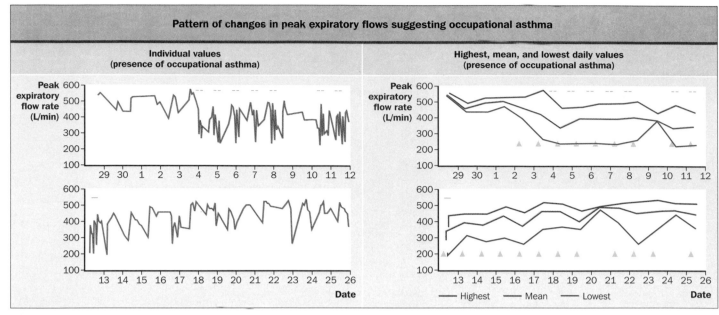

Figure 62.10 Pattern of changes in peak expiratory flows that suggest occupational asthma. The horizontal lines show the periods at work, while the triangles illustrate the need for an inhaled bronchodilator. [Adapted with permission from Malo et al.[18] (BMJ Publishing Group.).]

features of asthma[19]. In addition to measurements of lung function, assessment of impairment includes the degree of nonallergic bronchial hyperresponsiveness or airways reversibility, the minimum amount of medication required to maintain control of asthma, and the effects of asthma on the quality of life. When a change in clinical status occurs, reassessment is recommended.

CLINICAL COURSE

Subjects who have OA deteriorate if they continue in the same job without protection[20]. Fatality has been reported in a subject who had isocyanate-induced asthma and who died while working and exposed to the same agent[6]. A scheme of the progressive natural history of OA is shown in Figure 62.11.

The majority of patients who have OA improve, but do not recover completely even several years after removal from exposure[22]. Figure 62.12 shows some of the studies. The proportion

of subjects followed up in these studies is high, which suggests that the high rate of persistence of asthma is not the result of bias, that is 'sick' ones return for the follow-up examination. Follow-up studies of patients who have various types of OA show that those subjects who became asymptomatic after no further exposure had higher lung function and lower degree of nonallergic bronchial hyperresponsiveness at the time of diagnosis, and a shorter duration of exposure after the onset of symptoms. These findings suggest that they were diagnosed at an earlier stage of the diseases. Early diagnosis and removal from exposure are essential to ensure recovery.

Although symptoms and lung function improve within 1 year after removal from exposure, it takes longer for nonallergic bronchial hyperresponsiveness to improve. Specific IgE antibodies decrease even more slowly, with no plateau after 5 years as shown in subjects who have asthma induced by snow crabs[23]. It has been recommended that assessment of permanent respiratory

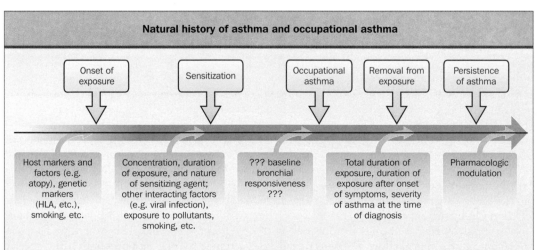

Figure 62.11 Natural history of asthma and occupational asthma. The boxes illustrate the steps, while the modifying factors before each step are listed under the horizontal line. (Reproduced with permission from Malo et al.[21])

Retrospective evidence for the persistence of symptoms and bronchial hyperresponsiveness after removal from the offending agent					
Agent	Number of cases	Duration of follow-up (years)	Persistence of symptoms (%)	Nonspecific bronchial hyperreactivity	
				Number	Percentage
Red cedar	38	0.5–4	29	38/38	100
	75	1–9	49	25/33	76
Colophony	20	1.3–3.8	90	7/20	35
Snow-crab	31	0.5–2	61	28/31	90
	31	4.8–6	100	26/31	84
Various	32	0.5–4	93	31/32	97
Isocyanates	12	1–3	66	7/12	58
	50	>4	82	12/19	63
	20	0.5–4	50	9/12	75
	22	1	77	17/22	77
Various	28	4–11	100	25/26	96

Figure 62.12 Retrospective evidence for the persistence of symptoms and bronchial hyperresponsiveness after removal of the offending agent. (Reproduced from Chan-Yeung and Malo[22] by courtesy of Marcel Dekker, Inc.)

impairment/disability should take place after at least 2 years of cessation of exposure[19].

The rate of decline in lung function of subjects who have OA with continuous exposure was greater than that of subjects who did not have asthma[24]. Moreover, specific bronchial reactivity to the offending occupational agents often persist after the subject has not been exposed for 2 or more years[25]. Thus, it is not advisable for these patients to return to the same job after they become asymptomatic.

The persistence of symptoms and nonallergic bronchial hyperresponsiveness in patients who have OA has a histologic basis. Higher total cell count and eosinophils in bronchoalveolar lavage fluid were found in subjects who had Western red cedar asthma and did not recover compared with those who recovered completely after removal from exposure. Saetta et al. documented improvement in airway wall remodeling (thickness of subepithelial fibrosis and number of subepithelial fibroblasts) 6 months after cessation of exposure in patients who had asthma induced by toluene di-isocyanate[26], but there was no improvement in bronchial inflammation and in the degree of nonallergic bronchial

hyperresponsiveness. However, the reasons for the persistence of symptoms, nonallergic bronchial hyperresponsiveness, and airway inflammation after removal from exposure are not known.

Some researchers have explored the possibility of 'curing' subjects who have OA using inhaled corticosteroids to reduce the degree of airways inflammation after the patients have permanently left the workplace[27]. While some improvements in various clinical and functional parameters were found, no case of cure from asthma was documented.

Since most cases of RADS occur in isolation, it is difficult to study the natural history using a series of such patients.

PITFALLS AND CONTROVERSIES

It is important to have objective evidence that the patient's asthma results from occupational exposure – confirmation of OA has many pitfalls. Lists of agents that cause OA published in articles and databases are useful to alert the physician, but the absence of an agent on such lists does not exclude the possibility of OA, as new chemicals are constantly being introduced into the market. Patients are often asked to leave the job when the diagnosis is suspected. However, one of the objective tests is to ask the patient to carry out serial monitoring of PEF for a period at work and a period away from work. Unless the patient has severe symptoms, it is best to obtain objective evidence first, before asking the patient to resign from his or her job. As discussed above, PEF monitoring also has limitations and must be measured according to a protocol and with a logging device, or together with serial measurement of nonallergic bronchial hyperresponsiveness. Specific-challenge tests have been said to be the 'gold standard' in diagnosis of OA, but these are not without pitfalls since both false positive and false negative results occur. When a new agent is suspected, investigators often uses several methods to confirm the diagnosis.

Although most people include RADS as a form of OA, others think that it is an entirely different condition because of differences in pathologic features. It is still very unclear whether exposure to a low level of irritant gases or fumes in the workplace or in the environment can actually induce asthma *de novo*. The long-term outcome of RADS has yet to be studied.

Despite a great deal that has been learned about OA over the past few years, much is still not known. Future research priorities should include further improvement in diagnostic and screening methods, as well as control of exposure to prevent development of the disease.

REFERENCES

1. Bernstein IL, Chan-Yeung M, Malo JL, Berstein D. Asthma in the workplace. New York: Marcel Dekker; 1993.
2. Chan-Yeung M, Malo JL. Epidemiology of occupational asthma. In: Busse W, Holgate S, eds. Rhinitis and asthma. Boston: Blackwell Scientific; 1994:44–57.
3. Blanc P. Occupational asthma in a national disability survey. Chest. 1987;92:613–7.
4. Tarlo SM, Broder I. Irritant-induced occupational asthma. Chest. 1989;96:297–300.
5. Mapp CE, Saetta M, Maestrelli P, et al. Mechanisms and pathology of occupational asthma. Eur Respir J. 1994;7:544–54.
6. Fabbri LM, Danieli D, Crescioli S, et al. Fatal asthma in a subject sensitized to toluene diisocyanate. Am Rev Respir Dis. 1988;137:1494–8.
7. Boulet LP, Boutet M, Laviolette M, et al. Airway inflammation after removal from the causal agent in occupational asthma due to high and low molecular weight agents. Eur Respir J. 1994;7:1567–75.
8. Lemiere C, Malo JL, Boulet LP, Boutet M. Reactive airways dysfunction syndrome induced by exposure to a mixture containing isocyanate: functional and histopathologic behaviour. Allergy. 1996;51:262–5.
9. Chan-Yeung M, Lam S, Kennedy SM, Frew AJ. Persistent asthma after repeated exposure to high concentrations of gases in pulpmills. Am J Respir Crit Care Med. 1994;149:1676–80.

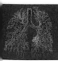
Occupational and Environmental Lung Diseases

10. Chan-Yeung M, Malo JL. Etiological agents in occupational asthma. Eur Respir J. 1994;7:346–71.
11. Chan-Yeung M, Malo J-L. Occupational asthma. N Engl J Med. 1995;333:107–12.
12. Lemiere C, Malo JL, Gautrin D. Nonsensitizing causes of occupational asthma. Med Clin North Am. 1996;80:749–74.
13. Chan-Yeung M. Occupational asthma. Chest. 1990;98:148S–61S.
14. Brooks SM, Weiss MA, Bernstein IL. Reactive airways dysfunction syndrome (RADS); persistent asthma syndrome after high level irritant exposures. Chest. 1985;88:376–84.
15. Malo JL, Cartier A, L'Archeveque J, et al. Prevalence of occupational asthma and immunologic sensitization to psyllium among health personnel in chronic care hospitals. Am Rev Respir Dis. 1990;142:1359–66.
16. Pepys J, Hutchcroft BJ. Bronchial provocation tests in etiologic diagnosis and analysis of asthma. Am Rev Respir Dis. 1975;112:829–59.
17. Burge PS. Single and serial measurements of lung function in the diagnosis of occupational asthma. Eur J Respir Dis. 1982;63 (Suppl. 123):47–59.
18. Malo JL, Côté J, Cartier A, Boulet LP, L'Archevêque J, Chan-Yeung M. How many times per day should peak expiratory flow rates be assessed when investigating occupational asthma? Thorax. 1993;48:1211–7.
19. American Thoracic Society. Ad Hoc Committee on Impairment/Disability Evaluation in Subjects with Asthma. Guidelines for the evaluation of impairment/disability in patients with asthma. Am Rev Respir Dis. 1993;147:1056–61.
20. Côté J, Kennedy S, Chan-Yeung M. Outcome of patients with cedar asthma with continuous exposure. Am Rev Respir Dis. 1990;141:373–6.
21. Malo JL, Ghezzo H, D'Aguino C, L'Archevêque J, Cartier A, Chan-Yeung M. Natural history of occupational asthma: relevance of type of agent and other factors in the rate of development of symptoms in affected subjects. J Allergy Clin Immunol. 1992;90:937–43.
22. Chan-Yeung M, Malo J-L. Natural history of occupational asthma. In: Bernstein IL, Chan-Yeung M, Malo JL, Berstein D, eds. Asthma in the workplace. New York: Marcel Dekker; 1993:299–322.
23. Malo JL, Cartier A, Ghezzo H, Lafrance M, McCants M, Lehrer SB. Patterns of improvement on spirometry, bronchial hyperresponsiveness, and specific IgE antibody levels after cessation of exposure in occupational asthma caused by snow-crab processing. Am Rev Respir Dis. 1988;138:807–12.
24. Lin FJ, Dimich-Ward H, Kennedy S, Chan-Yeung M. Longitudinal decline in lung function in patients with occupational asthma due to Western red cedar. Occup Environ Med. 1996;53:753–56.
25. Lemiere C, Cartier A, Dolovich J, et al. Outcome of specific bronchial responsiveness to occupational agents after removal from exposure. Am J Respir Crit Care Med. 1996;154:329–33.
26. Saetta M, Maestrelli P, DiStefano A, et al. Effect of cessation of exposure to toluene diisocyanate (TDI) on bronchial mucosa of subjects with TDI-induced asthma. Am Rev Respir Dis. 1992;145:169–74.
27. Malo JL, Cartier A, Côté J, et al. Influence of inhaled steroids on recovery from occupational asthma after cessation of exposure: an 18-month double-blind crossover study. Am J Respir Crit Care Med. 1996;153:953–60.

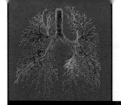
Chapter **63**	Air Pollution
	Helgo Magnussen

INTRODUCTION

The potential risk of environmental pollution to human health, particularly the effects of air pollution on the respiratory system, have been studied extensively during the past decades. Sulfur dioxide (SO_2) and particles form the most important components of smog during winter ('London-type' smog), whereas nitrogen dioxide (NO_2) and ozone (O_3) are the major components of photochemical smog during summer ('Los Angeles-type' smog). Particles are associated with both these types.

SULFUR DIOXIDE

Formation and exposure levels

Sulfur dioxide is produced mainly by the combustion of fossil fuels. Owing to the reduction in household coal burning and the increased number of large sources of emission, such as power plants, the distribution of emission sources has changed over the past decades. Currently, however, in most areas average annual ambient air concentrations are below 20 parts per billion (ppb) volume/volume. During episodes of air pollution, concentrations of more than 100ppb, with peaks exceeding 200ppb, may occur; in some places, particularly in eastern Europe, SO_2 concentrations may be as high as 500ppb. It has to be noted that the levels of SO_2 are often closely linked to those of particulate matter (PM).

Epidemiologic studies

Epidemiologic studies suggest that extremely high levels of SO_2 are associated with daily mortality, with a delay over days, and with respiratory morbidity due to asthma and bronchitis. These observations are in accordance with those made during the London smog episode in December 1952. The pollutant mixture encountered there contained high levels of SO_2 and suspended particles. Even at lower concentrations, subjects who have pre-existing respiratory and cardiovascular diseases appear to be at some increased risk from SO_2[1]. In addition, the Six Cities Study[2], which also referred to much lower levels of SO_2 and PM than occurred in the London smog episode, demonstrated that mortality was less closely related to SO_2 than to PM (see below).

Long-term exposure to SO_2 and particles may be associated with increased prevalence of cough and phlegm. However, recent data from reunified Germany showed that the higher levels of SO_2 and particles in the former East Germany were not associated with an increased prevalence of atopy, hay fever, or asthma in children or adults[3].

Exposure studies

Inhalation of SO_2 causes symptoms such as cough, chest tightness, and wheezing, which are closely related to air-flow obstruction.

Sulfur dioxide is a potent bronchoconstrictor in subjects with asthma[4], and about 20–25% of subjects who have nonspecific airway hyperresponsiveness show airway hyperresponsiveness to SO_2 (Fig. 63.1)[5]. The degree of bronchoconstriction is determined by minute ventilation and partially by the route of inhalation. In dry air or dry cold air, SO_2 responses are stronger than in humidified air. Although airway responsiveness to methacholine or histamine appears to be a prerequisite to hyperresponsiveness to SO_2[5], its degree does not correlate with the degree of responsiveness to SO_2. When SO_2 exposures are repeated within short time intervals, bronchoconstrictor responses are reduced. Apparently, SO_2 itself does not exert major effects on nonspecific airway responsiveness or allergen responsiveness in human subjects.

Mechanisms of action

Sulfur dioxide readily dissolves in the surface fluid layer of the airway epithelium and it undergoes a variety of chemical reactions to yield sulfuric acid, sulfites, bisulfites, and sulfates, which may induce harmful effects. Although SO_2 and its products interfere with disulfide bonds in biologic macromolecules, the mechanism that ultimately leads to cell damage is not known. After SO_2 exposure, release of inflammatory mediators may induce mucus hypersecretion and stimulate sensory nerve endings. Prolonged exposure to high concentrations of SO_2 may induce structural alterations that mimic those observed in chronic bronchitis.

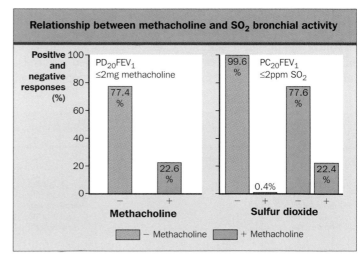

Figure 63.1 Relationship between methacholine and sulfur dioxide bronchial reactivity. Percentages of positive response to inhalation of SO_2 (right panel) in relation to airway responsiveness to methacholine (left panel) within a population-based sample ($n=780$) aged 20–44 years. Positive responses were defined as 20% falls in forced expiratory volume in 1 second (FEV_1) after inhalation of concentrations of 2ppm SO_2 (PC_{20}) and 2mg methacholine [provocative dose (PD_{20})]. (Data from Nowak et al.[5])

For clinical purposes, it is important to analyze the potential of drugs to protect against the effects of air pollution in subjects with asthma. It has been demonstrated that β_2-adrenoceptor agonists, disodium cromoglycate, nedocromil sodium, and theophylline either attenuate or block the bronchoconstrictor response to SO_2. In contrast, inhaled corticosteroids show only weak protection, and ipratropium bromide has no effect.

AEROSOLS AND PARTICLES

Recently, there has been increasing interest in health effects of PM. Acute and chronic exposure to inhalable particles have been found to be associated with adverse health effects, and increased mortality is closely related to exposure to particles, especially small size particles (Fig. 63.2)[1,6]. Clearly, the deposition of particles within the lower respiratory tract depends on particle diameter. Larger particles (diameter $>10\mu m$) are deposited in extrathoracic airways, whereas particles with an aerodynamic diameter $<10\mu m$ enter the lower airways. These particles have been defined as PM_{10}. The harmful effects of PM_{10} may also be related to the acidity carried by the particles.

Furthermore, it has been suggested that fine ($0.1–2.5\mu m$) and ultrafine ($0.01–0.1\mu m$) particles are even more strongly related to morbidity and mortality, in particular from cardiovascular diseases. It has been suggested that these particles, owing to their large number compared with their minor mass contribution, produce acute effects within the lung, which may be exaggerated through their oxidative properties, such as the catalytic actions of transition metals. These effects may ultimately change the viscosity of the blood, thereby increasing the cardiovascular risk in subjects affected by pre-existing cardiovascular diseases[7,8]. In addition, symptom scores and deterioration of lung function in subjects who have asthma are reported to be related to fine and ultrafine particles[9].

OZONE

Formation and exposure levels
Ozone is mainly generated from hydrocarbons and NO_2 under the presence of ultraviolet radiation. Average levels are smallest in winter and highest in summer. Concentrations normally peak in the afternoon. In most areas of the industrialized countries, annual average levels of O_3 range between 20 and 40ppb. Annual and daily cycles, however, are often associated with concentrations that reach or exceed 100ppb.

Background concentrations appear to have increased steadily during this century. It has been estimated for the USA in the 1980s that about half the population was living in areas with maximum concentrations of more than 120ppb. The situation in many parts of Europe is similar.

Epidemiologic studies
Epidemiologic studies have consistently demonstrated the occurrence of symptoms and a decline in spirometric volumes even after short-term exposures to O_3[10]. Furthermore, there is increasing evidence for an association between short-term O_3 levels and hospital admissions for respiratory disorders in subjects affected by pre-existing airway diseases[11]. In addition, symptoms of chronic respiratory disease and the annual rate of decline in forced expiratory volume in 1 second (FEV_1) have been found to be associated with long-term exposure to O_3.

Exposure studies
According to experimental exposure studies, O_3 causes pain on deep inspiration and a transient reduction in inspiratory capacity as reflected in FEV_1 or forced vital capacity (FVC). Parameters indicative of small airways narrowing can show longer-lasting or more exaggerated effects.

Compared with spirometric responses, changes in airway resistance are minor. Prolonged exposures over 6 hours with nearly continuous exercise have demonstrated that 80ppb of ozone is sufficient to elicit a response. Ozone responses are a function of concentration, minute ventilation, and time, with remarkably large individual variability. On average, subjects who have mild asthma show similar or only slightly greater lung function responses to O_3 than normal subjects. When O_3 exposures are repeated, a reduction in lung function responses occurs, which is called adaptation or tolerance.

Ozone causes transient increase in airway responsiveness to methacholine, which is probably not abolished in repeated exposures and does not correlate with changes in lung function. Exercise-induced asthma is not exaggerated by O_3, in contrast with allergen responses. Subjects who have allergic asthma exhibit increased bronchial allergen responsiveness after exposure to 120ppb O_3 for 1 hour at rest. Similarly, a significant increase in

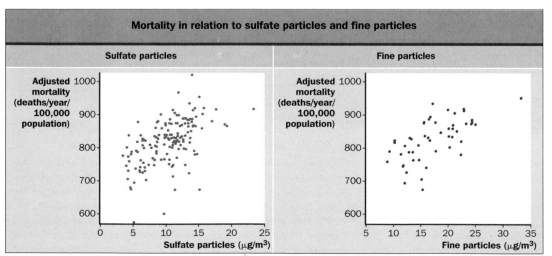

Figure 63.2 Mortality in relation to sulfate particles and fine particles. Relationship between mortality per year per 100,000 inhabitants adjusted for age, sex, and ethnic origin versus concentrations of sulfate particles and fine particles. The analysis is based on a comparison of 151 urban areas in 1980. (Data from Pope et al.[6])

bronchial allergen responsiveness has been found after 3 hours' exposure to 250ppb O_3, during intermittent moderate exercise (Fig. 63.3)[12]. There was also a slight bronchial allergen response following exposure to O_3 but not to filtered air in subjects who have allergic rhinitis. Furthermore, nasal allergen responses, in term of the concentrations of eosinophils and eosinophil cationic protein, were enhanced by O_3. It has, however, not been established whether the amplification of airway responses to allergen by O_3 acts under natural exposure conditions.

Cellular and biochemical effects
Ozone induces cellular and biochemical changes detectable within the bronchoalveolar lavage (BAL) fluid, with a neutrophil influx as a prominent feature. Airway inflammation occurs in the upper and lower airways and appears to be stronger in subjects who have asthma than it is in healthy subjects. Furthermore, responses are associated with elevated BAL fluid levels of prostanoids such as prostaglandins E_2 and $F_{2-\alpha}$ and thromboxane B_2 but not leukotrienes, and of cytokines and chemokines such as interleukin-6, interleukin-8, and granulocyte–monocyte colony-stimulating factor[13]. Levels of substance P and bradykinin in BAL fluid were elevated after O_3 exposure. In addition, O_3 causes cellular damage and an increase in epithelial permeability. Lung function responses to O_3 in terms of FEV_1 or FVC do not correlate with airway inflammation.

Mechanisms of action
Owing to its relatively low solubility in water, O_3 can penetrate into the lung periphery, causing lipid peroxidation and loss of functional groups of biomolecules. β_2-adrenoceptor agonists and atropine only prevent the O_3-induced increase in airway resistance. Indomethacin reduces O_3-induced decrements in spirometric volumes without effect on methacholine responsiveness. After treatment with budesonide, the increase in pulmonary

resistance and the neutrophil influx caused by O_3 in dogs are partially prevented but the increase in airway responsiveness is not prevented. It is not clear whether antioxidants affect the individual susceptibility to ozone in human subjects.

NITROGEN DIOXIDE

Formation and exposure levels
Nitrogen dioxide is derived predominantly from motor vehicles, power stations, and industrial processes. It also occurs in the work place and can contribute to indoor air pollution. Concentrations of NO_2 in urban areas are on average below 50ppb but may show peak values of 100–400ppb. Indoor concentrations exceeding 500ppb have been measured in kitchens when an unventilated gas stove was used.

Epidemiologic studies
Nitrogen dioxide has been found to be correlated with the frequency or duration of respiratory illness and functional impairment in children, even at low levels[14]. Results in adults and patients with respiratory diseases are less consistent. Some investigators have found an association between NO_2 levels and respiratory symptoms or peak flow rates in patients who have asthma, but there are conflicting reports. Most of these studies are confounded by the strong associations between different air pollutants.

Exposure studies
Experimental exposure studies have demonstrated that NO_2 does not affect lung function to a major extent in healthy subjects or subjects who have mild asthma, and data are conflicting in patients who suffer chronic obstructive pulmonary disease.

Subjects who have asthma may show enhanced airway responsiveness to histamine or methacholine after inhalation of NO_2[15]. In this respect, they are more sensitive than healthy subjects. Nitrogen dioxide has also been reported to enhance exercise-induced bronchoconstriction and the airway response to hyperventilation of cold air. However, there are also negative studies. The bronchoconstrictor response to hyperventilation of air containing a fixed concentration of SO_2 was found to be slightly enhanced by NO_2. It is likely that this enhancement was associated with the hyperventilation response and was not specific for SO_2. Nitrogen dioxide exposure may lead to enhanced bronchial allergen responses in subjects who have asthma in terms of both early and late phase responses (see Fig. 63.4)[16]. Other studies have found a tendency towards effects of NO_2 on allergen responsiveness but significant effects only when NO_2 was given in combination with SO_2. It appears that the effects of NO_2 in experimental studies are strongly influenced by the choice of subjects and the study protocol.

Cellular and biochemical effects
Bronchoalveolar lavage studies in healthy subjects have demonstrated that exposure to 3000–4000ppb of NO_2 causes a reduction in the inhibitory capacity of the α_1-proteinase inhibitor. Cell numbers in BAL fluid were altered in a concentration-dependent manner. Numbers of mast cells and lymphocytes were increased up to 1 day after exposure. In subjects who have mild asthma, exposure to 1000ppb NO_2 led to an increase in the concentration of thromboxane B_2 and prostaglandin D_2 and a

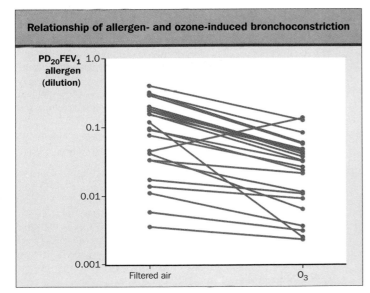

Figure 63.3 Inter-relationship of allergen- and ozone-induced bronchoconstriction. Individual values of cumulative doses of allergen ($PD_{20}FEV_1$) in subjects with mild asthma ($n=24$) that were needed to elicit a 20% fall in FEV_1, after previous exposure to filtered air or 250ppb O_3 for 3 hours of intermittent exercise. FEV_1, forced expiratory volume in 1 second. (Data from Jörres et al.[12])

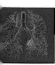

decrease in the concentration of 6-keto-prostaglandin-$F_{1-\alpha}$ without significant changes in cell counts[17]. Changes in alveolar permeability have been shown to occur with a delay of several hours.

Mechanisms of action

Bronchoconstriction experienced by subjects who have chronic bronchitis after inhalation of NO_2 can be attenuated by antihistamines, whereas atropine or β_2-adrenoceptor agonists are not effective. Owing to its oxidative properties, NO_2 may lead to lipid peroxidation and generate reaction products with constituents of the airway surface. Therefore, another way of achieving protection against NO_2 may be provided by antioxidants. Indeed, pretreatment with vitamins C and E has been shown to diminish the degree of lipid peroxidation in BAL fluid, and pretreatment with vitamin C to inhibit the increase in methacholine responsiveness induced by NO_2.

MIXTURES OF AIR POLLUTANTS

In daily life, air pollution is mostly the result of a complex mixture of components, whose harmful effects may also be modified by factors such as temperature and humidity. Therefore, studies on mixtures of air pollutants are important but difficult to perform. It has been shown that pre-exposure to NO_2 may exert a delayed effect on the spirometric response to O_3. Healthy subjects do not demonstrate significant synergism between the effects of O_3 and SO_2. In contrast, in patients who have asthma, sulfur-dioxide induced bronchoconstriction can be elicited after pre-exposure to a low dose of O_3, whereas simultaneous exposure to SO_2 and NO_2 did not indicate synergistic lung function effects. These results illustrate that the types of air pollutants, their concentrations, and the characteristics of the subjects are essential factors for the outcome of the studies. Furthermore, the time pattern of combined exposures may play a more important role than previously recognized (Fig. 63.5).

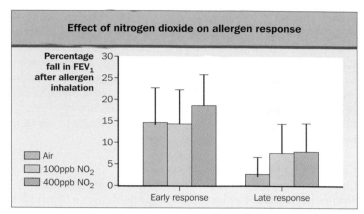

Figure 63.4 Inter-relationship of allergen and NO_2 bronchial reactivity. Mean values ($\pm$SD) of the percentage fall in forced expiratory volume in 1 seond (FEV_1) after allergen inhalation following exposure to clean air, 100ppb, or 400ppb NO_2 for 1 hour at rest. The study included eight subjects who had mild allergic asthma. (Data from Tunnicliffe et al.[16])

Actions of major components of air pollution regarding bronchoconstriction and airway inflammation		
Bronchoconstriction	SO_2	NO_2 and O_3
Healthy subjects	–	–
Subjects with asthma	+ +	–
Subjects with bronchitis	–	–
Airway inflammation		
Healthy subjects	+	+
Subjects with asthma	+	+ +
Subjects with bronchitis	–	–

Figure 63.5 Actions of major components of air pollution regarding bronchoconstriction and airway inflammation.

REFERENCES

1. Sunyer J, Saez M, Murillo C, et al. Air pollution and emergency room admissions for chronic obstructive pulmonary disease: A 5-year study. Am J Epidemiol. 1993;137:710–15.
2. Dockery DW, Pope CA, Xiping X, et al. An association between air pollution and mortality in six U.S. cities. N Engl J Med. 1993;329:1753–9.
3. Nowak D, Heinrich J, Jörres R, et al. Prevalence of respiratory symptoms, bronchial hyperresponsiveness and atopy among adults: West and East Germany. Eur Respir J. 1996;9:2541–52.
4. Sheppard D, Wong WS, Uehara CF, et al. Lower threshold and greater bronchomotor responsiveness of asthmatic subjects to sulfur dioxide. Am Rev Respir Dis. 1980;122:873–8.
5. Nowak D, Jörres R, Berger J, Claussen M, Magnussen H. Airway responsiveness to sulfur dioxide in an adult population sample. Am J Respir Crit Care Med. 1997;156:1151–6.
6. Pope CA III, Thun MJ, Namboodiri MM, et al. Particulate air pollution as a predictor of mortality in a prospective study of U.S. adults. Am J Respir Crit Care Med. 1995;151:669–74.
7. Seaton A, MacNee W, Donaldson K, Godden D. Particulate air pollution and acute health effects. Lancet. 1995;345:176–8.
8. Peters A, Döring A, Wichmann HE, Koenig W. Increased plasma viscosity during an air pollution episode. Lancet. 1997;349:1582–7.
9. Peters A, Wichmann HE, Tuch T, Heinrich J, Heyder J. Respiratory effects are associated with the number of ultrafine particles. Am J Respir Crit Care Med. 1997;155:1376–83.

10. Romieu I, Meneses F, Ruiz S, et al. Effects of air pollution on the respiratory health of asthmatic children living in Mexico City. Am J Respir Crit Care Med. 1996;154:300–7.
11. Burnett RT, Dales RE, Raizenne ME, et al. Effects of low ambient levels of ozone and sulfates on the frequency of respiratory admissions to Ontario hospitals. Environ Res. 1994;65:172–94.
12. Jörres R, Nowak D, Magnussen H. The effect of ozone exposure on allergen responsiveness in subjects with asthma or rhinitis. Am J Respir Crit Care Med. 1996;153:56–64.
13. Aris RM, Christian D, Hearne PQ, et al. Ozone-induced airway inflammation in human subjects as determined by airway lavage and biopsy. Am Rev Respir Dis. 1993;148:1363–72.
14. Braun-Fahrländer C, Ackermann-Liebrich U, Schwartz J, et al. Air pollution and respiratory symptoms in preschool children. Am Rev Respir Dis. 1992;145: 42–7.
15. Bylin G, Hedenstierna G, Lindvall T, Sundin B. Ambient nitrogen dioxide concentrations increase bronchial responsiveness in subjects with mild asthma. Eur Respir J. 1988;1:606–12.
16. Tunnicliffe WS, Burge PS, Ayres JG. Effect of domestic concentrations of nitrogen dioxide on airway responses to inhaled allergen in asthmatic patients. Lancet. 1994;344:1733–6.
17. Jörres R, Nowak D, Grimminger F, et al. The effect of 1ppm nitrogen dioxide on bronchoalveolar lavage cells in normal and asthmatic subjects. Eur Respir J. 1995;8:416–24.

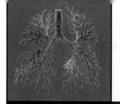

Section 12 Occupational and Environmental Lung Disease

Chapter 64 Berylliosis, Byssinosis, and Occupational Chronic Obstructive Pulmonary Disease

Anthony C Pickering

BERYLLIUM DISEASE

Introduction

Beryllium is a rare element used in industry for its properties of lightness and strength, and its resistance to high temperatures and corrosion. It is the lightest of all chemically stable substances. Beryllium alloys are widely and increasingly used in modern technology, such as the aerospace and nuclear industries, telecommunications, and the computer industry. Other industries could involve exposure to beryllium include the ceramic industry, dentistry (dental alloys), scrap metal reclamation, and metal machinists.

The majority of cases of beryllium disease occur in workers who are directly exposed because they handle beryllium alloys. It has also been described in vicinity workers, including a secretary, security guard, and cleaner, in the reclamation of nonferrous alloys and in the families of workers who return home wearing contaminated overalls.

Epidemiology, risk factors, and pathophysiology

Epidemiology

Chronic beryllium disease is a rare disease in the UK, with only seven new cases diagnosed by the medical respiratory boards under the Industrial Injuries Scheme in the UK between 1982 and 1996, and no claims for injury or disablement benefit since 1996. Epidemiologic studies in the ceramic and nuclear industries revealed sensitization and disease rates that vary between 2.9 and 15.8% in differing exposure categories[1,2]. A clearer idea of the incidence of the disease will be derived from the longitudinal studies now being conducted in the nuclear weapons industry in the USA.

Pathophysiology

The histopathology is characterized by the development of non-caseating granulomas in the lung parenchyma and hilar lymph nodes (Fig. 64.1). The granulomas consist of epithelioid cells, multinucleated giant cells, macrophages, and numerous lymphocytes. An alveolar wall infiltration by lymphocytes and histiocytes is a constant finding. The disease may progress to end-stage interstitial lung fibrosis with honeycomb changes. Granulomas may also be present in the skin, cervical, hilar, and abdominal lymph nodes, liver, spleen, kidneys, adrenals, and the central nervous system. The disease process is one of the development of a cell-mediated immune response to the beryllium antigen, which leads to the development of noncaseating granulomata. Helper T lymphocytes (CD4+) are the major lymphocyte population involved in the response to beryllium. Usually, 80–90% of the T lymphocytes from bronchoalveolar lavage (BAL) in patients who have beryllium disease are CD4+. The T-lymphocyte response is interleukin (IL)-2 dependent.

Clinical features

Two forms of pulmonary disease are recognized: acute and chronic berylliosis.

Acute berylliosis

Acute berylliosis follows an intense exposure to beryllium and is now rarely seen. The clinical features are those of a chemical pneumonitis associated with conjunctivitis, rhinitis, and tracheitis. Lower respiratory tract symptoms include a paroxysmal cough with occasionally bloodstained sputum and breathlessness on exertion. Fever, tachycardia, and inspiratory crackles throughout the lung fields may be present. The symptoms usually occur within 72 hours of exposure, although with low exposures the onset may be more insidious; berylliosis is regarded as acute if it occurs within 12 months of exposure.

Chronic berylliosis

Chronic berylliosis is a granulomatous disorder that predominantly affects the lungs – involvement of other organs can occur, but is rare. The clinical symptoms are those of a nonproductive cough with the insidious onset of exertional dyspnea and fatigue. These may be associated with nonspecific symptoms that include fever, anorexia, weight loss, lassitude, and malaise. In early, mild disease, the physical signs may be absent. As the disease progresses, bilateral basal inspiratory crackles develop, finger clubbing may be present (10–20% of cases), and signs of cor pulmonale ensue.

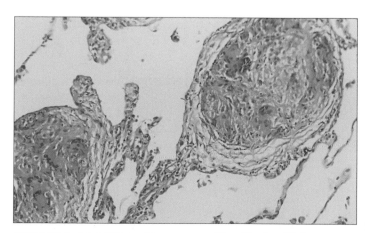

Figure 64.1 A lung biopsy from a case of berylliosis, with two areas of confluent granulomas surrounded by a rim of loose connective tissue. (Courtesy of Dr Alan Gibbs.)

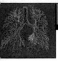

Diagnosis

The diagnosis of berylliosis is based on a history of exposure to beryllium salts, the clinical features, and the immunologic, radiologic, and physiologic findings.

Serology and bronchoalveolar lavage

The lymphocytic response in beryllium disease is specific to beryllium salts and has lead to the development of the beryllium lymphocyte proliferation assay (BeLT). The test is now reliable, reproducible, and is elevated on BAL lymphocytes in individuals who have beryllium disease and normal in unexposed subjects and in beryllium-exposed normal subjects[3]. Both BAL–BeLT and BAL lymphocytosis correlate with disease severity in berylliosis[4]. The picture may be obscured if the patient smokes cigarettes, which partially normalizes the BAL differential cell count. In some individuals, the blood BeLT may be abnormal in the face of negative lavage lymphocyte reactivity to beryllium. Follow-up studies of such individuals suggest a significant number (even in those who have left the industry) go on to develop pulmonary disease. Nevertheless, blood BeLT has a high positive predictive value in determining the presence or absence of chronic beryllium disease.

Radiology

The radiographic abnormalities of berylliosis may precede the onset of symptoms by a number of years. Characteristically, bilateral widespread opacities are initially predominantly round opacities, but become more irregular with disease progression (Fig. 64.2); accompanying hilar gland enlargement is uncommon and when present is modest in degree. High-resolution computed tomography (CT) scans identify the earliest radiographic changes when the plain chest radiograph is normal. The most frequent abnormalities described on CT scans are nodules, septal lines, areas of ground glass attenuation, and bronchial wall thickening[5].

Lung function

In the earliest stages of the disease (before the development of symptoms or radiologic changes), abnormalities in exercise physiology may be demonstrable, with reduced exercise tolerance, a rise in dead space to tidal volume ratio, and an increase in the difference between alveolar and arterial oxygen partial pressures. In more advanced disease, a mixed picture may be present of obstructive and restrictive lung defects with impaired gas transfer.

Differential diagnosis

The differential diagnosis of chronic beryllium disease includes all those conditions characterized by the formation of multi-organ noncaseating granulomas, especially sarcoidosis and, to a lesser extent, extrinsic allergic alveolitis. The features that may help to distinguish berylliosis from sarcoidosis are the absence of ocular, bone, and neurologic manifestations, normal tuberculin skin reactivity, and elevated levels of blood and BAL–BeLT.

Treatment

Acute disease is treated immediately with high-dose corticosteroids and, if indicated, oxygen. The majority of patients make a full recovery within 1–6 months, but a small proportion (17% in one series) progress to chronic disease.

The management of chronic beryllium disease is based on the concept that the suppression of granulomas prevents the development of fibrosis. It involves the early introduction of corticosteroids before significant fibrosis develops. Since beryllium is only slowly cleared from the lung, the treatment period is likely to be prolonged. In chronic disease, the initial treatment is with prednisolone 40mg on alternate days for 6 months, which is then reduced by 10mg/month until evidence of renewed disease activity is found. At the present time, it is not known whether the introduction of corticosteroids would be beneficial at a stage when evidence of lymphocyte sensitization is present, but no clinical evidence of disease. In the presence of end-stage disease, lung transplantation has been performed (Fig. 64.3).

Clinical course and prognosis

The prognosis of chronic beryllium disease is poorly documented. The longitudinal studies recently initiated in the nuclear weapons industry in the USA will provide this information. Preliminary results show sensitization in the absence of chronic beryllium disease[6], the progression of sensitization to clinical disease in a significant proportion of a small number of individuals followed up for 5 years, and in some cases progression of disease to increasing disability and death.

Pitfalls and controversies

The most important aspect of diagnosing berylliosis is to consider it as a possible diagnosis, and subsequently take an adequate occupational history (bearing in mind the possibility of a vicinity exposure).

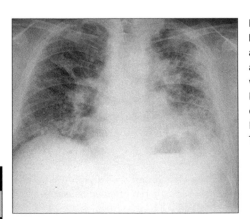

Figure 64.2 Chronic beryllium disease in a beryllium–copper alloy worker. Note the widespread small and large ill-defined opacities. (Courtesy of Professor AJ Newman Taylor.)

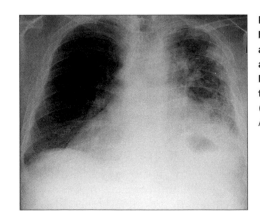

Figure 64.3 Chronic beryllium disease in a beryllium–copper alloy worker treated by single lung transplantation. (Courtesy of Professor AJ Newman Taylor.)

BYSSINOSIS AND ALLIED RESPIRATORY DISEASES

Introduction
The early description of respiratory symptoms in cotton workers reported 'work-related cough associated with a sensation of uneasiness beneath the sternum'. It was 14 years later, in 1845, that the specific periodicity of these symptoms, which characterize byssinosis, was described: 'all the workers have told us that the dust bothered them much less on the last days of the week than on Monday or Tuesday'[7]. The diagnosis remains based on a clinical history of work-related respiratory symptoms that are most severe on the first day of return to work after a period away from the workplace, such as a weekend or holiday.

In the past decade, a new terminology has been introduced in the literature – byssinosis has been divided into 'acute' and 'chronic' forms. Acute byssinosis refers to the acute airway response, to both cotton and flax dust, seen in subjects exposed to these dusts for the first time. This type of response may account for the substantial labor turnover observed over the first year of employment in cotton spinning mills. Chronic byssinosis is applied to the symptoms and disability reported in the early epidemiologic studies, which develop after many years of exposure to cotton dust.

Epidemiology, risk factors, and pathophysiology
Epidemiology
Epidemiologic studies in the UK have documented a progressive fall in the prevalence of byssinosis over the past 30 years. Schilling initially reported a 50% prevalence of byssinosis in the highest dust-exposure areas of cotton spinning[8]. This has fallen progressively to a current level of 3% in the Lancashire cotton spinning mills. However in the Middle and Far East, the prevalence rates of byssinosis in cotton mills remain high. Prevalence rates of 40% in Ethiopia, up to 50% in India, 30% in Indonesia, and 37% in the Sudan have been reported[9].

Pathogenesis
Both the mechanism(s) and the causative agent(s) of byssinosis remain a matter of speculation. The etiologic factor is likely to be water soluble, since washed cotton loses its ability to induce symptoms in affected individuals. Various mechanisms have been proposed, which include:
- antigen–antibody reactions (IgE- and non-IgE-mediated responses; neither is supported either by the pattern of disease development or by challenge testing);
- nonimmunologic release of histamine;
- bacterial endotoxin;
- fungal enzymes; and
- nonspecific pharmacologic release of mediators.

None of these factors individually fully explains all the clinical features of byssinosis.

Pathology
The pathologic features of byssinosis are poorly defined in published studies, which describe small numbers of workers and few nonsmokers. The main abnormalities include mucous gland hypertrophy and basement membrane thickening, features that do not differentiate byssinosis from chronic bronchitis or asthma. These studies have not shown an association between byssinosis and pulmonary emphysema or interstitial lung fibrosis.

Clinical features
Acute byssinosis
The results of artificial cardroom experiments that demonstrate acute airway responses to cotton dust on first exposure to that dust have been attributed to the individuals inherent airway reactivity. This is supported by a study of normal, cotton naive subjects in whom the response to cotton dust was significantly associated with their prechallenge airway reactivity, using a methacholine challenge system.

Cardroom experiments have shown a spectrum of responses in naive subjects, which vary between small asymptomatic falls in lung function to large changes (exceeding 30%), with associated symptoms following exposure to cotton dust. Since no longitudinal studies have been undertaken of workers from the time of their first employment in the industry, the fate of low-level responders is unknown. Longitudinal studies of cohorts of cotton workers suggest that cross-shift changes in lung function are associated with accelerated lung function decline (see Occupational chronic obstructive pulmonary disease). It is possible that this population of asymptomatic cotton-dust responders, identified by cardroom experiments, form a susceptible group of textile workers.

Chronic byssinosis
The classic form of byssinosis (chronic byssinosis) is characterized by a feeling of chest tightness and difficulty in breathing, which the worker experiences on his or her first day back at work after a period of absence from work. Additional symptoms that may be present include a cough, which is initially nonproductive and wheezing. Two patterns of symptomatology are seen in the workplace. Approximately half the workers experience their most severe symptoms during the first half of the working shift, developing symptoms shortly after starting work. The remainder are most affected over the second half of the shift. Most symptomatic workers experience a further exacerbation of their symptoms on leaving work in the evening, which may last through the evening and keep the individual awake during the night. A subjective improvement in symptoms occurs over subsequent days of the working week, with a further exacerbation of symptoms when cleaning procedures are undertaken at the end of the working week.

The periodicity of the symptoms formed the basis of Schilling's original classification of byssinosis, which has been widely used in epidemiologic studies of the textile industry. This grading system, however, does not take account of the irritant effects of cotton dust or the pulmonary function changes that may occur in the absence of symptoms. As a result of these deficiencies a new grading system has been proposed by the World Health Organization (WHO; see Fig. 64.4), which addresses these problems and includes the symptoms of byssinosis, chronic bronchitis, and physiologic measurement of cross-shift and permanent reductions in lung function[10].

In addition to the classic symptoms of byssinosis, studies of cotton workers report a number of work-related symptoms that do not have the characteristic periodicity of byssinosis; these include ocular and nasal irritation, cough, chest tightness, and wheeze.

Chronic bronchitis
Chronic bronchitis, defined as cough and sputum production, was first described in association with byssinosis in 1970[11]. Subsequently, the prevalence of bronchitis was found to be

World Health Organization grading system for byssinosis		
Classification		**Symptoms**
Byssinosis	Grade 0	No symptoms
	Grade B1	Chest tightness and/or shortness of breath (SOB) on most of first days back at work
	Grade B2	Chest tightness and/or SOB on the first and other days of the working week
Respiratory tract irritation	Grade RTI 1	Cough associated with dust exposure
	Grade RTI 2	Persistent phlegm (i.e. on most days during 3 months of the year) initiated or exacerbated by dust exposure
	Grade RTI 3	Persistent phlegm initiated or made worse by dust exposure either with exacerbations of chest illness or that persists for 2 years or more
Lung function	Acute changes	
	No effect	A consistent decline (decline occurs in at least 3 consecutive tests made after an absence from dust exposure of 2 days or more) in forced expiratory volume in 1 second (FEV_1) of <5% or an increase in FEV_1 during the work shift
	Mild effect	A consistent decline of between 5 and 10% in FEV_1 during the work shift
	Moderate effect	A consistent decline of between 10 and 20% in FEV_1 during the work shift
	Severe effect	A decline of 20% or more in FEV_1 during the work shift
	Chronic changes	
	No effect	FEV_1 value (by a preshift test after an absence from dust exposure of 2 days or more) – 80% of predicted (predicted values should be based on data obtained from local populations or similar ethnic and social class groups)
	Mild to moderate effect	FEV_1 (as above) – 60–79% of predicted value (as above)
	Severe effect	FEV_1 (as above) – <60% of predicted value (as above)

Figure 64.4 World Health Organization grading system for byssinosis[10].

greater in those who worked in cotton than in those who worked in man-made fiber mills (in males, 44.9% in cotton and 26% in man-made fiber mills)[12]. By 1997 the prevalence of bronchitis in the Lancashire cotton mills had fallen to 7.15%. Differentiating the relative contributions of cotton-dust exposure and cigarette smoking to the development of bronchitis in mill workers has been difficult, because of the small numbers of nonsmokers in the cotton industry. However, in a recent large study of 3000 textile workers, the role of cotton-dust exposure in the development of chronic bronchitis was clearly defined[13]. Chronic bronchitis is more prevalent in cotton workers than in those who work with man-made fiber, and exposure is additive to the effect of smoking. Effectively, the risk of developing chronic bronchitis for a nonsmoking cotton worker is the same as that for a man-made fiber worker who smokes. The diagnosis of chronic bronchitis is associated with a small but significant decrement in lung function.

Diagnosis

The diagnosis of byssinosis is based on a history of work-related respiratory symptoms (chest tightness and or breathing difficulty) which are most severe on the first day back at work after a break away from work. The diagnosis may be supported by measurement of lung function.

Acute cross-shift changes in lung function have frequently been demonstrated in byssinotic workers. The magnitude of change determines the grade of byssinosis. Serial measurements of lung function of workers in the industry demonstrate various patterns of lung function change. The clinical history of byssinosis is one of respiratory symptoms that are most severe on the first day back at work after a break. This, to some extent, is reflected in changes in lung function, in that the largest fall in lung function is seen to occur across the first working shift. Subsequent cross-shift falls over the remainder of the week are less marked and, although the overall level of airways obstruction may increase, the lowest measurement of lung function is recorded at the end of the working shift on the final working day. In other individuals, a progressive improvement in lung function occurs over the working week and is consistent with their clinical history. Whatever pattern of pulmonary change is recorded, the diurnal variation in lung function appears to be greatest on the first working day after a break from work.

In addition to abnormalities in lung function, cotton workers show changes in airway reactivity. The highest level of airway reactivity is found in byssinotics, workers who have nonspecific, work-related symptoms form an intermediate group, and asymptomatic workers have the lowest levels of airway reactivity. In one study of cotton textile workers[14], increased airway reactivity was seen in 78% of byssinotics, 37% of those with nonspecific symptoms, and 17% of asymptomatic workers.

No changes in gas transfer in workers exposed to hemp, flax, or cotton have been reported. A study of smoking and non-smoking byssinotic workers found changes in gas transfer only in the workers who smoked, and showed a dose–response relationship between the number of cigarettes smoked and the impairment of gas transfer. This finding, combined with pathologic studies of cotton workers, indicates that the development of emphysema in byssinotic workers is attributable to cigarette smoking habits rather than exposure to cotton dust.

Treatment

As with all forms of occupational lung disease, treatment consists of the early identification of disease and removal of the individual from exposure to the causative agent. In practice, in the textile industry this involves either moving the individual to an area of lower dust exposure or transfer from cotton spinning to man-made fiber production.

Clinical course and prevention

The assumption has been that with continued exposure to cotton dust the disease progressed from one grade to the next. However, two longitudinal studies suggest that this is not the case in all individuals. In both studies, cotton workers were recorded as initiating their disease at grade 2 or 3 without passing through the earlier grades. In addition, individuals have been reported in whom symptoms remitted despite continued exposure to cotton dust. This may reflect reduced levels of exposure to cotton dust or its contaminants. The end stage of byssinosis is one of fixed airways obstruction with associated disability.

The ultimate aim is to reduce dust exposure to a level that prevents disease development, which is achievable by investment in modern, enclosed machinery. The automation of the opening room and the enclosure of the blowing and carding processes is of particular importance in reducing dust exposure levels in the areas most frequently associated with lung disease (Figs 64.5 & 64.6).

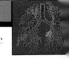

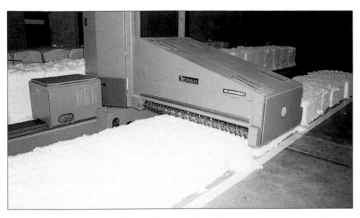

Figure 64.5 Automated opening and blending process previously conducted by manual feeding.

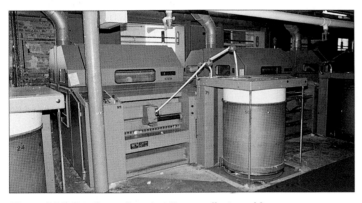

Figure 64.6 Totally enclosed cotton carding machine.

Pitfalls and controversies

The steady reduction in cotton dust exposure levels in Western countries has lead to the virtual disappearance of chronic byssinosis and to changes in the patterns of disease. It was believed that individuals progressed through the various stages of the Schilling classification; however, longitudinal studies have not confirmed this. In some individuals, symptoms of byssinosis may resolve despite continued exposure to cotton dust. Questions regarding the relationship between acute and chronic byssinosis, such as whether these are separate diseases or one is a continuation of the other remain unresolved. Longitudinal studies using the WHO classification will help to answer these questions. The etiologic agent that causes byssinosis remains unknown, although endotoxin is still the most likely agent.

OCCUPATIONAL CHRONIC OBSTRUCTIVE PULMONARY DISEASE

Chronic bronchitis, defined by the presence of regular cough and sputum, is well established as an occupational disease that is independent of cigarette smoking habits. The relationship between industrial exposures to dust or fumes and the development of obstructive airways disease in exposed workers is a source of considerable controversy. The methodologies of many of the studies that address these relationships have been criticized on the basis of small cohort numbers, inappropriate case controls, confounding of smoking habits, and lack of lung function data and of exposure data. Recent epidemiologic studies addressed these

criticisms and provide a clearer picture of the effects on the lung of chronic exposures to certain dusts and fumes, including coal dust (see Chapter 60), cadmium, welding fume, and cotton dust.

Cadmium

The inhalation of cadmium fumes at high concentrations may cause a chemical pneumonia. For many years, an association between fume exposure and the development of emphysema was suggested. In a case-control study of cadmium workers[15], a dose–response effect was demonstrated between cumulative exposures to cadmium and impairment of forced expiratory volume in 1 second (FEV_1) and diffusion coefficient. This decrement occurred independently of smoking habit and was consistent with the functional and radiologic changes of emphysema present in the workers.

Welding fume

Many studies of welders demonstrate an increased prevalence of chronic cough and sputum. A cross-sectional study of shipyard workers exposed to welding fume showed a small but significant impairment in FEV_1 of 250mL compared with nonexposed workers[16]. A 7-year follow-up study of these workers demonstrated an annual decline in FEV_1 of 16.2mL in nonsmoking, nonexposed workers, with declines attributable to smoking of 17.7mL/year and to welding fume of 16.4mL/year[17]. An interaction was noted between smoking and welding-fume exposure, with a disproportionate effect of fume on smokers compared with nonsmokers.

Cotton dust

Although chronic bronchitis associated with cotton-dust exposure was described 40 years ago, only in recent years has accelerated decline in lung function associated with cotton-dust exposure been definitely identified. A longitudinal study of cotton workers in the USA showed that the annual decline in FEV_1 in cotton workers is related to dust-exposure category. In the lowest exposure category ($150\mu g/m^3$), the annual decline in FEV_1 in nonsmokers is 18.4mL and in smokers 41.2mL. In the highest exposure category ($250\mu g/m^3$), the decline in nonsmokers is 34.6mL and in smokers 57.4ml[18]. The excess decline in lung function could be identified at mean annual cotton-dust exposures of only $200\mu g/m^3$ and by cross-shift changes in FEV_1 of 200mL. This study suggests that to prevent dust-related declines in lung function, exposures must be reduced to $100\mu g/m^3$ and smokers should be excluded from the high dust-exposure areas[19]. The current UK maximum exposure limit for cotton, using a personal sampling device, is $2.5mg/m^3$. Dust measurements in the USA are made using a different measuring device from that in the UK. At present time there have been no direct comparisons made between the different measuring devices.

Pitfalls and controversies

The physiologic significance of the excess rate of lung function decline reported in various industries has been challenged frequently. It seems likely that in any industrial population exposed to dust or fumes there may be a small number of 'sensitive' individuals who experience a significant loss of lung function. This is perhaps best demonstrated in cotton workers who, as a whole, have a low standardized mortality ratio(SMR) for respiratory disease compared with the general population, but an elevated SMR when byssinotics are studied as a separate group.

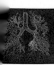
REFERENCES

1. Kreiss K, Wasserman S, Mroz MM, Newman LS. Beryllium disease screening in the ceramics industry. J Occup Med. 1993;35:267–74.

2. Kreiss K, Mroz MM, Zhen B, et al. Epidemiology of beryllium sensitization and disease in nuclear workers. Am Rev Respir Dis. 1993;148:985–91.

3. Newman LS. Beryllium disease and sarcoidosis: clinical and laboratory links. Sarcoidosis. 1995;12:7–19.

4. Newman LS, Bobka C, Schumacher B. Compartmentalized immune response reflects clinical severity of beryllium disease. Am J Respir Crit Care Med. 1994;150:135–42.

5. Newman LS, Buschman DL, Newell JD, Lynch DA. Beryllium disease: assessment with CT. Radiology. 1994;190:835–40.

6. Newman LS, Lloyd J, Daniloff E. The natural history of beryllium sensitisation and chronic beryllium disease. Environ Health Perspect. 1996;104(Suppl. 5):937–43.

7. Mareska J, Heyman J. Enquête sur le travail et la condition physique et morale des ouvriers employes dans les manufactures de coton, á Gand. Ann Soc Med Gand. 1845;16:199.

8. Schilling RSF. Byssinosis in cotton and other textile workers. Lancet. 1956;i:319–24.

9. Niven RMcL, Pickering CAC. Byssinosis: a review. Thorax. 1996;51:632–7.

10. World Health Organization. Recommended health-based occupational exposure limits for selected vegetable dusts. Report of a WHO study group. WHO technical report series 684. Geneva: World Health Organization; 1983.

11. Molyneux MKB, Tombleson JBL. An epidemiological study of respiratory symptoms in Lancashire mills, 1963–66. Br J Ind Med. 1970;27:225–34.

12. Berry G, Molyneux MKB, Tombleson JBL. Relationships between dust level and byssinosis and bronchitis in Lancashire cotton mills. Br J Ind Med. 1974;31:18–27.

13. Niven RMcL, Fletcher AM, Pickering CAC, et al. Chronic bronchitis in textile workers. Thorax. 1997;52:22–7.

14. Fishwick D, Pickering CAC. Byssinosis – a form of occupational asthma? Thorax. 1992;47:401–3.

15. Davison AG, Newman Taylor AJ, Darbyshire J, et al. Cadmium fume and emphysema. Lancet. 1988;1:663–7.

16. Cotes JE, Feinmann EL, Male VJ, et al. Respiratory symptoms and impairment in shipyard welders and caulker/burners. Br J Ind Med. 1989;46:292–301.

17. Chinn DJ, Stevenson IC, Cotes JE. Longitudinal respiratory survey of shipyard workers: effects of trade and atopic status. Br J Ind Med. 1990;47:83–90.

18. Glindmeyer HW, Lefante JJ, Jones RN, et al. Exposure-related declines in lung function of cotton textile workers. Am Rev Respir Med. 1991;144:675–83.

19. Glindmeyer HW, Lefante JJ, Jones RN, et al. Cotton dust and a cross-shift change in FEV_1 as predictors of annual change in FEV_1. Am J Respir Crit Care Med. 1994;149:584–90.

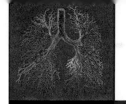

Section 13 Pleural Diseases

Chapter 65 Pneumothorax

Roland Vanderschueren

INTRODUCTION

Pneumothorax refers to the presence of free air between the visceral pleura and the parietal pleura[1]. Pneumothoraces are divided into spontaneous and iatrogenic; spontaneous pneumothorax has an unknown cause or occurs as a consequence of the natural course of a disease process.

Primary spontaneous pneumothoraces usually occur in apparently healthy people. Secondary spontaneous pneumothorax, however, is associated with underlying pulmonary pathology, usually chronic obstructive pulmonary disease (COPD), although acquired immune deficiency syndrome (AIDS) and *Pneumocystis carinii* infections appear to play an increasing role in the aetiology of primary spontaneous pneumothoraces[2].

Iatrogenic pneumothoraces occur as the result of diagnostic or therapeutic medical procedures. They can be intentional or a complication following pleural puncture.

Traumatic pneumothorax can follow any penetrating or non-penetrating chest trauma, with or without bronchial rupture (Fig. 65.1).

PRIMARY SPONTANEOUS PNEUMOTHORAX

Spontaneous pneumothorax mostly occurs in young male smokers aged between 20 and 40 years. The male:female ratio is about 5:1. Cigarette smoking is probably one of the most important risk factors.

Pathophysiology

There is no obvious underlying pulmonary disease in these patients. Thoracoscopic studies show that blebs and bullae play a role in pathogenesis and are frequently seen in patients who have spontaneous pneumothorax[3]. Pulmonary blebs (Fig. 65.2) are air-filled spaces between the lung parenchyma and the visceral pleura; in contrast, pulmonary bullae (Fig. 65.3) are air-filled spaces within the lung parenchyma itself. Blebs and bullae are also known as emphysema-like changes. The probable cause of the pneumothorax is rupture of an apical bleb or bulla, because the compliance of blebs and bullae in the apices is low compared with that of similar lesions situated in the lower parts of the lungs. It is often hard to assess whether bullae are the sites of leakage and where the site of rupture of the visceral pleura is[4]. Smoking causes a nine-fold increase in the relative risk of a pneumothorax in females and a 22-fold increase in males, with a dose–response relationship between the number of cigarettes smoked per day and the occurrence of primary spontaneous pneumothorax[5].

Classification of pneumothoraces	
Spontaneous pneumothoraces	**Iatrogenic pneumothoraces**
Primary idiopathic spontaneous pneumothorax	Traumatic pneumothorax
	Diagnostic (intentional) pneumothorax
Secondary spontaneous pneumothorax	Inadvertent pneumothorax

Fig. 65.1 Classification of pneumothoraces.

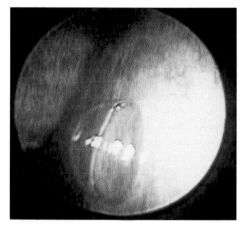

Fig. 65.2
Thoracoscopic view
of a bleb.

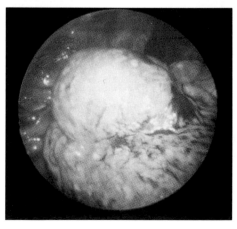

Fig. 65.3
Thoracoscopic view
of a bulla.

Clinical features

Symptoms are not always present and sometimes a small apical pneumothorax is found on routine chest radiography. In the majority of cases, however, the patient develops sudden unilateral chest pain and dyspnea, which is related to the size of the pneumothorax. Physical examination reveals hyperresonant percussion and reduced breath sounds. In left-sided pneumothorax, Haman's

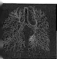

sign may be heard, i.e. a 'clicking' sound synchronous with the heartbeat. Another symptom is dry cough. In rare cases subcutaneous emphysema may be obvious on inspection of the neck, face, or chest. In a tension pneumothorax, breathlessness can be severe and there may be hypotension with cardiac tamponade.

Diagnosis

Spontaneous pneumothorax is usually suggested by the history and physical examination. A chest radiograph is needed to establish the diagnosis. If a small pneumothorax is suspected but not apparent on the chest radiograph, another film taken in complete expiration will often demonstrate the lesion, because during expiration air is expelled into the pleural cavity, making the pneumothorax more obvious. When there are adhesions between the pleurae the lung cannot collapse completely and a partial pneumothorax is seen (Fig. 65.4). Often there is some displacement of the mediastinum toward the normal side. Mediastinal emphysema and subcutaneous emphysema are rare.

Treatment

The choice of the best treatment method is still somewhat controversial. Several choices are available:

- rest and oxygen therapy;
- needle aspiration;
- simple intercostal drainage;
- medical thoracoscopy with talc poudrage;
- video-assisted thoracic surgery (VATS) with pleural abrasion or partial pleurectomy and bullectomy; and
- full thoracotomy.

The choice of initial treatment should depend on the presentation (Fig. 65.5). The size of the pneumothorax and the presence and extent of bullae are important. In a fit young person who is not distressed, the management should be conservative with weekly outpatient radiographs. If the patient is breathless, then needle aspiration through the second intercostal space anteriorly should be performed. Up to 2.5L of air can be aspirated with a 50mL syringe and a three-way tap. If the lung re-expands and the patient is comfortable, overnight observation is advised with a view to discharge and weekly follow-up. However, if the pneumothorax does not respond to aspiration, an intercostal tube should be inserted. If the lung is totally collapsed at presentation, aspiration should still be the first choice of treatment. If an intercostal tube is inserted, high concentrations of inspired oxygen may encourage re-expansion by the washout of nitrogen in the pleural cavity.

A recurrence of a spontaneous pneumothorax is an indication for more invasive therapy, such as pleural drainage with a chemical pleurodesis or surgical intervention[6].

Chemical pleurodesis

Needle aspiration, intercostal tube drainage and the use of a Heimlich flutter valve have proved to be safe procedures in the treatment of primary spontaneous pneumothorax, with few side effects, but most studies report a recurrence rate of 30–50%[7]. On recurrence, talc or 3g of tetracycline have proved to be effective sclerosing agents and can be instilled via an intercostal tube. In the case of talc poudrage, 4–6g of talc are insufflated by means of a talc atomizer or disposable single-use spray canister (Fig. 65.6), but this is best done under direct vision at VATS or thoracotomy for the best results. Chemical pleurodesis with talc slurry or tetracycline is very painful, and

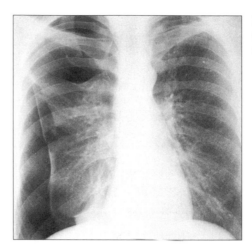

Fig. 65.4 Partial pneumothorax with adhesions.

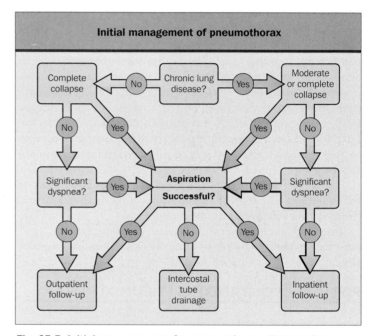

Fig. 65.5 Initial management of a pneumothorax. (Adapted from Miller AC, Harvey JE. Guidelines for the management of spontaneous pneumothorax. Br Med J. 1993;307:114–16.)

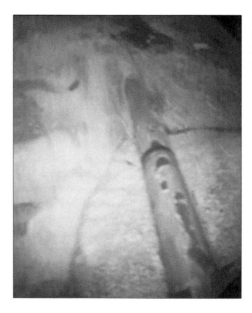

Fig. 65.6 Thoracoscopic view after pleural talc poudrage.

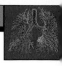

100–200mg lidocaine (lignocaine) should be added to the sclerosing solution. Sedation or parenteral analgesia is also recommended[8]. In general, pleurodesis via an intercostal drain is not as effective as pleurodesis performed under direct vision, and reviews report a recurrence rate of 8% in 1030 patients[9].

There has been concern over the safety of pleurodesis with talc, especially over the possibility of talc slurry causing acute pneumonitis and adult respiratory distress syndrome. However, this seems to occur only if more than 10g of talc is administered or if vascular injury is present[10]. No evidence of mesothelioma was found in two studies that followed patients for up to 35 years after talc pleurodesis, although some pleural thickening and calcification were seen[11,12].

Surgical treatment

There has been rapid development of minimally invasive surgery, particularly VATS, and a recent review of 805 patients who had spontaneous pneumothorax treated by VATS had a mean recurrence rate of 4%, which was higher than that after conventional surgical therapy (where the level was 1.5%)[5]. During VATS, bullae can be stapled with endostaplers, or resected by neodymium yttrium–aluminum–garnet (Nd:YAG) laser. In addition, tetracycline or talc is usually instilled or a pleural abrasion performed. Nowadays, thoracotomy is indicated only if thoracoscopy and VATS is not available or in cases of failure or recurrence after treatment with sclerosing agents or VATS, or both.

SECONDARY SPONTANEOUS PNEUMOTHORAX

Patients with secondary pneumothorax have an underlying pulmonary disease, often with diminished lung function, making the symptoms worse than those in primary spontaneous pneumothorax and sometimes life-threatening.

A summary of the most frequent underlying causes and diseases is given in Figure 65.7. The most common underlying association is COPD; infection with *P. carinii* in patients who have AIDS is becoming more important.

Clinical features

The symptoms are identical to these of primary spontaneous pneumothorax but are frequently disproportionate to the size of the pneumothorax. In some patients clinical deterioration occurs suddenly and rapidly, and fatal episodes have been documented[13]. Patients with COPD already have been hyperexpanded lungs, so physical examination will be less helpful than in patients with primary spontaneous pneumothorax because a contralateral difference in physical examination may not be apparent.

Diagnosis

The diagnosis is established by the chest radiograph. In patients who have COPD there are emphysematous changes in both lungs and often hyperlucent or bullous areas, which could be confounded with the appearance of a pneumothorax. The recognition of a visceral pleural line on the radiograph is essential. In uncertain cases computed tomography can be helpful although it is not good at differentiating a large bulla from a pneumothorax unless there are strands of tissue seen running within the bulla.

Causes of pneumothorax	
Iatrogenic	**Spontaneous**
Penetrating chest wounds	Primary (most common in young men)
Iatrogenic – including chest aspiration, intercostal nerve block, subclavian cannulation, transbronchial biopsy, needle aspiration lung biopsy, positive pressure ventilation	Secondary
	Chronic obstructive pulmonary disease
	Asthma
	Congenital cysts and bullae
	Pleural malignancy
	Interstitial lung fibrosing diseases
	Bacterial pneumonia
	Tuberculosis
	Whooping cough
Chest compression injury – including external cardiac massage	Cystic fibrosis
	Histiocytosis X
	Tuberous sclerosis
	Lymphangiomyomatosis
	Endometriosis of the pleura
	Marfan syndrome
	Sarcoidosis
	Esophageal rupture
	Pneumocystis carinii pneumonia

Fig. 65.7 Causes of pneumothorax.

Treatment

Treatment options in primary and secondary spontaneous pneumothorax are similar, but because of the more severe symptoms and the impaired lung function in secondary spontaneous pneumothorax, more of these patients will require treatment by intercostal tube thoracostomy. In the event of the pneumothorax recurring, pleurodesis should be done. As many of these patients have underlying lung disease and are not fit for surgery (even VATS), the pleurodesis is likely to be 'medical' (i.e. talc or tetracycline administered via an intercostal tube). However, if the patient is a possible candidate for lung transplantation, thoracoscopy with Nd:YAG treatment of blebs and stapling of bullae is preferable.

In patients who have AIDS and *P. carinii* infection, the occurrence of pneumothorax is an ominous prognostic sign[14]. Pneumothorax in these patients is mostly caused by a rupture of subpleural necrotic cavity. Simple tube thoracostomy is seldom successful and the simplest alternative seems to use a Heimlich valve, which allows the patient to be discharged from the hospital. If the fistula does not close then talc slurry should be used before invasive treatment such as VATS or thoracotomy.

CATAMENIAL PNEUMOTHORAX

This type of pneumothorax occurs in conjunction with menstruation and is mostly recurrent (see Fig. 65.8). The pathogenesis is still unclear. One of the hypotheses is that during menstruation air enters the peritoneal cavity and also the pleural cavity through a defect in the diaphragm. However, these defects are not always seen in patients treated for catamenial pneumothorax. Pleural or diaphragmatic endometriosis could also be of importance. The diagnosis of catamenial pneumothorax is obvious and, if they are recurrent, treatment should be the administration of ovulation-suppressing drugs. In cases where this treatment is not wanted or tolerated, thoracoscopy and pleurodesis are advised[15].

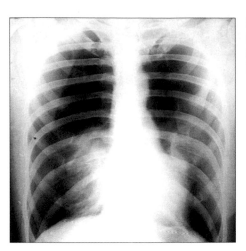

**Fig. 65.8
Catamenial
pneumothorax
(bilateral).**

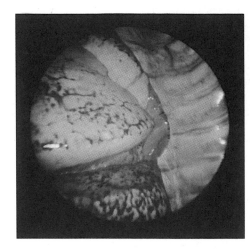

**Fig. 65.9 Idiopathic
spontaneous
pneumothorax.**
Thoracoscopic image
of a normal lung in a
patient with idiopathic
spontaneous
pneumothorax.

PITFALLS AND CONTROVERSIES

The primary treatment of pneumothorax is still controversial. The ideal treatment should aim at expanding the lung rapidly and completely, with restoration (or improvement) of pulmonary function. It should also have minimal morbidity and mortality with low cost and a short hospital stay. It is known that after conservative treatment (i.e. rest, simple aspiration, or drainage) of a first pneumothorax the recurrence rate is as high as 30–50%.

Thoracoscopy is performed more routinely nowadays for first pneumothoraces (in some cases) and for recurrent pneumothorax (in most cases). At thoracoscopy, radiologically occult anomalies (e.g. blebs or cysts) can be identified and a more effective subsequent surgical repair is possible. If the pleura and lung are normal at thoracoscopy (Fig. 65.9) in a young patient, pleurodesis is the best method of treatment, with a

recurrence rate of 6–8%[16]. Other patients need surgical treatment, either by VATS or thoracotomy, in which the usual procedure is pleurodesis by abrasion after repair of any lung abnormality. Pleurectomy should be performed in patients with secondary pneumothorax if pleurodesis fails.

In cases of life-threatening pneumothorax, the findings at physical examinations are usually sufficient to make the diagnosis. The most important step is to insert a large bore needle to evacuate the pneumothorax. The definitive treatment procedure can then be performed later. In a young patient with severe underlying disease who may be a candidate for lung transplantation, pleurodesis and thoracotomy should be avoided. The profession of the patient can also be of importance in choosing the type of treatment (e.g. pilots, construction workers), as a pneumothorax may put them or those they have a responsibility for at risk

REFERENCES

1. Light RW. Pneumothorax. In: Light RW, ed. Pleural diseases, 3rd ed. Baltimore: Williams and Wilkins; 1995:242–77.
2. Wait MA, Esterera A. Changing clinical spectrum of spontaneous pneumothorax. Am J Surg. 1992;164:528–31.
3. Vanderschueren RG. Le talcage pleural dans le pneumothorax spontané. Poumon Coeur. 1981;37:273–6.
4. Schramel FMNH, Postmus PE, Vanderschueren RGJRA. Current aspects of spontaneaous pneumothorax. Eur Respir J. 1997;10:1372–9.
5. Bense L, Eklund G, Wiman LG. Smoking and the increased risk of contracting spontaneous pneumothorax. Chest 1970;57:65–8.
6. van de Brekel JA, Duurkens VAM, Vanderschueren RGJRA. Pneumothorax: results of thoracoscopy and pleurodesis with talpoudrage and thoracotomy. Chest. 1993;103:345–7.
7. Light RW, O'Hara VS, Moritx TE, et al. Intrapleural tetracycline for the prevention of recurrent spontaeous pneumothorax. JAMA. 1990;264:2224–30.
8. Light RW. Pleural diseases, 3rd edn. Baltimore: Williams and Wilkins; 1995.
9. Milanez JR, Vargas FS, Tarcisio L, et al. Intrapleural talc for the prevention of recurrent pneumothorax. Chest. 1994;106:1162–5.
10. Bouchema A, Chastre J, Gaudichet A, Soler P, Gilbert C. Acute pneumonitis with bilateral pleural effusion after talc pleurodesis. Chest. 1984;86:795–7.
11. Lange P, Mortensen J, Groth S. Lung function 22–35 years after treatment of idiopathic spontaneous pneumothorax with talc poudrage or simple drainage. Thorax. 1988;43:559–61.
12. Research Committee of the British Thoracic Association and the Medical Research Council Pneumoconiosis Unit. A survey of long-term effects of talc and kaolin pleurodesis. Br J Dis Chest. 1997;73:285–8.
13. George RB, Herbert SJ, Shames JM, et al. Pneumothorax complicating pulmonary emphysema. JAMA. 1975;234:389–93.
14. Renzi PM, Corbeil C, Chasse M, Braidy J, Matar N. Bilateral pneumothoraces hasten mortality in AIDS patients receiving secondary prophylaxis with aerosolized pentamidine; association with a lower DCO prior to receiving aerosolized pentamidine. Chest. 1992;102:491–6.
15. Wilhelm JL, Scommegna A. Catamenial pneumothorax: bilateral occurrence while on suppressive therapy. Obstet Gynecol. 1977;50:223–31.
16. Almind M, Lange P, Viskum K. Spontaneous pneumothorax: comparison of simple drainage, talc pleurodesis and tetracycline pleurodesis. Thorax. 1989;44:627–30.

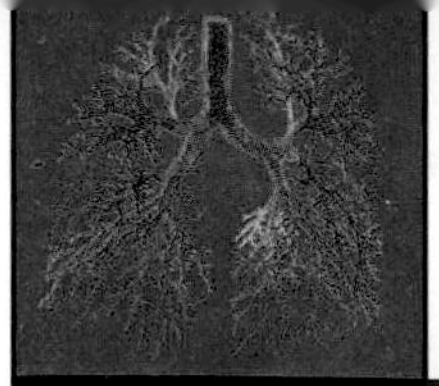

Chapter
66
Pleural Effusion

Robert Loddenkemper

Pleural effusion is defined as accumulation of fluid in the pleural space that exceeds the physiologic amounts of 10–20mL. Pleural effusion develops either when the formation of pleural fluid is excessive and/or when fluid resorption is disturbed. Pleural effusions may represent a primary manifestation of many diseases, but most often they are observed as secondary manifestation or complication of other diseases[1].

EPIDEMIOLOGY AND PATHOPHYSIOLOGY

Epidemiology
Pleural effusion is found in almost 10% of patients who have internal diseases, and the main cause in 30–40% of these is cardiac failure (Fig. 66.1). Among the noncardiac effusions, parapneumonic effusions are the most common at 48%, of which approximately 75% are of bacterial and 25% of viral origin. Malignant pleural effusions follow with 24% of cases, more than half of which are caused by lung or breast cancer. Pleural effusion is secondary to pulmonary embolism in 18% of noncardiac cases, to liver cirrhosis in 6%, and to gastrointestinal diseases, mainly pancreatitis, in 3% of cases. Many other possible causes, albeit extremely rare, play an important role in differential diagnosis. The discrepancy between these estimated incidences and the frequency distribution in the respiratory literature, in which malignant causes are the most common at 42% followed by infectious causes at 29% and idiopathic effusions at 15%, most probably results from patient selection (Fig. 66.2)[2]. Conversely, it may be concluded that, apart from cardiac effusions, effusions as sequelae of pneumonia, pulmonary embolism, and gastrointestinal diseases are easy to diagnose and therefore less frequently referred to the pulmonary specialist.

Pathophysiology
Pleural effusion may result from a number of pathophysiologic mechanisms, all of which disturb the physiologic balance between the formation and removal of pleural fluid. Transudative effusions are either caused by increased hydrostatic pressure (e.g. in cardiac failure) or by reduced plasma oncotic pressure because of protein deficiency (e.g. liver cirrhosis, nephrotic syndrome)[8]. The pleura itself remains intact. In contrast, pathologic changes in the pleura result in exudation caused by a diffuse increase of capillary permeability, to localized ruptures (e.g. blood vessels, lymphatic vessels, lung abscess, esophagus), or to disturbed absorption (e.g. lymphatic blockage).

A wide spectrum of diseases may be associated with pleural effusion. Figure 66.3 shows the relevant etiologic groups together with their most important characteristics, such as appearance, protein and cell content, and other possible features. In some diseases, the pleural effusion may either be an exudate or a transudate[9].

Approximate annual incidence of various types of pleural effusions in the USA			
Etiology	Number	Percentage	Percentage of noncardiac effusions
Congestive heart failure	500,000	37.5	
Other causes		63.5	
Pneumonia	400,000		48.0
Malignant disease	200,000		24.0
Pulmonary embolism	150,000		18.0
Cirrhosis with ascites	50,000		6.0
Gastrointestinal disease	25,000		3.0
Collagen vascular disease	6,000		0.7
Tuberculosis	2,500		0.3
Asbestos pleuritis	2,000		0.25
Mesothelioma	1,500		0.2
Total	1,337,000	100.0	100.0

Figure 66.1 Approximate annual incidence of various types of pleural effusions in the USA. (Adapted with permission from Light[1].)

Frequency distribution of noncardiac effusions					
Authors	Number	Neoplastic (%)	Infectious (%)	Various (%)	Idiopathic (%)
Storey et al.[3]	115	56	6	16	22
Hirsch et al.[4]	295	39	31	9	21
Lamy et al.[5]	194	46	33.5	12	20
Engel[6]	646	34.5	26.5	15	12.5
Loddenkemper[7]	250	34	39	18	9
Total	1500	42	29	14	15

Figure 66.2 Frequency distribution of noncardiac effusions.

CLINICAL FEATURES

Pleural effusion may be present at all ages, but is mainly found in adults. Malignant pleural effusions are observed mainly in patients over 60 years of age. The most common presentations are dyspnea and chest pain, and those of the individual underlying diseases. Physical examination reveals dullness on percussion, usually at the base of the thorax, and decreased breath sounds.

Imaging techniques
Pleural effusion may be demonstrated by a number of techniques with different sensitivities. The demonstration by percussion

Etiologic disease groups	Disease	Results of pleural fluid examination; those in brackets to be clarified			
		Appearance	Protein content (exudate >30g/L; transudate <30g/L)	Cells (if relatively typical)	Other features
Oncotic and hydrostatic disturbances	Cardiac insufficiency	Serous	Transudate	–	Pseudoexudate possible
	Superior vena cava obstruction	Serous	Transudate	–	–
	Constrictive pericarditis	Serous	Transudate	–	–
	Liver cirrhosis with ascites	Serous	Transudate	–	–
	Hypoalbuminemia	Serous	Transudate	–	–
	Salt retention syndrome	Serous	Transudate	–	–
	Peritoneal dialysis	Serous	Transudate	–	–
	Hydronephrosis	Serous	Transudate	–	–
	Nephrotic syndrome	Serous	Transudate	–	–
Infectious	Tuberculosis	Serous, hemorrhagic, purulent, chylous	Exudate	Lymphocytes (neutrophilic granulocytes)	Rarely, microscopic detection of bacteria, elevated adenosine deaminase, glucose decrease possible
	Viruses and mycoplasmas	Serous, (hemorrhagic)	Exudate	Lymphocytes	Giant cells possible
	Parapneumonic	Serous, (hemorrhagic)	Exudate	Neutrophilic granulocytes +	Bacteria +
	Nonspecific empyema	Purulent, (serous)	Exudate	Neutrophilic granulocytes + +	Bacteria +, glucose and pH decreased
	Fungi and parasites	Serous, (hemorrhagic)	Exudate	–	Infecting organisms microscopically or in culture
Neoplastic	Diffuse malignant mesothelioma	Serous, hemorrhagic	Exudate, (transudate)	Tumor cells	–
	Metastatic extrathoracic tumor	Serous, hemorrhagic, chylous	Exudate, (transudate)	Tumor cells	(Tumor markers) (Chromosome analysis)
	Bronchial carcinoma	Serous, hemorrhagic, chylous	Exudate, (transudate)	Tumor cells	Low glucose possible
	Lymphomas and leukemia	Serous, hemorrhagic, chylous	Exudate, transudate	Tumor cells	–
	Localized pleural tumors	Serous, (hemorrhagic)	Exudate, transudate	–	–
	Kaposi's sarcoma (AIDS)	Hemorrhagic	Exudate	–	–
	Chest wall tumors	Serous, hemorrhagic	Exudate	Tumor cells	–
	Accompanying effusion in tumors	Serous	Exudate, transudate	–	–
Vascular	Pulmonary infarction	Hemorrhagic, serous	Exudate, transudate	–	–
	Collaterals in liver cirrhosis	Hemorrhagic, serous	Exudate, transudate	–	Markedly decreased
Autoimmune	Rheumatoid arthritis	Serous, chylous	Exudate	Lupus erythematosus cells	Glucose and C3/C4
	Systemic lupus erythematosus	Serous, (hemorrhagic)	Exudate	–	–
	Sjögren's syndrome	Serous	Exudate, (transudate)	–	–
	Mixed connective tissue disease	Serous	Exudate	–	–
Originating from the abdomen	Pancreatitis, pseudocyst	Serous, (hemorrhagic)	Exudate, (transudate)	–	Elevated amylase
	Subdiaphragmatic abscess	Serous, purulent	Exudate	Neutrophilic granulocytes	–
	Liver cirrhosis with ascites	Serous, (purulent)	Transudate, (exudate)	–	–
	Abdominal tumor with ascites	Serous	Transudate	–	–
	Meigs' syndrome	Serous	Transudate, (exudate)	–	–
	Cholohemothorax (biliary fistula)	Bilious	Exudate	–	Bilirubin
	Endometriosis	Hemorrhagic	Exudate	–	–
Traumatic	Hemothorax	Hemorrhagic	Exudate	Erythrocytes	High hemoglobin
	Chylothorax	Chylous	Transudate, (exudate)	–	Chylomicrons, elevated triglycerides
	Esophageal perforation	Purulent	Exudate	Neutrophilic granulocytes	Elevated amylase, low pH
	Surgery (thorax, abdomen)	Serous, hemorrhagic	Exudate, transudate	–	–
	Seropneumothorax	Serous, (hemorrhagic)	Exudate	–	–
Miscellaneous	Uremic pleuritis	Serous, (hemorrhagic)	Exudate	–	–
	Myxedema	Serous	Transudate	–	–
	Yellow nail syndrome	Serous, (chylous)	Exudate	–	–
	Postmyocardial infarction syndrome	Serous, (hemorrhagic)	Exudate	–	–
	Periarteritis nodosa	Serous	Exudate	–	–
	Sarcoidosis	Serous, (hemorrhagic)	Transudate, (exudate)	–	–
	Familial Mediterranean fever	Serous	Exudate	–	–
	Benign asbestos effusion	Serous, (hemorrhagic)	Exudate	–	–
	Drug-induced	Serous	Exudate	–	–
	Radiation pneumonia	Serous, (hemorrhagic)	Exudate	–	–
	Lymphangioleiomyomatosis	Chylous	Transudate, (exudate)	–	–
	Tuberous sclerosis	Chylous	Transudate, (exudate)	–	–
	Cholesterol pleuritis (pseudochylothorax)	Chylous	Transudate, exudate	–	Cholesterol (crystals), low triglycerides
	Intrapleural infusion	Serous, (hemorrhagic)	Exudate, transudate	–	–
	Idiopathic	Serous, (hemorrhagic)	Exudate, transudate	Eosinophils	–

Figure 66.3 Etiology and characteristics of pleural effusions.
Parentheses denote that clarification is not fully validated as yet. + denotes neutrophilic granulocytes present in a moderate amount; + +, a considerable amount. (AIDS, acquired immune deficiency syndrome.)

requires at least 300–400mL of fluid, whereas at least 200–300mL is necessary for standard chest radiography. Smaller amounts can be recognized by lateral decubitus radiography, which also demonstrates whether the fluid is moving freely or not (Fig. 66.4). Ultrasound is able to demonstrate small effusions, and the sensitivity is almost 100% for volumes of 100mL and above. Computed tomography (CT) and magnetic resonance imaging have very similar sensitivities, but require a more advanced technology and are therefore much more expensive[2].

DIAGNOSIS

In the majority of cases, the etiology is based on the case history, clinical presentation, imaging techniques, and examination of the pleural fluid.

Diagnostic approach

The presence of a pleural effusion is established only by thoracentesis. The site should be selected according to clinical examination and radiological investigations. If the effusion is small, thoracentesis can be performed under ultrasound guidance. Thoracentesis is indicated in all cases of pleural effusion of unknown origin, and in effusions that do not resolve after appropriate treatment. If the results of pleural fluid examination are not conclusive, thoracentesis may be repeated. However, additional biopsy procedures, such as closed pleural needle biopsy (see Chapter 7) or thoracoscopy (see below) may become necessary to confirm or exclude malignant or tuberculous causes. These are performed in a stepwise diagnostic approach (Fig. 66.5)[9].

Evaluation of the pleural fluid

Often, evaluation of the pleural fluid yields valuable diagnostic information or even permits a clear diagnosis. The most important criteria are appearance, protein content, and cellular components. For more specific diagnostic questions, routine measurement of the glucose content is supplemented by determination of further laboratory parameters and bacterial culture (Fig. 66.6)[1,2,10].

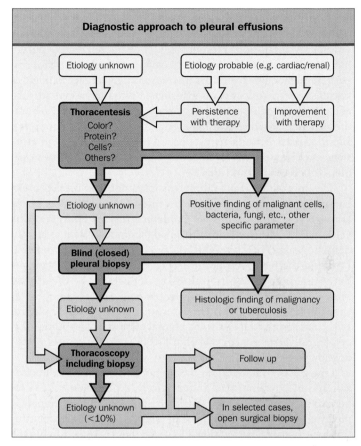

Figure 66.5 Diagnostic approach to pleural effusions

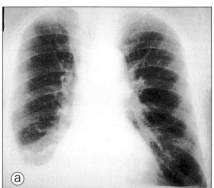

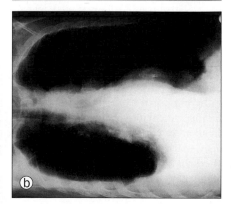

Figure 66.4 Right-sided basal pleural effusion.
(a) Posteroanterior view;
(b) right lateral decubitus view.

Investigative parameters of pleural effusion	
Obligatory	**Optional**
Appearance	Glucose (pH)
Total protein	Lactate dehydrogenase
Cell differentiation (cytology)	Cholesterol
	Triglycerides
	Amylase
	Bilirubin
	Creatinine
	Hematocrit
	Immunocytology
	Tumor markers
	Adenosine deaminase
	Lysozymes
	Antinuclear factor, rheumatoid factors, etc.
	Search for infecting organisms
	Tubercle bacilli
	Gram staining
	Anaerobic, aerobic bacteria
	Fungi, parasites

Figure 66.6 Investigative parameters of pleural effusion.

The appearance may be serous (light to dark, clear to turbid), serosanguineous (blood-tinged, in some cases because of thoracentesis!), hemorrhagic (bloody), purulent (fetid odor in anaerobic effusions), or chylous (milky). Bilious (cholothorax), brown (perforated amebic abscess), black (aspergillar infection), or yellowish green (rheumatoid pleuritis, pancreatic effusion) appearances are extremely rare. Blood-tinged effusions that occur with no trauma are mainly caused by tumors (hemorrhagic in 50%) or pulmonary infarction. Hemothorax is characterized by purely bloody effusions and hematocrit values that exceed those in peripheral blood by over 50%. Increased triglycerides distinguish chylous from pseudochylous effusions. Viscous effusions are rare and may indicate increased hyaluronic acid in malignant pleural mesothelioma, while ammonia odor may indicate urinothorax and food particles indicate esophageal perforation. Purulent effusions must be analyzed for infecting organisms (aerobic and anaerobic, tuberculous, and fungi).

The most important laboratory parameter is total protein content in the effusion, for which a threshold value of 30g/L separates a transudate from an exudate effusion. However, this value is not exclusive, and additional parameters such as lactate dehydrogenase (LDH; >200U/L) or cholesterol [>1.55mmol/L (>60mg/dL)] may be helpful (Fig. 66.7). The simultaneous determination of serum values is important, as these may strongly influence the values in the pleura. Thus, the quotient of total pleural protein and total serum protein (>0.5), pleural LDH and serum LDH (>0.6), pleural cholesterol (>60mg/dL), or pleural versus serum bilirubin (<0.6) permits a safer classification as exudate.

Low glucose values under 3.33mmol/L (60mg/dL) or an effusion:serum quotient <0.5 (alternatively, a pH value <7.3 with normal serum pH or LDH >1000U/L) may indicate rheumatoid pleuritis, lupus pleuritis, empyema, tuberculous or malignant effusion, or esophageal perforation. However, these entities differ in the frequency of decreased glucose values (Fig. 66.8).

The lowest glucose values <0.56mmol/L (<10mg/dL) are found in rheumatoid effusions and empyema. Parapneumonic effusions with values <2.22mmol/L (<40mg/dL) are frequently associated with bacterial infection. In tuberculous effusions, the chance of a positive culture improves markedly with decreased glucose concentrations. Low glucose content in malignant effusions indicates more extensive involvement and a poorer prognosis. A low pH reflects intensive, anaerobic metabolism of leukocytes, bacteria, or tumor cells.

Markedly elevated amylase values – higher and more persistently increased than in serum – are observed in acute pancreatitis and pancreatic pseudocysts (often >1,000U/L), esophageal perforation (salivary amylase, pH markedly decreased, down to 6.0), and occasionally in malignant effusions.

Triglyceride content >1.24mmol/L (>110mg/dL) strongly suggests a chylous effusion (intermediate values are further assessed by lipoprotein electrophoresis). As chylous effusions are not necessarily milky in appearance, triglycerides are determined in all effusions of uncertain etiology. Chylothorax is a rare cause of increased bilirubin in pleural effusions, while increased creatinine may be caused by urinothorax.

When pleural effusion is associated with rheumatoid arthritis or systemic lupus erythematosus, immunologic parameters (rheumatoid factor, antinuclear antibodies, lupus erythematosus cells, and complement values) are assessed in addition to the glucose levels.

Differentiation between transudate and exudate		
Parameter	Transudate	Exudate
Total protein (TP)	<30g/L	>30g/L
Ratio of TP pleura to TP serum	<0.5	>0.5
Lactate dehydrogenase (LDH)	<200U/L	>200U/L
Ratio of LDH pleura to LDH serum	<0.6	>0.6
Cholesterol	<1.55mmol/L (<60mg/dL)	>1.55mmol/L (>60mg/dL)
Bilirubin pleura:serum ratio	<0.6	>0.6

Figure 66.7 Differentiation between transudate and exudate.

Frequency of low glucose values in pleural effusions	
Entity	Frequency (%)
Rheumatoid pleuritis	85
Empyema	80
Malignant effusion	30
Tuberculous effusion	20
Lupus pleuritis	20

Figure 66.8 Frequency of low glucose values in pleural effusions. (Adapted with permission from Sahn[10]).

Although nonspecific, adenosine deaminase and lysozymes are frequently increased in tuberculous effusions.

The search for tumor cells focuses on analysis of the cellular components. In an analysis of 4000 cases of malignant effusions, the mean sensitivity of cytologic diagnostic procedures was 58% (range 41–88%, standard deviation ±14%). The results were partly improved by repeat analysis[11]. The sensitivity was also dependent on the tumor type and the primary tumor.

The red cell count and the relative and absolute numbers of lymphocytes, and neutrophilic and eosinophilic granulocytes, are rarely important in the differential diagnosis. Although usually rich in lymphocytes, tuberculous effusions in the early stages may contain a preponderance of granulocytes, which is also typical of nonspecific bacterial effusions. Increased eosinophils are of no great diagnostic value, but are very frequently observed in effusions of uncertain etiology and in chronic effusions.

Diagnostic testing for the infecting organisms that cause pleural effusion is indicated in empyemas with aerobic and anaerobic cultures, and in suspected tuberculous, fungal, or parasitic effusions.

Thoracoscopy

Medical thoracoscopy is an invasive technique that may be used when other more simple methods fail[11]. The technique is similar to chest-tube insertion by means of a trocar, the difference being that, in addition, the pleural cavity can be visualized, and biopsies can be taken from all areas of the pleural cavity, including the chest wall, diaphragm, mediastinum, and lung (Fig. 66.9). The main advantage of medical thoracoscopy compared with surgical thoracoscopy, which is videoassisted thoracic surgery, is that the examination can be performed under local anesthetic and

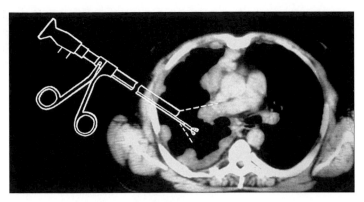

Figure 66.9 Technique of thoracoscopy. Computed tomography scan of a patient with malignant pleural effusion with large nodules on the chest wall and the mediastinum, onto whose hemithorax the thoracoscope with the biopsy forceps is projected (schematic representation only).

Sensitivity of medical thoracoscopy in malignant and tuberculous pleural effusions		
Biopsy procedure	Malignant; $n = 208$ (%)	Tuberculous; $n = 100$ (%)
Pleural effusion	62 (cytology)	28 (culture)
Closed needle biopsy	44	51
Effusion plus needle	74	61
Medical thoracoscopy	95	99
Effusion plus thoracoscopy	96	100
All materials	97	100

Figure 66.10 Sensitivity of medical thoracoscopy in malignant and tuberculous pleural effusions. Intrapatient comparison with pleural fluid examination and closed needle biopsy.

sedation after adequate premedication, and thus an anesthetist is not required. Furthermore, medical thoracoscopy is less expensive, as it may be safely performed with nondisposable instruments, and in an appropriate endoscopy room. One technique favors a single entry using a 9mm thoracoscope, with a working channel for accessory instruments and optical biopsy forceps, and local anesthetic. Another technique favors two entry sites using a 7mm trocar for the examination telescope and a 5mm trocar for accessory instruments, including the biopsy forceps, under sedative or (general) anesthetic.

Medical thoracoscopy is safe if the contraindications are observed and if certain standard criteria are fulfilled. An obliterated pleural space is an absolute contraindication. Relative contraindications include bleeding disorders, hypoxemia, an unstable cardiovascular state, and persistent, uncontrollable cough. Complications, such as benign cardiac arrhythmias, low-grade hypertension, or hypoxemia, can be minimized by oxygen administration. The most serious, but rare, complication is severe hemorrhage caused by blood vessel trauma during the procedure. However, this, and also lung perforation, can be avoided by using safe points of entry and a cautious biopsy technique. A serious complication of pneumothorax induction is air or gas embolism, which occurs very rarely (<0.1%). Several liters of fluid can be removed during thoracoscopy with little risk of pulmonary edema, because immediate equilibration of pressures is provided by direct entrance of air through the cannula into the pleural space.

Medical thoracoscopy is primarily a diagnostic procedure, but it can also be applied for therapeutic purposes. Pleural effusions are the leading indication for medical thoracoscopy, both for diagnosis and staging of diffuse malignant mesothelioma or lung cancer, and for treatment by talc pleurodesis in malignant or other recurrent effusions, or occasionally in empyema. If the facilities are available, medical thoracoscopy is performed in pleural effusions when the etiology remains undetermined after thoracentesis and closed pleural biopsy. This applies to at least 20–25% of effusions. Medical thoracoscopy has a sensitivity of about 95% in malignant pleural effusions and of almost 100% in tuberculous pleurisy (Fig. 66.10). In addition, it allows a fast and more definite biopsy diagnosis, including a higher yield in tuberculosis (TB) cultures, and the determination of hormone receptors in some malignancies. Underlying malignancy or TB is

excluded with high probability. Surgery, including surgical thoracoscopy, is not only much more invasive and expensive, but does not produce better results than medical thoracoscopy and is therefore reserved for carefully selected cases. In cases with effusions that are neither malignant nor tuberculous, thoracoscopy may give macroscopic clues to their etiology (e.g. in rheumatoid effusions, or effusions following pancreatitis, liver cirrhosis, extension from the abdominal cavity, or trauma, although in these entities the history, pleural fluid analysis, and other examinations are usually sufficient for diagnosis). When pleural effusion is secondary to the underlying primary lung diseases, such as pulmonary infarction or pneumonia, the diagnosis can frequently be made on macroscopic examination and be confirmed microscopically from lung biopsy specimens. Medical thoracoscopy is well suited to the diagnosis of benign, asbestos-related pleural effusions, which, by definition, are a diagnosis of exclusion. After thoracoscopy, the proportion of idiopathic pleural effusions usually falls below 10%.

Medical thoracoscopy can also be useful in the management of early empyema. In cases with multiple loculations, it is possible to open these spaces to remove the fibrinopurulent membranes by forceps and to create one single cavity, which can be drained and irrigated much more successfully. This treatment is carried out early in the course of empyema, before the adhesions become too fibrous and adherent. Thus, if an indication for placement of a chest tube is present and if the facilities are available, medical thoracoscopy is performed at the time of chest tube insertion. In general, the technique of medical thoracoscopy is similar to that of chest-tube placement, but allows the potential restoration of a single pleural cavity, and thus allows better local treatment. Thoracotomy or pleurectomy remains an option if these measures fail.

TREATMENT

Therapeutic aims in patients with pleural effusion are palliation of symptoms (pain, dyspnea), treatment of underlying diseases, prevention of pleural fibrosis with reduction of pulmonary function, and prevention of recurrences. The therapeutic approach depends on the availability of options for causal or only symptomatic treatment. Details are given in the descriptions of the specific disease entities.

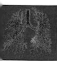
Pleurodesis

The aim of pleurodesis is to achieve fusion between visceral and parietal pleural layers, in order to prevent re-accumulation of fluid (or air) in the pleural space. Its main indications are malignant pleural effusions or, rarely, benign, recurrent pleural effusions when other treatments have failed (e.g. in liver cirrhosis, nephrotic syndrome, chylothorax, cardiac failure).

To achieve a complete pleural symphysis, several conditions need to be fulfilled[12]. In particular, the fluid must be removed completely from the pleural space to keep the visceral and parietal pleural layers in close contact. This is achieved with application of suction through appropriate drainage, provided a trapped lung (Fig. 66.11) and bronchial obstruction have been ruled out. Furthermore, to achieve complete fusion, the pleural surface needs to be irritated, either mechanically with pleural abrasion or through application of a sclerosing agent[13]. Various chemicals have been used in attempts to induce pleurodesis (Fig. 66.12). The most effective and also least expensive agent is talc, which has been used in most series via medical thoracoscopy. For thoracoscopic talc poudrage, general anesthetic or tracheal intubation are not necessary, but careful local anesthetic with parenteral analgesia is mandatory. If thoracoscopy is not available, many groups use a 'talc slurry' (talcum powder suspended in variable amounts of saline), with a reported overall success rate of 91%, which is comparable to that of talc insufflation, but fewer studies have been carried out using talc slurry than talc poudrage. A randomized trial is currently underway in North America to evaluate these two methods. Complications related to talc are rare, provided a sterile and asbestos-free form is used. Severe pain is usually less frequent than with tetracycline, and mild fever (probably related to the inflammatory process) can be observed for 2–3 days after the procedure. A few major complications have been reported, but these may be related to excessive dosages (doses of talc above 5g may be associated with acute respiratory failure) and/or other independent factors.

Tetracycline hydrochloride has a reportedly wide range of efficacy (45–77%). It requires heavy analgesia, but production of the parenteral form has been discontinued in the USA. Moreover, a relatively high rate of late recurrences has been reported. An alternative is doxycycline, but repeated dosages are frequently necessary. Minocycline has also been proposed as a replacement for tetracycline, but it may provoke vestibular symptoms when the dosages required for pleurodesis are used. The main drawbacks of bleomycin are cost and systemic absorption, with the risk of significant toxicity. Quinacrine (mepacrine) is frequently used in Scandinavia. It may provoke serious toxicity of the central nervous system, probably because of the high dosages required. *Corynebacterium parvum* is almost exclusively used in some European centers, and the average effectiveness of this agent has been reported to be 76%. However, in a randomized study with bleomycin, it was effective in only 32% of cases. The use of fibrin glue is controversial, because of the cost and lack of evidence of experimental effectiveness. Moreover, it has been demonstrated that failure of pleurodesis in malignant effusions is associated with increased pleural fibrinolysis, which could lead to rapid destruction of the fibrin glue.

In conclusion, if the facilities for medical thoracoscopy are available, talc poudrage is performed. This technique has many advantages, not only for diagnostic purposes, but also because large amounts of fluid can be removed immediately and completely during medical thoracoscopy with little risk of pulmonary edema

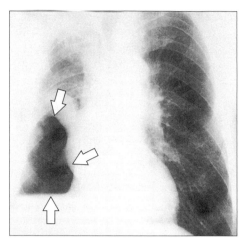

Figure 66.11 Radiograph of a patient with a trapped lung on the right side. The patient had an epidermoid bronchial carcinoma with massive pleural effusion on the right. Thoracoscopically, a trapped lower lobe was present after aspirating the effusion, leaving a hydropneumothorax (arrows) and the lung was unable to expand.

Complete success rates of commonly used pleurodesis agents			
Chemical agent	Total patients (n)	Successful (%)	Dose
Talc	165	93	2.5–10g
Corynebacterium parvum	169	76	3.5–14mg
Doxycycline	60	72	500mg (often multiple doses)
Tetracycline	359	67	500mg, up to 20mg/kg
Bleomycin	199	54	15–240 units

Figure 66.12 Complete success rates of commonly used pleurodesis agents. (Adapted with permission from Walker-Renard et al.[15])

because of the immediate equilibration of pressures by direct entrance of air into the pleural space. Furthermore, the re-expansion potential of the lung can be evaluated directly. In addition, the extent of intrapleural tumor spread can be identified. Talc poudrage is the best conservative option for pleurodesis, possibly because of even distribution of the talc to all parts of the pleura. Surgical pleurectomy is indicated rarely for pleurodesis, although it is the procedure of choice in units that do not have thoracoscopy if the patient is fit and, in the case of a malignant effusion, likely to survive months or years (e.g. breast cancer). The insertion of a pleuroperitoneal shunt is another important alternative if re-expansion of a trapped lung is impossible because of tumor and the effusion re-accumulates rapidly[14]. The fluid drains into the abdominal cavity with remarkably few complications.

SPECIFIC ENTITIES ASSOCIATED WITH PLEURAL EFFUSION

Oncotic and hydrostatic effusions

Causes of cardiac effusions

Cardiac effusions are predominantly caused by left ventricular failure, which leads to increased formation of pleural fluid through the visceral pleura, because of elevated pulmonary capillary pressure[1,8]. Right ventricular failure, which interferes in particular with lymphatic drainage through the parietal pleura because of increased venous pressure, is rarely the sole cause. Dyspnea predominates and, on auscultation, additional rales are often present because of left ventricular failure; furthermore, signs of right ventricular failure can be found. More than half of effusions are bilateral, and 27% are right-sided only and 15% left-sided only. Usually, the heart is enlarged. Chest radiography may reveal so-called pseudotumor, predominantly in the right horizontal or the oblique fissure, which disappears with diuretic treatment (Fig. 66.13).

Diagnostic thoracentesis is only indicated if cardiac treatment is not successful. Pleural effusions caused by heart failure are usually transudates; however, the protein content may be increased as a result of diuretic treatment (so-called pseudoexudate). In the differential diagnosis, constrictive pericarditis, pulmonary infarction, and pneumonia must also be considered.

The treatment of these effusions is that for heart failure, and therapeutic thoracentesis to relieve dyspnea is rarely necessary.

Hepatic and other abdominal causes of effusions

Pleural effusions secondary to liver cirrhosis are usually caused by the passage of ascitic fluid into the pleural cavity, or (less frequently) by decreased oncotic pressure caused by hypoalbuminemia[1]. Hemorrhage from congested collateral veins is another, extremely rare, cause. The clinical picture is of cirrhosis and ascites, and the diagnosis is based on thoracentesis and paracentesis with demonstration of transudates.

Differential diagnosis must exclude all other diseases, such as TB and pleural carcinomatosis secondary to cirrhosis-induced hepatic carcinoma, which may be associated with simultaneous ascites and pleural effusion. In women, Meigs' syndrome must be ruled out. Other rare causes of pleural effusion are viral hepatitis and intrahepatic abscess. Pleural effusion may rarely occur during peritoneal dialysis or abdominal surgery. Subphrenic abscess is associated with pleural effusion in over 50% of cases.

Approximately 20% of cases of acute pancreatitis develop pleural effusions, of which two thirds are left sided, while one third is right-sided or bilateral. Crucial diagnostic factors are amylase values in the effusion persistently above those in serum. The effusion may be serosanguineous or bloody. In cases of persistent effusion, a pancreatic abscess or pseudocyst must be excluded. In case of high amylase values, esophagus perforation must be excluded (salivary amylase).

Gallstone perforation into the pleura is extremely rare and results in a bilious effusion (cholothorax). Diaphragmatic hernia occurs most frequently on the left side following trauma and may resemble or, in cases of incarceration, even result in an effusion.

In the treatment of cirrhosis the goal is to remove ascites. Occasionally, therapeutic thoracentesis is indicated to relieve dyspnea. Pleurodesis may be attempted in therapy-resistant cases. In effusions from other abdominal causes, therapy is directed at the underlying disease.

Renal causes of effusions

Renal causes of pleural effusions are nephrotic syndrome, acute glomerulonephritis, uremia, and (rarely) hydronephrosis, which may result in retroperitoneal fluid collecting and causing a so-called urinothorax with increased creatinine values in the pleural fluid. The increased values are caused by retroperitoneal urinary leakage from trauma, retroperitoneal inflammatory, or malignant processes, failed nephrostomy, or even kidney biopsy[1]. The usually right-sided effusion observed in peritoneal dialysis corresponds chemically closely to dialysis fluid. Hemorrhagic effusion may develop during hemodialysis as a complication of anticoagulant treatment.

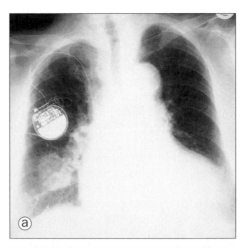

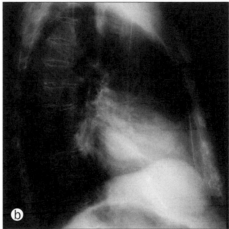

Figure 66.13
Pseudotumor of the lung.
(a) Posteroanterior and (b) lateral chest radiographs showing a mass caused by fluid trapped in a fissure.

Infectious pleurisy, empyema

Infections of the pleura usually result in an effusion[1,15]. However, initially only an inflammatory process that has no associated pleural fluid is possible (pleuritis sicca; dry pleurisy).

Pleuritis sicca is characterized by acute chest pain, in particular when breathing and coughing, which may radiate to the abdominal region or shoulder if the diaphragmatic pleura is involved, and thus make differential diagnosis more difficult. Clinical examination often reveals a circumscribed sensitivity to pressure, or pain on percussion in the area of the diseased pleura. On auscultation, inspiratory and expiratory pleural rub of different intensity may be present. The affected side of the chest may be less active in breathing, while further symptoms depend on the underlying disease. Chest radiography often reveals an elevation of the hemidiaphragm and rib crowding because of efforts to limit respiratory movement and pain.

In the exudative stage, the pleuritic pain disappears and dyspnea may develop. The effusion may be parapneumonic without infection (uncomplicated) or culture positive (complicated). Empyema is apparent by the macroscopic appearance of thick and turbid fluid (pus). The differentiation is important, as a complicated parapneumonic empyema usually requires tube thoracotomy.

Bacterial pneumonia is associated with an effusion in approximately 40% of cases, and is thus one of the main causes, although the frequency has been reduced by early antibiotic treatment. The spectrum of infecting organisms has also changed. In adults, anaerobic bacteria or a mixture of aerobic

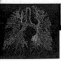

and anaerobic bacteria are found frequently. Among the aerobic bacteria, pneumococci predominate by more than 50%, and usually cause an uncomplicated effusion. Depending on the etiology of pneumonia, Gram-negative bacteria may play a role, in particular *Klebsiella pneumoniae* and *Pseudomonas aeruginosa*. In *Legionella* pneumonia, small pleural effusions occur in approximately 25% of patients. In children, pleurisy is mainly caused by staphylococci, pneumococci, or *Haemophilus influenzae*, while anaerobes are extremely rare.

The development of pleural effusion is correlated with the length of time that the pneumonia remains untreated, but has little influence on symptoms. If fever persists for more than 48 hours after initiation of antibiotic treatment, a complicating effusion (empyema) is likely. In contrast, patients who suffer anaerobic infections tend to have subacute symptoms over several days and can develop an effusion at any time.

Depending on the clinical picture and size of the effusion (more than 10mm thickness on the decubitus radiograph), a diagnostic thoracentesis is performed to ascertain bacterial contamination before the start of antibiotic treatment. The appearance (turbid, thick, putrid) and odor (foul in anaerobic infection) signal pleural empyema. Important parameters are Gram-stain, protein content, glucose, LDH, amylase pH, and leukocyte count. An uncharacteristic appearance, glucose values <2.22mmol/L (<40mg/dL), and pH values <7.2 suggest bacterial infection.

The antibiotic treatment of pneumonia with and without accompanying effusion is the same. However, empyema, which occurs in approximately 10% of pneumonias, may require additional pleural drainage.

Tuberculous pleurisy

Tuberculous pleurisy mainly affects younger patients and is twice as frequent in males than in females[16]. However, currently the trend is toward the development of tuberculous pleural effusions in older age groups. Tuberculous pleuritis usually occurs soon after the primary TB infection.

The onset of symptoms may be acute (severe pleuritic chest pain, nonproductive cough, high temperature, and dyspnea), or subacute (loss of appetite, weight loss, and night sweats). In many cases of acute onset, auscultation reveals only dry pleurisy, with the symptoms of effusion following later. Tuberculin skin tests are usually positive. The involvement of the lung parenchyma and lymph nodes found in 37–83% of patients is frequently not detected by radiography before the effusion disappears.

The old rule that any exudative pleural effusion of uncertain etiology and a positive tuberculin skin test must be considered and treated as tuberculous is no longer valid[12]. Tuberculosis can be proved by granulomata in a pleural biopsy specimen and from biopsy specimen culture. The effusion is usually clear and serous, and seldom turbid and serous. Predominantly, lymphocytes are present, but in the very early stages, neutrophils may be prominent. Low glucose values are found in only 20–50% of cases; however, the chances of a positive *Mycobacterium tuberculosis* culture from the exudate are higher in these cases. Adenosine deaminase is usually increased, but this is not diagnostic of TB. The transition to an empyema may be insidious. The most important diagnostic tools, closed pleural biopsy and thoracoscopy, permit a fast diagnosis based on histologic findings, and they also increase the chances of bacteriologic proof.

The treatment of TB is covered in Chapter 29.

Pleurisy caused by other organisms

Small pleural effusions are found in approximately 20% of infections by viruses, *Mycoplasma* spp., or *Rickettsia* spp., but do not necessarily affect the lungs[1]. The diagnosis is based mainly on the clinical picture, and on serum titers, virus culture, or virus antibodies in the pleural fluid. The exudate is characterized by lymphocytes and initially also by neutrophils. Thoracoscopy can be a valuable tool to exclude TB. Virus infections are frequently accompanied by pericarditis. Differential diagnosis must exclude pleurodynia (Bornholm's disease caused by coxsackievirus B6).

Although unusual, pleural effusion may occur in all mycotic lung diseases. The effusion is usually lymphocytic, but may also be eosinophilic. *Aspergillus fumigatus* infection is occasionally found after artificial pneumothorax treatment for TB, or postoperatively after lobectomy or pneumonectomy, especially in the presence of a bronchopleural fistula. Pleural effusion is observed in approximately 4% of blastomycoses and 20% of coccidioidomycosis. Cryptococci or other fungi are very rare causes of pleural effusion, but occur mainly in immunocompromised patients.

Parasitic pleural diseases are extremely rare and include amebiasis (perforation of a liver abscess into the pleural cavity!), echinococcosis, paragonimosis, and *Pneumocystis carinii* infection in relation to the acquired immunodeficiency syndrome.

Malignant pleural effusions other than mesothelioma

Malignant pleural diseases are mainly caused by hematogenic or lymphogenic metastases from extrathoracic primary tumors, or by direct tumor spread from adjacent organs[13]. However, increased asbestos exposure has also led to more cases of primary, diffuse, pleural mesothelioma (see Chapter 67). Tumor-related pleural effusions may have direct and indirect causes. Direct causes are increased capillary permeability caused by pleural metastases, obstruction of mesothelial capillaries, or disturbed reabsorption through insufficient lymphatic drainage caused by pleural metastases, involvement of mediastinal lymph nodes, or blockage of the thoracic duct. Indirect, paramalignant causes may be postobstructive pneumonia with pleuritis, atelectasis with decreased intrapleural pressure, pericardial involvement, vena cava syndrome, late effects of radiotherapy-induced pleuritis, pulmonary infarction, or hypoproteinemia. The distinction between these paramalignant and true malignant effusions is important when deciding on possible resection of bronchial carcinoma.

The majority of pleural tumors are not primary, but represent metastases or direct spread from adjacent organs. The most frequent primary tumors are bronchial (10–50%) and breast carcinoma (20–50%), followed by lymphomas, ovarian cancer, and others. Any malignant tumor, except for primary brain tumors, may metastasize into the pleura. In 20–50% of cases, the primary tumor cannot be localized. Pleural effusion develops in 8–15% of all patients who have bronchial carcinoma, with a rate of up to 27% in small-cell and up to 50% in metastasizing carcinomas. Malignant pleural effusion is found in approximately 7% of breast cancer patients at some point during their disease and is a first symptom of metastases in 43% of these. Between 5 and 33% of malignant lymphomas are associated with pleural effusion. Malignant effusions can be huge, filling the entire hemithorax, and shift the mediastinum to the unaffected side. Lung involvement and mediastinal lymph node

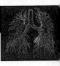

enlargement are best detected by CT. Cytologic investigation of the effusion and closed pleural biopsy yield success rates between 20 and 84%, depending on the primary tumor. Carcinoembryonic antigen is characteristically elevated with adenocarcinoma, but is not diagnostic of cancer. The safest diagnostic procedure, with a sensitivity of 90–98%, is medical thoracoscopy, in which biopsy specimens may also be taken from the lung. Histologic evaluation of large biopsy specimens additionally provides information on undetected primary tumors. Cytologic evaluation of the effusion is more successful for breast cancer than for other tumors. Histologic specimens for hormone-receptor determination may be taken during thoracoscopy. Malignant lymphomas are frequently accompanied by chylous effusions, for which cytologic evaluation and blind needle biopsy have low diagnostic sensitivities. Chromosome analysis and thoracoscopy are clearly superior in this respect. Benign ovarian tumors (Meigs' syndrome) and fibromyomas of the uterus are occasionally accompanied by pleural effusions. Pleural endometriosis is extremely rare.

Pleural effusions of other etiologies

Effusions may be observed in connection with autoimmune diseases, especially rheumatoid arthritis and systemic lupus erythematosus[1]. Sjögren's syndrome, dermatomyositis, scleroderma, 'mixed connective tissue disease', polyarteritis nodosa, and Wegener's granulomatosis are rarely associated with pleural effusion.

Pleural effusion is the most frequent thoracic manifestation of rheumatoid arthritis and occurs in 3–5% of cases, usually several years after the onset of arthritic symptoms. The effusion is characterized by very low glucose [<1.67mmol/L (< 30mg/dL)], low pH (< 7.2), increased LDH [11.7μkat/L (>700U/L)], elevated rheumatoid factor, and low complement levels. The course of rheumatoid pleurisy may vary, and spontaneous resorption is frequently observed. Recurrences are rare, but systemic corticosteroid therapy may be necessary. A chronic, sterile, therapy-resistant, pleural empyema may develop.

In systemic lupus erythematosus, the pleura is affected in approximately 50% of patients who have pleuritic symptoms and in 20–30% of cases by a pleural effusion, and is bilateral in more than half the cases. The frequent cardiac involvement is reflected by cardiomegaly. Antinuclear antibodies are typically increased in the pleural effusion; lupus erythematosus cells are characteristic if present. The changes of glucose, pH, and LDH values are less pronounced than in rheumatoid pleurisy. Corticosteroid treatment results in a rapid, satisfactory response.

Effusions caused by pulmonary infarction are nonspecific and may be exudative or transudative. Over 70% are blood-tinged, and approximately 20% are bloody.

Asbestos exposure may cause a bilateral, benign effusion that often recurs after spontaneous resorption. The exudate is sanguineous in over 30% of cases. The diagnosis must be based on at least 2 years of observation, following exclusion of other causes[17].

Exudative effusions may also be associated with familial Mediterranean fever, yellow-nail syndrome, sarcoidosis, radiation pneumonia, long-term medication [especially with nitrofurantoin, bromocriptine, procarbazine, methotrexate, mitomycin, amiodarone, methysergide, or practolol (now withdrawn)], or with drug-induced lupus erythematosus, Dressler's syndrome after myocardial infarction, cardiac surgery, and other diseases.

Approximately 15% of pleural effusions remain undiagnosed, particularly in young males, and eosinophils are frequently increased in these effusions, possibly because of virus infection. However, eosinophilia is also observed in other types of pleurisy.

Hemothorax

Hemothorax is mainly caused by trauma, pulmonary infarction, or tumors, and is characterized by hematocrit values over 50% above those in serum[1].

Traumatic hemothorax usually results from penetrating or contused thoracic injuries that lead to rib fracture and damage of intercostal or pulmonary vessels. The treatment depends on the clinical picture and on the severity of hemorrhage, which is monitored by intrapleural drainage. Thoracotomy is indicated if blood volumes exceed 100–200mL/hour. The prognosis depends largely on the patient's other injuries.

Chylothorax

Chylothorax is characterized by the direct passage of chyle from the thoracic duct into the pleural cavity. The pleural fluid is usually milky. The triglyceride content needs to be determined, as not all chylous effusions are milky in appearance, and as some milky effusions may be pseudochylous[18]. Triglyceride values >1.24mmol/L (>110mg/dL) indicate chylothorax, which may be excluded if the content is <0.56mmol/L (<50mg/dL). Results between these values need to be tested further for chylomicrons. Pseudochylothorax, which must be excluded in differential diagnosis, is characterized by high cholesterol values and by the absence of chylomicrons.

The cause in over 50% of cases are tumors, predominantly lymphomas. Approximately 25% are secondary to trauma to the thoracic duct, especially during surgery. Further, rare, causes are congenital defects, lymphangioleiomyomatosis, and tuberous sclerosis. The etiology remains unclear in 15% of patients.

The treatment of chylothorax depends on the cause. Irradiation of the mediastinum or systemic chemotherapy is indicated in cases of lymphoma or metastasizing tumor. Chylothorax following trauma is treated by pleural drainage. Pleurodesis may be successful in some patients. In individual cases, surgical ligature of the thoracic duct or pleurectomy may be indicated. A pleuroperitoneal shunt may be indicated if the effusions continue despite parenteral feeding followed by a fat-reduced diet with medium-chain fatty acids and surgery is not feasible. Currently, surgical ligation of the thoracic duct as it enters the chest through the esophageal hiatus is usually accomplished via videoassisted thoracic surgery.

Pleural thickening

The main cause of pleural thickening is fibrothorax, which may be secondary to empyema, tuberculous pleuritis, or hemothorax[1]. It can cause dyspnea, and the affected side of the chest may shrink and become distorted. The only possible treatment is decortication, which should be performed early whenever possible.

Asbestos exposure may lead to the formation of hyaline, sometimes sclerotic, pleural thickening (pleural plaques). This must be distinguished from other localized pleural thickenings, such as tumors, lipomas, lymphoma, and inflammatory changes. The much less frequent diffuse pleural fibrosis following asbestos exposure is often preceded by an asbestos effusion.

PITFALLS AND CONTROVERSIES

The indications for thoracentesis in pleural effusions is to differentiate between transudate and exudate. Cardiac effusions may become exudative after treatment. Another pitfall is the so-called pseudotumor (fluid in a fissure), which vanishes after cardiac failure treatment. In infectious pleural effusions, it is important to differentiate between uncomplicated and complicated parapneumonic effusions. The role of pH and glucose is helpful in this respect. In tuberculous pleurisy, the diagnosis may be made by biopsy of the pleura.

In malignant pleural effusions, the differentiation between true malignant and paramalignant effusions is essential, especially in lung cancer, where it changes the stage of the disease. Mesothelioma and adenocarcinoma of the pleura are often difficult to distinguish (see Chapter 67). Medical thoracoscopy plays an important role in the diagnostic approach to the evaluation of pleural effusions when the initial thoracocentesis is not diagnostic.

In the treatment of pleural effusions, the indications for drainage and fibrinolytic treatment in parapneumonic effusions are unclear. A good option for pleurodesis is talc poudrage. The alternatives are talc slurry and other sclerosing substances. A pleuroperitoneal shunt or surgery are indicated in selected cases where the lung fails to re-expand. The best timing for surgical decortication in empyema and fibrothorax is still unclear.

REFERENCES

1. Light RW. Pleural diseases. 3rd edn. Baltimore: Williams and Wilkins; 1995.
2. Loddenkemper R. Diagnostik der Pleuraergüsse. (Diagnosis of pleural effusions.) Dtsch med Wochenschr. 1992;117:1487–91.
3. Storey DD, Dines DE, Coles DT. Pleural effusion. A diagnostic dilemma. JAMA. 1976;236:2183–6.
4. Hirsch A, Ruffie P, Nebut M, Gignon J, Chrétien J. Pleural effusion: laboratory tests in 300 cases. Thorax. 1979;106–12.
5. Lamy P, Canet B, Martinet Y, Lamaze R. Evaluation des moyens diagnostiques dans les épanchements pleuraux. Poumon-Coeur. 1980;36:83–94.
6. Engel J. Häufigkeitsverteilung von Pleuraerkrankungen. Kongr Ber Wiss Tag Norddtsch Ges Lungen-u Bronchialheilk. 1980;16:181–3.
7. Loddenkemper R. Thoracoscopy: results in noncancerous and idiopathic pleural effusions. Poumon-Coeur. 1981;37:261–4.
8. Miserocchi G. Physiology and pathophysiology of pleural fluid turnover. Eur Respir J. 1997;10:219–25.
9. Loddenkemper R, Fabel H, Konietzko N, Magnussen H. Diagnostisches Vorgehen beim Pleuraerguß. (Diagnostic approach to pleural effusion.) Pneumol. 1994;48:278–280.
10. Sahn SA. The diagnostic value of pleural fluid analysis. Semin Respir Crit Care Med. 1995;16:269–78.
11. Loddenkemper R. Thoracoscopy – state of the art. Eur Respir J. 1998;11:213–21.
12. Rodriguez-Panadero F, Antony VB. Pleurodesis. State of the art. Eur Respir J. 1997;10:1648–54.
13. Walker-Renard PB, Vaughan LM, Sahn SA. Chemical pleurodesis for malignant pleural effusion. Ann Intern Med. 1994;120:56–64.
14. Petrou M, Kaplan D, Goldstraw P. The management of recurrent malignant pleural effusions: the complementary role of talc pleurodesis and pleuro-peritoneal shunting. Cancer. 1995;75:801–5.
15. Sahn SA. Management of complicated parapneumonic effusions. Am Rev Respir Dis. 1993;48:813–17.
16. Ferrer J. Pleural tuberculosis. Eur Respir J. 1997;10:942–7.
17. Epler GR, McLoud TC, Gaensler EA. Prevalence and incidence of benign asbestos pleural effusion in a working population. JAMA. 1982;247:617–22.
18. Staats BA, Ellefson RW, Budahn LL, Dines DE, Prakash UBS, Offord K. The lipoprotein profile of chylous and non-chylous pleural effusions. Mayo Clin Proc. 1980;55:700–4.

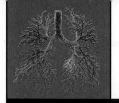

Section 13 Pleural Diseases

Chapter 67 Malignant Mesothelioma

James R Jett

INTRODUCTION

The acceptance of diffuse malignant mesothelioma as a distinct medical condition is based on numerous pathologic studies conducted in the first half of the 20th century. Mesothelioma originates from the lining cells (mesothelium) of a serous cavity. The tumor may be restricted to a small area, or involve the lining cells in a multifocal or continuous manner. One of the first epidemiologic studies to link malignant mesothelioma and asbestos was reported by Wagner et al., using data collected in 1960 among South African mine workers[1]. This connection has been confirmed by many subsequent studies.

EPIDEMIOLOGY, RISK FACTORS, AND PATHOLOGY

Epidemiology

There are an estimated 2000–3000 cases per year in the USA and it has been projected that the annual deaths from mesothelioma will peak at 3060 cases in the year 2002 and then start to diminish. The projections for mesothelioma mortality in Britain are similar, with a peak in about the year 2020 of 2700–3300 deaths[2]. A recent report estimating current trends was based on data from the Surveillance Epidemiology and End Results program for 1973–1992 in the USA[3] representing 9.5% of the US population. There was a virtually constant rate of mesothelioma for females and a consistently higher rate for males that increased during the study period. The growth rate for disease incidence among males was 14% for 1973–1974; this dropped to 0.4% for 1991–1992. There was no growth rate for females. The lifetime risk of mesothelioma peaks at 200 per 100,000 for men in the birth cohort for 1925–1929 and then decreases. The lifetime risk for females is essentially constant at 25 per 100,000. These data estimate the annual number of male mesothelioma cases will peak before the year 2000 at 2300 cases and are consistent with other estimates.

Etiology and risk factors

Asbestos is a naturally occurring fibrous silicate that is present everywhere in the soil. The main asbestos mineral groups are: serpentine fibers (long and curly) and amphibole fibers (straight or rod-like). Chrysotile, the only serpentine fiber, accounts for 95% of the asbestos used commercially. The distinction between the serpentine group and amphibole group is important as the serpentine fiber shape is more easily cleared from the respiratory tract. Fibers with the greatest length-to-diameter ratios have been shown to be the most carcinogenic. Epidemiologic data suggests that the amphibole crocidolite is associated with the highest risk of malignant mesothelioma

and chrysotile has the lowest risk. Another amphibole, amosite, carries an intermediate risk. Roggli et al. quantified the number of asbestos bodies in the lung tissue of:

- patients who died with asbestosis (fibrosis of the lung due to asbestos) without malignant pleural mesothelioma (MPM);
- patients with MPM but without asbestosis;
- 50 patients who died of other causes[4].

The lungs of patients with asbestosis but not MPM had the highest fiber counts and those with MPM but not asbestosis had an intermediate number of fibers. Some of the MPM patients had fiber counts that overlapped with the 50 patients who died of other causes. Therefore, it is uncertain whether a threshold of exposure to asbestos exists below which there is no risk of MPM, or whether some individuals are predisposed to the disease because of inherited or acquired genetic mutations.

Asbestos, especially the amphiboles, is the main cause of MPM, but does not account for all cases. Asbestos exposure is documented in only 50–70% of cases in some study series. Cases of MPM with no history of asbestos exposure are common. The most notable other causal factor is radiation exposure. In asbestos-related cases, the disease is diagnosed 35–40 years after the first exposure, and the incidence of MPM increases with greater exposure. Among a population of asbestos insulation workers from North America, 8% of deaths were due to mesothelioma. An increased incidence of MPM is also found among the wives of asbestos workers. Presumably, this was due to asbestos brought home on the hair or clothing of the spouse exposed to asbestos. To avoid this risk, work practices have been put in place since 1972 which state that asbestos workers must shower and change their clothing prior to leaving work.

Malignant mesothelioma cells frequently display multiple chromosomal changes, particularly losses or structural rearrangement of 1p, 3p, 6p, 9p, and 22. Homozygous deletions of the p16 gene or chromosome 9p 21–22 have been identified in 34 of 42 (85%) malignant mesothelioma cell lines, and in five of 23 (22%) primary tumors. The significance of these and other genetic mutations is uncertain, but the quest for a definitive tumor-suppressor gene continues.

Pathology

The four main histologic categories of MPM are:
- epithelial (tubulopapillary and epithelioid);
- sarcomatous (including desmoplastic);
- biphasic (mixed);
- poorly differentiated[5].

The epithelial type accounts for 50% of MPMs, 25% are biphasic, and 15% are sarcomatous; the remaining 10% are poorly differentiated. Partly because of its rarity, the histologic diagnosis of MPM is difficult, and considerable variation, as high as 50% in some studies, occurs in the diagnoses arrived at by different observers. Pathology panels have been formed in a number of countries to address this problem and for purposes of referral. The members of the North American Mesothelioma Panel reached a consensus of 75% or more on 70% of the referral material sent to them[6]. It is obvious, therefore, that even the experts do not always agree.

The main considerations in the differential diagnosis include mesothelial hyperplasia, metastatic adenocarcinoma, and sarcomas arising in adjacent structures. Histochemical stains for neutral mucin may be helpful in differentiating MPM from adenocarcinoma. Examples of the stains used are diastase-resistant periodic acid–Schiff and mucicarmine (hyaluronidase-resistant), which may be positive for adenocarcinoma and are usually negative for MPM. These stains do not help to differentiate sarcomatous mesothelioma from sarcoma. Electron microscopic evidence of long, thin, bushy surface microvilli has been found in epithelioid mesothelioma, while short, blunt microvilli are seen in adenocarcinomas. A length-to-diameter ratio of microvilli greater than 15 is considered to support strongly the diagnosis of MPM. Electron microscopy is less effective in the diagnosis of poorly differentiated epithelioid mesothelioma or in differentiating sarcomatous mesothelioma from sarcoma[5].

Monoclonal antibodies to molecules related to cell-differentiation have been the basis for immunohistochemical (IHC) studies to differentiate mesothelioma from those conditions that mimic it histologically. Cytokeratin is an intermediate filament and a marker for epithelial differentiation. A positive IHC test for cytokeratin helps differentiate a sarcomatoid mesothelioma, which is usually positive, from most sarcomas, which are usually negative. Adenocarcinomas also stain positive for cytokeratin. Perhaps the most useful of the IHC antibodies are those directed at specific glycoproteins that are more likely to be found in epithelium-derived tumors, particularly adenocarcinoma, than in mesotheliomas. The expression of these glycoproteins varies with the degree of differentiation and the site of origin of the adenocarcinoma. A panel approach is therefore recommended to increase the sensitivity of the testing procedure. The most common IHC antibodies used are carcinoembryonic antigen (CEA), Leu-MI (CD15), B72.3, and Ber-EP4[5]. One or more of these would typically be positive with adenocarcinoma and all should be negative with MPM. Unfortunately, none of these tests is absolutely fail-safe.

CLINICAL FEATURES

Primarily a disease of adults, MPM presents when the patient is about 60 years of age. Men account for 70–80% of cases[7,8]. Rarely have children been reported to develop this disease. The most common presentations are dyspnea, chest pain, or both. Figure 67.1 outlines the initial presentation of 90 cases of MPM and does not differ substantially from results that have appeared in other publications. The physical examination is usually unremarkable, except for dullness to percussion at one base of the lung caused by pleural effusion, and a tumor that infiltrates the pleural membranes. Palpable metastatic lymph nodes may occasionally be present and digital clubbing is observed in <10% of cases.

The tumor originates mainly on the parietal pleura, and progressively spreads to encase the lung surfaces and individual

Initial symptoms in 90 cases of malignant pleural mesothelioma		
Symptom	Number of cases	%
Pain	62	69
Nonpleuritic	56	–
Pleuritic	6	–
Shortness of breath	53	59
Fever, chills, or sweats	30	33
Weakness, fatigue, or malaise	30	33
Cough	24	27
Weight loss	22	24
Anorexia	10	11
Sensation of heaviness or fullness in chest	6	7
Hoarseness	3	3

Figure 67.1 Symptoms at initial presentation in 90 evaluable cases of malignant pleural mesothelioma. (Adapted, with permission, from Adams et al.[7]. Copyright 1986 American Cancer Society and Wiley-Liss Inc, a subsidiary of Wiley & Sons Inc.)

lobes by tracking along fissures. The tumor may reach several centimeters in thickness. It can penetrate into the chest wall, along needle tracts, infiltrate the diaphragm, invade mediastinal structures, and encase the heart and pericardium. Peritoneal involvement is found in about one third of cases coming to autopsy. Localized malignant mesotheliomas, sessile or pedunculated, can occur.

Radiologic findings
At the time of diagnosis, 78% of patients have a pleural effusion. The next most frequent indications on the chest radiograph are nodular thickening of the pleura and irregular thickening of the interlobar fissure (Fig. 67.2). A localized mass may be the only radiologic indication in 5–10% of individuals. Spontaneous pneumothorax has been reported occasionally. When the disease is more advanced, diffuse thickening of the pleura can decrease the volume of the affected hemithorax. Calcified or noncalcified plaques may also be identified. A prospective series followed over 1500 Swedish men who had pleural plaques for 16,000+ person-years and observed a risk of MPM of 1 in 1700 per year.

Computed tomography scans
Computed tomography (CT) provides more information on the extent of disease. Examination by CT of 50 patients with MPM showed pleural thickening that varied in extent and nodularity in 92% of patients[9] (Figs 67.3 & 67.4). Thickening of the interlobar fissure was seen in 86% of cases, pleural effusion in 74%, and, in 19 of 37 patients, the effusion affected more than one third of the hemithorax. Calcified pleural plaques were seen in 10 patients and affected the mesothelioma in 6 cases. Contraction of the involved hemithorax occurred in 42% of patients, but a mediastinal shift was present in only 7 (14%). Extension of the tumor into the chest wall and abdomen, as well as involvement of the mediastinal pleura, pericardium, and lymph nodes, was documented in some cases. Magnetic resonance imaging of the thorax with the use of multidimensional planes may be superior to CT scans for the evaluation of chest-wall and mediastinal involvement, and for evaluating the relationship of the tumor to the great vessels.

Staging
The literature contains at least six different staging systems for MPM, and the lack of a universal system has hindered comparison of reports. In 1992 the International Union Against Cancer

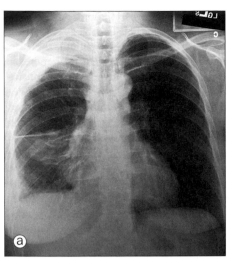

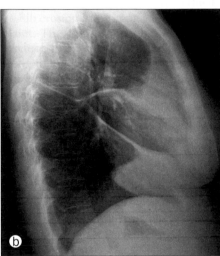

Figure 67.2 Chest radiographs of a patient who has malignant pleural mesothelioma.
(a) Posteroanterior.
(b) Lateral, in which thickening of the pleura of the major fissure is most clearly visible.

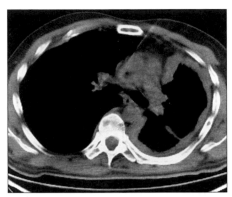

Figure 67.3 Computed tomography scan of the chest of a patient who has malignant pleural mesothelioma. Thickening of the entire circumferential pleura and invasion of the fissure can be seen on this cut. Note the associated loss of volume of the involved hemithorax.

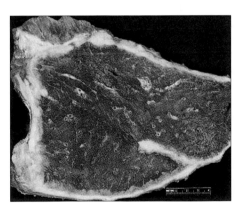

Figure 67.4 Pleural thickening. A cross-section of a lung removed at surgery by pleuropneumonectomy. This specimen was taken from the patient whose computed tomography scan is shown in Figure 67.3.

Tumor-nodes-metastasis staging system for malignant pleural mesothelioma	
Symbol	**Type of tumor (T)**
T1	T1a: tumor limited to the ipsilateral parietal pleura, including mediastinal and diaphragmatic pleura
	Visceral pleura not affected
	T1b: tumor affecting the ipsilateral parietal pleura, including mediastinal and diaphragmatic pleura
	Scattered foci of tumor also involving the visceral pleura
T2	Tumor affecting each of the ipsilateral pleural surfaces (parietal, mediastinal, diaphragmatic, and visceral) with at least one of the following features
	Diaphragmatic muscle affected
	Confluent visceral pleural tumor (including the fissures) or extension of tumor from visceral pleura into the underlying pulmonary parenchyma
T3	Describes locally advanced but potentially resectable tumor
	Tumor affecting all of the ipsilateral pleural surfaces (parietal, mediastinal, diaphragmatic, and visceral) with at least one of the following features
	Endothoracic fascia affected
	Extension into the mediastinal fat
	Solitary, completely resectable focus of tumor extending into the soft tissues of the chest wall
	Nontransmural involvement of the pericardium
T4	Describes locally advanced, technically unresectable tumor
	Tumor affecting all of the ipsilateral pleural surfaces (parietal, mediastinal, diaphragmatic, and visceral) with at least one of the following features
	Diffuse extension or multifocal masses of tumor in the chest wall, with or without associated rib destruction
	Direct transdiaphragmatic extension of tumor to the peritoneum
	Direct extension of tumor to the contralateral pleura
	Direct extension of tumor to one or more mediastinal organs
	Direct extension of tumor into the spine
	Tumor extending through to the internal surface of the pericardium with or without a pericardial effusion, or tumor involving the myocardium
Lymph nodes (N)	
NX	Regional lymph nodes cannot be assessed
N0	No regional lymph node metastases
N1	Metastases in the ipsilateral bronchopulmonary or hilar lymph nodes
N2	Metastases in the subcarinal or the ipsilateral mediastinal lymph nodes, including the ipsilateral internal mammary nodes
N3	Metastases in the contralateral mediastinal, contralateral internal mammary, ipsilateral, or contralateral supraclavicular lymph nodes
Metastases (M)	
MX	Presence of distant metastases cannot be assessed
M0	No distant metastasis
M1	Distant metastasis present

and the American Joint Committee of Cancer developed a TNM [primary tumor (T), regional nodes (N), and metastasis (M)] staging system, but its value for assessing prognosis is unclear. Recently, the International Mesothelioma Interest Group proposed a modified staging system (Fig. 67. 5 and see Fig. 67. 6) to reconcile and update previous systems[10]. These staging categories have been validated on a series of 131 patients from the Memorial Sloan–Kettering Cancer Center, but further validation based on many patients from different centers is needed to confirm and refine this new staging system.

Figure 67.5 Tumor-nodes-metastasis staging system for malignant pleural mesothelioma. This system was developed by the International Mesothelioma Interest Group to reconcile and update previous systems. (Adapted, with permission, from American College of Chest Physicians[10].)

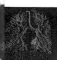

REFERENCES

1. Wagner JC, Sleggs CA, Marchand P. Diffuse pleural mesothelioma and asbestos exposure in the North Western Cape Province. Br J Ind Med. 1960;17:260–71.

2. Peto J, Hodgson J, Matthews F, et al. Continuing increase in mesothelioma mortality in Britain. Lancet. 1995;345:535–9.

3. Price B. Analysis of current trends in United States mesothelioma incidence. Am J Epidemiol. 1997;145:211–18.

4. Roggli VL, McGavran MH, Subach J, et al. Pulmonary asbestos body counts and electron probe analysis of asbestos body cores in patients with mesothelioma. Cancer. 1982;50:2423–32.

5. Battifora H, McCaughey WTE. Diffuse malignant mesothelioma. In: Battifora H, McCaughey WTE, eds. Tumors of the serosal membrane. Armed Forces Institute of Pathology, Fascicle. 15, 1995:17–88.

6. McCaughey WTE, Colby TV, Battifora H, et al. Diagnosis of diffuse malignant mesothelioma: experience of the US/Canadian Mesothelioma Panel. Modern Pathol. 1991;4:342–53.

7. Adams VI, Unni KK, Muhm JR, et al. Diffuse malignant mesothelioma of pleura. Cancer. 1986;58:1540–51.

8. Ruffie P, Feld R, Cormier Y, et al. Diffuse malignant mesothelioma of the pleura in Ontario, Quebec: a retrospective study of 332 patients. J Clin Oncol. 1989;7:1157–68.

9. Kawashima A, Libshitz HI. Malignant pleural mesothelioma: CT manifestations in 50 cases. AJR. 1990;155:965–9.

10. International Mesothelioma Interest Group. A proposed new international TNM staging system for malignant pleural mesothelioma. Chest. 1995;108:1122–8.

11. Boutin C, Rey F. Thorascopy in pleural malignant mesothelioma: a prospective study of 188 consecutive patients (diagnosis). Cancer. 1993;72:389–93.

12. Law MR, Gregor A, Hodson ME, et al. Malignant mesothelioma of the pleura: a study of 52 treated and 64 untreated patients. Thorax. 1984;39:255–9.

13. Sugarbaker DJ, Strauss GM, Lynch TJ, et al. Node status has prognostic significance in the multimodality therapy of diffuse malignant mesothelioma. J Clin Oncol. 1993;11:1172–8.

14. Rusch V, Saltz L, Venkatraman E, et al. A phase II trial of pleurectomy/decortication followed by intrapleural and systemic chemotherapy for malignant pleural mesothelioma. J Clin Oncol. 1994;12: 1156–73.

15. Ball DL, Cruickshank DG. The treatment of malignant mesothelioma of the pleura: a review of a 5 year experience with special reference to radiotherapy. Am J Clin Oncol. 1990;13:4–9.

16. Boutin C, Rey F, Viallat JR. Prevention of malignant seeding after invasive diagnostic procedures in patients with pleural mesothelioma. Chest. 1995;108:754–8.

17. Ong ST, Vogelzang NJ. Chemotherapy in malignant pleural mesothelioma: a review. J Clin Oncol. 1996;14:1007–17.

18. Boutin C, Nussbaum E, Monnet I, et al. Intrapleural treatment with recombinant gamma-interferon in early stage malignant pleural mesothelioma. Cancer. 1994;74:2460–7.

Chapter 68

Management of Chest Trauma

Patrick J Offner and Ernest E Moore

Thoracic injuries are a leading cause of death in trauma patients; they account for 25% of all trauma deaths, and are a contributing factor in another 25% of deaths[1]. With improved resuscitation and prehospital care, more patients who have critical chest injuries survive long enough to present to the hospital emergency department[2]. Airway obstruction and respiratory complications are common in these patients.

Only a small percentage of patients who suffer blunt thoracic trauma require operative intervention. Many can be managed with simple maneuvers, such as administration of supplemental oxygen, closed-tube thoracostomy, meticulous attention to clearance of secretions, and appropriate analgesia. With increased survival from improved initial management, more of these patients require prolonged intensive care.

The spectrum of chest trauma is broad and encompasses multiple organ systems (Fig. 68.1). The focus of this chapter is the initial management of patients who have suffered from a chest injury.

EPIDEMIOLOGY, RISK FACTORS, AND PATHOLOGY

Although chest injuries are common, modern epidemiologic data are sparse. The rate of thoracic injury in the USA is 12 patients per million persons per day, of whom one third require hospital admission[3]. Approximately 16,000 deaths/year are attributable to chest trauma[1]. Mortality statistics, however, markedly underestimate the societal impact of trauma. For instance, patients

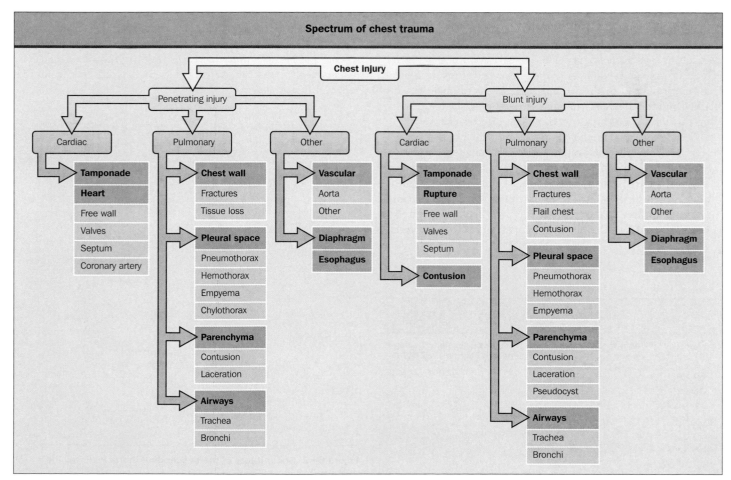

Figure 68.1 The spectrum of chest trauma. Chest injuries can occur by blunt and penetrating mechanisms. Multiple organ systems are often involved.

who suffer major chest injuries and flail chest have a major risk of disability. Moreover, over 50% may never return to work[4].

Mechanisms responsible for chest trauma vary with location of the trauma center. Furthermore, they reflect social change as well. Urban trauma centers treat increasing numbers of penetrating chest injuries, including those related to semiautomatic weapons. Over a 6-year period 2316 patients were admitted for acute chest trauma to Denver Health Medical Center (a large, urban, level I trauma center in Colorado). Of these, 1162 patients (58%) sustained penetrating wounds (828 as stab wounds and 334 as gunshot wounds), and 835 had blunt trauma (most resulting from motor vehicle accidents)[5,6]. Severe blunt chest injuries may have a penetrating component as well, as fractured ribs can lead to soft tissue and pulmonary parenchymal lacerations.

The types and distributions of chest injuries are remarkably similar in European and North American series. In Lausanne, Switzerland, over a 10-year period, Beeson and Saegesser reported more than 1500 patients who sustained chest trauma[7]. Although the North American Major Trauma Outcome Study analyzed all types of trauma, important information on subgroups of patients resulted. As of 1987, data became available on almost 50,000 patients from 60 hospitals, of whom 15,047 had chest injuries, of which 70% were blunt[1]. The distribution of injuries from each study is shown in Figure 68.2.

There are two basic mechanisms of lung injury – blunt and penetrating. Both cause injury by kinetic energy transfer. Penetrating wounds have direct injury from the wounding agent itself (i.e. knife or bullet), as well as injury caused by energy transfer to the tissue, which is largely related to the velocity of the wounding agent. High-velocity gunshot wounds can result in devastating soft-tissue injury related to cavitation, a 'shock-wave' effect. Low-velocity wounds (handgun or knife) result in localized injury limited to the wound path. Projectile ballistics can markedly influence the nature and amount of tissue injury; however, this topic is too broad to be covered in this chapter.

The predominant mechanism of injury in blunt trauma is acceleration and deceleration, in which skeletal inertia and organ inertia differ considerably. These differences result in shear injury to organs that are partially fixed to the skeletal system. A prime example of this mechanism is injury to the aorta. The descending aorta is not free to move where it is attached to the vertebral column. In contrast, the heart and aortic arch can move freely.

With deceleration from a frontal collision, or acceleration from a lateral impact, shear injury develops where the tethered and untethered portions meet (Fig. 68.3).

CLINICAL FEATURES

Given the multiple organ systems that may be involved in chest injuries, it is not surprising that the clinical presentation is varied. Additionally, chest trauma, in particular blunt trauma, rarely occurs as an isolated injury. Some findings, however, are seen throughout the entire spectrum of chest injuries. Hypoxemia is a frequent problem. The most common cause of shock and/or hypotension in trauma patients is hypovolemia from hemorrhage, although tension pneumothorax and pericardial tamponade need to be considered in all patients who suffer chest injuries. Findings on the initial presentation may have important diagnostic implications (Fig. 68.4).

Chest wall injuries

The most common type of thoracic injury is to the chest wall. The spectrum of chest wall injuries ranges from minor, isolated rib fractures to flail chest. Serious disability after major chest wall injuries is common, with important societal and economic effects.

Rib fractures are the most common injury following blunt chest trauma, and are more commonly seen in adults than in children because of the greater elasticity of the pediatric chest wall. As such, multiple rib fractures in children are a marker of severe injury, and are associated with high mortality[8].

Although rib fractures are rarely life threatening in and of themselves, they are frequently associated with other important injuries. When three or more ribs are fractured, the incidence of splenic and hepatic injury increases (relative risk of 6.2 and 3.6, respectively). This subgroup of patients should be considered for level I trauma center care[9].

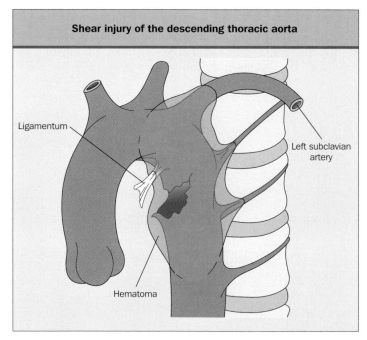

Shear injury of the descending thoracic aorta

Ligamentum

Left subclavian artery

Hematoma

Figure 68.3 Shear injury of the descending thoracic aorta. The descending aorta is fixed to the vertebral column. Deceleration or acceleration can result in shear injury where the tethered descending aorta joins the freely mobile heart and aortic arch.

Types of thoracic organ injury		
	Switzerland, n = 1500 (%)	**North American Major Trauma Outcome Study, n = 15,047 (%)**
Chest wall	54	56
Flail chest	13	5
Pneumothorax	20	20
Hemothorax	21	25
Pulmonary parenchyma	21	26
Miscellaneous	18	21

Figure 68.2 Types of thoracic organ injury. The distribution of thoracic injuries is remarkably similar in these geographically diverse populations.

Diagnostic implications of patient presentation	
Clinical presentation	**Diagnostic implication**
Chest wall pain and tenderness	Rib or sternal fractures
Persistent air leak from chest tube	Tracheobronchial injury, pulmonary laceration
Progressive infiltrates and hypoxemia	Acute respiratory distress syndrome, pulmonary contusion, pneumonia
Hemodynamic instability	Hemorrhagic shock, tension pneumothorax, massive hemothorax, blunt cardiac injury with or without tamponade
Sepsis syndrome	Missed esophageal injury, pneumonia, empyema, infected post-traumatic pulmonary pseudocyst
Unresolving pneumonia	Bronchial injury

Figure 68.4 Diagnostic implications of patient presentation.

The pattern of rib fracture may be suggestive of specific associated injuries. Rib fracture fragments may directly damage the underlying pleura or lung, which results in pneumothorax, hemothorax, pulmonary contusion, and/or parenchymal laceration. Other associated, potentially life-threatening intrathoracic injuries include blunt cardiac rupture, bronchial disruption, and major vascular tears. Fractures of the lower ribs are uncommon because of their mobility, but when found they raise concern for associated liver, spleen, or kidney injury. The first and second ribs are short, thick, and well protected by adjacent musculoskeletal structures. Accordingly, considerable force is required to fracture these ribs and associated injuries are quite common. Although early studies recommended mandatory angiography in patients whose first and second ribs are fractured, more recent studies do not[10,11]. Currently, angiography is indicated in the following circumstances:
- clinical evidence of vascular injury, such as distal vascular insufficiency;
- radiographic evidence of possible aortic injury (e.g. widened mediastinum, silhouetting of the aortic knob);
- large apical hematoma;
- associated brachial plexus injury; and
- substantial displacement of fracture fragments.

The primary symptom of rib fracture is pain that is worse with deep inspiration or sternal compression. Point tenderness and associated crepitus may be present. The pain may be severe enough to restrict ventilation on the injured side, which leads to atelectasis and decreased breath sounds on auscultation.

Flail chest is common, and occurs in 5–13% of adults hospitalized for blunt chest injury (Fig. 68.5). This injury usually results from a direct impact, of which motor vehicle accidents and falls are most common. Flail chest is uncommon in children because of their compliant chest wall. Flail chest can be defined as three or more adjacent ribs fractured in at least two places, that is the flail segment has lost continuity with the remaining chest wall and moves paradoxically with inspiration and expiration. Anatomically, flail chest can be categorized by location as anterior, lateral, or posterior (Fig. 68.5). Anterior flail chest (also termed sternal flail) results when the sternum is separated from the costochondral joints or adjacent ribs. Associated injuries may include blunt cardiac injury, great vessel disruption, and pulmonary parenchymal injury. Lateral flail chest may be associated with hepatic and splenic injury.

Other chest wall injuries include scapular and sternal fractures, which usually present with localized pain and tenderness. Sternal

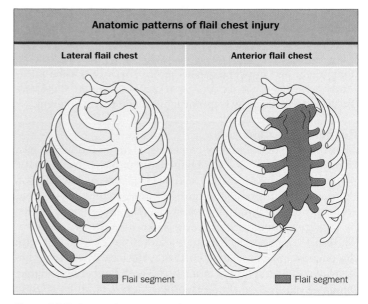

Figure 68.5 Anatomic patterns of flail chest injury. Flail chest can be categorized as anterior, lateral, or posterior. Anterior flail chest is also termed sternal flail chest.

fractures may have overlying ecchymosis and palpable deformity. Both of these injuries should trigger a search for more serious associated injuries. Although sternal fractures were once considered to be potentially life-threatening, more recent studies refute this idea[12].

Pleural space

A pneumothorax is defined as air within the pleural space, which results in loss of apposition between the parietal and visceral pleura, and some element of pulmonary parenchymal collapse. Mechanisms for pneumothorax include pulmonary laceration from penetrating injury or rib fracture, shear injury of the lung from deceleration, and increased intrathoracic pressure that results in regional lung overexpansion and alveolar rupture. Pneumothoraces are classified as tension, open, or simple. Tension pneumothorax occurs when there is a 'ball–valve effect' such that air enters the pleural space with each inhalation and has no means of escape. This leads to progressive collapse of the lung, displacement of the mediastinum and trachea away from the affected side, and impairment of venous return to the heart. Open pneumothorax is the classic 'sucking chest wound' and results from large chest-wall defects. With rapid equilibration of atmospheric and intrathoracic pressure, effective ventilation is impaired.

Physical findings may be scarce depending on the extent of the pneumothorax. Occasionally, pneumothoraces may be found on chest computed tomography (CT) obtained for other reasons, even though they are not evident on plain radiographs. Patients who suffer tension pneumothorax have hemodynamic instability related to the impaired central venous return. Breath sounds are usually diminished on the affected side. The involved hemithorax may be hyper- or hyporesonant to percussion, depending on the presence and volume of any associated hemothorax. Similarly, jugular venous distension may or may not be apparent, depending on the patient's volume status.

Hemothorax is defined as blood in the pleural space. Bleeding may arise from lacerations of chest wall vessels (intercostal or internal mammary) or the pulmonary parenchyma, or from injured great

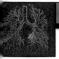

vessels. Massive hemothorax is defined as >1500cm³ of blood in the hemithorax. Physical findings include dullness to percussion and decreased breath sounds on auscultation. Massive hemothorax typically presents with hemodynamic instability, on the basis of both hemorrhage and impaired venous return. As with tension pneumothorax, jugular venous distension may or may not be evident. Tracheal deviation away from the injured side may be present.

Pulmonary parenchyma

The spectrum of pulmonary parenchymal injury following chest trauma varies from isolated pulmonary contusion to traumatic pseudocysts, frank laceration, and intraparenchymal hematoma. Pulmonary contusion is the most common finding (10–20% of adults hospitalized for blunt chest trauma) and is characterized by localized interstitial and alveolar hemorrhage with edema. The most common mechanism is a motor vehicle accident with direct chest impact. Characteristically, the patient worsens clinically and radiographically in the first 24–48 hours following the injury. The contusion slowly resolves unless it becomes complicated by infection, cavitation, or the acute respiratory distress syndrome (ARDS)[13]. Associated injuries are found in 40–60% of patients, and are directly related to outcome.

Basically, a pulmonary contusion is a bruise of the lung. Direct impact results in small vessel and alveolar disruption, which leads to both interstitial and alveolar hemorrhage and edema. Early after injury, the contused lung is poorly perfused and shunt is minimal. Tissue inflammation rapidly follows, and a zone of surrounding pulmonary edema is formed. This alters regional compliance and regional airway resistance, which results in localized ventilation–perfusion mismatch that progresses over 24–48 hours.

Pulmonary contusion is a well-recognized risk factor for ARDS. Although contrecoup injuries occasionally occur, experimental models suggest that abnormalities in the uninjured lung are the result of the systemic inflammatory response to injury. Whether inflammatory mediators originate from the injured lung or from an extrathoracic site is unclear[13].

Pulmonary contusion should be suspected in any patient who has a major chest wall injury. The classic radiographic finding is an irregular infiltrate that may correspond to the area of external wall injury. The infiltrate may range from discrete nodular densities to a diffuse patchy pattern, and is usually nonlobar in distribution. In many cases, the infiltrates only become apparent or progress significantly with fluid resuscitation (Figs 68.6 & 68.7). The nonanatomic nature of the infiltrate and frequently associated chest wall injury help to distinguish pulmonary contusion from aspiration. Clinically, the patient may manifest signs of associated chest wall injury with pain, tenderness, and crepitus on palpation. Lung contusion may result in early hypoxemia, and patients are frequently hypocapneic.

Post-traumatic pulmonary pseudocyst represents an unusual complication of blunt chest trauma. These pseudocysts typically evolve over the first week from a dense pulmonary contusion into an air- and/or fluid-filled loculation seen on plain radiographs (Fig. 68.8). Although these have long been recognized as benign processes in children that progressively resolve over several months, the authors' experience in adults is that they are found in the setting of severe pulmonary contusion with associated shock and other injuries. Under these circumstances, post-traumatic pulmonary pseudocysts can progress into a lung abscess, which may be refractory to noninvasive management such that, on occasion, resection of necrotic lung may be indicated (Fig. 68.9). In adults who suffer major chest injury and persistent sepsis, a CT scan is mandatory to seek a potentially infected pseudocyst (Fig. 68.10)[13].

Airways

Tracheal and bronchial injuries are uncommon, with an estimated incidence of between 1 and 9%, depending on the mechanism. More importantly, these injuries are life threatening, as illustrated by a series of >1000 trauma deaths, of which 33 involved tracheobronchial injuries. Of these 33 patients, 27 (82%) died at the scene, whereas 5 of the remaining 6 patients died within 2 hours of hospital admission[14]. With improved prehospital care and trauma systems, however, more of these patients now reach the hospital alive but in extremis. Early diagnosis and treatment are essential to prevent subsequent morbidity.

The trachea is the most anterior structure in the neck and is, therefore, vulnerable to direct injury. Associated injury to the esophagus and great vessels is common because of their close anatomic continuity. Tracheoesophageal injuries can be particularly difficult to manage.

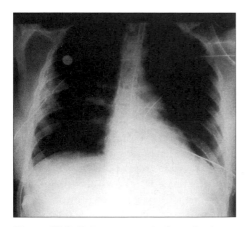

Figure 68.6 Pulmonary contusion prior to fluid resuscitation. Radiographic evidence of pulmonary contusion may not be apparent on the initial chest radiograph.

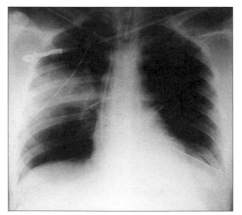

Figure 68.7 Pulmonary contusion following fluid resuscitation. This radiograph is of the same patient as in Figure 68.6 after volume resuscitation. The appearance of radiographic infiltrates does not follow normal anatomic patterns.

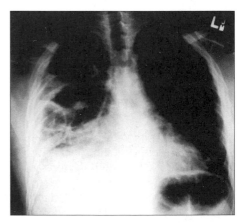

Figure 68.8 Post-traumatic pulmonary pseudocyst. The appearance of an air- and/or fluid-filled cavity in an area of previous pulmonary contusion is characteristic.

The trachea is tethered at the carotid cartilage such that rapid deceleration generates a shear force and results in injury. Similarly, shear forces from widening of the angle of the carina can result in mainstem bronchus injury. Obviously, a direct blow to the trachea can cause a rupture. Sudden increases in intratracheal pressure from a chest impact can result in a 'blow-out' injury of the trachea, which usually involves the membranous, posterior wall.

Of blunt tracheobronchial injuries, 80% occur within 2cm of the carina. Tracheobronchial injuries can have a highly variable clinical presentation, which may include cough, stridor, dyspnea, hemoptysis, and voice changes. Cervical subcutaneous emphysema and crepitus are often present. Auscultation may reveal a mediastinal crunch from air in the mediastinal soft tissue. Chest radiographs may show subcutaneous and/or mediastinal emphysema, persistent atelectasis, or pneumothorax. It is important to remember that a pneumothorax may not be present, depending on the location of the injury and the integrity of the mediastinal pleura. The 'fallen-lung sign', in which the hilum is displaced caudally, is considered diagnostic for bronchial disruption (Fig. 68.11). A large or persistent air leak and failure to re-expand a pneumothorax suggests bronchial injury. Occasionally, bronchial injuries present late with persistent cough, stridor, or recurrent, unresolving infections.

DIAGNOSIS

A brief and appropriately focused history of the injury, as well as the patient's past medical history, is crucial to the care of the patient. Knowledge of the injury mechanism can raise the index of suspicion for specific injuries and lead to appropriate diagnostic studies. Similarly, comorbidity (such as cardiac disease, chronic obstructive pulmonary disease, and cirrhosis) and the patient's medication history may clearly affect therapeutic decision-making.

Although diagnostic modalities such as chest radiograph and chest CT are sensitive and accurate, the physical examination must not be delayed as some injuries (e.g. tension pneumothorax, massive hemothorax) demand immediate treatment and cannot wait for adjunctive diagnostic studies. Obviously, the patient's clinical presentation may suggest specific diagnoses (see Fig. 68.4).

A standard anterior–posterior chest radiograph must be obtained as soon as possible, as the thorax represents a major potential site for occult intracavity hemorrhage. The images must be carefully examined in a consistent and systematic fashion to avoid overlooking associated injuries. Many radiographic abnormalities have important diagnostic and therapeutic implications (see Fig. 68.12).

The position of tubes and presence of other foreign bodies is noted. Importantly, many pulmonary processes are delayed in onset or evolve over the patient's resuscitation course, and so serial chest radiographs are important in some cases. In hemodynamically stable patients, inspiratory and expiratory views, as well as a lateral view, may help elucidate abnormalities found on an initial anteroposterior film.

A standard diagnostic technique for the evaluation of head and abdominal injuries is CT. More recently, studies suggest that CT has an increased role in selected patients who suffer blunt chest injury, as unsuspected thoracic injuries are sometimes detected by abdominal CT scans in patients who have blunt torso trauma[15]. The ability of CT to identify potentially life-threatening injuries that are not evident on plain radiographs has lead some investigators to recommend the routine use of emergent chest CT in all patients who suffer major blunt chest trauma[16]. Other investigators argue that

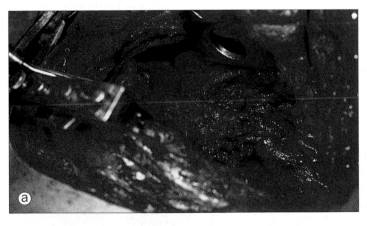

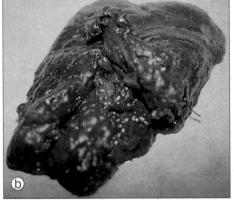

Figure 68.9 Necrotic right middle lobe. In adults, post-traumatic pulmonary pseudocysts may become infected or may be associated with significant pulmonary necrosis that requires thoracotomy and resection. (a) *In situ*. (b) Resected.

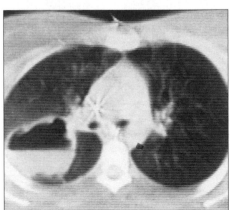

Figure 68.10 Post-traumatic pulmonary pseudocyst. Computed tomography (CT) scan is indicated in patients who have a post-traumatic pulmonary pseudocyst and signs of persistent sepsis. This CT scan from the patient shown in Figure 68.9 reveals a large cavity with an obvious air–fluid level.

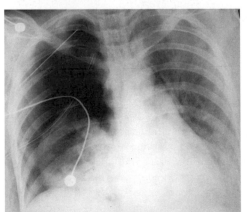

Figure 68.11 Radiographic sign of bronchial disruption. Caudal displacement of the hilum indicates a bronchial disruption.

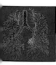

Diagnostic implications of chest radiography findings	
Radiographic abnormality	**Diagnostic implication**
Rib fractures	Flail chest, underlying visceral injury
Soft-tissue air	Pneumothorax
Air/fluid in pleural space	Pneumothorax, hemothorax
Persistent pneumothorax/ mediastinal air	Tracheobronchial tear, pulmonary laceration
Pulmonary infiltrate	Pulmonary contusion
Indistinct diaphragm	Ruptured diaphragm
Abnormal mediastinum	Thoracic aortic injury

Figure 68.12 Diagnostic implications of chest radiography findings.

chest CT scans alone rarely alter patient management[17,18]. The authors employ chest CT scanning in selected patients (e.g. patients who have unusual or unclear findings on standard radiographs), and feels that the routine use of CT as a screening study is not cost-effective. The authors do, however, use dynamic contrast CT scanning to screen for intimal defects or periaortic hematoma when aortic dissections are considered.

Ultrasound is commonly used in the evaluation of blunt trauma in Europe and Japan, and has been for more than a decade. Only recently, however, has it been adopted in the USA to identify intra-abdominal fluid in trauma patients. Ultrasound has also proved useful in the identification of hemopericardium and hemothorax following chest injury[19]. The technique is noninvasive, the equipment is portable, and studies can be repeated easily.

Bronchoscopy is an integral part of the initial evaluation of injuries to the tracheobronchial tree[20]. It aids the diagnosis of airway injury and facilitates safe endotracheal intubation. Moreover, bronchoscopy delineates the anatomy of the injury and assists in planning the repair. The possibility of cervical spine injury must not be overlooked when preparing for the procedure. Bronchoscopy may also be useful in the diagnosis and removal of tracheobronchial foreign bodies.

The efficacy of bronchoscopy in the treatment of lobar collapse remains unclear. Studies have failed to show a distinct advantage of bronchoscopy with suction of retained secretions over aggressive chest physical therapy. Patients who suffered severe chest injuries, however, have generally been excluded from such studies because they are unable to tolerate or effectively participate in aggressive pulmonary care[21]. Chest physical therapy may be less important than deep inhalation to clear secretions, but this, too, may be limited in patients who have chest trauma. Of additional concern is that if pain, contusion, or any other problem limits deep inhalation and/or coughing, the underlying pathophysiology that led to the collapse remains, such that the problem is likely to recur even if bronchoscopy is successful.

The authors use early bronchoscopy in intubated patients once oxygenation and ventilation have been stabilized. Nonintubated patients are treated with aggressive respiratory therapy. If no significant improvement is seen within 24 hours, bronchoscopy is performed to facilitate secretion removal and to exclude tracheobronchial injury or aspirated foreign bodies.

Recent improvements in technology have led to an increased use of video-assisted thoracoscopic surgery (VATS) in the evaluation and management of thoracic injury[22]. This technique allows

inspection of the diaphragm for injury, early evacuation of clotted hemothorax, and control of chest wall bleeding in selected patients. In addition, VATS may help manage postinjury empyemas that are inadequately treated using chest tube drainage[23].

TREATMENT

The initial management of the patient who has chest trauma is identical to that for any injured patient and follows the Advanced Trauma Life Support guidelines prepared by the American College of Surgeons Committee on Trauma. Immediate priorities include to establish a patent airway, maintain adequate ventilation, and diagnose and treat shock.

Ensuring an adequate airway has the highest priority, as without this all other resuscitative efforts are futile. Common causes of airway obstruction in trauma patients include posterior displacement of the tongue, soft tissue edema, blood, and foreign bodies (such as teeth or vomitus). Agitation in the trauma patient may signal hypoxia and an obstructed airway. The possibility of cervical spine injury must be kept in mind and appropriate precautions taken when the airway is secured.

Once an adequate airway has been secured, oxygenation and ventilation are assessed. All patients who have thoracic injury receive supplemental oxygen. Particular care is taken to identify the presence of tension pneumothorax, flail chest, open hemothorax, and massive hemothorax.

The circulatory system is assessed next, to seek the presence of shock. Hemorrhage is the most the common cause of shock in trauma patients; however, cardiogenic shock from cardiac tamponade, tension pneumothorax, or blunt cardiac injury can also occur. Major trauma victims should have two large-bore intravenous catheters placed to allow rapid resuscitation. Central venous access may be useful in selected patients. A low central venous pressure usually reflects hypovolemic tamponade, whereas a high central venous pressure may reflect cardiac tamponade.

Bleeding from wounds is best treated initially by direct pressure. Scalp wounds may be difficult to control using pressure alone. Placement of Michel clips or a continuous suture along the wound edge may be necessary in this situation.

Volume resuscitation is instituted with a warmed, balanced, crystalloid solution, such as Ringer's lactate. In adults, a bolus of 2L is administered and the patient's response is monitored. Patients who do not respond are given blood. Failure to respond also triggers a search for other causes of shock, in particular cardiac tamponade, tension pneumothorax, and massive hemothorax. When found, these require immediate treatment.

Once all conditions that are immediately life-threatening have been identified and treated, and the patient is stable, a more complete 'head-to-toe' evaluation can be undertaken. At times, this may not be possible until after the patient has undergone an operation.

Tension pneumothorax is easily treated with closed-tube thoracostomy. Trauma chest tubes are generally large bore (≥ 32 French) and placed through the fifth or sixth intercostal space, between the mid- and anterior axillary line. The placement and management of chest tubes is discussed in detail elsewhere (see Chapter 9). Unstable patients who have tension pneumothorax can be quickly treated initially by needle thoracostomy. Once the patient has stabilized, chest-tube placement can follow in a more deliberate fashion. Needle thoracostomy is performed on the affected side using a large-bore needle (≥ 16 gauge). The needle is inserted over the top of the rib in the second intercostal space at the midclavicular line.

Simple and open pneumothoraces are also treated using large-bore, chest-tube placement. Open pneumothorax also requires closure of the chest-wall defect. This can be accomplished initially using an occlusive dressing, but ultimately requires an operation.

Closed-tube thoracostomy is also indicated in patients who have a hemothorax. Complete evacuation and re-expansion of the lung are essential to stop further bleeding and minimize the occurrence of post-traumatic empyema. Radiographs are obtained following chest-tube placement to confirm complete evacuation and re-expansion. If the initial chest tube output exceeds 1500cm³, or if the output exceeds 250cm³/h for longer than 3 consecutive hours, urgent thoracotomy is indicated. An earlier recommendation to clamp the chest tube in setting of massive hemothorax has recently been challenged[24]. Autotransfusion of shed blood is a viable option in these patients and should be kept in mind.

Flail chest and pulmonary contusion frequently occur together. In the past, fluid restriction and diuresis have been advocated to prevent lung edema associated with pulmonary contusion. Subsequently, it was shown that edema with pulmonary contusion is the result of the direct lung injury and is not related to intravascular volume. Bongard and Lewis observed that oxygenation in both survivors and nonsurvivors of multiple trauma with pulmonary contusion did not correlate with plasma oncotic pressure and edema formation. These authors concluded that forced dehydration and intentional hypovolemic resuscitation in patients who have pulmonary contusion should be discontinued[25]. The authors believe that prompt crystalloid resuscitation is imperative to restore optimal organ perfusion and tissue oxygenation, and to limit postinjury multiple organ failure.

Historically, mandatory endotracheal intubation and mechanical ventilation were recommended in all patients who had flail chest. The rationale for this approach was that volume ventilation provided 'internal pneumatic stabilization' of the flail segment. With recognition that the underlying pulmonary contusion is largely responsible for gas-exchange problems in flail chest, selective intubation and mechanical ventilation has become standard practice, with the indications for intubation and ventilation being

the same as for any other trauma patient (e.g. respiratory failure, severe shock, severe head injury, airway obstruction, and associated injuries that require operation under general anesthetic). Similarly, standard weaning and extubation criteria apply. Resolution of the flail chest is not needed.

Operative stabilization of the chest wall is still used in selected patients. Prospective, randomized trials that compare operative and nonoperative management are currently lacking. Operative stabilization may be appropriate in selected subsets of patients, for instance those whose flail segments are particularly large or those who have difficulty weaning from the ventilator.

It is vital to prevent muscular splinting, regional hypoventilation, and accumulation of secretions in such patients, and to avoid atelectasis, pneumonia, and potentially avoidable respiratory failure. Accordingly, appropriate pain control is vital as it facilitates mobilization, deep breathing, and clearance of secretions. Clinical assessment of pain in patients who have major chest trauma is difficult. Frequently, atelectasis, lobar collapse, and other problems may develop in absence of complaints of pain. Several techniques are available to provide pain relief depending on the clinical scenario. Patients who suffer simple rib fracture can usually be managed using oral narcotics. More serious injuries may require parenteral narcotics. Patient-controlled analgesia may be effective in this regard, and avoids the wide swings in serum concentration associated with traditional intramuscular administration. Parenteral narcotics may cause respiratory depression, however, and interfere with the patient's respiratory care.

Direct pain control can also be achieved using an intercostal nerve block of the involved ribs, including two interspaces above and below the affected area. Another technique involves the placement of an intercostal catheter into the extrapleural space for intermittent administration of local anesthetic (Fig. 68.13). The authors prospectively evaluated this technique in 15 patients and documented significant improvement in pain during cough and deep breathing (assessed by standard visual analog scale). Moreover, inspiratory volumes increased significantly (before, 0.77 ± 0.09L; after, 1.3 ± 0.13L; $p < 0.05$). No procedure-related complications occurred[26].

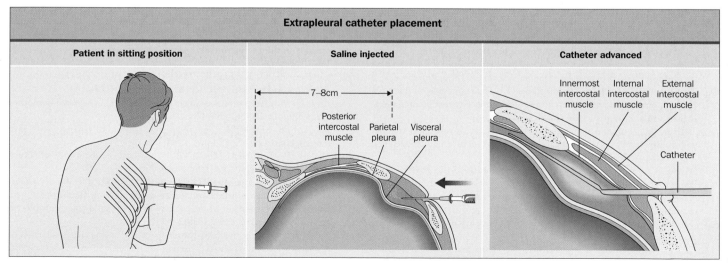

Figure 68.13 Extrapleural catheter placement. With the patient in a sitting position, a needle is introduced at the inferior margin of the most cephalad rib fracture. Saline (5mL) is injected to disrupt the pleura from the chest wall. A catheter is advanced through the needle into an extrapleural position.

More recently, the use of continuous epidural analgesic has become an important treatment modality in patients who have severe chest injury. This technique was shown to provide superior pain relief and restoration of ventilatory function compared with intravenous analgesia[27] and intrapleural catheter analgesia[28].

Early ambulation, coughing, and deep breathing are important components of respiratory care in such patients. Incentive spirometry is particularly useful because of its effectiveness, ease of use, and the minimal supervision required. It may also serve as an effective monitoring tool of a patient's progress. An abrupt decrease in volume may indicate inadequate pain control, or development or progression of an underlying pulmonary process. Intermittent positive-pressure breathing is another technique that may be useful in selected patients.

PITFALLS AND CONTROVERSIES

It is vitally important to obtain a secure airway in thoracic trauma patients. Proper endotracheal tube position is radiographically documented as auscultation of bilateral breath sounds does not always equate to proper endotracheal tube positioning. Excessive ventilator pressures must be avoided. Patients who clinically deteriorate after endotracheal intubation and positive-pressure ventilation are quickly evaluated for tension pneumothorax. If tension pneumothorax is excluded, systemic arterial air embolism is considered, but this diagnosis can be difficult to make. Sudden cardiovascular collapse or new, focal neurologic findings following endotracheal intubation and mechanical ventilation are classic indicators.

It is important to emphasize that the diagnosis of tension pneumothorax is a clinical one – to wait for radiographic confirmation prior to treatment is an error.

Central venous catheters can be helpful tools in monitoring patients who have blunt chest injury. If indicated, central line placement is carried out on the injured side. Procedure-related pneumothorax or hemothorax on the patient's uninjured side may have dire consequences.

Another common pitfall is the insertion of chest tubes that are too small to drain a hemothorax – 36 French chest tubes are preferred. Similarly, needle thoracentesis is rarely, if ever, adequate to drain a hemothorax.

The use of prophylactic antibiotics in patients who undergo tube thoracostomy remains controversial. Several trials have reported mixed results. A consensus has been difficult to reach because of differences in patient populations (trauma versus elective operations), differences in definition of empyema, and small numbers of patients. A recent meta-analysis suggests that prophylactic antibiotics can reduce the occurrence of empyema following chest-tube placement for trauma[29]. Currently, the authors do not routinely place patients on antibiotics for chest tubes.

REFERENCES

1. LaCicero J, Mattox KL. Epidemiology of chest trauma. Surg Clin North Am. 1989;69:15–19.
2. Shackford SR. Blunt chest trauma: the intensivist's perspective. J Intensive Care Med. 1986;1:125–36.
3. Mattox KL, Wall MJ, Pickard LR. Thoracic trauma: general considerations and indications for thoracotomy. In: Feliciano DV, Moore EE, Mattox KL, eds. Trauma, 3rd edn. Stamford: Appleton & Lange; 1996;345–54.
4. Landercasper J, Cogbill TA, Lindesmith LA. Long term disability after flail chest. J Trauma. 1984;24:410–14.
5. Mansour MA, Moore EE, Moore FA, Read RR. Exigent postinjury thoracotomy analysis of blunt versus penetrating trauma. Surg Gynecol Obstet. 1992;175:97–101.
6. Shorr RM, Crittenden M, Indeck M, et al. Blunt thoracic trauma: analysis of 515 patients. Ann Surg. 1987;206:200–5.
7. Beeson A, Saegesser F. Color atlas of chest trauma and associated injuries, Vol. 1. Oradell: Medical Economics Books; 1983.
8. Garcia VF, Gotschall CS, Eichelberger MR, Bowman LM. Rib fractures in children: a marker of severe trauma. J Trauma. 1990;30:695–700.
9. Lee RB, Bass SM, Morris JA, MacKenzie EJ. Three or more rib fractures as an indicator for transfer to a Level I Trauma Center: a population-based study. J Trauma. 1990;30:689–94.
10. Wilson JM, Thomas AN, Goodman PC, Lewis FR. Severe chest trauma: morbidity implication of first and second rib fracture in 120 patients. Arch Surg. 1978;113:846–9.
11. Poole GV. Fracture of the upper ribs and injury to the great vessels. Surg Gynecol Obstet. 1989;169:275–82.
12. Hills MW, Delprado AM, Deane SA. Sternal fractures: associated injuries and management. J Trauma. 1993;35:55–60.
13. Moore FA, Haenel JB, Moore EE. Blunt pulmonary injury. Adv Trauma Crit Care. 1993;8:1–28.
14. Bertelsen S, Howitz P. Injuries of the trachea and bronchi. Thorax. 1972;27:188–94.
15. Rhea JT, Novelline RA, Lawrason J, et al. The frequency and significance of thoracic injuries detected on abdominal CT scans of multiple trauma patients. J Trauma. 1989;29:502–5.
16. McGonigal MD, Schwab CW, Karder DR, et al. Supplemental emergent chest computed tomography in the management of blunt torso trauma. J Trauma. 1990;30:1431–4.
17. Poole GV, Morgan DB, Cranston PE, et al. Computed tomography in the management of blunt thoracic trauma. J Trauma. 1993;35:296–302.
18. Kiev J, Kerstein MD. Role of three hour roentgenogram of the chest in penetrating and nonpenetrating injuries of the chest. Surg Gynecol Obstet. 1992;175:249–53.
19. Röthlin MA, Nat R, Amigwerd M, et al. Ultrasound in blunt abdominal and thoracic trauma. J Trauma. 1993;34:488–95.
20. Hara KS, Prakash UBS. Fiberoptic bronchoscopy in the evaluation of acute chest and upper airway trauma. Chest. 1989;96:627–30.
21. Marini JJ, Pierson DJ, Hudson LD. Acute lobar atelectasis: a prospective comparison of fiberoptic bronchoscopy and respiratory therapy. Am Rev Respir Dis. 1979;119:971–8.
22. Smith RS, Fry WR, Tsai EKM, et al. Preliminary report on video thoracoscopy in the evaluation and treatment of thoracic injury. Am J Surg. 1993;166:690–5.
23. Landreneau RJ, Kennan RJ, Hazelrigg SR, et al. Thoracoscopy for empyema and hemothorax. Chest. 1995;109:18–24.
24. Ali J, Qi W. Effectiveness of chest tube clamping in massive hemothorax. J Trauma. 1995;38:59–63.
25. Bongard FS, Lewis FR. Crystalloid resuscitation of patients with pulmonary contusion. Am J Surg. 1984;148:145–51.
26. Haenel JB, Moore FA, Moore EE. Pulmonary consequences of severe chest trauma. Respir Care Clin North Am. 1996;2:401–24.
27. Mackersie RC, Karagianes TG, Hoyt DB, Davis JW. Prospective evaluation of epidural and intravenous administration of fentanyl for pain control and restoration of ventilatory function following multiple rib fractures. J Trauma. 1991;31:443–451.
28. Luchette FA, Radasher SM, Kaiser R, et al. Prospective evaluation of epidural versus intrapleural catheters for analgesia in chest wall trauma. J Trauma. 1994;36:865–70.
29. Fallon WF, Wears RL. Prophylactic antibiotics for prevention of infectious complications including empyema following tube thoracostomy for trauma: results of meta-analysis. J Trauma. 1992;33:110–16.

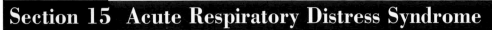

Chapter 69 Acute Respiratory Distress Syndrome

Luciano Gattinoni, Paolo Pelosi, Luca Brazzi, and Franco Valenza

Since its first description, more than 25 years ago in 12 patients[1], the acute respiratory distress syndrome (ARDS; originally known as the adult respiratory distress syndrome) has received more attention than any single entity in critical care medicine. The syndrome consists of an acute, severe alteration in lung structure and function characterized by hypoxemia, low respiratory system compliance, low functional residual capacity, and diffuse radiographic infiltrates, along with increased lung endothelial and alveolar epithelial permeability.

EPIDEMIOLOGY, RISK FACTORS, AND PATHOPHYSIOLOGY

Epidemiology

As a consequence of the different definitions of ARDS (see below), it has always been difficult to estimate the true incidence. The 1972 report of the National Heart, Lung, and Blood Institute[2] (NIH) suggested that about 150,000 cases of ARDS occurred per year in the USA[2], which represents an incidence of 60/100,000 population per year. This figure has been challenged in a number of reports (Fig. 69.1), all of which give an incidence that is an order of magnitude lower than the NIH estimates. Two points must be stressed, however. First, different ARDS definitions play an obvious role when its incidence is estimated. As shown in two articles[6,7], defining ARDS according to more or less strict criteria results in incidence estimates that differ by more than 100%. Second, some studies suffer from substantial methodologic problems. Despite this, it is likely that the true incidence of acute lung injury (ALI) and/or ARDS (ALI/ARDS) is closer to the most recent reported figures rather than to NIH estimates.

Risk factors

ARDS occurs following a variety of risk factors. The results of a systematic overview of the incidence and risk factors for ARDS were recently reported by Garber et al.[9], who reviewed 77 articles. The strongest evidence supporting a cause-and-effect relationship between ARDS and a risk factor was identified for sepsis, trauma, multiple transfusions, aspiration of gastric contents, pulmonary contusion, pneumonia, and smoke inhalation. The weakest evidence was identified for disseminated intravascular coagulation, fat embolism, and cardiopulmonary bypass.

Pathophysiology

Whenever an insult is applied to the lung, a host response is triggered, which is characterized by a close interplay of cells and humoral factors that results in lung inflammation (Fig. 69.2). Epithelium and endothelium are both involved, although injury to one or the other barrier may predominate. It is useful to consider two pathways – the effect of the insult directly on the lung (direct insult), and pulmonary lesions that result from an acute systemic inflammatory response (indirect insult). This distinction is important, as the pathway may govern the expression of the pulmonary abnormalities.

Incidence and mortality of acute respiratory distress syndrome			
Author	**Patient number**	**Incidence (100,000 population/year)**	**Mortality rate (%)**
National Heart, Lung, and Blood Institute[2]	–	60	–
Fowler[3]	88	5.2	65
Webster[4]	139	4.5	38
Evans[5]	62	25	60
Villar[6]	30/74	1.5/3.5	70/50
Thomsen[7]	110/83	8.3/4.8	–
Lewandowski[8]	17	3	58.8

Figure 69.1 Incidence and mortality of acute respiratory distress syndrome (ARDS). Data in Villar and Slutsky[6] and Thomsen and Morris[7] are reported according to two different definitions for ARDS.

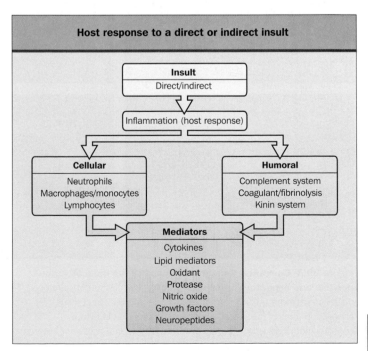

Figure 69.2 Host response to a direct or indirect insult.

Direct insult

Lung injury has been reproduced in animal models by direct application of the insult to the alveoli (as with intratracheal instillation of endotoxin or live bacteria, complement, tumor necrosis factor, etc.). Pulmonary epithelium was thus subjected to the initial injury, with activation of alveolar macrophages. These, in turn, activate the inflammatory network, which leads to pulmonary inflammation. Importantly, the prevalent damage following the direct insult is intra-alveolar, with alveolar filling by edema, fibrin, collagen, neutrophilic aggregates, and/or blood, and is often described as 'pulmonary consolidation'.

Indirect insult

Pulmonary lesions may also originate indirectly by mediators released from extrapulmonary foci into the blood, as during peritonitis, pancreatitis, and various abdominal diseases. The primary target in such cases is the pulmonary endothelial cell. The activation of the inflammatory network results in increased permeability of the endothelial barrier and recruitment of monocytes, polymorphonuclear neutrophil leukocytes, platelets, and other cells. Consequently, the prevalent damage is represented by microvessel congestion and interstitial edema, while intra-alveolar spaces are relatively spared.

It is likely that direct and indirect insults can coexist. This may occur, for example, in patients who have pneumonia when one lung is initially directly affected, and the other is indirectly injured hours or days later as the inflammation spreads by means of loss of compartmentalization (indirect insult).

It is important to differentiate between direct and indirect pathophysiologic pathways, as the underlying pathology (i.e. predominantly consolidation versus interstitial edema and collapse) seems to be different in the two conditions, at least during the early phases, and this may affect the approach to treatment. Figure 69.3, taken from the first report of the effect of positive end-expiratory pressure (PEEP) in ARDS studied using computed tomography (CT) scans, clearly emphasizes the point. Application of PEEP overdistended previously inflated lung regions in one patient, and resulted in a remarkable lung recruitment in the second. Intuitively, the different responses of the respiratory system to the same perturbation suggests different underlying conditions.

Models of acute respiratory distress syndrome

Before the introduction of CT scan technology, imaging of ARDS was limited to the chest radiograph, which showed (and was part of the ARDS definition) a widespread and bilateral appearance of 'pulmonary infiltrates'. Thus, ARDS was considered to be a homogeneous alteration of the lung parenchyma, with reduced gas content, characterized by an abnormal stiffness. The CT scan completely changed this model, as it has been consistently observed that the densities, which reflect the ratio of gas volume to the total lung volume [i.e. gas volume/(tissue volume + gas volume)] are primarily distributed in dependent lung regions such that nondependent lung regions are relatively normally inflated, while the intermediate regions are poorly inflated (Fig. 69.4)[10,11]. Typically, the normally inflated volume of lung tissue

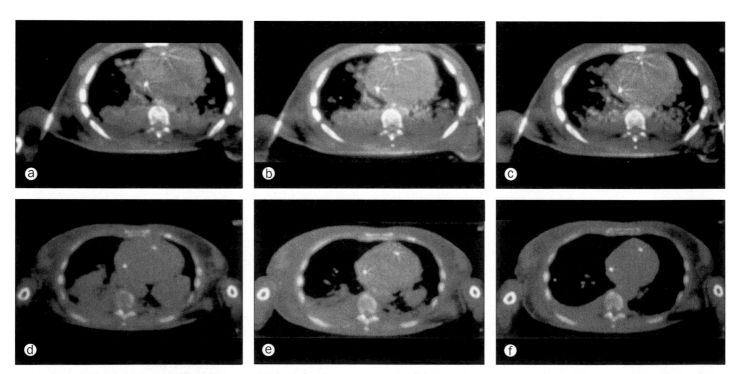

Figure 69.3 Computed tomography scans of the base at various positive end-expiratory pressures (PEEP). (a)–(c) Acute respiratory distress syndrome (ARDS) from bacterial pneumonia (direct insult). No changes in density (i.e. airspace collapse and/or parenchymal consolidation) and arterial partial pressure of oxygen (Pao_2) are observed with increasing levels of PEEP. (a) At 5cmH$_2$O, Pao_2 is 12.9kPa (97mmHg), density 59%; (b) At 10cmH$_2$O, Pao_2 is 13.7kPa (103mmHg), density 56%; (c) At 15cmH$_2$O, Pao_2 is 13.8kPa (104mmHg), density 53%. (d)–(f) ARDS from sepsis caused by peritonitis (indirect insult). Substantial clearing of the densities (which, in this instance, seem to represent airspace collapse) with changes in PEEP. (d) At 5cmH$_2$O, Pao_2 is 4.5kPa (34mmHg), density 70%; (e) At 10cmH$_2$O, Pao_2 is 6.5kPa (49mmHg), density 52%; (f) At 15cmH$_2$O, Pao_2 is 16.1kPa (121mmHg), density 32%. (10cmH$_2$O = 1kPa.)

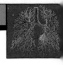

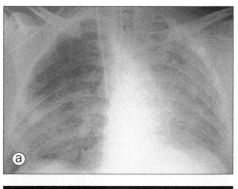
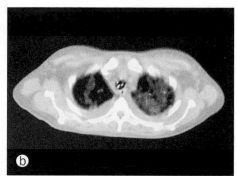
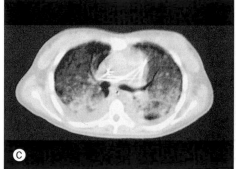
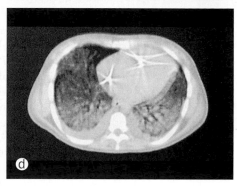

Figure 69.4 Acute respiratory distress syndrome in the early phase. (a) Chest radiograph, (b) computed tomography (CT) scan in the apical lung region, (c) CT scan at hilum, and (d) CT scan in the basilar lung region. All the images are at 10cmH$_2$O positive end-expiratory pressure. While the chest radiograph shows mainly a diffuse involvement, the CT scans clearly demonstrate a predominantly dependent distribution of the densities.

in patients who have ARDS approximates 200–400g in lungs that weigh as much as 2000–4000g (compared with 1000–1200g for a normal lung)[12].

These observations led to the model of the 'baby lung', since the amount of residual, normally inflated lung had the volume of a lung of a 5- or 6-year-old child. The baby lung presents the following characteristics:

- small and normal or near-normal compliance;
- located in the nondependent lung regions; and
- associated with a variable amount of abnormal lung, in part poorly inflated and in part collapsed or consolidated.

Accordingly, the ARDS lung could be modeled as a mixture of three zones:

- normally inflated (the baby lung, nondependent);
- recruitable (i.e. collapsed lung that could be opened with adequate inflation pressure); and
- consolidated lung (i.e. lung consists of alveolar filling such that it cannot be opened by increased alveolar pressure).

This model implies that the lung in the nondependent regions is spared by the disease process. However, when the patients are studied in the prone position a redistribution of densities from dorsal to ventral is frequently observed (Fig. 69.5)[13]. Accordingly,

the original baby lung model does not hold true, as although the inflated tissue (the baby lung) is nondependent, the repositioning effected change.

The most important finding of regional chest CT analysis is that the excess tissue mass, which probably derives from edema, is not gravity dependent, but is evenly distributed throughout the parenchyma, from ventral to dorsal in the supine position. Thus, the ALI/ARDS lung is characterized by diffuse, increased permeability (the whole lung is diseased), and the edema increases at each level, as a sponge soaks up water. The increased lung mass in a gravitational field, however, means an increased lung weight, and the most dependent levels are compressed by the increased weight of the levels above. In other words, if it is assumed that the lung behaves as a fluid, each lung level, from sternum to vertebra when in the supine position, is compressed by the pressure exerted by the levels above. This pressure, called 'superimposed pressure', equals, as in a fluid model, the density times the height of the superimposed lung. As shown in Figure 69.6, in the absence of gravity the lung would have pulmonary units of equal size, and each level would have the same gas/tissue ratio. In a gravitational field, on the other hand, the superimposed pressure causes compression (the lung becomes poorly inflated) and/or collapse (the lung is noninflated)

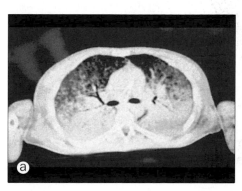
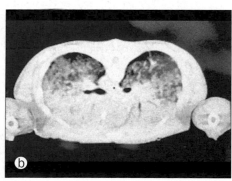

Figure 69.5 Redistribution of the lung densities. (a) Patient lying supine, (b) same patient turned prone.

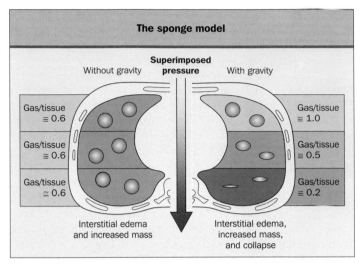

Figure 69.6 The sponge model. The edema is homogeneously distributed throughout the lung. In the absence of gravity, the lung would have pulmonary units of equal size (i.e. same gas/tissue ratio). In the presence of gravity, the superimposed pressure causes a size reduction and collapse of the dependent lung regions.

of the units in the dependent regions, with resultant atelectasis. This model accounts for the density redistribution seen in the prone position, as the gravitational forces compress the previously open ventral regions, while the dorsal regions inflate. Therefore, the sponge model suggests the following:
- the whole lung is altered;
- normally inflated tissue (baby lung) still occurs in the nondependent regions; and
- baby lung is not an anatomic reality, but a functional concept.

The sponge model seems most appropriate when ARDS results from an indirect insult to the lung, such that the diffuse increase in permeability leads to widespread interstitial edema and collapse. This model, however, is less applicable to ARDS caused by a direct insult, in which the primary problem is consolidation with alveolar filling and the amount of recruitable lung (i.e. previously collapsed lung) is small.

The sponge model is also limited because many patients have little or no reversal of lung density on turning prone, which implies that other factors contribute to the positional differences in the extent of lung collapse. Possibilities include the generally triangular shape of the lung, the effect of the weight of the heart on the dorsal lung units, the effect of differences in ventral and dorsal aspects of the diaphragm with regard to the transmission of abdominal pressure to the lung, and/or regional differences in chest wall compliance.

Mechanisms of action of positive end-expiratory pressure
Keeping the lung open
The primary role of PEEP in ARDS is to keep pulmonary units open at end-expiration when they would otherwise collapse. For years, the 'best PEEP' has been sought, on the assumption that for each ARDS lung there is an ideal level of PEEP. That such a level does not exist is clearly shown by CT scans, and PEEP is always a compromise between lung distension and lung recruitment. Indeed, in a study using PEEP levels from 0 to $20cmH_2O$ ($10cmH_2O = 1kPa$), regional quantitative analysis of the gas/tissue ratio showed, as expected from the sponge model, that the various levels of the same lung, from sternum to vertebra, require different levels of PEEP to stay open[14].

According to the sponge model, the superimposed pressure over a given lung level is a function of the density of the levels above times their height. It follows that the level of PEEP required to keep ventral regions open (in the supine position) is $0cmH_2O$ (no compression, no atelectasis). In the middle of the lung, the PEEP needed to counteract the superimposed pressure is higher, and it is highest in the most dependent lung regions. It also follows that, to keep the most dorsal regions open, the most ventral regions must be overexpanded, and consequently the PEEP level chosen is not 'best', but always a compromise (Fig. 69.7).

In the sponge model, the superimposed pressure causes compression atelectasis as a function of density and lung height, and accordingly:
- body size (a larger person has a larger lung) is an important variable to consider when deciding what PEEP level is appropriate to counteract superimposed pressure; and
- baseline lung density decreases with age, such that in neonates the baseline density is almost twice that in adults (thus, high levels of PEEP are sometimes required to keep the lung open in a small child who has ALI/ARDS).

Redistribution of ventilation/perfusion
While explaining the effect of PEEP on lung inflation is quite straightforward using the sponge model, explaining its beneficial

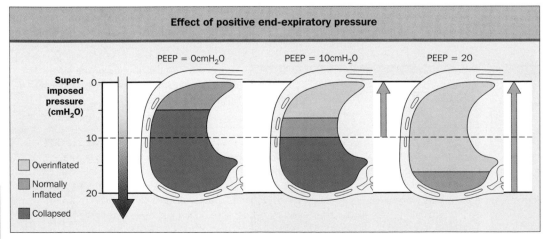

Figure 69.7 Effect of positive end-expiratory pressure (PEEP). Since PEEP acts as a counter force to the superimposed pressure over a given lung level (indicated by arrows), at zero EEP the superimposed pressure is 0 in the ventral regions and $20cmH_2O$ in the dorsal ones. To counterbalance $20cmH_2O$ of superimposed pressure (dependent lung regions) a PEEP of $20cmH_2O$ is necessary. However, while dependent lung regions are kept open, the nondependent ones become overinflated. ($10cmH_2O = 1kPa$.)

effects on oxygenation is more difficult. Compression atelectasis is much less prevalent in late-phase ARDS and in ARDS that results from primary lung injury. Accordingly, the ability to obtain recruitment with PEEP is limited. Although not proven, we suggest that the mechanism of PEEP in this setting is not the prevention of air-space closure at end exhalation, but possibly involves redistributing ventilation from ventral to dorsal regions. Overstretching the nondependent regions with PEEP decreases the compliance of these region such that ventilation may be diverted toward the more regions, increasing the ventilation/perfusion ($\dot{V}/\dot{Q}$) ratio of the poorly inflated regions. Unfortunately, no data are available on regional distribution of blood flow in humans, and thus a real understanding of the ventilation and perfusion redistribution phenomena is not possible.

Mechanisms of lung opening

When delivering a tidal volume (VT) in ARDS, two phenomena may occur – inflation and recruitment. Recruitment is defined as the inflation of previously noninflated regions. The pressures required to inflate the lung are known to be greater than those required to keep the lung open. Importantly, two kinds of collapse may coexist: one is collapse of the small airways, and the other is alveolar collapse from complete reabsorption of gases.

When the small airways collapse, some gas remains trapped behind the region of closure. If the small airways collapse persists, it evolves into alveolar collapse. The distinction between small airways and alveolar collapse is important, as the transpulmonary pressures required for opening may be greatly different: 10–20cmH$_2$O to open small airways, and 30–35cmH$_2$O to re-expand alveoli that have collapsed because of gas reabsorption[15]. Consequently, as shown in Figure 69.8, a complete range of opening pressures is found in ARDS, from 0–1cmH$_2$O to inflate open units (not exactly an opening pressure), to 10–20cmH$_2$O to counteract the small airways collapse (a pressure normally reached during normal tidal ventilation), and up to 30–35cmH$_2$O transmural pressure to open areas of alveolar collapse (pressures

not normally generated during normal tidal ventilation). At the end of the spectrum is consolidation in which opening is impossible because the air spaces are occupied with inflammatory exudate and cells.

Mechanisms of distribution of tidal volume

Distribution of the inspiratory volume is a function of two factors – airways resistance and regional respiratory system compliance. The CT scan, taken in static conditions, enables inferences to be made regarding variations in regional compliance. In ARDS, the distribution of the VT is a function of PEEP. In fact, on increasing PEEP from 0 to 20cmH$_2$O, the fraction of VT distributed to nondependent lung, compared with that distributed to dependent lung, decreases from 2.5:1 to approximately 1:1 (i.e. the ventilation becomes more homogeneous). This phenomenon has always been associated with better oxygenation[16]. The mechanism by which the VT is redistributed with PEEP is as follows:

- in the most ventral regions, which are already open, increasing PEEP causes a progressive stretching of the lung with a decrease of the regional compliance; and
- in the most dorsal regions, PEEP maintains recruitment of otherwise collapsing lung, and thus increases the compliance of this region as more pulmonary units become available for inflation.

The final effect depends on the balance between the overstretching and recruitment phenomena (Fig. 69.9).

Positioning

An important maneuver that is increasingly being used in ARDS is to place the patients in the prone position[17]. In Figure 69.5, the effects on density redistribution from dorsal to ventral are shown. This effect does not arise from a variable distribution of edema. In ARDS, the interstitial edema, rich in proteins, is not 'free' to move throughout the lung parenchyma. Instead, the density redistribution, according to the sponge model, results from 'squeezing' out the gas from the dependent lung regions because of the superimposed pressure.

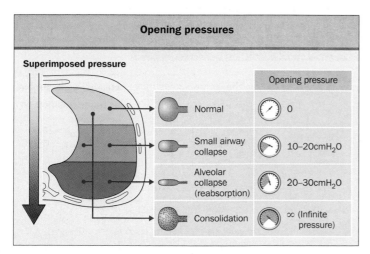

Figure 69.8 Opening pressures. The lung with acute respiratory distress syndrome is composed of normally inflated lung regions, consolidated lung regions, and collapsed (atelectatic) lung regions. Atelectasis may be caused by both compression atelectasis (needing up to 10–20cmH$_2$O of transpulmonary pressure to reopen) and reabsorption atelectasis (which needs up to 20–30cmH$_2$O of transpulmonary pressure to reopen). (10cmH$_2$O = 1kPa.)

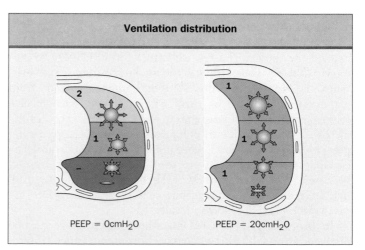

Figure 69.9 Effects of positive end-expiratory pressure (PEEP) on distribution of ventilation. At zero end-expiratory pressure, the distribution of ventilation is preferentially distributed to the nondependent lung region (2:1:0) since the dependent regions are partially collapsed at end expiration. At high PEEP, the distribution of ventilation is more homogeneous (1:1:1) because of overstretching of nondependent units and recruitment of the dependent ones. (10cmH$_2$O = 1kPa.)

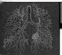

Acute Respiratory Distress Syndrome

The redistribution of lung density induced by the prone position is more pronounced in ARDS caused by extrapulmonary disease. In ARDS due to pulmonary disease, densities change much less on going from the supine to the prone position (Fig. 69.10). The prone position is associated with increased oxygenation in about 60–70% of ARDS patients. Several mechanisms are likely to be involved, and important differences may arise when ARDS occurs as a result of pulmonary versus extrapulmonary disease. In the latter, as atelectasis depends on lung density and height, a larger volume of lung opens in the prone position. In ARDS resulting from pulmonary disease, changes in thoracic compliance play a substantial role. In the prone position, for anatomic reasons, the dorsal component of the chest wall is stiffer than the anterior wall, and the V_T is distributed more toward the ventral and abdominal regions, where higher lung densities predominate (Fig. 69.11)[18]. Indeed, human and animal studies conclude that a more homogeneous inflation and/or ventilation is the main mechanism of oxygenation improvement in the prone position.

Chest wall compliance

Most of the available data on respiratory mechanics in ARDS relate to the respiratory system (i.e. the lung and the chest wall). The mechanical alterations observed were mainly attributed to the lung as chest wall compliance was considered to be normal. The few studies that investigated chest wall compliance *per se* found it to be decreased. More recently, it has become clear that in ARDS caused by pulmonary disease, chest wall compliance is normal, while in that caused by extrapulmonary disease it is greatly decreased[19]. It is more convenient to use the elastance (the reciprocal of compliance) to discuss the partitioning of compliance between chest and lung, as the elastance of the respiratory system is the sum of chest wall and lung elastances.

Elastance is the pressure required to keep the respiratory system inflated. Part of this pressure is spent to keep the lung inflated, and part to keep the thoracic cage (which includes the abdominal wall) expanded. Normally, lung and chest wall elastances are similar, such that half of the applied pressure keeps the lung inflated and half expands the thoracic cage when inflated. In ARDS caused by extrapulmonary disease, however, more pressure is required to expand the thorax. The reverse is true for ARDS due to pulmonary disease. Thus, although the total respiratory system elastance is similar in ARDS from pulmonary and from extrapulmonary disease, its partitioning is different. This explains, for instance, why heart size tends to remain normal when PEEP is increased in ARDS due to pulmonary disease (i.e. low pleural pressure around the heart), while it decreases in ARDS caused by extrapulmonary disease (i.e. progressively higher pleural pressure, because of the relative stiffness of the thorax). Accordingly, PEEP may have different hemodynamic consequences in ARDS that results from direct or indirect insults.

In this context, the issue of intra-abdominal pressure must be discussed. Normally, intra-abdominal pressure measured through the bladder is in the range 5–10cmH$_2$O. In ARDS caused by extrapulmonary diseases (most of which arise in the abdomen) intra-abdominal pressure is greatly increased. The authors found a strict correlation between abdominal pressure and chest wall elastance (i.e. increasing the abdominal pressure increases chest wall elastance, which reflects an increased stiffness of the thoracic cage). As the importance of chest wall elastance is becoming increasingly clear, the measurement of intra-abdominal pressure should be part of the assessment of ARDS patients (both for respiratory treatment and hemodynamic consequences).

Pulmonary circulation

The ARDS lung is usually characterized by increased pulmonary artery pressure and increased pulmonary vascular resistance. A mean pulmonary artery pressure ≥ 4.0kPa (≥ 30mmHg) is a universal hallmark of ARDS, regardless of etiology[20]. A single mechanism is unlikely to explain the increased resistance. Moreover, the causes of the pulmonary hypertension may change over time. Indirect evidence suggests that a generalized vasoconstriction exists in ARDS and that this can be modulated with vasodilatation. Moreover, inhaled nitric oxide may selectively dilate vessels in ventilated areas, which suggests that hypoxemia (arterial and mixed venous) is not the cause of the observed functional vasoconstriction.

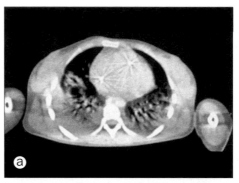
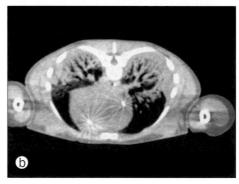

Figure 69.10 Distribution of lung densities that arise from consolidation, not collapse. Change of position from (a) supine to (b) prone does not affect the distribution of lung densities. Compare with Figure 69.5.

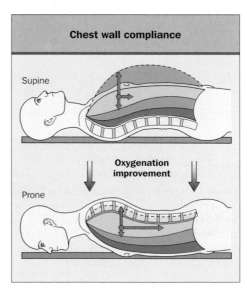

Figure 69.11 Effect of prone position on ventilation distribution. In the supine position the distribution of ventilation is preferentially distributed to the ventral regions. When the patient is prone, the stiffness of the dorsal chest wall favors the distribution of ventilation to the dorsal regions, facilitating reinflation in this area.

Chest wall compliance

Supine

Oxygenation improvement

Prone

Eicosanoids and other mediators are likely to be responsible. A second possible mechanism is vessel compression by the increased lung weight and superimposed perivascular pressure. The authors found, *in vivo*, that every increase of 0.13kPa (1mmHg) of pulmonary artery pressure is associated with a 14% increase of the original lung weight[21]. Unfortunately, it will not be possible to determine if this is an independent variable as, if it is possible that edema causes vessel compression, it is also possible that increased pulmonary artery pressure increases the interstitial edema, through increased microfiltration. Anatomic alterations in the vascular wall have also been described, such as swelling of the endothelial cells and, with time, medial hypertrophy. Finally, evidence of fibrin clot and cellular obstruction within the capillaries is found in 20–30% of ARDS patients. With time, the collapsed and/or obstructed vessels undergo remodeling or become completely obliterated by fibrotic processes, which lead to microvascular destruction. A summary of alterations in the pulmonary circulation is presented in Figure 69.12.

In considering the overall circulatory function, however, it is noteworthy that in ARDS, despite the generalized vasoconstriction, collapsed lung regions are appropriately underperfused compared with the inflated regions. Indeed, it is common to find 50–60% of collapsed lung associated with a shunt fraction (i.e. the flow through the collapsed regions) of 20–30% of the cardiac output, which suggests that a somewhat appropriate flow diversion is still occurring.

The physiopathologic consequences of elevated pulmonary vascular resistance depend on the cardiac reserve of each patient. If the right ventricle is able to increase its work, the hemodynamic consequences are nil. If right ventricular dysfunction is present, numerous systemic consequences arise.

Gas exchange alterations

The main alteration of gas exchange in ARDS is hypoxemia due to shunt, and is usually associated with normo- or hypo-capnia. However, while the hypoxemia persists, a progressive rise in arterial partial pressure of carbon dioxide ($PaCO_2$) occurs over time if the minute ventilation is maintained constant. Gas exchange is the final consequence of the match between ventilation and perfusion, which in turn depends on the anatomic structure of the lung (which changes with time and with the prevalent underlying pathology). An attempt to correlate lung structure with gas exchange alterations is given in Figure 69.13.

Early acute lung injury/acute respiratory distress syndrome, indirect insult

In early ALI/ARDS caused by an indirect insult, the lung architecture is preserved, and the primary pathophysiologic abnormality is edema with consequent collapse of dependent regions. The pulmonary blood flow through these regions is the main cause of shunt. The midlung regions are poorly inflated and, if perfused, could contribute to hypoxemia because of low $\dot{V}/\dot{Q}$. The nondependent regions are open and likely to be hyperventilated, because of the preferential distribution of VT to these regions. Thus, carbon dioxide elimination is not a problem. The application of PEEP may keep open the otherwise collapsing regions and increase ventilation of the poorly inflated regions to the extent that shunt decreases and low $\dot{V}/\dot{Q}$ may be corrected. If the PEEP level is excessive, however, the upper regions are kept open, but are overstretched, with less capability for ventilation. Oxygen may be exchanged, but the carbon dioxide clearance is impaired. This is one possible explanation why, with excessive PEEP, shunt decreases but the $PaCO_2$ may increase.

Early acute respiratory distress syndrome, direct insult

In early ALI/ARDS caused by a direct insult, the overall lung architecture is preserved, but the prevalent damage is intra-alveolar, with edema and collapse being secondary phenomena, and quantitatively more important than in ARDS from an indirect insult. The consolidated regions, if perfused, cause shunt just as if they were collapsed. It is likely that PEEP works by keeping the otherwise collapsing regions open. It is possible, however, that PEEP also works by redistributing VT from nondependent to dependent regions, thus improving the ventilation of low $\dot{V}/\dot{Q}$ regions. The shunt decrease may also be associated with a $PaCO_2$ increase in this instance, which suggests a ventilation diversion with PEEP.

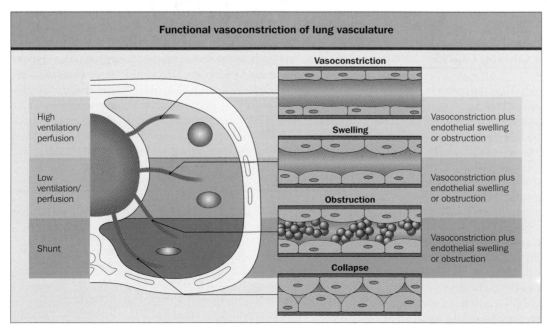

Functional vasoconstriction of lung vasculature

High ventilation/perfusion

Low ventilation/perfusion

Shunt

Vasoconstriction

Swelling

Obstruction

Collapse

Vasoconstriction plus endothelial swelling or obstruction

Vasoconstriction plus endothelial swelling or obstruction

Vasoconstriction plus endothelial swelling or obstruction

Figure 69.12 All the lung vasculature is functionally vasoconstricted. Moreover, endothelial swelling and obliteration may further increase pulmonary vascular resistance. In the dependent lung regions, vessel compression may be also present.

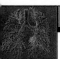
Gas exchange					
Acute respiratory distress syndrome	Lung injury	Lung structure	Pulmonary circulation	Mechanism of gas exchange	Corrections (other then fraction of inspired oxygen)
Early	Direct	Collapse in the dependent regions	Vasoconstriction and partial collapse	Shunt	Positive end-expiratory pressure (PEEP; re-expansion)
		Poorly inflated in middle regions	Vasoconstriction	Low ventilation/ perfusion ($\dot{V}/\dot{Q}$)?	PEEP (normalizing inflation)
		Inflated in upper regions	Vasoconstriction	High $\dot{V}/\dot{Q}$	Nitric oxide (increasing perfusion) Inhaled prostaglandin
		Consolidation and collapse in dependent regions	Vasoconstriction plus possible collapse	Shunt	PEEP (re-expansion)
	Indirect	Possible consolidation foci in middle regions	Vasoconstriction and low $\dot{V}/\dot{Q}$?	Shunt in consolidated area and low $\dot{V}/\dot{Q}$?	PEEP (?)
		Possible consolidation foci in nondependent regions	Vasoconstriction and high $\dot{V}/\dot{Q}$	Shunt in consolidated area	PEEP [ventilation redistribution to lower regions (?) by stretching upper regions?] plus nitric oxide – prostaglandins
		Consolidation	Vasoconstriction	Shunt	PEEP (ventilation redistribution to lower regions?)
Late	Widespread lesions	Fibrosis	Microvessel destruction and obliteration	Diffusion impairment?	No recruitment evident
		Bullae and emphysema-like alterations	–	Increased dead space	Nitric oxide?

Figure 69.13 Gas exchange in acute respiratory distress syndrome. ? indicates uncertainty.

Late phase acute lung injury/acute respiratory distress syndrome

The situation is likely to be different in the late stage of ALI/ARDS, in which the lung architecture is markedly altered because of fibrosis, capillary destruction, and emphysema-like lesions. In such conditions, PEEP is still required to maintain oxygenation, but it does not work by 'keeping open' the recruited units, since collapse is scarce, if any. Redistribution of ventilation and/or perfusion is a possible mechanism. Moreover, the structural changes of the lung may contribute to hypoxemia by some impairment of oxygen diffusion (fibrosis and interstitial thickening), while the emphysema-like lesions are likely to be the anatomic basis for carbon dioxide retention.

CLINICAL FEATURES AND DEFINITIONS

Originally, Ashbaugh et al.[1] defined ARDS as the presence of severe dyspnea, tachypnea, hypoxemia refractory to oxygen therapy, reduced lung compliance, and diffuse alveolar infiltration seen on chest radiographs, but they made no attempt to suggest quantitative values for these alterations. Bone et al.[22] in 1976 used a PaO_2/[fraction of inspired oxygen (FIO_2)] ratio <150 to characterize ARDS. In 1979, the NIH[23], introduced criteria based on time (fast and slow) and threshold oxygenation values at defined levels of FIO_2 and positive expiratory pressure. The explicit exclusion of cardiogenic pulmonary edema was formally introduced by Pepe et al.[24], who proposed a quantitative threshold for pulmonary wedge capillary pressure. Fowler et al.[25] introduced a quantitative measurement of respiratory system compliance. In 1988 a new approach was proposed by Murray et al.[26], who developed a 'lung injury score' to quantify, albeit roughly, the presence, severity, and evolution of acute and chronic damage involving lung parenchyma.

Recently, the American–European Consensus Conference on ARDS[27] recommended that ARDS be described as a particularly severe subset of ALI, which, in turn, was defined as a 'syndrome of inflammation and increased permeability that is associated with a constellation of clinical, radiologic and physiologic abnormalities that cannot be explained by, but may coexist with, left atrial or pulmonary capillary hypertension'. A summary of ALI/ARDS definitions is presented in Figure 69.14.

The definitions of ALI/ARDS are not of merely academic interest, as testing new treatments requires trials in which the homogeneity of the study population plays a substantial role. Interestingly, considering the evolution of ARDS definitions, it is clear that more extensive and quantitative criteria were added over the years to define a more homogeneous population, but the recent American–European Conference almost represents a return to the original, very simple definition. The dilemma is still unsolved – simple criteria mean that a large trial with a very inhomogeneous population is feasible; strict criteria result in a homogeneous population and a large trial becomes unfeasible. Work is still required to find the best compromise between these opposing needs.

DIAGNOSIS

The diagnosis of ALI/ARDS is simple, according to its current definition, as it requires a known predisposing factor, bilateral pulmonary infiltrates on the chest radiograph, and a threshold PaO_2 value normalized for the FIO_2 in use.

An accurate patient history is of paramount importance to infer the etiology and pathogenesis of ALI/ARDS, and assessment of traditional signs must be carried out despite the availability of newer technology. Respiratory frequency, dyspnea, symmetry or

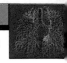

Acute respiratory distress syndrome definitions					
Reference	Clinical	Oxygenation threshold	Bilateral infiltrates	Respiratory system compliance	Threshold wedge pressure
Ashbaugh et al.[1]	1	None	Yes	None	Clinical judgment
Bone et al.[22]	1	Partial pressure of arterial oxygen (PaO_2)/fraction of inspired oxygen (FIO_2) $\leq 21kPa$ ($\leq 150mmHg$)	Yes	None	Clinical judgment
Zapol et al.[23]	1	$PaO_2 <6.6kPa$ ($<50mmHg$) 100% FIO_2 after 2h 60% FIO_2 after 24h Positive end-expiratory pressure (PEEP) $5cmH_2O$	Yes	None	Clinical judgment
Pepe et al.[24]	1	$PaO_2 <10.0kPa$ ($<75mmHg$) $FIO_2 \geq 50\%$	Yes	None	$>2.4kPa$ ($>18mmHg$)
Bell et al.[28] and Fein et al.[29]	1	$PaO_2 \geq 6.6kPa$ ($50mmHg$) $FIO_2 \geq 50\%$	Yes	None	$>2.0kPa$ ($>15mmHg$)
Fowler et al.[25]	1	PaO_2/alveolar $PO_2 <0.2$	Yes	$>50mL/cmH_2O$	$>1.6kPa$ ($>12mmHg$)
Murray et al.[26]	+	PaO_2/FIO_2 score 0–4 PEEP score 0–4	Chest radiograph score 0–4	Compliance score 0–4	Clinical judgment
Bernard et al.[27]	+	$PaO_2/FIO_2 <26.6kPa$ ($<200mmHg$), acute respiratory distress syndrome $PaO_2/FIO_2 <40kPa$ ($<300mmHg$), acute lung injury	Yes	None	Clinical judgment

Figure 69.14 Definitions of acute respiratory distress syndrome.

asymmetry of thoracic movements, percussion, and auscultation may provide insights into the etiology, and prevalent underlying pathology, and may also indicate the patient's ability to deal with the respiratory distress (as an example, signs of muscle fatigue must be carefully sought so as not to delay initiating mechanical ventilatory support if this is found).

Etiologic diagnosis

In most instances, the risk factor that leads to ALI/ARDS is clear, as in aspiration or lung contusion. In some patients, however, the etiology is not apparent. In patients who have ALI/ARDS and signs of sepsis, a systematic search for all the possible foci of infection must be carried out, using all available techniques.

Pathogenic diagnosis

Our recent findings suggest that ALI/ARDS should be separated into pulmonary and extrapulmonary causes. In most circumstances, this is an easy distinction based on an accurate history and clinical assessment. Such a distinction is more useful in the early phases of ALI/ARDS. With time, and with the structural changes that occur in the lung, the pathophysiologies of the two processes are likely to overlap.

Pathophysiologic characterization

Together with etiologic and pathogenic screening, every patient who has ALI/ARDS must be carefully investigated to define the specific pathophysiologic characteristics, as this enables treatment to be tailored more precisely.

Gas exchange

Characterization of the degree of gas-exchange impairment is the most common way of defining the severity of ALI/ARDS. It is always useful to observe the oxygenation response at different FIO_2 values (including a brief test with FIO_2 of 1.0), and to conduct a

formal PEEP trial (e.g. 5, 10, and $15cmH_2O$). Changes in FIO_2 may markedly affect the PaO_2/FIO_2 ratio, and the response may suggest the presence of $\dot{V}/\dot{Q}$ mismatch. The PEEP trial (in which hemodynamic status is controlled) may enable the effect of recruitment maneuvers to be estimated. The $PaCO_2$ response during the PEEP trial (in which minute ventilation is kept constant) may also be informative. An increase in PaO_2 with a decrease in the $PaCO_2$ indicates effective recruitment. An increase in PaO_2 with an increase in $PaCO_2$ could indicate overstretching of the nondependent lung (in addition to recruitment).

In some circumstances, it may be necessary to measure mixed venous (or central venous) blood gases. This is particularly true when cardiac output is low, since the fraction of shunt flow is directly related to the cardiac output. In some cases, an increase in PaO_2 occurs simply because of a decrease in cardiac output, with no improvement in lung function.

Imaging

It is important to obtain both routine chest radiographs and CT scans in all ALI/ARDS patients. In a series of 74 ALI/ARDS patients, 24 had pneumothoraces and in 37% of the these the pneumothorax was ventral in location and only detected by CT scan. Although not well studied, cross-table lateral films may have discovered many of these. Moreover, in 60% of the cases the CT scan provided additional clinical information compared with conventional radiology, and in 22% the findings resulted in a change in the clinical management[30]. These and other data emphasize the importance of this technology in the routine clinical management. Also, CT scans are the best tool with which to discriminate between recruitment and consolidation, and the authors routinely perform a PEEP trial during the CT scan, taking images at different pressures. This may be of great help when tailoring the respiratory support, as the potential of recruitment in a given patient is assessed precisely. Unfortunately, the pathology and physiology targets of a number of clinical trials that have been conducted on patients who have ALI/ARDS or sepsis. Some strategies were based on blocking the trigger of the inflammatory response (e.g. anti-LPS antibodies), or focused on single elements of the inflammatory network (e.g. antitumor necrosis factor antibodies, soluble tumor necrosis factor receptors, interleukin-1 receptor antagonist), and/or modified neutrophil function (liposomal prostaglandin E_1, antioxidants), and others addressed the consequences of inflammation such as hemodynamic imbalances (e.g. inhibitors of nitric oxide synthase, prostaglandin E_1). A summary of these trials is given in Figure 69.18. Almost all the studies found either no major benefit or that the intervention was actually harmful. Given the complexity of the inflammatory network, perhaps multiple sites should be blocked or potentiated simultaneously as opposed to the selective blocking of single events or mediators of the overall process.

Timing may be a key point in such a therapeutic philosophy. For example, corticosteroids have not been found helpful in the early phases of ALI/ARDS, but may prove beneficial during later phases, possibly preventing or limiting the fibrotic evolution of the ALI/ARDS lung.

Symptomatic treatment

Symptomatic (i.e. supportive) treatment is currently the cornerstone of ARDS therapy. The possible changes in mortality of ALI/ARDS over time that have recently been reported by some groups may result from differences in supportive treatment, or from differences in the iatrogenic nature of the treatments.

Arterial blood gas targets

In the past few years, the 'lung rest' philosophy (i.e. permissive hypercapnia) has become more accepted, which has lead to the acceptance of arterial blood gas tensions that are markedly abnormal with respect to $PaCO_2$. Although it may be reasonable to accept a high $PaCO_2$, we believe that the PaO_2 should be maintained around 10.6kPa (80mmHg), instead of 8.0kPa (60mmHg) as suggested by other investigators, to avoid the risk of sudden deterioration of oxygen saturation.

Lung opening

Irrespective of the prevalent damage that underlies ALI/ARDS, some degree of lung collapse is always present when the patient is referred to the intensive care unit (ICU). For hours or days before admission to the ICU, most patients are likely to have increased secretions, high respiratory frequency, and/or low V_T, which are all risk factors for atelectasis. To reach the goal of an open, expanded lung, airways patency must be assured (consider bronchoscopy) and atelectasis reversed if possible. Although formal rules to recruit as much lung as possible are not established, transpulmonary pressure and respiratory system compliance must be considered.

Clinical trials directed at the pathogenesis										
Strategy	**Author**	**Study characteristics present**						**Number of patients**	**Diagnosis**	**Results**	
		p	r	d1	d2	c	n			Overall	Stratified
Antilipopolysaccharide	McCloskey et al.[36]	No	Yes	Yes	No	Yes	No	2199	Sepsis	=	na
	Ziegler et al.[37]	No	Yes	Yes	No	No	No	543	Sepsis	=	+
Interleukin-1 receptor antagonist	Fisher et al.[38]	Yes	No	No	Yes	Yes	No	99	Sepsis/shock	+	na
	Fisher et al.[39]	No	No	Yes	No	No	No	893	Sepsis	=	+
	Opal et al.[40]	Yes	Yes	Yes	No	Yes	No	696	Sepsis stratified	=	na
Antibodies against tumor necrosis factor (TNF)-α	Abraham et al.[41]	No	No	No	Yes	No	No	994	>50% acute lung injury	=	+
	Cohen and Carlet[42]	Yes	Yes	No	Yes	Yes	Yes	553	Sepsis/shock	=	+
	Reinhart et al.[43]	Yes	Yes	No	Yes	Yes	Yes	122	Sepsis/shock	=	+
Antibodies against soluble TNF receptor	Abraham et al.[44]	Yes	Yes	Yes	Yes	Yes	Yes	498	Sepsis/shock	=	+
Cortisone	Bernard et al.[45]	Yes	Yes	Yes	No	No	No	99	Acute respiratory distress syndrome (ARDS)	=	na
	Bone et al.[46]	Yes	Yes	Yes	No	Yes	No	382	ARDS	=	na
	Luce et al.[47]	Yes	Yes	Yes	No	No	No	87	ARDS	=	na
	Meduri et al.[48]	Yes	Yes	Yes	No	Yes	No	24	ARDS (late)	+	na
Liposomal prostaglandin E_1	Abraham et al.[49]	Yes	Yes	Yes	No	Yes	No	25	ARDS	=	na
Prostaglandin E_1	Bone et al.[50]	Yes	Yes	Yes	No	No	No	100	ARDS	=	na
	Holcroft et al.[51]	Yes	Yes	Yes	No	No	No	41	ARDS	+	na
Antioxidants	Jepsen et al.[52]	Yes	Yes	Yes	No	No	No	66	ARDS	=	na
	Suter et al.[53]	No	No	No	Yes	No	No	61	ARDS	=	na
	Bernard et al.[54]	Yes	Yes	Yes	No	Yes	No	48	ARDS	=	na
Inducible nitric oxide synthase	Petros et al.[55]	No	Yes	Yes	No	No	No	12	Sepsis	=	na
Anticyclo-oxygenase	Haupt et al.[56]	No	Yes	Yes	No	Yes	No	29	Sepsis	=	na
	Yu and Tomasa[57]	Yes	Yes	Yes	No	No	No	54	Sepsis	+	na

p, prospective; r, randomized; d1, double-blind; d2, dose ranging (more than one dose tested); c, multicenter; n, multinational
=, no positive result; +, positive result; na, not available

Figure 69.18 Clinical trials directed at the pathogenesis of acute lung injury/acute respiratory distress syndrome.

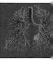

Transpulmonary pressure

The airspace opening pressure is expressed as a transpulmonary pressure (i.e. the difference between intra-alveolar and pleural pressure). Transpulmonary pressure is a function of the pressure applied to the airways and of the elastances of the lung and chest wall, according to equation (69.1), in which P_{AW} is the applied airways pressure, E_L is the elastance of the lung, and E_W is the elastance of the chest wall.

■ EQUATION 69.1

$$\text{Transpulmonary pressure} = P_{AW} \times [E_L/(E_L + E_W)]$$

Normally, E_L equals E_W, and the transpulmonary pressure, as an average, would be approximately half of the pressure applied to the airways. However, as previously discussed, in ALI/ARDS caused by direct or indirect insult, the $E_L/(E_L + E_W)$ value may be very different. For example, in ARDS from direct insult the ratio is >1 for patients who have extrapulmonary disease. It follows that, to achieve the same opening transpulmonary pressure, a higher P_{AW} is required in ARDS that arises from extrapulmonary problems than in ARDS from pulmonary conditions.

Respiratory system compliance

The recruitment maneuver may be difficult when respiratory system compliance is relatively good (as in moderate ALI), or when one lung has a good compliance compared with the other. In such conditions, it is difficult to achieve an adequate transpulmonary pressure, unless volumes up to 2L or more are insufflated. Artificially reducing the total respiratory system compliance (by applying external compression or turning the patient prone) may help to reach the required transpulmonary pressure without insufflating excessive volumes.

Once opened, the lung must be kept open and PEEP is the leading strategy used to prevent lung collapse. The level of PEEP is a compromise between that required to keep the lung open and that which results in overstretching, as noted above.

Iatrogenic cost of mechanical ventilation

Inspired oxygen fraction

The suggestion that a high F_{IO_2} (i.e. >0.60) causes lung damage is based on experimental studies carried out on normal animals, in which, in most cases, the inspired air was not appropriately humidified. No consistent evidence shows that high F_{IO_2} is dangerous in ALI/ARDS as there is worldwide experience with patients treated for days or weeks with 100% oxygen who ultimately survive[58].

Plateau pressures and pressure swings

It has been suggested that $35cmH_2O$ of plateau airway pressure is the safe upper threshold for mechanical ventilation. However, pressure *per se* is not dangerous (e.g. a diver may have an alveolar pressure of several atmospheres!). What is important is the transpulmonary pressure, and possibly the difference in pressure between end-expiration and end-inhalation. A plateau pressure of $35cmH_2O$ may be associated with a wide range of transpulmonary pressures, depending on the relationship between the lung and chest wall elastances and, in nonparalyzed patients, on the action of respiratory muscles.

The effect of high inflation pressures differs markedly depending on the starting inflation pressure or, more specifically, the lung volume present at end-exhalation.

Intratidal collapse and reinflation

Intratidal collapse and reinflation is a form of barotrauma that may be most likely to occur when compression atelectasis is the primary type of lung damage. In fact, during inspiration, even low plateau pressures ($20–25cmH_2O$) are sufficient to open the dependent lung regions when compression atelectasia, and small airways collapse, occurs. If the PEEP level is not adequate these dependent lung regions will recollapse at end-expiration. To avoid this phenomenon, a PEEP level sufficient to counteract the lung weight is required. As above, however, a single PEEP value cannot overcome the continuum of lung weight, at least in supine patients. Accordingly, a single 'best' pattern of ventilatory support does not exist for all patients who have ALI/ARDS. To clarify and understand the differences between the various strategies, it is useful to start from the equation of motion for the respiratory system, equation (69.2).

■ EQUATION 69.2

$$\text{Muscle pressure} + \text{ventilator pressure} = (V_T \times \text{elastance}) + (\text{resistance} \times \text{flow})$$

Respiratory support may thus be applied in three ways:
- a driving pressure needed to overcome the elastic and resistive load of the respiratory system is provided by the ventilator (i.e. the patient's muscle pressure equals zero);
- a driving pressure is provided by a combination of muscle pressure and ventilator pressure; or
- a driving pressure is totally provided by the patient's respiratory muscles (i.e. the ventilator pressure equals zero).

Driving pressure provided by the ventilator only (controlled mechanical ventilation)

The mode chosen to deliver the ventilation may be volume or pressure targeted. In the volume preset modes, V_T is delivered with a predefined inspiratory flow–time profile. As seen from equation (69.2), the pressure that the ventilator must generate depends on the mechanics of the respiratory system. The higher the elastance, the greater the ventilation pressure needed. During pressure-preset ventilation, the ventilator applies a predefined pressure to the airways. In this case, the higher the elastance the lower the V_T.

Driving pressure provided by both respiratory muscles and ventilator

Generally, ventilators deliver a positive pressure breath at a preset V_T (assisted ventilation), or a preset pressure (pressure-support), and the muscles of respiration activate the ventilator-delivered breath. A combination of pressure–volume targets is synchronized with intermittent mandatory ventilation. This is generally given along with pressure support, in which a low rate, volume-targeted V_T is associated with pressure-supported spontaneous ventilation. Some types of combined modality support may be delivered without intubation (i.e. noninvasive positive-pressure ventilation).

Driving pressure provided exclusively by respiratory muscles

When the driving pressure is provided exclusively by respiratory muscles the mode is more a respiratory support than a

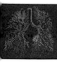
23. Zapol WM, Snider MT, Hill JD, et al. Extracorporeal membrane oxygenation in severe acute respiratory failure. A randomized prospective study. JAMA. 1979;242:2193–6.

24. Pepe PE, Potkin RT, Reus DH, Hudson LD, Carrico CJ. Clinical predictors of the Adult Respiratory Distress Syndrome. Am J Surg. 1982;144:124–30.

25. Fowler AA, Hamman F, Zerbe GO, Benson KN, Hyers TM. Adult Respiratory Distress Syndrome. Prognosis after onset. Am Rev Respir Dis. 1985;132:472–8.

26. Murray JF, Matthay MA, Luce JM, Flick R. An expanded definition of the Adult Respiratory Distress Syndrome. Am Rev Respir Dis. 1988;138:720–3.

27. Bernard GR, Artigas A, Brigham KL, et al. The American–European Consensus Conference on ARDS. Definitions, mechanisms, relevant outcomes, and clinical trial coordination. Am J Respir Crit Care Med. 1994;149:818–24.

28. Bell RC, Coalson JJ, Smith JD, Johanson WJ Jr. Multiple organ system failure and infection in Adult Respiratory Distress Syndrome. Ann Intern Med. 1983;99:293–8.

29. Fein AL, Lippmann M, Holtzman H, Eliraz A, Goldberg SK. The risk factors, incidence, and prognosis of ARDS following septicemia. Chest. 1983;83:40–2.

30. Tagliabue M, Casella TC, Zincone GE, Fumagalli R, Salvini E. CT and chest radiography in the evaluation of adult respiratory distress syndrome. Acta Radiol. 1994;35:230–4.

31. Mancebo J, Artigas A. A clinical study of the Adult Respiratory Distress Syndrome. Crit Care Med. 1987;15:243–6.

32. Suchyta MR, Clemmer TP, Elliot CG, Orme JF, Weaver LK. The adult respiratory distress syndrome. A report of survival and modifying factors. Chest. 1992;101:1074–9.

33. Hudson LD, Milberg JA, Anardi D, Mauder RJ. Clinical risk for development of the Acute Respiratory Distress Syndrome. Am J Respir Crit Care Med. 1995;151:293–301.

34. Milberg JA, Davis DR, Steinberg KP, Hudson LD. Improved survival of patients with Acute Respiratory Distress Syndrome (ARDS):1983–1993. JAMA. 1995;273:306–9.

35. Heffner. JE, Brown LK, Barbieri CA, Harpel KS, DeLeo J. Prospective validation of an Acute Respiratory Distress Syndrome Predictive Score. Am J Respir Crit Care Med. 1995;152:1518–26.

36. McCloskey RV, Straube RC, Sanders C, Smith SM, Smith CR. Treatment of septic shock with human monoclonal antibody HA–1A. A randomized, double-blind, placebo-controlled trial. CHESS Trial Study Group. Ann Intern Med. 1994;121:1–5.

37. Ziegler EJ, Fischer CJ Jr, Sprung CL, et al. Treatment of gram-negative bacteremia and septic shock with HA-1A human monoclonal antibody against endotoxin. A randomized, double blind, placebo-controlled trial. The Ha-1A Sepsis Study Group. N Engl J Med. 1991;324:429–36.

38. Fischer CJ, Slotman GJ, Opal SM, et al. Initial evaluation of human recombinant interleukin-1 receptor antagonist in the treatment of sepsis syndrome: a randomized, open-label, placebo-controlled, multicenter trial. The IL-1RA Sepsis Syndrome Study Group. Crit Care Med 1994;22:12–21.

39. Fischer CJ Jr, Dhainaut JF, Opal SM, et al. Recombinant human interleukin 1 receptor antagonist in the treatment of patients with sepsis syndrome. Results from a randomized, double-blind, placebo-controlled trial. Phase III rhIL-1ra Sepsis Syndrome Study Group. JAMA. 1994;271:1836–43.

40. Opal SM, Fischer CJ, Dhainaut JF, et al. Confirmatory interleukin-1 receptor antagonist trial in severe sepsis: a phase III, randomized double-blind, placebo-controlled, multicenter trial. The interlukin-1 Receptor Antagonist Sepsis Investigator Group. Crit Care Med. 1997;25:1115–24.

41. Abraham E, Wunderink R, Silverman H, et al. Efficacy and safety of monoclonal antibody to human tumor necrosis factor α in patients with sepsis syndrome. A randomized, double-blind, multicenter clinical trial. TNF-α Mab Sepsis Study Group. JAMA. 1995;273:934–41.

42. Cohen J, Carlet J. INTERSEPT: an international, multicenter, placebo-controlled trial of monoclonal antibody to human tumor necrosis factor-α in patients with sepsis. International Sepsis Study Group. Crit Care Med. 1996;24:1431–40.

43. Reinhart K, Wiegand-Lohnert C, Grimminger F, et al. Assessment of the safety and efficacy of the monoclonal anti-tumor necrosis factor antibody-fragment, MAK 195F, in patients with sepsis and septic shock: A multicenter, randomized, placebo-controlled, dose-ranging study. Crit Care Med. 1996;24:733–42.

44. Abraham E, Glauser MP, Butler T, et al. P55 tumor necrosis factor receptor fusion protein in the treatment of patients with severe sepsis and septic shock. A randomized controlled multicenter trial. Ro 45–2081 Study Group. JAMA. 1997;277:1531–8.

45. Bernard GR, Luce JM, Sprung CL, et al. High-dose corticosteroids in patients with the adult respiratory distress syndrome. N Engl J Med. 1987;317:1565–70.

46. Bone RC, Fischer CJ Jr, Clemmer TP, Slotman GJ, Metz CA and the Methylprednisolone Severe Sepsis Study Group. Early methylprednisolone treatment for septic syndrome and the adult respiratory distress syndrome. Chest. 1987;92:1032–6.

47. Luce JM, Montgomery AB, Marks JD, Turnur J, Metz CA, Murray JF. Ineffectiveness of high-dose Methylprednisolone in preventing parenchymal lung injury and improving mortality in patients with septic shock. Am Rev Respir Dis. 1988;138:62–8.

48. Meduri GU, Headley AS, Golden E, et al. Effects of prolonged methyprednisolone therapy in unresolving acute respiratory distress syndrome: a randomized controlled trial. JAMA. 1998;280:159–65.

49. Abraham E, Park YC, Covingron P, Conrad SA, Schwartz M. Liposomal prostaglandin E$_1$ in acute respiratory distress syndrome: a placebo-controlled, randomized, double-blind, multicenter clinical trial. Crit Care Med. 1996;24:10-15.

50. Bone RC, Slotman G, Maunder R, et al. Randomized double-blind, multicenter study of prostaglandin E1 in patients with the adult respiratory distress syndrome. Prostaglandin E1 Study Group. Chest 1989;96:114–19.

51. Holcroft JW, Vassar MJ, Weber CJ. Prostaglandin E1 and survival in patients with the adult respiratory distress syndrome. A prospective trial. Ann Surg. 1986;203:371–8.

52. Jepsen S, Herlevsen P, Knudsen P, Bud MI, Klausen NO. Antioxidant treatment with N-acetylcysteine during adult respiratory distress syndrome: a prospective, randomized, placebo-controlled study. Crit Care Med. 1992;20:918–23.

53. Suter PM, Domenighetti G, Schaller M, Laverrière M, Ritz R, Perret C. N-Acetylcysteine enhances recovery from Acute Lung Injury in man. Chest. 1994;105:190–4.

54. Bernard GR, Wheeler AP, Arons MM, et al. A trial of antioxydant N-Acetylcysteine and Procysteine in ARDS. Chest. 1997;112:164–72.

55. Petros A, Lamb G, Leane A, Moncada S, Bennett D, Vallance P. Effects of nitric oxide synthase inhibitor in humans with septic shock. Cardiovasc Res. 1994;28:34–9.

56. Haupt MT, Jastremski MS, Clemmer TP, Metz CA, Goris GB. The Ibuprofen Study Group. Crit Care Med. 1991;19:1339–47.

57. Yu.M, Tomasa G. A double-blind, prospective, randomized trial of Ketoconazole, a thromboxame synthase inhibitor, in the prophylaxis of the adult respiratory distress syndrome. Crit Care Med. 1993;21:1635–42.

58. Artigas A, Bernard GR, Carlet J, et al. American–European Consensus Conference on ARDS, Part II. Ventilatory, pharmacologic, supportive therapy, study design strategies and issues related to recovery and remodelling. Intensive Care Med. 1998;24:378–98.

59. Gattinoni L, Bombino M, Pelosi P, et al. Lung structure and function in different stages of severe adult respiratory distress syndrome. JAMA. 1994;271:1772–9.

60. Krafft P, Fridrich P, Pernerstorfer T, et al. The adult respiratory distress syndrome: definitions, severity and clinical outcome. Intens Care Med. 1996;22:519–29.

61. D'Amico R, Pifferi S, Leonetti C, Torri V, Tinazzi A, Liberati A, on behalf of the study investigators. Effectiveness of antibiotic prophylaxis in critically ill adult patients: systematic review of randomised controlled trials. Br Med J. 1998;316:1275–85.

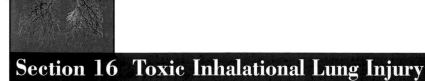
Chapter 70

Toxic Inhalational Lung Injury

Lee S Newman and Lisa A Maier

INTRODUCTION

A variety of chemicals when liberated into the atmosphere as gases, fumes, or mist can cause irritant lung injury or asphyxiation. As summarized in Figure 70.1, any level of the respiratory tract can be the target for toxins, which produce a wide range of disorders from tracheitis and bronchitis to pulmonary edema.

EPIDEMIOLOGY, RISK FACTORS, AND PATHOLOGY

Epidemiology

Smoke inhalation is common among the general population. The use of potentially toxic chemicals in industry continues to rise, and accidental spills, explosions, and fires can result in complex exposures for which little is known of the health consequences. It is challenging to estimate the potential magnitude of the health effects produced by inhaled toxins. For example, in the USA alone, more than 500,000 workers are at risk of exposure to ammonia (NH_3) and other gases such as sulfur dioxide (SO_2). More than 100,000 individuals have potential exposure to hydrogen sulfide (H_2S). Tens of thousands risk smoke inhalation from household fires. The number of people environmentally exposed to potentially hazardous levels of air pollutants such as ozone can be estimated in the tens of millions.

Etiology and risk factors

Major risk factors for inhalational exposure and injury are related to the environment and not to the host. Exposures occur randomly in the general environment, such as when a chemical spill occurs on a highway or railroad, carbon monoxide (CO) leaks in a home, or a person incorrectly mixes household chemicals together and releases a gas or aerosol[1]. Smoke that comprises the pyrolysis products of synthetic materials is a common cause of injury to the respiratory tract, as well as a cause of pulmonary insufficiency and death from fires. Occupational injuries are more common, and occur especially when workers handle chemicals, work in areas that are inadequately ventilated, or enter exposed areas with improper protective equipment[2]. Sources of occupational exposure to major chemical causes of irritant lung injury and asphyxiation are given in Figure 70.2.

Factors that influence the acute effects of toxic chemicals include solubility, particle size, concentration, duration of exposure, chemical properties, and host factors such as minute ventilation of the exposed individual. The more water-soluble compounds dissolve in the upper respiratory tract and airways,

Range of toxicity produced by inhaled agents	
Example of toxins	**Effect**
Carbon monoxide, cyanide, hydrogen sulfide	Asphyxiation
Ammonia	Mucous membrane irritation and sloughing
Ammonia, phosgene, hydrogen sulfide	Laryngeal edema and obstruction
Hydrogen chloride, chlorine	Tracheobronchitis
Ammonia	Bronchiectasis
Sulfur dioxide, hydrogen chloride, oxides of nitrogen, ozone	Bronchoconstriction, airway edema, asthma
Oxides of nitrogen, sulfur oxides	Bronchiolitis obliterans
Hydrogen fluoride, mustard gas	Chemical pneumonitis
Chlorine, phosgene	Adult respiratory distress syndrome
Hydrogen sulfide	Bacterial pneumonia
Ammonia	Pulmonary interstitial fibrosis
Hydrofluoric acid	Systemic effects, hypocalcemia, hypomagnesemia
Nitric oxide	Systemic effects, methemoglobinemia

Figure 70.1 Range of toxicity produced by inhaled agents.

Sources of exposure to inhalational toxins	
Toxin	**Sources of exposure**
Ammonia	Agriculture, explosives, plastics
Hydrogen chloride	Fertilizers, textiles, dyes, rubber manufacture
Hydrofluoric acid	Fertilizers, insecticides, glass and ceramic etching, masonry, metal working, pharmaceuticals, chemical manufacture
Sulfur dioxide	Air pollution, smelting, power plants, chemical manufacture, paper manufacture, food preparation
Chlorine	Household cleaners, paper, textiles, sewage treatment, swimming pools
Oxides of nitrogen	Air pollution, welding, hockey rinks, chemical and dye manufacture, agriculture
Phosgene	Firefighters, paint strippers, chemical, pharmaceutical, and dye manufacture, and chemical warfare
Mustard gas	Chemical warfare
Ozone	Welding, air pollution, high altitude, chemical manufacture
Carbon monoxide	Firefighters, smoke inhalation, smelters, miners, transportation, home furnaces
Hydrogen cyanide	Metallurgy, electroplating, plastics, polyurethane manufacture
Hydrogen sulfide	Metallurgy, chemical manufacture, waste-water treatment, natural gas and oil drilling, paper mills, coke ovens, rayon manufacture, rubber vulcanization

Figure 70.2 Sources of exposure to inhalational toxins.

encountered in the manufacture of fertilizers, textiles, rubber, and dyes, acute exposure causes mucous membrane irritation of the eyes and airways at levels as low at 5–10 parts per million (p.p.m.). Acute higher levels of exposure can cause acute airflow obstruction and gas exchange abnormalities. Meat wrappers become exposed to hydrogen chloride when using heated polyvinyl chloride film.

Hydrofluoric acid

Hydrofluoric acid (HF) is highly corrosive, and the majority of health effects from hydrofluoric acid involve dermal injury to the hands. Hydrofluoric acid releases free hydrogen ions that penetrate and corrode the skin, potentially down to bone, and even produce bone demineralization and necrosis. The respiratory effects parallel those of the skin, except that in the lungs the effects have a very rapid onset and patients present with acute respiratory distress. Hydrofluoric acid is water soluble and thus exerts its predominant effects on the upper airways, which results in the rapid onset of tissue damage and bronchoconstriction, and sometimes even leads to chemical pneumonitis, delayed onset pulmonary edema, and death.

Sulfur dioxide

Sulfur dioxide and sulfuric acid (H_2SO_4) aerosols are produced by fossil fuel combustion. They are encountered in power plants and in various industrial processes such as smelting, chemical manufacture, paper manufacture, food preservation, metal and ore refining, and refrigeration. Past sulfur dioxide air pollution catastrophes have been associated with increased death rates for patients with chronic lung disease and the elderly.

As little as 0.5 p.p.m. of sulfur dioxide can be detected in air from its characteristic odor. At levels of 6–10 p.p.m., immediate irritation of eyes and nasopharynx are reported. High exposures ($\geq$ 50 p.p.m.) injure the larynx, trachea, bronchi, and alveoli. A wide range of individual variability in the response to this substance is found, but atopics and asthmatics show the most susceptibility. Prior exposure to ozone may potentiate the effect of sulfur dioxide in asthmatics. Classically, patients first experience a burning of the eyes, nose, and throat (with associated cough, chest pain, chest tightness, and dyspnea), along with conjunctivitis, corneal burns, and pharyngeal edema, followed hours later by pulmonary edema. Individuals can develop bronchiolitis obliterans 2–3 weeks after exposure. Persistent airflow obstruction has been observed in smelter workers up to 4 years after overexposure, probably because of bronchiolitis obliterans.

Treatment is symptomatic. Systemic corticosteroids may be beneficial in acute toxicity. Bronchospasm in asthmatics may reverse spontaneously after removal from exposure, or may require administration of bronchodilators and inhaled corticosteroids.

Chlorine

Chlorine is of intermediate solubility, and liberates hydrogen chloride and oxygen free-radicals when it contacts water. The result is dose-dependent epithelial cell injury. At low levels of exposure, the upper airways and eyes are irritated. Increasing levels of exposure injure the nasopharynx and larynx. Higher exposures result in pulmonary edema within 6–24 hours. Pulmonary function tests typically show airflow obstruction and air trapping. Long-term consequences include persistent airflow obstruction in some survivors. Clinical management is supportive. Even symptomatic individuals who have negative physical

examinations and laboratory tests must be observed for at least 6 hours because of the potential for a delay in the onset of significant airway toxicity. If symptoms persist, corticosteroids may improve outcome[9].

Oxides of nitrogen

The oxides of nitrogen (NO, NO_2, N_2O_4) can produce fatal respiratory injury for some of the millions of workers who come into contact with these gases. Occupations at risk include coal miners following firing of explosives, welders who work with acetylene torches in confined spaces, hockey rink workers, and chemical workers who may be exposed to by-product fumes in the manufacture of dyes, lacquers, and nitric acid (HNO_3). 'Silo-filler's disease' is caused by inhalation of nitrogen dioxide that forms when corn or alfalfa stored in a silo ferments. The risk is greatest in the first few weeks after the silo is filled[10]. Since the oxides of nitrogen have low water solubility, the lower respiratory tract can be exposed to these potent oxidizers with little warning. Nitrogen dioxide reacts with water in the lung to form nitric and nitrous (HNO_2) acids. The oxides dissociate into oxygen free-radicals, nitrates, and nitrites, which cause tissue inflammation, lipid peroxidation, and impairment of surfactant activity (among other cellular changes). Notably, nitric oxide has a high affinity for hemoglobin, and so causes methemoglobinemia.

With exposures of 15–25 p.p.m., acute mucous membrane irritation affects the eyes and throat. At exposure levels of 25–100 p.p.m., toxic pneumonitis and bronchiolitis can develop, often with a smothering sensation and dyspnea. Exposures above 150 p.p.m. are often fatal, and associated with bronchiolitis obliterans, chemical pneumonitis, and pulmonary edema. Nitrogen oxide and nitrogen dioxide produce the greatest degree of toxicity, which includes pulmonary edema and subsequent bronchiolitis obliterans. Symptom onset may be delayed and patients are also cautioned that relapses can occur 3–6 weeks after initial exposure, with symptoms of cough, chills, fever, and shortness of breath. Some individuals develop persistent obstructive lung disease and chronic bronchitis. Case reports suggest improvement after corticosteroids in those who manifest bronchiolar inflammation.

Phosgene

Also called carbonyl chloride, phosgene replaced chlorine as the preferred chemical weapon of World War I, and resulted in the majority of gas attack fatalities. Phosgene is an intermediate product in the manufacture of isocyanates, pesticides, dyes, and pharmaceuticals. It has a low odor threshold at 1 p.p.m., and produces a characteristic smell of musty hay. As a result of its poor water solubility, phosgene causes only mild upper airway and eye irritant symptoms, and deposits distally in the lung where it hydrolyzes to form hydrochloric acid (aqueous HCl) and carbon dioxide. At high levels of exposure, dyspnea, chest tightness, and cough occur. Acute exposure produces necrosis and sloughing of tracheal, bronchial, and bronchiolar mucosa with associated edema, hemorrhage, and atelectasis. Progressive respiratory failure and ARDS may follow.

Mustard gas

Sulfur mustard gas was first used as a chemical warfare agent in Europe in 1917. Mustard agents are not gases, but liquids at environmental temperatures. They are volatile, enter vapor phase at ambient temperatures, and have low water solubility. Exposure to sulfur mustard produces eye irritation and swelling within 2–3 hours. With higher exposure, blurred vision, conjunctival edema, and iritis can occur, with potential for corneal ulceration. The skin becomes pruritic, erythematous, and, 4–16 hours later, forms blisters. Acute respiratory damage in this setting may be evident within a few hours or, more commonly, several days later. Chemical pneumonitis and pulmonary edema can also occur, with upper airway irritation, sneezing, hoarseness, epistaxis, cough, and dyspnea. Acute injury includes edema, inflammation, and destruction of the airway epithelium, with pseudomembranes developing that are similar to those seen with diphtheria. Secondary complications include infection and airway stenosis. The long-term effects include death caused by respiratory infections, chronic bronchitis, and accelerated longitudinal decline in airflow.

Ozone

Ozone is a light blue gas with an acrid 'electric' odor. It occurs naturally in the stratosphere, where it is produced by the interaction between oxygen and ultraviolet light. In the troposphere, it is produced as a result of photochemical reactions between oxides of nitrogen and volatile organic compounds. Ozone is a major component of environmental air pollution and remains a serious pollutant for urban populations worldwide. Its low water solubility means that ozone principally affects the lower respiratory tract. In healthy individuals exposed to low concentrations of ozone, acute increases in airway resistance and decreases in FEV_1 and forced vital capacity have been reported, probably through a neural reflex mechanism. With acute exposures to low concentrations, patients can develop chest pain, dyspnea, and cough. Exposure to concentrations as low as 0.08 p.p.m. for 6 hours with intermittent exercise has been shown to cause lung function and inflammatory changes. Exposure to 0.12 p.p.m. for 1 hour is the US Environmental Protection Agency Air Quality Standard.

Chemical asphyxiants

Nitrous oxide, carbon monoxide, hydrogen cyanide (HCN), and hydrogen sulfide interfere with oxygen delivery, which results in asphyxiation. Others, such as methane, ethane (C_2H_6), argon (Ar), and helium (He_2), are more innocuous at low concentrations, but at high exposure levels can displace oxygen or block the reaction of cytochrome oxidase or hemoglobin, impairing cellular respiration and oxygen transport. Several important asphyxiants are discussed below.

Carbon monoxide

Carbon monoxide is colorless, tasteless, and odorless, and is the major cause of death by poisoning in the USA and most industrialized countries. Exposure results from incomplete combustion of carbon-containing materials such as gasoline, coal, and wood. Home exposures occur from furnace gas leaks or fire smoke inhalation. Methylene chloride (CH_2Cl_2), which is used in paint strippers and as a household solvent, metabolizes into carbon monoxide and can be deadly if handled in poorly ventilated areas[11].

Severe forms of carbon monoxide poisoning are characterized by unconsciousness, seizures, syncope, coma, neurologic deficits, pulmonary edema, myocardial ischemia, and metabolic acidosis. Lower exposures produce symptoms of headache, nausea, weakness, giddiness, and tinnitus. Confusion typically occurs at carboxyhemoglobin levels >30%, with coma ensuing at 35–45%, and death at 50%. In addition to acute toxic effects, victims are at risk for delayed neuropsychologic effects. Carboxyhemoglobin levels correlate poorly with the clinical severity of neurologic sequelae. Carbon monoxide half-life in individuals at rest is approximately 4 hours and can be reduced to 60–90 minutes by breathing 100% oxygen by face mask or to <60 minutes with oxygen administered by manual bag-assisted ventilation.

Nonrandomized studies have found that hyperbaric oxygen reverses the acute effects of carbon monoxide poisoning and is the most rapid means of reversing acute poisoning. Additional treatments may improve acute neurologic defects. Results of controlled trials are unclear as to the efficacy of hyperbaric oxygen as a treatment for the delayed neuropsychologic symptoms. Cardiac monitoring is warranted for individuals who have carboxyhemoglobin levels >25%, because of the risk of arrhythmias and myocardial infarction[5].

Hydrogen cyanide

Individuals exposed to smoke generated by the combustion or pyrolysis of plastics and polyurethanes are at particular risk of hydrogen cyanide toxicity. The fumes are absorbed through the skin and respiratory tract. By binding to the cytochrome A–cytochrome A_3 subcomplex, hydrogen cyanide blocks oxidative phosphorylation and mitochondrial oxygen utilization, which results in lactic acidosis.

Symptoms produced by exposures to 50 p.p.m. of cyanide gas include headache, tachycardia, tachypnea, and dizziness. Exposures >100 p.p.m. can cause confusion, apnea, and seizures. The patient may emit a bitter almond odor, but this is not a reliable or consistent marker of exposure. The key to diagnosis rests with the occupational and environmental history. Venous blood appears hyperoxygenated and the patient may have a distinctive red appearance prior to respiratory insufficiency, although, as in carbon monoxide poisoning, this is not a reliable clinical sign. Carboxyhemoglobin levels are measured to help separate cyanide intoxication from carbon monoxide poisoning. Treatment focuses on life-support measures and detoxification. Early mechanical ventilation, hyperoxygenation, and treatment of metabolic acidosis are critical. Amyl nitrate followed by sodium nitrite is recommended. Amyl nitrate and sodium nitrite form methemoglobin. Sodium thiosulfate binds the cyanide and can also be used following amyl nitrate.

Hydrogen sulfide

Hydrogen sulfide is both a respiratory irritant and asphyxiant. As a colorless, naturally occurring gas, it is found in marshes, sulfur springs, and as a decay product of organic matter. It is known for its typical 'rotten-egg' odor. Occupational exposure occurs in the manufacture of chemicals and metals, and in petroleum refineries, natural gas plants, coke ovens, paper mills, rubber vulcanization, rayon manufacture, and tanneries. Heavier than air, hydrogen sulfide accumulates in low-lying areas; it causes poisoning during oil drilling and waste-water treatment and as a result of natural gas field leaks. The hydrogen sulfide reaction with metalloenzymes, such as cytochrome oxidase, accounts for much of its toxicity in humans.

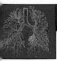

The odor threshold for this gas is low (0.13 p.p.m.). At concentrations of 50 p.p.m., hydrogen sulfide is a mucous membrane irritant. Above 100 p.p.m., the gas fatigues the sense of olfaction, which makes individuals insensitive to its continued presence. When inhaled, it preferentially affects the lower respiratory tract. At concentrations of 250 p.p.m., pulmonary edema can occur. At 500 p.p.m., systemic and neurologic effects develop, with sudden loss of consciousness seen above 700 p.p.m. At >1000 p.p.m., the gas produces hyperpnea and apnea, which paralyzes respiratory drive centers. Thus, death caused by asphyxia can result at 1000 p.p.m. or above.

Prolonged low level (50 p.p.m.) exposures can cause respiratory tract inflammation and drying; typical symptoms of cough, sore throat, hoarseness, rhinitis, and chest tightness occur between 50 and 250 p.p.m. At higher acute exposure levels, such symptoms may not manifest because of the rapid absorption of the gas through the lung into the blood stream.

Management is generally supportive, with prompt endotracheal intubation and mechanical ventilation for severe cases of intoxication. Oxygen enhances sulfide metabolism and benefits hypoxic tissue. As the mechanism of toxicity is similar to that of cyanide, induction of methemoglobinemia with infusion of 3% sodium nitrite or inhalation of amyl nitrate is recommended. Hyperbaric oxygen therapy may be beneficial.

PITFALLS AND CONTROVERSIES

Many of the uncertainties in this arena of pulmonary medicine pertain to the management and treatment of inhalational injury, for which a few general comments apply. In cases of severe inhalational injury, intubation may be required for airway protection. Careful observation, preferably in an intensive-care setting, is recommended for suspected cases of significant inhalational injury. Direct laryngoscopy or fiberoptic bronchoscopy is advocated by some investigators to assess for laryngeal edema. However, no clear guidelines are available to direct clinicians as to when intubation, laryngoscopy, or bronchoscopy is warranted. While many clinicians may empirically prescribe corticosteroids, such medications have not been proved efficacious. We are dependent on case reports and small case series to justify the use of corticosteroids.

A common clinical pitfall is prematurely to dismiss patients who may be at risk for delayed-onset respiratory disorders such as asthma, bronchiolitis obliterans, chemical pneumonitis, or pulmonary edema. Given sufficient dose and solubility, most acutely inhaled substances pose a risk for immediate or delayed-onset pulmonary edema, which warrants careful observation. Even those toxin victims who are thought to be stable and ready for discharge from the emergency room must be given detailed instructions about the warning signs of delayed-onset respiratory tract injury.

REFERENCES

1. Blanc PD, Galbo M, Hiatt P, Olson KR. Morbidity following acute irritant inhalation in a population-based study. JAMA. 1991; 266:664–9.
2. Newman LS. Current concepts: occupational illness. N Engl J Med. 1995;333:1128–34.
3. King TE Jr. Bronchiolitis. In: Schwarz MI, King TE Jr, eds. Interstitial lung disease, 3rd edn. Hamilton: BC Decker; 1998:645–84.
4. Colby TV, Swensen SJ. Anatomic distribution and histopathologic patterns in interstitial lung disease. In: Schwarz MI, King TE Jr, eds. Interstitial lung disease, 3rd edn. Hamilton: BC Decker; 1998:31–49.
5. Rorison DG, McPherson SJ. Acute toxic inhalations. Emerg Med Clin North Am. 1992;10:409–35.
6. Chan-Yeung M, Malo J-L. Current concepts: occupational asthma. N Engl J Med. 1995;33:107–12.
7. Becklake MR. Chronic airflow limitation: its relationship to work in dusty occupations. Chest. 1985;88:608–17.
8. Kennedy SM. Acquired airway hyperresponsiveness from non-immunogenic irritant exposure. In: Beckett WS, Bascome R, eds. Occupational medicine: state of the art reviews. Philadelphia: Hanley and Belfus; 1992:287–300.
9. Chester EH, Kaimal PH, Payne CB Jr, Kohn PM. Pulmonary injury following exposure to chlorine gas. Chest. 1977;72:247–50.
10. Douglas WW, Hepper NGG, Colby TV. Silo-filler's disease. Mayo Clin Proc. 1989;64:291–304.
11. Stewart RD, Hake CL. Paint-remover hazard. JAMA. 1976;235:398–401.

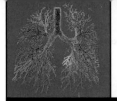

Section 17 Chest Wall Disorders

Chapter 71

Scoliosis and Kyphoscoliosis

Anita K Simonds

INTRODUCTION

Spinal curvature is the most common cause of chest wall deformity. A scoliosis describes lateral curvature of the spine (Fig. 71.1). Kyphosis indicates backward and lordosis forward curvature in an anteroposterior (median) plane. Many patients who have a thoracic scoliosis are mistakenly described as having a kyphoscoliosis, because the rib angle prominence is misinterpreted as a kyphotic component. In fact, most idiopathic thoracic scolioses incorporate a lordotic and rotatory element. The degree of lateral curvature is expressed by the Cobb angle, which is calculated from a radiograph as shown in Figure 71.2.

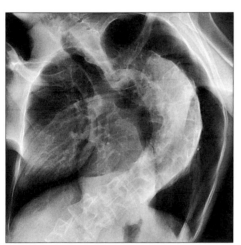

Figure 71.1 Early onset thoracic scoliosis caused by arthrogryposis.

Calculation of Cobb angle

Cobb angle

Figure 71.2 Method of calculation of Cobb angle. From the vertebral bodies at the top and bottom of the curve lines are drawn parallel to the planes of the vertebral bodies. Perpendicular lines to these are then drawn and the Cobb angle is found at the intersection.

EPIDEMIOLOGY, RISK FACTORS, AND PATHOPHYSIOLOGY

The causes of chest wall deformity are shown in Figure 71.3. By far the most common form of scoliosis is the idiopathic variety, which accounts for approximately 80% of cases. Scoliotic curves of more than 35° affect 1/1000 of the population and those that exceed 70° are estimated to occur at a rate of 0.1/1000[1]; females are at greater risk of severe curves than are males. Idiopathic scoliosis occurs more often with increasing maternal age and in higher socioeconomic groups, but there is no association between the incidence of scoliosis and birth order, or season of birth[2].

Marfan syndrome affects 1/5000 of the population and around 63% of affected individuals develop a spinal deformity. Diagnosis can be confirmed by linkage to the Marfan syndrome gene MFS1, which produces fibrillin. Related syndromes may result from mutations in microfibrils that interact with fibrillin in the extracellular matrix[3]. Congenital arachnodactyly (Beals' syndrome), in which scoliosis is common, has also been shown to be caused by fibrillin deficiency. The genetic basis of idiopathic scoliosis remains unclear and causation may be shown to be polygenic

Classification of spinal deformity	
Idiopathic deformities	**Associated with neuromuscular disease**
Idiopathic scoliosis	Cerebral palsy
Idiopathic kyphosis	Poliomyelitis
Congenital deformities	Muscular dystrophies
Bone	Myopathies
Scoliosis	Hereditary sensory motor neuropathies
Kyphosis	Friedreich's ataxia
Cord	Syringomyelia
Myelodysplasia	**Acquired deformity caused by**
Syndromes in which scoliosis is common	Surgery/trauma
	Infection
Neurofibromatosis	Pyogenic
Marfan syndrome	Tuberculosis (Pott's kyphosis)
Osteogenesis imperfecta	Radiotherapy
Klippel–Feil syndrome	Tumor
Muccopolysaccharidoses	Neuroblastoma
Treacher Collins syndrome	Osteoma
Goldenhar's syndrome	Hemangioma
Apert's syndrome	Chordoma
Ehlers–Danlos syndrome	Eosinophilic granuloma
Vertebral and epiphyseal dysplasias	
Arthrogryposis	

Figure 71.3 Classification of spinal deformity.

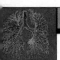

and multifactorial, in that particular growth patterns may exacerbate a genetic predisposition.

Spinal curvature is acquired in neuromuscular disorders that involve the chest wall and thoracic musculature before skeletal maturity occurs. Up to 50% of boys who have Duchenne's muscular dystrophy develop a scoliosis, and spinal curvature is common in many of the other congenital muscular dystrophies, myopathies, and conditions such as types I and II spinal muscular atrophy. A scoliosis often develops after a thoracotomy carried out in childhood or young adulthood.

Kyphosis

Idiopathic kyphosis is rare (see Fig. 71.3). An increase in thoracic kyphosis occurs with age and is exacerbated by factors that increase a tendency to osteoporosis such as oral corticosteroid therapy. Pott's tuberculosis (TB) of the spine is still a common cause of acquired kyphosis.

Effects of chest wall deformity on respiratory and cardiac function

Chest wall disorders affect respiratory function and cause a restrictive ventilatory defect. Any significant scoliosis or kyphosis results in a loss of height, so that arm span is used to predict normal lung volumes. As a rule of thumb, patients who have a thoracic curve >70° are subject to significant ventilatory limitation[1].

Lung volumes

While both scoliosis and kyphosis diminish lung volumes, which results in a restrictive ventilatory defect, lateral curvature has a more profound effect on chest wall mechanics. Total lung capacity is reduced in all chest wall disorders. In a pure scoliosis, both vital capacity (VC) and expiratory reserve volume are decreased with relative preservation of residual volume (Fig. 71.4). An obstructive ventilatory defect is rare in scoliosis and kyphosis, unless the individual is a smoker.

The relationship between pulmonary impairment and the deformity is complex and cannot be predicted accurately from the Cobb angle alone[4]. The four major determinants of a reduced VC are the number of vertebrae involved in the curve, cephalad position of the curve, Cobb angle, and the degree of loss of normal thoracic kyphosis.

In paralytic scoliosis, lung volumes are reduced not only by chest wall restriction, but also by respiratory muscle weakness.

Chest wall mechanics

Chest wall compliance (Ccw) is an important determinant of lung volumes and the work of breathing. Individuals with a Cobb angle of <50° experience a minimal reduction in Ccw, whereas Ccw is likely to be significantly reduced if the Cobb angle is >100°. A direct relationship between Cobb angle and Ccw is not seen in patients who have neuromuscular disorders, as respiratory muscle weakness contributes independently to chest wall stiffness. Alteration in chest wall properties cannot solely be attributed to the mechanical deformity of scoliosis, as Estenne et al.[5] have demonstrated a decrease in Ccw in 75% of patients (VC <60% predicted) affected by chronic respiratory muscle weakness in the absence of a scoliosis.

Lung compliance

Although lung expansion is compromised by chest wall properties, primary pulmonary pathology is unusual in patients who have idiopathic scoliosis. However, lung compliance is reduced because of a shift in the pressure–volume curve to the right. These changes in pulmonary characteristics largely arise from an alteration in alveolar forces caused by chronic hypoventilation. In neuromuscular patients, micro- and macroatelectasis may complicate the picture. Microatelectasis seems relatively rare, however, as fine-section computed tomography scans have shown areas of atelectasis in only a minority of patients affected by respiratory muscle weakness[6]. Recurrent aspiration pneumonia may occur in neuromuscular patients who have bulbar weakness. Pulmonary fibrosis is also seen in patients who have old TB, and these individuals may have areas of bronchiectasis. Cystic lung changes affect some individuals with neurofibromatosis.

Gas transfer coefficient tends to be raised in scoliotic patients in the presence of a low transfer factor (see Fig. 71.4), because extrathoracic compression squeezes more air than blood out of the lungs, and thereby decreases accessible alveolar volume.

Respiratory muscles/thoracic pump during sleep

Impaired respiratory muscle function might be expected in idiopathic scoliosis, as the respiratory muscles work at a mechanical disadvantage when chest wall shape is altered. Lisboa et al.[7] showed reduced transdiaphragmatic pressure in patients who have scoliosis. Other workers have confirmed a reduction in static respiratory mouth pressure in patients who suffer scoliosis[8] and thoracoplasty[9]. These findings tend to support the contention that the efficiency of the respiratory muscles may be affected by relatively small degrees of chest wall deformity. Respiratory muscle action is further reduced by the loss of intercostal muscle tone during rapid eye movement (REM) sleep, and a reduced ability to compensate for added respiratory load. This explains why early features of ventilatory failure during sleep predate the development of diurnal ventilatory failure.

Control of breathing

Impaired hypercapnic ventilatory drive is usually secondary to chronic carbon dioxide retention in scoliotic patients. However, primary drive disorders may complicate some neuromuscular conditions, and may be acquired in patients who have poliomyelitis that affects brainstem control mechanisms. Generally, however, ventilatory drive is increased in neuromuscular patients to compensate for respiratory muscle insufficiency.

Typical pulmonary function results in idiopathic thoracic scoliosis	
Parameter	**Effect**
Forced expiratory volume in 1s (FEV_1)	Reduced
Forced vital capacity (FVC)	Reduced
FEV_1/FVC	Normal
Residual volume	Normal
Total lung capacity	Reduced
Transfer factor for carbon monoxide (DLCO)	Reduced
Transfer coefficient (DLCO /accessible alveolar volume; KCO)	Supranormal

Figure 71.4 Typical pulmonary function results in idiopathic thoracic scoliosis. Transfer coefficient is usually supranormal, but it is reduced in the presence of pulmonary hypertension.

Pulmonary and cardiac hemodynamics

Cor pulmonale is the end-stage result of severe, untreated chest wall deformity. The pulmonary artery pressure becomes elevated at rest with an inverse correlation between pulmonary artery pressure and arterial oxygen tensions.

An additional stress on hemodynamics is the effect of nocturnal hypoventilation on pulmonary artery pressure. The exact level of nocturnal hypoxemia that generates pulmonary hypertension is unknown, but severe, nocturnal arterial blood gas disturbances inevitably lead to daytime problems if untreated.

CLINICAL FEATURES

Spinal abnormalities are best understood by describing the age of onset, etiology, and location of the curve (e.g. adolescent onset, idiopathic thoracic scoliosis). During physical examination accompanying features should be sought, such as café-au-lait spots and neurofibromata. Marfan syndrome is a clinical diagnosis that requires the involvement of two out of three main systems (ocular, cardiac, and skeletal). A careful search for cardiac lesions is mandatory in early-onset scoliosis, which has an increased incidence of congenital heart disease. Lesions demonstrated radiologically, such as hemivertebrae and rib fusion, suggest the presence of a congenital scoliosis.

Patients are observed in the standing position and viewed bending forward to obtain an indication of the degree of lateral rib hump deformity. The lower back is examined for hairy tufts and other cutaneous stigmata of spinal dysraphism.

Progression of curvature

Only one in five curves that are <20° progress[10]. Detailed studies of the natural history of untreated idiopathic scoliosis are rare, but the younger the age at presentation, the greater the potential for progression as more of the growth spurt needs to be accommodated, and spinal growth continues until at least the age of 25 years. High and low thoracic curves together with thoracolumbar curves seem to be more unstable than lumbar deformities. Curves most likely to progress include those caused by congenital failure of segmentation, infantile idiopathic scoliosis, the angular curve of neurofibromatosis, pronounced paralytic curves, and scoliosis associated with progressive childhood neuromuscular conditions[10].

DIAGNOSIS

Cardiopulmonary decompensation – identification of high-risk cases

The vast majority of patients who have a thoracic spinal curvature do not develop cardiorespiratory problems and therefore do not require long-term respiratory follow up. However, it is important to be able to identify the minority at risk of problems so that appropriate therapeutic intervention be carried out.

Cor pulmonale was the primary cause of death in a series of 102 untreated idiopathic thoracic scoliosis patients[11]. Age at onset of the scoliosis is crucial. Branthwaite showed that in patients who developed cardiorespiratory problems attributable to their scoliosis, 90% had an early-onset curvature (i.e. onset before the age of 5 years)[12].

A VC of 50% predicted is an important cut-off figure, as those with a VC of <50% predicted at presentation are much more likely to develop respiratory decompensation than those who have larger lung volumes.

The mean age of patients in respiratory failure who presented for ventilatory support was 49 years in idiopathic scoliosis patients, 51 years in patients who had previous poliomyelitis, and 62 years in those who suffered sequelae of pulmonary TB. Pehrsson et al. followed lung function over for a period of 20 years in idiopathic scoliosis patients[13]. Respiratory failure occurred in 25%, all of whom had a VC <45% predicted and a thoracic Cobb angle >110°.

Monitoring high-risk patients

Pulmonary function, arterial blood gas tensions, and assessment of respiratory muscle strength using mouth pressures is helpful, particularly in the group who have neuromuscular disease. A fall in VC of >15% on assuming the supine position indicates significant diaphragm weakness. Braun et al. showed that daytime hypercapnia is associated with mouth pressure <30% predicted[14].

As well as inquiries about breathlessness and exercise tolerance, patients are asked about symptoms of nocturnal hypoventilation (morning headache, poor sleep quality, frequent arousals, nocturnal confusion, and morning anorexia), and if any are present the patient should undergo monitoring of respiration during sleep. A characteristic picture of nocturnal hypoventilation is usually found with episodes of desaturation and carbon dioxide retention, most pronounced in REM sleep (Fig. 71.5).

TREATMENT

Management of spinal deformity
Conservative management

The success of a conservative approach depends on the age of the patient, the curve size at presentation, and its propensity to progression.

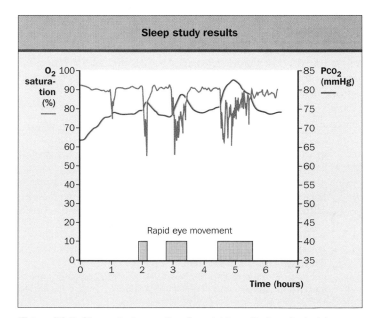

Figure 71.5 Sleep study results. Overnight monitoring of arterial oxygen saturation and transcutaneous carbon dioxide in an individual who has congenital scoliosis that presented with morning headaches. Note the marked desaturation and carbon dioxide retention during episodes of rapid eye movement sleep.

Surgery for scoliosis

In general, surgery is performed to correct unacceptable deformity and prevent progression. It is not carried out to improve ventilatory function.

Thoracic scolioses >45° are usually judged unacceptable[10]. However, a lesser curve associated with a greater degree of rotation may create a rib hump, which is just as concerning to the patient. It is a surgical maxim that even the best operative technique does not completely straighten a spine. About a 50% correction of the Cobb angle in smaller curves can be expected from a Harrington rod procedure[10]. The best guide to a successful result is the initial amount of spinal flexibility. Also, the greater the degree of rotation, the greater the inflexibility of the curve.

Spinal fusion followed by casting has now been superceded in many situations by Harrington rod instrumentation. The system provides distraction to the concave side of the spine and compression to the convex side, which enhances stabilization and reduces any rotational tendency.

Ventilatory impairment

Optimization of respiratory function

Patients must be advised about smoking and obesity. The influenza and pneumococcal vaccine are recommended for those who have ventilatory limitation.

Hormone replacement therapy reduces the risk of osteoporosis in postmenopausal females. Care should be taken not to miss the reactivation of TB in patients with a thoracoplasty. Patients who suffer Marfan syndrome may require β-blocker therapy to reduce the risk of aortic dissection.

Exercise is encouraged, apart from for those who have pulmonary hypertension and in individuals with Marfan syndrome.

Pulmonary rehabilitation programs suggest that exercise and a reduction in deconditioning is just as valuable in restrictive disease as in chronic obstructive pulmonary disease[15].

Treatment of ventilatory insufficiency

In patients who experience a progressive fall in lung volumes, positive pressure hyperinflation carried out with a portable device several times a day may reverse this trend. Protriptyline at low dose (5–10mg at night) may reduce mild-to-moderate nocturnal hypoventilation and act as a holding therapy until ventilatory support is required.

Ventilatory failure

The evidence now clearly shows that ventilatory failure in patients who have chest wall disease can be successfully treated using noninvasive ventilation at night. Negative pressure devices are effective, but have been largely supplanted by nasal positive-pressure ventilation (NIPPV). In scoliotic patients who receive NIPPV 5-year survival is around 80%, with figures of 100% in patients with previous poliomyelitis and over 90% in those with post-tuberculous conditions[16,17]. It seems increasingly likely that individuals who have nonprogressive disorders may live a normal or near-normal life span, provided NIPPV is introduced before the development of intractable pulmonary hypertension. Patients report good quality of life using NIPPV, and many are able to return to work.

Also, NIPPV can be used to palliate symptoms of breathlessness and cor pulmonale in patients who have progressive disorders, and will alter the natural history of these conditions. Early work suggests that 5-year survival as high as 73% can be achieved in Duchenne's muscular dystrophy[18].

REFERENCES

1. Bergofsky EH. Thoracic deformities. In: Roussos C, ed. The Thorax. Part C: disease, 2nd edn. New York: Marcel Dekker, Inc; 1995;66:1915–49.
2. Ryan MD, Nachemson A. Thoracic idiopathic scoliosis: perinatal and environmental aspects in a Swedish population and their relationship to curve severity. J Pediatr Orthop. 1987;7:72–7.
3. Child A. Marfan syndrome – current medical and genetic knowledge: how to treat and when. J Card Surg. 1997;12(Suppl.):131–6.
4. Kearon C, Guillermo RV, Kirkly A, Killian KJ. Factors determining pulmonary function in adolescent idiopathic thoracic scoliosis. Am Rev Respir Dis. 1993;148:288–94.
5. Estenne M, Heilporn A, Delhez L, Yernault J-C, De Troyer A. Chest wall stiffness in patients with chronic respiratory muscle weakness. Am Rev Respir Dis. 1983;128:1002–7.
6. Kinnear W, Gevenois PA, Estenne M, De Troyer A. Reduced pulmonary compliance in quadriplegic patients – the role of microatelectasis. Am Rev Respir Dis. 1991;143:A166.
7. Lisboa C, Moreno R, Fava M, Ferretti R, Cruz E. Inspiratory muscle function in patients with severe kyphoscoliosis. Am Rev Respir Dis. 1985;132:48–52.
8. Cooper DM, Rojas JV, Mellins RB, Keim HA, Mansell AL. Respiratory mechanics in adolescents with idiopathic scoliosis. Am Rev Respir Dis. 1984;130:16–22.
9. Shneerson JM. Deformities of the thoracic cage. II Acquired deformities. In: Emerson P, ed. Thoracic medicine, 1st edn. London: Butterworths; 1981:363–4.
10. Leatherman KD, Dickson RA, Leatherman KDDRA. Basic principles. In: Leatherman KD, Dickson RA, Leatherman KDDRA, eds. The management of spinal deformities, 1st edn. 1988;1–27.
11. Freyschuss V, Nilsonne U, Lundgren KD. Idiopathic scoliosis in old age. 1. Respiratory function. Arch Med Scand. 1968;184:365.
12. Branthwaite MA. Cardiorespiratory consequences of unfused idiopathic scoliosis. Br J Dis Chest. 1986;80:360–9.
13. Pehrsson K, Bake B, Larsson S, Nachemson A. Lung function in adult idiopathic scoliosis: a 20 year follow up. Thorax. 1991;46:474–8.
14. Braun NMT, Rochester DF. Muscular weakness and respiratory failure. Am Rev Respir Dis. 1979;119(Suppl.):123–5.
15. Simonds AK. Pulmonary rehabilitation in non-COPD disorders. In: Simonds AK, Muir JF, Pierson DJ, eds. Pulmonary rehabilitation, 1st edn. London: BMJ Publishing Group; 1996:212–35.
16. Simonds AK, Elliott MW. Outcome of domiciliary nasal intermittent positive pressure ventilation in restrictive and obstructive disorders. Thorax. 1995;50:604–9.
17. Leger P, Bedicam JM, Cornette A, et al. Nasal intermittent positive pressure ventilation. Long term follow-up in patients with severe chronic respiratory insufficiency. Chest. 1994;105:100–5.
18. Simonds AK, Fielding S, Muntoni F. Impact of nasal ventilation on survival in hypercapnic Duchenne muscular dystrophy (DMD) patients. Eur Respir J. 1997;10:35.

Chapter 72
Acute and Chronic Neuromuscular Disorders

Jean-William Fitting

PATHOPHYSIOLOGY

The exchange of carbon dioxide and oxygen between the blood and the atmosphere results from an integrated process that involves the ventilatory pump and the lungs. The ventilatory pump is complex and extends from the central nervous system to the chest wall, the engines of which are the respiratory muscles. A variety of neuromuscular disorders may affect the ventilatory pump at different sites (Fig. 72.1). When severe, acute neuromuscular disorders result in respiratory failure. Chronic neuromuscular disorders manifest by progressive respiratory insufficiency, but may also present as acute respiratory failure as the initial manifestation, an intercurrent complication, or the terminal event. With few exceptions, these disorders induce respiratory muscle weakness, which itself results in alveolar hypoventilation and impaired cough.

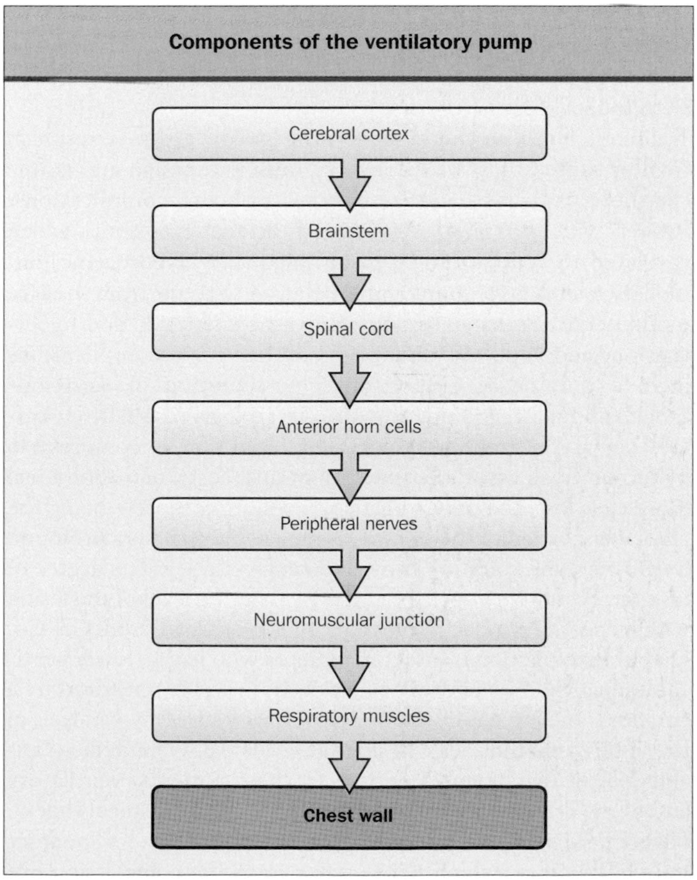

Lung volumes

Weakness of inspiratory and expiratory muscles cause a reduction of vital capacity (VC) and of its components. The end-expiratory lung volume, or functional residual capacity (FRC), is decreased, whereas residual volume (RV) may be normal or increased (Fig. 72.2)[1-3]. As a consequence of the sigmoidal shape of the pressure–volume relationship of the respiratory system, large changes in inspiratory pressure exerted near total lung capacity (TLC), or large changes in expiratory pressure exerted near RV, produce only small changes in lung volume. Nevertheless, the actual loss of lung volume is always higher than expected for a given loss of muscle strength in neuromuscular disorders, because of alterations of lung and chest wall mechanics, which are present even in the absence of associated scoliosis[4].

Lung and chest wall mechanics

Acute respiratory muscle weakness results in loss of lung volume without change in compliance. In contrast, long-standing respiratory muscle weakness is associated with a modification of the lung pressure–volume relationship; the lung elastic recoil pressure is lower than normal at TLC (which is itself reduced), but is higher than normal at any absolute lung volume, and the lung compliance is reduced. The likely causes of these alterations in lung mechanics are a reduced number of alveoli in

---

Components of the ventilatory pump

Cerebral cortex

↓

Brainstem

↓

Spinal cord

↓

Anterior horn cells

↓

Peripheral nerves

↓

Neuromuscular junction

↓

Respiratory muscles

↓

Chest wall

Figure 72.1 Components of the ventilatory pump.

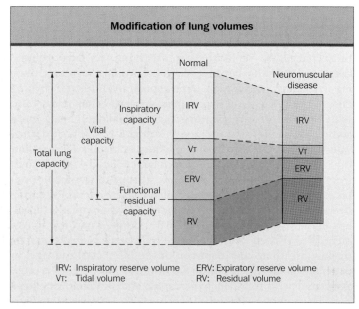

Modification of lung volumes

IRV: Inspiratory reserve volume   ERV: Expiratory reserve volume
VT: Tidal volume   RV: Residual volume

Figure 72.2 Modification of lung volumes in neuromuscular diseases.

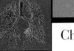

patients suffering from neuromuscular disorders from early childhood, and a stiffening of lung elastic fibers induced by shallow breathing. Areas of microatelectasis are an additional contributing factor, but are present only in a minority of patients[4].

Chest wall compliance is also lower than normal in chronic neuromuscular disorders, because of a stiffening of costosternal and costovertebral joints, tendons, and ligaments. The stiffening of the lung and chest wall are responsible for the lower level of the equilibrium position of the respiratory system (i.e. FRC) and contribute with respiratory muscle weakness to the drop in TLC and VC[4].

Forced expiration and cough

Expiratory muscle weakness modifies the contour of the flow–volume curve during a forced expiration, with a slower rise of flow, a smaller peak expiratory flow, and an abrupt cessation of flow at end-expiration. However, because maximum expiratory flow requires only a low driving pressure over most of VC, the ratio of forced expiratory volume in 1s to forced vital capacity (FEV_1/FVC) is usually normal or may be supranormal despite expiratory muscle weakness. In contrast, cough is generally inefficient because expiratory muscles are unable to produce the high positive pleural pressure that normally induces dynamic compression of central airways and transient acceleration of flow. This anomaly leads to frequent pulmonary infections[4].

Dyspnea

Although their physical activity is much reduced, patients who have neuromuscular disorders often complain of dyspnea. Dyspnea can be defined as a sensation of difficult breathing and is subserved, at least in part, by the sensation of respiratory effort[5]. The latter increases when the ratio between tidal inspiratory pressure and maximal inspiratory pressure (PI/PImax) increases. In neuromuscular disorders, PI may be elevated because of lower lung and chest wall compliance, and PImax is reduced because of inspiratory muscle weakness. When muscle weakness is reversible, the sensation of dyspnea may fluctuate markedly (Fig. 72.3).

Respiratory failure

With progressive respiratory muscle weakness, the breathing pattern changes to rapid shallow breathing. As tidal volume decreases, the ratio of dead space to tidal volume increases, causing alveolar hypoventilation, hypercapnia, and ultimately hypoxemia. The prevalence of hypercapnic respiratory failure increases with the extent of respiratory muscle weakness, being more common when respiratory muscle strength is <30% of normal values. However, considerable individual variability occurs, and the risk of respiratory failure cannot be predicted with certainty from measurement of VC or PImax. Part of this variability can be explained by the occurrence of respiratory troubles during sleep. Nocturnal studies show that alveolar hypoventilation develops initially at night, and particularly during rapid eye movement (REM) sleep. This sleep stage is normally characterized by shallow breathing and inhibition of the intercostal muscles. In patients who have neuromuscular disorders, REM sleep is often associated with transient hypercapnia and profound desaturation. These nocturnal anomalies precede and predispose to diurnal respiratory failure[4].

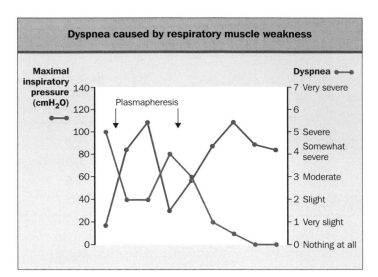

Figure 72.3 **Dyspnea caused by respiratory muscle weakness in a patient who has myasthenia gravis.**

EPIDEMIOLOGY AND CLINICAL FEATURES

A variety of neurologic disorders can affect respiration. The most important are presented here according to the anatomic level of the lesion. They are classified as acute or chronic, but some acute disorders have permanent consequences, and some chronic disorders may manifest with acute respiratory failure (Fig. 72.4).

Central nervous system
Acute disorders
Head and spinal cord injury
Traumatic injury to the brain and the spinal cord may result in total or subtotal loss of respiratory muscle function and is furthermore associated with a number of acute complications. Patients with brain injury develop early arterial hypoxemia, which is related to ventilation–perfusion inequality. Neurogenic pulmonary edema is frequent and is believed to result from massive α-adrenergic discharge, pulmonary vasoconstriction and hypertension, and capillary disruption. Other early complications include pulmonary embolism, hypersecretion of tenacious bronchial mucus, and pneumonia[6]. Tetraplegia results from cervical spinal cord trauma, spinal artery infarction, or compression by tumor. In all cases, the function of intercostal and abdominal muscles is lost, the only remaining expiratory muscle being the clavicular portion of the pectoralis major. This means a profound impairment in expiratory force and cough efficacy. The degree of inspiratory muscle impairment depends on the level of the lesion with respect to phrenic nerve roots, which originate from C3–C5. Diaphragm function is intact in patients who have a lower cervical lesion. Their inspiratory function is, however, impaired by a paradoxic movement of the upper rib cage caused by paralysis of the intercostal muscles[4]. Lesions at levels C3–C5 induce a variable loss of diaphragm function. In these patients, ventilatory autonomy often improves after the initial phase of spinal shock[7]. Higher cord injuries result in a nearly complete loss of respiratory muscle function, which necessitates immediate and long-term ventilatory assistance.

Acute and chronic neuromuscular disorders that cause respiratory failure		
Level of lesion	**Acute disorders**	**Chronic disorders**
Central nervous system	Head and spinal cord injury Stroke Tetanus	Multiple sclerosis Parkinson's disease Shy–Drager syndrome
Anterior horn cells	Paralytic poliomyelitis Rabies Flavivirus encephalomyelitis	Amyotrophic lateral sclerosis Spinal muscular atrophies Postpoliomyelitis atrophy
Peripheral nerves	Guillain–Barré syndrome Critical illness polyneuropathy Diphtheria Herpes zoster Neuralgic amyotrophy Phrenic nerve injury Metabolic and toxic causes	Hereditary neuropathies
Neuromuscular junction	Botulism Organophosphate poisoning Snake bite, tick paralysis	Myasthenia gravis Lambert–Eaton syndrome
Muscles	Acute corticosteroid myopathy Electrolyte disorders	Duchenne's muscular dystrophy Myotonic dystrophy Facioscapulohumeral disease Limb girdle dystrophy Congenital myopathies Acid maltase deficiency Mitochondrial myopathies Inflammatory myopathies

Figure 72.4 Acute and chronic neuromuscular disorders that cause respiratory failure.

Stroke

Hemispheric strokes affect the voluntary pathway of respiration, with elevation and decreased voluntary activation of the contralateral hemidiaphragm. Cheyne–Stokes breathing may develop, in particular with bilateral hemispheric lesions. However, these alterations have only modest clinical consequences because the automatic pathway is preserved. Brainstem strokes may affect respiratory rhythm in various ways. Lesions of the dorsolateral medulla result in fatal apnea. In contrast, injuries that spare the dorsolateral medulla do not impair automatic respiratory rhythm, even in extensive strokes leading to a locked-in syndrome. Lateral medullary strokes that result from occlusion of a distal vertebral artery induce the loss of automatic breathing, or Ondine's curse. While breathing is maintained during wakefulness, potentially fatal hypoventilation and central apnea develop during sleep. This must be differentiated from obstructive apnea, which may also be associated with lateral medullary strokes and which results from paralysis of pharyngeal muscles[7,8].

Tetanus

Tetanus toxin produced by *Clostridium tetani* reaches the central nervous system by retrograde axonal transport and blocks the synaptic release of inhibitory transmitters. Localized or generalized spasms develop through loss of central inhibition and death results from respiratory failure, because of laryngospasm or generalized spasms, including of the respiratory muscles. Specific therapy includes antibiotics, human tetanus immune globulin, muscle relaxants, or neuromuscular blockade, and intubation and mechanical ventilation[9].

Chronic disorders
Multiple sclerosis

Multiple sclerosis is an inflammatory, demyelinating disease that can affect almost any area of the central nervous system. Depending on the location of lesions, different types of respiratory anomalies may develop, and occasionally can be life threatening. Respiratory control can be affected by loss of automatic breathing, voluntary breathing, or both. Bulbar dysfunction increases the risk of respiratory failure caused by aspiration and pneumonia. Respiratory muscle weakness is usually moderate, but may become severe and includes diaphragmatic paralysis during relapses of the disease. Patients are particularly at risk of acute respiratory failure when infection and fever accompany an exacerbation. In these circumstances, severe respiratory muscle weakness can occur acutely, because of a conduction block of demyelinated fibers[10].

Extrapyramidal diseases

Parkinson's disease is associated with frequent respiratory complications, which include pneumonia (the most common cause of death in these patients). Abnormal control of breathing is frequently present, with tachypnea accompanied by dyspnea. Respiratory muscle weakness manifests by reduced lung volumes, impaired ability to clear secretions, and a delay in achieving peak expiratory flow. Finally, some patients with Parkinson's disease present with a dynamic instability of upper airway patency, which is recognized as a saw-tooth pattern on both inspiratory and expiratory flow–volume curves[11,12]. Respiratory dysfunction can also be induced by L-dopa therapy in patients who have Parkinson's disease. Within 1 hour of drug administration, some patients develop dyskinesias associated with tachypnea and dyspnea, which may be result from choreiform movements and rigidity–akinesis of respiratory muscles[13].

Shy–Drager syndrome is a multiple system atrophy that manifests by parkinsonism and autonomic failure. It is often associated with abnormal control of breathing, including irregular respiratory rate and tidal volume, central apneas, Cheyne–Stokes breathing, apneustic breathing, or central hypoventilation. The most dangerous anomaly lies in bilateral vocal cord abductor paralysis, which can result in obstructive sleep apnea and death[13].

Anterior horn cells
Acute disorders
Paralytic poliomyelitis

Before the advent of poliovirus vaccines, poliomyelitis was the most frequent neuromuscular disorder to result in respiratory failure. It is now rare, and usually attributed to live, attenuated polio vaccines. The acute infection has few symptoms, with fever and myalgia in adults, and upper airway infection in children. Only a minority of infected persons develop paralysis, which is widely and asymmetrically distributed. Respiratory complications include irregular breathing and apneas, upper airway obstruction, aspiration, and respiratory muscle weakness or paralysis. About 25% of patients require ventilatory assistance during the acute infection, but ventilatory autonomy is often recovered within months through reinnervation of denervated fibers[7,9,14].

Rabies

Rabies is an almost universally fatal disorder. The virus is transported along the peripheral nerves and enters the central nervous system, where it induces inflammation most often in the brain. In 20% of cases, the inflammation is predominant in the spinal cord and presents as paralytic rabies. In this form, a progressive, ascending paralysis develops, which may be indistinguishable from the Guillain–Barré syndrome (GBS), and which leads to respiratory muscle weakness and eventual respiratory arrest. Immediate prophylaxis is mandatory for subjects likely to be exposed to rabies and consists of human rabies immune globulin and rabies vaccine[9].

Flavivirus encephalomyelitis

Tick-born encephalitis is caused by a flavivirus and is endemic in Central Europe. In a minority of patients acute myelitis develops, in which paralysis and areflexia predominate in upper limbs. Severe weakness of respiratory muscles may be associated, and requires prolonged mechanical ventilation.

Chronic disorders
Amyotrophic lateral sclerosis

Amyotrophic lateral sclerosis (ALS) is a progressive degenerative disorder characterized by loss of both upper and lower motor neurons. With an incidence of 1–2/100,000 persons, ALS is the most frequent motor neuron disorder in developed countries. It affects predominantly middle aged to older subjects, with a male-to-female ratio of 2:1. Its cause is unknown, but a familial form exists in 5–10% of cases, usually with autosomal dominant transmission, caused by a defect localized in chromosome 21. The prognosis is very poor in ALS, with 50% of patients dying within 3 years and 80% within 5 years, usually of respiratory failure.

However, clinical features are not uniform. Loss of lower motor neurons often predominates, resulting in fasciculations, amyotrophy, and weakness, whereas loss of upper motor neurons manifests by spasticity and hyperreflexia. In the majority of cases, weakness initially develops in the extremities, whereas in a minority the bulbar lesions are prominent from the onset of disease. Similarly, respiratory muscle dysfunction is quite variable during the course of ALS. In some patients, respiratory muscle strength and lung volumes are relatively preserved, even when peripheral muscle weakness has progressed to the point where they are wheel-chair bound. Abdominal muscle dysfunction usually occurs before diaphragmatic dysfunction, leading to a predominantly expiratory muscle weakness. However, in rare cases, the initial manifestation may be severe respiratory weakness because of predominant phrenic motor neuron lesions. Ultimately, most patients suffer from alveolar hypoventilation unless ventilatory support is initiated. Death most commonly occurs after bronchial aspiration, pulmonary infection, and acute respiratory failure[4,14,15].

Spinal muscular atrophies

The spinal muscular atrophies (SMAs) are inherited in an autosomal recessive mode and arise from an anomaly of chromosome 5. All are characterized by weakness and amyotrophy, which predominates in the proximal muscles and begins in the lower limbs. Respiratory muscle weakness is caused by paralysis of intercostal muscles, whereas the diaphragm is preserved. The SMA are classified into three types according to the age of onset; types I and II are also termed Werdnig–Hoffmann disease, and type III Kugelberg–Welander disease. Type I SMA begins before the age of 6 months, and results in death from respiratory failure before the age of 2 years. Type II begins before the age of 18 months, progresses more slowly, and leads to death in late childhood, as a result of both respiratory muscle weakness and scoliosis. Type III begins after 18 months and is associated with late respiratory complications, resulting mainly from kyphoscoliosis[14,16].

Postpoliomyelitis muscular atrophy

Approximately 25% of patients with previous poliomyelitis can present with new problems 20–40 years after the initial episode. These include further muscular weakness attributed to degeneration of reinnervated motor units. In patients who have respiratory muscle sequelae and kyphoscoliosis, further dysfunction of respiratory muscles may induce alveolar hypoventilation. However, the loss of muscle strength is gradual and can be detected by appropriate tests before respiratory failure develops[14].

Peripheral nerves
Acute disorders
Guillan–Barré syndrome

An acute, multifocal, demyelinating polyradiculoneuropathy, GBS is of uncertain pathogenesis. In about half of cases, GBS follows a viral infection (varicella-zoster virus, cytomegalovirus, Epstein–Barr virus, human immunodeficiency virus), *Mycoplasma pneumoniae* infection, influenza vaccine, surgery, or malignancy (lymphomas). Cerebrospinal fluid is characterized by elevated proteins and a cell count of 10 or fewer mononuclear leukocytes per cubic millimeter. Muscle weakness and paralysis commonly begin in the lower extremities and progress in an ascending pattern to include the respiratory muscles. Maximum weakness is attained within 2 weeks in 50% of cases, and within 4 weeks in 90%. Respiratory failure develops as a result of both respiratory muscle weakness and pulmonary infections caused by aspiration. Of these patients, 15–30% require mechanical ventilation. Sensory impairment is minor, but autonomic dysfunction may be severe, and includes arrythmias and hyper- or hypotension. Presently, specific therapy is limited to plasmapheresis, which may limit progression of the disease and accelerate recovery when given early. Corticosteroids are ineffective and may be harmful. Most patients recover fully from GBS, but 15% manifest residual weakness and 5% develop a chronic form with relapsing episodes of demyelination[7,9,14].

Critical illness polyneuropathy

Patients who stay for longer than 5 days in the intensive care unit, and who suffer from sepsis and failure of two or more organs, are at high risk of developing critical illness polyneuropathy. This is an acute and reversible axonal neuropathy, manifested by symmetric and predominantly distal weakness or paralysis. Cerebrospinal fluid is unremarkable, in contrast with that of GBS. Electrophysiologic examination shows normal conduction velocities, but low or absent action potential amplitude. Neural biopsies show the absence of inflammation. The resulting respiratory muscle weakness is a frequent cause of prolonged and difficult weaning from mechanical ventilation. However, electrophysiologic and clinical recovery is complete within 6–12 months[17,18].

Diphtheria

Diphtheria, caused by *Corynebacterium diphtheriae*, is characterized by a pharyngeal and tracheal inflammatory membrane. In

20% of cases an exotoxin provokes cardiac and neurologic complications, which begin with palatal paralysis. A demyelinating polyneuropathy develops 6 weeks after the initial infection and can result in respiratory failure if the respiratory muscles are involved. Neurologic symptoms progress over 1–2 weeks, then stabilize, and regress over several months. Antitoxin is the only specific therapy and must be administered as early as possible[9,14].

Herpes zoster
Herpes zoster is caused by the reactivation of varicella-zoster virus and generally affects sensory nerves, with unilateral vesicular eruption that involves a single dermatome. Motor neurons may occasionally be affected, with resultant flaccid paralysis. The phrenic nerve may be involved in midcervical lesions, which induces complete and permanent hemidiaphragm paralysis – a cause of dyspnea, but not of respiratory failure. Since herpes zoster is not invariably accompanied by a cutaneous eruption, it may remain undetected in cases of unexplained, usually unilateral, diaphragm paralysis[4,14].

Neuralgic amyotrophy
Neuralgic amyotrophy (Parsonage–Turner syndrome) is an acute neuritis that affects cervical roots and is manifest by sudden onset of neck and shoulder pain, followed by sensory and motor impairment with prominent weakness and amyotrophy of shoulder and arm muscles. A recent history of viral infection or immunization is present in a minority of patients. Diaphragmatic paralysis, commonly bilateral, may ensue and induce dyspnea and orthopnea (Fig. 72.5). The diaphragm function appears to recover slowly and only in a minority of patients[19].

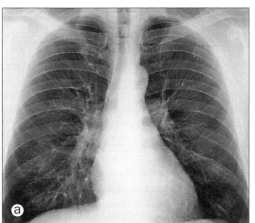
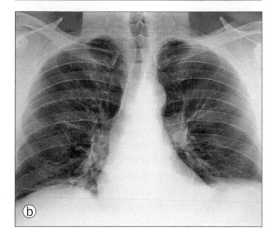

Figure 72.5 Bilateral diaphragmatic paralysis.
(a) Normal diaphragmatic location. (b) Chest radiograph during acute neuralgic amyotrophy with elevation of both hemidiaphragms.

Phrenic nerve injury
Damage to the phrenic nerves induces unilateral or bilateral diaphragmatic paralysis. Such injury can be caused by trauma, surgery, mediastinal tumors, pleural space infections, or forceful manipulation of the neck. Diaphragmatic paralysis is a common complication of open-heart surgery and results from cold or stretch injury to the nerve. This dysfunction is reversible, with recovery of 80% of cases within 6 months, and 90% within 1 year[14].

Metabolic and toxic causes
Acute intermittent porphyria causes an axonal neuropathy, which may be severe enough to induce respiratory failure. Acute hyperkalemic paralysis, commonly triggered by drugs in patients who suffer renal failure or adrenal insufficiency, is frequently complicated by respiratory failure. Other causes of acute neuropathy that result in respiratory muscle paralysis include poisoning with ciguatoxin (produced by protozoan algae and transmitted by fish), saxitoxin (transmitted by shellfish), tetrodotoxin (elaborated by the pufferfish), and thallium[7,9].

Chronic disorders
Hereditary neuropathies
Hereditary motor and sensory neuropathies represent a group of autosomal dominantly or recessively inherited disorders characterized by chronic degeneration of the peripheral nerves and roots. Muscle weakness affects the extremities, but may also progress to diaphragmatic paralysis after a long evolution[14].

Neuromuscular junction
Acute disorders
Botulism
Botulism is caused by an exotoxin elaborated by C. *botulinum*, a Gram-positive, spore-forming anaerobe widely present in the soil. The disease occurs in three syndromes – food-borne botulism from the consumption of improperly cooked food that contains the spores and toxin, infantile botulism caused by colonization of the gastrointestinal tract in the first 6 months of life, and wound botulism secondary to injuries or the use of injectable drugs, either intravenously or subcutaneously. The toxin is hematogenously disseminated, enters the neurons via endocytosis, binds irreversibly to calcium channels, and blocks acetylcholine release at the neuromuscular junction and at postganglionic parasympathetic nerve terminals. The incubation period lasts hours to days in food-borne disease, and days to 2 weeks in wound botulism. Gastrointestinal symptoms appear first with nausea and vomiting, followed by blurred vision, diplopia, and a descending paralysis, which includes respiratory muscles. Mortality is <10% with the use of mechanical ventilation, which may be required for up to 3 months in severe cases. Respiratory muscles appear to recover more slowly than other muscle groups. The diagnosis is from the isolation of toxin or the organism in food, gastric aspirate, stools, and serum in food-borne botulism, and in serum and wound tissue in wound botulism. Specific therapy includes enemas and gastric lavage, surgical debridement of wounds, high-dose penicillin, and antitoxin within the first days[9,20].

Organophosphate poisoning
Poisoning occurs with ingestion, inhalation or absorption via mucous membranes of organophosphate insecticides. The latter compounds are anticholinesterases, which induce a cholinergic

crisis and skeletal muscle weakness from dysfunction of post-synaptic neuromuscular junctions. The acute intoxication presents as a potentially fatal cholinergic crisis. An intermediate form may develop 1–4 days after intoxication, and is characterized by cranial and proximal muscle weakness and respiratory failure. Specific therapy includes atropine and cholinesterase reactivator pralidoxime[9].

Snake bite, tick paralysis

Snake neurotoxins act by preventing the release of acetylcholine at the neuromuscular junction. Paralysis develops 6–12 hours after the bite, with ptosis, diplopia, blurred vision, dysphagia, proximal muscle paralysis, and respiratory failure. After mechanical ventilation is initiated, paralysis usually regresses in 2–3 days. Specific therapy includes monovalent or polyvalent antivenin. Tick paralysis is also caused by a neurotoxin blocking the release of acetylcholine. After a 5-day latent period, a rapidly ascending paralysis develops and leads to respiratory failure. Removal of the tick reverses the process[9].

Chronic disorders

Myasthenia gravis

Myasthenia gravis is the most common disorder of the neuromuscular junction and is mediated by antibodies against acetylcholine receptors. Muscle weakness, which is exacerbated by exercise, is due to a reduction of available acetylcholine receptors. The onset of the disease is usually insidious, but may be abrupt. Weakness most commonly affects extraocular muscles (ptosis, diplopia), but also affects facial muscles, bulbar muscles (bronchial aspiration), laryngeal muscles (stridor), and truncal and limb muscles. Exacerbation of symptoms may occur with exertion, infection, surgery, or a variety of drugs [most commonly the neuromuscular blocking agents, aminoglycosides, clindamycin, tetracycline, propranolol, quinidine, procainamide, lidocaine (lignocaine), corticosteroids, chlorpromazine, and phenytoin]. Treatment of myasthenia gravis includes cholinesterase inhibitors, immunosuppression, thymectomy, and plasmapheresis.

Acute respiratory failure develops in crises of the disease. A myasthenic crisis is a rapid worsening of symptoms caused by a triggering factor, like surgery, infection, stress, or drugs. A cholinergic crisis results from an excess of anticholinesterase agents. Weakness worsens because of a cholinergic block and is associated with muscarinic symptoms, which include hypersalivation, increased bronchial secretions, bradycardia, nausea, and vomiting. A mixed or brittle crisis comprises both myasthenic and cholinergic symptoms. Since the respiratory muscles are usually affected less severely, they may suffer cholinergic block when other muscles require more anticholinesterase agents. Apart from mechanical ventilation, the treatment of acute respiratory failure includes corticosteroids and plasmapheresis, and temporary discontinuation of anticholinesterase medication. An insidious form of respiratory failure may develop in those who have long-standing, generalized muscle weakness[9,14,21].

The Lambert–Eaton myasthenic syndrome occurs in association with small-cell carcinoma in 50% of presentations. Weakness is caused by a reduction of acetylcholine release, and predominates in the pelvic girdle and thigh muscles. Some respiratory muscle weakness is frequent, but respiratory failure is rare[14,21]. It can precede the presentation of the tumor by several months.

Diseases of muscle

Acute disorders

Acute corticosteroid myopathy

Severe generalized weakness may develop in critically ill patients treated with high-dose corticosteroids and neuromuscular blocking agents. Rhabdomyolysis can be detected by increased serum creatine kinase levels and myoglobinuria. Histologic changes are found with widespread muscle necrosis and atrophy, and with loss of myosin filaments. This syndrome is often observed in patients treated by mechanical ventilation, and severe respiratory muscle weakness may prolong weaning, or even necessitate long-term ventilatory support[22,23].

Electrolyte disorders

Hypophosphatemia is common in chronic alcoholism, diabetic ketoacidosis, or Gram-negative infections and induces generalized weakness, hypotonia, and areflexia. Acute respiratory failure can occur in hypophosphatemic patients, and is rapidly reversed by phosphate administration. Failure is caused respiratory muscle weakness because the diaphragm strength is impaired in this situation, but increases after phosphate infusion[24]. Severe hypokalemia is another cause of muscle weakness. Respiratory failure can result from acute hypokalemic paralysis, as a complication of treatment for diabetic ketoacidosis, of barium sulfide poisoning, or of ureterosigmoidostomy[9].

Chronic disorders

Duchenne's muscular dystrophy

Duchenne's muscular dystrophy (DMD) is an X-linked recessive disorder caused by mutations of the gene for the protein dystrophin. Weakness, clumsiness, and waddling gait are observed in early childhood. With progressive muscle weakness, most patients are wheelchair dependent by the age of 12 years. Absolute values of VC increase until 10–12 years, then plateau, and inexorably diminish. From this age on, the ventilatory decline is further aggravated by the development of scoliosis. Patients who have DMD may remain clinically stable despite considerable loss of lung volume. Eventually, they develop nocturnal hypoxemia, hypercapnia, and commonly die of acute respiratory failure secondary to pulmonary infection when 20–25 years of age. Congestive heart failure may be associated, because of left ventricular fibrosis. Surgical correction of scoliosis improves comfort, but not the lung volumes. Noninvasive or invasive home mechanical ventilation should be considered before the stage of terminal respiratory failure[14,22].

Myotonic dystrophy

Myotonic dystrophy is the most common muscle dystrophy in adults, with an incidence of 1 in 8000. It is inherited in an autosomal dominant pattern, and is characterized by myotonia (delayed muscular relaxation), progressive muscle weakness, cardiac conduction defects, endocrine abnormalities, cataract, ptosis, frontal baldness, and temporal wasting. Respiratory failure is frequent because of weakness that predominantly affects the respiratory muscles. Aggravating factors include central or obstructive sleep apnea, and pharyngeal and laryngeal dysfunction that leads to aspiration. Rarely, severe dyspnea may result from myotonia of the respiratory muscles; this can be alleviated by antimyotonic therapy. Patients affected by myotonic dystrophy manifest a high susceptibility to anesthetic agents and respiratory depressants. When surgery is needed, close postoperative monitoring is mandatory for at least 24 hours. Congenital myotonic dystrophy occurs in the offspring of 15% of affected mothers. It is manifested by hypotonia, severe facial weakness, and frequent respiratory failure that necessitates mechanical ventilation. The prognosis is good for those who survive respiratory complications of the neonatal period[14,22].

Other adult muscular dystrophies

Facioscapulohumeral disease is an autosomal dominant dystrophy that affects the face and arm muscles. In 20% of cases, trunk muscles are involved and respiratory failure develops. Limb girdle dystrophy is a group of autosomal and recessive dystrophies that can lead to respiratory failure[22].

Congenital myopathies

Congenital myopathies are characterized by definite abnormalities on muscle biopsy. The form most often associated with respiratory failure is nemaline myopathy, characterized by accumulation of rod-like bodies in muscle fibers – it can appear in the neonatal period, in childhood, or in adults. Centronuclear myopathy affects mainly slow-twitch oxidative fibers (type I). An X-linked recessive form often requires mechanical ventilation at birth. Autosomal dominant forms develop in childhood and adulthood, but rarely lead to respiratory failure[22].

Metabolic myopathies

Acid maltase deficiency causes glycogen storage disease. In the infantile form, all organs accumulate glycogen and death ensues from cardiorespiratory failure by the age of 2 years. In the childhood form, organomegaly is variable and respiratory failure is common because of severe muscle weakness. In the adult form, organomegaly is rare, and nocturnal hypoxemia and respiratory failure are frequent and caused by predominant dysfunction of the diaphragm.

Mitochondrial myopathies represent a group of systemic diseases in which mitochondrial disorders are recognized in muscle biopsies by the presence of 'ragged, red fibers'. Three mitochondrial myopathies are associated with respiratory failure, either initial or precipitated by anesthesia or respiratory depressants:
- Kearns–Sayre syndrome;
- myoclonic epilepsy and ragged-red fibers (known as MERRF);
- mitochondrial myopathy, encephalopathy, lactic acidosis, and stroke-like episodes (known as MELAS).

Depressed ventilatory response to hypoxia and hypercapnia may occur independently of respiratory muscle weakness[16,22].

Inflammatory myopathies

Polymyositis, dematomyositis, and inclusion body myositis are characterized by lymphocytic infiltrates of muscles. Respiratory muscle weakness is frequent, but ventilatory failure is relatively rare. Interstitial lung disease is present in up to 30% of cases and is often associated with antibodies to histidyl–transfer RNA synthetase (Jo-1 antigen). Systemic lupus erythematosus (SLE) is frequently associated with respiratory muscle weakness without signs of generalized muscle involvement. The 'shrinking lung syndrome' observed in patients who have SLE results from dysfunction and elevation of the diaphragm, caused by both muscle atrophy and fibrosis[14,22].

DIAGNOSIS

History

The clinical setting is thoroughly assessed. Often, the cause of respiratory failure is a long-standing neuromuscular disorder. If not, evidence of trauma, wounds, infection, exposure to insects, drugs, or toxic agents is sought. Clues of an underlying neuromuscular disorder may be found in the history – fatigability on repetitive tasks, difficulty in arising from a chair or in performing tasks with the arms elevated, difficulty with speech or swallowing liquids, tracheal aspiration, or impaired cough.

Dyspnea is a common symptom of respiratory insufficiency, although obviously not specific. Typically, dyspnea occurs on exertion, but may be masked in patients whose exercise capacity is severely restricted by limb weakness. Dyspnea at rest is an alarm signal of ongoing or imminent acute respiratory failure. Bilateral diaphragmatic paralysis causes orthopnea, which can be severe enough to prevent normal sleep and to necessitate nocturnal ventilatory support. In neuromuscular disorders, nocturnal hypoventilation commonly develops before the onset of diurnal hypercapnia, and may be recognized by the presence of early morning headache and daytime sleepiness[3].

Physical examination

Patients who complain of dyspnea of unexplained origin, or for whom a neuromuscular disorder is suspected, are given a detailed neurologic examination. This includes assessment of the presence and distribution of muscle atrophy and weakness, fasciculation, spasticity, and abnormal tendon reflexes.

The clinical examination is often unremarkable when weakness is mild or even moderate. Rapid, shallow breathing typically accompanies more severe muscle weakness. Signs of diaphragmatic paralysis are sought in the supine position – elevation of respiratory rate, prominent contraction of the sternocleidomastoid and scalene muscles, and abdominal paradox. The last sign consists of an indrawing of abdominal wall during inspiration, instead of the normal synchronized outward movement of both rib cage and abdomen (see Fig. 72.6). The signs of spinal cord injury vary according to the level of lesion. Patients injured above the C3–C5 level are extremely dyspneic and tachypneic, heavily recruit inspiratory neck muscles, and show abdominal paradox. Diaphragmatic function is preserved in lesions below C5 – during inspiration, these patients show a normal expansion of the abdomen, but often a paradoxic indrawing of the upper rib cage because of paralysis of the inspiratory rib cage muscles[3,4].

Imaging

The chest radiograph may help in severe diaphragmatic dysfunction. Elevation of one hemidiaphragm suggests paralysis on that side, but other causes must be eliminated, such as atelectasis or subpulmonary pleural effusion. Elevation of both hemidiaphragms is compatible with diaphragmatic paralysis, but can also result from inadequate inspiration or diffuse interstitial lung disease. Comparison with previous radiographs is most helpful (see Fig. 72.5). Examination under fluoroscopy of diaphragm movements in the supine position may help. During sniffing, both hemidiaphragms normally show a brisk caudad displacement. In hemidiaphragm paralysis, the corresponding side shows a paradoxic cephalad movement. In bilateral paralysis, both hemidiaphragms

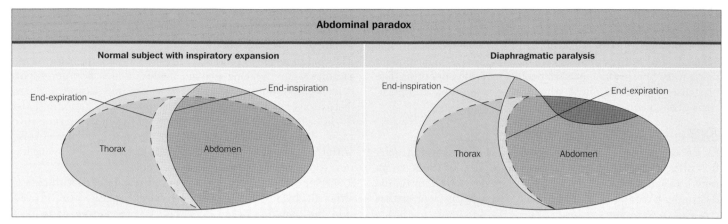

Abdominal paradox

| Normal subject with inspiratory expansion | Diaphragmatic paralysis |

Figure 72.6 Abdominal paradox caused by severe dysfunction or paralysis of the diaphragm. Normal subject with inspiratory expansion of both the thorax and abdomen (left). Diaphragmatic paralysis with marked expansion of the thorax, and paradoxic motion of the diaphragm and abdomen (right). Abdominal paradox should be looked for in the supine position.

show this paradoxic shift. The hemidiaphragm movement can also be seen with ultrasound, which avoids irradiation[25].

Arterial blood gases

The hallmark of significant respiratory muscle weakness is hypercapnia and hypoxemia. Diaphragmatic paralysis does not cause hypercapnia, unless it is associated with an increased load caused by a lung or chest wall anomaly. When caused by respiratory muscle weakness, hypercapnia is a late sign and develops only when respiratory muscle strength is reduced to 30% of predicted. In acute disorders or decompensations, hypercapnia is associated with an elevated bicarbonate and a low pH. In chronic disorders, global respiratory muscle weakness results in progressive hypercapnia with markedly elevated bicarbonates and a normal pH. Initially, alveolar hypoventilation develops only during the night, in particular during REM sleep. Such episodes can be detected by falls in arterial oxygen saturation during nocturnal pulse oximetry[3,26].

Pulmonary function tests

In the absence of associated lung or skeletal disease, a reduction of VC suggests respiratory muscle weakness. However, this simple test is not sensitive in mild neuromuscular disorders because VC only falls significantly when respiratory muscle strength is reduced by 50%. Normally, VC decreases by 5–10% when moving from an upright to a supine position, whereas a 30–50% fall strongly suggests diaphragm weakness or paralysis. In neuromuscular disorders, FRC is normal or decreased, RV is normal or increased, and TLC is decreased. The RV/TLC ratio is increased and does not reflect obstructive lung disease in this setting.

The flow–volume loop may show several anomalies – a delay in reaching peak expiratory flow, a truncation of peak expiratory and peak inspiratory flow, and an abrupt drop of expiratory flow at the end of expiration. In contrast with normal subjects, the forced inspiratory volume in 1s is often smaller than FEV_1, because of muscle weakness and/or bulbar involvement with upper airway obstruction.

Gas transfer (DLCO) is reduced with respiratory muscle weakness, but less than lung volumes. Thus, DLCO corrected for alveolar volume (KCO) is typically raised[3,26].

Respiratory muscle function

Maximal respiratory pressures

Since loss of lung volume is neither sensitive nor specific for respiratory muscle weakness, the direct measurement of respiratory muscle strength is clearly often needed in patients who have neuromuscular disorders. This is classically performed by measuring PImax and maximal expiratory pressure (PEmax) at the mouth during volitional efforts against a near-complete occlusion (a small leak is left open to avoid recording pressures generated by orofacial muscles). By convention, PImax and PEmax represent the maximal pressure sustained for 1s, which can now be computed by portable devices (Fig. 72.7). The best (largest pressure) of at least three maneuvers is recorded. A standard, flanged mouthpiece is convenient for most patients, but does not prevent air leaks when orofacial muscle weakness is present. Traditionally, PImax is measured from RV, and PEmax from TLC[27]. However, pressures recorded under these circumstances include the recoil pressure of the respiratory system. In contrast, PImax and PEmax measured at FRC reflect only muscle strength. The main limitation of maximal respiratory pressures is their difficulty for the subject. As a consequence, low values are difficult to interpret, because, while they reflect true muscle weakness, they can also be found in normal subjects (see lower limits of normal values, Fig. 72.8). In

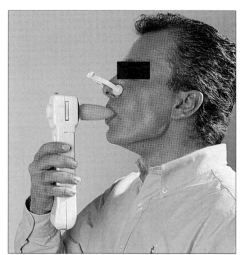

Figure 72.7 The technique of measurement of maximal pressures. The subject holds a portable device and performs a maximal inspiratory effort against a near-complete occlusion to generate maximal inspiratory pressure. The same device allows the measurement of maximal expiratory pressure.

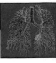

Maximal respiratory pressures					
Age (years)	Sniff nasal inspiratory pressure; functional residual capacity (cmH$_2$O)	Maximal inspiratory pressure; functional residual capacity (cmH$_2$O)	Maximal inspiratory pressure; residual volume (cmH$_2$O)	Maximal expiratory pressure; functional residual capacity (cmH$_2$O)	Maximal expiratory pressure; total lung capacity (cmH$_2$O)
Men[a] 20–65	111 (63–159)	106 (60–152)	115 (67–163)	130 (72–188)	146 (72–220)
66–80	91 (48–134)	82 (37–127)	90 (40–140)	102 (38–166)	118 (40–196)
Women[a] 20–65	87 (51–123)	83 (45–121)	84 (46–122)	86 (46–126)	101 (45–157)
66–80	75 (53–97)	58 (26–90)	67 (33–101)	69 (33–105)	79 (37–121)
Boys[b] 7–17	–	–	75 (29–121)	–	96 (50–142)
Girls[b] 7–17	–	–	63 (21–105)	–	80 (38–122)

[a]From Uldry and Fitting[28]; [b]From Wilson et al.[27].

Figure 72.8 Normal values of maximal respiratory pressures. Sniff nasal inspiratory pressure is performed from functional residual capacity (FRC). Maximal inspiratory pressure is performed from FRC or from residual volume. Maximal expiratory pressure is performed from FRC or from total lung capacity. Values are means and normal ranges (mean ± 2SD). Data reproduced from Wilson et al.[27] and Uldry and Fitting[28] with permission from the BMJ Publishing Group.

contrast, PImax >7.8kPa (80cmH$_2$O) in men and >6.9kPa (70cmH$_2$O) in women excludes significant inspiratory muscle weakness[25]. Values of PImax and PEmax are approximately 10% lower in the supine than in the sitting position.

Sniff nasal inspiratory pressure

Inspiratory muscle strength can be assessed by sniff nasal inspiratory pressure (SNIP), which is measured in one occluded nostril during a maximal sniff performed through the contralateral nostril (Fig. 72.9)[29]. The best (largest) of 10 values obtained from FRC is recorded. This test is easy to perform for most subjects and is not hampered by orofacial muscle weakness. However, it cannot be performed accurately with severe nasal obstruction. The SNIP can be measured using portable devices that record peak instantaneous pressure. Normal values of SNIP are similar or slightly higher than for PImax (see Fig. 72.8), and are similar in sitting and supine positions[28].

Sniff transdiaphragmatic pressure

The formal evaluation of diaphragm strength requires specialized equipment. The transdiaphragmatic pressure (Pdi) is the pressure difference created across the diaphragm during a contraction, and is computed by measuring esophageal (Pes) and gastric pressures with balloon or catheter systems. Diaphragmatic strength is most reliably measured during maximal sniffs from FRC. Values of sniff Pdi below 9.8kPa (100cmH$_2$O) in men and 7.8kPa (80cmH$_2$O) in women suggest diaphragm weakness[30,31].

Phrenic nerve stimulation

The use of a nonvolitional test is necessary if a patient cannot cooperate. Stimulation of the phrenic nerves measures the twitch Pdi, which represents only a fraction of the sniff Pdi, but can be used to detect or monitor diaphragm weakness. In contrast with electrical stimulation, the technique of magnetic stimulation of the phrenic nerves is easy and painless, and is preferred[25]. The test is performed by applying a coil to the neck region, usually over the C6–C7 spinous processes (see Fig. 72.10). Magnetic stimulation can measure diaphragm strength noninvasively by recording twitch mouth pressure (Pm), the latter reflecting twitch Pes. Values below 1.8kPa (19cmH$_2$O) for twitch Pdi and below 1.08kPa (11cmH$_2$O) for twitch Pm suggest diaphragm weakness.

In summary, the respiratory evaluation of a patient who has a known or suspected neuromuscular disorder should include history, physical examination, chest imaging, lung function tests,

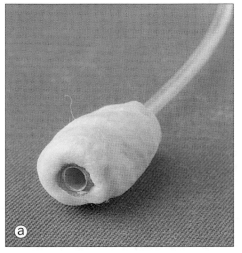

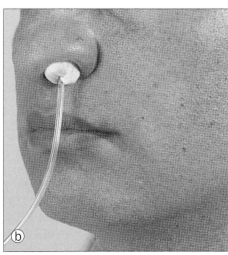

Figure 72.9 Method for performing sniff nasal inspiratory pressure. (a) A plug made of two-to-three waxed ear plugs is hand-fitted around the tip of a catheter. (b) The plug and catheter are inserted into one nostril, which enables the measurement of sniff nasal inspiratory pressure while the subject performs a maximal sniff through the contralateral nostril.

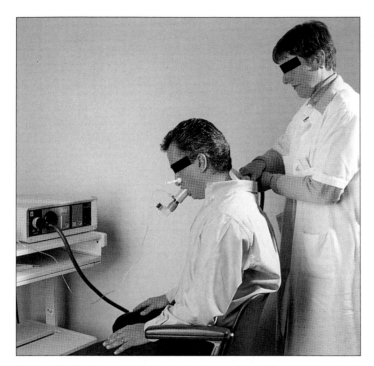

Figure 72.10 The method of phrenic nerve stimulation. Using cervical magnetic stimulation, the experimenter applies the coil of the stimulator on the C6–C7 area. In this example, twitch mouth pressure is recorded as a noninvasive measure of diaphragm strength.

Respiratory assessment in neuromuscular disorders	
Type	**Notes**
Clinical assessment	History – dyspnea, orthopnea, difficulty in coughing or swallowing, early morning headache, daytime somnolence
	Examination – tachypnea, cyanosis, abdominal or rib cage paradox, contraction of abdominal or neck muscles, amyotrophy
Imaging	Static – chest radiography
	Dynamic – fluoroscopy, ultrasound
Functional assessment	Simple tests
	Sitting and supine vital capacities
	Lung volumes
	Flow–volume loop
	Arterial blood gases
	Nocturnal oximetry
	Maximal inspiratory pressure, maximal expiratory pressure, sniff nasal inspiratory pressure
	Specialized tests
	Sniff transdiaphragmatic pressure
	Phrenic nerve stimulation
	Twitch transdiaphragmatic pressure, twitch mouth pressure
	Conduction time

Figure 73.11 Respiratory evaluation of patients who have neuromuscular disorders.

arterial blood-gas tension estimation, and simple tests of respiratory muscle strength. If in doubt or if diaphragm function is to be specifically assessed, the patient should be referred to a specialized laboratory (Fig. 72.11). Simple and noninvasive tests of lung function and respiratory muscle strength are preferred to monitor the evolution over time (Fig. 72.12).

TREATMENT

Indications for mechanical ventilation

Whenever possible, specific treatment of the causal neurologic process is applied. However, this is not available for some neuromuscular disorders, and is often not adequate to prevent respiratory failure in others. In many cases, the primary therapeutic option is ventilatory support. The methods of invasive and noninvasive mechanical ventilation are described in Chapters 3.11 and 3.12.

Patients who have neuromuscular disorders are at high risk of acute respiratory failure, in particular during upper airway or pulmonary infections. Mechanical ventilation is indicated when the patient develops severe dyspnea, tachypnea, and acute carbon dioxide retention. Endotracheal intubation is mandatory if the patient cannot protect the airway, if retention of secretions occurs, or any associated acute dysfunction is present. Otherwise, noninvasive mechanical ventilation may be tried if the patient is cooperative. In other patients, chronic respiratory failure develops with no or only few symptoms, such as mild dyspnea, increased fatigability, and daytime somnolence. The time at which ventilatory assistance must be initiated in this setting is not clear, and many patients may not accept this therapy without subjective benefit. Nevertheless, nocturnal ventilatory assistance should be initiated with unequivocal symptoms of chronic hypoventilation or when daytime arterial carbon dioxide tension exceeds 6.6kPa (50mmHg). Noninvasive positive-pressure ventilation is the mode of choice in these circumstances. However, patients who have severe respiratory muscle weakness that necessitates >16 hours of ventilatory assistance per day generally require invasive mechanical ventilation via a tracheostomy[32].

Mechanical ventilation in specific disorders
Acute respiratory failure
In spinal cord injury, the degree of ventilator dependence is mainly determined by the level of the lesion with respect to phrenic nerve roots. Endotracheal mechanical ventilation is initiated after the acute injury, but weaning or transfer to noninvasive mechanical ventilation is often possible later, because of partial neurologic recovery, conditioning of the diaphragm, and decreased flaccidity of the chest wall.

Patients who have GBS are intubated when their VC falls below 15–20mL/kg, and they can be weaned when this value is exceeded during recovery. Intubation may be necessary earlier to protect the airway. Prolonged mechanical ventilation is common, and tracheostomy should be considered early. However, nearly all patients eventually wean from the ventilator. Myasthenia gravis can lead to acute respiratory failure. Intubation is often indicated, especially because of pharyngeal muscle dysfunction. However, the duration of mechanical ventilation is usually short and tracheostomy is often not necessary.

Chronic respiratory failure
Patients who have muscular dystrophies and progressive myopathies develop chronic respiratory insufficiency at some point, starting

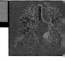

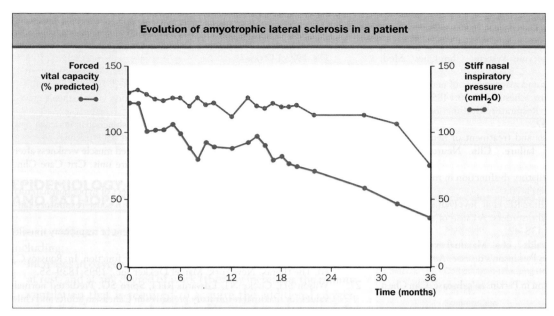

Figure 72.12 Evolution of amyotrophic lateral sclerosis in a patient. In this case, forced vital capacity remains initially stable and drops after 30 months. In contrast, sniff nasal inspiratory pressure falls early, heralding progression of the disease.

with nocturnal hypoventilation and hypoxemia. Noninvasive positive-pressure ventilation is the preferred mode of treatment and is initially used only during the night. With progressive muscular weakness, ventilatory support is extended to the daytime. Ultimately, survival can only be prolonged by positive-pressure ventilation via a tracheostomy.

In selected cases, ALS may represent an indication for mechanical ventilation. Noninvasive positive-pressure ventilation can relieve dyspnea or symptoms of nocturnal hypoventilation in patients who do not have significant bulbar involvement. However, with progressive respiratory and bulbar muscle weakness, tracheostomy becomes the only way of providing mechanical ventilation. This prolongs survival while the disease progresses to complete paralysis. Thus, this option must be discussed in advance to allow the patient to make a considered choice. Under these circumstances, only about 10% of patients opt for tracheostomy[32].

Diaphragmatic pacing

Patients who are ventilator dependent because of a high cervical-cord lesion or central alveolar hypoventilation are potential candidates for diaphragmatic pacing. This technique consists of stimulating the phrenic nerves via intrathoracic implanted electrodes, the receiver being activated by radiofrequency waves generated by an external power. Diaphragmatic pacing is an effective method of supporting ventilation in patients who have good phrenic nerve and diaphragm function, but its use is limited by high costs and the required specialized skills.

PITFALLS AND CONTROVERSIES

In the presence of a neuromuscular disorder, the main omission is to miss the diagnosis and fail to appreciate the likelihood of respiratory failure, which is easily done by wrongly attributing symptoms to other more common diseases. Thus, in the absence of evidence of cardiac or pulmonary disease, dyspnea should not automatically be attributed to a psychogenic cause. Orthopnea is a frequent symptom of left heart failure, but may herald diaphragmatic paralysis. Unexplained fatigue and lack of concentration should not simply be attributed to age, but should raise the suspicion of alveolar hypoventilation.

The physical examination of the respiratory system should not be performed only in the sitting position – abdominal paradox, which accompanies diaphragmatic paresis or paralysis, can only be recognized when supine. On the chest radiograph, small but normal lungs may not reflect poor inspiratory effort, but true inspiratory muscle weakness. Hypercapnia should not always be ascribed to chronic obstructive pulmonary disease, even with a positive smoking history or a mild degree of airflow limitation.

In summary, the main danger is to fail to think of respiratory muscle dysfunction and not make the appropriate measurements. A loss of respiratory muscle strength can only be diagnosed if it is measured. Thus, once the suspicion of respiratory muscle weakness is raised, simple tests such as FVC, PImax, PEmax, and SNIP must be performed. The second danger is to minimize the risk of acute respiratory failure. In a patient who has a neuromuscular disorder, hypercapnia should be sought and must be considered as a sign of imminent ventilatory failure.

REFERENCES

1. Gibson GJ, Pride NB, Newsom Davis J, Loh LC. Pulmonary mechanics in patients with respiratory muscle weakness. Am Rev Respir Dis. 1977;115:389–95.
2. De Troyer A, Borenstein S, Cordier R. Analysis of lung volume restriction in patients with respiratory muscle weakness. Thorax. 1980;35:603–10.
3. Rochester DF, Esau SA. Assessment of ventilatory function in patients with neuromuscular disease. Clin Chest Med. 1994;15:751–63.
4. De Troyer A, Estenne M. The respiratory system in neuromuscular disorders. In: Roussos C, ed. The thorax. New York: Marcel Dekker Inc.; 1995:2177–212.

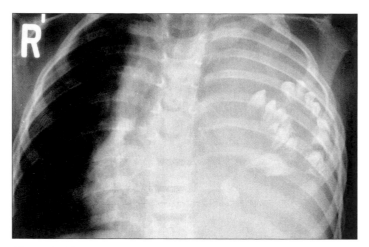

Figure 74.10 **Posteroanterior chest radiograph of a mature teratoma.** A large, anterior mediastinal mass occupies the entire left hemithorax, with mass effect on the mediastinum. Well-formed teeth within the mass are diagnostic of a teratoma.

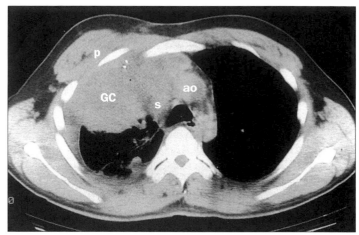

Figure 74.11 **Nonseminomatous, malignant germ-cell tumor.** A large, predominantly right-sided, anterior mediastinal neoplasm (GC) is intimately associated with the superior vena cava (s) and aorta (ao), and invades the chest wall and pectoral muscles (p). A small right pleural effusion is present.

Nonseminomatous, malignant germ-cell tumors

Nonseminomatous, malignant germ-cell tumors affect young, symptomatic men and include choriocarcinoma, embryonal cell carcinoma, endodermal sinus (yolk sac) tumor, and mixed germ-cell tumors[3,14]. The tumor markers AFP and HCG are elevated in the majority of patients[3]. A significantly increased AFP level is usually found in endodermal sinus tumor and embryonal cell carcinoma, whereas HCG is typically increased in choriocarcinoma[6]. Nonseminatomatous, malignant germ-cell tumors may be associated with various hematologic neoplasms, such as acute leukemia or myelodysplastic syndrome, and up to 20% of patients have Klinefelter's syndrome[3,14]. These tumors manifest radiologically as large, irregular, heterogeneous neoplasms with central necrosis, hemorrhage, and cyst formation (frequently with invasion of adjacent structures), pleural and pericardial effusions, and lymph node and distant metastases (Fig. 74.11).

The standard therapy involves systemic chemotherapy with cisplatin-containing regimens, followed by surgical resection of residual tumor if a positive response is achieved[14]. The response to therapy may be followed by serum tumor markers, which are expected to normalize after treatment. Compared with seminoma, the prognosis is less favorable; however, complete remission rates of 50–70% and a 5-year survival rate of approximately 50% can be achieved[14].

Intrathoracic goiter

Most mediastinal goiters are extensions from cervical goiters in asymptomatic women[4]. Rarely, compression of the trachea or esophagus may cause symptoms such as dyspnea or dysphagia. The risk of malignant degeneration is small[3]. The majority of intrathoracic goiters are located in the anterior–superior mediastinum on the left, but other compartments may be affected. Completely intrathoracic goiter with no cervical component is rare. The chest radiograph often reveals a cervicothoracic mass with tracheal deviation. On CT, these are lobulated, encapsulated lesions with heterogeneous attenuation from hemorrhage, cystic changes, intrinsic iodine, and calcification (Fig. 74.12)[9]. Intense and sustained contrast enhancement is common. In functioning goiters, uptake of radioactive iodine (^{123}I or ^{131}I) and technetium (^{99m}Tc pertechnetate) is diagnostic, but scan results do not change the management. Symptomatic or large goiters may be surgically excised.

Parathyroid adenoma

Mediastinal ectopic parathyroid glands are usually located within or near the thymus gland[3]. The majority are encapsulated, functioning, benign adenomas, most commonly seen in older women who have persistent hyperparathyroidism following cervical parathyroidectomy[4]. As a result of their small size, they are rarely detected on chest radiographs and frequently mimic a lymph node on CT. Localization is achieved by ^{99m}Tc sestamibi scintigraphy, which is more sensitive than dual isotope digital subtraction imaging using ^{99m}Tc pertechnetate and thallium-201 chloride. Selective venous sampling for parathyroid hormone levels may be necessary. Surgical excision is the treatment of choice.

DISEASES OF THE MIDDLE MEDIASTINUM

Nonlymphomatous lymph-node enlargement
Benign mediastinal lymphadenopathy

Infectious and noninfectious granulomatous diseases may involve the mediastinal lymph nodes. Infectious granulomatous diseases include tuberculosis and fungal infections, such as histoplasmosis and coccidioidomycosis[3]. The most important noninfectious diseases include sarcoidosis and silicosis. Lymphadenopathy associated with granulomatous infection is usually unilateral and asymmetric, in contrast to bilateral and symmetric lymph-node enlargement observed in sarcoidosis. On radiologic imaging, many of these disorders cause nodal calcification, which may have an 'eggshell' configuration, characteristic of silicosis, or less commonly sarcoidosis. Although calcified lymph nodes generally represent a benign process, differentiation from malignant lymphadenopathy by CT is frequently impossible and histologic examination may be required.

Several other causes of benign lymph-node enlargement include reactive hyperplasia from bacterial and viral lung infections, amyloidosis, drugs such as phenytoin, and Castleman's

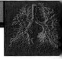

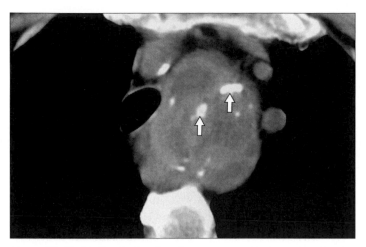

Figure 74.12 Mediastinal goiter. Chest computed tomography without contrast demonstrates a heterogeneous mass with large calcifications (arrows) and displacement of the trachea.

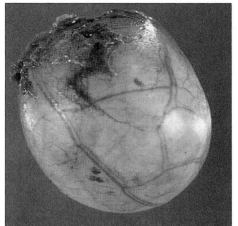

Figure 74.13 Bronchogenic cyst. Gross specimen of a spheric, bronchogenic cyst reveals clear fluid contents confined by a thin wall, with smalll vessels.

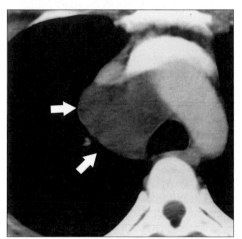

Figure 74.14 Bronchogenic cyst. Chest computed tomography demonstrates a bronchogenic cyst (arrows) with an imperceptible wall, water attenuation contents, and close proximity to the tracheal carina.

disease, also termed angiofollicular lymphoid hyperplasia or giant lymph-node hyperplasia. Castleman's disease usually manifests in young, asymptomatic adults as incidental, large, well-circumscribed, mediastinal lymph nodes, most commonly located in the anterior mediastinum[3].

Metastatic disease

Primary lung, breast, renal cell, gastrointestinal, and prostate carcinomas, as well as malignant melanoma, can metastasize to mediastinal lymph nodes. Diagnosis is established by history of a known primary malignancy confirmed by biopsy. The treatment depends on the underlying disease.

Mediastinal cysts

Foregut cysts

Congenital foregut cysts represent 20% of mediastinal masses, and 50–60% of these are bronchogenic cysts[5]; enterogenous cysts, which include esophageal duplication and neurenteric cysts, account for approximately 10–15%. Up to 20% of foregut cysts cannot be histologically classified and hence are termed nonspecific or indeterminate cysts[13].

Bronchogenic cysts

Bronchogenic cysts are thought to originate from abnormal budding of the ventral foregut. The majority are located in the mediastinum, most commonly in subcarinal or paratracheal locations, and nearly 15% arise in the pulmonary parenchyma; other locations are rare. These cysts are lined by the pseudostratified, columnar, ciliated respiratory epithelium and may contain serous fluid, mucus, milk of calcium, blood, or purulent material (Fig. 74.13)[13].

Bronchogenic cysts are usually seen in adults, but can be found in all age groups; males and females are equally affected. Patients are commonly asymptomatic, but infection or bleeding eventually causes symptoms in up to two thirds of cases. Radiologic imaging usually reveals a well-circumscribed, spheric, mediastinal mass. On CT, these cysts are typically homogeneous, do not enhance, and may have variable attenuation depending on fluid content (Fig. 74.14)[13]. The cyst wall may enhance and contain calcifications. A gas–fluid level within the cyst is a rare finding and may indicate communication with the airways or infection[13].

Large cysts in children may compress the airways, which results in atelectasis, bronchopneumonia, or air trapping. When a bronchogenic cyst exhibits characteristic radiologic features, diagnosis can be made by bronchoscopic or thoracoscopic needle drainage of cyst fluid, which contains mucus and bronchial epithelial cells. Treatment of choice is surgical resection (even in the absence of symptoms), although incidental cysts in asymptomatic adults have been followed clinically and radiologically. Needle drainage is an alternative in patients who are at high risk for surgical complications.

Enterogenous cysts

Enterogenous (esophageal duplication and neurenteric) cysts originate from the dorsal foregut, the majority are located in the middle or posterior mediastinum[13], and they typically manifest in childhood. Enterogenous cysts are lined by squamous or enteric epithelium and may contain gastric mucosa and/or pancreatic and neural tissue. The cyst walls have two well-defined, smooth muscle layers with myenteric plexus. Esophageal duplication cysts almost always adhere to the esophagus or are located within its wall and can be associated·with gastrointestinal malformations. Similarly, neurenteric cysts may be associated with gastrointestinal and/or cervical or upper thoracic vertebral anomalies, occasionally with a fibrous attachment to the spine or intraspinal extension[13].

Most enterogenous cysts are discovered during childhood because of the symptoms. Hemorrhage or rupture may occur, especially when gastric epithelium or pancreatic tissue is present.

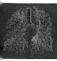
Their radiologic features are similar to those of bronchogenic cysts[13]. Esophageal duplication cysts are usually located close to the distal esophagus on the right. Most neurenteric cysts are located in the posterior mediastinum, above the level of the carina on the right, and approximately half are associated with scoliosis, anterior spina bifida, vertebral fusion, hemivertebrae, and other vertebral anomalies. Surgical excision is the treatment of choice, but to exclude intraspinal extension, MRI should be performed preoperatively[13]. Prognosis following complete resection is excellent.

Pericardial cysts

Pericardial cysts, also termed 'spring water' or 'clear water' cysts because of their clear fluid contents, are uncommon developmental lesions of the middle mediastinum[4,6]. The vast majority are discovered incidentally in asymptomatic middle-aged adults. These cysts are well circumscribed and usually abut the heart, diaphragm, and the anterior chest wall, typically in the right cardiophrenic angle[13]. A nonenhancing cystic mass of water attenuation and an imperceptible wall are demonstrated on CT (Fig. 74.15)[13]. Unless significant symptoms or atypical imaging features are found, pericardial cysts are followed clinically and radiologically.

Vascular lesions

Vascular lesions constitute approximately 10% of all mediastinal masses and may originate from the arterial or venous portions of the systemic or pulmonary circulation. They may mimic neoplasms on chest radiographs and should be considered in the differential diagnosis before biopsy is performed. The diagnosis is usually established with contrast-enhanced CT, MRI, and/or angiography.

Diaphragmatic hernias

Hiatal hernias are common and result when an abdominal structure, usually the stomach, extends through the diaphragmatic esophageal hiatus into the thorax and manifest as a retrocardiac mass. Congenital defects in the diaphragm, with herniation of the omentum or other abdominal contents into the thorax, include foramen of Morgagni hernias, which manifest as a right cardiophrenic angle mass, and Bochdalek's hernias, which may protrude into the posterior mediastinum. Diagnosis can be

established by a gastrointestinal barium study or CT. Treatment of symptomatic cases is surgical.

DISEASES OF THE POSTERIOR MEDIASTINUM

Neurogenic tumors

Neurogenic tumors constitute 15–20% of all adult and 40% of pediatric mediastinal neoplasms[2,4,6,15]. Approximately 90% occur in the posterior mediastinum. A neurogenic tumor is the most common cause of a posterior mediastinal mass and accounts for 75% of primary posterior mediastinal neoplasms. Approximately 50% of neurogenic tumors in children are malignant, whereas in adults the majority are benign[3,15]. Half of the patients are asymptomatic[6]. Neurogenic tumors are generally grouped into three categories[4] – peripheral nerve tumors, sympathetic ganglia tumors, and paraganglionic tumors.

Peripheral nerve tumors
Schwannoma and neurofibroma
Schwannoma (also termed neurilemoma) and neurofibroma are the most common mediastinal neurogenic tumors[6]. Over 90% are benign and 10% are multiple[15]. They are slow-growing neoplasms and usually arise from a posterior spinal nerve root, but can involve any nerve in the thorax[4-6]. Schwannoma and solitary neurofibroma affect men and women equally, in the third and fourth decades. While these tumors can attain large sizes, most patients are asymptomatic[15]. Approximately 30–45% of neurofibromas occur in individuals who have neurofibromatosis (von Recklinghausen's disease)[4]. The presence of multiple neurofibromas or a single plexiform neurofibroma is pathognomonic of this disorder[16]. Patients who have neurofibromatosis and mediastinal neurogenic tumors are at increased risk for malignant transformation of a pre-existing neurofibroma. Malignant transformation of a schwannoma is extremely rare.

Radiologically, schwannomas and neurofibromas are sharply marginated, spheric, and occasionally lobulated posterior mediastinal masses, which usually span one to two rib interspaces, but can attain large sizes[4,15]. Up to half of the cases cause benign splaying and pressure erosion of the ribs, vertebral bodies, and neural foramina[13]. Of schwannomas and neurofibromas, 10% grow through and widen adjacent intervertebral foramina and expand on either end with a 'dumbbell' or 'hourglass' configuration (Fig. 74.16)[15]. Typically, CT reveals a heterogeneous mass, which may contain punctate calcification or low attenuation areas[13]. The treatment of choice is surgery, but to identify intraspinal extension, MRI should be performed preoperatively (Fig. 74.17). Recurrences are uncommon, even when excision is incomplete[15].

Malignant tumor of nerve sheath origin
Malignant tumors of nerve sheath origin are a rare group of spindle cell sarcomas thought to represent the malignant counterparts of schwannomas and neurofibromas. They occur equally in men and women in the third to fifth decades[16], and approximately half occur in individuals who have neurofibromatosis. The incidence of sarcomatous degeneration in neurofibromatosis is approximately 5%. A malignant tumor of nerve sheath origin can also occur sporadically or be induced by radiation[16]. While pain and an enlarging mass are common presentations, diagnosis of malignancy is difficult and often delayed.

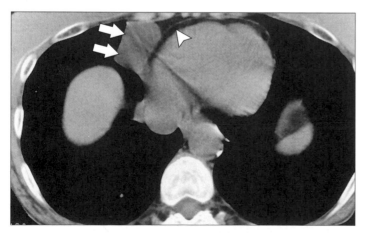

Figure 74.15 Pericardial cyst. Chest computed tomography reveals a sharply marginated pericardial cyst in the right cardiophrenic angle (arrows). The cyst has low attenuation contents with an imperceptible wall and abuts the anterior chest wall, pericardium (arrowhead), and diaphragm.

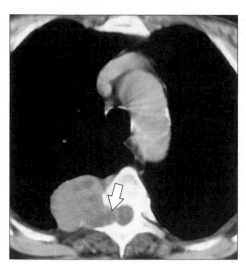

Figure 74.16 Chest computed tomography of neurofibroma. Heterogeneous attenuation, intraspinal extension (arrow), and pressure erosion of the neural foramina are demonstrated.

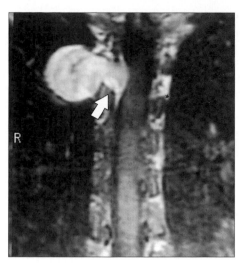

Figure 74.17 Gadolinium-enhanced, coronal magnetic resonance image of neurofibroma. Intraspinal extension (arrow) and effacement of the spinal cord.

Sympathetic ganglia tumors

Sympathetic ganglia tumors are common neoplasms of the posterior mediastinum in children, but are rare in adults[15]. Ganglioneuroma and ganglioneuroblastoma occur most commonly in sympathetic ganglia in the posterior mediastinum, whereas approximately half of neuroblastomas arise from the adrenal glands, and one third are located in the mediastinum, the most common extra-abdominal location.

Ganglioneuroma

Ganglioneuromas are benign tumors that equally affect male and female patients over 3 years of age to young adults. Half of the patients are symptomatic from local effects of the tumor or intraspinal extension[15]. Radiologically, they are well circumscribed, oblong, paraspinal masses that usually span three to five vertebrae, and may exhibit skeletal displacement or pressure erosion[13]. To exclude intraspinal extension, MRI is warranted. Surgical excision is the treatment of choice, and may necessitate a combined thoracic and neurosurgical approach[15].

Ganglioneuroblastoma

Ganglioneuroblastomas are tumors that usually occur in children under the age of 10 years, have no gender predilection, are malignant, and demonstrate composite histologic, biologic, and radiologic features of both ganglioneuromas and neuroblastomas[15]. Symptoms, when present, are caused by local mass effect, invasion of adjacent structures, or metastases. Staging and treatment are the same as for neuroblastomas.

Neuroblastoma

Neuroblastoma affects young children, 70–90% under the age of 5 years, and typically affects boys[15]. Neuroblastoma in patients over 5 years affects boys and girls equally. Two thirds of patients have constitutional symptoms, pain, cough, dyspnea, paraplegia, opsomyoclonus, and Horner's syndrome[3,15]. Systemic symptoms, such as hypertension, tachycardia, perspiration, flushing, and severe watery diarrhea, may occur because of elevated catecholamine and vasoactive intestinal peptide levels. Radiologically, the masses are paraspinous, occasionally with local invasion, contralateral extension, and/or skeletal erosion[15]. Approximately one third contain extensive calcifications apparent on radiographs. On CT, the tumors are heterogeneous because of hemorrhage and

necrosis, and calcification can be detected in 80% of cases[13]. For the detection of intraspinal extension and vascular or skeletal involvement, MRI is helpful. Metaiodobenzylguanidine scintigraphy (^{123}I or ^{131}I) may demonstrate uptake in both primary and metastatic neuroblastoma[13].

Neuroblastoma and ganglioneuroblastoma are treated with surgical resection. Adjuvant chemotherapy and irradiation are used for residual disease or as a primary treatment modality in advanced cases. Radiotherapy in children can lead to delayed complications such as myelitis and scoliosis[15]. The prognosis depends upon the age at diagnosis, the size, differentiation, and stage of the tumor, and is generally poor.

Paraganglionic tumors
Pheochromocytoma

Pheochromocytomas are functioning paraganglionic tumors that most commonly arise from the adrenal glands, and are seen more frequently in men in the third to fourth decades of life[15]. Approximately 10% of pheochromocytomas are extra-adrenal, and <2% are intrathoracic[15]; the latter tend to be more malignant and multicentric. Symptoms relate to systemic catecholamine excess or local mass effect. Pheochromocytomas can be part of a multisystem endocrine syndrome, such as type 2a or 2b multiple endocrine neoplasia syndrome. Diagnosis can be established by measurement of urine catecholamines and their metabolites (vanillyl mandelic acid, homovanillic acid, metanephrine, and normetanephrine). Typically, CT and MRI reveal a well-delineated, enhancing, posterior mediastinal mass. The neoplasm is typically ^{123}I and ^{123}I-metaiodobenzylguanidine avid[13]. Treatment includes sympathetic α- and β-blockade for 1–2 weeks followed by surgical excision. Chemotherapy and/or radiotherapy can be used for metastatic disease.

Paraganglioma

Paraganglioma are rare tumors of paraganglionic tissue[3,4], the majority of which are benign, asymptomatic, and nonfunctioning. Radiologically, they typically manifest as a sharply marginated, middle or posterior mediastinal nodule or mass, usually located adjacent to the aorta, pulmonary arteries, heart, or costovertebral sulci, or within the left atrial wall. They are hypervascular lesions and demonstrate marked contrast enhancement[13]. The treatment is surgical excision.

Lateral thoracic meningocele

Lateral thoracic meningocele is a rare lesion that consists of redundant meninges which protrude through the intervertebral foramen and contain cerebrospinal fluid. They represent the most common posterior mediastinal lesion in neurofibromatosis, and has no sex predilection. The diagnosis is usually established in an asymptomatic patient in the fourth to fifth decades of life. Radiologic studies demonstrate a well-circumscribed, paraspinous, cystic lesion, frequently associated with vertebral abnormalities such as erosion, kyphoscoliosis, and widening of neural foramina. Continuity with the thecal sac may be demonstrated by CT or MRI[13]. Symptomatic lesions are treated with surgical excision.

MISCELLANEOUS DISORDERS OF THE MEDIASTINUM

Mediastinitis

Mediastinitis describes a variety of infectious and inflammatory conditions. Acute mediastinitis is more common than the chronic form and may be caused by esophageal or tracheobronchial perforation, penetrating chest trauma, postoperative sternal wound infection, extension of an oropharyngeal infection, a paravertebral or vertebral abscess, radiation therapy, malignancy, and rarely anthrax.

Patients who have acute mediastinitis usually present with sudden onset of high fever, chills, chest pain, dyspnea, and dysphagia. Physical examination may reveal systemic toxicity, respiratory distress, Hamman's sign, subcutaneous emphysema, chest-wall tenderness, and edema. Chest radiography and CT show mediastinal widening, pneumomediastinum, mediastinal air–fluid levels or fluid collection, and pleural effusions. An esophagram may reveal perforation. Acute mediastinitis is generally diffuse, but may be localized when secondary to sternal wound infection. The treatment includes surgical drainage, debridement, repair of the source of infection, and broad-spectrum antibiotics. The mortality rate is high, especially when the diagnosis is delayed.

Chronic mediastinitis, also termed fibrosing mediastinitis or granulomatous mediastinitis, is caused by various infectious and inflammatory processes. Histoplasmosis and tuberculosis account for most cases. Noninfectious causes include sarcoidosis, silicosis, prior mediastinal hematoma, radiation therapy, and drugs such as methysergide and hydralazine. Chronic mediastinitis can be associated with various idiopathic and autoimmune diseases, such as retroperitoneal fibrosis, Riedel's thyroiditis, pseudotumor of the orbit, sclerosing cholangitis, systemic lupus erythematosus, and rheumatoid arthritis. Dense fibrous tissue, most commonly located in the paratracheal, carinal, and hilar regions, compresses and strangulates mediastinal structures such as the superior vena cava, pulmonary vessels, airways, and esophagus. Superior vena cava syndrome is the most common clinical manifestation. Chest radiographs, CT, MRI, and perfusion scintigraphy, in addition to endoscopy, help to suggest the diagnosis. Typical is a CT finding of mediastinal calcification with coexistent pulmonary or hepatosplenic granulomatous disease. Histologic examination of mediastinal tissue may be necessary to exclude a neoplastic process or active infection. Treatment is ineffective and mostly palliative; the benefit of corticosteroids is controversial. In the presence of viable fungal organisms or rising serum antibody titers, antifungal agents can be administered. With superior vena cava syndrome, long-term anticoagulation and vascular bypass procedures can be considered.

Pneumomediastinum

Pneumomediastinum is typically caused by alveolar overdistention and rupture from increased intrathoracic volume or pressure caused by mechanical ventilation, trauma, an acute attack of asthma, or spontaneous rupture. Air dissects into the pulmonary interstitium, peribronchovascular tissues, and mediastinum (see Fig. 1.77), and frequently decompresses into the soft tissues of the neck[17]. Less commonly, pneumomediastinum can be secondary to tracheobronchial or esophageal perforation, traumatic entry of air directly through the chest wall, cervical emphysema, or pneumoperitoneum that tracks into the mediastinum, or a gas-forming infection.

REFERENCES

1. Fraser RS, Paré JAP, Fraser RG, Paré PD. The normal chest. In: Fraser RS, Paré JAP, Fraser RG, Paré PD, eds. Synopsis of diseases of the chest, 2nd ed. Philadelphia: WB Saunders; 1994:1–116.
2. Azarow KS, Pearl RH, Zurcher R, Edwards FH, Cohen AJ. Primary mediastinal masses. J Thorac Cardiovasc Surg. 1993;106:67–72.
3. Hoffman OA, Gillespie DJ, Aughenbaugh GL, Brown LR. Primary mediastinal neoplasms (other than thymomas). Mayo Clin Proc. 1993;68:880–91.
4. Wychulis AR, Payne WS, Clagett OT, Woolner LB. Surgical treatment of mediastinal tumors. J Thorac Cardiovasc Surg. 1971;62:379–91.
5. Cohen AJ, Thompson L, Edwards FH, Bellamy RF. Primary cysts and tumors of the mediastinum. Ann Thorac Surg. 1991;51:378–86.
6. Davis RD, Oldham HN, Sabiston DC. Primary cysts and neoplasms of the mediastinum: recent changes in clinical presentation, methods of diagnosis, management and results. Ann Thorac Surg. 1987;44:229–37.
7. Lewis JE, Wick MR, Scheithauer BW, Bernatz PE, Taylor WF. Thymoma: a clinicopathologic review. Cancer. 1987;60:2727–43.
8. Morgenthaler TI, Brown LR, Colby TV, Harper Jr CM, Coles DT. Thymoma. Mayo Clin Proc. 1993;68:1110–23.
9. Strollo DC, Rosado de Christenson ML, Jett JR. Primary mediastinal tumors. Part I. Tumors of the anterior mediastinum. Chest. 1997;112:511–22.
10. Drachman DB. Myasthenia gravis. N Engl J Med. 1994;330:1797–810.
11. Suster S, Rosai J. Thymic carcinoma. Cancer. 1991;67:1025–32.
12. Ryu JH, Habermann TM. Pulmonary lymphoma: primary and systemic disease. Semin Respir Crit Care Med. 1997;18:341–52.
13. Strollo DC, Rosado de Christenson ML, Jett JR. Primary mediastinal tumors. Part II. Tumors of the middle and posterior mediastinum. Chest. 1997;112:1344–57.
14. Nichols CR. Mediastinal germ cell tumors: clinical features and biologic correlates. Chest. 1991;99:472–9.
15. Shields TW, Reynolds M. Neurogenic tumors of the thorax. Surg Clin North Am. 1988;68:645–68.
16. Swanson PE. Soft tissue neoplasms of the mediastinum. Semin Diagn Pathol. 1991;8:14–34.
17. Maunder RJ, Pierson DJ, Hudson LD. Subcutaneous and mediastinal emphysema: pathophysiology, diagnosis, and management. Arch Intern Med. 1984;144:1447–53.

Chapter 75

Obstructive Sleep Apnea

Charles W Atwood, Jr and Patrick J Strollo, Jr

INTRODUCTION

Obstructive sleep apnea (OSA) is a disorder characterized by collapse of the pharyngeal airway during sleep accompanied by arousal from sleep. An apnea is defined as a complete cessation of airflow for at least 10 seconds[1]. The presence of continued ventilatory effort characterizes it as an obstructive apnea compared with a central apnea, in which airflow and ventilatory effort are both absent. A hypopnea, a related term, is a reduction in airflow by a defined amount, usually by less than 50%, accompanied by a desaturation of at least 4% and/or an arousal from sleep. Sleep-disordered breathing (SDB) is a more general term used to encompass both sleep apneas and hypopneas. The term sleep apnea–hypopnea syndrome (SAHS) is used to define patients who have a sleep-study based diagnosis of sleep apneas and hypopneas associated with clinical symptoms of the disorder. Severe SAHS occurs when there are more than 50 apneas and/or hypopneas in an hour [apnea/hypopnea index (AHI)]. Patients who have mild or moderate SAHS have AHIs of 10–30 and 31–50, respectively. Examples of sleep apneas and hypopneas are shown in Figure 75.1.

EPIDEMIOLOGY, RISK FACTORS, AND PATHOPHYSIOLOGY

Epidemiology

A recent, large epidemiologic study of the prevalence of SDB in middle-aged Americans in Wisconsin found that 4% of men and 2% of women had symptomatic disease, and had SAHS (which is quite common)[2]. Using a conservative definition of the significant number apneas and hypopneas (>5 apneas or hypopneas per hour of sleep), Young et al. reported sleep study abnormalities with no clinical symptoms in 9% of men and 4% of women[2], although most laboratories take an AHI of >10 to be significant (half the Wisconsin incidence). An Australian questionnaire survey of the prevalence of SDB in 35- to 69-year-olds found that 3.6% of the sample had an AHI >15 (5.7% in men and 1.2% in women). The incidence of snorers was 60%, but the questionnaire used was biased toward the identification of snorers[3]. The significance of SDB with no clinical symptoms is not known.

Risk factors

Several conditions appear to predispose an individual to sleep apnea; it tends to increase with age, male gender, obesity, increased neck circumference, use of alcohol or sedative/hypnotic medications, and craniofacial abnormalities such as retrognathia[1,4]. Certain craniofacial abnormalities, which include retrognathia and a decreased intermolar distance (resulting in a high, arched palate), are strongly

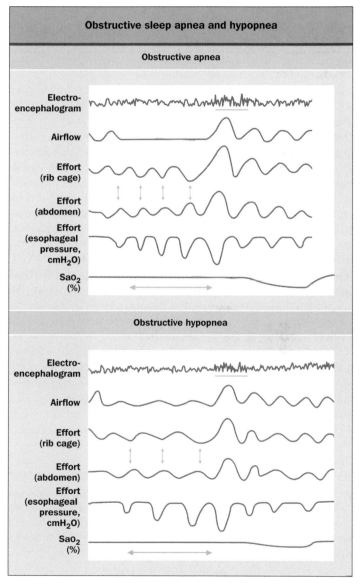

Obstructive sleep apnea and hypopnea

Obstructive apnea

Electro-encephalogram
Airflow
Effort (rib cage)
Effort (abdomen)
Effort (esophageal pressure, cmH$_2$O)
SaO$_2$ (%)

Obstructive hypopnea

Electro-encephalogram
Airflow
Effort (rib cage)
Effort (abdomen)
Effort (esophageal pressure, cmH$_2$O)
SaO$_2$ (%)

Figure 75.1 Obstructive sleep apnea and hypopnea. (Top) Example of key elements of obstructive sleep apnea. Note cessation of airflow for at least 10 seconds, out-of-phase (paradoxic) movement of thoracic and abdominal respiratory effort signal, increasingly negative deflections of esophageal pressure (which indicates increasing airway resistance), oxygen desaturation, and arousal from sleep. (Bottom) Example of key elements of obstructive sleep hypopnea. Note reduction (but not cessation) in airflow for at least 10 seconds, out-of-phase (paradoxic) movement of thoracic and abdominal respiratory effort signals, increasingly negative esophageal pressure deflections (which indicates increased airway resistance), oxygen desaturation, and arousal from sleep. 10cmH$_2$O = 1kPa.

predictive of SDB when combined with the body mass index (BMI; kg/m^2)[5]. However, the relative importance of the contributions of each of these variables to an individual's risk of developing sleep apnea is not known.

Alcohol before sleep appears to predispose to SDB, probably because of a greater relaxation effect on the upper airway dilator muscles, such as the genioglossus, compared with its effect on the diaphragm, which results in a more negative upper-airway pressure generated during inspiration than can be defended against by activation of pharyngeal dilator muscles.

The precise risks of SDB for an individual are uncertain, although hypertension, coronary heart disease, and stroke have been identified as being more common in subjects who have OSA, particularly severe OSA; these increases are confounded by the effects of age, gender, BMI, alcohol consumption, and smoking. All these factors lower the odds ratio for OSA being a major risk factor and large, long-term studies are needed before the precise risk of OSA itself can be clarified.

Pathophysiology

The pathophysiology of OSA is complex and incompletely understood[6]. Anatomic features of the upper airway (such as pharyngeal diameter, the presence of tonsils, hyoid bone position, and relative upper and lower jaw structure) interact with 'neuromuscular factors' (such as resting muscle tone of the pharyngeal dilator muscle group) and the effects of state (sleep versus wakefulness) to determine upper airway caliber[6]. Upper airway tone and patency is a dynamic process.

Upper airway size is an important determinant of OSA. A smaller airway is more prone to closure for a given degree of upper airway tone than a larger airway, since the amount of narrowing required to complete closure is less than for a larger airway. Tonsils or other intraluminal, soft-tissue obstruction can contribute to pharyngeal narrowing at specific airway sites.

Upper airway muscle tone and function is dynamic and is important in the pathophysiology of OSAs. In patients who do not have sleep apnea, the tone of the genioglossus, the chief pharyngeal dilator muscle, increases during inspiration and decreases during exhalation, a function that is maintained during nonrapid eye movement (REM) sleep. Furthermore, in normal humans, during wakefulness the genioglossus contracts in response to sudden negative intrapharyngeal pressure. This airway reflex is normally decreased during non-REM sleep (Fig. 75.2), a finding that may predispose to upper airway collapse[8]. In patients who have OSA, resting genioglossal tone is generally increased during wakefulness, which may result from the need for greater neuromuscular compensation for the smaller pharyngeal airway present in these patients. Obstructive apneas occur when the smaller-than-normal airway narrows further during sleep, as the increased genioglossal tone present during wakefulness is significantly decreased[6].

In addition to differences in genioglossus tone during sleep, anatomic factors such as neck soft-tissue mass, parapharyngeal fat, upper airway vascular engorgement, and intraluminal adhesive surface forces, all of which favor pharyngeal narrowing, are likely to play a role in the development of OSA. As airflow through the narrowed pharynx becomes turbulent, vibrations occur in the soft tissues of the pharynx. As pharyngeal intraluminal pressure becomes negative with each inspiratory effort, the likelihood of airway collapse increases, and apneas and hypopneas occur as a result (Fig. 75.3).

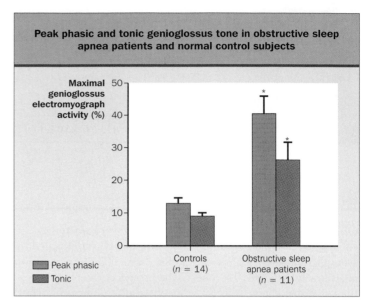

Figure 75.2 Peak phasic and tonic genioglossus tone in obstructive sleep apnea (OSA) patients and normal control subjects. Mean data from all subjects demonstrate that both peak phasic and tonic genioglossal electromyogram activity are higher in OSA patients than in normal subjects. Asterisks denote $p < 0.005$ versus controls. (Adapted from Mezzanote et al.[7] by copyright permission of The American Society for Clinical Investigation.)

A common feature of sleep apnea is the patient's lack of awareness of it. Frequently, patients who have moderate SAHS deny a problem with sleep or daytime functioning, and make excuses for actions or behaviors ultimately attributable to sleep apnea. A concerned spouse or partner may motivate the patient to seek clinical attention. The patient may not realize until after the OSA has been treated how impaired he or she was. Not surprisingly, the time from onset of symptoms to clinical diagnosis and treatment is frequently many years.

CLINICAL FEATURES

Important clinical features of SDB are shown in Figure 75.4. Snoring is frequently associated with sleep apnea but may occur independently. Many patients are unaware of the effects of sleep apnea on the quality of their sleep, and awaken feeling unrefreshed without realizing why. This leads to daytime sleepiness, and frequently measurable effects on cognitive functioning. Sleep fragmentation from repetitive arousals from sleep appear to be the main cause of daytime hypersomnolence, although influences from oxyhemoglobin desaturation may be important.

Hypersomnolence

The daytime somnolence of SDB is important to recognize. Sleepiness that results in decrements in work performance, concentration lapses, inattention, and decreased reaction times have been well documented. Depending on the patient's occupation, this may lead to unacceptable risks to the patient and the general public. For example, in truck drivers or school bus drivers, untreated sleep apnea with excessive daytime sleepiness may cause catastrophic accidents[1]. Disabling daytime sleepiness may lead to disciplinary actions against employees who fall asleep at work. Loss of productive time and errors caused by sleepiness decrease productivity.

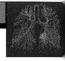

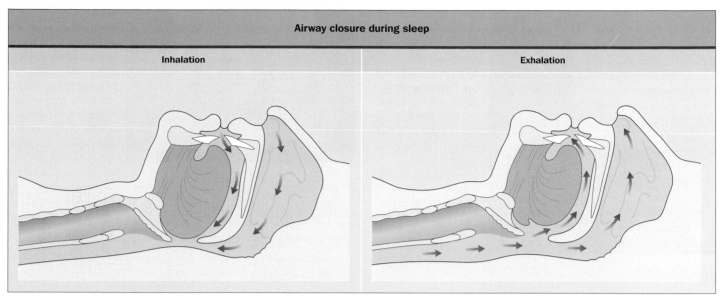

Figure 75.3 Airway closure during sleep. Demonstrates an upper airway segment that is narrowed and susceptible to airway closure during inhalation, when pharyngeal intraluminal pressure is negative. During exhalation, the segment remains narrowed and unstable, which sets up the upper airway segment for a repeat cycle of closure with the next inhalation.

Clinical features of obstructive sleep apnea	
Symptoms	**Signs**
Excessive daytime sleepiness	Snoring
Unrefreshing sleep	Nocturnal choking
Restless sleep	Nocturnal cardiac arrhythmia
Morning dry mouth	Sleeping at inappropriate times
Morning headache	Cor pulmonale
Difficulty concentrating	Polycythemia
Irritability, mood changes	

Figure 75.4 Important symptoms and signs of obstructive sleep apnea.

Hypoxemia

Nocturnal hypoxemia is another important feature of sleep apnea. The extent and frequency of oxygen desaturation is commonly used to classify severity of sleep apnea; the deeper and more frequent the desaturation, the greater the severity of the disorder.

The physiologic impact of desaturation in sleep apnea is not completely understood. In severe cases, it is associated with polycythemia and the possible development of pulmonary hypertension. It may also contribute to the development of neurocognitive deficits. However, isolation of the effect of desaturation from other aspects of sleep apnea, such as sleep fragmentation and changes in activation of the sympathetic nervous system, is difficult. Clinically, most patients who suffer sleep apnea have most if not all physiologic perturbations, which are all treated simultaneously.

Obesity

Patients who have sleep apnea are frequently obese, although severe forms of the disorder can occur in individuals of normal body weight. Severity of sleep apnea tends to increase with increasing weight. The typical male obesity pattern of central or truncal weight distribution is more common than the typical female pattern of obesity, which has a more peripheral distribution. Neck circumference is strongly predictive of sleep apnea, even more so than BMI in some studies[4].

Myxedema, acromegaly, Down's syndrome, and other causes of macroglossia are all strongly associated with OSA and must be excluded.

Craniofacial and airway abnormalities

In patients who are not obese, craniofacial structural abnormalities may contribute to sleep apnea. A retrognathic mandible and an inferiorly displaced hyoid bone have been associated with sleep apnea[1]. Since these abnormalities tend to occur over time, it is not known whether they are causative of sleep apnea or reflect changes in facial structure that result from sleep apnea. These and other craniofacial structural features can be assessed using a lateral cephalometric radiograph (see Fig. 75.5). These radiographs may help in the management of sleep apnea, especially if reconstructive upper-airway surgery is contemplated. In selected cases, other forms of upper airway imaging, such as computed tomography or magnetic resonance imaging, may help.

Some patients who suffer sleep apnea have large palatine tonsils that may partially obstruct the pharyngeal lumen (see Fig. 75.6). This tends to occur in younger patients, but may be seen occasionally in adults. Surgical removal of palatine tonsils is not uniformly successful in the treatment of sleep apnea. Caution is recommended before proceeding with using this surgery alone to treat OSA. Sleep apnea occurs in patients who have acquired immunodeficiency syndrome caused by tonsilar hypertrophy related to human immunodeficiency virus[9].

Overlap syndrome

One subset of OSA patients that appears to be at increased risk for pulmonary hypertension, and perhaps other serious complication, is the patient who has overlap syndrome, which is the coincidence of OSA and chronic obstructive pulmonary disease (COPD), with consequent diurnal and nocturnal hypoxemia[10]. The overlap syn-

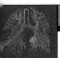

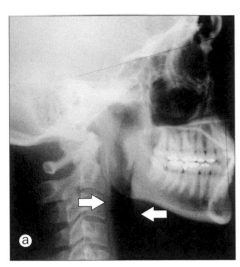

Figure 75.5 Lateral cephalometric radiographs. (a) From a normal subject. (b) From a patient who has obstructive sleep apnea, which shows a narrowed posterior airway space (thin dark line immediately posterior to the mandible) and steeper plane of mandible compared with those of the normal subject (arrows).

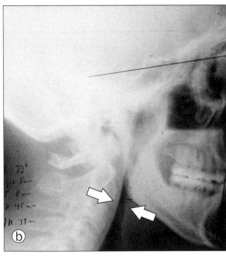

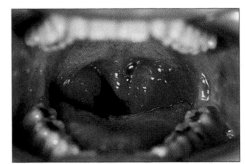

Figure 75.6 Obstructing palatine tonsils. Example of palatine tonsils that nearly obstruct the posterior oropharyngeal airway. Surgical removal of tonsils is not always curative of obstructive sleep apnea.

What to assess in a sleep history	
General problem area	**Particular difficulties**
Daytime sleepiness	Sleep at work or other inappropriate times or places Difficulty driving a car because of sleepiness Daytime napping
Bed habits and behaviors	Bedtime – restlessness throughout night Out-of-bed time – can be substantial Number of awakenings Insomnia
Snoring and apneas	Patient history of snoring and apneas given by partner Patient awakenings with choking, gasping, or dyspnea
Habits	Alcohol ⎤ Cigarettes ⎥ all worsen obstructive sleep apnea Caffeine ⎦
Other medical history	Hypertension ⎤ may be made worse Cardiopulmonary disorders ⎥ by obstructive sleep Cerebrovascular disease ⎦ apnea

Figure 75.7 Aspects of sleep history key to the clinical evaluation of obstructive sleep apnea.

drome is relatively common, as was demonstrated in one study in which 30 of 265 patients who had OSA with a AHI >20 also had a forced expiratory volume in 1 second to vital capacity ratio (FEV_1/VC) of <60%, indicating moderate to severe COPD. These patients were older than the rest of the study population and were all men. Their BMI was not different, but their resting arterial partial pressure of oxygen (PaO_2) was lower and $PaCO_2$ higher than those of the patients who had OSA only. The pulmonary artery pressure was also higher at rest and on exercise in the overlap syndrome patients; thus, the risk of developing respiratory insufficiency and cor pulmonale appears to be higher with this combination[10]. Typically, these problems are not noticed for many years and right-sided ventricular failure may be the presenting complication of the two conditions. It is not uncommon for patients who have overlap syndrome to come to medical attention with acute respiratory failure that requires intubation and mechanical ventilation. Pulmonary hypertension is common in these patients; its response to oxygen for diurnal hypoxemia and treatment of sleep apnea is variable, but some improvements usually occur.

DIAGNOSIS

History
The diagnosis of SDB begins with a thorough medical history, with emphasis on sleep habits and behaviors. Important aspects of the sleep history are shown in Figure 75.7. The diagnosis of

OSA is often obvious from the history in severely affected patients; however, in milder cases it is not so clear. Studies of the sensitivity and predictive value of sleep history to detect sleep apnea have given various results. In the population of a sleep-disorders clinic (i.e. those already selected by the referral process), the sleep history may be quite predictive of sleep apnea, but in a general medical population, the history is easily overlooked or not considered.

Physical examination
The physical examination of patients who have sleep apnea must note any general obesity, which together with BMI is associated with and predictive of sleep apnea. A neck circumference of more than 42cm for a man and 40cm for a woman is also strongly associated with sleep apnea.

Other aspects of the general medical examination must include the oral cavity, size of the tongue, presence of tonsils, and position of the posterior portion of the soft palate. Obstructing tonsils similarly may contribute to upper airway narrowing.

General craniofacial structure and the degree of retrognathia is noted. Deviation of the nasal septum may contribute to snoring and make positive airway pressure (PAP) therapy for OSA uncomfortable. Examination of the soft and hard palate and oral cavity may reveal a narrowed intermolar distance and a high-arched hard palate, suggestive of abnormal craniofacial features that are closely associated with an increased risk for sleep apnea[5].

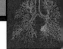
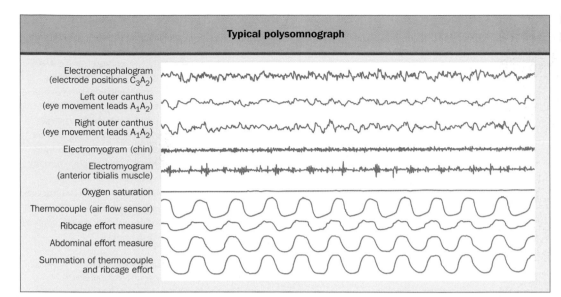

Typical polysomnograph

Electroencephalogram (electrode positions C_3A_2)

Left outer canthus (eye movement leads A_1A_2)

Right outer canthus (eye movement leads A_1A_2)

Electromyogram (chin)

Electromyogram (anterior tibialis muscle)

Oxygen saturation

Thermocouple (air flow sensor)

Ribcage effort measure

Abdominal effort measure

Summation of thermocouple and ribcage effort

Figure 75.8 A typical polysomnogram.

Chronic peripheral edema may be a clue to severe right-sided ventricular failure associated with significant and untreated sleep apnea. Left-sided ventricular failure and the presence of congestive heart failure have been associated with an increased likelihood of SDB. The presence of concomitant pulmonary disease is determined because of the likelihood of more serious desaturation during sleep apneas and hypopneas.

Sleep laboratory diagnosis

The diagnosis of sleep apnea requires measurement of the abnormal breathing patterns and associated abnormalities that define the syndrome. The indications for an overnight sleep study include:

- patients who snore but have a low probability of SDB, for whom SDB can be eliminated and perhaps the snoring treated by surgery;
- patients likely to have SDB, with typical symptoms and the appearance of a subject who has OSA;
- assess response to therapy for SDB;
- detect nocturnal hypoxemia, particularly in patients who have chronic lung disorders, such as COPD and kyphoscoliosis; and
- identify other unexplained sleeping disorders for which the history is not clear or helpful (e.g. restless leg syndrome, narcolepsy, poor sleep hygiene, and sleep pattern).

Traditionally, a sleep study entails a full polysomnogram that measures a large number of physiologic signals during sleep (Figs 75.8 & 75.9). Polysomnography requires trained technicians, and is labor intensive and costly. However, it provides an enormous amount of useful data to the clinician about the patient's sleep, whether SDB is present and its severity, as well as other physiologic data. A variety of sleep disorders not related to breathing also show characteristic findings on polysomnography.

As polysomnographic technology has advanced and become miniaturized, the absolute requirement to monitor in a sleep laboratory has decreased and high-quality studies are now possible outside the sleep laboratory. Recordings may be performed using miniaturized multichannel recorders at the patient's home or in other settings.

Another diagnostic approach that has been adopted in some centers is to record a fewer number of variables overall, but focus on the key respiratory variables that define SAHS, which include oronasal air flow, respiratory effort, pulse oximetry, and heart

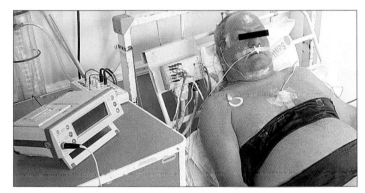

Figure 75.9 Polysomnography. Example of a patient set-up to undergo polysomnography.

rate. Variables such as electroencephalogram and electromyelogram are omitted and sleep stages are not recorded. Sleep apnea disease burden is measured in terms of apnea and hypopnea frequency and desaturations, with no reference to the effect on sleep. These sleep apnea diagnostic systems are easily portable, relatively simple to operate, and provide minimal but frequently sufficient results on SDB to diagnose sleep apnea.

Simple screening studies in patients who almost certainly just snore, or clearly have OSA, are perfectly adequate for clinical management. Several simple systems are available, often with a videocamera, microphone, oximeter, heart rate recorder, and a means to detect body movement. Often the oximeter tracing alone reveals the classic pattern of OSA (see Fig. 75.10).

TREATMENT

Medical therapy

A variety of simple medical therapies have been described. Body position (i.e. the patient sleeps on his or her side) is useful when sleep apnea is documented to occur only when the patient sleeps supine. A tennis ball placed in a pocket on the back of pajamas occasionally works. Weight loss has been shown to be effective as a primary therapy for sleep apnea, but is difficult to achieve[11]. No alcohol in the evenings, no night sedation, and avoidance of late meals may help. Stopping smoking may reduce pharyngeal congestion and improve nasal patency.

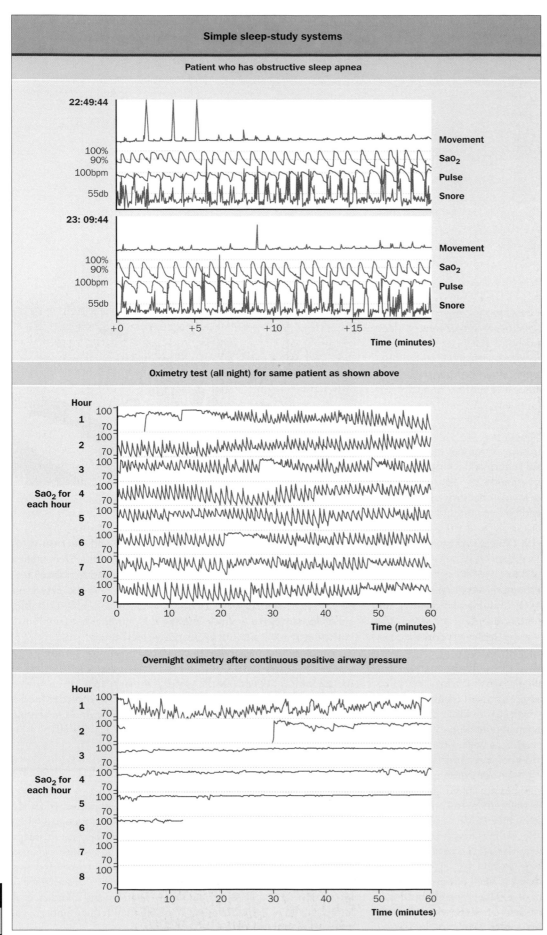

Figure 75.10 Simpler sleep-study systems. (Top) Recording of body movement (movement), oximetry (Sao₂), heart rate (pulse), and snoring (snore, in decibels) which clearly shows obstructive sleep apnea (OSA). (Middle) The same patient's oximetry trace is shown for the whole night with desaturation throughout the night, i.e. severe OSA. (Bottom) Oximetry for 4 hours after commencing continuous positive airway pressure (following a 1 hour period of observation), with complete control of the OSA.

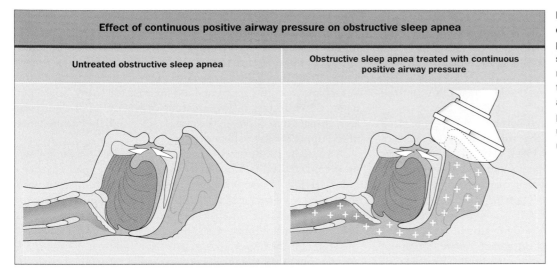

Effect of continuous positive airway pressure on obstructive sleep apnea

| Untreated obstructive sleep apnea | Obstructive sleep apnea treated with continuous positive airway pressure |

Figure 75.11 Effect of continuous positive airway pressure (CPAP) on obstructive sleep apnea (OSA). The chief mechanism of CPAP in the treatment of OSA is airway splinting and dilatation of obstructed pharyngeal segments. Both untreated OSA and OSA treated using CPAP are shown.

Medications that have been tried as therapy for OSA include protriptyline, fluoxetine, and progesterone, but none has demonstrated unequivocal efficacy.

Positive airway pressure

A variety of medical and surgical treatments for SAHS have been described. The mainstay of treatment, however, is PAP therapy[1]. The most widely used of the PAP therapies is nasal continuous positive airway pressure (CPAP). Nasal CPAP treats OSA by pneumatically dilating the upper airway, which prevents its closure (Fig. 75.11).

A wide range of comfortable silicone CPAP masks that fit tightly over the nose with no leakage are now available. The pressure required to overcome the upper airway narrowing is usually about $10cmH_2O$. Most patients need to try the system during daytime hours, with help and advice from sleep technicians before a nighttime study. 'Intelligent' CPAP machines adjust the airway pressure breath by breath during the night and an average is taken to reach the optimal, most comfortable pressure. Usually one or two study nights are required before a patient is ready to take a CPAP device home. It is only necessary to repeat a CPAP sleep study if the patient's symptoms are not adequately controlled or return. Occasionally it is worth repeating the study if the patient has lost a considerable amount of weight and thinks the OSA has improved dramatically.

Compliance studies all show that only those who suffer the most severe daytime somnolence use the equipment regularly. Overall, the average nighttime use is 4–5 hours, and about 20–40% of patients stop using CPAP within 3 months. Many patients claim good symptomatic improvement with just 5 hours use per night, but (in general), the lower the initial AHI and the milder the symptoms, the less likely that the subject is compliant. Factors that adversely affect compliance and that can be influenced include mask discomfort, particularly when the nasal bridge is affected, and nasal blockage and stuffiness.

Bilevel PAP is an alternative to CPAP for OSA. It operates on the principle that a higher level of PAP is required to open the obstructed pharyngeal airway segment than is required to maintain its patency. Therefore, during bilevel PAP therapy, the inspiratory pressure is higher than the expiratory pressure. Some patients who complain about exhaling against an elevated pressure during CPAP therapy find bilevel PAP more comfortable to use.

Oral appliances

Oral appliances, or mandibular advancement splints (MASs), have emerged as an effective alternative to palatal surgery and CPAP for the treatment of snoring. Previous studies also suggest that MASs are nearly as effective as CPAP for the treatment of mild and moderate OSA[12]. These devices are individually fitted to the upper and lower incisors, and usually are hinged to allow the subject to breathe through the mouth during sleep. The effect a MAS is to pull the mandible forward a few millimeters (Fig. 75.12). They have not been adequately tested for severe OSA, but when used in mild or moderate OSA, patients generally prefer MAS to CPAP. These appliances may have an important role in the management of all but the most severe cases of OSA.

Surgical therapy

Surgical treatments for OSA seek to alter the upper airway anatomy to eliminate sites of obstruction. Studies have shown that the upper airway tends to be diffusely affected in the majority of cases, rather than having segments of discrete obstruction that might be amenable to traditional surgical correction using uvulopalatopharyngoplasty (UPPP)[13].

Tracheostomy is an effective treatment for SAHS, but is disfiguring and is unacceptable to many patients. In the early 1980s, UPPP was developed as a better alternative to tracheostomy[14]. Despite initial enthusiasm for the procedure, subsequent studies have shown a response rate of <50% in unselected patients[15]. The diffuse nature of pharyngeal involvement in OSA probably accounts for the poor success rate of UPPP[16]. Even when patients are selected on the basis that the obstruction is at the level of the soft

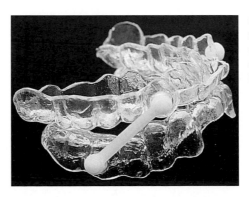

Figure 75.12 A mandibular advancement splint – inserted before sleep.

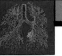
palate, which should be correctable using UPPP, cure rates are still lower than ideal. Furthermore, no clear consensus exists among surgeons as the best way to evaluate and select candidates for UPPP.

Laser-assisted uvuloplasty (LAUP) was developed in Europe to treat snoring, and does so very successfully for uncomplicated snoring. Over time, LAUP has been used to treat OSA, but the results have not been as successful[14].

Increasingly, the approach favored by surgeons expert in sleep apnea therapy is to use procedures that treat multiple segments of the upper airway obstruction seen in OSA. These newer approaches consider the finding that the majority of patients who suffer SAHS have upper airway collapse at more than one segment[17].

A geniohyoid advancement procedure with or without a traditional UPPP may be curative of SAHS in approximately 70% of patients. In this procedure, the genioglossus is advanced through a mandibular osteotomy at the geniotubercle, the site of genioglossus insertion on the anterior mandible. This 'plug' of bone and tongue-muscle insertion is advanced several millimeters and resecured to the mandible. The hyoid bone is then resuspended, using a suture or fascia, in a higher (cephalad) position relative to the mandible. The overall effect is to advance the anterior pharyngeal wall from the level of the base of the tongue to the lower part of the hypopharynx (just above the epiglottis). A more anterior tongue position also decreases its opportunity to obstruct the airway while sleeping supine (Fig. 75.13).

An additional surgical option for OSA is maxillomandibular advancement. In this procedure, the maxilla and mandible are both advanced through an intentional facial fracture and then plated into a new position (Fig. 75.14). This procedure has been used when other surgical procedures have not successfully alleviated sleep apnea[17].

CLINICAL COURSE

Information on the natural history of OSA once established is scanty. Loud snoring often precedes the onset of daytime somnolence and, by inference, OSA. A 5-year follow-up of 58 patients who had OSA and refused any treatment showed no changes in AHI or nocturnal hypoxemia, and weight gain did not appear to cause the syndrome to worsen[18]. This broadly agrees with the observation that if successful treatment for OSA is stopped, the condition recurs within a few days. Other studies, however, report a deterioration in AHI of untreated patients, but the prediction of deterioration remains difficult. The mechanisms that cause this deterioration may include trauma to the nasopharynx from recurrent loud snoring for many hours per night, which results in myxomatous degeneration of the uvula; also, changes may occur in the muscle fibers and the maintenance of the upper airway caliber during sleep[19].

A study in 1988, however, showed that in an 8-year follow-up period, mortality was higher in patients who had an apnea index (AI) >20 and who refused treatment, compared with those who were successfully treated[20]. Cardiovascular mortality was also higher (Fig. 75.15). This was a retrospective study and subject to considerable bias. Nonetheless, the implications of this study for the importance of detection and treatment of OSA are considerable if the results are verified in subsequent trials. In fact, a prospective population-based study in Sweden looked at the health consequences of snoring with and without excessive daytime somnolence (EDS) in men aged 30–69 years. The combination of snoring and EDS was associated with a significant increase in mortality, but this disappeared in men over the age of 60. The risk of cardiovascular mortality was 2.9 for subjects with both snoring and EDS, whilst snoring without EDS had no increased mortality risk[21]. Thus, the combination of snoring and EDS appears to be associated with an increased mortality rate but the effects seem to be age dependent.

PITFALLS AND CONTROVERSIES

Although OSA is a common disorder the morbidity and mortality have been difficult to quantify because of confounding factors. It has generally been appreciated that OSA impairs automobile driving and is associated with an increased risk of crashes. Less clear is the degree of medical risk associated with OSA.

Cardiovascular risks have been postulated for untreated OSA, but clinical evidence of an increase in cardiovascular morbidity and mortality is unclear. Of the relationships between OSA and cardiovascular disease studied to date, the strongest evidence links OSA to hypertension.

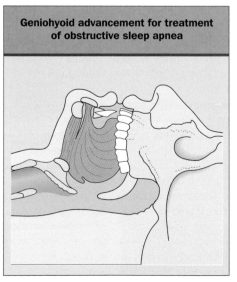

Geniohyoid advancement for treatment of obstructive sleep apnea

Figure 75.13 Geniohyoid advancement to treat obstructive sleep apnea. The geniotubercle (insertion site of the genioglossus) is advanced following a small mandibular osteotomy. The hyoid bone is resuspended in a more superior and anterior position, which results in advancement of the anterior pharyngeal wall and an increase in the posterior pharyngeal airway diameter.

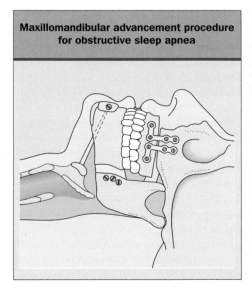

Maxillomandibular advancement procedure for obstructive sleep apnea

Figure 75.14 Maxillomandibular advancement procedure for obstructive sleep apnea. A maxillary and mandibular LeFort 1 osteotomy is performed. Both maxilla and mandible are advanced by 6–8mm and refixed in a forward position. In this example, note the prior geniotubercle advancement and hyoid suspension.

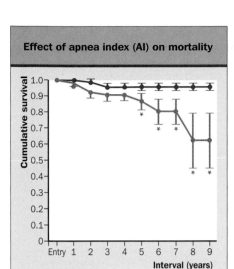

Figure 75.15 Effect of apnea index (AI) on mortality. Cumulative survival of untreated obstructive sleep apnea (OSA) patients based on initial AI. The study was retrospective and subject to bias, but does suggest that untreated OSA with an AI >20 may be associated with earlier mortality. Asterisks denote $p < 0.05$ for the comparison between the two survival curves at each point. The error bars represent standard error. (Adapted with permission from He et al.[20])

Community-based studies looking at sleep apnea have suggested an association between OSA and systemic hypertension, independent of age, body-mass index, or other recognized confounders. There is evidence of increased muscle sympathetic nerve activity during both sleep and wakefulness in subjects with OSA, with surges of sympathetic nerve activity at the end of each apnea, with large rises in systemic arterial blood pressure. Also, these increases in activity diminish with nasal CPAP. There is also some evidence that subjects with significant OSA show an abnormal pressor response to isocapnic hypoxia, which is not seen in normotensive subjects with no OSA[21].

Whilst the incidence of SDB is lower in women, it has been reported to be as high as 4.9% in those aged 30–49 years, and the 5 year survival is significantly poorer in women with OSA than in a similar population of men[22]. It has been assumed that premenopausal women are protected from SDB by their greater central chemoreceptor drive, especially during the luteal phase of the menstrual cycle. Ventilatory response to hypercapnia is increased during this phase. However, cardiovascular variability has also been shown to occur in this group if they have OSA, and this is accentuated during the luteal phase of the menstrual cycle. Premenopausal women with OSA may be another, as yet, unidentified group with an increased risk of developing adverse cardiovascular events – much as occurs in younger female diabetics who have a 19-fold increased risk of cardiovascular disease compared with healthy premenopausal women.

The lack of clinical awareness of sleep disorders is the largest pitfall to overcome in the evaluation and treatment of patients who have various conditions. Both physician and public information about sleep is needed to highlight the importance of this area.

Compliance with treatment remains a problem. Patients who suffer severe OSA are usually pleased with the improvements experienced on CPAP, but the equipment is cumbersome and unattractive, and unlikely to be the answer for most patients who have mild or moderate OSA and who are sleepy but not badly affected enough to tolerate CPAP. Newer, non-invasive treatments are needed and oral appliances may prove a useful alternative.

UPPER AIRWAY RESISTANCE SYNDROME

Introduction
Upper airway resistance syndrome (UARS) is a form of SDB characterized by daytime hypersomnia, increased upper airway resistance during sleep, and the absence of hypopneas and apneas on a polysomnogram.

Epidemiology, risk factors, and pathophysiology
Epidemiology
To extrapolate the prevalence of UARS from large, epidemiologic studies of OSA is difficult, because UARS is not easy to detect by standard polysomnography. Similarly, the epidemiology of excessive sleepiness does not give a true estimate of the frequency of UARS in a population, since excessive daytime sleepiness is itself difficult to measure.

Risk factors
Patients who have UARS tend to be younger and have a lower body weight (usually in the normal range) than those who have OSA. Snoring is variable in UARS, although frequently present.

The male predominance associated with OSA may not apply to UARS, for example a high prevalence of SDB is found in nonobese women who have certain craniofacial structural disproportions[7]. Although the women examined had negative sleep studies by conventional criteria, they demonstrated objective improvement in daytime sleepiness following CPAP therapy, which suggests that reductions in upper airway resistance and the corresponding arousals resulted in improved sleep quality and reduced daytime sleepiness.

Pathophysiology
Increased upper airway resistance is the central pathophysiologic event in UARS. In certain patients, the increased upper airway resistance leads to brief arousals for 3–15 seconds. The mechanisms that link increased pharyngeal airway resistance with arousal from sleep may be associated with increases in intrathoracic pressure during inspiratory effort against a partially obstructed upper airway. Arousals related to large, negative pressure changes in intrathoracic pressure are generally considered to be part of the pathophysiology of OSA. It is likely that UARS and OSA represent opposite ends of the clinical spectrum of SDB.

Clinical features
Hypersomnia is the chief clinical feature of UARS. The mean Multiple Sleep Latency Test score (the time taken to fall asleep during the day in a quiet room) is reduced, which indicates a high degree of daytime somnolence, and snoring is common.

Diagnosis
Since UARS is a clinical diagnosis, it should be considered in patients who present with daytime hypersomnia. Although the diagnosis may be likely on the basis of clinical features, polysomnography is necessary (see Fig. 75.16). First, OSA must be excluded and, second, frequent brief electoencephalogram arousals associated with increases in upper airway resistance must be detected. An increasing number of laboratories are using sensitive airflow monitoring techniques, such as nasal cannula pneumotachograph systems, to detect flow changes in relation to increased respiratory effort. With an improved technical capability to detect inspiratory airflow limitation, more cases of UARS may be detected.

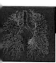

A final diagnostic approach for UARS in practice is to use a therapeutic trial of CPAP therapy in patients who have daytime somnolence but no OSA (and no evidence of other causes of excessive daytime somnolence). If the patient's daytime sleepiness improves, UARS is considered likely.

Treatment
Treatment options for UARS include positive airway pressure therapy (CPAP or bilevel PAP), upper airway surgery, and oral appliances.

Clinical course and prevention
Daytime sleepiness associated with UARS is likely to continue unless treated, although no studies that address the long-term outcome of patients affected by UARS have been performed. Whether UARS can be prevented is unclear. Factors such as obesity may contribute to the risk, although most patients appear to have normal body weight. Factors such as craniofacial structural abnormalities may require surgical intervention.

Pitfalls and controversies
One of the most controversial types of SDB is UARS. Lack of a clinically useful definition makes clinical detection more difficult. Moreover, a definite diagnosis requires application of sleep laboratory tools and techniques not routinely available in all sleep laboratories.

One area that remains unclear is the optimal treatment of UARS. Nasal CPAP has been shown to be effective in alleviating daytime hypersomnia, but long-term adherence to this therapy is open to question. Surgical therapy and oral appliances may be options in the future.

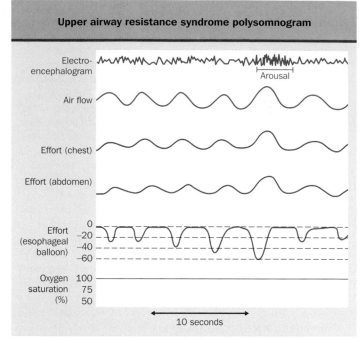

Figure 75.16 Example of upper airway resistance syndrome polysomnograph. Note that air flow is only minimally perturbed by an increase in upper airway resistance. Respiratory effort recorded in chest and abdomen belts is similarly minimally affected. Respiratory effort as recorded by esophageal pressure shows increasingly negative pleural pressure deflections, which indicate increased respiratory effort because of elevated upper airway resistance. The progression of increasing respiratory effort culminates in an arousal, shown in the electrocardiogram channel.

REFERENCES

1. Strollo PJ, Rogers, RM. Obstructive sleep apnea. N Eng J Med. 1996;334:99–104.
2. Young T, Palta M, Dempsey J, Skatrud J, Weber S, Badr S. The occurence of sleep-disordered breathing among middle-aged adults. N Engl J Med. 1993;328:1230–5.
3. Olsen LG, King MT, Hensley MJ, Saunders NA. A community study of snoring and sleep-disordered breathing. Am J Respir Crit Care Med. 1995;52:711–16.
4. Strohl K, Redline S. Recognition of obstructive sleep apnea. Am J Respir Crit Care Med. 1996;154:279–89.
5. Kushida C, Efron B, Guilleminault C. A predictive morphometric model for the obstructive sleep apnea syndrome. Ann Intern Med. 1997;127:581–7.
6. White D. Pathophysiology of obstructive sleep apnea. Thorax. 1995;50:797–804.
7. Mezzanote WS, Tangel DJ, White DP. Waking genioglossal electromyogram in sleep apnea patients versus normal controls (a neuromuscular compensatory mechanism). J Clin Invest. 1992;89;1571–9.
8. Wheatley J, Mezzanote WS, Tangel DJ, White DP. Influence of sleep on genioglossal muscle activation by negative pressure in normal man. Am Rev Respir Dis. 1993;148:597–605.
9. Epstein L, Strollo PJ, Donegan RB, Delmar JU, Hendrix C, Westbrook PR. Obstructive sleep apnea in patients with human immunodeficiency virus (HIV) disease. Sleep. 1995;18:368–76.
10. Chaouat A, Weitzenbaum E, Kreiger J, et al. Association of chronic obstructive pulmonary disease and sleep apnea syndrome Am J Crit Care Med. 1995;151:82–6.
11. Smith P, Gold AR, Meyers DA, Haponik EF, Bleecker ER. Weight loss in mildly to moderately obese patients with obstructive sleep apnea. Ann Intern Med. 1985;103:850–5.
12. Schmidt-Nowara W, Meade TE, Hays MB. Treatment of snoring and obstructive sleep apnea with a dental orthosis. Chest. 1991;99:1378–85.
13. Launois S, Feroah TR, Campbell WN, et al. Site of pharyngeal narrowing predicts outcome of surgery of obstructive sleep apnea. Am Rev Respir Dis. 1993;147:182–9.
14. Atwood C, Sanders MH, Strollo PJ. Palatal and nonpalatal surgery for sleep apnea hypopnea syndrome. Clin Pulmonary Med. 1997;4:205–12.
15. Sher A, Schechtman KB, Piccirillo JF. The efficacy of surgical modification of the upper airway in adults with obstructive sleep apnea syndrome. Sleep. 1996;19:156–77.
16. Shepard J, Thawley SE. Localization of upper airway collapse during sleep in patients with obstructive sleep apnea. Am Rev Respir Dis. 1990;141:1350–5.
17. Riley R, Powell NB, Guilleminault C. Obstructive sleep apnea syndrome: a review of 306 consecutively treated surgical patients. Otolaryngol Head Neck Surg. 1993;108:117–25.
18. Sforza E, Addati G, Cirignotta F, Lugaresi E. Natural evolution of the sleep apnea syndrome: a five year longitudinal study. Eur Respir J. 1994;7:1765–70.
19. Calverley PMA. Obstructive sleep apnea: a progressive disorder? Thorax. 1997;52:843–4.
20. He J, Kryger MH, Zorick FJ, Conway W, Roth T. Mortality and apnea index in obstructive sleep apnea. Chest. 1988;88:9–14.
21. Lindberg E, Janson C, Svärdsudd K, et al. Increased mortality among sleepy snorers: a prospective population-based study. Thorax. 1998;53:631–7.
22. Sullivan CE, McNamara SG. Sleep apnea and snoring: potential links with vascular disease. Thorax. 1998;53(suppl 3) S8–11.

Chapter 76

Central Sleep Apnea and Other Forms of Sleep-Disordered Breathing

Charles W Atwood, Jr and Patrick J Strollo, Jr

CENTRAL SLEEP APNEA

Epidemiology, risk factors, and pathophysiology

Epidemiology

Central sleep apnea (CSA) occurs in 5 to 10% of all patients who have sleep-disordered breathing (SDB)[1]. The problem appears due to a failure of ventilatory drive, and there are many known (secondary) causes. The primary or idiopathic form is less common than secondary causes such as congestive heart failure (CHF), in which it can occur in 40–50% of such patients[2], or neurologic conditions such as cerebrovascular disease.

Risk factors

Risk factors include CHF and neurologic disease, and ascent to high altitude (particularly in individuals who have spent little previous time at altitudes >2500m).

Pathophysiology

Transient withdrawal of central respiratory drive to respiratory muscles results in CSA; this mechanism occurs in a number of ways (Fig. 76.1).

In considering the pathophysiology of CSA, three subtypes can be described.

Mechanisms of central sleep apnea	
Mechanism	**Clinical example**
Central hypoventilation	Primary central hypoventilation Brainstem infarction Encephalitis Arnold–Chiari malformation
Neuromuscular respiratory dysfunction	Muscular dystrophy Spinal atrophy Amyotrophic lateral sclerosis
Instability of central respiratory drive	Sleep onset (transient instability) Hyperventilation-induced hypocapnia Hypoxia (pulmonary disease, high altitude) Congestive heart failure Disorders of the central nervous system

Figure 76.1 Mechanisms in the pathophysiology of central sleep apnea (CSA). Three primary mechanisms by which CSA occurs are described and clinical examples of each mechanism given. Central hypoventilation is discussed later in this chapter and neuromuscular diseases are discussed in Chapter 72.

Central hypoventilation

Central hypoventilation occurs when respiratory drive to the ventilatory muscles is inadequate. This can occur by several mechanisms. First brainstem lesions affecting the respiratory centers and the metabolic control of breathing result in CSA. These lesions may be the result of critically placed infarctions, infections, or tumors. A rare primary form of central hypoventilation (congenital central hypoventilation syndrome) has been described as well (central hypoventilation is discussed in greater detail later in this chapter).

Neuromuscular respiratory dysfunction

Patients with a variety of neuromuscular diseases may develop CSA due to the inability of the respiratory pump to respond to central respiratory drive. Central sleep apnea is a variable manifestation of neuromuscular disease. It may be seen in patients with postpolio syndrome, amyotrophic lateral sclerosis, and muscular and myotonic dystrophies. Clinically, patients with neuromuscular disease-related CSA are usually hypercapnic and have advanced degrees of other symptoms (e.g. muscle weakness). Daytime somnolence, lethargy, and morning headache are other common symptoms in these patients.

Instability of central respiratory drive

Instability of the central respiratory drive can precipitate CSA. This variant of CSA can be encountered in a number of clinical situations. The first is CSA associated with sleep onset. Sleep onset CSA is usually transient and asymptomatic. It is seen on polysomnograms done for evaluation of many different sleep disorders and is thought to reflect the normal transition from the behavioral respiratory control system, which predominates during wakefulness, to the metabolic control system that regulates ventilation during sleep. Sleep onset CSA becomes a clinical problem only if repeated arousals with the CSA occur that delay sleep onset. At sleep onset, a central apnea occurs if the arterial partial pressure of carbon dioxide ($PaCO_2$) is below the apnea threshold, the $PaCO_2$ at which the respiratory control centers in the brainstem are stimulated to initiate ventilation. During sleep, ventilation is stimulated as long as the $PaCO_2$ is above the apnea threshold; when $PaCO_2$ is below the apnea threshold, apnea occurs until $PaCO_2$ increases to a level at or above the threshold.

The other clinical situations where instability of central respiratory drive is thought to be important are in patients with CHF and Cheyne-Stokes respiration (CSR) and in patients with neurological diseases, such as cerebral infarctions. In these two conditions, the mechanism of instability of central respiratory drive is not well understood. In the case of CHF-related CSA (CSR), intrinsic properties of the central respiratory drive appear to be the main factor

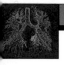

contributing to the CSR breathing pattern of central apnea – hyper-nea – central apnea. Arterial P_{CO_2} also appears to be an important determinant of the disorder; patients with lower $PaCO_2$ have CSR more commonly than patients with normal $PaCO_2$. A correlation with decreased left ventricle (LV) function and CSA exists as well. This association between LV function and CSA has been thought to be based on delay of blood circulation to respiratory control sensors as a result of poor cardiac pump function. While contributory, it does not account for the degree of abnormality encountered in CHF patients, thus implicating other mechanisms.

Patients with neurological diseases, particularly cerebral infarctions, also appear to have an increased prevalence of CSA. The specific mechanisms in these patients are not known. It is possible that the CSA is the result of direct neuronal damage or death resulting in abnormal central respiratory drive, although, in many cases, the site of infarction is not obviously in the brainstem, the site of the respiratory controller.

Role of arousals

The sensitivity of the arousal mechanism in CSA is important but difficult to quantify. In all forms of CSA, if an arousal from sleep does not occur, the apnea–arousal cycle is broken. Some studies have found that sedative medications may be useful in increasing the arousal threshold and decreasing sleep onset arousal. The role of such medications in practice is unclear because of the potential for dependence, concern about precipitating falls in a frail population, and the potential for worsening any underlying obstructive sleep apnea (OSA).

Clinical features

Hypercapnia associated with CSA is usually the result of a central hypoventilation disorder or neuromuscular respiratory disease. Such patients may have little sensation of dyspnea associated with respiratory insufficiency and hypercapnia, although patients who have neuromuscular respiratory disease may complain of dyspnea as the condition progresses. Restless sleep, daytime somnolence, and morning headache may be seen in all forms of hypercapnic CSA. Right heart failure and polycythemia may develop at an advanced stage. Overt respiratory failure that requires mechanical ventilation is occasionally the presenting complaint, and usually occurs after another medical problem, such as bronchitis or pneumonia, has disrupted the existing physiologic homeostasis.

Although the symptoms of CSA and OSA differ, some overlap occurs (Fig. 76.2).

Patients who have eucapnic or hypocapnic forms of CSA are typically older, have a more normal body weight, and have coexistent cardiac or neurologic diseases. This is true of the idiopathic form as well as secondary forms associated with CHF. Such patients tend to hyperventilate during wakefulness, and therefore the $PaCO_2$ is lower than that in patients who have CHF.

Symptoms of insomnia, nocturnal dyspnea, and daytime sleepiness (because of sleep fragmentation and frequent arousals) are common, although daytime hypersomnia is less frequent in this group of patients. Cor pulmonale and polycythemia are also uncommon in hypocapnic CSA[1].

Diagnosis

Regardless of its type, a high clinical suspicion is essential for the diagnosis of CSA, and polysomnography is necessary (Fig.

Signs and symptoms of central sleep apnea versus obstructive sleep apnea		
Sign or symptom	**Central sleep apnea**	**Obstructive sleep apnea**
Daytime sleepiness	Yes	Yes
Restless sleep	Yes	Yes
Snoring	No	Yes
Nocturnal choking	No	Yes
Nocturnal dyspnea	Variable	No
Morning headache	Variable	Variable
Insomnia	Yes	Variable
Nocturnal desaturation	Yes	Yes
Hypercapnia	Variable	Variable

Figure 76.2 Comparison of common signs and symptoms of central sleep apnea versus obstructive sleep apnea.

76.3). Central apneas are distinguished from obstructive apneas by the lack of respiratory effort during the apnea.

The potential for underlying cardiovascular and cerebrovascular disease must be assessed. Figure 76.4 provides an approach to the diagnostic evaluation of patients who have CSA.

Treatment

Patients who have hypercapnic CSA are treated for any underlying central nervous system (CNS) or peripheral neuromuscular conditions. These treatments include supplemental oxygen, nasal continuous positive airway pressure (CPAP), bilevel positive airway pressure (BiPAP), respiratory stimulant medications, or a combination of these.

If the hypercapnic CSA results from central hypoventilation or neuromuscular respiratory conditions, the patient benefits most from nocturnal ventilatory assistance, which may be carried out through a tracheostomy or noninvasively by mask ventilation. Patients must avoid benzodiazepines, narcotics, and other sedatives that may suppress respiratory drive.

Supplemental oxygen is useful for alleviating nocturnal hypoxemia, provided it does not induce hypercapnia.

The optimal treatment for nonhypercapnic CSA has not been defined. Treatment of the underlying cause is the first step (e.g. CHF). Therapy can also include supplemental oxygen, respiratory stimulants, and positive pressure therapy. At present, supplemental oxygen therapy is the mainstay of therapy as it 'stabilizes' the respiratory control centers, although the mechanisms by which this is accomplished are not clear. Acetazolamide has been used successfully to alleviate abnormal respiratory patterns in altitude sickness. Its mechanism of action is to induce a mild degree of metabolic acidosis and increase respiratory drive by inducing a bicarbonate diuresis.

Clinically important improvements in left ventricular function have resulted from CPAP in patients who suffer CHF[4], but the number of such patients treated successfully with CPAP are small. In one study, the benefit of CPAP therapy was limited to the group of patients who had higher [>1.6kPa (>12mmHg)] pulmonary capillary wedge pressures (PCWPs). By contrast, the lower PCWP group [<1.6kPa (<12mmHg)] showed a reduction in cardiac index. The mechanism by which CPAP improves CSA

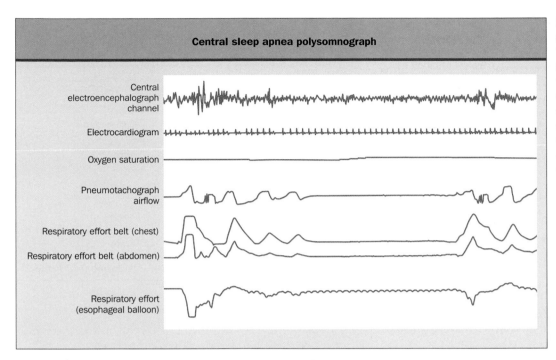

Central sleep apnea polysomnograph

Central electroencephalograph channel

Electrocardiogram

Oxygen saturation

Pneumotachograph airflow

Respiratory effort belt (chest)

Respiratory effort belt (abdomen)

Respiratory effort (esophageal balloon)

Figure 76.3 Example of central sleep apnea polysomnograph. The sleep epoch shown is 30 seconds. The patient is awake at the beginning of the tracing. A sleep-onset central apnea, characterized by absence of air flow and respiratory effort, occurs as stage 1 sleep is entered. An arousal at the end of the epoch ends the apnea.

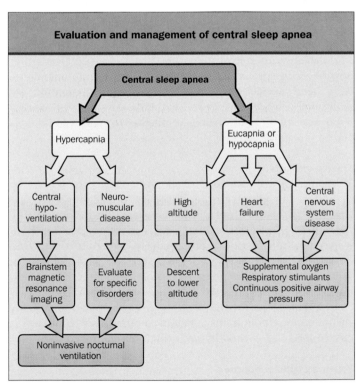

Evaluation and management of central sleep apnea

Central sleep apnea

Hypercapnia

Eucapnia or hypocapnia

Central hypo-ventilation

Neuro-muscular disease

High altitude

Heart failure

Central nervous system disease

Brainstem magnetic resonance imaging

Evaluate for specific disorders

Descent to lower altitude

Supplemental oxygen
Respiratory stimulants
Continuous positive airway pressure

Noninvasive nocturnal ventilation

Figure 76.4 Evaluation and management of central sleep apnea.

appears related to its improvement in oxygen saturation and a slight elevation in $PaCO_2$, which moves ambient $PaCO_2$ closer to the apnea threshold[5].

Clinical course

Where CSA is secondary to another condition, such as CHF, the clinical outcome is related to the severity of the underlying disorder. Cheyne–Stokes respiration, for example, is thought to be a poor prognostic sign for patients who have CHF[6].

In most cases, treatment of CSA, whether with positive pressure ventilation, respiratory stimulants, supplemental oxygen, or a combination of these therapies, improves clinical symptoms. If severely fragmented sleep can be consolidated and nocturnal dyspnea prevented, the patient almost certainly benefits from the therapy.

Pitfalls and controversies

Compared with OSA, primary (idiopathic) CSA is uncommon. Clinicians managing CSA should be aware that the secondary form of CSA (CSR) may be present in a large fraction of these patients. Although the significance of CSA in CHF is not known with certainty, awareness of the problem is important for clinicians who manage these patients. The long-term clinical benefit of treating CSA in CHF patients is not known.

OTHER FORMS OF CENTRAL HYPOVENTILATION

Disorders of central hypoventilation are a heterogeneous and uncommon group of disorders characterized by the inability of the central respiratory centers to provide adequate output to the respiratory pump. The hallmark is hypercapnia, and as effective treatment to optimize ventilatory function and quality of life is available and involves the provision of ventilatory support, respiratory physicians manage these patients.

Epidemiology, risk factors, and pathophysiology
Epidemiology and risk factors
Figure 76.5 lists the conditions associated with central hypoventilation. Trauma accounts for most spinal cord injuries and is the leading cause of central hypoventilation, with approximately 10,000 new cervical spinal injuries each year in the USA. In addition, the prevalence of this disorder is approximately 400,000[8].

Although no longer a public health or important clinical problem in the developed world, poliomyelitis continues to be a significant public health problem in developing nations. Patients

Classification of disorders of central hypoventilation	
Type of neuron	**Disorder**
Brainstem motoneurons	Primary central hypoventilation
	Congenital malformations (Chiari malformations; syringomyelia)
	Trauma
	Infarction
	Encephalitis
	Tumors
	Chronic metabolic alkalosis
	Multiple sclerosis
	Sarcoidosis
Spinal neurons	Poliomyelitis
	High cervical cord trauma

Figure 76.5 Classification of disorders of central hypoventilation by site of primary defect in the central nervous system.

Comparison of clinical features of central hypoventilation and neuromuscular disease		
Clinical feature	**Central hypoventilation**	**Neuromuscular respiratory disease**
Frequency	Uncommon	Common
Ages affected	Infants through adults	Primarily adults
Hypercapnia	Yes	Yes
Hypoxia	Yes	Yes
Dyspnea	No	Yes
Respiratory mechanics	Normal	Impaired
Ability to hyperventilate	Normal	Impaired
Therapy	Oxygen	Oxygen
	Chronic ventilator support	Chronic ventilator support
	Diaphragm pacing	Disease modifying drugs

Figure 76.6 Comparison of clinical features of central hypoventilation and neuromuscular disease.

who have chronic ventilatory failure from the polio epidemics in the 1950s still require treatment.

Syringomyelia and Chiari malformations are examples of congenital brain lesions that may result in central hypoventilation. Brain injury and neuronal loss from acute encephalitis, multiple sclerosis, and multiple system atrophy (Shy–Drager syndrome) are examples of rare acquired disorders that may lead to central hypoventilation. Structural lesions caused by brainstem infarctions, neoplasms, or postencephalitis are rare, but are the most common nontraumatic causes. These conditions result in severe clinical sequelae and the outcomes tend to be poor.

Neurologic conditions, such as multiple sclerosis, multiple system atrophy, or demyelinating disorders, can result in clinically significant hypoventilation, but respiratory failure is rare.

Pathophysiology

Central hypoventilation can occur as a congenital disorder in the first several hours of life or as an acquired disorder in adulthood, usually as the result of significant brainstem injury. The basic defect is the inability to transduce afferent input from central and/or peripheral chemoreceptors into the efferent limb of the respiratory system. Flat or very decreased respiratory responses to respiratory chemostimuli, such as hypercapnia and hypoxia, may occur. While awake, behavioral control of breathing mechanisms work and chemosensory mechanisms play a limited role in maintaining ventilatory rhythm. However, during sleep the automaticity of breathing is deficient, although partial defects of ventilatory control occur in other respiratory conditions such as chronic obstructive pulmonary disease (COPD), sleep apnea syndrome, and asthma.

Clinical features

Hypercapnia and hypoxemia are the hallmark signs of central hypoventilation syndromes, regardless of etiology[9]. Hypercapnia can range from mild [$P_{CO_2}<6.6kPa$ ($<50mmHg$)] to severe [$P_{CO_2}>8.5kPa$ ($>65mmHg$)]. Symptoms may also include progressive lethargy and easy fatigability, daytime hypersomnia, and headache. Dyspnea is variable, but is generally minimal with central hypoventilation, which may be a differentiating feature from neuromuscular or chest wall disorders that cause

respiratory failure, but have an otherwise similar presentation (Fig. 76.6).

Diagnosis

The diagnosis of central hypoventilation is made after other possible explanations, such as neuromuscular respiratory failure, have been excluded by history, physical examination, or additional physiologic tests. Patients affected by central hypoventilation have impaired ventilatory responses to hypoxia and hypercapnia[10].

Physiologic tests

Ventilatory sensitivity to hypercapnia[11] and hypoxia[12] can be determined by plotting respiratory rate, tidal volume, inspiratory flow rate, and mouth occlusion pressures in the first 0.1 seconds of inspiration against progressively higher levels of inspired carbon dioxide or progressively lower levels of oxygen saturation over time. Increases in respiratory rate and minute ventilation occur in response to the ventilatory stimulus given, but the variability in these measurements in normal subjects is considerable[11,12]. However, if a response curve with a markedly shallow slope is found, insensitivity to ventilatory stimulants is determined and central hypoventilation must be considered.

Voluntary hyperventilation

To distinguish between central and peripheral causes of hypoventilation, the ability to hyperventilate voluntarily and decrease carbon dioxide by 1.3kPa (10mmHg) or more can be measured. In central hypoventilation, maximal voluntary hyperventilation is accomplished easily for short periods of time, as the respiratory pump is not affected. If the cause of hypoventilation is peripheral (i.e. respiratory muscle weakness), the patient may be unable to lower the carbon dioxide by voluntary hyperpnea.

Imaging studies

Magnetic resonance imaging (MRI) is the procedure of choice for imaging the brainstem and upper spinal cord. Contrast enhancement may be necessary to detect arteriovenous malformations or other small, critically placed lesions. Congenital malformations, such as Chiari malformations or a syrinx, are shown very well using MRI (Fig. 76.7.).

Treatment

Treatment of central hypoventilation depends on its severity, degree of impairment of other systems (e.g. level of mental status, degree of muscle paralysis), and the patient's willingness to use what may be lifelong supportive therapy, such as home ventilation or diaphragmatic pacing[13].

Treatment for milder cases includes ventilatory stimulants, such as progesterone and methylxanthines, which may successfully delay progression of ventilatory insufficiency[14]. Supplemental oxygen therapy is important for all patients who have documented hypoxemia, and may reduce the severity of complications such as polycythemia, pulmonary hypertension, and heart failure, and retard progression in respiratory insufficiency.

Diaphragm pacing

The rationale for diaphragmatic pacing is that electric stimulation of the muscle, either directly or via the phrenic nerve, substitutes for the intrinsic respiratory-center output. Considerable commitment from the patient and medical team is required for this approach to work optimally.

Nocturnal ventilation

Nocturnal ventilation augments ventilation during sleep, a time of increased vulnerability of the respiratory system because of the normal hypoventilation associated with sleep. Nocturnal ventilation can be invasive or noninvasive, and the aim is to augment ventilation during sleep, to rest ventilatory muscles, and to improve gas exchange.

Invasive ventilation

Invasive nocturnal ventilation requires a tracheostomy. Prior to the development of noninvasive ventilation techniques that use face masks, this was standard treatment. As effective noninvasive techniques are now available, the need for a permanent tracheostomy in the management of chronic ventilatory insufficiency has decreased.

Noninvasive ventilation

Ventilation of patients without the need for a surgical airway can be accomplished using either a negative or positive pressure system. Negative pressure systems, such as an iron lung or a cuirass, were the first type of noninvasive ventilators and their main advantage over positive pressure ventilators is that a nasal or oronasal mask, which some patients find uncomfortable, is not needed. Many disadvantages exist, however. Negative pressure ventilators are usually bulky and cumbersome to use and assistance climbing in and out of them is also sometimes required. The most important problem is that such ventilators tend to induce upper airway collapse and thus cause OSA.

Positive pressure, noninvasive ventilators are now the mainstay of nocturnal ventilation. They are small, easily portable, and relatively inexpensive. Both pressure-cycled and volume-cycled versions are available. Which type of positive pressure ventilator to choose is less important than the ability of the patient to learn to use it successfully.

Noninvasive nocturnal positive pressure ventilation may improve daytime hypersomnia, daytime gas exchange, and polycythemia. It may delay the need for a tracheostomy in patients who have progressive hypoventilation disorders and it eliminates the need for tracheostomy in patients who have stable forms of hypoventilation, depending on other factors such as secretion control. Swallowing and speech are preserved, which enhances quality of life[15].

Long-term ventilatory support

In patients who have severely compromised ventilatory function and in those who have difficulty clearing secretions, supplemental ventilatory support may be required long term if the patient desires to live with his or her disease. In cases of encephalitis, brainstem infarction, or arteriovenous malformations that affect the brainstem respiratory centers, nocturnal ventilation alone may not be a viable option – permanent, continuous ventilatory support may be needed. Permanent tracheostomy with mechanical ventilatory support is indicated here. Patients who receive continuous ventilator therapy at home require large and sustained amounts of support from family and outside caregivers. Nonetheless, reasonable quality of life can be achieved for motivated patients and their families.

Clinical course

The clinical course is variable and depends on the etiology and severity of the hypoventilation, its complications, and other comorbidities. The age of onset of primary central hypoventilation ranges from infancy in congenital cases to the seventh decade of life[16]. The average age of onset is about the third to fourth decade

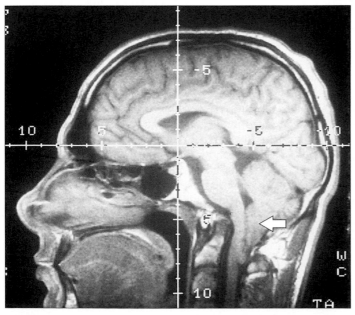

Figure 76.7 Contrast-enhanced magnetic resonance image of an Arnold–Chiari deformity. This 21-year-old man has progressive, nocturnal central hypoventilation as a result of the Chiari type 1 malformation demonstrated. Note the cerebellar tonsil descent into the spinal canal with impingement of brainstem structures (arrow).

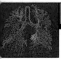
and in half of 30 cases it is an acquired disorder. Causes include encephalitis, meningitis, parkinsonism, syringomyelia, vascular malformation, and mental retardation.

Congenital brainstem abnormalities, such as Arnold–Chiari malformations (Fig. 76.7), have a prognosis that depends on the degree of neurologic damage associated with the descent of cerebellar tissue into the upper spinal canal, the degree of medullary and spinal cord compression, and associated neurologic conditions such as hydrocephalus or meningocele. These may be detected in infancy or adulthood. The cause of respiratory symptoms is central apnea as a result of impingement of the brainstem respiratory centers at the foramen magnum or through adduction of vocal cords with subsequent inspiratory stridor. Both complications are more common in younger patients.

Secondary causes of central hypoventilation

Only a minority of patients who have poliomyelitis develop the paralytic form. Survivors of the outbreaks in the 1950s are still alive, and some require permanent home-ventilator support. The postpolio syndrome is a late sequela, and such patients develop progressive muscle weakness, fatigue, and joint pain after 20–40 years of stability. How often this leads to respiratory muscle dysfunction is not known, but a heightened index of suspicion for this late complication must be maintained.

Spinal cord trauma has a variable course. In a population-based sample of 358 patients who had spinal cord injuries, the case-fatality rate was <4%. Of cervical cord injuries, 36% experienced neurologic improvement compared with the initial severity of injury and over 95% of all patients who had spinal cord injury were discharged home. Unfortunately, respiratory dysfunction remains a significant problem for most patients who have cervical cord injury, despite improvement in other areas of function[8].

The outcome after other CNS injuries, such as severe encephalitis, infarctions that involve the brainstem respiratory centers, and CNS neoplasms, is usually poor. Involvement of the reticular activating system may result in permanent coma, and patients afflicted with such disorders and their family members must be involved in discussions about therapy, as often the only therapy is support using chronic mechanical ventilation.

Complications of central hypoventilation

Complications of central hypoventilation include pulmonary hypertension, polycythemia, right and left heart failure, and respiratory failure. Complications related to treatment of this disorder, such as ventilator-associated lung and bronchial infections, must be considered as well.

Pitfalls and controversies

Disorders of central hypoventilation are rare, and their pathophysiology is poorly understood. Central hypoventilation may be primary (congenital) or secondary (acquired). Development of these disorders typically occurs after a serious brain injury – a severe encephalitis, a neoplasm, or an infarction of the area of the respiratory centers of the medulla. Congenital cases of pure central hypoventilation may also occur, albeit rarely. The prognosis of these conditions is poor. Nonetheless, successful clinical management with either noninvasive ventilation or ventilation through a permanent tracheostomy is possible.

SLEEP-DISORDERED BREATHING IN CHRONIC LUNG DISEASE

Epidemiology and risk factors
Epidemiology
Poor quality sleep is a common complaint with COPD. Most patients do not have OSA, but a fraction have oxygen desaturations <85%. The size of the subpopulation of these patients who have nocturnal desaturation is unknown, since measurements of nocturnal oxygen saturation are not routinely carried out.

Risk factors
Risk factors for nocturnal hypoxemia include severity and type of pulmonary disease, amount of rapid eye movement sleep over the course of a night, and body weight. Patients who have obstructive airways disease appear to be at greater risk of nocturnal desaturation than patients who suffer interstitial disease. If thoracic wall, neuromuscular disease or diaphragmatic paralysis is also present, nocturnal hypoxemia is likely to be worse for a given degree of COPD.

Diagnosis
Detecting SDB in patients who have COPD and other forms of lung disease is important, and sleep studies must be carried out for those who show symptoms of SDB. Patients in whom cor pulmonale or polycythemia develops despite medical management must undergo sleep studies to detect occult sleep apnea or severe desaturations.

Treatment
All patients who suffer lung disease and qualify for supplemental oxygen at night must have continuous oxygen therapy. Some centers empirically increase the oxygen flow by 1 or 2L/minute during sleep. If OSA or other forms of SDB are detected, these patients are treated with CPAP or BiPAP. Such patients frequently are unable to tolerate CPAP therapy, especially if the OSA is mild, and may complain about difficulty exhaling against the expiratory pressures of CPAP. Bilevel pressure devices may be an option in such cases; these may be better tolerated because of lower expiratory pressures. Occasionally, dramatic improvements in dyspnea and quality of life are seen with nocturnal ventilatory assistance; however, predicting who is likely to benefit is difficult. Clinical trials that examined various methods of nocturnal ventilatory support using positive pressure breathing delivered by mask were frequently positive in the short term, but were not able to sustain positive results after approximately 3 months of use.

Clinical course
Nocturnal desaturation in patients who have lung disease complicates the medical care of these patients as it necessitates oxygen therapy, and may decrease quality of life. Continuous home oxygen therapy for severe hypoxemic lung disease has been shown to prolong life in two large randomized clinical trials conducted in the early 1980s[17,18]. When patients have only nocturnal desaturation, the benefit of oxygen therapy is less clear. One study compared survival over an average of 70 months between two groups of COPD patients, one of which had less than the expected amount of nocturnal desaturation

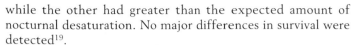
while the other had greater than the expected amount of nocturnal desaturation. No major differences in survival were detected[19].

The combination of OSA and COPD can be debilitating, and has been termed the overlap syndrome. Cor pulmonale, chronic respiratory insufficiency, and polycythemia characterize this syndrome. Treatment is directed at both disorders, with the chief aim being to maintain normal oxygen saturation. Noninvasive ventilation is considered not only to treat OSA, but also to treat respiratory insufficiency and hypercapnia. Without therapy, these patients are expected to have a high degree of morbidity and early mortality.

REFERENCES

1. White D. Central sleep apnea. In: Kryger R, Dement W, eds. Principles and practice of sleep medicine. Philadelphia: WB Saunders; 1994:513–24.
2. Javaheri S, Parker TJ, Wexler L, et al. Occult sleep-disordered breathing in stable congestive heart failure. Ann Intern Med. 1995;122:487–92.
3. Bradley T, Phillipson EA. Central sleep apnea. Clin Chest Med. 1992;13:493–505.
4. Bradley T, Holloway RM, McLaughlin PR, Ross BL, Walters J, Liu PP. Cardiac output response to continuous positive airway pressure in congestive heart failure. Am Rev Respir Dis. 1992;145:377–82.
5. Naughton MBD, Rutherford R, Bradley TD. Effect of continuous positive airway pressure on central sleep apnea and nocturnal PCO_2 in heart failure. Am J Respir Crit Care Med. 1994;150:1598–604.
6. Hanly P, Zuberi N, Gray R. Pathogenesis of Cheyne–Stokes respiration in patients with congestive heart failure. Chest. 1993;104:1079–84.
7. Guilleminault C, Stoohs R, Kim Y, Chervin R, Black J, Clerk A. Upper airway sleep-disordered breathing in women. Ann Intern Med. 1995;122:493–501.
8. Gerhart K. Spinal cord injury outcomes in a population-based sample. J Trauma. 1991;31:1529–35.
9. Weinberger S, Schwartzstein RM, Weiss JW. Hypercapnia. N Eng J Med. 1989;321:1223–31.
10. McNicholas W, Carter JL, Rutherford R, Zamel N, Phillipson EA. Beneficial effect of oxygen in primary alveolar hypoventilation with central sleep apnea. Am Rev Respir Dis. 1982;125:773–5.
11. Read D. A clinical method for assessing the ventilatory responses to carbon dioxide. Australas Ann Med. 1967;16:20–32.
12. Rebuck A, Campbell EJM. A clinical method for assessing the ventilatory responses to hypoxia. Am Rev Respir Dis. 1974;109:345–50.
13. Hyland R, Jones NL, Poles ACP, Link SCM, Vanderlinden RG, Epstein SW. Primary alveolar hypoventilation treated with nocturnal electrophrenic respiration. Am Rev Respir Dis. 1978;117:165–72.
14. Lyons H, Hwang CT. Therapeutic use of progesterone in alveolar hypoventilation associated with obesity. Am J Med. 1968;44:881–8.
15. Hillberg R, Johnson DC. Noninvasive ventilation. N Eng J Med. 1997;337:1746–52.
16. Mellins R, Balfour HH Jr, Turino GM, Winters RW. Failure of automatic control of ventilation (Ondine's curse). Medicine. 1970;49:487–504.
17. Nocturnal Oxygen Treatment Trail Group. Continuous or nocturnal oxygen therapy in hypoxemic chronic obstructive lung disease. Ann Intern Med. 1980;93:391–8.
18. Medical Research Council Working Party. Long-term domiciliary oxygen therapy in chronic hypoxic cor pulmonale complicating chronic bronchitis and emphysema. Lancet. 1981;i:681–5.
19. Connaughton J, Catterall JR, Elton RA, Stradling JR, Douglas, NJ. Do sleep studies contribute to the management of patients with severe chronic obstructive pulmonary disease? Am Rev Respir Dis. 1988;138:341–4.

Drug-induced bronchospasm
Aspirin sensitivity
Aspirin
Nonsteroidal anti-inflammatory drugs
β-Adrenergic blockers
Contrast media
Neuromuscular blocking agents
Inhaled pentamidine
Adenosine
Sotalol
Dipyridamole (i.v.)

Figure 77.2 Drugs that induce bronchospasm.

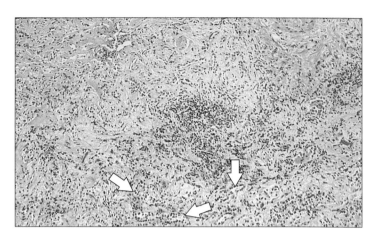

Figure 77.3 Atypical type II pneumocytes. This lung biopsy from a patient with bleomycin toxicity shows extensive fibrosis and inflammatory cell infiltrates. The alveoli are lined by hyperplastic cuboidal cells (arrows) that protrude in the lumen. These bizarre cells suggest drug-induced injury.

cuboidal, have large and hyperchromatic nuclei, unusual nuclear chromatic patterns, and prominent nucleoli (Fig. 77.3). These cells are often noted in the face of injury from cytotoxic therapy and are suggestive, but not diagnostic, of drug-related injury. With noncytotoxic, drug-induced, interstitial injury, fewer type II cells may be present or they may be absent. Also present are various degrees of fibrosis and mononuclear cell infiltration; occasionally, mononuclear cell infiltration predominates. The prognosis with interstitial pneumonitis and/or fibrosis is variable. In some cases, resolution or improvement occurs, but progressive fibrosis and respiratory failure can also occur. This type of pattern is most commonly associated with the cytotoxic drugs, but can also occur with cardiovascular agents and antimicrobial drugs.

Hypersensitivity pneumonitis
Drug-induced hypersensitivity pneumonitis is characterized by an acute-to-subacute presentation. Systemic symptoms with fever, fatigue, myalgias, and arthralgias are often present. Pulmonary symptoms are cough and dyspnea, but these appear after the systemic symptoms. Eosinophilia is present in 20–40% of cases. Chest radiographs typically show air-space disease, which may be focal, lobar, or diffuse in distribution; a peripheral predominance of infiltrates may be present. In some cases, Löffler's syndrome with transient patchy infiltrates is seen.

Pathologically, acute inflammation with neutrophils and eosinophils, as well as a prominent mononuclear cell infiltration, are seen. Two patterns occur: In one pattern, eosinophils are confluent in alveoli and heavily involve the interstitium, a pattern usually associated with a Löffler's-like syndrome. The second pattern shows fibrosis and a mixed mononuclear cell infiltrate with interstitial, but not alveolar, eosinophils. Prognosis is generally good with a Löffler's-like syndrome, but is more variable with the more chronic picture of fibrosis. This pattern of hypersensitivity pneumonitis is seen with a variety of drugs, but most commonly with gold and nitrofurantoin.

Noncardiogenic pulmonary edema
Noncardiogenic pulmonary edema presents with acute respiratory distress occurring over several hours. Chest radiographs show diffuse alveolar filling infiltrates with no cardiomegaly or pleural effusions. Prognosis is generally good if the offending agent is stopped and supportive care is given. This type of injury is commonly seen with aspirin and the opiates.

Acute pneumonia
Acute pneumonia presents with acute distress similar to noncardiogenic edema. Pathologic studies, however, also show the presence of interstitial and alveolar inflammation with some degree of fibrosis. Prognosis is variable and less favorable than that with noncardiogenic pulmonary edema. Although improvement often occurs, persistent respiratory impairment may remain and cause significant problems. This effect is most commonly seen with the combination of mitomycin and *Vinca* alkaloids.

Pulmonary veno-occlusive disease
Pulmonary veno-occlusive disease is characterized by occlusion of the pulmonary veins, which leads to pulmonary hypertension. The usual presentation is the insidious development of dyspnea. Chest radiographs may show Kerley-B lines in the absence of cardiomegaly. Pulmonary veno-occlusive disease has been reported to occur with several cytotoxic drugs and prognosis is poor.

Pulmonary renal syndrome
Pulmonary renal syndrome is a rare disorder similar to Goodpasture's syndrome. Patients present with dyspnea, hemoptysis, and hematuria. Pathologically, pulmonary hemorrhage is seen, but linear deposits of immunoglobulin are not seen. Pulmonary renal syndrome is seen with penicillamine.

Airway patterns
Bronchospasm
Bronchospasm can be induced by several drugs, most commonly aspirin, nonsteroidal anti-inflammatory drugs (NSAIDs), and β-blockers. This reaction usually occurs in patients who have underlying asthma or chronic obstructive airways disease. Bronchospasm occurs minutes to hours after ingestion of the offending drug; it may be severe and difficult to treat.

Cough
Angiotensin-converting enzyme (ACE) inhibitors can cause chronic cough in 5–15% of patients[4]. It occurs in women more frequently than men and usually after 1–2 months of treatment, but occasionally later. All ACE inhibitors can induce chronic

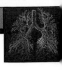

cough, but the direct angiotensin II antagonist losartan does not appear to do so. Those patients who suffer asthma are not at increased risk. Although airways irritation and bronchoconstriction are possible mechanisms, the mechanism of toxicity is unclear. Nonspecifically, blocking the metabolism of bradykinins and substance P leads to an increase of these neuropeptides, which have irritant and bronchoconstrictor effects. Also, ACE inhibitors may nonspecifically increase sensitivity to irritant-induced cough. Drug withdrawal results in improvement within a few weeks. Occasionally, a response to inhaled cromolyn occurs, which may help those patients in whom it is vital to continue ACE inhibitors.

Obliterative bronchiolitis

Obliterative bronchiolitis is a rare complication of drug therapy and has been described almost exclusively with penicillamine. Patients present with increasing dyspnea and cough, and physical examination may be normal or squeaks and crackles may be present. Chest radiographs show hyperinflation. Expiratory chest computed tomography (CT) shows air trapping and a mosaic pattern. Pathologically, obliteration of the small conducting airways by concentric luminal narrowing occurs because of an intense lymphocytic infiltration. The occluding plugs of granular tissue common in bronchiolitis obliterans (unrelated to drug therapy) are not usually found.

Drug-induced systemic lupus erythematosus

Some drugs cause a lupus-like syndrome. The incidence of renal and neurologic complications is low with drug-induced lupus, but that of pleuropulmonary complications is high. The drugs that most commonly cause this syndrome are hydralazine, procainamide, quinidine, isoniazid, and diphenylhydantoin. Isolated reports suggest that many other drugs cause this problem.

Neurologic disorders

Many drugs can inhibit neural drive, cause peripheral neuropathy, block neuromuscular functions, or produce myopathy (see Aldrich and Prezant[5] for a review of this subject).

MECHANISMS OF TOXICITY

Several mechanisms are proposed for drug-induced injury to the lungs, and more than one may be operative with any drug. The first is the creation of an imbalance in the oxidant–antioxidant system. Reactive oxygen metabolites, which are formed within phagocytic cells, help in host defense, but can produce multiple toxic effects. Antioxidants (such as superoxide dismutase, catalase, and glutathione) can detoxify these reactive molecules and maintain an acceptable balance. Some cytotoxic drugs are believed to alter the normal balance – bleomycin, cyclophosphamide, and carmustine. Interference with the oxidant–antioxidant system is an unusual mechanism for noncytotoxic drugs, but may play a role in toxicity caused by nitrofurantoin.

A second mechanism is an alteration in the fine immunologic balance that exists in the lung, which is open to the atmosphere, and that is designed to protect against invading pathogens, but also has mechanisms to prevent excessive reactions and self-destruction. This is an important mechanism of toxicity for many antimicrobials and anti-inflammatory agents. In some cases of drug toxicity, a marked influx of eosinophils occurs, which suggests an acute reaction to antigen and alteration of the immune balance. In many other cases in which eosinophils are not found, experimental evidence also favors immune alteration, as for noncytotoxic drugs such as gold, amiodarone, and nitrofurantoin and the cytotoxic agent methotrexate. Bronchoalveolar lavage in these cases shows an increase in lymphocytes, usually of the suppressor subtype. Enhanced lymphocyte blastogenesis and lymphokine release after exposure of cells to some drugs, notably gold and nitrofurantoin, have also been shown. With some drugs, such as bleomycin, lavage has shown an excess of neutrophils. Complement activation has been noted with the opiates and may also play a role in inducing toxicity. Finally, drugs can also alter pathways with effects on the lung, such as aspirin's inhibition of the cyclo-oxygenase pathway that leads to the bronchospasm.

Another possible mechanism of drug-induced injury is change in matrix repair by altering the balance between collagenosis and collagenolysis. Bleomycin, gold, and penicillamine may effect injury partially through this system. Finally, a neural effect of some drugs that causes increased permeability and leads to pulmonary edema has been suggested as a factor with opiates, major tranquilizers, and salicylates.

SPECIFIC DRUGS

Noncytotoxic drugs
Amiodarone

Amiodarone is used for serious ventricular arrhythmias and refractory supraventricular arrhythmias. Its use is often limited by toxicity, which can be ophthalmic, cutaneous, hepatic, thyroid related, or pulmonary. The incidence of pulmonary toxicity is 5% and is increased in those patients who receive more than 400mg/day. Three forms of pulmonary toxicity are found[6–8], of which interstitial pneumonitis is the most common. Patients present over weeks to months with cough, dyspnea, and weight loss. The second pattern is that of acute pneumonia, in which patients have the acute-to-subacute onset of fever, cough, and chest pain. In both types, the erythrocyte sedimentation rate (ESR) is elevated and a peripheral leukocytosis occurs. Episodes of acute, noncardiogenic pulmonary edema have been described as a serious third type of toxicity, which usually occurs after cardiac and noncardiac surgery, particularly pneumonectomy. A connection with use of high, inspired concentrations of oxygen during surgery is possible.

Chest radiographs show interstitial infiltrates in the chronic pneumonitis pattern, a mixture of interstitial and alveolar infiltrates with acute pneumonia, and diffuse infiltrates with noncardiogenic pulmonary edema. Although less common, focal or lobar infiltrates, pulmonary masses, and pleural effusions have been described. Areas of high density in amiodarone-associated infiltrates are shown by CT scans because large accumulations of macrophages contain amiodarone, which is high in iodine content. These areas of high attenuation are not, however, pathognomonic of amiodarone toxicity, but rather of use of the drug. Gallium scans are positive with amiodarone toxicity.

Pathologically, interstitial and alveolar inflammation and a variable amount of fibrosis is seen. Macrophages of foamy appearance are present in tissue (see Fig. 77.4); the foaminess results from phospholipid accumulation because amiodarone inhibits phospholipase. With acute pneumonia, intra-alveolar hemorrhage and hyaline membrane formation can also be seen. The diagnosis is suspected in any patient who develops respiratory distress while

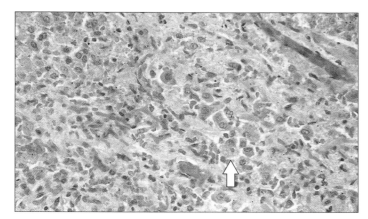

Figure 77.4 Lung histology associated with amiodarone pulmonary toxicity. An interstitial inflammatory infiltrate is seen with vacuolated macrophages. These 'foamy macrophages' contain a large amount of abundant, pale cytoplasm of foamy appearance. Although such macrophages are characteristically seen with amiodarone, they do not mean toxicity has occurred.

receiving the drug, although congestive heart failure usually needs to be excluded. Pulmonary function tests show a low diffusing capacity, but are nonspecific; a normal diffusing capacity, however, eliminates the diagnosis. A positive gallium scan and elevated ESR are suggestive findings. Treatment consists of discontinuing the drug. Corticosteroids are often given at a dose of 40–60mg/day, but resolution can take some time because the half life of the drug is long (up to 60 days). In cases where the drug cannot be stopped, a lower dose and concomitant corticosteroids may be useful. High doses of oxygen must be avoided in patients on amiodarone who undergo major surgery and a substitute drug used if possible.

Nitrofurantoin

The potential for pulmonary toxicity from nitrofurantoin used for urinary suppression has been recognized for many years. The incidence is <1%, but the drug is widely used. Nitrofurantoin causes both a hypersensitivity pneumonitis or, less commonly, a chronic pneumonitis[9]. The hypersensitivity pneumonitis is characterized by systemic symptoms of fever, arthralgias, chest pain, and a maculopapular rash that occurs with pulmonary symptoms of cough and dyspnea. The syndrome usually occurs within the first month of administration of the drug. Eosinophilia is present in most cases. Alveolar filling and interstitial infiltrates are seen and pleural effusions can occur. Some cases have a normal radiograph. Pathologically, interstitial inflammation, particularly by eosinophils, is seen. Chronic toxicity may occur after months to years of therapy and is not a sequelae of the acute type. Dyspnea and cough are seen and systemic symptoms are less common, although fatigue and weight loss may occur. Chest radiographs show interstitial infiltrates. Peripheral eosinophilia can occur, but is less common than with acute toxicity. Positive antinuclear antibodies and rheumatoid factors, and elevated immunoglobulins are often found. Biopsies show interstitial inflammation and fibrosis.

In most cases, a diagnosis is made clinically. The prognosis is good for the hypersensitivity pneumonitis on stopping the drug. With chronic toxicity, the outcome is less favorable – about 70% of cases do not improve or have some persistent abnormalities. Corticosteroids are used, but a beneficial effect has not been proven.

Gold

Gold is used to treat rheumatoid arthritis and other rheumatic diseases, and both parenchymal gold sodium thiomalate and oral gold (auranofin) can cause pulmonary toxicity. The most common presentation is a hypersensitivity pneumonitis, but occasionally bronchiolitis obliterans with organizing pneumonia (BOOP) and possibly obliterative bronchiolitis (OB) may be seen[10].

The incidence of gold toxicity is <1% and a genetic predisposition to its development is possible. It typically occurs after several months of therapy. Patients present with cough, dyspnea, and a rash, and approximately 40% have eosinophilia. Radiographs show diffuse reticular infiltrates. Pathologically, interstitial inflammation is seen. Gold deposits can be detected in the lung, but their role in toxicity is unknown. Bronchoalveolar lavage studies show increased lymphocytes with a predominance of suppressor or cytotoxic cells[11]. Prognosis is good with discontinuation of the agent and treatment with corticosteroids, which need to be tapered slowly over months. Another pattern of toxicity occasionally seen is BOOP, which also shows a good response to treatment with corticosteroids. Prognosis is variable, and not as favorable as for idiopathic BOOP.

D-Penicillamine

D-Penicillamine, used to treat rheumatic disorders and Wilson's disease, has been associated with OB (only in patients who have rheumatoid arthritis), hypersensitivity pneumonitis, and (rarely) a pulmonary renal syndrome[12]. Patients who have OB develop severe dyspnea as well as cough associated with obstructive and restrictive lung function abnormalities. Lung biopsies show infiltration of bronchiolar walls with inflammation and concentric luminal narrowing. The prognosis of OB is poor, with little response to bronchodilators and corticosteroids, but anecdotal reports indicate success with cyclophosphamide and azathioprine. The mechanism of this unusual airway toxicity is unclear; it is postulated that rheumatoid arthritis may induce the injury, but penicillamine interferes with matrix repair and so prolongs the injury and increases the frequency of this entity over that seen with rheumatoid arthritis alone.

Hypersensitivity pneumonitis secondary to D-penicillamine appears to have a good prognosis and presents in a similar pattern to that seen with other drugs. The pulmonary renal syndrome presents acutely with respiratory distress, and hemoptysis, similar to Goodpasture's syndrome. Prognosis is poor. Patients are treated with immunosuppression, including cyclophosphamide and azathioprine in addition to corticosteroids. The role of plasmapheresis in the treatment of pulnonary renal syndrome, although useful in Goodpasture's syndrome, is unproven.

Aspirin

Salicylates are associated with acute noncardiogenic edema and exacerbation of bronchospasm[13]. Pulmonary edema usually occurs when salicylate levels are >40mg/dL. Two groups of patients with this complication have been noted. The first consists of younger patients with planned overdoses as a suicide attempt. The second group consists of older individuals with multiple medical problems in whom the overdose is accidental. The clinical presentation includes confusion, focal neurologic findings, tachypnea, inspiratory crackles, proteinuria, primary respiratory alkalosis, and metabolic acidosis. The neurologic findings may lead to a delay in obtaining a history of aspirin ingestion. Treatment is with forced alkaline diuresis and supportive care. Prognosis is good if the diagnosis is made promptly[13].

Aspirin and other NSAIDs may precipitate bronchospasm in some asthmatics[14], and is often associated with conjunctivitis and rhinitis. The triad of nasal polyps, aspirin sensitivity, and asthma is known as Samter's syndrome. The frequency of aspirin-induced bronchospasm is between 5 and 10% of asthmatics and is more common in those who have perennial rhinitis or nasal polyps, but it occurs most frequently in young adults or adolescents. Occasionally, it appears after aspirin has been taken for some time. Bronchospasm usually happens within several hours of taking the drug, but it can occur within minutes. Overproduction of leukotrienes secondary to interference with the cyclo-oxygenase pathway is probably the mechanism of salicylate-induced bronchospasm. This is supported by the beneficial effect of the 5-lipoxygenase inhibitor zileuton on the syndrome. Aspirin and NSAID avoidance is recommended if possible. Desensitization has been successful in some cases.

Cytotoxic drugs

Bleomycin

Bleomycin is known to induce pulmonary fibrosis in both animal models and in patients who receive the drug for a variety of malignancies. The incidence of clinically significant toxicity is 4%; subclinical toxicity detected by pulmonary function tests has been found in 25% of cases[1]. Most cases present as interstitial pneumonitis and/or fibrosis, but acute pneumonia and hypersensitivity pneumonitis are also occasionally seen. Several risk factors have been identified for toxicity – age >70 years, total dose received, radiation to the chest, use of supplemental oxygen, renal insufficiency, and use of multidrug regimens. Studies suggest that although toxicity can occur even at low doses of bleomycin, the incidence increases significantly at doses >400 units (Fig. 77.5). Cases that occur at higher doses are also associated with increased mortality. The synergistic effect of both radiation and high inspired concentrations of oxygen have been documented in both animal models and clinical studies. There is no safe threshold dose of supplemental oxygen and its use must be avoided in all patients who receive the drug or have signs of toxicity.

Patients typically present with the subacute to insidious onset of dyspnea and dry cough. The physical examination characteristically shows bibasilar crackles, and chest radiographs initially show infiltrates at the bases peripherally (Fig. 77.6). With more advanced disease, diffuse interstitial infiltrates and small lung fields are seen. Chest CTs may help detect subpleural septal thickening and interstitial changes earlier than on radiograph (Fig. 77.7). Acinar infiltrates can be seen and are more common when hypersensitivity pneumonitis or acute pneumonia is present. Focal infiltrates and nodular densities are also described. Pathologically, atypical type II pneumocytes, alveolar and interstitial infiltration, and varying degrees of fibrosis are seen (see Fig. 77.4). Bronchoalveolar lavage studies in animal models and some human cases have shown increased polymorphonuclear cells.

Pulmonary function tests in patients who have bleomycin pulmonary toxicity show a decreased diffusing capacity and, in more advanced cases, a restrictive defect. Attempts have been made to use pulmonary function tests for screening, but no clear documentation of efficacy has been established. Such tests continue to be used clinically because of the serious nature of bleomycin toxicity. A significant decrease in diffusing capacity during treatment does not indicate definite toxicity, but is a cause of concern and

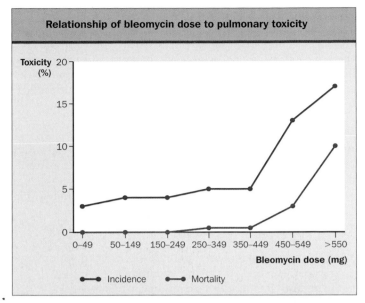

Figure 77.5 Relationship of bleomycin dose to pulmonary toxicity. Bleomycin toxicity occurs even at low doses, but the incidence and mortality increase as the dose exceeds 400 units. (Adapted from Blum et al.[15], ©1973 American Cancer Society, by permission of Wiley-Liss, Inc., a subsidiary of John Wiley & Sons, Inc.

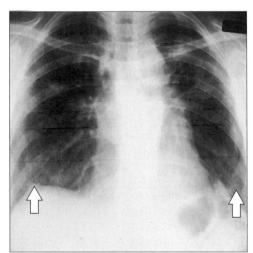

Figure 77.6 Chest radiograph in bleomycin toxicity. Fine bibasilar infiltrates are shown (arrows), suggestive of drug toxicity.

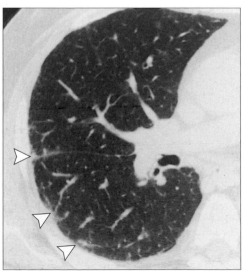

Figure 77.7 Bleomycin toxicity. In a patient receiving bleomycin who had a large decrease in the diffusing capacity, the chest computed tomography scan showed early changes of septal thickening and increased markings in the subpleural area (arrowheads). These changes are suggestive of drug toxicity.

may require further investigation to exclude that possibility. Treatment of bleomycin toxicity involves withdrawal of the drug, avoidance of supplemental oxygen, avoidance of chest radiation therapy, and use of corticosteroid therapy. Although clinical improvement occurs, often residual lung function abnormalities and respiratory symptoms occur. Mortality can be as high as 50% in those who have severe pneumonitis.

Mitomycin
Although not as well studied as bleomycin, mitomycin causes serious pulmonary toxicity in about 4% of cases. Three patterns of toxicity occur:
- most common is an acute pneumonitis seen when mitomycin is used with *Vinca* alkaloids;
- interstitial pneumonitis and/or fibrosis, similar to that seen with bleomycin; and
- rarely, cases of pulmonary infiltrates, associated with micro-angiopathic hemolytic anemia and uremia.

In the mitomycin–*Vinca* alkaloid reaction, patients develop severe episodes of respiratory distress usually several hours after they receive a dose of the *Vinca* alkaloid[16]. In some cases, the respiratory failure requires intubation. Radiographs show new bilateral interstitial infiltrates. With supportive care and, in most cases, corticosteroids, improvement occurs over several days. Unfortunately, approximately 50% of cases have residual pulmonary impairment similar to that seen with mitomycin-induced pulmonary fibrosis. Lung histology shows fibrosis and a mononuclear cell infiltration. No clear risk factors are identified and the mechanism of toxicity is unknown.

The interstitial pneumonitis and/or fibrosis syndrome presents in a similar manner to that seen with bleomycin toxicity, with the insidious onset of dyspnea. Chest radiographs show interstitial disease. In many cases, the response to corticosteroids is good. The rare entity of mitomycin-induced, microangiopathic hemolytic anemia occurs with pulmonary hemorrhage, which presents as diffuse pulmonary infiltrates, and sometimes respiratory failure. Prognosis is poor – corticosteroids and occasionally plasmapheresis are therapies that have been used.

Nitrosoureas
The nitrosoureas, carmustine and lomustine, are frequently used for brain tumors because of their penetration into the central nervous system. They have also been used in high doses as part of regimens prior to autologous marrow or peripheral stem-cell transplantation. Two patterns of injury have been noted, namely interstitial pneumonitis and/or fibrosis and acute pneumonia. The first pattern has been described after treatment of brain tumors and toxicity may not appear for months to years after treatment – in children respiratory failure may develop up to 10 years later[17]. Several risk factors have been identified – a dose relationship with increasing risk of toxicity (particularly at doses above 1500mg/m^2), pre-existing pulmonary disease, and use in multidrug regimens.

Patients present with the insidious onset of dyspnea and dry cough. Physical examination shows bibasilar crackles and occasionally rhonchi. Signs of consolidation have also been reported. Chest radiography can show a variety of findings, which include either upper-lobe infiltration or cystic changes, lower lobe infiltrates, bilateral alveolar filling infiltrates, patchy infiltrates, and nodular densities (Fig. 77.8). Pneumothorax has also been reported. Lung function shows restriction and occasionally

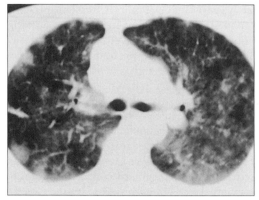

Figure 77.8 Carmustine toxicity. This computed tomography scan shows the patchy nature of fibrosis after use of carmustine. Respiratory failure developed over several years.

obstruction. Pathologic findings are similar to those found with other cytotoxic agents. Often, however, fibrosis is patchy and there is little inflammation. Treatment with corticosteroids is usually not effective and discontinuing the drug is the main stay of treatment. Prognosis is poor, with a reported mortality in up to 90% in severe cases.

An acute pneumonia-like pattern with the development of diffuse interstitial or alveolar infiltrates can occur several weeks after the use of high-dose carmustine. This form of toxicity is usually responsive to corticosteroids. In some cases in which lung function was monitored after high-dose chemotherapy, marked decreases in the diffusing capacity were noted, presumably because of carmustine toxicity; this improved with corticosteroids.

Methotrexate
The antimetabolite methotrexate is used in leukemia, lymphoma, osteogenic sarcoma, breast cancer, and a variety of inflammatory diseases. Methotrexate has caused a variety of pulmonary complications. The most common is hypersensitivity pneumonitis, but pulmonary fibrosis, noncardiogenic pulmonary edema, and pleuritis have also been described. The frequency of toxicity depends in part on its use in multidrug regimens, with some combinations reported to have rates of toxicity up to 40%. Other risk factors are adrenalectomy, corticosteroid tapering, and more frequent administration of methotrexate.

Typically, methotrexate toxicity presents as a subacute illness over several weeks with malaise, myalgias, fever, chills, dyspnea, and cough. A skin rash has been noted in some cases. The chest radiograph shows diffuse, bilateral, reticular, reticulonodular, nodular, or patchy alveolar filling infiltrates (Fig. 77.9).

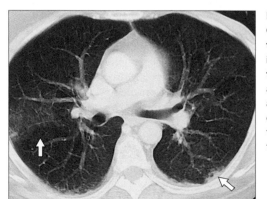

Figure 77.9 Computed tomography scan in methotrexate toxicity. Patchy acinar infiltrates are seen (arrows), consistent with this type of drug toxicity.

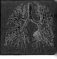

Eosinophilia is present in up to 40% of cases. Occasionally, a picture of interstitial fibrosis or noncardiogenic edema develops. Pathologically, lung biopsies show prominent mononuclear cell infiltration with lymphocytes as the predominating cells. A loosely formed granulomatous reaction may also be seen (Fig. 77.10). Overall prognosis is good and often the response to corticosteroids is dramatic. Occasionally, the syndrome resolves spontaneously, but some patients develop pulmonary fibrosis, although mortality is rare.

The presence of systemic symptoms and eosinophilia, and the response to corticosteroids suggest an immunologically mediated disorder, also supported by lavage findings that show a lymphocytic predominance with helper cells in some cases and suppressor cells in others. Occasionally, however, the lack of recurrence with a rechallenge is reported.

Cyclophosphamide
The alkylating agent cyclophosphamide is widely used to treat a variety of malignancies. Toxicity is rare and the usual pattern of pulmonary toxicity is interstitial pneumonitis and/or fibrosis. The presentation of toxicity is usually insidious and may develop slowly, after years of use. A more acute to subacute form of toxicity can occur after high-dose therapy. Risk factors have not been identified, partly because cyclophosphamide is almost always used in multidrug regimens with other known pulmonary toxins. Patients present with progressive dyspnea. Chest radiographs show patchy areas of fibrosis (Fig. 77.11). Pathologically, findings are similar to those of other cytotoxic drugs. The prognosis is generally poor, although some improvement of symptoms can be found with corticosteroids; the fibrosis tends to be progressive.

DIAGNOSIS

The diagnosis of drug toxicity is often difficult to confirm and must be made clinically. Rechallenge with recurrence is the gold standard, but is not practical in most cases as serious toxicity might be produced. Additionally, with cytotoxic and anti-inflammatory agents, multidrug regimens are often used and it can be difficult to ascribe the reaction to any specific drug. The underlying disease, such as some autoimmune diseases, may themselves cause pulmonary effects, which makes the diagnosis of a drug effect more difficult. Compounding factors may also affect the lung, such as intercurrent infection or progression of tumor, which may complicate the diagnosis of drug toxicity.

Unfortunately, radiographic findings are usually nonspecific for drug toxicity and pathology can be supportive, but not pathognomonic, of drug-induced injury. Whether to obtain tissue and if so whether a transbronchial biopsy will suffice or an open biopsy is needed depends on the individual situation. In cases where the differential diagnosis is broad, invasive procedures help eliminate other entities and so indicate pulmonary toxicity. In cases where an invasive procedure may carry a high risk, such as in cardiac patients, and where other means are available to diagnose or treat the other suspected problems, such as bacterial infection or congestive heart failure, a conservative approach is often taken.

The mainstay of diagnosis of drug-induced injury remains a strong clinical suspicion of drug toxicity and knowledge of the types of reactions seen.

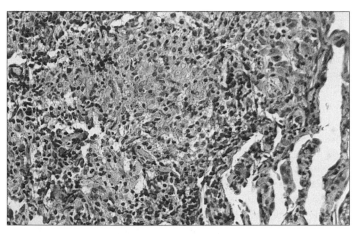

Figure 77.10 Methotrexate toxicity. This biopsy from a patient who had methotrexate pneumonitis shows extensive infiltration with lymphocytes and also loosely formed granulomas. Atypical type II pneumocytes are not seen.

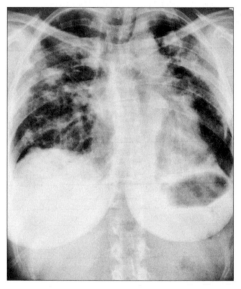

Figure 77.11 Cyclophosphamide toxicity. This patient received high-dose cyclophosphamide for lymphoma and a progressive restrictive disease associated with volume loss on chest radiography and patchy areas of fibrosis developed over several years. She ultimately required a lung transplant. Pathology of the native lung was consistent with a cytotoxicic drug injury.

Prevention
Although risk factors have been described for some drugs, in most cases it is not possible to prevent drug-induced toxicity. Use of antioxidants and antifibrotic agents is being studied in animal models and may have some relevance for prophylactic use with some cytotoxic agents, like bleomycin and mitomycin. The low incidence of toxicity and the potential side effects of these agents may hinder their use.

Lung function tests have been used to detect the earliest stages of toxicity with some drugs, and diffusing capacity is the most sensitive indicator of drug-induced injury. Such tests have not been found useful with methotrexate, which is understandable given the proposed immunologic mechanism and lack of dose relationship. They have also not been shown to be predictive in mitomycin toxicity and, although widely used, have not been proved to help prevent bleomycin pulmonary toxicity.

Use of supplemental oxygen increases the risk of toxicity with bleomycin. It is proposed that it could also exacerbate toxicity caused by mitomycin and carmustine. In anyone suspected of toxic reactions to these drugs, it is prudent to avoid any supplemental oxygen unless absolutely necessary. If a patient needs

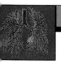

surgery, in which high concentrations of oxygen are routinely used during induction of anesthesia, it is important to be aware of the potential complications.

PITFALLS AND CONTROVERSIES

For drug-induced toxicity it is unclear whether screening pulmonary function tests should continue to be carried out. These are now performed almost exclusively for cytotoxic drug injury, usually with bleomycin and occasionally with mitomycin and carmustine. They are carried out regularly during therapy and a significant decrease in the gas transfer or vital capacity is taken as an indication of subclinical toxicity and the drug is stopped. Studies have not been undertaken to show the efficacy of this practice, but many oncologists believe that stopping the drug in some patients has prevented cases of toxicity. The use of diffusing capacity as a marker is also complicated because these cytotoxic drugs are known to affect epithelial or vascular cells that line the alveolar vascular interface, and can cause a decrease in the diffusing capacity without indicating the onset of interstitial inflammation or fibrosis. More sophisticated tests separate the vascular and membrane components of the diffusing capacity, but routine use of these is not practical. Better screening tests for toxicity are needed and if serum or bronchoalveolar biologic markers of fibrosis can be found and validated, they may prove a better method than lung function tests.

One of the most difficult decisions for a clinician in some cases is whether a given drug can be continued or restarted when the diagnosis of drug-induced toxicity is suspected but not clear. In some cases, no effective substitute agent is available. Each case must be considered individually, but as a general principle, drugs with a high propensity for fibrosis, such as bleomycin and mitomycin, or where the initial reaction itself was severe and life threatening, should not be given again, even if toxicity is not proved. In cases of less severe toxicity or in which irreversible fibrosis is unlikely, reinstitution can be considered, if essential. In some cases, as documented with methotrexate and amiodarone, a lower dose and/or corticosteroid cover may ameliorate or eliminate the reaction.

The greatest pitfall with drug-induced injury is the failure to consider the diagnosis. Except for some cytotoxic agents that have a well-recognized potential for fibrosis, drug-induced lung disease is uncommon, and often less common than many other possible pulmonary complications. A clinician may be personally familiar with only a limited number of reactions and cannot be expected to have detailed knowledge of reactions to all drugs. If the diagnosis is considered, however, information can be obtained and appropriate steps taken.

REFERENCES

1. Cooper JAD, White DA, Matthay RA. Drug induced pulmonary disease, Part 1: cytotoxic drugs. Am Rev Respir Dis. 1986;133:321–40.
2. Cooper JAD, White DA, Matthay RA. Drug induced pulmonary disease, Part 2: non cytotoxic drugs. Am Rev Respir Dis. 1986;133:488–505.
3. Rosenow EC II, Myers JL, Swensen SJ, Pisoni RJ. Drug induced pulmonary disease. An update. Chest. 1992;102:239–50.
4. Ravid D, Leshner M, Lang R, et al. Angiotensin-converting enzyme inhibitors and cough: a prospective evaluation in hypertension and in congestive heart failure. J Clin Pharmacol. 1994;34:1116–20.
5. Aldrich TK, Prezant DJ. Adverse effects of drugs on the respiratory muscles. Clin Chest Med. 1990;11:177–89.
6. Martin WJ II, Rosenow EC III. Amiodarone pulmonary toxicity: recognition and pathogenesis, Part I. Chest. 1988;93:1067–75.
7. Martin WJ II, Rosenow EC III. Amiodarone pulmonary toxicity: recognition and pathogenesis, Part II. Chest. 1988;93:1242–8.
8. Greenspan AJ, Kidwell GA, Hurley W, Mannion J. Amiodarone-related post operative adult respiratory distress syndrome. Circulation. 1991;84:407–15.
9. Holmberg L, Berman G. Pulmonary reactions to nitrofurantoin. Eur J Respir Dis. 1981;62:180–9.
10. Tomoika H, King TE Jr. Gold induced pulmonary disease: clinical features, outcomes and differentiation from rheumatoid lung disease. Am J Respir Crit Care Med. 1997;155:1011–20.
11. Zitnick RJ, Cooper JAD Jr. Pulmonary disease due to antirheumatic agents. Clin Chests Med. 1990;11:139–50.
12. Wolfer F, Schurle DR, Lin JJ, et al. Upper and lower airway disaster in penicillamine-treated patients with rheumatoid arthritis. J Rheumatol. 1983;10:406–10.
13. Heffner JE, Sahn SA. Salicylate-induced pulmonary edema: clinical features and prognosis. Ann Intern Med. 1981;95:405–9.
14. Meeker DP, Wiedeman HP. Drug induced bronchospasm. Clin Chest Med. 1990;11:163–75.
15. Blum RH, Carter SK, Agre K. A clinical review of bleomycin – a new antineoplastic agent. Cancer. 1973;31:903–14.
16. Rivera MP, Kris MG, Gralla RJ, White DA. Syndrome of acute dyspnea related to combined mitomycin plus vinca alkaloid chemotherapy. Am J Clin Oncol. 1995;18:245–50.
17. O'Drisoll BR, Hasleton PS, Taylor PM, et al. Active fibrosis up to 17 years after chemotherapy with carmustine (BCNU) in childhood. N Engl J Med. 1990;323:378–82.

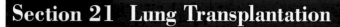

Chapter

78

Lung Transplantation: An Overview

Jim Dauber and Paul Corris

THE EVOLUTION OF CLINICAL LUNG TRANSPLANTATION

The modern era of lung transplantation began in 1981 with the achievement of prolonged survival for patients who received combined heart–lung transplants for pulmonary vascular disease. The major reason for this success was the development of cyclosporin A. Prior to this pharmacologic advance, immunosuppression consisted almost exclusively of high doses of corticosteroids, which resulted in poor wound healing and a variety of infections that uniformly lead to death in the first 6 months after surgery. For the next 7 years, the majority of patients transplanted for end-stage lung disease of any sort received a heart–lung transplant.

Thinking regarding isolated lung transplantation changed markedly around 1988 as a result of two new observations:
- a failing right ventricle could achieve normal function once the burden of pulmonary hypertension is lifted; and

- single lung allograft is sufficient to provide excellent function in patients who have severe air-flow limitation in the native lung.

Accordingly, it became possible to avoid heart–lung transplantation in the majority of patients who have pulmonary vascular disease, and to transplant a single lung only into most candidates. Improvements in surgical techniques, prophylaxis for infection, and control of rejection also reduced in-hospital mortality. These developments resulted in rapid growth in lung transplantation (Fig. 78.1).

Currently, however, limitation in the supply of donated lungs has caused the frequency of lung transplant to plateau at approximately 850 procedures per year in the USA, and no more than 1500 per year worldwide. As the number of candidates has continued to increase, the disparity between the sizes of the donor and candidate pools continues to widen and the waiting time for receipt of a transplant continues to lengthen (Fig. 78.2).

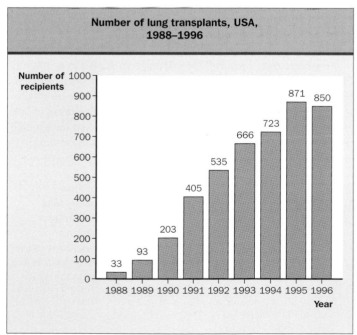

Figure 78.1 The number of lung transplants performed in the USA during 1988–1996. The rate seems to have reached a peak in 1995. These numbers were derived from the 1997 Annual Report from the United Network for Organ Sharing (UNOS)[1]. (The data and analyses reported in the 1996 and 1997 Annual Reports of the US Scientific Registry of Transplant Recipients and the Organ Procurement and Transplantation Network have been supplied by UNOS. The authors alone are responsible for the reporting and interpretation of the data in Figs 78.1–78.5.)

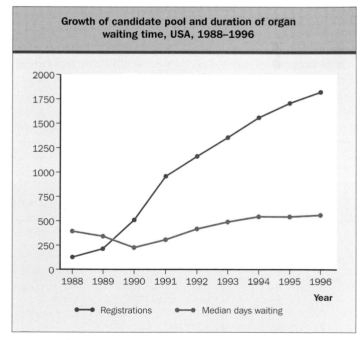

Figure 78.2 Growth of the candidate pool and duration of waiting time for an organ in the USA during 1988–1996. These numbers were derived from the 1997 Annual Report from the United Network for Organ Sharing (UNOS)[1].

OUTCOME AFTER LUNG TRANSPLANTATION

Although survival has improved over the past 10 years and, for many conditions, can exceed the survival of patients who do not receive a transplant, it still lags behind the survival of patients who receive liver or heart transplants (Fig. 78.3). Nonetheless, lung transplantation has become the accepted therapy for many end-stage pulmonary and pulmonary vascular diseases. The most common condition that results in lung transplantation is emphysema. The rates of lung transplantation for other conditions are shown in Figure 78.4. Important differences occur in disease-specific survival rates (Fig. 78.5).

In addition to increasing the length of life, lung transplantation improves the quality of life, as determined by standardized health-state measures[3]. Satisfaction studies indicate that over 90% of recipients would recommend a transplant to a family member or friend if they needed this intervention. The cost to achieve these results is not trivial, however, as the incremental cost for each quality-adjusted year of life gained was $176,817 in 1995[4].

THE 'CONTINUUM' OF LUNG TRANSPLANTATION

Phase 1 – 'making the list'
Referrals
For patients to be considered for lung transplantation they must have end-stage pulmonary parenchymal or vascular disease, and ideally a life expectancy of 2 years or less. Although survival can be predicted on the basis of various physiologic measurements with a reasonable degree of accuracy in patients who have cystic fibrosis, primary pulmonary hypertension, and interstitial fibrosis, for other conditions survival can be so prolonged, and patients can be so limited by dyspnea, that transplantation is considered on the basis of improvement of quality of life alone (e.g. emphysema).

Life expectancy in any single patient is difficult to predict, as is the duration of the waiting time to receive a suitable organ. Accordingly, most centers suggest that patients be referred earlier rather than later in their course. An early referral enhances the possibility that a patient will receive a transplant at the most opportune time.

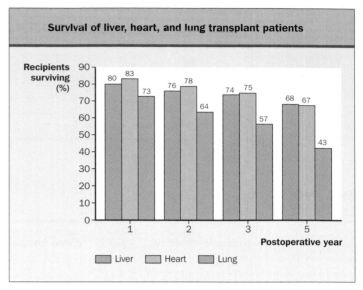

Figure 78.3 **Comparison of survival after 1, 3, and 5 years in recipients of a liver, heart, and lung transplant.** What is notable is the steeper rate of decline in survival for the lung recipients compared with heart and liver recipients. The main explanation for the lower long-term survival in lung recipients is chronic rejection[2].

Contraindications to transplantation
It is more practical to consider the exclusion criteria or contraindications to transplantation (Fig. 78.6) than it is to attempt to develop suitable inclusion criteria.

Most transplant centers do not consider simultaneous transplantation of the liver or kidney because of:
- logistic problems inherent in obtaining multiple allografts and coordinating the transplant teams; and
- difficulties associated with exposing patients to the prolonged anesthetic time required for grafting two organs in sequence.

The definition of active malignancy probably varies from center to center, but generally patients should have a tumor-free interval of at least 3 years for malignancies that have a low likelihood of late recurrence, and of at least 5 years for those known to have a high rate of late recurrences (e.g. breast and malignant melanoma).

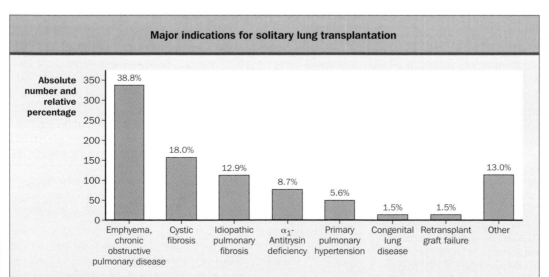

Figure 78.4 **The major indications for solitary lung transplantation.** Emphysema and/or chronic obstructive pulmonary disease accounts for more than a third of transplants and is twice as common as the next leading indication[1].

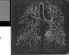

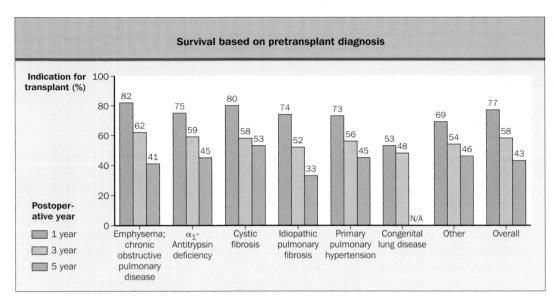

Figure 78.5 Survival based on pretransplant diagnosis. 1997 UNOS Annual Report for the cohort of transplants performed between October 1987 and December 1996[1].

Contraindications to lung transplantation

Unstable clinical status (including acute respiratory failure)
Severe dysfunction of major organs
  Kidney
  Liver
  Central nervous system
  Bone marrow
  Heart (left ventricular dysfunction)
Active malignancy
Infection with human immunodeficiency virus
Uncontrollable systemic or pulmonary infections
Unable to walk more than 180m (600ft) in 6 minutes or have no potential for rehabilitation
Ideal body weight <80% or >120%
Severe osteoporosis with compression fractures
Active tobacco abuse
Drug or alcohol dependency
History of poor adherence to medical regimens
Inadequate social and financial support

Figure 78.6 Contraindications to lung transplantation.

The candidate should not have uncontrolled pulmonary infection. Patients who have septic lung disease may be transplanted with a double-lung allograft if their chronic infection is controlled and if their bacterial flora are susceptible to at least two classes of antibiotics. As many patients affected by septic lung disease have or develop resistant flora (particularly those who have cystic fibrosis), it is important to monitor antibiotic sensitivities regularly during the preoperative course. When highly resistant strains are encountered, they must be tested for synergy between classes of antibiotics and for high-dose inhibition by aminoglycosides, which may be delivered by aerosol in the postoperative period. Transplants for patients infected with panresistant strains of *Pseudomonas aeruginosa* or *Burkholderia cepacia*, which is highly resistant, are controversial[5].

The potential for rehabilitation after lung transplantation is critical. Given the shortage of donors, transplants for patients

who will not be able to walk again, or who do not have the desire to walk again, are difficult to justify. The distance a subject walks in 6 minutes is an important benchmark for lung transplantation[6]. Failure to achieve 180m (600ft) is associated with an unacceptable postoperative mortality rate, and with a short preoperative survival[7]. Most centers demand that candidates achieve this distance before being listed for a transplant. Subjects who have severe limitation of cardiac output because of pulmonary vascular disease are generally considered to be exceptions to this rule, but the extent of their marked debilitation creates enormous challenges in the early postoperative period.

Malnutrition and muscle wasting are thought to be serious problems in patients whose body weight is <80% of ideal. These patients may have more difficulty withstanding the stress of transplantation. Weakness from muscle wasting greatly retards post-transplant rehabilitation, and a poor nutritional status may increase the risk of infection. Marked obesity also slows recovery after the transplant and failure to control weight preoperatively presages even greater problems postoperatively. Obesity also aggravates other disorders associated with immunosuppression, such as hypertension, hyperlipidemia, and diabetes mellitus.

Patients being considered for transplantation have often already been treated with corticosteroids for many years and their intrinsic disease has markedly reduced physical activity. These factors, along with age and hormonal deficiencies, frequently result in a substantial loss of bone mineral density. Immunosuppressive agents such as corticosteroids and cyclosporin accelerate loss of bone mineral. Accordingly, patients who have severe osteoporosis or those with a history of compression fractures in the pretransplant period are at high risk for the development or the recurrence of fractures postoperatively. Many centers do not accept severely osteoporotic patients unless therapy improves their bone density[8].

Many patients who suffer severe emphysema are strongly addicted to nicotine and find it nearly impossible to stop smoking. Recidivism in a lung recipient is not only bad public relations, but also puts the recipient at increased risk for pulmonary infection and accelerated cardiovascular disease. Most centers require at least 6 months of abstinence from smoking before evaluating the candidate. Addiction to narcotics is an equally important problem. Some patients with end-stage lung disease are given narcotics to treat dyspnea or a variety of chronic pain syndromes. Despite the marked improvement in lung function and overall physical status following a transplant, pain syndromes frequently recur and result in the recipient returning to narcotic use.

The importance of an adequate social support system cannot be overemphasized. Despite the treatment advancements and experience gained over the past 10 years, recipients still commonly experience life-threatening complications, and the emotional stresses associated with these can be substantial. Family members or close friends are routinely needed to help monitor the recipients, assist with their medications, transport them to health care facilities, and provide emotional support.

Financial support today is even more critical than it was in the early days, since the more prolonged survival results in a higher cost of continuing medical care. Standard postoperative immunosuppressive medications, outpatient clinic visits, and monitoring generally cost between $15,000 and $20,000 per year in the USA. Hospitalizations obviously increase this figure.

Some centers accept candidates as old as 67 years of age for a single lung transplant, but the usual cut off is 65. The limit for a double-lung allograft is more universal at 60 years of age, whereas for heart–lung transplantation it is usually 50. These limits are not rigid, particularly for single lung transplantation. Flexibility is needed for patients whose chronologic age exceeds their physiologic age and who have a strong desire to regain a more normal lifestyle.

Phase 2 – remaining on the list
Length of wait for lung transplantation
The time candidates must wait for a suitable organ varies widely within and between programs. At the University of Pittsburgh Medical Center, candidates who are AB positive may wait only a few weeks for a transplant, whereas candidates who are O positive generally have to wait 18–24 months. Predicting how long a candidate will have to wait is important since these estimates may markedly alter how the patient is managed prior to transplantation.

Medical management of lung candidates
The goals of preoperative management are to preserve existing lung function and improve the overall functional status of candidates. Some centers require that patients relocate to the area around the center, on the basis that the frequent follow-up and ready access to specialist health care providers increases the likelihood that candidates will be healthy enough to survive the surgery and recover quickly when the donor organ becomes available. This approach also assures that candidates can be at the transplant center on short notice. Centers that do not have strict residency rules usually require candidates to return at least annually for re-evaluation, or at shorter intervals when indicated.

Communication between the candidate's health care providers and the transplant center is essential. Transplant centers must be aware of changes in the condition of candidates, particularly if the candidates have accrued sufficient time on the waiting lists to be a potential recipient for a suitable donor lung. This approach identifies candidates who deteriorate to the point that transplantation is no longer feasible, as well as those who feel too well to undergo transplantation when an organ becomes available. In the latter instance, candidates are placed on an inactive list such that they no longer accrue time, but do not lose what they have accumulated.

If their condition deteriorates they are subsequently re-listed and usually undergo transplantation shortly thereafter.

Some centers strongly emphasize the need for pulmonary rehabilitation, reasoning that such programs improve patient's exercise tolerance and quality of life. In addition, pulmonary rehabilitation programs may contribute to weight loss in obese candidates, regenerate muscle and improve strength in cachectic candidates, and help to reverse osteoporosis. Delaying the listing of candidates whose waiting times will be short, but who have suboptimal physical conditioning, so that they can benefit from pulmonary rehabilitation before the transplant may be justified.

Another area of concern relates to the decision of whether to intubate a patient on the waiting list. Although success has been achieved in a number of such patients, transplantation in the mechanically ventilated patient is clearly a high risk procedure and should only be undertaken after careful consideration[9]. The critical shortage of donor lungs mitigates against intubating patients who develop progressive respiratory failure – most transplant centers advise the referring clinicians that ventilatory support via nasal intermittent positive pressure ventilation can be attempted, but that patients who slip into ever worsening respiratory failure as a result of chronic progressive irreversible lung disease should not be intubated. Clearly, patients who have advanced disease and who suffer an acute deterioration as a result of a reversible complication, such as pneumonia, present a different set of circumstances; these patients may be considered for temporary intubation.

Phase 3 – the transplant and early postoperative period
Matching procedure and candidate
Three types of lung transplantation are carried out: single-lung, double-lung and heart–lung allografting. Indications for each are given in Figure 78.7. Controversy still exists as to the use of a single lung in young subjects affected by pulmonary hypertension or in patients who have emphysema secondary to α_1-anti-trypsin deficiency. Double-lung allografts for candidates under 40 years of age who have these two diseases are justified if the longer waiting time does not jeopardize survival.

Criteria for the donor
Despite a considerable effort to increase the donor pool, the number of organs donated has increased little over the past 3 years. The rate of lung transplantation lags behind that of other organs because only one out of five donors who provide adequate kidneys, livers, and hearts provide a suitable lung. Recently, limits on age and function of the donor lung were relaxed[10], which has permitted growth in the number of transplants without diminishing early survival. The effects of this policy on long-term survival need to be evaluated. In addition, more vigorous efforts to increase the donor pool for lungs are needed. The present criteria for the donor are shown in Figure 78.8.

General considerations
No procedure in medicine depends as much as lung transplantation on a team approach from various disciplines, such as surgeons, respiratory physicians, microbiologists, physical therapists, and nurses, if success is to be achieved. To minimize any confusion and optimize patient care, it is essential to develop standard treatment protocols and to organize regular, multidisciplinary ward rounds on a daily basis.

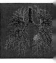
Matching diseases to procedures

Disease	Cause	Preferred procedure
Chronic obstructive lung disease	Cigarette induced	Single > double
	α_1-Antitrypsin deficiency	Single = double
	Bronchiolitis obliterans	
	Idiopathic (recurred in lung allograft)	Single
	Graft-versus-host disease from bone marrow transplantation	Single
	Post lung transplantation	Single
Interstitial lung disease	Idiopathic pulmonary fibrosis	Single
	Sarcoidosis (recurred in lung allograft)	Single
	Scleroderma, CREST syndrome (calcinosis cutis, Raynaud's phenomenon, esophageal dysfunction, sclerodactyly, and telangiectasia), rheumatoid arthritis, mixed connective tissue disease	Single
	Eosinophilic granuloma (recurred in lung allograft)	Single
	Pneumoconioses	
	Silicosis	Single
	Asbestosis	Single
	Heavy metal disease (recurred in lung allograft)	Single
	Lymphangiolyomyomatosis (recurred in lung allograft)	Single
Pulmonary vascular diseases	Primary pulmonary hypertension	Single = double
	Eisenmenger's syndrome with correctable cardiac defect	Single = double
	Eisenmenger's syndrome without correctable cardiac defect	Heart–lung
	Chronic left ventricular failure with reactive pulmonary hypertension	Heart–lung
Septic lung disease	Cystic fibrosis	Double
	Idiopathic bronchiectasis	Double

Figure 78.7 Matching diseases to procedures.

Criteria for donor selection

Function of donor lung

Clear chest radiograph

Adequate oxygenation [arterial partial pressure of oxygen (Pao_2) >46kPa (>350mmHg) on fraction of inspired oxygen (Fio_2) of 1, or Pao_2/Fio_2 >33kPa (>250mmHg)]

No abnormal findings at bronchoscopy

Normal gross appearance of the lungs at time of harvest

Demographics of suitable donors

Age <65 years

No history for clinically significant lung disease

Cigarette exposure of <30 pack-years

Figure 78.8 Criteria for donor selection.

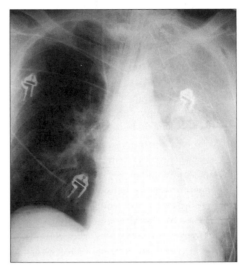

Figure 78.9 Chest radiograph showing typical features of acute lung injury in the immediate postoperative period after left single-lung transplantation.

Initial respiratory management

Although occasionally patients are extubated in the operating theater, the majority of patients are extubated 12–24 hours after surgery. They therefore arrive in the Intensive Care Unit mechanically ventilated via a single lumen endotracheal tube. The approach to ventilation is to minimize the risk of trauma, while ensuring adequate oxygenation on as low a fraction of inspired oxygen as possible. Volume controlled ventilation with tidal volumes up to 10mL/kg with 0.5kPa (5cmH$_2$O) positive end expiratory pressure usually suffices. Fluid intake is restricted in the early postoperative period and diuresis encouraged, to avoid accumulation of fluid in the lungs.

The current methods of donor lung preservation all result in a degree of pulmonary vascular injury, which leads to the development of protein-rich edema fluid and neutrophil accumulation[11]. This injury is usually regarded as a complication of reimplantation, but it is increasingly becoming clear that brain death itself can induce systemic and local cytokine responses in the donor lungs that lead to pulmonary vascular injury. The injury is manifest by dense parenchymal infiltrates and significant hypoxemia (Fig. 78.9). This may require much more aggressive ventilatory management and diuresis, and consideration of the use of inhaled nitric oxide[12,13]. When diuretics are used it is important to ensure that the circulating blood volume is not reduced sufficiently to impair adequate tissue perfusion. It is also important to avoid electrolyte abnormalities and prerenal uremia.

Chest drains must be monitored for evidence of mediastinal or pleural hemorrhage, and if this is persistent or massive surgical re-exploration is required. Significant hemorrhage occurs most commonly following cardiopulmonary bypass in patients who have extensive pleural adhesions. The frequency of surgical re-exploration for bleeding has decreased markedly over the years, in part because of improved intraoperative visualization of the entire pleural surface, including the posterior mediastinum. This has been achieved by the introduction of a transverse or clam-shell incision to perform bilateral sequential lung transplants in patients affected by suppurative lung disease. The increased use of aprotinin has also contributed[14].

One complication unique to single-lung transplantation for emphysema during mechanical ventilation via a single lumen endotracheal tube is that of gas trapping within the emphysematous native lung, which results in mediastinal shift with simultaneous atelectasis of the allograft and hyperinflation of the native lung (see Fig. 78.10)[15]. Split-lung ventilation and occasionally native lung volume reduction may be required in such cases[16]. Another early complication of lung transplantation is that of

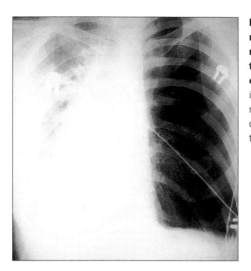

Figure 78.10 Chest radiograph following right single-lung transplantation for emphysema. Shown is overinflation of the native left lung and compression of the transplanted right lung.

phrenic nerve injury, which has been documented to occur in up to 30% of patients, most commonly following bilateral transplant procedures[17]. Phrenic nerve injury may significantly complicate weaning from mechanical ventilation, but in the majority of patients phrenic nerve paralysis is transient.

Infection prophylaxis

It is routine for patients to receive prophylactic antibiotics following surgery and it is the authors' routine practice to give floxacillin (flucloxacillin) and metronidazole for the first week, until healing of bronchial anastomosis has been identified. Other centers use ceftazidime and clindamycin as routine prophylaxis. Patients who have bronchiectasis, cystic fibrosis, and colonization of their lungs with *Pseudomonas* spp. receive appropriate antibiotic cover according to pretransplant cultures. Moreover, all donor lungs are lavaged, with samples sent to the microbiology laboratory before implantation so that further appropriate antibiotics may be started as early as possible to cover donor-acquired pulmonary sepsis.

A recent review of data in Newcastle, UK, from 112 consecutive lung donors demonstrates the presence of organisms in 62% of cases. Gram-negative organisms were often associated with poor initial graft function as a result of diffuse alveolar damage. Recipients with airways colonized by aspergilli are generally given prophylactic antifungal treatment to reduce the incidence of disseminated fungal infections, as well as infections at the bronchial anastomotic site. The risk of dissemination is of particular concern in patients who have a complicated postoperative course, and prophylactic nebulized amphotericin, 20mg q12h, can be given. Other options include low-dose intravenous amphotericin, liposomal amphotericin, or oral itraconazole. Itraconazole has some draw backs in the early postoperative period because it's absorption is difficult to predict, with an unpredictable gastric pH. It also has a significant effect of increasing cyclosporin levels. Some donor lung lavages show evidence of *Candida* spp., so prophylactic use of fluconazole may be warranted. If early complications necessitate continued mechanical ventilation beyond 48 hours, nebulized colistin (colomycin) may help prevent colonization of the lungs with Gram-negative organisms. The prophylaxis therapy used in the University of Pittsburgh center is summarized in Figure 78.11.

Pain control

Pain control is extremely important in the immediate postoperative period, because the aim is to extubate the patient as quickly as possible. In this period, physical therapy and early rehabilitation are important to reduce pooling of secretions in the lower respiratory tract, and thereby reduce the risk of pneumonia. The majority of patients benefit from effective analgesia via an epidural catheter to prevent chest pain associated with physical therapy and coughing. The importance of adequate pain control to prevent early infectious complications cannot be overemphasized.

Immunosuppression

Standard therapy is a three-drug regimen based on either cyclosporin A or tacrolimus (FK-506). The other components are corticosteroids and azathioprine. Immediately after surgery, all three drugs are given intravenously. The route of administration is subsequently converted to the oral one as the patient progresses. Many centers augment maintenance immunosuppression in the early postoperative period with antilymphocyte globulins. Such induction therapy may delay the onset, and reduce the overall prevalence, of acute rejection, but at the cost of an increased rate of infection[18].

Both tacrolimus and cyclosporin A are usually given twice a day, and their concentration in whole blood is measured just prior to the next dose to determine the trough level. Therapeutic trough levels for both are narrow. A trough <5ng/mL (measured by monoclonal immunoassay) for tacrolimus or a trough <100ng/mL (measured by monoclonal cyclosporin assay) for cyclosporin A is usually insufficient to prevent rejection. Troughs that exceed 20ng/mL or 400ng/mL, respectively, are associated with acute toxicity, principally to the kidneys and central nervous system. Rapid elevations in serum creatinine demand lower levels of these drugs.

The initial dose of azathioprine is 3mg/kg, but leukopenia often requires a reduction. Prednisolone is begun at 0.3–1.0mg/kg per day, and the dose is lowered during the first year if rejection is controlled, with a target of 0.1mg/kg per day. It is possible to wean recipients completely off corticosteroids, but most patients require 5–7.5mg/day to prevent rejection.

Both cyclosporin A and tacrolimus are metabolized in the liver such that interactions with a number of commonly used drugs may alter the concentration of both agents. Rapid elevations in levels because of drug interactions cause acute toxicity, whereas rapid reductions allow rejection to occur. Anticipation of drug interactions when starting and stopping new medications is critical (Fig. 78.12), and frequent monitoring of levels is required. Even in stable recipients, blood levels must be measured monthly to detect unexpected fluctuations, which can occur with both medications, and to monitor compliance with drug regimens.

Monitoring

After extubation, patients are commonly transferred from the Intensive Care Unit to a step-down ward. Central venous and arterial catheters may be removed and oxygen saturation is monitored continuously by an oximeter. Twice daily chest radiographs are taken during the first week and are monitored for ill-defined perihilar infiltrates and septal lines, which suggest acute rejection. Pleural effusions may occur in addition to parenchymal changes. If any clinical deterioration is seen, additional chest radiographs

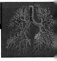

Prophylaxis for infection						
Organism	Peak prevalence postoperative day	Starting point postoperative day	Antimicrobial agents	Dosage	Duration	Comment
Bacteria	1–14	0	Ceftazidime	1g i.v. q8h	3–14 days	–
			Clindamycin	600mg i.v. q8h	3–14 days	–
Herpes simplex virus	1–7	1	Acyclovir	400mg p.o. q8h	3 months	Stop if ganciclovir given for cytomegalovirus Dosage adjustment required for renal insufficiency
Candida spp.	7–30	When organisms identified in donor trachea or isolated from lower airway of allograft	Amphotericin B	25mg i.v. daily	21 days	Dosage adjustment required for renal insufficiency
			5-Flucytosine	1g p.o. q12h	As for amphotericin	Dosage adjustment required for renal insufficiency Dosage adjustment required for leukopenia
			Fluconazole	400mg i.v./p.o. daily	4–6 weeks	–
Toxoplasma spp. (heart–lung transplant only)	7–60	Only for mismatch (positive donor to negative recipient)	Pyrimethamine	25mg p.o. daily	Initial 6 weeks	–
			Folinic acid	15mg p.o. daily	Initial 6 weeks	–
Cytomegalovirus (CMV)	30–40	5	Ganciclovir	5 mg/kg i.v. q12h	14 days	Role of CMV immunoglobulin and oral ganciclovir in prophylaxis is still under investigation Dosage adjustment required for renal insufficiency Dosage adjustment required for leukopenia
		During treatment of rejection with augmented immunosuppression	Ganciclovir	5mg/kg i.v. daily	Day 15–90 for serologically positive donors and serologically negative recipients Day 15–22 for serologically positive recipients	See text for comments on 'pre-emptive' treatment
Pneumocystis carinii	>90	30	Trimethoprim 160mg, sulfamethoxazole 800mg	1 tablet Monday, Wednesday, Friday; or twice daily for 7 days/month; or twice daily for 2 weeks every 3 months	Indefinite	–
			Dapsone	100mg p.o.3 days/week	Indefinite	Not the first-line drug for prophylaxis of P. carinii
Mycobacterium tuberculosis	?	Before transplant or immediately after surgery	Isoniazid	300mg p.o. daily	1 year	–

Figure 78.11 Prophylaxis for infection.

Drugs that alter the concentration of cyclosporin and tacrolimus in the blood	
Raise blood levels	Decrease blood levels
Calcium channel blockers: diltiazem, verapamil, nicardipine	Anticonvulsants: phenytoin, carbamazepine, phenobarbital
Methylprednisolone	Antibiotics: rifampin (rifampicin), nafcillin
Antifungal agents: ketoconazole, itraconazole, fluconazole	Other drugs: ticlopidine, octreotide
Macrolide antibiotics: erythromycin clarithromycin	
Whole grapefruit and grapefruit juice (tacrolimus only)	
Other drugs: allopurinol, bromocriptine, danazol, metoclopramide	

Figure 78.12 Drugs that alter the concentration of cyclosporin and tacrolimus in blood.

are performed. After the second week, the frequency of radiographic and other studies can be adjusted according to the patient's clinical status. Importantly, chest radiographs show normal appearances in 26% of cases of acute rejection during the first month. Spirometry must be performed as soon as practicable after surgery. Formal testing in a laboratory, including vital capacity, forced expiratory volume in 1 second (FEV_1), flow–volume curves, total lung capacity, and diffusing capacity using the single breath method, must be performed prior to discharge from hospital. Many transplant units teach patients to monitor their own lung function using a handheld, battery-operated spirometer[19]. The Papworth (UK) group report a 5% sustained reduction in FEV_1 or vital capacity to be a sensitive and specific marker of lung rejection or infection that warrants further investigation, even in the absence of clinical symptoms or chest radiographic abnormalities.

All patients who undergo single-lung transplantation are given a perfusion lung scan within the first week after transplantation.

The graft should have immediate preferential perfusion compared with the native lung and any evidence of hypoperfusion of the new lung raises the probability of a vascular anastomotic stricture or thrombosis. Vascular anastomotic complications are rare, but carry a high mortality. Pulmonary venous obstruction can lead to dense parenchymal infiltrates and both arterial and venous strictures or thromboses lead to persistent hypoxemia. The diagnosis requires a high index of suspicion and the use of transesophageal echocardiography isotope perfusion scanning and pulmonary angiography (Fig. 78.13). Treatment often requires surgery, although the careful use of thrombolytic agents has been described.

The principal problem in the early management of lung transplantation recipients is that clinically it is impossible to differentiate between opportunistic infections of the lung and lung rejection. Both complications present with identical respiratory symptoms and physical signs, which include fever, cough, shortness of breath, malaise, and crackles on auscultation. A pleural effusion may complicate both conditions. The chest radiograph also may be unhelpful because pulmonary infiltrates are common to both, and in the early postoperative period may also occur as a result of reimplantation injury.

Bronchoscopy

Fiberoptic bronchoscopy with bronchoalveolar lavage (BAL) and transbronchial biopsy (TBB) has a central role in the monitoring of a lung allograft. In the first 3 months after lung transplantation, bronchoscopy is carried out in response to a deterioration in clinical condition, a new infiltrate on chest radiograph, or a drop in lung function. Although TBB may have a 15–28% false negative rate for rejection, it remains the gold standard in practical terms for the diagnosis of acute lung rejection[20]. It is generally believed that four to six biopsies should be taken and that serial sections should be reported by a pathologist familiar with lung transplant pathology and graded using the guidelines established by the International Society of Heart and Lung Transplantation[21]. A deterioration in clinical condition in the first 3 months, of course, may also be caused by lung infection; moreover, a number of studies have shown that infection and rejection are commonly seen concurrently in the first 3 months after transplantation. For these reasons, it is important to perform BAL at the same time as TBB to provide samples for microbiologic examination. Studies must include cytology and culture for bacteria, fungi, and viruses.

Acute rejection

Acute rejection is seen in up to 40% of recipients within the first 30 days of transplantation. Episodes that occur in the first 2 weeks typically cause fever, chills, malaise, increasing tightness in the chest, cough, and worsening dyspnea. Physical examination reveals signs of pleural effusions and consolidation. A new leukocytosis or worsening of persistent leukocytosis is the rule. Pulmonary function studies show increasing restriction and widening of the alveolar–arterial oxygen gradient. Chest radiographs have new or worsening interstitial infiltrates, with or without pleural effusions.

The principle morphologic changes found in acute rejection are perivascular lymphocytic infiltrates, which may extend into alveolar septae at the later stages of rejection (Fig. 78.14). In addition, airways may show a lymphocytic infiltrate. It is usual to carry out two to three biopsies from each lobe of one lung, because rejection may be patchy and multiple biopsies from different lobes afford a greater chance of positive diagnosis. Many

studies have tried to establish reliable but less invasive methods of diagnosing rejection on blood or BAL cells and fluid. To date, none have proved sufficiently sensitive and specific for routine clinical use, although the Pittsburgh Group reported some success using the donor-specific primed lymphocyte response of BAL cells in a diagnosis of lung allograft rejection.

The grading of acute pulmonary rejection is based on the intensity of lymphocyte infiltrate and is given in Figure 78.15. Acute rejection is a complex, integrated immune response stimulated by the recognition of histocompatibility antigens on the surface of donor cells. The most important histocompatibility antigens are those of the major histocompatibility complex (MHC). T-cell recognition of foreign MHC occurs via complex interaction between the donor antigens and the T-cell antigen receptor and accessory or costimulatory molecules, including CD3, CD28, and adhesion molecules such as vascular cell adhesion molecule 1 and intercellular adhesion molecule 1. Following that interaction, the T cell becomes activated, a term which refers to a cascade of events that includes signal transduction, gene transcription, and release of cytokines.

Although the role of bronchoscopy with TBB in the investigation of a drop in lung function or deterioration in clinical state is well understood, the role of bronchoscopy with TBB in patients who have no pulmonary symptoms and a satisfactory lung function (i.e. true surveillance bronchoscopy) has not been established. Large transplant centers have different policies with respect to surveillance bronchoscopy. The Newcastle (UK) unit

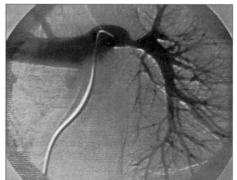

Figure 78.13 Pulmonary angiogram showing stenosis of pulmonary artery anastomosis after a left single lung transplantation.

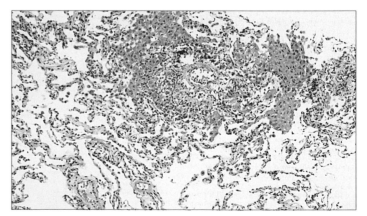

Figure 78.14 Transbronchial lung biopsy specimen showing acute rejection. The lymphocytes surround an arteriole and infiltrate surrounding alveolar walls (graded A3).

has demonstrated an incidence of 20% unexpected rejection on routine surveillance biopsies taken at 1 week, and 1, 3 and 6 months after transplantation. It is not clear, however, from any of the reported studies whether treating such episodes impacts on patient outcome, particularly with regard to the development of more chronic rejection as manifest by obliterative bronchiolitis. It must be noted, however, that an effective surveillance program requires that effective treatment be available, in addition to an ability to identify and detect occult rejection. The introduction of new, potentially more effective immunosuppressive agents in lung transplantation, such as tacrolimus, mycophenolate mofetil, and rapamicin, may eventually confirm the value of surveillance in reducing the incidence of obliterative bronchiolitis.

Episodes of acute vascular rejection are usually treated with pulsed methylprednisolone 10mg/kg intravenously for 3 days, followed by increased oral prednisolone for 1 month. Rejection episodes resistant to increased corticosteroids may be treated by intravenous murine monoclonal T-cell antibody (OKT3).

In general, the response to treatment is usually brisk and symptoms generally begin to improve within 24 hours of starting therapy. Within 1 week after completing therapy, allograft function should have improved dramatically – failure to achieve this end point warrants immediate re-evaluation. Even with an adequate clinical response, a transbronchial lung biopsy is performed within 3–6 weeks to confirm histologic improvement.

Infection

The principal cause of early postoperative death is infection. Bacterial pneumonia is common in the early postoperative period, and affects up to 35% of patients, and is also the major infectious complication in the intermediate and late postoperative periods[21]. The factors that influence the development of pneumonia include both immunosuppression and alterations in the natural defense mechanisms, such as a depressed cough reflex and reduced clearance, in part because of depressed ciliary beat frequency. The initial approach to determine the appearance of consolidation on the chest radiograph in a patient who has received a lung allograft is not different to that in any other immunocompromised patient. Transbronchial lung biopsy, however, is usually carried out at an earlier stage, because acute rejection may present with identical clinical features – as discussed earlier.

Initially, any sputum is sent for Gram stain, and culture and blood cultures are taken. Fiberoptic bronchoscopy is carried out with lavage and protected brush specimens from the involved segments. The high incidence of pneumonia is caused by Gram-negative rods, such as *Pseudomonas* spp., but all transplant centers have reported typical pneumonia organisms such as *Streptococcus pneumoniae*, *Haemophilus influenzae*, *Mycoplasma pneumoniae*, *Legionella pneumophila*, and *Staphylococcus aureus*.

Although patients transplanted for cystic fibrosis do not have a higher frequency of pneumonia, they do have an increased frequency of *Pseudomonas* spp. isolated from sputum and lavage, and such patients benefit from prophylactic, nebulized colistin to prevent the development of pneumonia.

Cytomegalovirus (CMV) is the most common viral pathogen (Fig. 78.16). A recipient negative for CMV antibody who receives an organ from an antibody positive donor has the potential for the most severe disease[23]. Antibody-positive patients who receive lungs from either antibody-positive or -negative donors may also develop CMV disease, but the risk is not as great as in the former category. Antibody-negative patients who receive lungs from antibody-negative donors have a negligible risk, provided they receive seronegative blood products.

Much literature has been published concerning the prophylaxis and management of CMV disease in lung transplant recipients. The high incidence of CMV disease in antibody-negative recipients of lungs from positive donors has led to a number of strategies for prophylaxis, and practice varies widely. Some groups use intravenous high titer anti-CMV immunoglobulin, given at intervals for up to 6 weeks after transplantation until the recipient seroconverts. Other groups include oral ganciclovir 1g q8h for various periods from 2 weeks to 3 months after transplantation. Ganciclovir is an effective agent, but has significant toxicity to bone marrow and reproductive organs, particularly in males. It is virus static rather than virucidal, and so infection may recur when prophylaxis is discontinued. The advantage of delaying the onset of CMV disease is that immunosuppression is usually less at the later date, and so the host may be more able to deal with the pathogen. In some centers, combination prophylaxis with both CMV hyperimmunoglobulin and ganciclovir is used.

The third approach is to use pre-emptive therapy with ganciclovir based on weekly testing for antigenemia in at-risk patients.

Histologic grading of acute cellular rejection		
Grade	Nominal severity	Extent of perivascular infiltrates
A0	No rejection	No significant abnormality
A1	Minimal	Infrequent perivascular mononuclear cell infiltrates mainly surrounding venules with a thickness of just a few cells
A2	Mild	More frequent infiltrates that involve veins and arteries which are more than several cells thick
A3	Moderate	More exuberant mononuclear cell infiltrates which extend from the perivascular space into the alveolar interstitium
A4	Severe	Infiltrates extend into the alveolar space with pneumonocyte damage; there may necrosis of vessels and lung parenchyma

Figure 78.15 Histologic grading of acute cellular rejection. (Adapted from Yousem et al.[22])

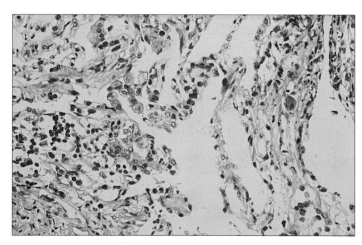

Figure 78.16 Transbronchial lung biopsy showing cytomegalovirus pneumonia. A typical owl's eye inclusion body is shown.

This is conceptually more scientific, but by nature relies on repeated blood sampling and the availability of a reliable antigenemia testing service, which may not be practical after patients have been discharged from hospital. The sensitivity and positive predictive value of antigenemia testing in the prediction of CMV disease in CMV antibody-negative recipients who receive lungs from antibody-positive donors is unclear. The role of prophylaxis in antibody-positive recipients is also debated. With an incidence of disease in that group ranging from 15 to 30%, potential gains of prophylaxis need to be weighed carefully against cost and toxicity of the available agents.

Ganciclovir (5mg/kg intravenously q12h for 2–3 weeks) is the treatment of choice for established infections. The dose must be adjusted for renal insufficiency and leukopenia. Failure to respond raises the possibility of resistance, in which case foscarnet should be given. Despite effective therapy, CMV remains an important cause of mortality.

Herpes virus pneumonia was reported as a common problem in early heart–lung transplant recipients and for that reason acyclovir prophylaxis has traditionally been given for 6–12 weeks after transplantation in patients who do not receive ganciclovir prophylaxis. Either of these drugs virtually eliminates the threat of serious herpes simplex disease.

Pneumocystis carinii is one of the potential opportunistic infections following lung transplantation, but is virtually eliminated by the widespread use of prophylaxis. Without it, infection was reported in up to 88% of heart–lung transplant recipients. It is rare before 6 months after transplantation, but prophylaxis is usually started within the first month. Prophylactic treatment is taken twice daily for 3 days each week using trimethoprim 160mg and sulfamethoxazole 800mg in combination. It is unclear how long prophylaxis needs to be continued and no prospective studies have evaluated this need. Trimethoprim–sulfamethoxazole (co-trimethoxazole) probably has a much broader impact than simply *Pneum. carinii* prophylaxis, and the drug is generally well tolerated in the doses suggested above. It has been the authors' policy to continue it indefinitely; however, if prophylaxis is stopped it should be restarted during periods of augmented immunosuppression.

Infection with *Candida* spp. is likely when these organisms are isolated from the airway of the donor lung at harvest, or from the recipient lung at explant. Bronchoscopic evaluation of the allograft in the first 4–7 days is indicated in such instances. A grayish membrane over the air-way anastomosis suggests invasion, which should be confirmed by endobronchial biopsy. The terminal ring of cartilage from the telescoped donor airway is a prime target for invasion. Therapy is the same as outlined in Figure 78.11 for prophylaxis, but the treatment is continued until the anastomosis heals completely. Invasion of parenchyma of the transplanted lung is unusual, but may occur in highly immunosuppressed recipients who have been treated with broad-spectrum antibiotics and have a heavy burden of fungal organisms. This problem requires prolonged treatment with intravenous amphotericin supplemented with 5-flucytosine.

Aspergillus spp. also invade the bronchial anastomosis in the early postoperative period, typically in recipients whose respiratory tracts were colonized with the fungus preoperatively. The organisms infect not only devitalized tissue at the anastomosis, but also ischemic areas of the adjacent bronchus with the potential to cause life-threatening hemorrhage from invasion of the bronchial arteries in the distal donor bronchus. It is mandatory to take a biopsy of devitalized tissue that overlies the anastomosis in recipients who were colonized with aspergilli before or at the time of transplant.

Air-way complications

Dehiscence of the air-way anastomosis is occasionally encountered. Surgical intervention is rarely undertaken for such cases, since meticulous supportive care leads to survival in most cases. Obstruction secondary to exuberant granulation tissue may occur at this time, but it can be relieved by laser ablation. Stenosis secondary to scarring usually does not occur until several months after surgery. Balloon dilatation and placement of expandable wire stents are promising therapies for this complication[24,25].

Causes of death in the early post-transplant period

Causes of death in the early post-transplant period are given in Figure 78.17. Despite marked improvements in the prevention and control, infection is still the leading cause of death. Acute rejection is a relatively rare cause of death, but the need to augment immunosuppression to control this very common complication contributes greatly to the risk of, and response to, infection.

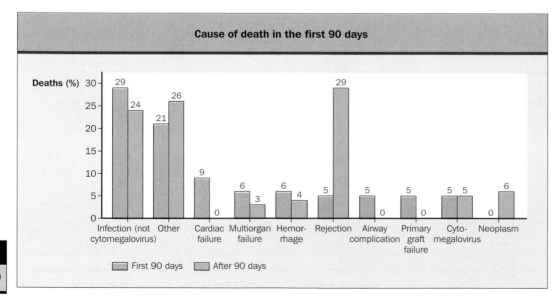

Cause of death in the first 90 days

Figure 78.17 Cause of death in the first 90 days. (Adapted from the April 1996 report of the St Louis International Lung Transplant Registry[26].)

Transition to outpatient management

Until recently, even healthy recipients remained in hospital for 3–6 weeks after transplant for surveillance and for physical therapy. Health-care reform has led to a marked reduction in the postoperative length of stay, which has created the need for alternative methods of patient education and rehabilitation. Recipients who have achieved a sufficient level of independence may be discharged to housing that is adjacent to the medical center, where they may continue their postoperative training and rehabilitation for days or weeks before returning home. During this period, they return daily to the transplant center for education and intravenous drug therapy while gaining additional independence. Highly deconditioned recipients benefit greatly from therapy on an acute rehabilitation unit.

Phase 4 – management of the recipient as an outpatient

Introduction

With about 850 new transplants being performed each year, and with improving rates of survival, the number of lung recipients continues to grow. Consequently, practicing pulmonologists are expected to play an increasing role in their management. Practitioners must be aware, however, of when to refer the recipient back to the transplant center. The major complications encountered after 90 days are similar to those encountered earlier, namely rejection and infection, but differences in the presentation of rejection and in the causes of infection occur. In addition, a number of other disorders associated with immune suppression are seen, and these require sound management to allow the recipient to realize the maximum potential from the transplant.

Rejection

The incidence of acute rejection is greatest in the first 6 months and declines markedly thereafter. More than two thirds of recipients experience at least one episode of acute rejection within the first 2 years and the majority are treated for at least two episodes[27]. After 6 months another form of allograft dysfunction, called chronic rejection or bronchiolitis obliterans syndrome (BOS), begins to emerge. Eventually, up to two thirds of all long-term survivors experience chronic rejection[28,29]. With such a high prevalence, careful monitoring of the allograft for rejection is essential to permit early detection and treatment.

Symptoms of acute rejection that occur 2–3 months after transplant are often not as intense as those encountered early in the postoperative period. Accordingly, other methods are needed to detect allograft dysfunction. Most centers rely on monthly pulmonary function testing. A documented decline of 10% in forced vital capacity (FVC) or FEV_1 mandates patient evaluation at the transplant center. Rejection does not always cause a decline in lung volumes or flow rates[30]. This is particularly true for acute rejection in double lung recipients during the first 6 months, when increases in spirometric values occur because of improved chest wall mechanics, despite the presence of histologically significant acute rejection.

Many transplant centers perform surveillance bronchoscopy, which includes transbronchial biopsies at predetermined intervals, as discussed earlier. Some investigators suggest that this approach is justifiable, particularly in the first postoperative year, as conditions that require a change in management may be found in as many as 50% of patients[31,32]. Other investigators counter this opinion, however, as altering therapy in response to finding

subclinical evidence of rejection on these biopsies provides no marked clinical utility. Unexpected findings are much lower in succeeding years, during which time most centers perform bronchoscopy only when required by clinical indications (Fig 78.18).

Differences in acute and chronic rejection are outlined in Figure 78.19. Two points deserve attention:

- histologic changes of acute and chronic rejection may be detected in the same TBB specimen; and
- biopsy specimens from up to one third of recipients with chronic rejection do not demonstrate bronchiolitis obliterans[33].

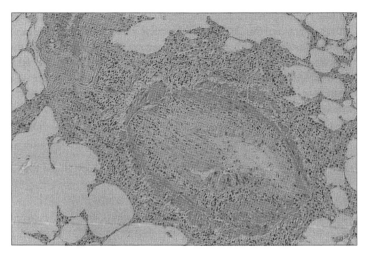

Figure 78.18 Open lung biopsy specimen showing obliterative bronchiolitis. Bronchiolar lumen is obliterated by organizing fibrin, myofibroblasts, and lymphocytes.

Comparison of acute and chronic rejection		
Feature	**Acute rejection**	**Chronic rejection**
Peak frequency	First 6 months	Years 1–4
Onset	Abrupt to subacute	Usually subtle
Symptoms	Tightness in chest (immediate postoperative period) Cough (usually nonproductive) Dyspnea	Dyspnea with heavy exertion Cough (usually productive)
Physiologic	Restrictive impairment Desaturation of arterial blood	Obstructive impairment Normoxia until late
Radiologic	Diffuse interstitial infiltrates Pleural effusions	No abnormality until disorder is far advanced Computed tomography evidence of bronchiectasis and mosaic pattern
Hematologic	Leukocytosis	Normal white blood cell count
Histologic	Perivascular mononuclear cell infiltrates Airway inflammation is variable	Obliterative bronchiolitis Phlebosclerosis Atherosclerosis of pulmonary arteries Perivascular mononuclear cell infiltrates
Response to treatment	Majority of cases improve rapidly with intravenous corticosteroid 'Refractory rejection' occurs in 10–15% of all recipients	Sustained response to corticosteroids is rare Increase in forced expiratory volume in 1 second is not the rule Majority of recipients have progressive decline in allograft function

Figure 78.19 A comparison of acute and chronic rejection.

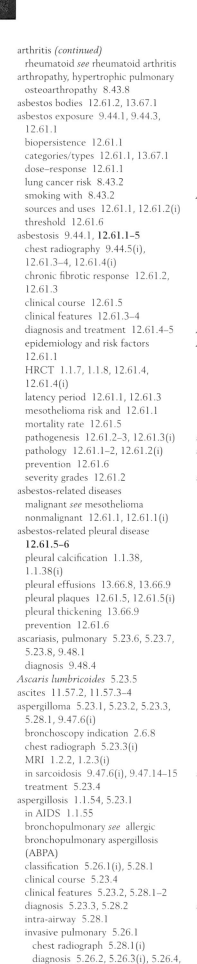

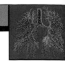

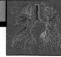

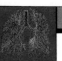

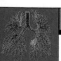